Library of Congress Cataloging in Publication Data
Main entry under title:

Pediatric neurosurgery.

Bibliography
Includes index.
1. Nervous system—Surgery. 2. Children—Surgery.
3. Pediatric neurology. I. American Association of
Neurological Surgeons. Section of Pediatric Neurosurgery.
[DNLM: 1. Neurosurgery—In infancy and childhood. WL 368
M478p]
RD593.P383 1982 617'.48059'088054 82-11881
ISBN 0-8089-1490-1

Grune & Stratton, Inc.
111 Fifth Avenue
New York, New York 10003

Distributed in the United Kingdom by
Academic Press Inc. (London) Ltd.
24/28 Oval Road, London NW 1

Library of Congress Catalog Number 82-11881
International Standard Book Number 0-8089-1490-1
Printed in the United States of America

Pediatric Neurosurgery

Surgery of the Developing Nervous System

SECTION OF
PEDIATRIC NEUROSURGERY OF THE
AMERICAN ASSOCIATION OF
NEUROLOGICAL SURGEONS

G&S

GRUNE & STRATTON
A Subsidiary of Harcourt Brace Jovanovich, Publishers
New York London
Paris San Diego San Francisco São Paulo
Sydney Tokyo Toronto

To Donald Darrow Matson, M.D.

Although Donald Darrow Matson was not the founder of pediatric neurosurgery, he was its undisputed champion for nearly two decades until his premature death in 1969. It is with the deepest admiration and respect that this volume is dedicated to his memory by those who have attempted to expand the frontiers that he originally explored.

Donald Matson was born in 1913 at Fort Hamilton, New York. His college education was obtained through a scholarship at Cornell University, and his medical education continued at Harvard. Except for a three-year distinguished period of service in the armed forces and a year as chief neurosurgical resident at Duke University, he remained at Harvard for the rest of his career.

The major part of his neurosurgical training was obtained at Peter Bent Brigham and Children's Hospitals where he developed an interest in pediatrics under the guidance of Dr. Franc Ingraham. Dr. Matson was invited to join Dr. Ingraham after completing his medical training. This alliance resulted in an impressive productivity of laboratory investigation and clinical progress relating to pediatric neurosurgery. One of the by-products of their work was a textbook published in 1954, *Neurosurgery of Infancy and Childhood.* Following Dr. Ingraham's retirement, Dr. Matson became the first Ingraham Professor of Neurosurgery at Harvard, a chair he held until his death.

In addition to his dedication to pediatric neurosurgery, he was equally committed to teaching and the improvement of neurosurgical training. He was a superb teacher himself, not didactic, but rather he set forth a method of approaching, investigating, and resolving clinical problems. Although his knowledge was not overwhelming, his ability to reach the correct diagnostic and therapeutic answers was uncanny. Dr. Matson's interest in neurosurgical training was not confined to his own program; throughout his term on the American Board of Neurological Surgery he attempted to exert an impact on all programs to improve standards of training and medical care.

Dr. Matson's experience in pediatric neurosurgery was eloquently recorded in his volume, *Neurosurgery of Infancy and Childhood* (2nd ed), published in 1969, the year of his death. This textbook has remained the most complete and influential work in the field. The authors of this book, therefore, humbly dedicate this effort to the principle of excellence in pediatric neurosurgery which Donald Matson so clearly defined.

Robert L. McLaurin, M.D.

To Kenneth Shulman, M.D.

Kenneth Shulman was born on September 6, 1928. He was first introduced to medicine while working in the family drugstore where his father was a pharmacist.

Ken Shulman graduated from Clark University, with Honors, in 1952, and from Washington University School of Medicine, with Honors, in 1954. He received his neurosurgical training at the Neurological Institute in New York City, under the guidance of J. Lawrence Pool, M.D. Dr. Shulman first became seriously interested in the evolving subspecialty of pediatric neurosurgery toward the end of his residency training, and he spent 3 months with Dr. Donald Matson at the Children's Hospital in Boston, Massachusetts. In 1961 Dr. Shulman became the director of the pediatric neurosurgical service at New York University Medical Center, where he spent 3 years. From 1964 to 1967 he was the Director of Pediatric Neurosurgery at the Children's Hospital of Philadelphia. He returned to New York in 1967 at the Albert Einstein College of Medicine where he ultimately became Professor and Chairman of the Department of Neurological Surgery.

One of Dr. Shulman's accomplishments was his early research, which reflected his complete commitment to pediatric neurosurgery. He also was a leader in the organization and establishment of the Pediatric Section of the American Association of Neurological Surgeons, of which he was President pro-tem from 1971 to 1972 and Chairman from 1975 to 1976. More recently, he supervised a large laboratory complex within his department that was investigating intracranial pressure, brain tissue pressure, and brain edema and its biomechanics.

Dr. Shulman had a brilliant mind as well. He was capable of expressing his thoughts succinctly and thereby imparting knowledge to all who either worked with him or attended his many lectures. His gift for poetic and philosophical thought brought an additional dimension to his scientific contributions. Most of all, he was a sensitive and compassionate human being who was admired, respected, and regarded with affection by everyone who had the opportunity to know him.

With Dr. Shulman's death we have lost a teacher, colleague, and friend; yet we are all the better for having been associated with him. It is in the spirit of friendship and respect that we acknowledge the masterful and talented contributions he made to pediatric neurosurgery and to the publication of this volume.

Fred Epstein, M.D.

Contents

PART II HYDROCEPHALUS AND INTRACRANIAL HYPERTENSION

PART III TRAUMA

Foreword

The Pediatric Section of the American Association of Neurological Surgeons came into being in 1972. This occurred in response to the burgeoning knowledge and experience in pediatric neurosurgery and to the increasing number of individuals devoting themselves, either exclusively or predominantly, to that field. It soon became apparent that there was a need for an up-to-date volume on this specialty for trainees and practitioners in neurosurgery, as well as other physicians whose practice includes care of infants and children. The classical masterpiece, *Neurosurgery of Infancy and Childhood* (2nd ed), by Dr. Donald Matson was the most comprehensive volume extant, but it suffered from the inevitable fate of all medical publications in this day of rapid expansion of knowledge and technical development. It also was evident that the field had become sufficiently extensive and complex that a single-authored treatise was bound to have numerous deficits. The Pediatric Section, therefore, embarked on the project that resulted in this volume.

An effort was made to enlist those authors who have demonstrated the greatest expertise in the individual topics. The chapters dealing with clinical problems encountered by the neurosurgeon have been provided by Pediatric Section neurosurgeons in order to achieve the desired result of producing a volume of practical information useful to the student or practitioner. Chapters dealing with material that is tangential, but nevertheless essential, to the practice of pediatric neurosurgery have been offered by other specialists. It is hoped that the result is a volume with a base of fundamental knowledge on which is superimposed the application of that knowledge to clinical situations. It is fully recognized, however, that although this project represents the state-of-the-art today, the flourishing field of pediatric neurosurgery will undoubtedly require future revisions if it is to achieve its intended purpose.

This work is not intended to be an atlas of neurosurgical procedures and operations. Although several chapters touch on the technical aspects of neurosurgery, the emphasis has been on considerations of fundamental pathologic anatomy and physiology, diagnostic considerations, and the application of the various modalities of treatment to the conditions encountered by the neurosurgeons.

Sir Winston Churchill stated: "Writing a book was an adventure. To begin with it was a toy, an amusement; then it became a mistress, then a master, and then a tyrant." The chief editor of this volume admits to periodic agreement with this analysis. Although a little tyranny may have been an essential ingredient, the cooperation received by the multiple authors, by my secretary Mrs. Peggy Roberts, and by the publisher has been deeply appreciated.

Robert L. McLaurin, M.D.

Contributors

A. Loren Amacher, M.D., F.R.C.S. (C), F.A.C.S.
Associate Professor
Department of Clinical Neurological Sciences, Pediatrics, and Surgery
University of Western Ontario
London, Ontario, Canada

Frank M. Anderson, M.D.
Clinical Professor
Division of Neurosurgery
University of Southern California School of Medicine and
Senior Attending Staff
Division of Neurosurgery
Children's Hospital of Los Angeles
Los Angeles, California

Diane S. Babcock, M.D.
Assistant Professor
Departments of Pediatrics and Radiology
Children's Hospital Medical Center
University of Cincinnati College of Medicine
Cincinnati, Ohio

Alex Berenstein, M.D.
Assistant Professor of Radiology
New York University Medical Center
New York, New York

Derek A. Bruce, M.B., Ch.B.
Associate Neurosurgeon
Children's Hospital of Philadelphia and
Associate Professor of Neurosurgery and Pediatrics
University of Pennsylvania School of Medicine
Philadelphia, Pennsylvania

Leonard Bruno, M.D.
Assistant Professor of Neurosurgery
University of Pennsylvania School of Medicine
Philadelphia, Pennsylvania

C. Dennis Bucko, M.D.
Clinical Assistant Professor
Section of Plastic Surgery
University of California
San Diego, California

Peter W. Carmel, M.D.
Associate Professor
Department of Neurosurgery
College of Physicians and Surgeons
Columbia University
New York, New York

William R. Cheek, M.D.
Chief, Department of Neurosurgery
Texas Children's Hospital
St. Luke's Episcopal Hospital and
Assistant Professor
Baylor College of Medicine
Houston, Texas

David R. Cook, M.D.
Associate Professor
Department of Anesthesiology
Children's Hospital of Pittsburgh and
The University of Pittsburgh School of Medicine
Pittsburgh, Pennsylvania

Rolando F. Del Maestro, M.D., Ph.D., F.R.C.S. (C)
Assistant Professor
Department of Clinical Neurological Sciences, Pediatrics, and Surgery
University of Western Ontario
Victoria Hospital
London, Ontario, Canada

Robert M. Ehrlich, M.D., F.R.C.P. (C)
Department of Pediatrics
The Hospital for Sick Children and
Professor of Pediatrics
The University of Toronto
Toronto, Ontario, Canada

Howard M. Eisenberg, M.D.
Professor of Surgery
Chief of Neurosurgery
University of Texas Medical Branch
Galveston, Texas

A. B. Eisenbrey, M.D.
Associate Clinical Professor
Department of Neurological Surgery
Wayne State University and
Chief, Section of Neurological Surgery
Children's Hospital of Michigan
Detroit, Michigan

Fred Epstein, M.D.
Associate Professor of Neurosurgery
New York University Medical Center
New York, New York

Nancy Epstein, M.D.
Clinical Instructor of Neurosurgery
New York University Medical Center
New York, New York

Peter T. Frame, M.D.
Associate Professor of Clinical Medicine
Department of Medicine
Division of Infectious Diseases
University of Cincinnati College of Medicine
Cincinnati, Ohio

Bokyung K. Han, M.D.
Assistant Professor
Departments of Pediatrics and Radiology
Children's Hospital Medical Center
University of Cincinnati College of Medicine
Cincinnati, Ohio

E. Bruce Hendrick, M.D.
Professor of Surgery
University of Toronto and
Neurosurgeon-in-Chief
The Hospital for Sick Children
Toronto, Ontario, Canada

Harold J. Hoffman, M.D.
Professor of Surgery
Division of Neurosurgery
University of Toronto and
Neurosurgeon, Division of Neurosurgery
The Hospital for Sick Children
Toronto, Ontario, Canada

Jack Holland, M.B., M.R.C.P., F.R.C.P. (C)
Research Institute
Hospital for Sick Children and
Assistant Professor of Pediatrics
University of Toronto
Toronto, Ontario, Canada

Robin P. Humphreys, M.D.
Associate Professor of Surgery
University of Toronto and
Neurosurgeon, Division of Neurosurgery
The Hospital for Sick Children
Toronto, Ontario, Canada

Glenn W. Kindt, M.D.
Professor and Head
Division of Neurosurgery
University of Colorado Medical School
Denver, Colorado

David M. Klein, M.D., F.A.C.S.
Associate Professor (Neurosurgery)
State University of New York School of Medicine and
Chief, Department of Neurosurgery
Children's Hospital
Buffalo, New York

Sanford J. Larson, M.D., Ph.D.

Professor and Chairman
Department of Neurosurgery
Medical College of Wisconsin
Milwaukee, Wisconsin

Ronald J. Lemire, M.D.

Professor of Pediatrics
University of Washington School of Medicine and
Director of Inpatient Services
Children's Orthopedic Hospital and Medical Center
Seattle, Washington

Abraham Lieberman, M.D.

Professor of Neurology
New York University Medical Center
New York, New York

Joseph H. Marcy, M.D.

Professor, Department of Anesthesiology
Children's Hospital of Pittsburgh and
The University of Pittsburgh School of Medicine
Pittsburgh, Pennsylvania

Anthony Marmarou, Ph.D.

Associate Professor of Neurological Surgery
Albert Einstein College of Medicine
Bronx, New York

J. Gordon McComb, M.D.

Associate Professor
Division of Neurological Surgery
University of Southern California School of Medicine
Los Angeles, California

Robert L. McLaurin, M.D.

Professor and Head
Division of Neurosurgery
Children's Hospital Medical Center
University of Cincinnati College of Medicine
Cincinnati, Ohio

David G. McLone, M.D., Ph.D., F.A.C.S.

Chairman, Pediatric Neurosurgery
Children's Memorial Hospital and
Associate Professor
Northwestern University Medical School
Chicago, Illinois

John Mealey, Jr., M.D.

Professor of Surgery
Division of Neurosurgery
Indiana University School of Medicine
Indianapolis, Indiana

Peter H. Mestad, M.D.

Assistant Professor of Anesthesiology/Pediatrics
Department of Anesthesiology
Children's Hospital of Pittsburgh and
The University of Pittsburgh School of Medicine
Pittsburgh, Pennsylvania

Thomas H. Milhorat, M.D.

Professor and Chairman
Department of Neurosurgery
Downstate Medical Center
Brooklyn, New York

Ian R. Munro, M.D.

Associate Professor of Surgery
University of Toronto and
Plastic Surgeon
Division of Plastic Surgery
The Hospital for Sick Children
Toronto, Ontario, Canada

Frank E. Nulsen, M.D.

Professor of Neurological Surgery
Case Western Reserve University School of Medicine and
Neurosurgeon, University Hospital of Cleveland
Cleveland, Ohio

Mark S. O'Brien, M.D.

Professor of Surgery
Emory University School of Medicine and
Chief, Section of Neurosurgery
Henrietta Egleston Hospital for Children
Atlanta, Georgia

Shizuo Oi, M.D.

Chairman, Department of Neurosurgery
The National Kagawa Children's Hospital
Kagawa, Japan

Harold D. Portnoy, M.D.

Attending Neurosurgeon
Crittenton Hospital and
Clinical Professor of Medical Physics
Department of Health Sciences
Oakland University
Rochester, Michigan, and
St. Joseph Mercy Hospital and
Pontiac General Hospital
Pontiac, Michigan

Anthony J. Raimondi, M.D.

Professor and Chairman
Division of Neurological Surgery
Northwestern University Medical School
Chicago, Illinois

Donald H. Reigel, M.D., F.A.C.S.
Chief, Division of Neurosurgery
The Western Pennsylvania Hospital
Pittsburgh, Pennsylvania

Harold L. Rekate, M.D.
Assistant Professor of Neurological Surgery
Case Western Reserve University School of Medicine and
Associate Neurosurgeon
University Hospitals of Cleveland
Cleveland, Ohio

James H. Salmon, M.D.
Clinical Assistant Professor (Neurosurgery)
University of Pittsburgh and
Consultant, Children's Hospital
Pittsburgh, Pennsylvania

Martin Peter Sayers, M.D.
Clinical Professor of Surgery (Neurosurgery)
College of Medicine
Ohio State University and
Chief, Department of Pediatric Neurosurgery
The Children's Hospital
Columbus, Ohio

Luis Schut, M.D.
Chief, Neurosurgical Services
Children's Hospital of Philadelphia and
Professor of Neurosurgery and Pediatrics
University of Pennsylvania School of Medicine
Philadelphia, Pennsylvania

James F. Schwartz, M.D.
Professor of Pediatrics and Neurology
Emory University School of Medicine and
Chief, Section of Neurology
Henrietta Egleston Hospital for Children
Atlanta, Georgia

Hervey D. Segall, M.D.
Professor of Radiology
University of Southern California School of Medicine and
Director, Department of Neuroradiology
Children's Hospital of Los Angeles and
Los Angeles County—University of Southern California Medical Center
Los Angeles, California

Kenneth Shapiro, M.D.
Assistant Professor of Neurosurgery
Assistant Professor of Pediatrics
Director of Pediatric Neurosurgery
Leo M. Davidoff Department of Neurological Surgery
Albert Einstein College of Medicine
Bronx, New York

William A. Shucart, M.D.
Professor and Chairman
Department of Neurosurgery
Tufts—New England Medical Center
Boston, Massachusetts

Kenneth Shulman, M.D. (deceased)
Professor and Chairman
Albert Einstein College of Medicine
Bronx, New York

Bennett M. Stein, M.D.
Byron Stookey Professor and Chairman
Neurological Surgery
College of Physicians and Surgeons
Columbia University and
Director of Service
Department of Neurosurgery
Columbia-Presbyterian Medical Center
New York, New York

Roy D. Strand, M.D.
Neuroradiologist
Associate Professor in Radiology
Harvard Medical School
Boston, Massachusetts

Suzie C. Tindall, M.D.
Neurosurgical Resident
Emory University School of Medicine
Atlanta, Georgia

Tadanori Tomita, M.D.
Associate Professor of Surgery (Neurosurgery)
Children's Memorial Hospital
Chicago, Illinois

Jose Manuel Velasco-Siles, M.D.
Hospital Infantil de Mexico
Mexico

Joan L. Venes, M.D., F.A.C.S.
Pediatric Neurosurgery
Texas Neurological Institute at Dallas, P.A.
Dallas, Texas

Steven L. Wald, M.D.
Assistant Professor of Surgery
Section of Neurosurgery
University of Vermont
Burlington, Vermont

Josef Warkany, M.D.
Professor of Research
Children's Hospital Medical Center and
Department of Pediatrics
University of Cincinnati College of Medicine
Cincinnati, Ohio

I DEVELOPMENTAL ABNORMALITIES

1. Normal Development of the Central Nervous System: Correlation with Selected Malformations

Ronald J. Lemire
Josef Warkany

METHODS OF STUDYING HUMAN CENTRAL NERVOUS SYSTEM DEVELOPMENT

The study of the development of the human nervous system has been from a descriptive viewpoint utilizing individual specimens or large collections of embryos and fetuses. While each specimen represents an important contribution, thus far it has not been possible to study human neurodevelopmental processes either in vivo or by explanation. The descriptions of the human central nervous system (CNS), therefore, must reference important experimental studies in animals if the dynamic processes of development are to be fully understood. Most such studies have been done in amphibians, although recently more information has been obtained from rodents and subhuman primates.

This chapter, while emphasizing human CNS development, will liberally include experimental information derived from both embryologic and teratologic studies. Previous works that extensively cover normal CNS development in humans[1–5] and in animals[6] provide reference sources for the reader interested in more detailed information. Emphasis will be on early CNS development as most structural anomalies arise during the first few months of gestation.

STAGES OF EMBRYONIC GROWTH

The timing of development in the human embryo is based on 23 stages, each of which encompasses 2–31 days.[7–9] Many of the specific landmarks in the development of the early neural tube are correlated with these stages. Table 1-1

The authors greatly appreciate the manuscript preparation by Mrs. Paula Livesley. Drs. David B. Shurtleff and Irvin Emanuel have also been most helpful and we wish to thank them.

Table 1-1
Stage of Embryonic Development Related to Size and Age

Stage	Crown-Rump Length (mm)	Gestational Age (Days)
1		1
2		2–3
3		4–5
4		5–6
5	0.1–0.2	7–12
6	0.2	13–15
7	0.4	15–17
8	1.0–1.5	17–19
9	1.5–2.5	19–21
10	2.0–3.5	22–23
11	2.5–4.5	23–26
12	3–5	26–30
13	4–6	28–32
14	5–7	31–35
15	7–9	35–38
16	8–11	37–42
17	11–14	42–44
18	13–17	44–48
19	16–18	48–51
20	18–22	51–53
21	22–24	53–54
22	23–28	54–56
23	27–31	56–60

depicts these developmental stages as correlated with both crown–rump (CR) length and the approximate gestational age (the latter based on the work of Jirásek).[10]

Prior to the staging system for human embryos, most descriptions relied on CR length, and therefore some errors existed in correlating developmental information over the past century. Another problem lies in interfacing the stages of human development with those in animals but some accurate correlations are available.[11,12]

FETAL AND POSTNATAL GROWTH

Staging of fetal growth has not been done to date and therefore most references are based on the CR length of the fetus. While this approach permits discrepancies, it is the most practical method even though fetal foot length correlations are more accurate. During the last three months of gestation and after birth, the reference is again shifted to gestational weeks, and later to days, weeks, months, and years.

The main concept in CNS development is that, like other developmental processes, it is a continuum. Among the major organ systems in the body, it is one of the first to be recognized in the embryo (Stage 8) and one of the last to finish significant development after birth. Although the emphasis in this chapter will be on early development, many questions relating to CNS development originate later.

EARLY CNS DEVELOPMENT

Induction and Experimental Studies

It is now known how the human CNS is induced, but studies on experimental animals provide some clues to the process in general. The chordomesoderm (notochord and mesoderm), underlying the presumptive neural plate, appears to be instrumental in activating the ectoderm both initially to form neural plate and then to transform it into various structures.[13,14] In chick embryos regular indentations of overlying neural plate by notochord have been demonstrated.[15] The ratio of neuroectodermal cells to mesodermal cells is important in determining the type of structure that will develop.[16,17] If there is an increase in the ratio of neuroectoderm to mesoderm, more rostral structures develop, whereas increasing the mesodermal component causes differentiation of caudal structures. The mechanism by which the induction occurs is not known but evidence exists that both cellular contact and diffusion of material may be important.[6]

Cellular Kinetics

While the developing neural tube is generally divided into ependymal, mantle, and marginal layers, the main cellular division takes place in the ependyma (the germinal layer). The early observations of F.C. Sauer[18–21] showed that early neural tubes consisted entirely of germinal cells arranged in a pseudostratified epithelium. The nuclei of these cells moved freely through the cytoplasm from periphery to central canal—a to-and-fro cycle. Later studies confirmed and extended his observations.[22–27] It is now known that this interkinetic germinal cell cycle has four general phases as follows:

M phase In the mitotic phase the nucleus is located at the luminal surface.

G1 phase The G stands for "gap." In this first gap daughter nuclei are moving back toward the periphery and thymidine incorporation is beginning.

S phase Nuclei are located peripherally, thymidine is continuing to be incorporated, and most of the synthesis of DNA occurs.

G2 phase The second gap phase has some thymidine incorporation and DNA synthesis. The nuclei are now moving back toward the lumen.

The generation time for the entire cycle to be completed varies according to species and also regions of the brain.[6]

Neurulation in Animals

The process by which the neural tube initially folds is called neurulation.[28] Because it occurs very early, it is vitally important to the developing embryo, and although it has been well studied, many of the mechanisms remain unclear. Controversy exists as to whether the neuroepithelium, the surrounding mesoderm, or both are responsible for the processes of neurulation: Are the effective factors within the neuroepithelium, related to cell division,[29–31] due to a differential water gradient,[32–35] to differential contractile tensions across the neural plate,[36] or to contractile filaments?[37] Interaction between neuroepithelium and mesoderm has been suggested by some studies;[31,35] and more recently, with the help of the scanning electron microscope, cytoplasmic blebs, short microvilli, microfilaments, cytoplasmic threads, and lamellapodia have all been identified as factors that may be involved in the process of neurulation.[38–40]

Neurulation in Humans

Discussion of neurulation in human embryos can be related to the staging system previously discussed (Table 1-1), and then correlations made with the estimated gestational age and CR length. Primary orientation of the embryo arises in Stage 6 when the primitive streak and Hensen's node are present. Shortly thereafter (Stage 7) a cellular process (the notochord) is found extending rostrally from Hensen's node. We previously mentioned that the notochord is thought to play a role in induction of the neural plate, and while this is not known in humans, the neural plate does appear and is in contact with the notochord in Stage 8. This is perhaps the first definable period of neurulation from the standpoint or morphology alone. Over the following 10 days one of the most critical phases of embryonic development occurs—the folding and closure of the neural tube. Somites (lateral mesodermal condensations) begin to appear in Stage 9 and the neural folding process begins. The embryo is 1.5–2.5 mm in CR length and about 20 days old. Over the next two days, when there are six to seven somites, fusion of the neural folds occurs (Stage 10). The initial site of fusion is at the level of the third of fourth somite,[8] which correlates with future rhombencephalon (hindbrain).

After the initial fusion occurs, there are unfused rostral neural folds and unfused caudal neural folds. At what time these become known as the anterior and posterior neuropores, respectively, is somewhat arbitrary. Fusion continues caudally near the most recently formed somite. By early Stage 11 (the 13–15 somites) the younger embryos have fused neural folds to the level of the colliculi rostrally. Closure of the anterior neuropore is completed during this stage, around the 25th day of gestation. The primordia of the thalamus and corpus striatum distort the final hole and may be involved in the closure. At this time the only contact between the neuroectoderm and the amniotic cavity is through the posterior neuropore.

Neurulation is completed during Stage 12 (3–5 mm CR length; 26–30 days gestational age). The final site of closure has not been determined, but most likely it is around the future midlumbar level. There are 21–29 somites in Stage 12, and if one subtracts the four somites that are incorporated into the occipital bone and 20 for the cervical and thoracic vertebrae, a rough correlation can be made regarding the closure site. Two important factors should be noted at this time. First, there is no longer contact between the amniotic fluid and the neuroectoderm, and second, more segments of spinal cord and vertebrae need to be formed. Table 1-2 summarizes the events regarding neurulation in the human embryo.

Abnormal Neurulation

Classification

In recent years emphasis has been placed on the concept of neural tube defects (NTD), and yet the distinction with neurulation defects is usually unclear. In the general sense any developmental defect of the CNS can be called a neural tube defect, and within that context neurulation defects are a subgroup. One manner in which this distinction can be made is on the basis of whether or not the lesion is covered with skin. As noted above the neuroectoderm is no longer in contact with the amniotic cavity after Stage 12 because neurulation has been completed and surface ectoderm (future skin) separates neural tube from the outside. Table 1-3 gives examples of the distinction between defects of neurula-

Table 1-2
Stages Relating to Neurulation in Human Embryos

Stage	CR Length (mm)	Gestational Age (Days)	Somites	Event
7	0.4	15–17		Hensen's node
8	1.0–1.5	17–19		Neural plate
9	1.5–2.5	19–21	1–3	Neural folds
10	2.0–3.5	22–23	4–12	First fusion
11	2.5–4.5	23–26	13–20	Anterior neuropore closes
12	3–5	26–30	21–29	Posterior neuropore closes

Table 1-3
Examples of Neural Tube Defects

	Neurulation Defects	Postneurulation Defects
Craniospinal	Craniorachischisis	Iniencephalus clausus
Cranial	Anencephaly	Encephalocele
Spinal	Meningomyelocele	Myelocystocele

tion and those arising beyond Stage 12 (and which will be discussed later in this chapter).

The classification of neurulation defects falls into three general categories: (1) those involving the brain and spinal cord. (2) those involving the brain alone, and (3) those involving the spinal cord alone. When both the brain and spinal column fail to undergo proper neurulation, a condition of total dysrhaphism (or craniorachischis) results (Figs. 1-1 and 1-2). If the brain alone fails to close, then anencephaly is found. The varying nomenclatures of anencephaly have recently been reviewed[41] but most cases can be subdivided into holoacrania, if the defect extends to involve the foramen magnum (Fig. 1-3), or meroacrania, if the foramen magnum is not involved (Fig. 1-4). A significant number of those

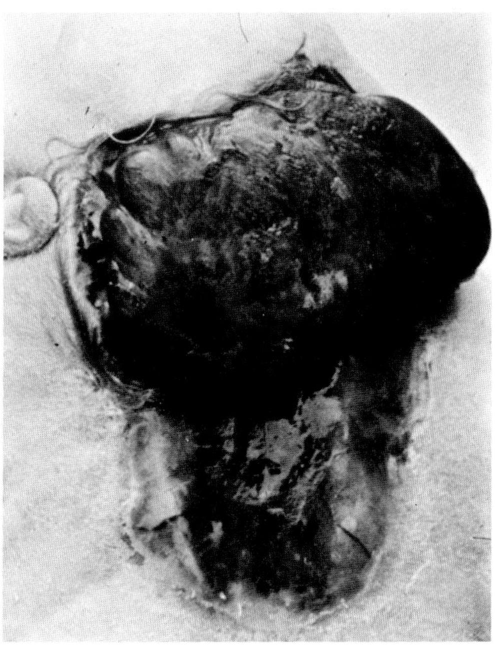

Figure 1-1. Posterior view of human fetus with craniorachischisis. All of the brain is exposed, as is much of the spinal cord. (Reprinted with permission from Lemire RJ, Loeser JD, Leech RW, et al.: Normal and Abnormal Development of the Human Nervous System. Hagerstown, Harper & Row, 1975.)

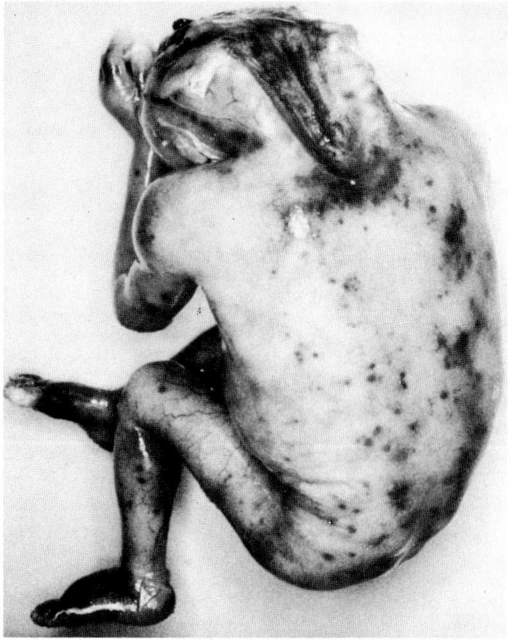

Figure 1-2. Young human fetus with holoacrania and rachischisis of the cervical and upper thoracic cord. (Reprinted with permission from Lemire RJ, Loeser RD, Leech RW, et al: Normal and Abnormal Development of the Human Nervous System. Hagerstown, Harper & Row, 1975.)

specimens with holoacrania have also a spinal rachischisis involving the upper cervical vertebrae and some have marked spinal retroflexion.[42] The latter condition, spinal retroflexion, is not unique to anencephaly and is discussed elsewhere relative to its overlap with other conditions.[43,44]

Caudally defective neurulation results in myelocele if the lesion is flat (Fig. 1-5), or meningomyelocele if an enlarged subarachnoid space ventral to the dysplastic cord is present (Fig. 1-6).

The correlation of these anatomic locations with the probable stages in which they arise in human embryos is shown in Table 1-4.

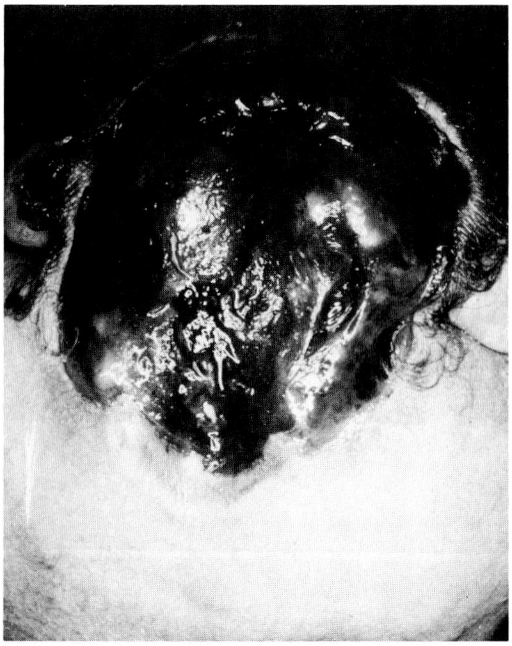

Figure 1-3. Human specimen with holoacrania. The defect includes the foramen magnum. (Reprinted with permission from Lemire RJ, Loeser RD, Leech RW, et al: Normal and Abnormal Development of the Human Nervous System. Hagerstown, Harper & Row, 1975.)

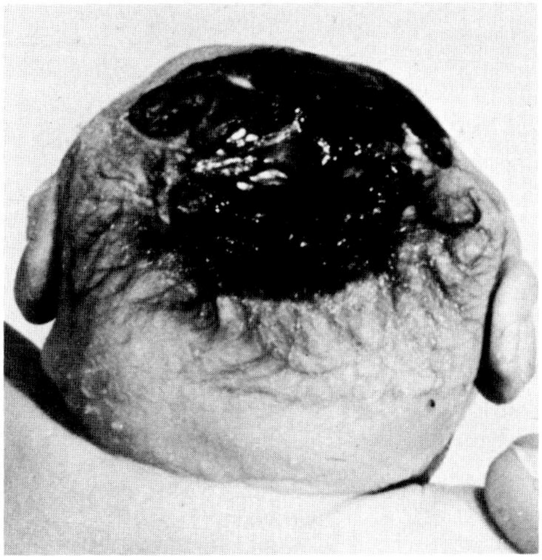

Figure 1-4. Human specimen with meroacrania. The open defect in the brain does not extend to the foramen magnum. (Reprinted with permission from Lemire RJ, Loeser RD, Leech RW, et al: Normal and Abnormal Development of the Human Nervous System. Hagerstown, Harper & Row, 1975.)

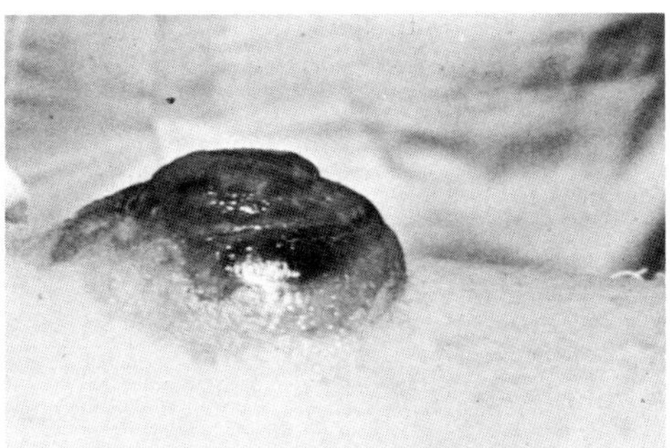

Figure 1-5. Myelocele in a newborn. The central portion is exposed spinal cord and a small subarachnoid enlargement ventral to the cord is beginning to create a sac. (Reprinted with permission from Lemire RJ, Loeser RD, Leech RW, et al: Normal and Abnormal Development of the Human Nervous System. Hagerstown, Harper & Row, 1975.)

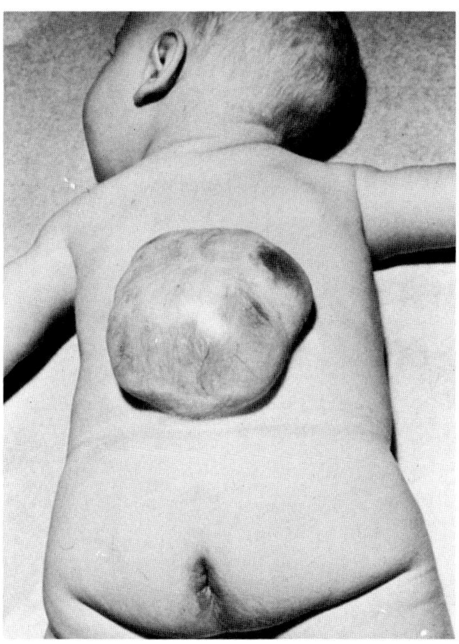

Figure 1-6. Epithelialized meningomyelocele, which now has the appearance of a skin-covered lesion but is actually a neurulation defect. (Reprinted with permission from Lemire RJ, Loeser RD, Leech RW, et al: Normal and Abnormal Development of the Human Nervous System. Hagerstown, Harper & Row, 1975.)

Table 1-4
Association of Embryonic Stage with Neurulation Defect

Stage(s)	Neurulation Defect
8–10	Craniorachischisis
11	Anencephaly
12	Meningomyelocele

Pathogenesis: Human Studies

Evidence bearing on many aspects of the pathogenesis of neurulation defects is mentioned below on studies dealing with experimental production of these defects. Most theories can be grouped into two main categories as follows: (1) the neural folds never fuse and the primary defect is in the neuroepithelium[45] or in the mesoderm[46] or (2) the neural folds normally fuse and then reopen either secondary to increased intraluminal pressure[47] or a primary defect in the neuroepithelium.[48]

Nonclosure of neural folds was first suggested in 1886 by Recklinghausen[49] as the mechanism of neural tube dysraphism. On the basis of studies of human embryos and two fetuses, Patten[45] suggested that the reason neurulation was inhibited was because of overgrowth of neuroepithelium. While many human embryos definitely support the concept that the neural tube never closed, not all exhibit the phenomenon of neural overgrowth.[50–53] Neural overgrowth clearly seen in some experimentally induced spina bifidas is probably the result and not the cause of dysraphism.

Reopening of a closed neural tube has been suggested as a mechanism for dysraphism. Gardner[47,54] related this to increased pressure within the neural tube lumen with subsequent blowout at sites of weakness—the last portions to close. Based on observations of one monkey and 100 human embryos, Padget[48,55] proposed that a "neuroschisis" occurs on the dorsal neuroepithelium following which a "neuroschistic bleb" forms, which can subsequently enlarge and rupture through the surface ectoderm.

The common spina bifida aperta or cystica, the lesion best known to neurosurgeons, frequently concurs with other anomalies of the central nervous system. In fact, the association with the Arnold–Chiari malformation, aqueduct stenosis, and hydrocephaly is usually considered a complex and attempts have been made to explain these anomalies as sequences of the spina bifida. The downward placement of parts of the medulla and cerebellum through the occipital foramen into the cervical spinal canal, the Arnold–Chiari malformation, has been explained by fixation or tethering of the dysraphic caudal spinal cord, which does not permit the normal ascent of the cord within the spinal canal in fetal life, thus leading to the low position of the medulla and cerebellum. An alternative theory contends that the hydrocephalus, which is present in a high percentage of patients with spina bifida, pushes the tentorium downward and displaces the hindbrain and the cerebellum into the cervical spinal canal. A third theory considers the Arnold–Chiari malformation, aqueduct stenosis, and hydrocephaly as coordinated and independent anomalies occurring in cases of spina bifida like microgyria, overgrowth of parts, and heterotopias. From a review of the literature and animal experiments, it appears that the association of spina bifida with the Arnold–Chiari malformation is very close, whereas hydrocephaly and aqueduct stenosis develop more independently in postnatal life as parallel phenomena.

Other theories and descriptions of human specimens have recently been

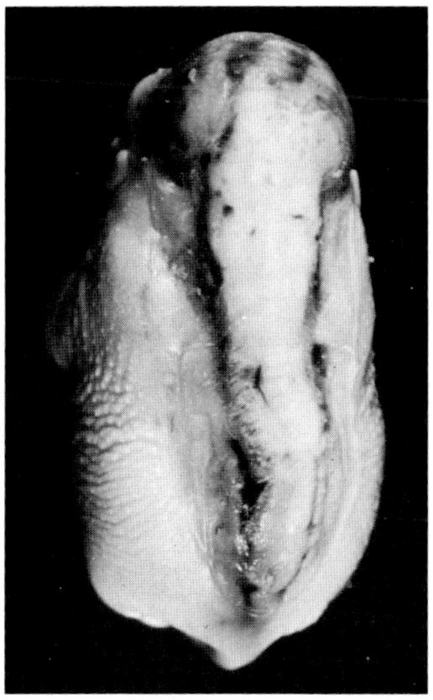

Figure 1-7. A 21-day rat fetus. Rear view shows complete craniorachischisis: the brain as well as the spinal cord are dysraphic and exposed on the animal's dorsum (produced by aspirin administered to the mother on tenth day of gestation).

discussed in depth for those wishing to pursue this further.[41] Because most evidence relative to this problem has been gained from experimental studies, this will now be reviewed.

Pathogenesis: Experimental Studies

There are many methods of producing exencephaly, spina bifida, and other forms of neural dysraphism in experimental animals (Figs. 1-7–1-10). Trypan blue, x-irradiation, hypervitaminosis A, salicylates, antimetabolites, hypoxia, hyperthermia, and others have been used to produce exencephaly and spina bifida, which has made possible studies of the abnormal morphogenesis of these lesions.[41] In addition, genetically determined neural tube anomalies occurring in inbred strains of mice can serve as models of exencephaly and spina bifida. By examining affected fetuses and embryos, one can see the lesions in early stages

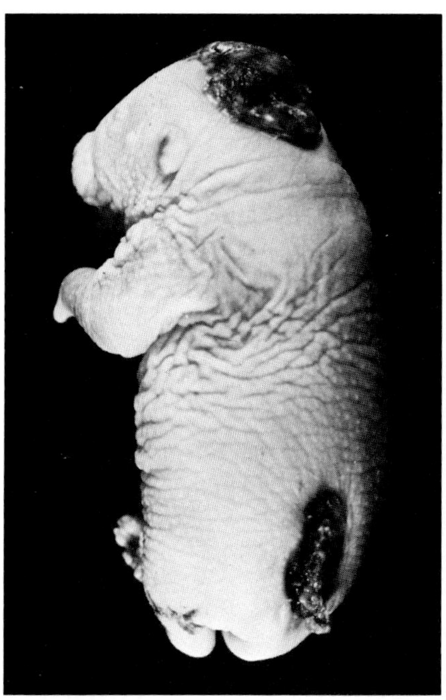

Figure 1-8. A 21-day fetus showing exencephaly and spina bifida produced by aspirin administered to the mother on days 2–9 of gestation.

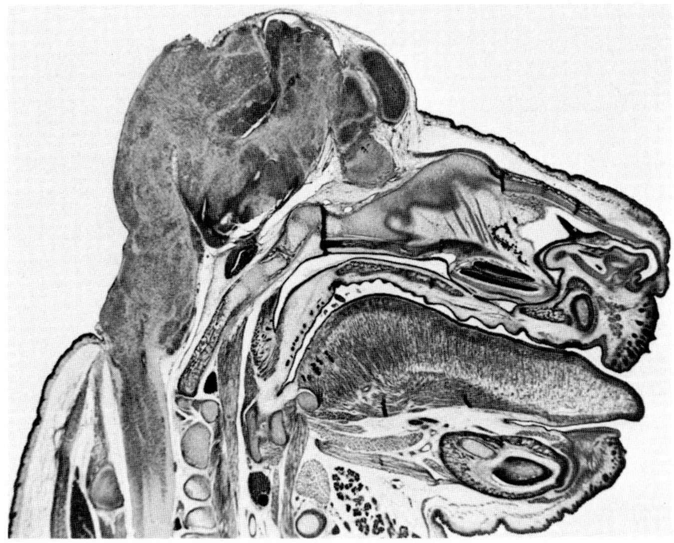

Figure 1-9. Sagittal section through the head of a rat fetus showing exencephaly produced by sodium salicylate. The brain lies without skin and bone cover on the cranial basis, exposed to amniotic fluid. As pregnancy progresses, the brain structures deteriorate and slough off. The exencephaly is converted into anencephaly.

and follow their development until term. Removal of fetuses before term yields specimens in good stages of preservation, histologic sections can be obtained in series, and skeletal anomalies can be studied in cleared specimens. Observation of animal fetuses, therefore, is superior in some respects to examination of human fetal specimens. On the other hand, there may be specific changes in human fetuses that are not present in animals. But in principal questions neural tube defects in humans and animals are in agreement; they are due to failure of closure of the neural plate in early embryonic life, resulting in exencephaly–anencephaly if the defect is rostral and in spina bifida if the defect is caudal.

Incidence and Etiology

Incidences of neural tube defects—that is, numbers of cases present at birth—vary according to geography, ethnic and familial factors, sex, and definition of terms. One can think of 1/1000 deliveries as a starting figure, but must remember that variations are remarkable. Neural tube defects thus are notoriously frequent in Ireland where 5/1000 can be cited as an average figure, whereas 0.5/1000 or less are recorded in Japan, Norway, Hungary, and other countries. In a comparative study in 24 cities of 16 countries, Stevenson, Johnson, Stewart et al.[56] found a 40-fold difference in the frequencies of anencephaly between the highest, in Belfast (Ireland), and the lowest, in Bogota (Colombia)

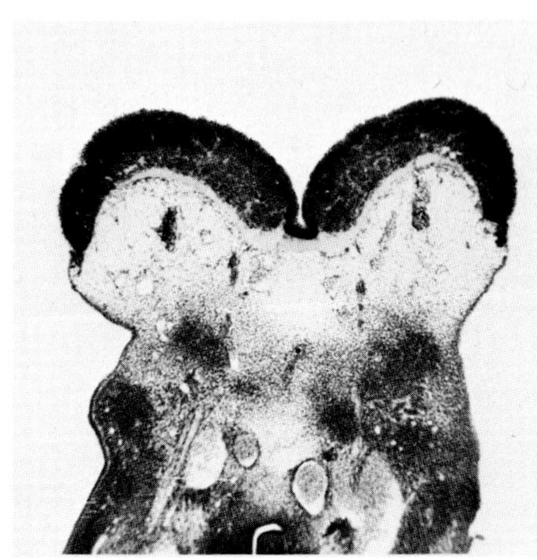

Figure 1-10. Transverse section through spina bifida (open neural plate) of a rat fetus whose mother was treated with trypan blue on days 8–10 of gestation. There is a wide-open trough as the central canal has not formed and the lateral portions of the neural plate failed to close dorsally in the midline. The neural tissue exposed to amniotic fluid will be eroded and reduced to an area medullovasculosa present at birth.

and Lubljana (Yugoslavia). In the same publication the difference between the highest frequency of spina bifida in Belfast (2.5 percent/1000) and the lowest in Manila (0.03/1000) is even more striking. Some of the incidence variations of anencephaly have been discussed in detail by Lemire et al.[41]

Etiologies of neural tube defects are complex.[41] There is a common form that includes most cases of anencephaly, spina bifida, and encephalocele (the last often complicated by hydrocephaly); this type shows a familial tendency but recurrence rates that do not correspond to Mendelian rules are expressed as empiric risk figures, and causation is said to be "multifactorial." A genetic tendency is assumed with a long list of environmental factors cited as secondary causes. A small number of neural tube defects that are accompanied by other malformations can be attributed to abnormal genes, chromosome, or aberrant tissue bands.

Postneurulation Development of the Caudal Neural Tube

When the posterior neurpore closes in Stage 12, there are approximately 25 segments of neural and vertebral development. While this actually is a simplified statement of a complex developmental process, it is intended to call attention to the fact that the spinal cord and spinal column still have more segmentation to acquire. Because neurulation has been completed, the additional lengthening must take place by a different process that has been described in animals but is poorly understood in humans.

The notochord and caudal end of the neural tube blend into an undifferentiated mass of cells, which can be called the "caudal cell mass." This cellular mass can differentiate in many ways and some cells are destined to become spinal cord. The manner in which the tail elongates, and new cord is formed, has been described experimentally[57–60] and in humans.[61] In some manner vacuoles appear and become surrounded by cells that orient around them. These vacuoles eventually coalesce and then make contact with the existing spinal cord, causing elongation of the neural tube. This growth, poorly understood in humans, occurs during Stages 13–20, and results in numerous accessory lumens (Figs. 1-11 and 1-12).[62,63] The overall process of elongation of the caudal neural tube is referred to as "canalization" (as opposed to neurulation).

The third phase of caudal neural tube development overlaps with canalization. Too many spinal and vertebral segments are formed and sometime around Stages 18–20 a regression of the more caudal segments occurs. This phenomenon, termed "retrogressive differentiation" by Streeter,[64] results in the formation

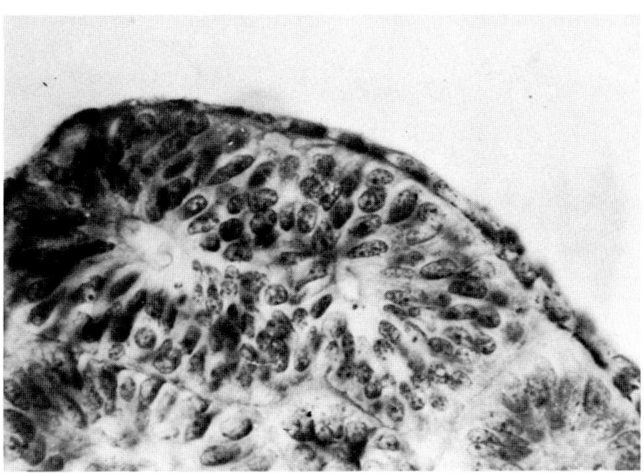

Figure 1-11. Photomicrograph of section through the caudal end of a human embryo showing multiple lumens found during the canalization phase of spinal cord development. (Reprinted with permission from Lemire RJ, Loeser RD, Leech RW, et al: Normal and Abnormal Development of the Human Nervous System. Hagerstown, Harper & Row, 1975.)

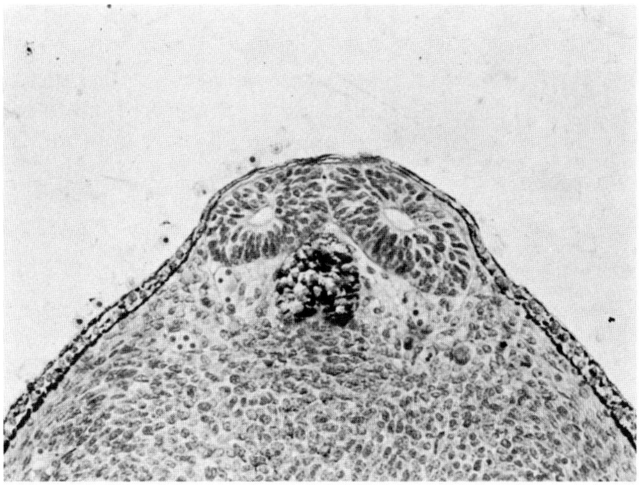

Figure 1-12. Photomicrograph of section through the caudal end of a human embryo. The two lumens are each surrounded by neural cells that are oriented around them. The ventral structure is the notochord.

of the filum terminale, conus medullaris, and its cavity, the ventriculus terminalis.[65] the ascent of the caudal end of the spinal cord continues throughout gestation.

Skin-Covered Defects of the Caudal Neural Tube

Malformations of the caudal neural tube and vertebrae that arise after closure of the posterior neuropore are covered with skin (Fig. 1-13). In most cases it is difficult to determine whether or not these anomalies originate during the canalization or retrogressive differentiation phase. Because the caudal cell mass has been shown experimentally to contain totipotent cells (cells that can differentiate into many different tissues depending on inductive influences), it is not surprising that a variety of malformations arise from this area.[66,67] Table 1-5 lists several conditions that probably arise from abnormal caudal neural tube and vertebral differentiation.

DEVELOPMENT OF THE CEPHALIC NEURAL TUBE

Cerebral Cortex

Normal Development

Following closure of the anterior neuropore in Stage 11, there is an interval before the first indication of differentiation of the telencephalon takes place in human embryos. In Stage 15 bilateral cerebral vesicles appear; their connections

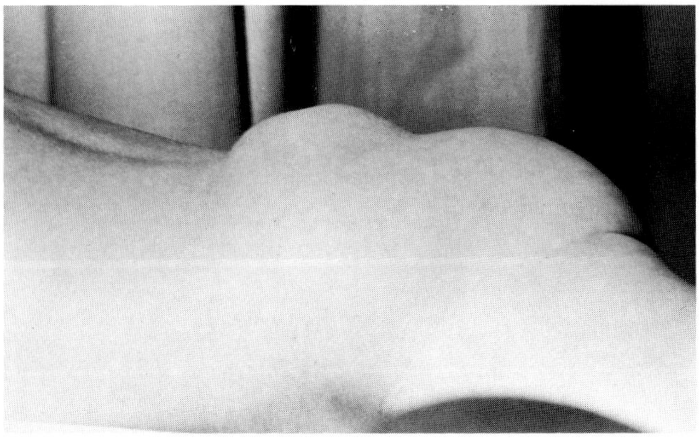

Figure 1-13. Lateral view of a skin-covered lumbosacral lipoma in an infant.

Table 1-5
Skin-Covered Sacrococcygeal Lesions*

Condition	Pathology	Possible Origin	Associated Features and Comments	References
Myelocystocele	Multicystic ependyma-lined cavities	Ventriculus terminalis	Cloacal exstrophy Vertebral defects	Von Recklinghausen[49] Lemire, Loiser, Leech, et al.[3]
Diastematomyelia	Two cords with or without separate dural sheaths	Canalization phase (some)	Myelocele or incidental finding	James and Lassman[91] Cohen and Sledge[92]
Lumbosacral lipoma	Subcutaneous lipoma communicating by fibrous stalk to intraspinal lipoma	Fetal period of retrogressive differentiation	Usually none Can occur with myelocele	Lassman and James[93] Dubowitz, Lorber, and Zuchary[94] Barson[95] Emery and Lendon[96]
Meningocele	Prolapsed dura mater and arachnoid through incomplete posterior arch	Unknown	Rare without associated lipoma	Lemire et al.[3]
Sacrococcygeal teratoma	Numerous cellular types from many tissues; neural tissue prominent feature	Ependymal rests in coccyx; germ cells	Female predominance; malignant transformation after infancy	Ashley[97]
Chordoma	Resembles notochord; solid, soft, or gelatinous	Notochord	Adult onset usual	Steegman[98]
Anomalies of sacrum	Varied from segmentation anomalies to agenesis	Retrogressive differentiation	Maternal diabetes	Warkany[83]

*Other lesions in this region include hemangioma, duplication of the rectum, bone tumors, epidermoid (dermoid) cysts, chrondroma, neurobastoma, glioma.

with the existing neural tube later become termed the foramina of Monro. The midline lamina terminalis forms a keel for these enlarging structures, and by Stage 17 areas that will become frontal and parietal lobes are identifiable. Primordia of occipital pole are present in Stage 19 and temporal pole in Stage 23.[2,4,68] These areas have no resemblance to final form as the main differentiation of cerebral cortex takes place throughout gestation, especially during the latter half.

Development of other structures also takes place during this time. During Stage 16 the primordium of the corpus striatum is present, and in Stage 18 the wall of the cerebral vesicle begins to differentiate into mantle layer. The first indication of cortical gray matter is when neuroblasts migrate from the ependymal zone into this mantle layer in Stage 22. Four defined cell layers are present by the end of the embryonic period, Stage 23. These do not correspond to the later layers and include (1) the innermost ependymal layer, (2) the mantle layer, (3) a layer of cells (the "intermediate") that has migrated to form the primordium of the cortical cellular layer, and (4) the marginal veil of His, a relatively acellular layer. The intermediate layer subdivides into two layers when the fetus is 46 mm CR length, a fiber layer and inner nuclear layer (spongioblasts and neuroblasts). By 95 mm CR length, primordia of three of the final cell layers are present; precursors of layers IV, V, and VI. Obviously, the differentiation of the cytoarchitecture of the cerebral cortex is very complex and has regional variation. The interested reader wishing to pursue this further is referred to the works of Bolton and Moyes,[69] Brun,[70] Conel,[71] Duckett and Pearse,[72] and Streeter.[73] Jacobson[6] reviews experimental observations of cytoarchitectonic development.

The external surfaces of the developing brain can provide some clues as to the gestational age. Because of the fissures and sulci, most of the cortical surface becomes buried once development of the gyri begins. Hesdorffer and Scammon,[68] Larroche,[74] Dorovini-Zis and Dolman,[75] and Chi, Dooling, and Gilles[76] have extensively studied development of the external patterns (Fig. 1-13). Timing has not yet been determined with the precision of embryonic staging and some morphologic variability exists between specimens that are supposedly the same age. Therefore, rather than centering on a given gyrus or sulcus, the overall pattern may be assessed and guide the viewer to an approximate age. While there will not be further discussion in the present chapter about important factors involved in these morphologic variations, a normal "brain growth spurt" as proposed by Dobbing[77] is undoubtedly a major influence on form as well as function.

Other changes within the forebrain can be identified specifically in the young fetus. For example, the internal capsule fibers first present at Stage 19 have almost completely separated the caudate nucleus from the lentiform nucleus by 70 mm CR length. The separation of cellular areas, fiber tracts, and nuclear groups takes place over a long period, yet myelination is a relatively late event, beginning in the fourth to fifth gestational month and continuing for several years after birth.[78] While the diencephalon is developing independently, there are obvious interrelationships with the forebrain that must take place. Development of these deep nuclei has been discussed elsewhere and are beyond the scope of this chapter.[3] Each aspect of fetal CNS development is a dynamic process that does not yet conveniently fit into stages such as found in the embryo.

Abnormalities of the Brain

In addition to anencephaly and exencephaly, discussed previously as neural tube defects, many malformations of the brain can be attributed to abnormal prenatal development. *Micrencephaly* is a small brain enclosed in a small skull. Abnormal genes and chromosomes, as well as prenatal environmental interferences, can reduce brain growth to varying sizes. Known causes are too numerous to be listed here, but it should be mentioned that family history or associated malformations sometimes permit an etiologic classification. Micrencephaly is seldom a neurosurgical problem except that some forms of craniosynostoses or encephaloceles may have to be considered in the differential diagnosis. *Congenital hydrocephaly,* an increased amount of fluid in the cranial cavity, is relatively rare compared with the forms that develop after birth. Some hydrocephalic children who are born with augmented amounts of fluid within the ventricular system show no enlargement of the head at birth. This at first subclinical hydrocephaly is due to subnormal development of the brain, which is often associated with other congenital malformations and results in postnatal psychomotor retardation. Many types of hydrocephaly that become manifest in postnatal life only have prenatal origins, such as spina bifida cystica, Arnold–Chiari malformation, congenital atresia of the foramina of Luschka and Magendie, and tumors. Some are gene-determined, few are due to chromosomal abnormalities, and some can be caused by prenatal infections such as cytomegalic inclusion disease and toxoplasmosis. Some forms of congenital hydrocephalus originate by primary maldevelopment of the brain whereas others are due to secondary destructive processes in an originally normal brain. The extreme form of the latter type is *hydranencephaly,* an anomaly characterized by absence of the cerebral hemispheres in the presence of intact meninges and a rather normal skull. The thin-walled sac of meninges that replaces the hemispheres is filled with cerebrospinal fluid. Children with this severe malformation of the brain may be encountered by neurosurgeons who are asked for a differential diagnosis.

Schizencephaly is a kind of hydranencephaly in which there are no signs of encephaloclastic processes. It is a developmental anomaly that results in large symmetric clefts or gaps of the cortex formed at early stages of brain development.[79]

Porencephaly, another cerebral defect that involves cortical tissue and penetrates the white matter into the ventricular system, is probably of later origin and a secondary anomaly following circulatory disturbances. The lesion can be unilateral or bilateral; it is lined by connective and glial tissue and covered externally by dura that takes a normal course over the surface of the brain. The central gyri and the island of Reil are common sites, but the defects can occur in any lobe.

Lissencephaly is the term applied to a brain with a smooth surface, without convolutions (agyria), that resembles to a certain extent the brain of a 4–5-month-old fetus. When found in postnatal life, the anomaly is attributed to failure of migration of neuroblasts to the surface. The superficial cellular stratum contains neurons that arrived early in development; they were not moved inward by subsequent immigration to become deeper layers.[80] In complete lissencephaly the convexities of the hemispheres are smooth and only the sylvian fissures and traces of other fissures are present. In pachygyria the gyri are wider than normal; the sulci are shallow and poorly formed but the major fissures are better defined than in lissencephaly. Both lissencephalic and pachygyric brains are usually reduced in size and weight. The white matter is always underdeveloped but subcortical structures of the diencephalon and telencephalon can appear normal. The lateral ventricles remain large as in fetal stages owing to lack of development of the white matter. Lissencephaly can occur in familial syndromes that include ocular, cardiac, renal, hepatic and skeletal anomalies.[81]

Failure of brain development in the transverse direction leads to *cyclopia* with one median eye or to a series of less marked malformations such as ethmocephaly, cebocephaly, and trigoncephaly. The milder forms are seen by neurosurgeons. *Holoprosencephaly* refers to the cerebral changes of the cyclopia series: the prosencephalon fails to cleave sagittally into cerebral hemispheres with inadequate development of telencephalon, diencephalon, and olfactory and optic bulbs. Underdevelopment of the olfactory parts of the brain in these malformations has been emphasized and has led to the term *arhinencephaly.* In alobar holoprosencephaly, the most severe form, there is a single ventricle without hemispheric division, corpus callosum, and septum pellucidum. Micrencephaly and microcephaly are usually present in fetuses with arhinencephaly.

Exencephaly means an exposed brain without skin and bone cover. It is the forerunner of anencephaly. Encephalocele (Fig. 1-14) is the term for a brain hernia protruding through a congenital opening of the skull; if covered by meninges and skin, the lesion is compatible with life and is operable. There are occipital, parietal, frontal, nasal, and nasopharyngeal forms that vary greatly in size. Large encephaloceles may contain only fluid whereas small lesions can harbor a portion of the brain. Presence or absence of brain in the hernia determines the prognosis of operated cases. Hydrocephaly and microcephaly may be associated with encephaloceles.

The *corpus callosum* develops relatively late in normal brains; it can be absent or underdeveloped in brains that otherwise are free of malformations and go unnoticed in such cases throughout a normal life. But it can also be absent in severely abnormal brains with midline defects that cause serious disturbances of psychomotor functions. In humans the corpus callosum develops in the lamina terminalis and remains small and limited to the rostral part of the brain to the fourth fetal month. From the fifth month on it grows rapidly caudad until it reaches the extent known in the adult brain. Agenesis of the corpus callosum may be complete or partial, with the defect limited to the posterior portions. In some instances the anterior commissure, fornix, and the septum pellucidum are also absent but the longitudinal callosal bundle is formed. Among the severe cerebral malformations associated with agenesis of the corpus callosum are those of the cyclopia series and parietal encephaloceles. Callosal defects usually are sporadic but the anomaly can also occur as a recessively inherited trait in families in which epilepsy is manifest. The malformation is always present in trisomy 13 and occasionally in other chromosomal disease pictures.

Cerebrovascular malformations are among the most important congenital anomalies encountered by neurosurgeons. They are often compatible with a normal postnatal life and occur in persons who do not have associated malformations. It is not unusual, therefore, for neurosurgeons to treat patients in their 40s or 50s because of complications of congenital cerebrovascular malformations that in themselves were symptomless for decades. The cerebral vasculature is first represented by a network of endothelium-lined channels from which

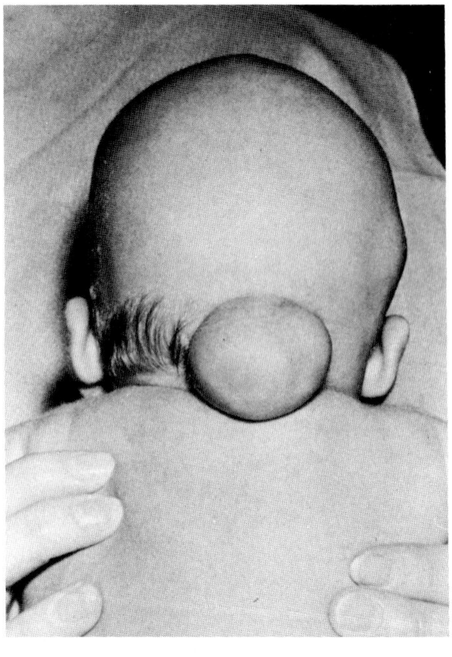

Figure 1-14. Occipital encephalocele in an infant. The lesion is completely covered with skin. (Reprinted with permission from Lemire RJ, Loeser RD, Leech RW, et al: Normal and Abnormal Development of the Human Nervous System. Hagerstown, Harper & Row, 1975.)

arteries, veins, and capillaries are derived in Stages 10 and 11 (2–4.5 mm CR length). At the end of this period the first circulation of the head is established.[3] After the cerebral vasculature is separated from the external and dural strata, the cerebral blood vessels are formed by retrogression of some and growth and differentiation of other channels that form the permanent arteries, capillaries, and veins. The stems of origin of all cerebral arteries in the 2-month-old embryo already are similar to those of the adult but the veins attain their adult distribution somewhat later, in the 3-month-old embryo.[82] Errors in the connections of the arterial and venous systems in the early months of fetal life can result in arteriovenous malformations that manifest themselves in children and, more often, in adults. Faulty differentiation of vessel walls may lead to formation of intracranial aneurysms. Although aneurysms encountered in later life can be acquired by atherosclerosis, infection, or hypertension, *congenital* berry or saccular aneurysms do occur as evidenced by cases in children and families and by associated malformations (e.g., polycystic kidneys). The aneurysms are seen at points of division of arteries and lie initially in the subarachnoid space but extension into the brain substance or the subdural space can occur.[83] Cerebral aneurysms in children and their surgical treatment were discussed by Amacher and Drake.[84]

Cerebellum

Normal Development

Although the rhombencephalon comprises a significant portion of the early embryonic brain, it is not until Stage 14 that the cerebellar plates can be identified. At this same time the pontine flexure is found.[5] Figure 1-15 follows

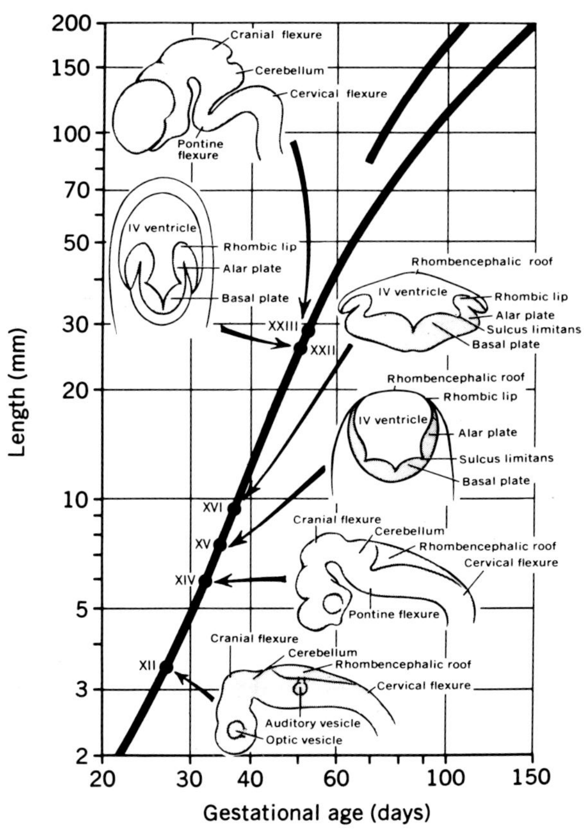

Figure 1-15. Cerebellum lateral and coronal news. Schematic representation of early development of the human cerebellum as correlated with developmental stage (Roman numerals), gestational age, and crown–rump length. (Reprinted with permission from Lemire RJ, Loeser RD, Leech RW, et al: Normal and Abnormal Development of the Human Nervous System. Hagerstown, Harper & Row, 1975.)

subsequent early development through the remainder of the embryonic stages. By the end of this period, the cerebellum is very primitive and most of its growth takes place during the fetal period. The best way to illustrate this is by looking at the timing of appearance of various portions of the midline vermis (Table 1-6). The sequential growth of the cerebellum throughout fetal life has been studied extensively and fairly accurate assessments of developmental age can be made grossly and histologically.[85–89]

Table 1-6
Appearance of Lobules and Fissures in the Cerebellar Vermis

Structure	CR Length (mm)	Estimated Gestational Age (Days)
Anterior medullary velum	60	70
Lingula	105	92
Precentral fissure	105	92
Central lobule	105	92
Preculminate fissure	78	80
Culmen	78	80
Primary fissure	72	75
Declive	130	105
Posterior superior fissure	130	105
Folium	130	105
Horizontal fissure	132	106
Tuber	132	106
Prepyramidal fissure	87	83
Pyramis	105	92
Secondary fissure	105	92
Uvula	105	92
Posterolateral fissure	45	62
Nodulus	105	92
Posterior medullary velum	127	102

Cerebellar Malformations

Cerebellar aplasia or *hypoplasia* sometimes has been found at necropsy in normal persons who had no or only minimal motor disturbances during life. But such defects can also occur associated with more or less severe malformations of the central nervous system, such as anencephaly, cyclopia, Dandy–Walker syndrome, and Arnold–Chiari malformation. In patients with cerebellar underdevelopment who have spastic diplegia, cerebral palsy, or mental retardation, clinical manifestations are probably due to associated cerebral anomalies. Agenesis and hypoplasia cerebelli can be limited to the vermis, or to one hemisphere; they can be unilateral or bilateral. Malformations of individual folia have been observed.[3,90] *Clefts of the cerebellum* (dysraphism) affect the inferior vermis and the velum medullare posterius. Closure of the cerebellar area proceeds in the rostro-caudal direction; it can be delayed and a resulting cleft can be combined with incomplete development of the occipital bone and the cervical spine, resulting in a cerebellomeningocele. Clefts can also be associated with cerebellar cysts, syringobulbia, or syringomyelia. Hyperplasia of the cerebellum sometimes occurs with megalencephaly. Cerebellar hypoplasia can be a recessively inherited trait. In children with trisomy 13, trisomy 18, or trisomy 21, developmental anomalies of various degrees have been reported and some cases have been attributed to environmental injuries during fetal life.[83]

REFERENCES

1. Hochstetter F: Beitrage zur Entwicklungsgeschichte des Menschlichen Gehirns. Vienna, Deuticke, part I, 1–168S; part II, 1–206S, 1919–1929
2. Streeter GL: The development of the nervous system, in Keibel F, Mall FP (eds): Manual of Human Embryology, vol II. Philadelphia, JB Lippincott, 1912, pp 1–156
3. Lemire RJ, Loeser JD, Leech RW, et al: Normal and Abnormal Development of the Human Nervous System. Hagerstown, Harper & Row, 1975
4. Bartelmez GW, Dekaban AS: The early development of the human brain. Contrib Embryol 37:13–32, 1962
5. O'Rahilly R, Gardner E: The timing and sequence of events in the development of the human nervous system during the embryonic period proper. Z Anat Entwickl-Gesch 134:1–12, 1971
6. Jacobson M: Developmental Neurobiology (ed 2) New York, Plenum Press, 1978
7. Streeter GL: Developmental Horizons in Human Embryos. Age Groups XI–XXIII, Embryology Reprint, vol II, Carnegie Inst Wash, Washington DC, 1951
8. Heuser CH, Corner GW: Developmental horizons in human embryos. Description of age group X, 4 to 12 somites. Contrib Embryol 36:29–39, 1957
9. O'Rahilly R: Developmental Stages in Human Embryos, Part A: Embryos of the First Three Weeks (Stages 1 to 9). Carnegie Inst Wash, Washington, D.C., 1973
10. Jirásek JE: In Cohen MM Jr (ed): Development of the Genital System and Male Pseudohermaphroditism. Baltimore, Johns Hopkins Press, 1971
11. Witschi E: Development of Vertebrates. Philadelphia, WB Saunders, 1956
12. Shepard TH: Catalog of Teratogenic Agents (ed 3). Baltimore, Johns Hopkins University Press, 1980
13. Grabowski CT: The induction of secondary embryos in the early chick blastoderm by grafts from Hensen's node. Am J Anat 101:101–134, 1957
14. Grabowski CT: Neural induction and notochord formation by mesoderm from the node area of the early chick blastoderm. J Exp Zool 150:233–246, 1962
15. Jurand A: The development of the notochord in chick embryos. J Embryol Exp Morphol 10:602–621, 1962
16. Saxen L, Toivonen S: The two-gradient hypothesis in primary induction: The combined effect of two types of inductors mixed in different ratios. J Embryol Exp Morphol 9:514–533, 1961
17. Toivonen S, Saxen L: Morphogenetic interaction of presumptive neural and mesodermal cells mixed in different ratios. Science 159:539–540, 1968
18. Sauer FC: Mitosis in the neural tube. J Comp Neurol 62:377–405, 1935a
19. Sauer FC: The cellular structure of the neural tube. J Comp Neurol 63:13–23, 1935b
20. Sauer FC: The interkinetic migration of embryonic epithelial nuclei. J Morphol 60:1–11, 1936
21. Sauer FC: Some factors in the morphogenesis of vertebrate embryonic epithelium. J Morphol 61:563–579, 1937
22. Watterston RL: Structure and mitotic behavior of the early neural tube, in DeHaan RL, Ursprung H (eds): Organogenesis. New York, Holt, Rinehart & Winston, 1965, pp 129–159
23. Sidman RL: Cellular proliferation and migration in the developing brain, in Drugs and Poisons in Relation to the Developing Nervous System, Public Health Service Publication 1791, 1967, pp 5–11
24. Adrian EK Jr, Walker BE: Incorporation of thymidine-H^3 by cells in the normal and injured mouse spinal cord. J Neuropath Exp Neurol 21:597–609, 1962
25. Fugita S: Kinetics of cellular proliferation. Exp Cell Res 28:52–60, 1962
26. Martin A, Langman J: The development of the spinal cord examined by autoradiography. J Embryol Exp Morphol 14:25–35, 1965
27. Rakic P, Sidman RL: Supravital DNA synthesis in the developing human and mouse brain. J Neuropath Exp Neurol 27:246–276, 1968

28. Karfunkel P: The mechanisms of neural tube formation. Int Rev Cytol 38:245–271, 1974
29. Burt AS: Neurulation in mechanically and chemically inhibited amblystoma. Biol Bull 85:103–115, 1943
30. Jelínek R, Friebova Z: Influence of mitotic activity on neurulation movements. Nature 209:822–823, 1966
31. Davis JO: Photochemical analysis of neural tube formation. Biol Bull 87:73–95, 1944
32. Glaser OC: On the mechanism of morphological differentiation in the nervous system. I. The transformation of a neural plate into a neural tube. Anat Rec 8:525–551, 1914
33. Glaser OC: The theory of autonomous folding in embryogenesis. Science 44:505–509, 1916
34. Hobson LB: On the ultrastructure of the neural plate of the early chick embryo, with notes on the effects of dehydration. J Exp Zool 88:107–134, 1941
35. Jacobson C-O: Cell migration in the neural plate and the process of neurulation in the axolotl larva. Zool Bidr Uppsala 35:433–449, 1962
36. Lewis WH: Mechanisms of invagination. Anat Rec 97:139–156, 1947
37. Baker PC, Schroeder TE: Cytoplasmic filaments and morphogenetic movement in the amphibian neural tube. Dev Biol 15:432–450, 1967
38. Bancroft M, Bellairs R: Differentiation of the neural plate and neural tube in the young chick embryo. A study by scanning and transmission electron microscopy. Anat Embryol 147:309–335, 1975
39. Portch PA, Barson AJ: Scanning electron microscopy of neurulation in the chick. J Anat 117:341–350, 1974
40. Waterman RE: Topographical changes along the neural fold associated with neurulation in the hamster and mouse. Am J Anat 146:151–172, 1976
41. Lemire RJ, Beckwith JB, Warkany J: Anencephaly. New York, Raven Press, 1978
42. Ballantyne JW: Manual of Antenatal Pathology and Hygiene. II. The Embryo. New York, William Wood, 1905
43. Lemire RJ, Beckwith JB, Shepard TH: Iniencephaly and anencephaly with spinal retroflexion. A comparative study of eight human specimens. Teratology 6:27–36, 1972
44. Bowden RA, Stephens TD, Lemire RJ: The association of spinal retroflexion with limb anomalies. Teratology 21:53–59, 1980
45. Patten BM: Overgrowth of the neural tube in young human embryos. Anat Rec 113:381–393, 1952
46. Marin-Padilla M, Ferm VH: Somite necrosis and developmental malformations induced by vitamin A in the golden hamster. J Embryol Exp Morphol 13:1–8, 1965
47. Gardner WJ: Rupture of the neural tube; the cause of myelomeningocele. Arch Neurol 4:1–7, 1961
48. Padget DH: Spina bifida and embryonic neuroschisis—A causal relationship. Johns Hopkins Med J 123:233–252, 1968
49. Recklinghausen F von: Untersuchunger über die Spina Bifida. Berlin, Druck und Verlag von Georg Reimer, 1886
50. Dekaban AS: Anencephaly in young human embryos. J Neuropath Exp Neurol 22:533–548, 1963
51. Dekaban AS, Bartelmez GW: Complete dysraphism in a 14 somite human embyro. Am J Anat 115:27–42, 1964
52. Lemire RJ, Shepard TH, Alvord EC Jr: Caudal myeloschisis (lumbosacral spina bifida cystica) in a five millimeter (horizon XIV) human embryo. Anat Rec 152:9–16, 1965
53. Nishimura H, Takano K, Tanimura T, et al: High incidence of several malformations in the early human embryos as compared with infants. Biol Neonate 10:93–107, 1966
54. Gardner WJ: The Dysraphic States: From Syringomyelia to Anencephaly. Amsterdam, Excerpta Medica, 1973

55. Padget DH: Neuroschisis and human embryonic maldevelopment. J Neuropath Exp Neurol 29:192–216, 1970
56. Stevenson AC, Johnston HA, Stewart MIP, et al: Congenital malformations—A report of a series of consecutive births in 24 centres. Bull WHO 34:1–127, 1966
57. Gaertner RA: Development of the posterior trunk and tail of the chick embryo. J Exp Zool 111:157–174, 1949
58. Seichert V, Jelinek R: Tissue shifts in the end and tail bud of the chick embryo. Folia Morphol (Prague) 16:436–446, 1968
59. Jelínek R, Seichert V, Klika E: Mechanism of morphogenesis of the caudal neural tube in the chick embryo. Folia Morphol (Prague) 17:355–367, 1969
60. Klika E, Jelínek R: The structure of the end and tail bud of the chick embryo. Folia Morphol (Prague) 17:29–40, 1969
61. Kunitomo K: The development and reduction of the tail and of the caudal end of the spinal cord. Contrib Embryol 8:161–198, 1918
62. Bolli P: Sekundare Lumenbildungen im Neuralrohr und Ruckenmark menschlicher Embryonen. Acta Anat 64:48–81, 1966
63. Lemire RJ: Variations in development of the caudal neural tube in human embryos (horizons XIV–XXI). Teratology 2:361–370, 1969
64. Streeter GL: Factors involved in the formation of the filum terminale. Am J Anat 25:1–11, 1919
65. Kernohan JW: The ventriculus terminalis: Its growth and development. J Comp Neurol 38:107–125, 1925
66. Werner JL, Taybi H: Presacral masses in childhood. Am J Roentgenol Radium Ther Nucl Med 109:403–410, 1970
67. Lemire RJ, Graham CB, Beckwith JB: Skin-covered sacrococcygeal masses in infants and children. J Pediatr 79:948–954, 1971
68. Hesdorffer MB, Scammon RE: Growth of human nervous system. I. Growth of cerebral surface. Proc Soc Exp Biol Med 33:415–418, 1935
69. Bolton JS, Moyes JM: The cytoarchitecture of the cerebral cortex of a human foetus of 18 weeks. Brain 35:1–25, 1912
70. Brun A: The subpial granular layer of the foetal cerebral cortex in man: Its ontogeny and significance in congenital cortical malformation. Acta Pathol Microbiol Scand 179(suppl):1–98, 1965
71. Conel JL: The Postnatal Development of the Human Cerebral Cortex (7 vols). Cambridge, Harvard University Press, 1939–1963
72. Duckett S, Pearse AGE: The cells of Cajal–Retzius in the developing human brain. J Anat 102:183–187, 1968
73. Streeter GL: The cortex of the brain in the human embryo during the 4th month, with special reference to the so-called "Papillae of Retzius." Am J Anat 7:337–344, 1907
74. Larroche J-C: The development of the central nervous system during intrauterine life, in Falkner F (ed) Human Development. Philadelphia, WB Saunders, 1966, pp 257–276
75. Dorovini-Zis K, Dolman CL: Gestational development of brain. Arch Path Lab Med 101:192–195, 1977
76. Chi JG, Dooling EC, Gilles FH: Gyral development of the human brain. Ann Neurol 1:86–93, 1977
77. Dobbing J: The later development of the brain and its vulnerability, in Davis JA, Dobbing J (eds): Scientific Foundations of Paediatrics. London, William Heinemann, 1974, pp 565–577
78. Yakovlev PI, LeCours AR: The myelogenetic cycles of regional maturation of the brain, in Minowski A (ed): Regional Development of the Brain in Early Life. Oxford, Blackwell, 1967, pp 3–70
79. Yakovlev PI, Wadsworth RC: Schizencephalies: A study of congenital clefts in the cerebral mantle. I. Clefts with fused lips. II. Clefts with hydrocephalus and lips separated. J Neuropathol Exp Neurol 5:116–130, 169–206, 1946
80. Stewart RM, Richman DP, Caviness VS Jr: Lissencephaly and pachygyria. Acta Neuropathol 31:1–12, 1975

81. Dieker H, Edwards RH, ZuRhein G, et al: The lissencephaly syndrome. Birth Defects Orig Art Series 5:53–64, 1969
82. Kaplan HA, Aronson SM, Browder EJ: Vascular malformations of the brain. An anatomical study. J Neurosurg 18:630–635, 1961
83. Warkany J: Congenital Malformations: Notes and Comments. Chicago, Year Book Medical Publishers, 1971
84. Amacher AL, Drake CG: The results of operating upon cerebral aneurysms and angiomas in children and adults. Child's Brain 5:151–165, 1979
85. Bradley OC: On the development and homology of the mammalian cerebellar fissures. J Anat Physiol 37:448–475, 1903
86. Langelaan J: On the development of the external form of the human cerebellum. Brain 42:130–170, 1919
87. Larsell O: Morphogenesis and evolution of the cerebellum. Arch Neurol Psychiat 31:373–395, 1934
88. Larsell O: The development of the cerebellum in man in relation to its comparative anatomy. J Comp Neurol 87:85–129, 1947
89. Loeser JD, Lemire RJ, Alvord EC Jr: The development of the folia in the human cerebellar vermis. Anat Rec 173:109–114, 1972
90. Dow RS, Moruzzi G: Physiology and Pathology of the Cerebellum. Minneapolis, University of Minnesota Press, 1958
91. James CCM, Lassman LP: Spinal Dysraphism: Spina Bifida Occulta. New York, Appleton–Century–Crofts, 1972
92. Cohen J, Sledge CG: Diastematomyelia. Am J Dis Child 100:257–263, 1960
93. Lassman LP, James CCM: Lumbosacral lipomas: Critical survey of 26 cases submitted to laminectomy. J Neurol Neurosurg Psychiat 30:174–181, 1967
94. Dubowitz V, Lorber J, Zachary RB: Lipoma of the cauda equina. Arch Dis Child 40:207–213, 1965
95. Barson AJ: Symptomless intradural spinal lipomas in infancy. J Pathol 104:141–144, 1971
96. Emery JL, Lendon RG: Lipomas of the cauda equina related to neurospinal dysraphism. Develop Med Child Neurol 20(suppl):62–70, 1969
97. Ashley DJB: Origin of teratomas. Cancer 32:390–394, 1973
98. Steegman AT: Chordomas, in Minkler J (ed): Pathology of the Nervous System, vol 2. New York, McGraw–Hill, 1971, pp 1917–1927

2. Spina Bifida

Donald H. Reigel

Spina bifida is a term used to describe a birth defect resulting from abnormal fusion of the posterior neural tube. The etiology is unclear and the genetics are multifactorial. Characteristically the change ranges from one or more vertebrae being incompletely developed with a minimal abnormality such as an absent spinous process and associated dorsal intralaminar cleft, to the more profound changes of absence of the dorsal half of the vertebrae at multiple levels, abnormal vertebral bodies, and high-degree kyphosis. In its full expression, such as myelomeningocele, the entire central nervous system is involved, and there are associated multisystem anomalies. In discussions of myelomeningocele, authors have emphasized the spinal cord lesion but have frequently failed to describe the profound changes in the cerebral hemispheres and the brain stem, which further contribute to the enormous effect upon the patient. During the past 15 years, the care of children with spina bifida has excited the emotions of neurosurgeons and catalyzed medical ethics discussions more than any other birth defect.

TERMINOLOGY

Spina bifida occulta refers to a vertebral anomaly consisting of the absence of a spinous process and varying amounts of the associated lamina. Usually the central nervous system (CNS), cauda equina, and meninges are involved. The neurologic examination is normal. Most frequently the skin is normal over the vertebral defect; however, associated dimples, sinuses, hypertrichosis, and hemangiomata may indicate the presence of occult lesions such as lipoma, dermoid, diastematomyelia, and tethered spinal cord. Spina bifida occulta is usually discovered by incidental spina x-rays and occurs in perhaps 20 to 30 percent of the population. The most important aspect of spina bifida occulta is an awareness of its presence and the slightly increased risk of occult intraspinal lesion for these patients.

Meningocele (spina bifida cystica, spina bifida aperta) becomes evident at birth with observation of a cystic skin-covered midline mass over the lumbodorsal area. About 10 percent of patients with spina bifida will have meningocele.[1] The dorsal half of one or more vertebrae is absent and the sac is composed of cerebrospinal fluid (CSF), meninges, and skin. Ganglion cells have been identified in the sac, but the spinal cord and cauda equina are usually normal. As with spina bifida occulta, a high suspicion for associated occult intraspinal lesions must be maintained. Generally the remainder of the CNS is not involved, and the prognosis for development is excellent. There is increased association of hydrocephalus with meningocele, but it does not reach the 80–90 percent association observed with myelomeningocele.

Myelomeningocele is the most severe form of spina bifida. The midline mass, in addition to CSF and meninges, contains spinal cord and cauda equina (Fig. 2-1). All of these patients will have Arnold–Chiari malformation and most will develop hydrocephalus. Frequently there are changes in the cerebral cortex such as polymicrogyria. There is sensory motor loss distal to the lesion, which produces neurogenic bladder and varying degrees of weakness in the lower extremities. Orthopedic deformity and other system anomalies are commonly present.

Spina bifida cystica usually defines those patients with meningocele or myelomeningocele.[2]

Lipomeningocele or lipomyelomeningocele refers to lesions as described above that are associated with a lipoma. This may be extradural and/or intradural and involve the cauda equina and the conus medullaris (Fig. 2-2).

Anterior meningocele most commonly refers to a pelvic mass that communicates with the spinal subarachnoid space through a small opening in the anterior sacrum. The content of the mass is usually limited to cerebrospinal fluid. Anterior meningocele has also been observed in the thoracic area.

Spinal dysraphism is a general term used for the above-described forms of spina bifida. There is a varying degree of abnormal fusion of the neural, mesodermal, and ectodermal tissues in the dorsal medial region of the developing fetus.[3]

Arnold–Chiari malformation is a congenital anomaly of the hindbrain, which is usually associated with myelomeningocele. The medulla oblongata and pons are elongated and distorted, and the cerebellar vermis is displaced into the

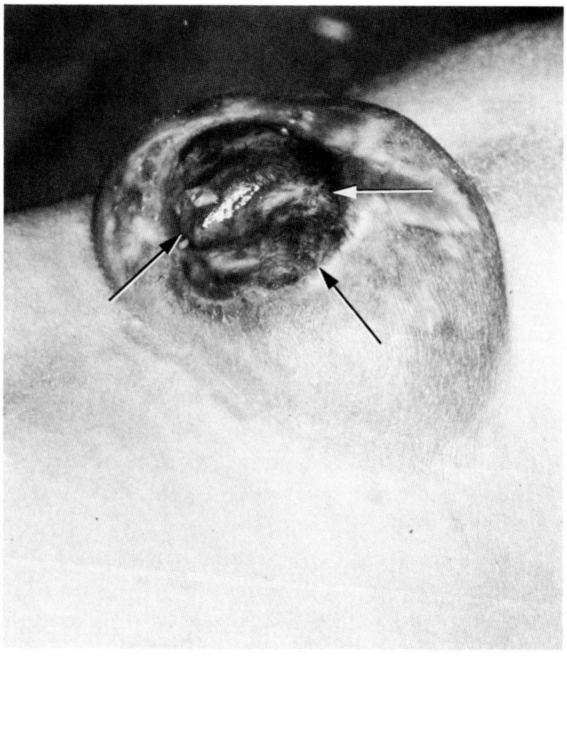

Figure 2-1. External appearance of lumbar myelomeningocele. Black arrow points to central canal and white arrow to neural plaque.

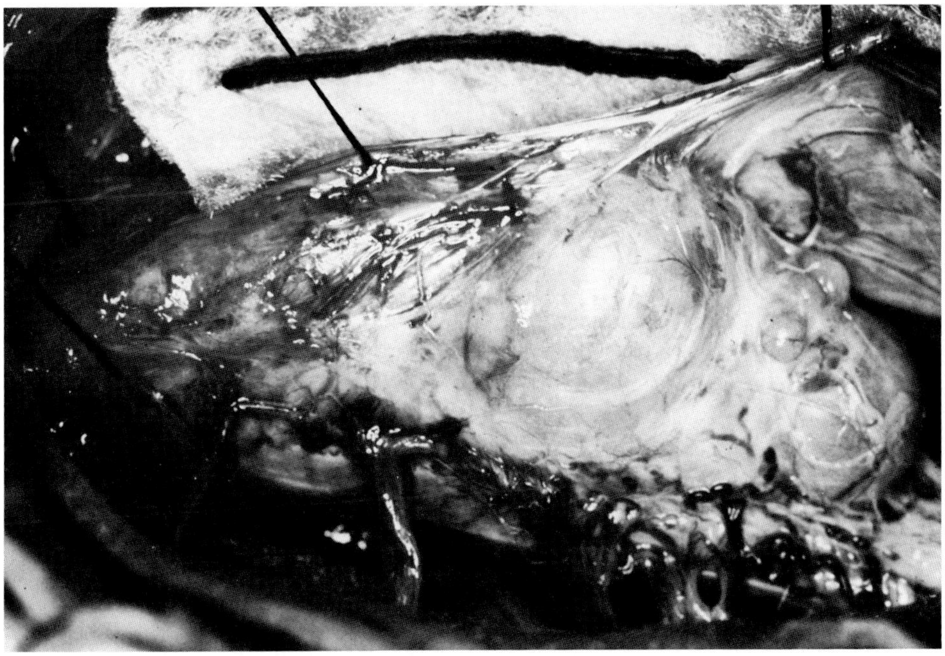

Figure 2-2. Lipomyel-omeningocele.

cervical spinal canal. Abnormalities of the skull, dura, midbrain, cerebellum, hemispheres, cisterns, and ventricles have been described with Arnold–Chiari malformation.[4–6]

Rachischisis describes a failure of ectodermal and mesodermal closure that results in the brain and spinal cord being exposed to the environment. It is identified at birth and is incompatible with survival.

INCIDENCE AND EPIDEMIOLOGY

In North America spina bifida occulta occurs in 20–30 percent of the people. The risk of spina bifida with meningocele or myelomeningocele is one to two per 1000 live births.[2,7]

There are geographic variations with the highest incidence being reported at four to five per 1000 live births in some regions of Ireland.[8] In addition regional differences have been reported in Great Britain, Europe, Canada, and the United States. Declining frequency occurs from east to west on the North American continent.[9] The rate of spina bifida is much lower in blacks than in caucasians.[9] Unexplained seasonal and yearly frequency variations of spina bifida have been described. The suggestion that there are variations in the frequency of spina bifida related to socioeconomic status does not seem to have adequate supporting data. The data to suggest that the maternal age or parity is related to the incidence of spina bifida are incomplete.[10,11]

GENETICS

There is a familial tendency or predisposition to the occurrence of spina bifida. The statistics do not fit Mendelian transmission. The hereditary predisposition for spina bifida has been described as multifactorial. Environmental factors, familial tendency, declining risk with increasing distance of relatives, and the fact that when one or more siblings are affected there is marked increase in risk for subsequent siblings to be affected, has been cited as evidence to support multifactorial inheritance.[9] In North America the risk of having a child with spina bifida is about 0.1 to 0.2 percent. If there is one sibling with spina bifida, however, the risk increases to about 5 percent; if there are two, the risk increases to approximately 12–15 percent.[12] Twinning, consanguinity, and seasonal variation studies have produced little further information to determine genetic inheritance.[9,13]

Recently Fineman, Jorde, Martin, et al.[14] suggested that spina bifida occulta and spina bifida cystica may be related to an autosomal dominant gene with a 75 percent penetrance. Their data also indicated that spina bifida occulta and spina bifida cystica may be different phenotypic expressions of the same gene. Further analysis, however, will be required to test this thesis.[14]

Regardless of the genetic forms of inheritance, genetic counseling should be offered to all parents and close relatives of children with spina bifida. A detailed listing of facilities offering these services may be obtained from the National Foundation of the March of Dimes.[15]

ETIOLOGY

There has been great interest in identifying etiologic factors of spina bifida, which would then lead to prevention. Perhaps one of the most popular theories was proposed by Renwick in 1972.[16] He suggested that a teratogenic substance existed in blighted potatoes that caused anencephaly and spina bifida. This thesis has never been verified, however, and studies have shown no statistical difference in exposure to potatoes between groups of mothers of children with spina bifida and control groups.[17] Furthermore trials of potato avoidance have failed to reduce the incidence of spina bifida.[18]

Numerous deficiency states, including folic acid and zinc, have been suggested as etiologic factors. Recently it has been reported that periconceptional vitamin supplementation was associated with a statistically significant reduction in neural tube defects when compared with a similar unsupplemented group.[19]

Nocturnal fever, viruses, hypervitaminosis A, hormonal and ovulatory changes, and dextromorphan have been suggested as etiologic factors.[9,20–24] Despite the abundance of suggested teratogens for spina bifida, conclusive supporting data for a causal factor continue to be missing.

EMBRYOLOGY

Most investigators agree that the area of the posterior neuropore is the site of embryologic abnormality. Differing forms of spina bifida may be related to the phases of development of the caudal neural tube. These include neurulation, canalization, and retrogressive differentiation.[25] The timing of the intrauterine occurrence of spina bifida is controversial because of conflict about embryogenesis.

Von Rechlinghausen proposed failure of the embryonic neural plate to close in tubular form at 25–28 days of gestation,[26] which was then followed by the associated mesodermal and ectodermal changes of spina bifida.[25]

Gardner has proposed overdistention of the neural tube by CSF as the single cause of rupture of the caudal neural sac leading to spina bifida.[27] This would occur at 2–3 months of intrauterine life. The background work of Morgagni[28] and Weed[29] has been important in the development of this theory.

Patten observed overgrowth of the dorsal caudal neural plate in chick and human embryos and suggested that this was the primary event leading to failure of the neural tube to close.[30–32] Whether overgrowth is a primary abnormal embryologic event or secondary to failed fusion remains to be determined.

More recently Padget[33–35] and Padget and Lindenberg[36] suggested the appearance of a cleft in the neural tube that permitted a "bleb" of proteinacious material to protrude into surrounding mesodermal and ectodermal tissues, resulting in changes in the neural plate, mesoderm, and ectoderm. Blebs may appear at any location and could explain the variable forms of spina bifida. This theory is attractive because it preserves the nonclosure theory of embryogenesis. Recently Osaka, Tanimura, Hirayama, et al.[37] challenged the theory on the basis of human fetus studies.

None of the embryogenesis theories adequately explain all of the neuropathologic changes observed with spina bifida, and the need for continuing investigation remains.

PATHOLOGY

Although the pathologic abnormalities observed at the site of the neuroplaque may be the most obvious, additional change is frequently found throughout the entire central and peripheral nervous system. The variations and combinations are numerous, and awareness of this potential contributes to more comprehensive understanding in the care of the patient and on the part of the patient's family.

Brain

Lobar agenesis, polymicrogyria, holoprosencephaly, and cerebellar dysgenesis are commonly observed. Hydrocephalus and associated anomalies of the aqueduct and cerebrospinal fluid pathways occur at a very high frequency. The Arnold–Chiari malformation is invariably present. Agenesis of the corpus collosum, cysts of the septum pellucidum, midline lipoma, and arachnoid cysts have been observed.[38]

Spinal Cord

The site of the spinal cord lesion is most frequently at the distal thoracic, lumbar, or sacral areas. Over 70 percent of meningoceles and myelomeningoceles will be found here. Approximately 10 percent of meningoceles will be in the cervical area as opposed to 3 percent of myelomeningoceles. Occasionally more than one lesion will be observed in the same patient, and up to three have been reported.[39]

In about one third of the patients the neuroplaque will demonstrate an open-book appearance with the central canal in the center (myeloschisis). About one third will have varying forms of diastematomyelia or hemicord-like structures. Frequently both the anterior and posterior nerve roots appear to emanate from the anterior half of the spinal cord. The angle of departure of the nerve roots will often be more tangential. Arachnoid forming the cystic component of the lesion is adherent to the neural plaque, dura, and skin. The anterior columns of the spinal cord are frequently intact, whereas there are varying degrees of dorsal column destruction.[40] Hydromyelia and syringomyelia may be present in 40 percent of patients. The incidence of hydrocephalus is not reported in these studies, however, and a high frequency of uncontrolled hydrocephalus may

Table 2-1
Systemic Anomolies Associated with Spina Bifida

Skeletal	Gastrointestinal	Pulmonary	Craniofacial	Cardiovascular	Genitourinary
Clubfeet	Inguinal hernia	Tracheoesophageal fistula	Synostosis	Ventriculo-septal defect (VSD)	Hydronephrosis
Hip dislocation	Mickel's diverticulum	Situs inversus	Cleft palate	Atrial-septal defect (ASD)	Hydroureter
Rib anomalies	Malrotation		Strabismus	Patent ductus	Horseshoe kidney
Kyphoscoliosis	Omphalocele		Low-set ears	Coarctation	Undescended testes
Pectus excavatum	Imperforate anus		Hypertelorism		Hydrocele
Snydactaly					Malrotation
					Exstrophy

artificially inflate the frequency figures for hydromyelia. Both extradural and intradural lipoma, dermoid, and fibrolipomas may be associated with all forms of spina bifida. Neuron counts in the lumbosacral spinal cords from children with myelomeningocele have demonstrated reductions related to the degree of cord damage or deformity present. Normal rostral spinal cord segments contained normal neuron numbers.[41] Studies of the peripheral nervous system of newborn children with myelomeningocele have demonstrated reduction in the size of peripheral nerves. Preservation of part or all of the fibers of nerves distal to the plaque have been demonstrated, however.[42]

There is a high incidence of other system congenital malformations with spina bifida. A study of 434 patients with spina bifida demonstrated an average of 2.2 associated defects per patient.[43] Skeletal malformations are the most frequent, with clubfeet and hip dislocation being the most common. Table 2-1 lists generally associated systemic anomalies.

NEUROPHYSIOLOGY

In the past it was commonly thought that the motor lesion of myelomeningocele patients was at the level of the anterior horn cell. Clinical observations, however, have revealed upper motor neuron lesions in patients with functioning isolated distal cord segments.[44] Stark and Drummond[45] have demonstrated that neuroplaque stimulation results in involuntary contraction of 80–100 percent of paralyzed muscles of the lower extremities. The magnitude of contraction was similar to that observed following peripheral nerve stimulation of normal infants. Absence of fibrillation potentials further led Stark and Drummond to conclude that paralysis associated with myelomeningocele was secondary to an upper motor neuron lesion. They postulated that the lesion was either within the plaque itself or just rostral to the plaque.[45] The etiology of the upper motor neuron lesion remains undetermined. Possible explanations include abnormal development and change occurring in the neuroplaque before, during, or after birth.

Somatosensory evoked potential studies of newborn children with myelomeningocele have demonstrated intact sensory nerves to and from the neuroplaque. In 2 of 7 patients studied, afferent integrity through the plaque was observed.[46] Interference with afferent conduction, therefore, appears to be located at the level of the neuroplaque.

The observation of functioning motor and sensory systems within the neuroplaque provides further support for meticulous protection and preservation of the neuroplaque during early care of the myelomeningocele patient. Furthermore these findings, coupled with Lendon's[41] observation of normal neuronal populations in the rostral spinal cord, have provided the background data to justify cauda equina reconstruction, as described by Epstein, Spielholz, Battista, et al.,[47] in which proximal intercostal nerves are anastamosed to nerve roots distal to the lesion. Early electromyographic observations have indicated reinnervation of muscle groups within the lower extremities. This exciting technique offers the possibility of bypassing the afferent and efferent interruption that occurs at the level of the plaque.[41,47]

HISTORY OF TREATMENT

Although the condition of spina bifida may have been recognized by Hippocrates and medieval Arab physicians, credit has been given to Nicholai Talpius for providing one of the earliest descriptions in 1685.[48,49] In 1857 Athol[50] described a sacral mass associated with the meninges and Virchow[51] introduced the popular term spina bifida occulta in 1875. Doran and Guthkelch[49] indicated that Morgagni (1769) was the first to describe the association of hydrocephalus and spina bifida and credits Marsh, Gould, Clutton, et al.[52] and Von Recklinghausen[26] for detailing the varieties of spina bifida.

Although operative treatment for spina bifida may have occurred as early as 1610 when Forestus ligated a sac, significant attempts to repair the condition did not occur until the 20th century.[53] With the advent of aseptic surgical technique and antibiotics, an increasing number of surgeons began to consider operative closure of spina bifida. Care in selecting candidates for surgery was exercised and often extensive paralysis and hydrocephalus were contraindications to operation. Operative delay was recommended in order to permit epithelialization of the lesion.[54,55] The operative mortality during the early 20th century was reduced from 50 percent to about 10 percent.

Prior to the 1950s, infection and hydrocephalus were the leading causes of death; however, with the development of CSF shunts and antibiotics, the results of active treatment of infants began to improve along with enthusiasm for more inclusive therapy.

In 1962 Sharrard, Zachary, Lorber, et al.[56] reported that 40 infants whom they had operated upon during the first 48 hours of life had improved muscle function and decreased morbidity (meningitis) compared with unoperated patients. They concluded that operative closure should be an emergency.[56] During the 1960s the group at Sheffield became the example of aggressive comprehensive care of the newborn. The introduction of antibiotics, CSF shunts, modern anesthesia, and improved neonatal care provided new hope for these patients.

In 1969 Matson[2] was discussing the problem of spina bifida on the "basis of study and treatment of more than 1500 hospitalized patients." He emphasized the variable expressions of this birth defect and the importance of considering the uniqueness of each child. Although he supported withholding operations in early infancy if the patient was totally paralyzed below the upper lumbar level, he also emphasized that these children should not be abandoned. If satisfactory development occurred, later repair was offered to the child at the age of 2–6 years.It probably can be safely stated that Matson was concerned with those who would live in distinction to selecting children to die. Clearly his work emphasized the special considerations and needs of each child.[2]

In 1971 Lorber[57] catalyzed an ethical controversy when he suggested that children with extensive paralysis, severe hydrocephalus, kyphosis, and major associated anomalies should be selected for no treatment and that death would uniformly follow. Since then numerous reports have indicated that significant numbers of children selected for no treatment will survive (8–35 percent). Unfortunately many believe that the history of the development of care and personal observations indicate that the untreated survivors are significantly more impaired than they would have been if treated.[58] Lorber's experience occurred in 1960s, and since then there has been a definite decline in mortality figures from his reported 50 percent.[59–61] Our experience and that of others is that early active treatment today leads to 95 percent survival within the first two years.[62,63] Cost analysis plays a significant role in Lorber's advocacy for selection; however, recent studies have indicated that selection is more expensive than comprehensive care.[62,64] The reliability of the criteria for predicting mental outcome and physical abilities has been unacceptable and has led many to conclude that the vast majority of infants with spina bifida should be treated.[58,65,66] A thoughtful review and analysis of the issues surrounding selected treatment for myelomeningocele has been given by Black.[67] Recently Leonard and Freeman[62] suggested that the outlook for children with spina bifida may have changed from one of hopelessness and despair to one where children may grow to become productive participating citizens. If this is true, we must look very closely at outdated suggestions that we select certain children to die in distinction to offering comprehensive care to all.

CLINICAL ASSESSMENT

Meningocele and myelomeningocele are usually evident at birth. With the use of amniocentesis for alpha-fetoprotein and ultrasound, an increased number of children are being diagnosed during intrauterine life. Most pediatricians and neurosurgeons now agree that prompt closure of open lesions is associated with decreased mortality and morbidity. The neurosurgeon therefore will often be consulted early, and perhaps from the delivery room. Routine neonatal care should be instituted. The child should not be fed and should be kept in an environment that maintains normal thermia. Lesions should be covered with sterile saline-moistened, nonadherent dressings, and the patient should be kept in the prone or decubitus position to protect exposed neural tissues. The initial purposes of evaluation are to obtain a prompt opinion of the child's general pediatric condition and the degree of neurologic deficit.[68] With the aid of the neonatologist or pediatrician, associated cardiopulmonary, gastrointestinal, and genitourinary conditions that would interfere with an early contemplated surgical procedure should be identified. Occasionally delivery will have been complicated by unexpected abnormal fetal presentation or hydrocephalus. Initial observation thus should also include a search for trauma. After general neurologic examination of the newborn, the lesion is carefully observed for size and location. The rostral level of cord involvement will provide a general opinion of the level of the spinal cord lesion. The sensory motor examination of a child with myelomeningocele is complicated by the presence of numerous normal and abnormal reflexes.[44,45,69] Understanding of this phenomenon is mandatory for protecting the parents and medical staff from developing overly optimistic opinions of motor potential. It is also important for the surgeon, since the disappearance of reflex activities following operation may be misinterpreted as significant loss of function. Neuroplaque stimulation, motion, and sound will elicit abnormal reflex activities in the lower extremities that may have no bearing upon volitional motor function. The sensory motor examination requires that the child be relaxed and quiet. The cutaneous dermatomes are stimulated sharply from distal to proximal until one identifies the dermatome that produces facial or upper extremity response characteristic of pain perception. The motor examination is also done with the child at rest, and is begun with stimulation of the torso or upper extremities with observation for voluntary motion below the level of the lesion. Hip flexion requires the innervation of L1–L3 and adduction requires L2–L4, as does knee extension. Hip abduction, hip extension, and knee flexion require the presence of L5–S2. Plantor flexion and intrinsic muscle action of the feet require the preservation of the sacral roots.[70] Orthopedic deformities may also provide clues to the motor level. Patients with levels above T12, for example, will often have flaccid hips and feet, whereas patients with lesions below L1 and 2 will have flail feet. Sharrard[70–73] has described the limb and spinal deformities associated with neurologic deficit in detail. Additional aid in identifying the sensory level may come in the future with the application of somatosensory evoked potentials.[74]

Over 90 percent of patients with myelomeningocele will have a form of neurogenic bladder. It is extremely difficult to predict the type of bladder dysfunction an infant will display at the time of neonatal examination. Because of the presence of abnormal reflexes, anal wink and tone cannot be used as a reliable indication of perineal sensation. One is left with observing for the preservation of spontaneous voiding and the nature of the urinary stream. Those children with lower motor neuron defect (approximately 30 percent) will be easy to credé and often remain dry, whereas those patients with sphincter or bladder spasticity may be extremely difficult to credé, and this maneuver will lead to ureteral reflex and subsequent infection. Reliable determination of bladder function may not be possible for months after operation. The important factor is that the high incidence of neurogenic bladder be recognized and that the appropriate steps be taken to ensure that the bladder intermittently is emptied completely. Usually bowel incontinence is associated with bladder incontinence; and, generally, lower motor neuron lesions produce anal relaxation and prolapse. Contrary to bladder control, however, bowel training and now biofeedback offer the possibility that many of these children will achieve continence.[75]

OPERATIVE TECHNIQUE

Once the initial evaluation of the infant has been completed, we recommend early repair of all patients unless there are pediatric contraindications or death is imminent. If the lesions is open and draining CSF and operation cannot be performed within 24 hours, or if the lesion is closed and operation cannot be performed in 48 hours, we delay operation until three negative, consecutive 24-hour cultures are obtained from the surface of the lesion. The lesion can usually be sterilized with good local care. If signs of sepsis or ventriculitis develop, we treat with external ventricular draining and systemic and intrathecal antibiotics until sterilization of the cerebrospinal fluid and lesion is achieved.[76]

The purposes of operation are to preserve intellectual, motor, and sensory function by restoring the spinal cord to its normal environment and to prevent infection. Meningitis and ventriculitis produce intellectual and developmental delay. An additional purpose is to restore the normal contour of the back, which contributes to ease of care and future bracing.

The operative technique for primary closure of myelomeningocele has been described by many; modern methods include the use of the microscope and kyphectomy.[2,77–79] The general guidelines for closure include protection and preservation of exposed neural tissue and a five-layer closure. Potentially neurotoxic scrubs and topical antibiotics are avoided. The five-layer closure

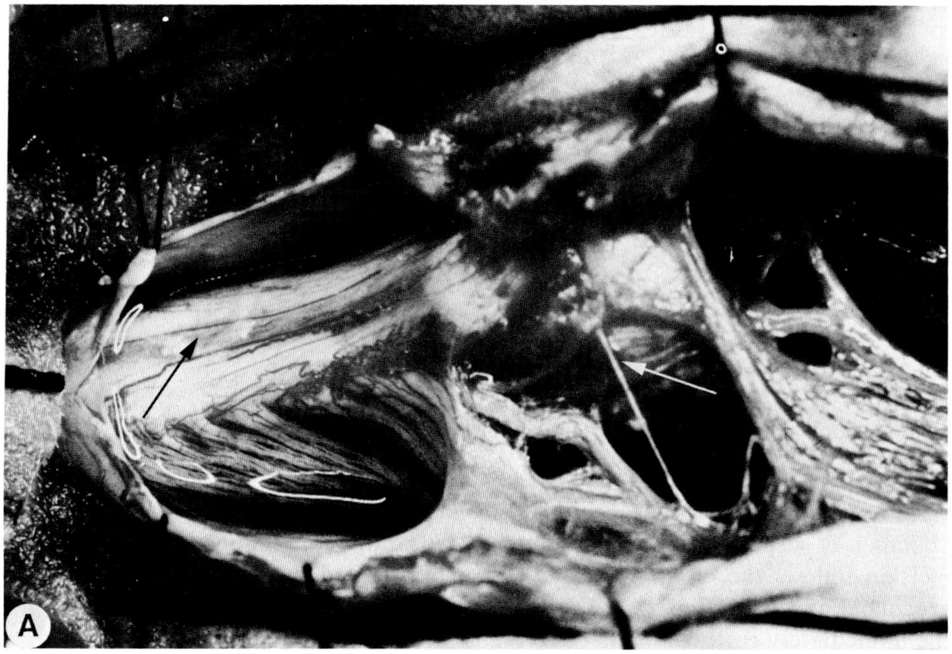

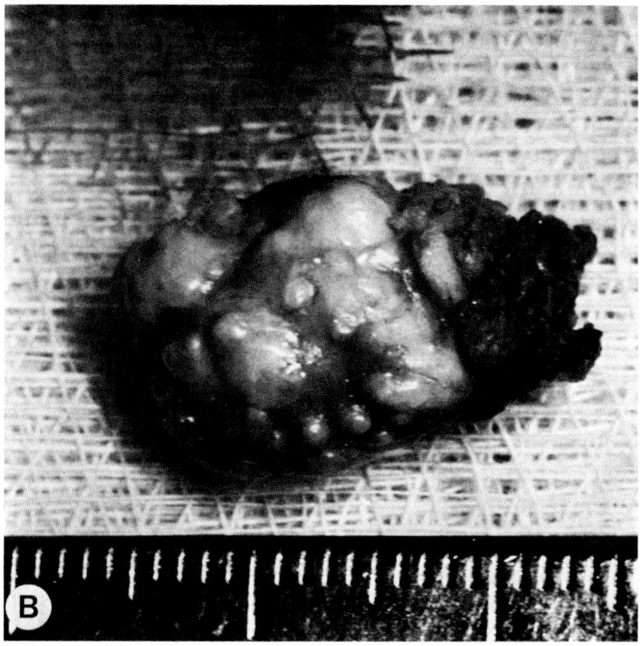

Figure 2-4. A. Dermoid at site of repair within conus. White arrow—dermoid; dark arrow—rostral spinal cord. B. Typical dermoid. C. Spinal cord following removal.

thoracolumbar kyphosis (Fig. 2–5A). The width of the vertebral bodies is increased and they may actually protrude posterior to the dermal surface of the back. The natural course of this defect with growth and development is that of progressive angulation and deformity. The presence of kyphosis complicates early repair in that it is difficult to obtain adequate subcutaneous tissue and skin coverage over the defect. Frequently there may be skin necrosis, leading to postoperative infection and ventriculitis. A variety of plastic surgical procedures have been described to obtain adequate skin coverage.[2,80,81] Even in the presence of adequate skin coverage, however, progression of the underlying kyphosis leads to the recurring complication of skin ulceration and vertebral angulation. Life expectancy is often reduced because of associated progressive cardiopulmonary complications. Bracing becomes difficult and ambulatory capacity declines.

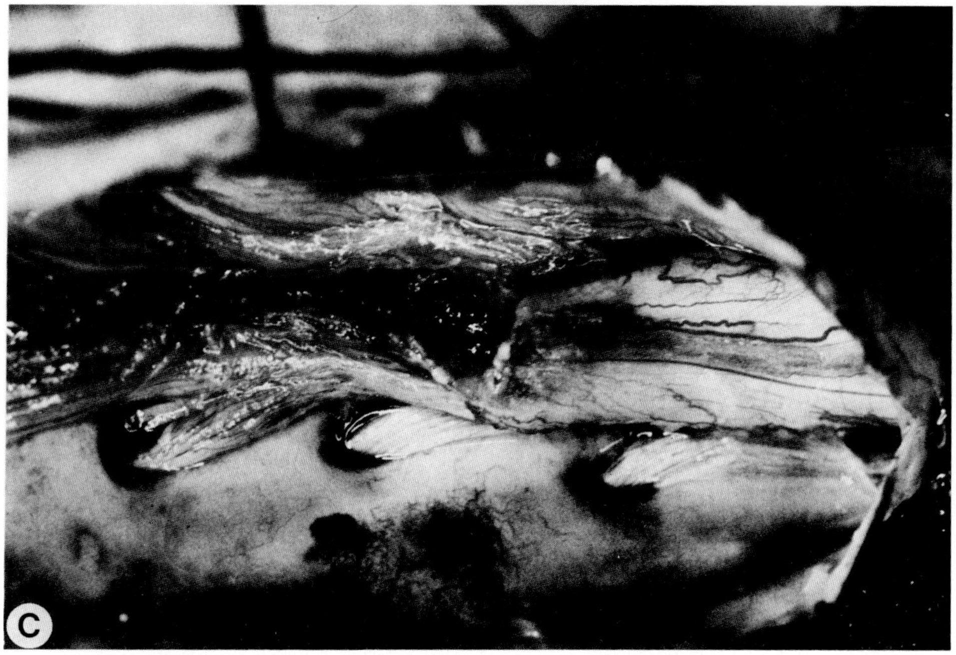

Primary spinal osteotomy for kyphosis associated with myelomeningocele was proposed by Sharrard in 1968. He was able partially to correct the deformity and obtain good skin coverage.[82] We have found that kyphectomy can be done safely at birth during the time of primary operation, and it enables one to obtain good skin coverage and vertebral alignment leading to reduced hospitalization time and early ambulation (Fig. 2–5B).[79]

Following operation the infant is returned to the isolette with no restriction on positioning. Prophylactic antibiotics are not used. As soon as bowel sounds are present, routine infant feeding programs are started.

The wound is observed closely for signs of infection and wound breakdown. If an early meticulous five-layer closure has been achieved, it is unlikely that superficial infection or necrosis will be followed by meningitis and attendant ventriculitis. Cellulitis and wound breakdown, however, will delay insertion of a CSF shunt for hydrocephalus. If wound infection develops, the patient should be treated with appropriate local drainage, surgical scrubs, and high-dose systemic antibiotics selected on the basis of cultures and sensitivity studies. If ventriculitis develops in the presence of hydrocephalus, we have found prompt clearing of the infection and control of the hydrocephalus with the use of external ventricular drainage and the addition of intrathecal antibiotics.[76] Ventricular taps for control of hydrocephalus and treatment of infection are not recommended, since they are known to cause porencephaly.

Meticulous closure as described is associated with a significant reduction in the incidence of postoperative CSF leak or fistula. In the event that fistula does occur, we have found that there is a marked reduction in the morbidity if secondary closure is performed immediately rather than hopeful observation for spontaneous closure. External ventricular drainage of hydrocephalus has been proposed to control leaks, but it predisposes to secondary infection with meningitis and ventriculitis. Insertion of a shunt is ill advised in the presence of CSF leak, since the incidence of infection may be increased because of the failure to recognize early infection at the site of the leak.

Although the etiology of hydrocephalus associated with myelomeningocele has been ascribed to aqueductal stenosis, many surgeons have noted exacerbation of hydrocephalus following repair of myelomeningocele. Perhaps as few as 15

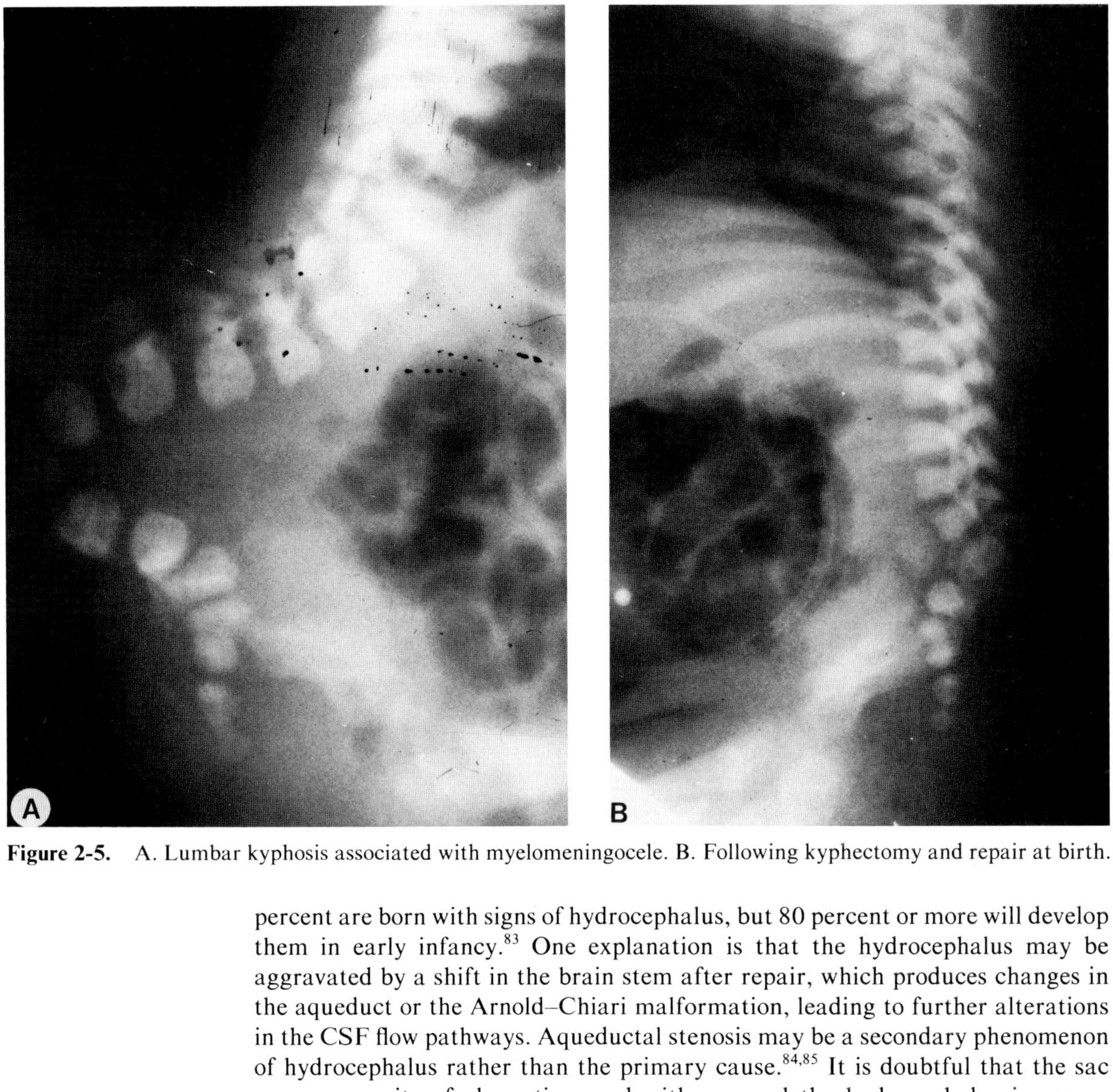

Figure 2-5. A. Lumbar kyphosis associated with myelomeningocele. B. Following kyphectomy and repair at birth.

percent are born with signs of hydrocephalus, but 80 percent or more will develop them in early infancy.[83] One explanation is that the hydrocephalus may be aggravated by a shift in the brain stem after repair, which produces changes in the aqueduct or the Arnold–Chiari malformation, leading to further alterations in the CSF flow pathways. Aqueductal stenosis may be a secondary phenomenon of hydrocephalus rather than the primary cause.[84,85] It is doubtful that the sac serves as a site of absorption; and with removal the hydrocephalus is aggravated.

Intermittent short periods of apnea, decreased spontaneous activity, and poor feeding patterns may suggest early hydrocephalus. The onset of hydrocephalus can usually be verified by serial examinations, transcephalic impedance, and ultrasound.[86,87] Marked hydrocephalus may be present with only minimal cranial enlargement. These children thus should rarely be discharged without a computerized tomographic (CT) scan.[83] As soon as clinical suspicion is high that progressive hydrocephalus is present, CT scan should be performed. If clinical examination indicates the absence of wound infection and signs and symptoms of meningitis or ventriculitis, we recommend insertion of a ventriculoperitoneal shunt because of its described advantages over ventriculoatrial shunts.[88,89] We do not predispose a child to porencephaly by ventricular taps preoperatively for CSF culture. In the rare event that cultures and analysis of CSF obtained at the time of shunt insertion indicate ventriculitis, we externalize the shunt and treat with systemic and intrathecal antibiotics. McLaurin[90] has demonstrated successful treatment with only high-dose intravenous and intrathecal antibiotics.

RESULTS

Survival rates have been steadily improving over the past decade and now may be as high as 80–95 percent in the first two years of life.[59,62,63] Early repair has been shown to contribute to these improvements in survival.[91,92] The higher the lesion, the greater the morbidity and mortality. The single most important factor associated with reduced survival is the presence or absence of hydrocephalus. The most common cause of early death remains infection, such as meningitis, ventriculitis, and pneumonia. Shunt complications significantly contribute to increased mortality and morbidity. Over the long term, renal failure begins to takes its toll. It is difficult to predict intellectual outcome for an individual; however, it appears that the group of children with only myelomeningocele have higher intelligence quotients (87 percent greater than 80) than those with myelomeningocele and hydrocephalus (63 percent greater than 80).[93] There appears to be no correlation between the degree of hydrocephalus prior to insertion of the shunt and subsequent IQ.[94] Lacunar skull deformity also cannot be equated with intellectual potential.[95] All children with myelomeningocele appear to have perceptual motor deficit, and it is not necessarily related to IQ, although other factors may be involved, including length of hospitalization.[93] Perceptual motor deficits therefore should not be interpreted as retardation. Recent studies have suggested that the reductions in IQs observed in children with hydrocephalus and myelomeningocele may be related to complications such as infection and ventriculitis. The authors concluded that irrespective of the degree of hydrocephalus, a child born with myelomeningocele could expect normal intellect, provided infection did not develop.[96] The findings are consistent with Zachary's conclusion[97] that in the past the development of capability and personality of these children has been neglected and that continued progress may be anticipated in these areas.

Ambulatory potential and capacity are related to many factors, including intelligence, orthopedic deformity, and such complications as trophic ulcer. With proper orthopedic management, orthoses, and crutches, however, most children will walk.[98]

The management of urinary continence has now been markedly altered with the advent of pharamocologic treatment of neurogenic bladder and the introduction of nonsterile intermittent catheterization.[99–104] Intelligent management of urinary incontinence permits the development of social relationships.[105]

The sacral (S2–S4) innervation is required for erection and ejaculation. An individual's ability in these areas is highly variable, and with certain lesions reflex erection and ejaculation are possible. Shurtleff and Sousa[106] have indicated that 18 percent of a group of 60, aged 16–24, were sexually active. Sexual counseling has been urged for all of these patients.[106,107]

Clearly the major handicap imposed upon children with myelomeningocele is that of psychosocial problems originating within themselves, their families, and society. Educational mainstreaming, special counseling, improved understanding of the patient's potential, and increased public awareness of spina bifida contribute to reduction in this form of stress.

MENINGOCELE

In addition to the routine assessment described with myelomeningocele, we have frequently recommended preoperative metrizamide myelography and/or CT to identify dermoid, diastematomyelia, lipoma, or tethered cord. After complete evaluation we recommend operation to prevent infection and to restore continuity of the back. Delay of operation to an older age predisposes the child to neurologic deficit and psychologic trauma. We therefore encourage operation at the time of diagnosis, which is usually at birth. The child can then begin a healthy normal developmental process with the parents and family.

The operative technique follows the guidelines described for myelomeningocele. The neck of the dural sac is often significantly smaller than the sac and may be surprisingly narrow. Occasionally nerve roots or the filum terminale may be involved within the sac. Nerve roots should be replaced and the filum sectioned. The spinal cord is normal. Excessive dura is excised and the remainder is closed. The fascia and skin closure are similar to those for myelomeningocele. The postoperative management requires all of the same precautions and observations as with the child with myelomeningocele—but the incidence of hydrocephalus is markedly reduced, and the prognosis for normal development is very good.

Anterior Sacral Meningocele

This form of meningocele extends anteriorly into the presacral retroperitoneal space and usually communicates with the sacral subarachnoid space through a narrow anterior sacral defect. The sacral canal may be abnormally enlarged secondary to lipoma, dermoid, teratoma, or intrasacral meningocele. These lesions may present as problems with constipation, obstetric complications, or pelvic masses.[108–110] Incontinence, recurrent genitourinary tract infections, headache, and radicular pain may also alert one to the diagnosis. The mass may be palpated by abdominal, rectal, or pelvic examination. The differential diagnosis includes most pelvic tumors. Plain x-rays of the sacrum show the posterior apsect of the pelvis to be intact and the classical "scimitar" (sickle-shaped) sacrum.[111] Intravenous pyelogram may show changes in the bladder and ureters. The diagnosis is established by metrizamide myelography. Ultrasound and CT may also assist in confirmation of the diagnosis.[112]

With operative obliteration of the dural communication, the pelvic mass will disappear. Generally sacral laminectomy has been recommended because it permits visualization of the intraspinal space and direct suture of the opening into the sacral canal. Occasionally, dural graft may be required to close the meningocele.[108] Barring complications such as infection, the results should be gratifying.

DELAYED COMPLICATIONS

Even with improved care and prognosis, it has become evident that spina bifida is a dynamic disease of the central nervous system and that optimal development of the child requires serial neurologic examination for delayed complications. These may include seizure disorder, shunt malfunction, cervical–medullary compression from Arnold–Chiari malformation, tethered spinal cord, and occult tumor such as dermoid, lipoma, diastematomyelia, and hydromyelia. Aggressive management of these complications leads to enhanced development and performance.

Seizure Disorder

Approximately 30–35 percent of our patients have developed seizure disorder requiring anticonvulsants. Retrospective studies of hydrocephalic children have shown similar results.[113] Prompt recognition and treatment are associated with improved intellectual development. We have also found that exacerbation may be observed with occult infection and insidious shunt malfunction. Prompt revision of the CSF shunt is usually associated with recovery of seizure control with minimal medication.

Cerebrospinal Fluid Malfunction

Computed tomography has demonstrated that shunt failure may be relatively silent to common diseases of childhood such as viremia or psychosocial stresses. Serial examination and routine scanning programs will identify these patients and lead to shunt revision and improved intellectual development. Asymptomatic hydrocephalus ("arrested hydrocephalus") may be an insidious disease leading to progressive intellectual and personality deterioration. Some of these patients will develop sudden deterioration and precipitous demise unless their shunt function is maintained.[114]

Arnold–Chiari Malformation

This malformation is present to varying degrees in almost all patients with myelomeningocele. It may be associated with medullary and spinal cord compression and cause changes in level of consciousness, apnea, laryngeal nerve palsy and stridor, and aspriation, and changes in upper extremity sensation and strength. These changes may be precipitous and lead to sudden death. The anatomy, pathology, diagnosis, and management of this problem are discussed in Chapter 4.

Tethered Spinal Cord

Progressive subtle neuromuscular deterioration may be observed in patients with spina bifida who were previously thought to have static neurologic deficit. This deterioration is frequently secondary to delayed spinal complications as outlined in Table 2-2. The complaints and findings on examination are shown in Table 2-3. Serial somatosensory evoked potentials may demonstrate progressive delay in the latency of the response, suggesting pathologic change of the spinal cord.[115] New neurologic deficit or change in somatosensory evoked potentials may suggest tethered spinal cord. Confirmation of the diagnosis requires metrizamide myelography with the capability of combining CT scanning of the spine (Fig. 2–6). Prior to myelography, however, we recommend a cerebral CT scan to evaluate shunt function, since lumbar puncture in the presence of large

Table 2-2
Delayed Spinal Complications of Spina Bifida

Tethered Spinal Cord
Conus
Filum
Tethered Spinal Cord Combined with Tumor
Lipoma
Dermoid
Neurenteric cyst
Fibroma
Diastematomyelia
Arachnoiditis
Hydromyelia
Dermal Sinus and Stalks

Table 2-3
Complaints and Findings of 74 Patients

On Examination:	Months
Mean age	120
Duration of symptoms	9
Neonatal repair of myelomeningocele	65
Sacral sensory—Motor level	43
Low lumbar sensory—Motor level	31
Hydrocephalus	35
Flexed posture	21
Gait disturbance or weakness	33
Foot deformity	31
By History:	
Motor weakness, gait change, spasticity	46
Paresthesia and pain	23
Orthopedic deformity (extremity or spine)	21
Change in bowel or bladder control	6
Flexed posture	6
Sensory change	4

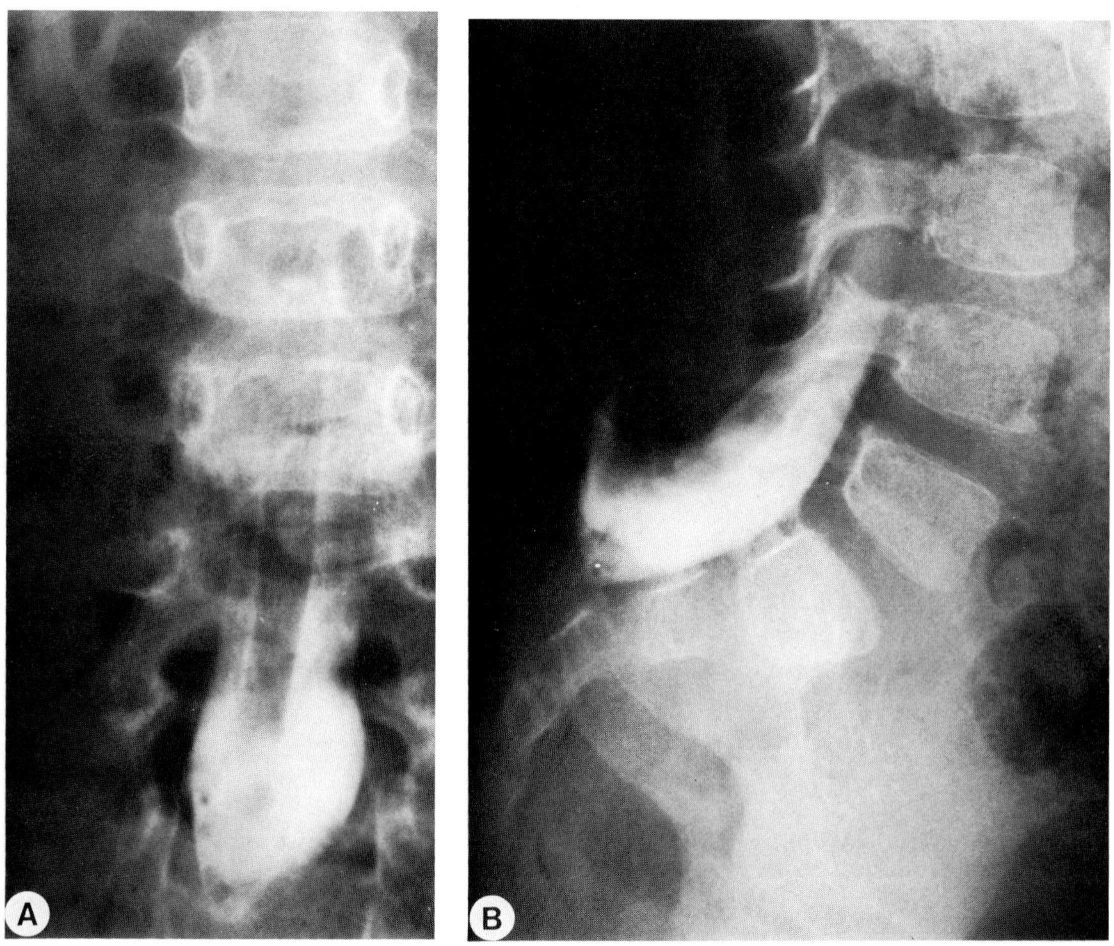

Figure 2-6. A. Anteroposterior metrizamide myelogram of tethered cord to S2. B. Lateral view.

ventricles may precipitate cervical–medullary compression secondary to the Arnold–Chiari malformation. The myelographic abnormalities observed with tethered spinal cord frequently include dorsal termination of the spinal cord at the level caudal to L4. The cord is elongated and decreases in diameter toward its termination. The angle of the nerve roots departing from the spinal cord increases toward perpendicular and may actually be reversed.[116] There may be a sessile termination of the cord, suggesting arachnoid scar or tumor. The incidence of occult spinal tumor such as lipoma, dermoid, and fibroma may approximate 50 percent.[117]

The indications for laminectomy and release of the spinal cord are relief of pain, interruption of neurologic deterioration, and recovery or maintenance of function. Hoffman, Hendrick, and Humphreys[118] have demonstrated arrest of scoliosis following release of tethered spinal cord. Intraoperative evoked potentials have indicated that the adherent termination of the spinal cord in patients with previous operations for myelomeningocele is nonfunctional,[115] and thus we have used sharp microtransection of the cord at the point of the attachment without evidence of postoperative deterioration (Fig. 2-7). Occult tumors, hydromyelia, and diastematomyelia are treated as described elsewhere in this text.

The results of operation on 74 of our patients are shown in Table 2-4. Surgical observations of attenuated dorsal spinal cord vessels, absence of spinal cord pulsation, and a pale, ischemic-appearing spinal cord suggest that vascular insufficiency may play a role in the pathophysiology of this problem. The observation that these abnormalities may be accented by pelvic flexion prior to the release of the spinal cord further suggests that alternating traction forces may contribute to the functional change in the distal spinal cord.

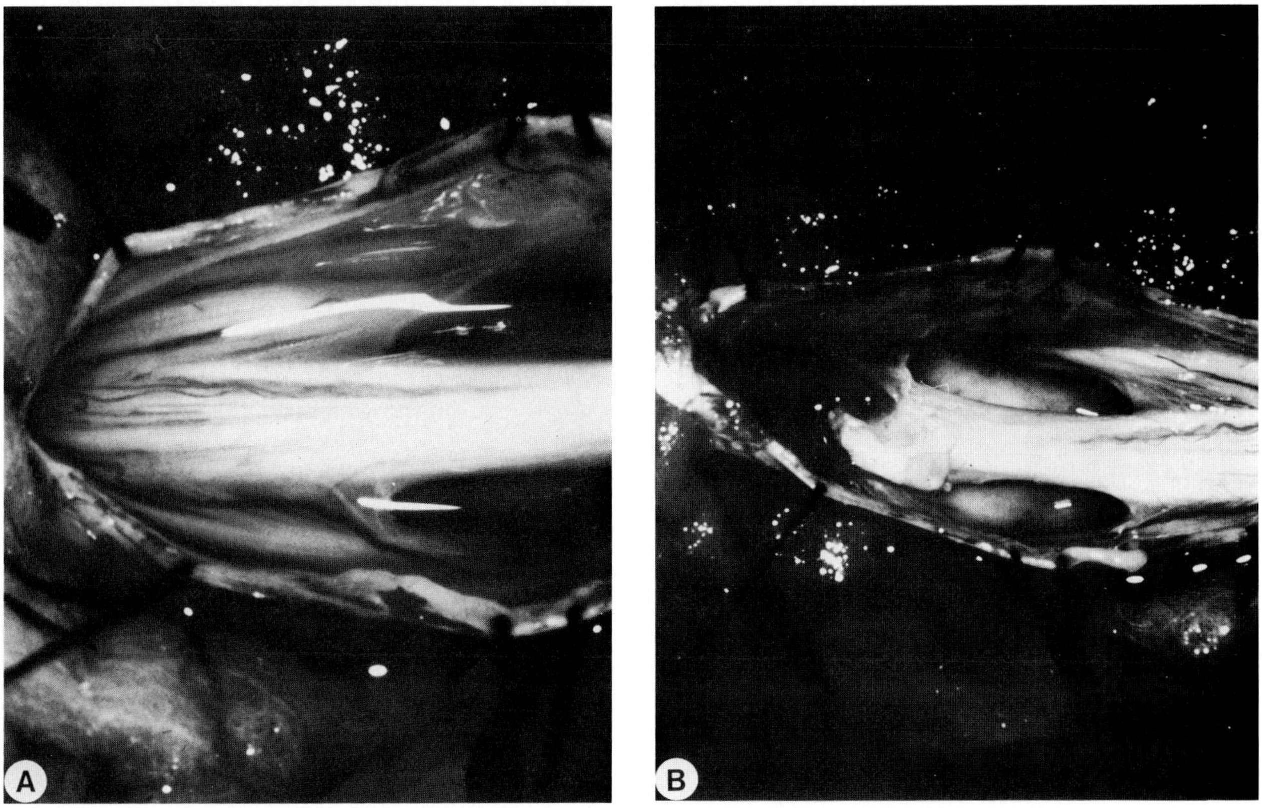

Figure 2-7. A. Tethered spinal cord prerelease. Note narrow cord and linear vasculature. B. Postrelease. Note serpentine vessels and width of spinal cord.

Table 2-4
Results of Operation

	Number	Improved	Same	Worse
Flexed Posture	21	14	7	0
Bladder Control				
Incontinent Group	58	3	55	0
Normal bladder 6/16 developed neurogenic changes	16	4	11	1
Foot deformity	29	7	20	2
Lower-Extremity Weakness or Spasticity	46	42	4	0
Orthopedic Deformity	31	12	19	?
Progressive Spinal Deformity	8	0	8	0
Pain	23	21	2	0

The recognition of subtle neuromuscular deterioration leading to diagnosis of tethered spinal cord followed by prompt surgical correction results in the recovery or maintenance of function and maximal ambulation.

Hydromyelia

Progressive upper and/or lower extremity weakness along with kyphosciolosis may result from hydromyelia.[119,120] Myelography, radioisotope ventriculògraphy, and spinal CT are used to establish the diagnosis. When the findings indicate hydrocephalus and hydromyelia, shunt revision should be the primary treatment. Gardner[121] has recommended occlusion of the obex as further treatment. Generally the incidence of hydromyelia is markedly reduced if ventricular size is maintained at or near normal.

ANTENATAL DIAGNOSIS

Open neural tubes can be diagnosed with a high degree of accuracy within the first 16 weeks of pregnancy with the use of ultrasonography and alpha-fetoprotein analysis of amniotic fluid.[122–125] Some 5 to 20 percent of neural tube abnormalities will be closed, and alpha-fetoprotein will not be elevated.[124] Separate collaborative studies in the United Kindgom and the United States have shown maternal serum alpha-fetoprotein assays to be an effective way to screen for identification of a fetus with an open neural tube defect.[125,126] Mothers with positive serum alpha-fetoprotein screenings are candidates for ultrasound and amniocentesis.[126]

Screening programs may lead to reductions in the frequency of spina bifida; however, there will always be those who refuse to consider interruption of a pregnancy because of its presence. Furthermore 90 percent or more of all patients with neural tube defects are born to families without previously affected children. Neurosurgeons should be prepared to inform parents and relatives of children with spina bifida of the availability of screening and diagnostic techniques and of centers for genetic counseling.

CONCLUSIONS

The prognosis for newborn infants with myelomeningocele is better at this time than at any time in history. New operative methods for closure of the neuroplaque and initial kyphectomy have reduced the incidence of wound breakdown and infection. The development of new shunting systems and diagnostic tools such as ultrasound and CT scans have enabled critical determination of shunt function leading to earlier revision and thus preventing irreversible change of the brain. Multimodality neuropsychologic testing has confirmed normal intellectual performance in many of these children. Intermittent, clean catheterization has drastically reduced the incidence of unrelenting urinary tract infection and the need for diversion. Advances in selection of orthopedic procedures and improved techniques have led to most children with myelomeningocele being able to achieve ambulation. Quality and prognosis appear to be directly related to comprehensive health care. Advances in community understanding and interaction have enabled children with myelomeningocele to attain social acceptance, educational advances, and reward.

REFERENCES

1. Laurence KM, Tew BJ: Natural history of spina bifida cystica and cranium bifidum cysticum. Arch Dis Child 46:127–138, 1971
2. Matson DD: Neurosurgery of Infancy and Childhood (ed 2). Springfield, Charles C Thomas, 1969
3. Lichtenstein BW: Spina dysraphism (spina bifida and myelodysplasia). Arch Neurol Psychiatr 99:792–810, 1940
4. Nadich TP, Publowski RM, Nadich JB, et al: Computed tomographic signs of the Chiari II malformation. Part I: Skull and dural partitions. Radiology 134:65–71, 1980
5. Nadich TP, Publowski RM, Nadich JB: Computed tomographic signs of Chiari II malformation. II: Midbrain and cerebellum. Radiology 134:391–398, 1980
6. Nadich TP, Publowski RM, Nadich JB: Computed tomographic signs of Chiari II malformation III: Ventricles and cisterns. Radiology 134:657–663, 1980
7. McLaughlin JF, Shurtleff DB: Management of the newborn with myelodysplasia. Clin Pediatr 18:463–476, 1979
8. Elwood JH: Major central nervous system malformations notified in Northern Ireland 1964–1968. Dev Med Child Neurol 14:731–739, 1972
9. Thompson MW, Rudd NL: The genetics of spinal dysraphism, in Morley TP (ed): Current Controversies in Neurosurgery, Philadelphia, WB Saunders, 1976, pp 126–146
10. Carter CO, Evans KA: Spina bifida and anencephalus in greater London. J Med Genet 10:209–234, 1973
11. Till K: Paediatric Neurosurgery. London, Blackwell, 1975
12. Fraser F: Genetic counselling in some common paediatric diseases. Am J Hum Genet 26:636–659, 1974
13. Laurence KM, Carter CO, David PA: Major central nervous system malformations in South Wales II: Pregnancy factors, seasonal variation, and social class effects. Br J Prev Soc Med 22:212–222, 1968
14. Fineman RM, Jorde LB, Martin RA, et al: The inheritance of spinal dysraphia as an autosomal dominant defect in four families. Am J Med Genet (to appear)
15. Birth Defects. Genetic Services International Directory (ed 4). The National Foundation–March of Dimes, 1974
16. Renwick JH: Hypothesis: Anencephaly and spina bifida are usually preventable by avoidance of a specific but unidentified substance present in certain potato tubers. Br J Prev Soc Med 26:67–88, 1972
17. Clarke CA, McKendrick OM, Sheppard PM: Spina bifida and potatoes. Br Med J 3:251, 1973
18. Nevin NC, Merrett JD: Potato avoidance during pregnancy in women with a previous infant with either anencephaly or spina bifida. Br J Prev Soc Med 29:111, 1975
19. Smithells RW, Sheppard S, Schorah CJ: Possible prevention of neural-tube defects by periconceptional vitamin supplementation. Lancet i:647, 1980
20. Janerich DT: Influenza and neural-tube defects. Lancet i:551–552, 1971

21. Layde PM, Edmonds LD, Erickson JD: Maternal fever and neural tube defects. Teratology 21:105–108, 1980
22. Miller P, Smith DW, Shepart TH: Maternal hyperthermia as a possible cause of anencephaly. Lancet i:519, 1978
23. Leck I: Maternal hyperthermia and anencephaly. Lancet i:671, 1978
24. Leck I, Hay S, Witte JJ, et al: Malformations recorded on birth certificates following A2 influenza epidemics. Pub Health Rep 84:971, 1969
25. Warkany J: Morphogenesis of spina bifida, in McLaurin R (ed): Myelomeningocele. New York, Grune & Stratton, 1977, pp 31–35
26. Rechlinghausen F von: Virchows Arch Path Anat 105:243, 1886
27. Gardner WJ: Etiology and pathogenesis of the development of myelomeningocele, in McLaurin RL (ed): Myelomeningocele. New York, Grune & Stratton, 1977, pp 3–30
28. Morgagni JB: The Seats and Causes of Diseases Investigated by Anatomy (3 vols), translated by Benjamin Alexander. London, A Millar and T Caldwell, 1769
29. Weed LH: The development of cerebro-spinal spaces in pig and in man. Cont Embryol Carnegie Inst 5:1–116, 1971
30. Patten BM: Embryological stages in the development of spina bifida and myeloschisis. Anat Rec 94:487, 1946
31. Patten BM: Overgrowth of the neural tube in young embryos. Anat Rec 113:381–393, 1952
32. Patten BM: Embryological states in the establishment of myeloschisis with spina bifida. Am J Anat 93:365–395, 1953
33. Padget DH: Spina bifida and embryonic neuroschisis—A causal relationship; definition of postnatal confirmations involving a bifid spine. John Hopkins Med J 128:233–252, 1968
34. Padget DH: Neuroschisis and human embryonic maldevelopment: New evidence on anencephaly, spina bifida and diverse mammalian defects. J Neuropath Exp Neurol 29:192–216, 1970
35. Padget DH: Development of so-called dysraphism; with embryologic evidence of clinical Arnold–Chiaria and Dandy–Walker malformations. Johns Hopkins Med J 130:127–165, 1972
36. Padget DH, Lindenberg R: Inverse cerebellum morphogenetically related to Dandy–Walker and Arnold–Chiaria syndromes: Bizarre malformed brain with occipital encephalocele. Johns Hopkins Med J 131:228–246, 1972
37. Osaka K, Tanimura T, Hirayama A, et al: Myelomeningocele before birth. J Neurosurg 49:711–724, 1978
38. Dooling EC, Barlow JF, Murphy JV, et al: Cyst of the cavum septi pellucidi. Arch Neurol 27:79–84, 1972
39. Tryfonas G: Three spina bifida defects in one child. J Pediatr Surg 8:75–76, 1973
40. Emery JL, Lendon RG: Clinical implications of cord lesions in neurospinal dysraphism. Dev Med Child Neurol 14:45–51, 1972
41. Lendon RG: Neuron population in the lumbosacral cord of myelomeningocele children. Dev Med Child Neurol 20(suppl): 82–85, 1969
42. Ralis J, Ralis HM: Morphology of peripheral nerves in children with spina bifida. Dev Med Child Neurol 109:101–104, 1972
43. Brown SF: Congenital malformations associated with myelomeningocele. J. Iowa Med Soc. LXV (No. 3):101–104, 1975
44. Stark GD, Baker GCW: The neurological involvement of the lower limbs in myelomeningocele. Dev Med Child Neurol 9:732–744, 1967
45. Stark GD, Drummond M: The spinal cord lesion in myelomeningocele. Dev Med Child Neurol 13:1–14, 1971
46. Reigel DH, Dallman DE, Scarff TB, et al: Intra-operative evoked potential studies of newborn infants with myelomeningocele. Dev Med Child Neurol 18:42–49, 1977
47. Epstein F, Spielholz N, Battista A, et al: Delayed cauda equina reconstruction in meningomyelocele. Neurosurgery 6:540–541, 1980
48. Christopher F: Spina bifida occulta; with report of a case. Surg Gynec Obstet 33:1–7, 1921
49. Doran PA, Guthkelch AN: Studies in spina bifida cystica I. General survey and reassessment of the problem J Neurol Neurosurg Psychiat 24:331–345, 1961

50. Athol J: Fatty tumor from the sacrum of a child connected with the spinal membranes. Trans Pathol Soc Lond viii 16:28, 1857
51. Virchow: Ein fall von hypertrichosis circumscripta mediana Kombiniert mit spina bifida. Ztschr Ethnol vii:279, 1875
52. Marsh H, Gould AP, Clutton HH, et al: Trans Clin Soc London 18:339, 1885
53. Forestus: Obs Chir, Libri V, Lib III, Obs VII, 1610
54. Moore JE: Spina bifida with a report of 385 cases treated by excision. Surg Gynec Obstet 1:137–140, 1905
55. Ingram FD, Swan H: Spina bifida and cranium bifidum. I: A survey of five hundred forty-six cases. N Engl J Med 228:559–563, 1943
56. Sharrard JW, Zachary RB, Lorber J, et al: A controlled trial of immediate and delayed closure of spina bifida cystica. Arch Dis Child 38:18–22, 1963
57. Lorber J: Results of treatment of myelomeningocele: An analysis of 524 unselected cases with special references to possible selection for treatment. Dev Med Child Neurol 13:279–303, 1971
58. Freeman JM: To treat or not to treat: Ethical dilemmas of treating the infant with a myelomeningocele. Clin Neurosurg 20:134–146, 1973
59. Ames MD, Schut L: Results of treatment of 171 consecutive myelomeningoceles—1963 to 1968. Pediatrics 50:466–470, 1972
60. Mawdsley T, Rickham PP: Further follow-up study of early operation for open myelomeningocele. Dev Med Child Neurol 20(suppl): 8–12, 1969
61. Rickham PP: The swing of the pendulum: The indications for operating on myelomeningoceles. Med J Aust 2:743–746, 1976
62. Leonard CO, Freeman KM: Spina bifida. A new disease. Pediatrics 68:136–137, 1981
63. McLone D, Raimondi AJ, Sommers R: The results of early treatment of 100 consecutive newborns with myelomeningocele. Kinder Chir 34(2):115–117, 1981
64. Shurtleff DB, Lamers J: Clinical considerations in the treatment of myelodysplasia, in Crandell B, Brazier MAB (eds): Prevention of Nueral Tube Defects—The role of Alphafetoprotein. New York, Academic Press, 1978, p 103
65. Page L: Editorial comment on Black P: Selective treatment of infants with myelomeningocele. Neurosurgery 5:338, 1979
66. Foltz EL, Kronnal R, Shurtleff DB: To treat or not to treat: A neurosurgeon's perspective of myelodysplasia. Clin Neurosurg 20:147, 1973
67. Black P: Selective treatment of infants with myelomeningocele. Neurosurgery 5:334–338, 1979
68. Prechtl H, Beintema D (eds): The Neurological Examination of the Full Term Newborn Infant. England, Lavenham Press, 1965.
69. Guthkelch AN: The indications and contraindications for early operation in myelomeningocele, in Morley TP (ed): Current Controversies in Neurosurgery. Philadelphia, WB Saunders, 1976, pp 147–155
70. Sharrard WJW: The mechanism of paralytic deformity in spina bifida. Dev Med Child Neurol 4:310–313, 1962
71. Sharrard WJW: The segmental innervation of the lower limb muscles in man. Ann Roy Coll Surg Engl 35:106–122, 1964
72. Sharrard WJW: Neuromotor evaluation of the newborn, in American Academy of Orthopaedic Surgeons: Symposium on Myelomeningocele. St. Louis, CV Mosby, 1972, pp 26–40
73. Sharrard WJW: Assessment of the myelomeningocele child, in McLaurin RL (ed): Myelomeningocele. New York, Grune & Stratton, 1977, pp 389–410
74. Scarff TB, Toleikis JR, Bunch WH, et al: Dermatomal somatosensory evoked potentials in children with myelomeningocele. Z Kinderchir 28:384–386, 1979
75. Wald A: Use of biofeedback in treatment of fecal incontinence in patients with meningomyelocele. Pediatrics 68:45–49, 1981
76. Scarff TB, Nelson P, Reigel DH: External drainage for ventricular infection following cerebrospinal fluid shunts. Child's Brain 5:129–136, 1978
77. Amacher L: The microsurgical anatomy of lumbar rachischisis. Adv Ophthamol 37:197–202, 1978
78. McLone DG: Technique for closure of myelomeningocele. Child's Brain 6:65–73, 1980

79. Reigel DH: Kyphectomy and myelomeningocele repair. Modern techniques in surgery. Neurosurgery 13:1–9, 1979
80. Curtin JW: Reconstructive surgical procedures in myelodysplasia. South Med J 67:406–411, 1974
81. Zook EG, Dzenitis AJ, Bennett JE: Repair of large myelomeningoceles. Arch Surg 98:41–43, 1969
82. Sharrard WJW: Spinal osteotomy for congenital kyphosis in myelomeningocele. J Bone Jt Surg 50B:466–471, 1968
83. Stein SC, Schut L: Hydrocephalus in myelomeningocele. Child's Brain 5:413–419, 1979
84. McMillan JJ, Williams B: Aqueduct stenosis: Case review and discussion. J Neurol Neurosurg Psychiatr 40:521–532, 1977
85. Williams B: Is aqueduct stenosis the result of hydrocephalus? Brain 96:399–412, 1973
86. Sauerbrei EE, Harrison PB, Ling E, et al: Neonatal intracranial pathology demonstrated by high-frequency linear array ultrasound. J Clin Ultrasound 9:33–36, 1981
87. Reigel DH, Dallmann DE, Scarff TB, et al: Transcephalic impedance measurement during infancy. Dev Med Child Neurol 19:295–304, 1977
88. Stark GD, Drummond MB, Poneprasert S, et al: Primary ventriculo-peritoneal shunts in treatment of hydrocephalus associated with myelomeningocele. Arch Dis Childh 49:112–117, 1974
89. Robertson JS, Maraqa MI, Jennett B: Ventriculoperitoneal shunting for hydrocephalus. Br Med J 2:289–292, 1973
90. McLaurin RL: Treatment of infected ventricular shunts. Child's Brain 1:306–310, 1975
91. Heimberger RF: Early repair of myelomeningocele (spina bifida cystica) J Neurosurg 37:594–600, 1972
92. Stark GD, Drummond M: Results of selective early operation in myelomeningocele. Arch Dis Child 48:676–682, 1973
93. Soare P, Raimondi AJ: Intellectual and perceptual-motor characteristics of treated myelomeningocele children. Am J Dis Child 131:199–204, 1977
94. Raimondi AJ, Soare P: Intellectual development in shunted hydrocephalus children. Am J Dis Child 127:664–671, 1974
95. Stein S, Schut L, Borns P: Lacunar skull deformity (Luckenschadel) and intelligence in myelomeningocele. J Neurosurg 41:10–13, 1974.
96. McLone D, Czyzewski D, Raimondi AJ: The effects of complications on intellectual function in 173 children with myelomeningocele. J Pediatr (to appear)
97. Zachary RB: The improving prognosis in spina bifida. Clin Pediatr 11:11–14, 1972
98. Krupka J, Geddes N, Carroll NC: Comprehensive management in the child with spina bifida. Orthoped Clin N Am 9:97, 1978
99. Action Committee of Myelodysplasia, Section of Urology: Current approaches to evaluation and management of children with myelomeningocele. Pediatrics 63:663, 1979
100. Awad SA, Downie J, Kiruluta H: Pharmacologic treatment of disorders of bladder and urethra: A review. Canad J Surg 22:515, 1979
101. Lapides J, Deoatno AC, Lowe BS, et al: Follow-up of unsterile intermittent self-catheterization. J Urol 111:184, 1974
102. Hannigan KF: Teaching intermittent self-catheterization to young children with myelodysplasia. Dev Med Child Neurol 21:365, 1979
103. Scott FB, Bradley WE, Timm GW: Treatment of urinary incontinence by an implantable prosthetic sphincter. Urology 1:252, 1973
104. Whitehead WE, Parker LH, Masek BJ, et al: Biofeedback treatment of fecal incontinence in myelomeningocele. Dev Med Child Neurol (in press)
105. Laurence KM, Deresford A: Continence, friends, marriage and children in 51 adults with spina bifida. Dev Med Child Neurol 17:123–128, 1975
106. Shurtleff DB, Sousa JC: The adolescent with myelodysplasia: Development, achievement, sex and deterioration, in McLaurin RL (ed): Myelomeningocele. New York, Grune & Stratton, 1977, pp 809–835

107. Comarr AE: Neurological disturbances of sexual function among patients with myelodysplasia, in McLaurin, RL (ed): Myelomeningocele. New York, Grune & Stratton, 1977, pp 797–808

108. Anderson TM, Burke BL: Anterior sacral meningocele. A presentation of three cases. JAMA 237:39–42, 1977

109. Oren M, Lorber B, Lee SH, et al: Anterior sacral meningocele: Report of five cases and review of the literature. Dis Colon Rectum 20:492–505, 1977

110. Vogel EH: Anterior sacral meningocele as a gynecologic problem: Report of a case. Obstet Gynec 36:766–768, 1970

111. Silvis RS, Riddle LR, Clark GG: Anterior sacral meningocele. Am Surg 22:554–566, 1956

112. Walpert SM, Scott RM, Carter BL: Computed tomography in spinal dysraphism. Surg Neurol 8:199–206, 1977

113. Hosking GP: Fits in hydrocephalic children. Arch Dis Child 49:633–635, 1974

114. James HE, Schut L: Pitfalls in the diagnosis of arrested hydrocephalus. Acta Neurochir 43:13–17, 1978

115. Reigel DH, Scarff TB, Woodford JE: Surgery for tethered spinal cord in myelomeningocele patients. American Association of Neurological Surgeons, April 1976. Dev Med Child Neurol 18 (suppl 37):165, 1977

116. Heinz ER, Rosenbaum AE, Scarff TB, et al: Tethered spinal cord following meningomyelocele repair. Radiology 131:153–160, 1979

117. Reigel DH: Personal experience

118. Hoffman HJ, Hendrick EB, Humphreys RP: The tethered spinal cord: Its protean manifestations, diagnosis and surgical correction. Child's Brain 2:145–155, 1976

119. Hall PV, Campbell RL, Kalsbeck JE: Meningomyelocele and progressive hydromyelia. J Neurosurg 43:457–463, 1975

120. Cameron AH: The Arnold–Chiari and other neuroanatomical malformations associated with spina bifida. J Pathol Bact 73:195–211, 1957

121. Gardner WJ: Hydrodynamic mechanism of syringomyelia: Its relationship to myelocele. J Neurol Neurosurg Psychiat 28:247–259, 165

122. Globus MS, Loughman WD, Epstein CJ, et al: Prenatal genetic diagnosis in 3000 amniocenteses. N Engl J Med 300:157–163, 1979

123. Powledge TM, Fletcher J: Guidelines for the ethical, social and legal issues in prenatal diagnosis. N Engl J Med 300:168–172, 1979

124. Brock DJH, Sutcliffe RG: Alpha-fetoprotein in the antenatal diagnosis of anencephaly and spina bifida. Lancet 2:197, 1972

125. Wald NJ, Cuckle H, Brock JH, et al: Maternal serum-alpha-fetoprotein measurement in antenatal screening for anencephaly and spina bifida in early pregnancy (Report of United Kingdom collaborative study on alpha-fetoprotein in relation to neural tube defects). Lancet 1:1323–1332, 1977

126. Milunsky A, Alpert E, Neff RK, et al: Prenatal diagnosis of neural tube defects IV: Maternal serum alpha-fetoprotein screening. Obstet Gynec 55:60–66, 1980

3. Encephalocele

Donald H. Reigel

The deformity of encephalocele was first illustrated in medieval art and archaic sculpture.[1] And, according to Emery and Kalhan, the first medical report appeared in the 16th century.[2] Encephalocele has been defined as an extracranial protrusion of intracranial tissue through an abnormal congenital midline opening. Occasionally, cranial contents may extrude through one of the normal openings, such as the optic foramen or sphenoid fissure.[3] The mass usually contains meninges, and cerebrospinal fluid, and it may or may not contain cerebral tissue.[4–6] Encephalocele most commonly occurs posteriorly at the occiput, but it is also observed anteriorly in the region of the forehead, nose, and base of the skull.

The frequency of anterior and posterior location of encephalocele varies from the Eastern to the Western world. In Thailand, Burma, and India, encephalocele is most commonly located anteriorly and has been reported to occur as often as 1 in 5000.[7–9] In America and Europe, the incidence of encephalocele has been reported as 1–3 per 10,000 live births.[10–12] Of these 70 percent are located in the occipital area. The remainder are divided equally among the anterior cranium (frontal and parietal) and the nasal, pharyngeal, and sphenoidal areas.[13] The incidence of anterior basal encephaloceles has been estimated as 1 in 35,000 live births.[14] Encephalocele is reported to constitute 10–20 percent of all cranial–spinal malformations.[12,13] The ratio of spinal to cranial malformations in the western world is the reverse of that in the East.[4]

The classifications of encephalocele have been developed in relation to their anatomic content, the site of the lesion at surgery, and the site of the cranial defect. The classification on the basis of contents includes cranial meningocele—meninges only; encephalocystocele—meninges, cerebrospinal fluid, and choroid plexus; encephalomeningocele—meninges and brain.[4] A surgical classification given by Matson includes, in order of frequency, occipital, parietal, frontal, nasophayrngeal, and nasal.[13] The classification developed by Suwanwela, based on location of the cranial defect as determined by postmortem dissection, is illustrated in Figure 3-1.[15]

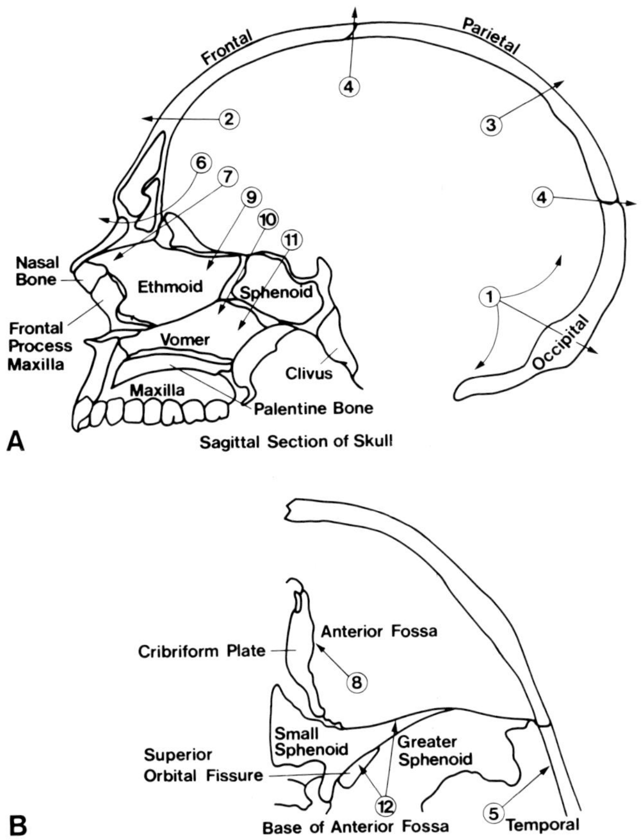

I. CRANIAL VAULT
1. Occipital 70%
2. Interfrontal
3. Parietal 10%
4. Anterior or Posterior Fontanel
5. Temporal

II. FRONTAL ETHMOIDAL (SINCIPITAL) 15%
6. Naso Frontal
7. Naso Ethmoidal
8. Naso Orbital

III. BASAL ENCEPHALOCELE 1.5%
9. Transethmoidal
10. Sphenoethmoidal
11. Transphenoidal

C 12. Frontosphenoidal or spheno - orbital

Figure 3-1. Cranial defects as described by Suwanwela.[15] A, B. Location of defects. C. Classification of defects.

PATHOLOGY

Occipital Encephalocele

The neuropathologic change may range from a large leptomeningeal cyst containing cerebrospinal fluid and choroid plexus to displacement of the entire brain into the occipital sac. Brain tissue has been found in the sac in 25–80 percent of patients at the time of operation.[12] In addition to a variable portion of of the cerebral hemispheres being located in the occipital sac, the relationship of the remaining brain to the cranial fossa may be markedly distorted, with displacement of the frontal lobe to the middle fossa and the temporal lobe to the posterior fossa. Microgyria, holoprosencephaly, heterotopia, and agenesis have been described. There is a high frequency of structural change of the hippocampus and amygdala. Optic pathway dysgenesis is common. The cerebellum may be partly or completely within the cyst. Cerebellar aplasia, absence, and inversion have also been described.[16,17] Marked alteration in cerebrospinal fluid pathways may occur and frequently leads to the development of hydrocephalus. The lateral, third, and fourth ventricles have been identified within encephaloceles. The ventricular system may show abnormal communications and contours. Aqueduct change is common.[18] The hypothalamus, thalamus, and brain stem are affected to varying degrees. Cellularity and fusion defects have been demonstrated.

The position, nuclear structure, and size of the brain stem have been reported to be abnormal. Spinal cord distortion, hydromyelia, and change in the posterior columns have frequently been described. Variable distortion and agenesis of the cerebral vascular tree, along with persistence of the fetal vasculature, has also been observed. Demonstrable pyramidal tract hypoplasia may explain the frequent clinical observation of spasticity.[1,11,18,19] Many patients with occipital encephalocele will have Arnold–Chiari malformation, and association of Dandy–Walker cyst has also been described.[18,20]

Frontoethmoidal and Basal Encephalocele

With anterior encephalocele varying amounts of frontal lobe are usually displaced outside the cranium. The anterior lateral and third ventricle may extend into the encephalocele.[15,21] Changes in the cortex, thalamus, hypothalamus, commissures, optic pathways, brain stem, and aqueduct as described above have also been observed with anterior encephaloceles.[4,15] Some of the systemic anomalies frequently associated with encephalocele are listed in Table 3-1.

EMBRYOLOGY

The embryologic development of encephalocele has often been compared to that of myelomeningocele. Traditionally, the genesis of encephalocele has been ascribed to failure of the neural tube to fuse at the level of the anterior neuropore on approximately the 25th day of gestation[20,22] (see also Chapter 1). Neural tissue overgrowth and viral infections have been suggested as causes of persistent openings in the neural tube.[23,24]

Gardner has proposed that the neural tube reopens after closure rather than fails to close.[25] He suggests that this occurs during about the eighth week of gestation because of a permeability defect in the roof of the fourth ventricle. Cerebrospinal fluid, he says, then accumulates within the neural tube and results in a "hydrocephalomyelia," which produces rupture of the neural tube and the changes observed in encephalocele. The reports of myelomeningocele in the human fetus prior to formation of the choroid plexus challenge the validity of this hydrocephalomyelia theory.[26]

Leong and Shaw have described displacement and herniation of the mesencephalon in patients with occipital encephalocele, which corresponds to the area of the anterior neuropore.[1] Only in the most severe case, however, was there schisis of the mesencephalon. They therefore proposed that the primary defect may be in the tissues overlying the mesencephalon and that subsequent growth and movement of the brain determine the content of the sac. Whether a neural tube fusion failure initiates this change remains undetermined, and thus the controversy regarding the development of lesions continues to be between those who are suggesting that the encephalocele occurs as a result of neural tube failure and those who suggest that the tube closes normally, reopens, and then proceeds abnormally. In Chapter 1 Lemire and Warkany emphasize the importance of this debate in relationship to teratogens. Radiation, hyperthermia, hypervitaminosis, salicylates, trypan blue, hypoxia, and numerous other agents have been reported as causing encephalocele in experimental animals.[4,20]

Table 3-1
Systemic Abnormalities[12,14,18,29,35]

Facial cleft	Polydactyly
Klippel–Feil and other vertebral deformities	Laryngomalacia
Spina bifida	Cradiac defects—dextrocardia
Diastematomyelia	Pulmonary hypoplasia
Dysplastic extremities	Renal agenesis

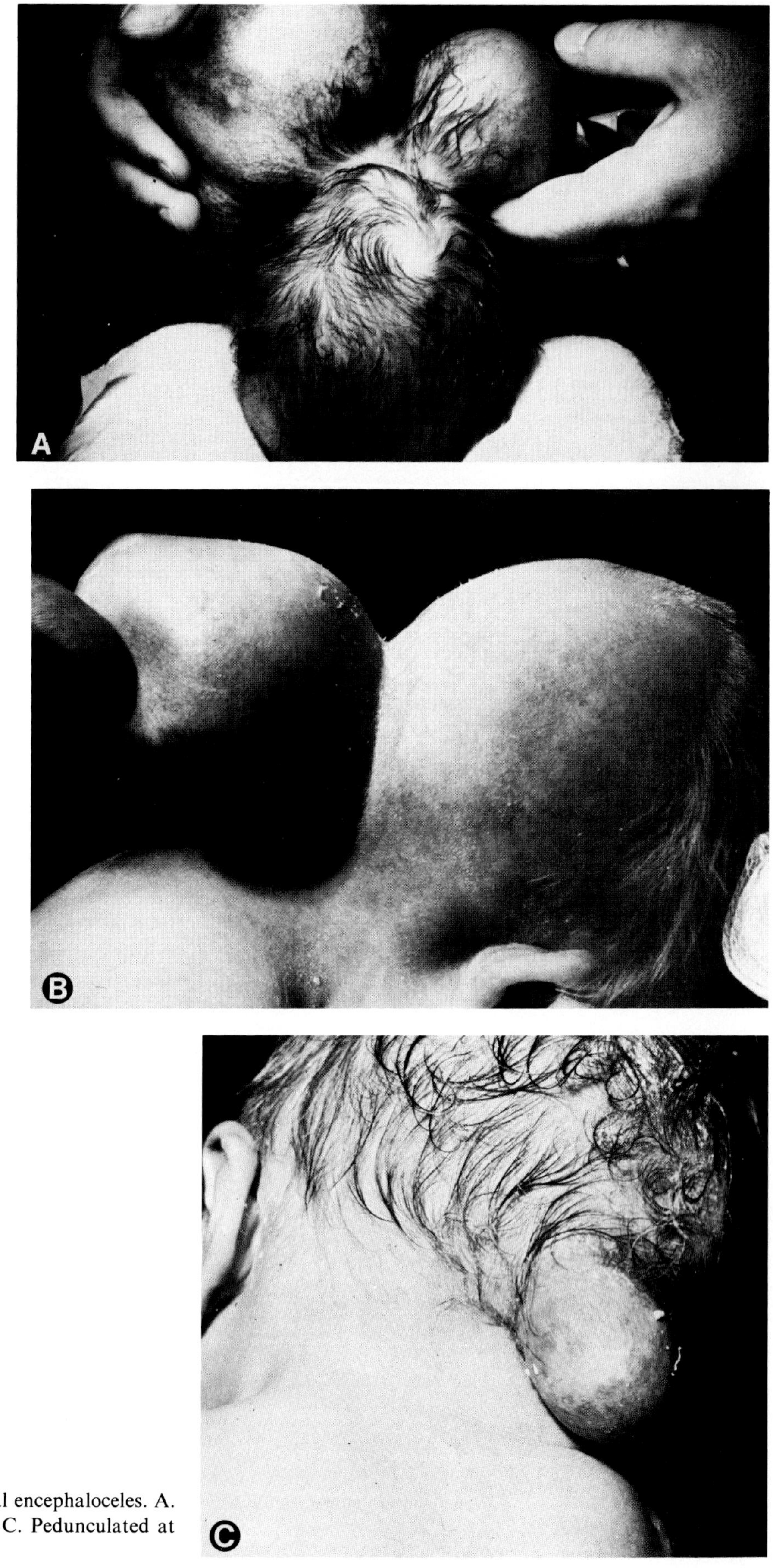

Figure 3-2. Variety of occipital encephaloceles. A. Bilobed and sessile. B. Sessile. C. Pedunculated at the cervical–occipital junction.

The embryology and etiology of encephalocele remain unclear, and the relationship of neuroectoderm to mesoderm in its genesis has not yet been identified.

CLINICAL FEATURES

Occipital, parietal, and temporal encephalocele are usually discovered at the time of birth.[13,20] Their size and content are highly variable, and the skin coverage may be partial or complete, and may display hypertrichosis and capillary hemangiomata (Figs. 3-2, 3-3, and 3-4). Size cannot be used as a reliable indicator of content or prognosis (Fig. 3-3). Matson has described sessile and pedunculated occipital encephaloceles[13] (Figs. 3-2 and 3-4). Palpation and transillumination may assist the examiner in determining the presence of brain tissue. The observation of microcephaly and a large sac may further suggest brain content within the sac. This combination is frequently associated with a poor prognosis.

The neurologic examination is often normal. Associated brain and spinal cord abnormalities, however, may result in cranial nerve deficit, visual impariment, spasticity, and focal motor weakness. The signs of hydrocephalus may be present at birth or may develop shortly thereafter. The general physical examination may be normal, but patients should be evaluated for associated defects, as listed in Table 3-1.

Diagnostic aspiration for identification of cerebrospinal fluid within encephaloceles has been advocated. But, this should be discouraged because of the risk of cerebrospinal leak and infection.[8]

Anterior encephaloceles may be obvious at birth and display the content and size variability associated with occipital encephaloceles[15,27] (Fig. 3-5). Anterior encephaloceles may be divided into two groups: sincipital—those appearing at the root of the nose, and basal—those that appear in the orbit, nose, or pharynx. Intraorbital encephalocele may produce unilateral or bilateral exophthalmos.[13,28] Nasal encephaloceles may be observed at the bridge of the nose or within the nostrils and may cause airway obstruction[29] (Fig. 3-5B). It has been suggested that nasal encephaloceles are generally medial within the nose, whereas polyps are lateral. A pulsatile intranasal mass that increases in size with crying may indicate continuity with the interior of the cranium.[21] The diagnosis of anterior basal encephalocele may be delayed and may only become evident because of cerebrospinal leak and recurrent meningitis.[30] In addition to nasal polyps, the differential diagnosis of nasal encephalocele includes nasal glioma, dermoid cyst, sinus pericranium, teratoma, neurofibroma, lymphangioma, hemangioma, and ethmoid meningoma.[31,32]

Plain x-rays and tomography may establish the size, location, and shape of the cranial defect, which is usually smooth, well circumscribed, and without sclerosis. Occipital defects are easily visualized; however, the anterior encephalocele defect may require special views such as the occipital-mental view.[33] Computerized tomography may enable sharp identification of bony defects, hydrocephalus, and associated brain deformity. Combined with density determinations, it helps to identify the content of the sac. The visualization of abnormalities in the cerebrovascular tree, however, still requires angiography.[34] Hypothalamic–pituitary dysfunction has been documented in patients with basal encephalocele and should be considered in all of these patients.[5]

Recently, visual evoked respones have been used to study the visual systems of children with occipital encephalocele.[10] The ability to obtain a visual response from the surface of the sac may indicate the presence of visual cortex within the sac, whereas the absence of a response over the occipital area and sac may

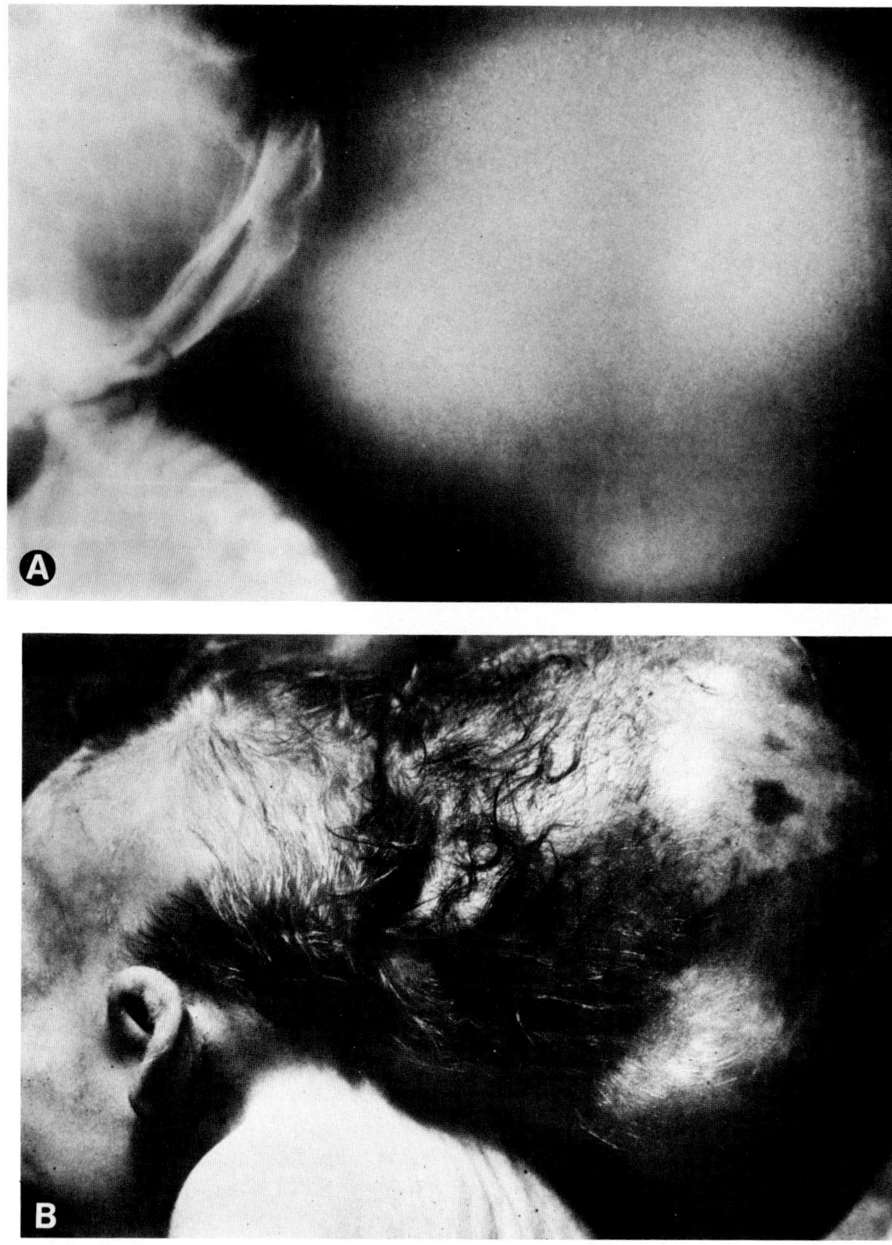

Figure 3-3. A. Lateral skull x-ray of large occipital encephalocele. B. Lateral profile of the child. C. Small amount of dysmorphic brain (white arrow), which is connected to the intracranial brain by a small (pedunculated) stalk. Dura preserved for closure (black arrow). (D) Dural closure (arrow). Note small cranial defect associated with large occipital encephalocele.

indicate pathologic change within the visual pathways and/or absence of visual cortex within the encephalocele. This information may be helpful in contemplated surgical treatment.

TREATMENT

Matson recommends operative treatment for all patients with encephalocele, except those who are terminal. He has described tenuous skin coverage and cerebrospinal fluid leak as indications for urgent operation,[13] and has emphasized

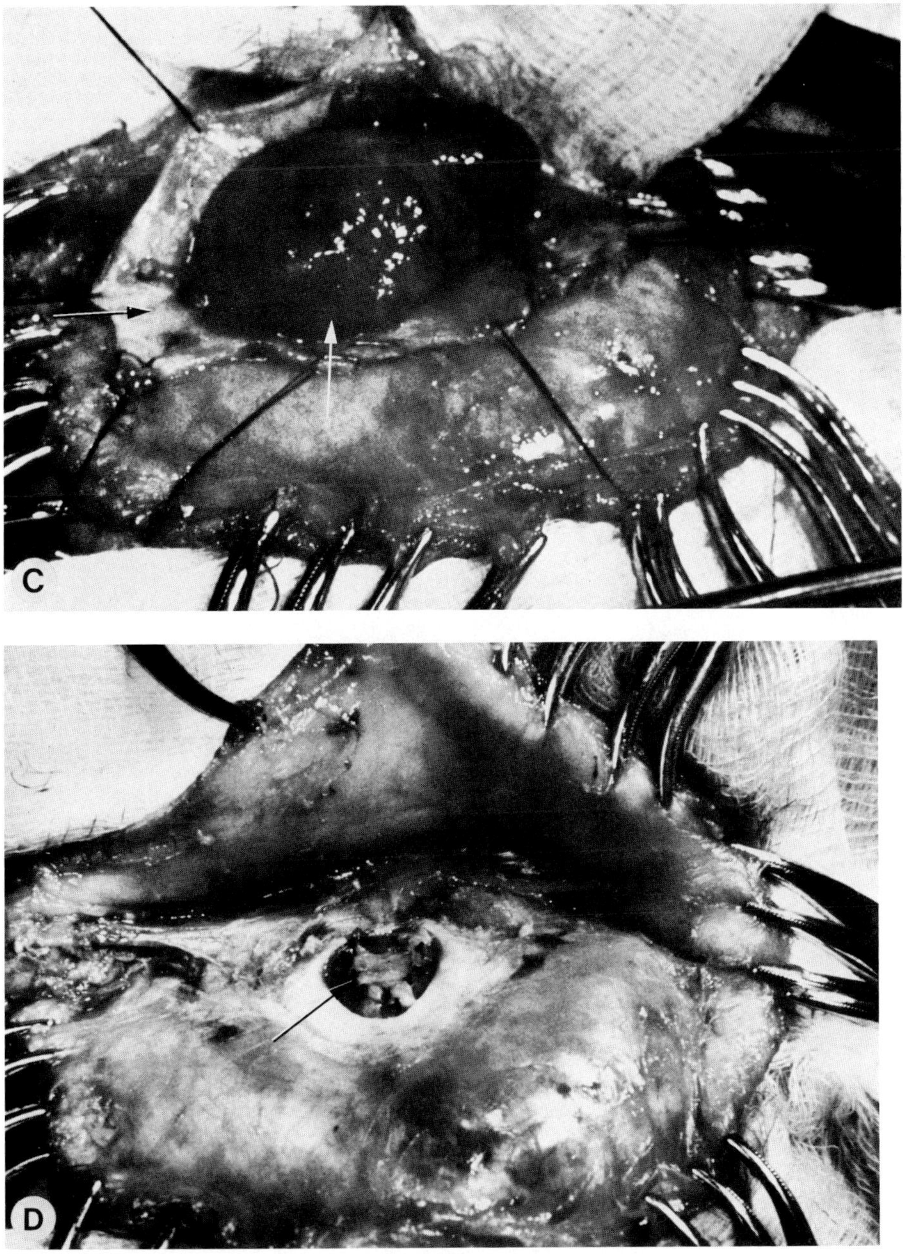

that ease of care and diminution of parental psychic trauma are also considerations. Developmental prognosis is not considered in the decision to recommend operation. Prevention of infection and preservation of function have also been used as indications for operation. Untreated encephaloceles may continue to enlarge because of increasing brain herniation and increased deficit may follow. Early operation may prevent this complication.[15]

Others, however, have suggested that patients with microcephaly and large amounts of brain within the encephalocele may have a poor prognosis and should not have operative treatment.[7,35]

The primary goals of operation for encephalocele are closure of the dura at the level of the cranium, replacement and/or removal of extracranial cerebral tissue, and restoration of cranial contour with good skin coverage. These goals are not always achievable.

For operation, patients are placed in the prone position with the head

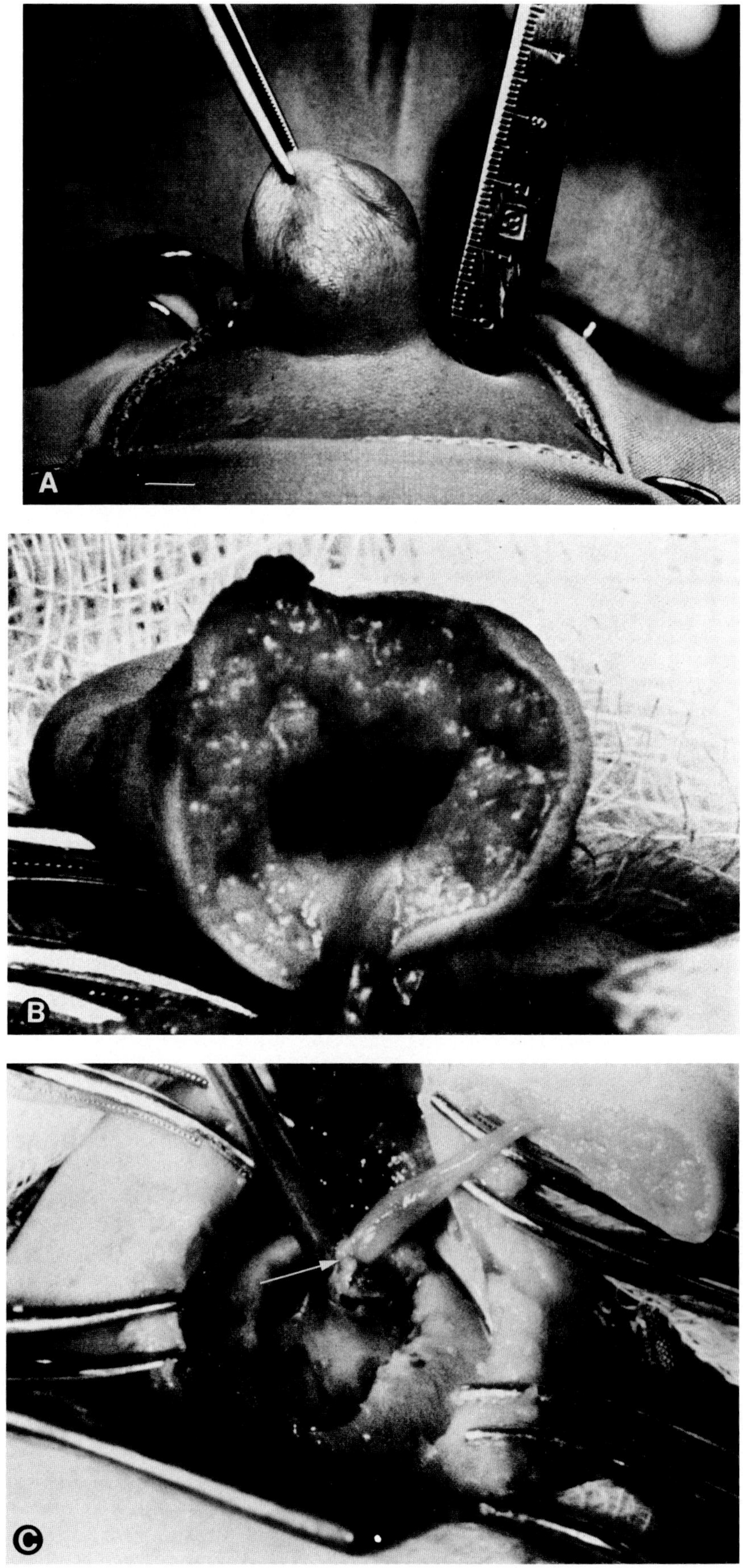

Figure 3-4. A. Pedunculated occipital encephalocele. B. Interior of the sac. C. Small dural stalk with no cerebral content (arrow).

suspended in a well-padded cerebellar head rest. Aspiration of cerebrospinal fluid in large encephaloceles prior to skin incision may reduce the bulk of the mass and contribute to the ease of dissection and operative removal (Fig. 3–3B). Suspension of the mass with an instrument as described by Hendrick may also make dissection easier.[29] The skin incision is usually a transverse ellipse planned so as to leave adequate skin for closure. Unlike the closure of a myelomeningocele, this is generally not a problem here.[13] The pericranium is identified and separated from the overlying tissue and then is incised at a sufficient distance from the cranial defect to permit adequate inspection and dissection of the contents (Fig. 3–3C). If visual evoked potentials have been demonstrated over the sac, preservation of cerebral tissue is mandatory. Every effort should be made to conserve cerebral tissue; however, occasionally it will be necessary to amputate tissue demonstrating abnormal morphology or necrosis in order to achieve closure. In the future, intraoperative recording of visual and somatosensory evoked potentials may be useful in identifying functional tissue. Dissection of the dura and brain should always be tempered by the knowledge that there may be abnormal sinus locations and venous connections to the torcula, straight sinus, and occipital sinus. Occasionally the cranial defect will need to be enlarged in order to ensure safety of dissection and replacement of intracranial contents. Following excision of the mass, the dura is closed meticulously and dural graft may be required (Fig. 3–3D). No attempt is made during infancy to close the cranial defect.[12,13,29] In older children the cranial defect may be closed with autogenous bone or acrylic. It is desirable to attempt periosteal closure. The skin is then closed over the defect. The postoperative period may be complicated by an acute increase in hydrocephalus and this should be treated promptly with a cerebrospinal fluid shunt. Seizure is frequently associated with encephalocele and should be vigorously controlled.

The closure and repair for temporal and parietal encephalocele are similar to the considerations described for occipital encephalocele.[20,36]

The risk of meningitis occurring with anterior encephalocele because of the potential of cerebrospinal fluid fistula, and/or proximity to contaminated areas such as the sinuses, nose, and mouth, makes tight dural closure of paramount

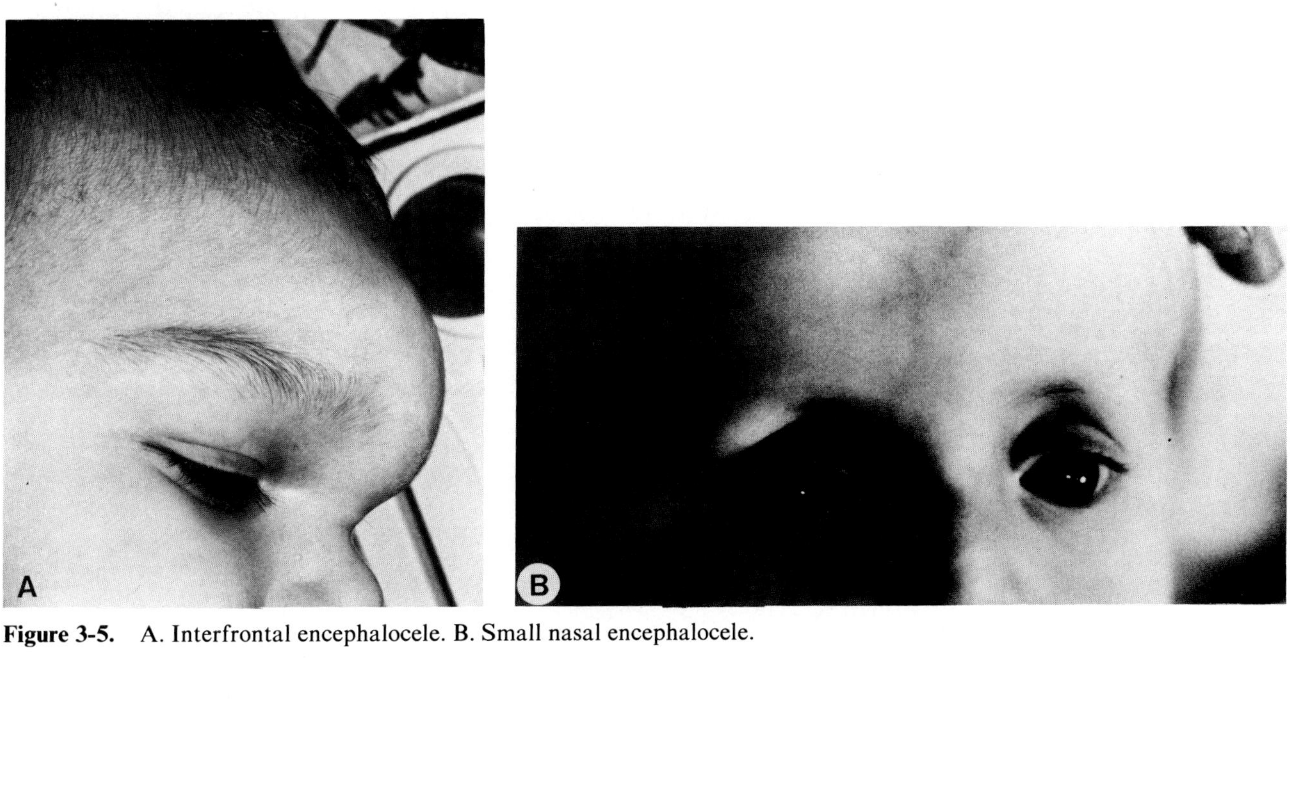

Figure 3-5. A. Interfrontal encephalocele. B. Small nasal encephalocele.

importance. Most surgeons therefore recommend intracranial operation for treatment of these lesions.[7–9,13,30] Extracranial operations often require transversing contaminated areas and are associated with difficult dural closure. Matson recommends coronal incision for repair.[13] Orbital encephaloceles are repaired by intracranial dural operation. Autogenous dural graft may be required to achieve watertight closure of anterior encephaloceles. Sphenoidal and cribiform defects are generally repaired from the intradural space. Contrary to the case with orbital encephalocele where the cerebral extension is amputated and withdrawn prior to dural closure, no attempt is made to remove the amputated tissue associated with nasal, pharyngeal, or sphenoidal extensions.[13,31] Frequently, this remaining cerebral tissue will atrophy and disappear.[29] Most authors recommend closure with autogenous bone, regardless of the location of the bony defect. Plastic and reconstructive operations are delayed to a secondary stage and often include correction of hypertelorism. Suwanwela and co-workers recommend extracranial operation only when the lesion is located at the forehead or the root of the nose and is associated with a short canal with the intracranial portion being accessible through the defect. The advantage is that removal of the extradural tissue, closure of the dura, and plastic reconstruction may be accomplished at the same operation.[27]

PROGNOSIS

Generally, the prognosis for motor and intellectual development is less favorable for infants with occiptial encephalocele than for those with anterior encephalocele.[13] Children with occipital encephalocele containing brain and who develop hydrocephalus have a poor prognosis. Perhaps only 20–30 percent achieve normal intellectual development. In the absence of hydrocephalus, this improves to 40 percent; however, many will have physical disability.[12] When the sac contains only cerebrospinal fluid, and there is no hydrocephalus, there may be normal intellect in as many as 86 percent, but if this group develops hydrocephalus, that number will be only 30 percent.[12,13,18,25] Mealey has suggested that 50 percent of patients with occipital encephalocele are at risk of developing hydrocephalus.[12] Contrary to the prognosis for occipital encephalocele, that for children with anterior encephalocele is excellent. In the absence of the complications of infection and hydrocephalus, one may anticipate normal intellectual development for these children.[12,13,31]

REFERENCES

1. Leong AYS, Shaw CM: The pathology of occipital encephalocele and a discussion of the pathogenesis. Pathology 11:223–234, 1979
2. Emery JL, Kalhan SC: The pathology of exencephalus. Dev Med Child Neurology 22:51–64, 1970
3. Leone CR Jr, Malowe JF: Orbital presentation of an ethmoidal encephalocele. Arch Ophthal 83:445–447, 1970
4. Suwanwela, C: Craniomeningocele and encephalomeningocele, in Sano K, Ishii S (eds): Recent Progress in Neurological Surgery, Proceedings of the Symposia of the Fifth International Congress of Neurological Surgery, Toyko, October 7–13, 1973. Amsterdam, Excerpta Medica, 1974, pp 49–55
5. Lieblich JM, Rosen SW, Guyda H, et al: The syndrome of basal encephalocele and hypothalamic-pituitary dysfunction. Ann Int Med 89:910–916, 1978

6. Modesti LM, Glasauer FE, Terplan KL: Sphenoethmoidal encephalocele. Child's Brain 3:140–153, 1977
7. Suwanwela C, Chaturaporn H: Fronto-ethmoidal encephalocele. J Neurosurg 25:172–182, 1966
8. Whatmore WJ: Sincipital encephalomeningoceles. Br J Surg 60:261–270, 1973
9. Tandon PN: Meningoencephalocoeles. Acta Neurol Scand 46:369–383, 1970
10. Engel R, Buchan GC: Occipital encephaloceles with and without visual evoked potentials. Arch Neurol 30:314–318, 1974
11. Karch SB, Urich H: Occipital encephalocele: A morphological study. J Neurol Sci 15:89–112, 1972
12. Mealey J Jr, Dzenitis AJ, Hockey AA: The prognosis of encephaloceles. J Neurosurg 32:209–218, 1970
13. Matson DD: Neurosurgery of Infancy and Childhood (ed 2). Springfield, Ill, Charles C Thomas, 1969, pp 61–75
14. Van Nouhuys JM, Bruyn GW: Nasopharyngeal transsphenoidal encephalocele, cratelike hole in the optic disc and agenesis of the corpus callosum; pneumoencephalographic visualization in a case. Psychiat Neurol Neurochir 67:243–258, 1964
15. Suwanwela C, Suwanwela N: A morphological classification of sincipital encephalomeningocele. J Neurosurg 36:201–211, 1972
16. Smith MT, Huntington HW: Inverse cerebellum and occipital encephalocele: A dorsal fusion defect uniting the Arnold-Chiari and Dandy–Walker spectrum. Neurology 27:246–251, 1977
17. Friede RL: Uncommon syndromes of cerebellar vermis aplasia. II. Tecto-cerebellar dysraphia with occipital encephalocele. Dev Med Child Neurol 20:764–772, 1978
18. Hutchison JW, Stovring J, Turner PT: Occipital encephalocele with holoprosencephaly and aqueduct stenosis. Surg Neurol 12:331–335, 1979
19. Caviness VS Jr, Evrard P: Occipital encephalocele: A pathologic and anatomic analysis. Acta Neuropath (Berlin) 32:245–255, 1975
20. McLaurin RL: Parietal cephaloceles. Neurology 14:764–772, 1964
21. Luyendijk W: Intranasal encephaloceles: A survey of 8 neurosurgically treated cases. Psychiat Neurol Neurochir 72:77–87, 1969
22. Campbell JB: Congenital anomalies of the neural axis. Am J Surg 75:231–256, 1948
23. Patten BM: Embryological states in the establishing of myeloschisis with spina bifida. Am J Anat 93:365–395, 1953
24. Williamson AP, Blattner RJ, Robertson GG: The relationship of viral antigen to virus-induced defects in chick embryo: Newcastle-disease virus. Dev Biol 12:498–519, 1965
25. Gardner WJ: Etiology and pathogenesis of the development of myelomeningocele, in McLaurin RL (ed): Myelomeningocele. New York, Grune & Stratton, 1977, pp 3–30
26. Alvord EC, Shaw C-M, Sumi SM: Central nervous system developmental abnormalities, in Thompson RA, Green JR (eds): Pediatric Neurology and Neurosurgery. New York, SP Medical & Scientific Books, 1978, p 102
27. Suwanwela C, Sukabote C, Suwanwela N: Frontoencephalomeningocele. Surgery 69:617–625, 1971
28. Chohan BS, Parmar IPS, Bhatia JN: Anterior orbital meningoecephalocele. Am J Ophthal 68:144–146, 1969
29. Hendrick EB, Hoffman HJ, Hugenholtz H: in Sano K, Ishii S (eds): Recent Progress in Neurological Surgery, Proceedings of the Symposia of the Fifth International Congress of Neurological Surgery, Toyko, October 7–13, 1973. Amsterdam, Excerpta Medica, 1974, p 56
30. Copty M, Verret S, Langelier R, et al: Intranasal meningoencephalocele with recurrent meningitis. Surg Neurol 12:49–52, 1979
31. Nakamura T, Grant JA, Hubbard RE: Nasoethmoidal meningoencephalocele. Arch Otolaryngol 100:62–64, 1974

32. Griffith BH: Frontonasal tumors: Their diagnosis and management. Plastic Reconstruct Surg 57:692–699, 1976
33. Harverson G, Bailey IC, Kiryabwire WM: The radiological diagnosis of anterior encephalocoeles. Clin Radiol 25:317–322, 1974
34. Gilmor RL, Kalsbeck JE, Goodman JM, et al: Angiographic assessment of occipital encephaloceles. Radiology 103:127–130, 1972
35. Guthkelch AN: Occipital cranium bifidum. Arch Dis Childhood 45:104–109, 1970
36. Nagulich I, Borne G, Georgevich Z: Temporal meningocele. J Neurosurg 27:433–440, 1967

4. The Arnold–Chiari Malformation

Peter W. Carmel

The hindbrain malformations that are commonly, but incorrectly, grouped under the term "Arnold–Chiari malformation" remain poorly understood. There is great controversy concerning the definition of these anomalies, their embryogenesis, pathogenesis, and surgical treatment. It is unfortunate that a single term has been coined to describe these various abnormalities. At the time of Chiari's first paper in 1891, it was apparent that there was a *spectrum* of abnormalities of increasing severity, and Chiari subdivided these into three groups.[1] Combining all groups into a single eponimic term has muddled thinking about the malformations, and often has confused appropriate therapy for these disorders.

DESCRIPTION OF THE ARNOLD–CHIARI MALFORMATIONS

Perhaps the first description of one of this group of hindbrain deformities, now called the Arnold–Chiari malformation, was by John Cleland, in a paper published in 1883.[2] This was fully eight years before the first of Chiari's two papers on this subject. Cleland described the pathologic findings in nine infants at autopsy and two chick embryos. The first of these cases was of greatest interest to Cleland, who felt that it offered insight into the developmental nature of the anomaly. This was a full-term infant who had spina bifida and who apparently had severe craniolacunae ("the frontal bones were much perforated"). The brain stem was elongated, and the fourth ventricle extended into the upper cervical canal (Fig. 4-1). Cleland particularly noted distortion of the "inferior vermiform process, which extends so far that what appears to be the pyrimid touches the corpora quadrigemina, while the uvula looks backward and the laminated tubercle hangs down from an exaggerated velum posticum as an appendix ¾ of

The author thanks Professor Dr. Herbert Hunger—Generalsekrtar, Osterreichische Akademie der Wissenschaften—for permission to reproduce Figures 4-2 and 4-3 from Chiari's 1896 article and Professor David Sinclair—Editor, Journal of Anatomy—for permission to reproduce Figure 4-1 from Cleland's 1883 article.

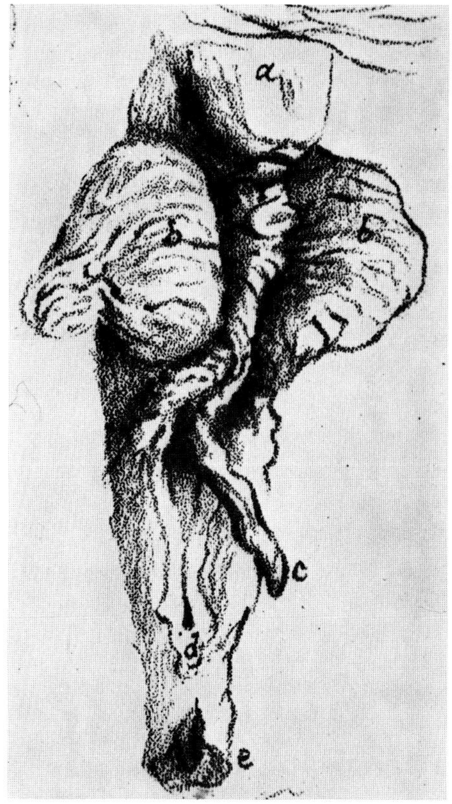

Figure 4-1. Drawing of Cleland's case 1. The inferior vermis (c) protrudes downward into the cervical canal, as does the fourth ventricle. The level of the obex (d) is also inferiorly displaced. Distortion of the tectum is indicated at (a). (Reprinted with permission from Cleland J: Contribution to the study of spinal bifida, encephalocele, and anencephalus. J Anat Physiol 17:255–266, 1958.)

an inch in length, lying in the fourth ventricle." This description fits into the Chiari Type II, or "true" Arnold–Chiari malformation. Cleland noted in particular the distortion of the vermis, both in the rostral and caudal directions. Chiari made similar observations in his 1896 article,[3] but he was apparently unaware of Cleland's earlier report.

In 1891 Chiari described three types of hindbrain anomaly associated with hydrocephalus and illustrated each of these types with a single case.[1] A further report was published in 1896, in which clinical and autopsy findings were described for 24 cases.[3] Each of these was profusely illustrated and the illustrations have become a source of great information. They help to resolve the confusion that has arisen over the exact definition of Chiari's two most important types of malformations.

CHIARI'S ANOMALIES

Type I

In the Type I anomaly Chiari described "peg-like elongation of the tonsils and medial part of the inferior lobes of the cerebellum which go along the medulla into the cervical canal." The abnormality in this type is restricted to the cerebellum. A number of authors, however, have translated Chiari's definition as defining cerebellar tonsils which "accompany the medulla oblongata into the spinal."[4] This would imply a caudal displacement of the medulla into the cervical canal. Examination of Chiari's illustrations of 14 cases of Type I anomaly shows that the medulla is not dislocated caudally, the lower cranial nerves are not elongated, and the upper cervical nerves do not run upward to their foramina (Fig. 4-2). These findings indicate that the brain stem is *not* involved in Chiari's definition of Type I.

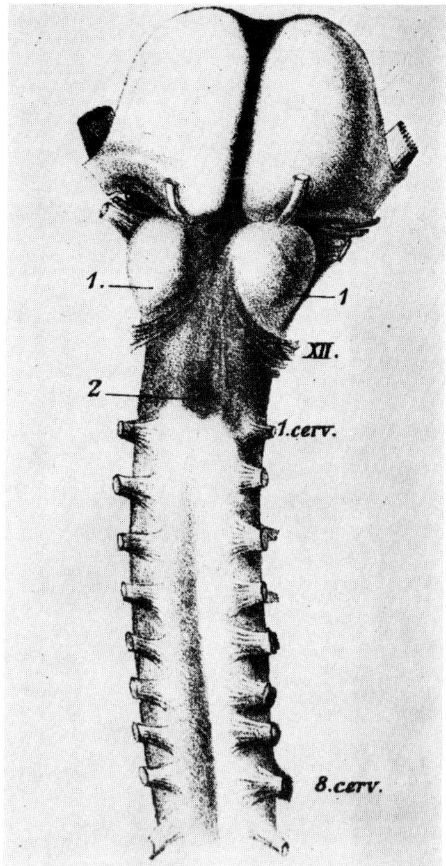

Figure 4-2. Illustration of ventral surface of brain stem and upper cervical cord of Chiari Type I anomaly, taken from Chiari's 1896 paper.[3] The XIIth cranial nerve runs *downward* to its foramina and the upper cervical nerves do *not* run upward to their foramina, indicating that the medulla is not caudally displaced. The impression of the dens is seen in the ventral surface of the cord above C_1 (2). (Reprinted with permission from Chiari H: Veber veranderungen des Kleinhirns, des pons und der medulla oblongata in folge von congenitaler hydrocephalie des grosshixns. Deuschr Akad Wiss Wien 63:71–116, 1896.)

In 1894, three years after Chiari's first paper, Arnold described multiple abnormalities in a newborn infant.[5] Most of this paper was devoted to visceral and lung abnormalities and only scant attention was given to the brain stem. He did note that parts of the cerebellum and fourth ventricle were herniated through the foramen magnum, but the medulla was described as being normal. This description is consistent with Chiari's Type I anomaly.

Type II

In his initial description Chiari defined Type II as "displacement of the parts of the cerebellum and the elongated fourth ventricle which reach the cervical canal." By the time his fuller description was published, however, Chiari had changed this to read, "displacement of part of the lower vermis, displacement of the pons and displacement of the medulla oblongata into the cervical canal and elongation of the fourth ventricle into the cervical canal." This change emphasized brain-stem displacement and cerebellar dysplasia as the major components of the malformation. Chiari had also come to understand that the cerebellar anomaly was quite different from the usual form of tonsillar herniation, and that there was malformation of the inferior vermis as well (Fig. 4-3).

THE ARNOLD–CHIARI MALFORMATION

In 1907 Schwalbe and Gredig gratuitously added Arnold's name to Chiari's Type II malformation, and coined the term "Arnold–Chiari malformation."[6] It must be noted that they were working in Arnold's laboratory in Heidelberg at the time. Nevertheless, this attempt to curry favor with their boss has confused

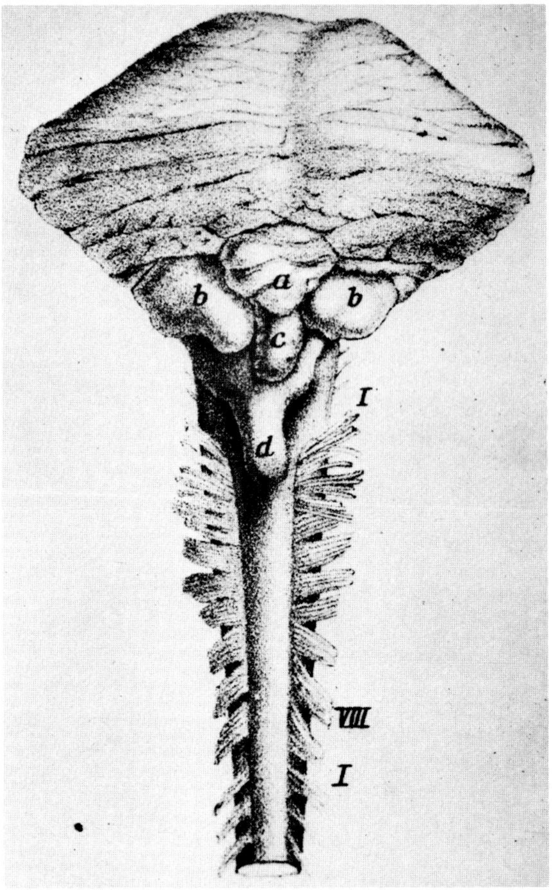

Figure 4-3. Illustration of the Type II anomaly as it appeared in Chiari's 1896 paper.[3] Both the tonsils (b) and the inferior portion of the vermis (c) are elongated caudally. The fourth ventricle (d) is displaced into the upper cervical region, and in this case is imperforate. Because of the caudal displacement of the cervico–medullary junction, the upper cervical nerve roots (I) have a rostral course to their exit foramina. (Reprinted with permission from Chiari H: Veber veranderungen des Kleinhirns, des pons und der medulla oblongata in folge von congenitaler hydrocephalie des grosshixns. Deuschr Akad Wiss Wien 63:71–116, 1896.)

discussion of the Chiari malformations ever since. Schwalbe and Gredig further distinguished the cerebellar malformation as Arnold's malformation. This incorrect characterization has carried over into contemporary literature.[7–9] These authors did make a significant contribution with their description of the cervical–medullary junction changes in the Type II anomaly. The junction between brain stem and spinal cord could be shifted without changing the contour of the hindbrain, or the hindbrain could override the upper cervical cord. This "kink" should not be called the Chiari deformity, and it was not found in all of the Type II cases in Chiari's description. The term Arnold–Chiari malformation should probably be reserved for the Type II anomaly. Use of this term to describe tonsilar herniation, either congenital or acquired, is erroneous.

Peach[10,11] has defined the Arnold–Chiari malformation as "a variable displacement of a tongue of tissue, derived from the inferior cerebellar vermis, to the upper cervical canal accompanied by a similar caudal dislocation of the medulla and fourth ventricle, the medulla often showing a 'kink-like' deformity." Although it is likely that there is a wide spectrum of malformations of the hindbrain and cerebellum and that some cases will not fit into Chiari's classifications, separation of the Type I and Type II anomalies should always be attempted. The Type II anomaly is largely found in infants, is almost invariably associated with hydrocephalus, and is initially treated by a shunting procedure. The Type I anomaly most often becomes apparent in later years, usually the adolescent or early adult period, and is frequently found without concomitant hydrocephalus. In addition to these obvious dissimilarities, the two types have quite different implications as to the presence of other central nervous system malformations, bone anomalies, and prognosis. Some of the distinguishing features of Type I and Type II are given in Table 4-1.

Table 4-1
Comparison of Chiari's Type 1 and Type 2 Anomalies

Anomaly	Type 1	Type 2
Caudal dislocation of medulla	No	Yes
Caudal dislocation of inferior vermis	No	Yes
Spina bifida	May be present	Rarely absent
Hydrocephalus	May be absent	Rarely absent
Medullary "kink"	Absent	Present in 55%
Course of upper cervical nerve roots	Usually normal	Usually cephalad

Type III

The Type III anomaly was the highest degree of displacement of posterior fossa neural structures found by Chiari. In this type the cerebellum herniated through the foramen magnum into a bifid cervical canal. The posterior fossa was dysraphic and open, with the cerebellum forming a sac-like encephalocele. This severe degree of anomaly is rarely compatible with postnatal life, and is occasionally associated with a caudal myelomeningocele. Gardner[4] considers this condition a severe form of Klippel–Feil syndrome. Association between the Chiari malformation Type III and Klippel–Feil syndrome seems to be confirmed by the following case.

CASE REPORT

B. P. was a full-term infant girl, born to a primiparous 24-year-old mother after an unremarkable pregnancy. Both parents were from Peru, S. A., and had emigrated to the United States 2½ years earlier. Apgar at 2 minutes was 5, and there was some initial respiratory difficulty.

Examination revealed the head to be fixed in a hyperextended position in relationship to the thorax (Fig. 4-4). In the suboccipital region a soft, pulsatile bulge was felt, which ran downward to the thoracic spine. The skull was open, and bifid lamina were palpable caudal to the sac. Hair and skin covered the entire sac and no neural elements were seen. Both the chest and abdominal cavities appeared shortened in their rostral–caudal extent.

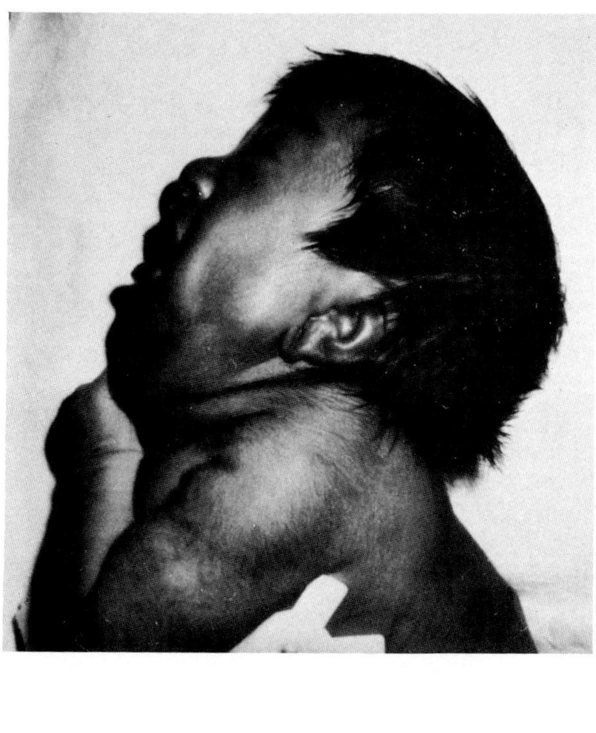

Figure 4-4. Child with Chiari Type III anomaly. A large sac-like protrusion extends from the head to the upper portion of the thoracic region (covered with hair). The head is extremely extended and is fixed in this position.

Neurologic examination revealed good movement of arms and legs, and appreciation of pinprick throughout. Cranial nerves were intact, except for diminished gag reflex. There was stridor on crying, an attempt at laryngoscopy was not successful. The child had diminished suck, and occasional reflux of milk through the nose was noted.

Chest x-rays revealed diminished lung volume. Skull and spine films confirmed both cranium and spina bifidum (Fig. 4-5). A computerized tomography (CT) scan

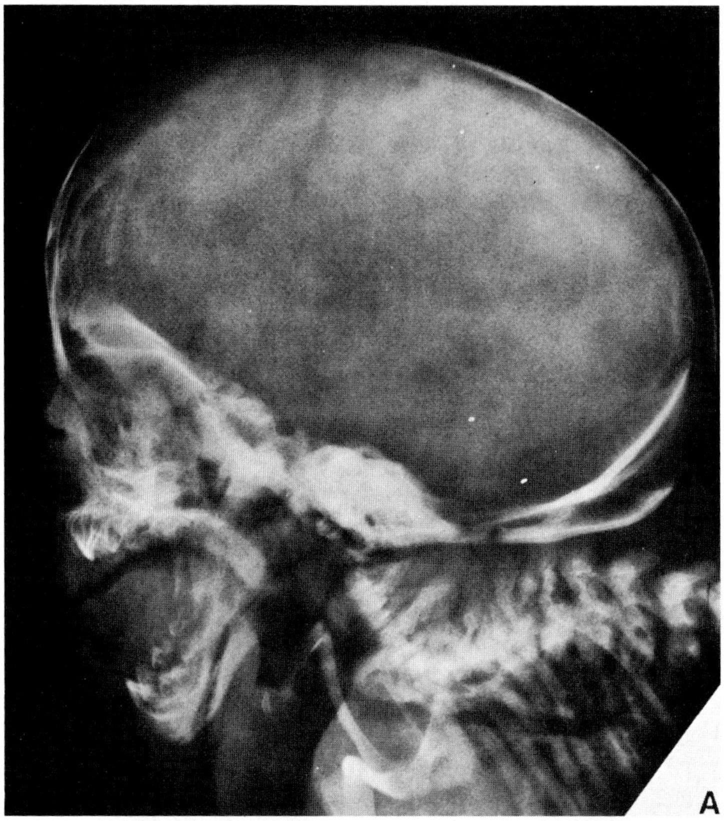

A

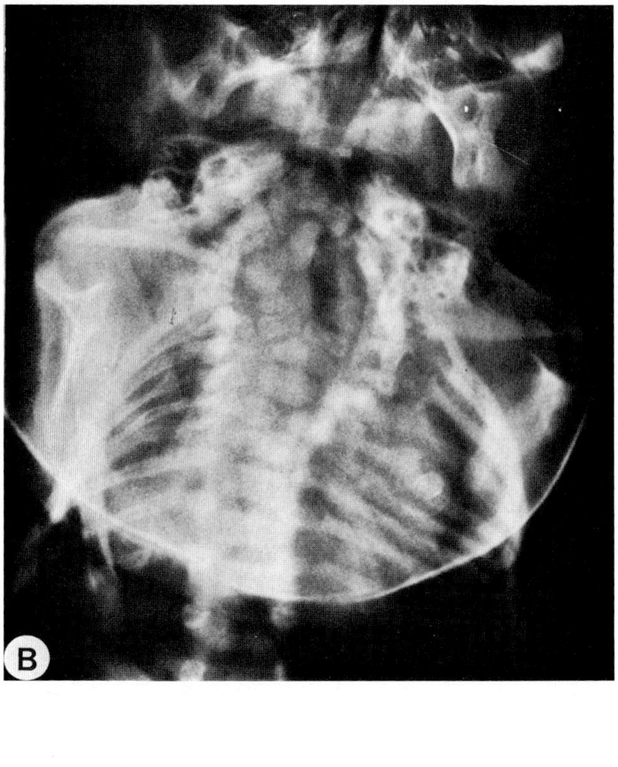

B

Figure 4-5. X-rays of the child in Figure 4-4. The small posterior fossa is open and the foramen magnum is widened. The cervical and upper thoracic spines are bifid. Most of the cervical vertebral bodies are fused into several large blocks, and there is fusion of several laminae. These changes are much the same as those seen in Klippel–Feil malformation. A. Lateral view, B. Anteroposterior view.

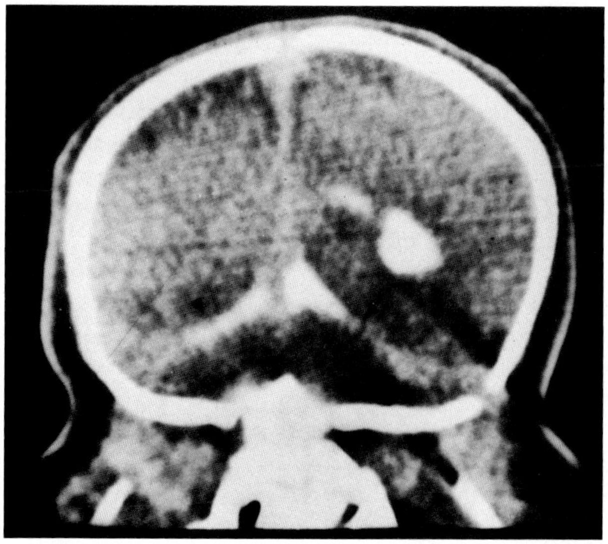

Figure 4-6. CT scan in the coronal plane following intrathecal injection of metrizamide. Contrast material is seen beneath the tentorium (arrows), and the small size of the posterior fossa is demonstrated.

was carried out after intrathecal injection of metrizamide, and demonstrated a small posterior fossa (Fig. 4-6) with migration of neural structures through the bifid foramen magnum and into the upper spinal canal.

Respiratory difficulties became progressively worse, and the child died at age 3 weeks. The neural anomalies described above were confirmed at autopsy.

EMBRYOGENESIS

Cleland attributed the malformation that he described to a primary dysgenesis of the brain stem. In this opinion he was strongly influenced by studies of the chick embryo published by Lebedeff in 1881.[12] Here embryos in which the medullary blastoma appeared to be overdeveloped, resulting in thickening and plication of all or part of the brain stem, were described. Cleland connected this anomaly to the human malformation. He discounted hydrocephalus as a causative factor and stated that "hydrocephalus was obviously of much later origin, when the different parts of the brain were already formed."

Chiari attributed the presence of all three types of anomalies to hydrocephalus of the cerebrum.[3] He attributed the downward caudal herniation of the posterior fossa contents to an increasing hydrocephalus of the cerebrum.

The hydrocephalus theory has been restated in recent years by Gardner, who has proposed that failure of the primitive rombic roof to be permeable during fetal development results in dilatation of both the cephalic and spinal portions of the closed neural tube.[4,13] The resultant enlargement of the primitive ventricles causes caudal migration of the hindbrain. This hydrocephalus, in turn, causes the tentorium to migrate too far caudally in early life. The difference between the Type I and Type II anomalies is attributed by Gardner to an opposing Bering effect of the posterior choroid plexus in the Type I anomaly. In Type II, because of the myeloschisis, this opposing effect is lost as the ventricular pulse generated by the beating of the posterior plexus is expended in spurting through the caudal opening of the neural tube. This leads to a greater posterior migration of the tentorium.

Although this ingenious theory is stimulating, reports of Arnold–Chiari malformations without hydrocephalus indicate that hydrocephalus is not the sole causative factor.[10,14] In addition, reported cases of the Type II anomaly without the presence of a myelomeningocele,[9,15–17] which would have no caudal exit to dampen a Bering pulse, and yet have typical brain-stem caudal displacement, do not support Gardner's theory. Finally, the absence of these brain-stem anomalies from the large number of cases of congenital hydrocephalus of all types, including those that appear to have occurred very early in fetal development, make hydrocephalus unlikely to be the sole causative factor of the malformations.

A "tethering" theory of the Type II malformation has been proposed by Penfield and Coburn[18] and by Lichtenstein.[7] These authors felt that traction on the cord tethered at the level of the myelomeningocele resulted in caudal displacement of the brain stem and cerebellum. If this were the mechanism, however, the abnormal direction of nerve roots should be greatest closest to the tether and be dissipated higher up in the cord, which is not the case. In addition, a traction mechanism would not explain those cases in which the cord is not tethered, which would include most of the Type I cases. The tethering theory must now be regarded as discredited.

Most contemporary writers seem to agree with Cleland that primary dysgenesis of the brain stem is the cause of the malformation. There is marked disagreement, however, as to the nature of this dysgenesis. The cause of the anomaly was attributed to a local overgrowth of the brain stem and generalized overgrowth of the cereberum by Patten[19] and by Barry, Patten, and Stewart.[20] This theory recalls that proposed by Lebedeff a century ago.[12] Because of this overgrowth, excessive volume of the cerebrum causes caudal displacement of the tentorium, which results in an abnormally small posterior fossa. In addition, overgrowth of the cerebellum and medulla forces these structures to protrude gradually through the foramen magnum down into the cervical canal. This herniation in turn eventually blocks the subarachnoid space and progressive hydrocephalus results. The theory of overgrowth of the entire central nervous system as a cause for the Chiari malformations has not met with wide acceptance.

Daniel and Strich carefully reviewed the pathologic features of 26 cases of Chiari Type II deformity.[21] Each of these 26 cases had an associated myelomeningocele. They stressed that the posterior fossa was unduely small in these cases, with remarkably low peripheral attachment of the tentorium. They attributed the hindbrain abnormality to failure of the pontine flexure to form in early embryonic life. Failure of this flexure would account for the marked elongation of the brain stem seen in this abnormality. Certain features of the anomaly, including beaking of the tectum and thickening of the intrathalmic connexsus, thus were related to upward movement of the brain stem; while herniation of the medulla and vermis into the upper cervical canal were related to elongation in a caudal direction. These authors were perhaps the first to concentrate on the thick fibrous tissue overlying the herniated vermis and tonsils. In the past this thickened band had been ascribed to a chronic meningitis. Daniel and Strich, however, felt that this tissue would have formed fibrous and vascular elements of the choroid plexus if it had invaginated into the roof of the fourth ventricle in the ordinary course of development.

In a carefully described series of 20 cases, and a thorough review of the literature, Peach reviewed the theories regarding embryogenesis of Arnold–Chiari malformation.[10,22] He pointed out the relative incidence of each of the distinctive features of the Type II abnormality, and concluded that the abnormality is the result of failure of the pontine flexure to form because of developmental arrest, a theory close to that of Daniel and Strich.

Careful examination of the concomitant anomalies with the Chiari Type II malformation reveals many other instances of arrested development and abnormal formation of central nervous system structures.[11,23] Within the cerebellum itself the folia are poorly myelinized and a reduction in the cellularity of the granular layer is noted. The dentate nuclei in particular maintain an infantile or neonatal configuration. Heterotopias in the form of nodules of cortical tissue are found commonly on a surface of the ventricles and occasionally in the subarachnoid space. The intrathalamic connection is abnormally thickened and hypoplasia of the falx is found in most cases. The cerebrum is not spared changes, and the ventricular surfaces often have a granular appearance of the ependymoma, while the cortical surfaces frequently reveal microgyria.

CLINICAL SYNDROMES

Because of the marked difference in the presentation, treatment, and course of the Type I and Type II anomalies, their clinical symptoms and presenting signs are discussed separately. As the Type II anomalies are found in early infancy, and are more obvious in their presentation, they are dealt with first.

Type II

The vast majority of Chiari Type II anomalies are found in children with myelomeningocele. Here the myelomeningocele comes first to the attention of the clinician, and the signs and symptoms noted are most often attributed to dysplasia of the spinal cord, or concomitant hydrocephalus.

More than 90 percent of children with Chiari Type II abnormalities go on to develop hydrocephalus.[24] Hydrocephalus becomes apparent within a variable period after correction of the spinal defect, with most appearing in the first three months following birth and more than 80% percent of those who will develop hydrocephalus becoming apparent before six months. These hydrocephalic syndromes usually have little to distinguish them clinically from other cases of congenital hydrocephalus.

Many other abnormalities of the spine are found in association with the Type II anomaly. In particular there is frequent association with bony malformations of the cervical–medullary junction, and assimilation of the atlas, platibasia, basilar impression, and Klippel–Feil deformity are frequent findings.[37]

A common syndrome specific to the Type II malformation is the presence of respiratory distress. This is demonstrated by laryngeal stridor, and weakness or paralysis of the vocal cords on laryngoscopy.[25,26] These symptoms appear first at feeding, washing, and crying. They are usually transient and generally disappear when the child is quiet. They can become permanent with frightening suddeness, however, and threaten the child with asphyxia and death.

Specific cranial nerve deficits have been related to this anomaly, with hypoplasia of the vagus nerve in particular and degeneration of the nuclei of the lower cranial nerves.[22,26,40] Hypotonia or spasticity of the upper limbs, above the level of the overt spinal defect, is frequently found as well.

Many of these symptoms will be ameliorated or disappear entirely following adequate decompression of hydrocephalus,[24,27] but in some children there are continued signs of brain-stem dysfunction even after adequate shunting of the hydrocephalus. These signs and symptoms are felt to be the result of direct brain-stem compression at the level of the upper cervical region and foramen magnum. It has been noted that in children with myelodysplasia, extensive surgery of the spine for correction of scoliosis is occasionally accompanied by a sudden impaction of the Arnold–Chiari malformation of the cervical region. This may lead to acute exacerbation of hydrocephalus or brain-stem compression and death.[26]

Hoffman, Hendrick, and Humphreys[27] have reported a group of 15 infants and children who required operation for Chiari malformation. In this group five infants were the most severely affected. These children had apneic spells, loss of gag reflex, and extremity weakness, which quickly progressed to quadriplegia. In four of these children hydrocephalus had been treated prior to posterior fossa surgery but the children had failed to respond. In the other child hydrocephalus became apparent after decompressive surgery and shunting was necessary. A similar situation was found among the children above one year of age, in whom decompression did not alleviate hydrocephalus. More than half were shown to have aquaductal stenosis, and when shunts blocked in these children they required shunt revision even after posterior fossa decompression.

Type I

The Type I malformation may become symptomatic at almost any age, but typically appears in older teenagers or young adults. Pain is the single most common presenting sign.[28,29] This is often suboccipital and cervical, but may be dermatomal when associated with syringomyelia. Sharp facial pain, akin to trigeminal neuralgia, is not rare.[23] Cranial nerve abnormalities may cause dysarthria, dysphagia, or diplopia.[29,39] Motor symptoms are usually unilateral weakness in an arm, or bilateral weakness or spasticity in the legs.[30,31] Complaints related to the Type I anomaly may be related to compression at the foramen magnum, obstruction of cerebrospinal fluid (CSF) flow, or syringomyelia.[38]

RADIOLOGIC EXAMINATION

Type II

Extensive radiologic examination of the child with a Type II anomaly frequently takes place only after the spinal defect has been closed, and in some cases after hydrocephalus has been treated by shunting. It is important to distinguish those radiologic features that reflect prior surgical intervention and those that do not.[32]

Skull films of the child with Chiari Type II malformation and hydrocephalus will show enlargement of the cranium and cephalo-facial disproportion typical of congenital hydrocephalus. Craniolacunia, or *luckenschadel,* are found in approximately 85 percent of children with the Chiari Type II malformation. These fenestrated areas in the frontal, parietal, and membrane occipital bones are seen on plain x-rays, or can be demonstrated by using the bone window of CT scans.

The shadow caused by the insertion of the tentorium and dural sinuses is unusually low and the posterior fossa appears quite small (Fig. 4-7). Measurement of the foramen magnum on skull radiographs and reveals that more than 70 percent of children with myelomeningoceles have enlargement of the foramen magnum and there is often elongation of the upper cervical laminar arches (Fig. 4-8). X-rays may also reveal platybasia, basillar impression, assimilation of the atlas, or Klippel–Feil deformity. Hemivertebra of the spine is found in at least 20 percent of reported cases.

Contrast x-ray studies performed on these children have included ventriculography, pneumoencephalography, myelography, and, more recently, contrast-enhanced CT scanning.[32] Ventriculography will demonstrate hydrocephalus as well as obstruction of the air flow at the upper end of the aqueduct or posterior third ventricle. Pneumoencephalography reveals the low-lying tonsils as well as the caudally displaced fourth ventricle in those cases where the air can penetrate into the ventricular system. Myelography, particularly in the supine position,

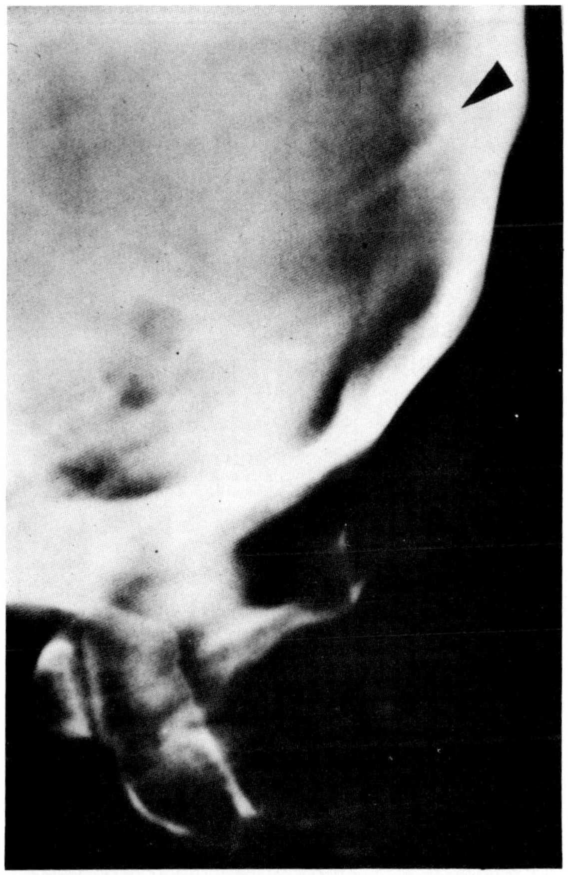

Figure 4-7. Lateral laminogram of the skull of child born with myelomeningocele. Arnold–Chiari Type II malformation was demonstrated by myelography. Arrow indicates the low insertion of the tentorium and the small size of the posterior fossa.

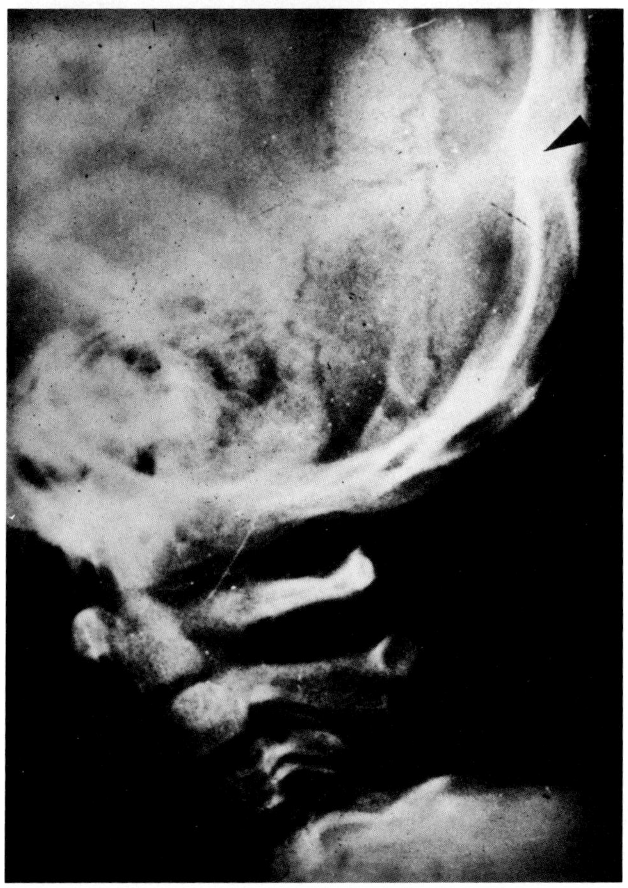

Figure 4-8. Lateral x-ray of child with myelomeningocele repaired shortly after birth. The posterior fossa is small, as outlined by bone density at transverse sinus, and insertion of tentorium is low (arrow). The foramen magnum is enlarged, and the laminae of C_1 and C_2 are elongated.

the CSF by blood and transudate. These patients experienced severe headache, neck stiffness, and fever with elevated spinal fluid protein content. This "posterior fossa syndrome" has been reviewed elsewhere.[34]

Mortality rates for decompressive operations range from 5 to 10 percent,[35] with respiratory compromise the major cause. Another major complication is tetraplegia, which is a consequence of excessive head flexion as the child is positioned for operation.

In patients who have an obstructive syndrome, with moderate or progressive hydrocephalus, a shunting procedure is the operation of choice and often relieves all symptoms. In several series patients who initially underwent shunting procedures required further postoperative decompression of the posterior fossa.[23,27,36] Patients with uncontrolled hydrocephalus have increased risk during the time of posterior fossa surgery.

REFERENCES

1. Chiari H: Ueber veranderungen des kleinhirns infolge von hydrocephalie des grosshirns. Deutsch Med Wschr 17:1172–1175, 1891
2. Cleland J: Contribution to the study of spina bifida, encephalocele, and anencephalus. J Anat Physiol 17:257–291, 1883
3. Chiari H: Ueber veranderungen des kleinhirns, des pons und der medulla oblongata in folge von congenitaler hydrocephalie des grosshirns. Denschr Akad Wiss Wien 63:71–116, 1896
4. Gardner WJ: The Dysraphic States. Amsterdam, Excerpta Medica, 1973
5. Arnold J: Myelocyste, transposition von gewebskeimen und sympodie. Beitr Path Anat 16:1–28, 1894
6. Schwalbe E, Gredig M: Uber entwicklungsstorungen des kleinhirns, hirnstamms und halsmarks bei spina bifida (Arnold'sche und Chiari'sche Missbildung). Beitr Pathol Anat u Allg Pathol 40:132–194, 1907
7. Lichenstein BW: Distant neuroanatomic complications of spina bifida (spinal dysraphism). Hydrocephalus, Arnold–Chiari deformity, stenosis of the aqueduct of Sylvius, etc: Pathogenesis and pathology. Arch Neurol Psychiat 47:195–214, 1942
8. List CF: Neurologic syndromes accompanying developmental anomalies of the occipital bone, atlas and axis. Arch Neurol Psychiat 45:577–616, 1941
9. Teng P, Papatheodorou G: Arnold–Chiari malformation with normal spine and cranium. Arch Neurol 12:622–624, 1965
10. Peach B: Arnold–Chiari malformation with normal spine. Arch Neurol 10:497–501, 1964
11. Peach B: Arnold–Chiari malformation: Morphogenesis. Arch Neurol 12:527–535, 1965
12. Lebedeff A: Ueber die entstehung der anencephalie und spina bifida bei vogeln und menschen. Virchow Arch 86:263–298, 1881
13. Gardner WJ: Anatomic features common to the Arnold–Chiari and the Dandy–Walker malformations suggest a common origin. Cleveland Clin Q 26:206–222, 1959
14. Carmel PW, Markesbery WR: Early descriptions of the Arnold–Chiari malformation. The contribution of John Cleland. J Neurosurg 37:543–547, 1972
15. Carmel PW, Markesbery WR: Arnold–Chiari malformation in an elderly woman. Arch Neurol 21:258–262, 1969
16. Swanson HS, Fincher EF: Arnold–Chiari deformity without bony anomalies. J Neurosurg 6:314–319, 1949
17. Verbiest H: The Arnold–Chiari malformation. J Neurol Neurosurg Psychiat 16:227–233, 1953
18. Penfield W, Coburn DF: Arnold–Chiari malformation and its operative treatment. Arch Neurol Psychiat 40:328–336, 1938
19. Patten BM: Embryological stages in establishing of myeloschisis with spina bifida. Am J Anat 93:365–395, 1953

20. Barry A, Patten BM, Stewart BH: Possible factors in the development of Arnold–Chiari malformation. J Neurosurg 14:285–301, 1957
21. Daniel PW, Strich SJ: Some observations on the congenital deformity of the central nervous system known as the Arnold–Chiari malformation. J Neuropath Exp Neurol 17:255–266, 1958
22. Peach B: Arnold–Chiari malformation: Anatomic features of 20 cases. Arch Neurol 12:613–621, 1965
23. Barnett HJM, Foster JB, Hudgson P: Syringomyelia. Philadelphia, WB Saunders, 1973
24. Mori K, Handa H, Okuno T, et al: Arnold–Chiari type II malformation. A clinicopathological study with special reference to its surgical treatment. Neurochirurgia 21:9–14, 1978
25. Kirsch WM, Duncan BR, Black FO, et al: Laryngeal palsy in association with myelomeningocele, hydrocephalus and Arnold–Chiari malformation. J Neurosurg 28:207–214, 1968
26. Schut L, Bruce DA: The Arnold–Chiari malformation. Orthoped Clin N Am 9:913–921, 1978
27. Hoffman HJ, Hendrick EB, Humphreys RP: Manifestations and management of Arnold–Chiari malformation in patients with myelomeningocele. Child's Brain 1:255–259, 1975
28. Appleby A, Foster JB, Hankinson J, et al: The Chiari anomalies in adult life. Brain 91:131–139, 1968
29. Mohr PD, Strang FA, Sambrook MA, et al: The clinical and surgical features in 40 patients with primary cerebellar ectopia (adult Chiari malformation). Q J Med 181:85–96, 1977
30. Gardner WJ, Goodall RJ: The surgical treatment of Arnold–Chiari malformation in adults. J Neurosurg 7:199–206, 1950
31. Malis LI, Cohen I, Gross SW: Arnold–Chiari malformation. Arch Surg 63:783–798, 1951
32. Naidich TP, Pudlowski RM, Naidich JB, et al: Computed tomographic signs of the Chiari II malformation. Part I: Skull and dural partitions. Radiology 134:65–71, 1980
33. Lapras C, Lotfi M: Surgical management of Chiari II malformation in children. Mod Probl Paediat 18:142–145, 1977
34. Carmel PW, Fraser RAR, Stein BM: Aseptic meningitis following posterior fossa surgery in children. J Neurosurg 41:44–48, 1974
35. Calliauw L, Dehaene I: The surgical risk in the treatment of Arnold–Chiari malformations. Acta Neurochir 39:173–179, 1977
36. Banerji NK, Millar JHD: Chiari malformation presenting in adult life. Its relationship to syringomyelia. Brain 97:157–168, 1974
37. Cameron AH: The Arnold–Chiari and other neuroanatomical malformations associated with spina bifida. J Path Bact 73:195–211, 1957
38. Rhoton AL Jr: Microsurgery of Arnold–Chiari malformation in adults with and without hydromyelia. J Neurosurg 45:473–483, 1976
39. Sieben RL, Hamida MB, Shulman K: Multiple cranial nerve deficits associated with the Arnold–Chiari malformation. Neurology 21:673–681, 1971
40. Venes JL: Multiple cranial nerve palsies in an infant with Arnold–Chiari malformation. Dev Med Child Neurol 16:817–820, 1974
41. Verbiest H: The Arnold–Chiari malformation in adults without concomitant anomalies of the skull or the vertebral column. Folia Psych Neurol Neuroch Neerl 56:544–551, 1953

5. Sacral Agenesis and Diastematomyelia

Donald H. Reigel

SACRAL AGENESIS

In 1852 Hohl described congenital absence of the sacrum and since that time more than 200 patients with varying degrees of dysplasia of the distal spinal cord, absence of the lumbar, sacral, coccygeal, and occasionally thoracic vertebrae, have been described in the medical literature.[1–5] Other terms used to describe this spinal agenesis include caudal dysplasia and caudal regression syndrome.[5] The incidence is said to be between 0.01 and 0.05 per 1000 live births and 0.05 to 0.1 percent of pediatric admissions. There is no sex preference.[1,4] Patients with extensive absence of caudal vertebral segments will be readily diagnosed at birth because of the appearance of the gluteal area, arthrogrypotic deformity of the lower extremities, and the inability to palpate the lumbosacral vertebrae. With mild expressions, however, the diagnosis may be less obvious and the only abnormality may be neurogenic bladder, which is not detected until later childhood.[6] Neurologic deficit distal to the remaining vertebral segment is variable but generally involves loss of motor function and a relative preservation of sensory function. Extensive lumbosacral agenesis is nearly always associated with anomalies of the visceral, genitourinary, cardiopulmonary, and musculoskeletal systems.[1,4,7,8]

Embryology and Etiology

In Chapter 1 Lemire and Warkany have suggested that sacral agenesis is a malformation of the caudal neural tube and may result from abnormal retrogressive differentiation as described by Streeter.[9] Ignelzi has suggested that the absence of vertebrae and the lack of distal skeletal muscle development may be secondary to developmental failure of the caudal notochord and spinal cord.[10] Although there have been isolated reports of familial sacral agenesis such as sex-linked dominant transmission, this disorder has not been considered hereditary.[10,11] Chromosome analyses of patients with sacral agenesis to date have been normal.[7,12] Breech delivery and intrauterine growth retardation commonly occur with sacral agenesis.[4,7] Maternal diabetes mellitus appears to predispose to sacral agenesis. Reports have indicated a 1 percent incidence of sacral agenesis among infants of diabetic mothers, and 15 percent of infants with sacral agenesis will have mothers with diabetes mellitus.[4,7] These statistics, however, do not support diabetes mellitus as a cause.[5] Numerous teratogenic agents such as trypan blue, ultraviolet light, insulin, pyrexia, lithium, fat solvents, and streptogrinin have been reported to produce the syndrome in embryos of experimental animals. Unfortunately, none of these teratogens explain the etiology of this dysplasia in humans.[5]

Neuropathology

Limited neuropathologic studies have demonstrated dysplasia and hypoplasia of the distal spinal cord and atrophy of the roots of the cauda equina. In the lower extremities the muscles supplied by these roots are absent and replaced by fat. The brain and rostral spinal cord have been reported to be normal.[5,7] The extent of neuropathologic change varies with the number of absent segments. With minimal sacral-coccygeal involvement, there may be only minor change in the sacral roots with no normal motor function of the lower extremities. The general pathology demonstrates the association of multisystem anomalies described below.

Clinical Features

Physical examination of the characteristic patient with multiple segment agenesis shows flattening of the buttocks, shortening of the gluteal cleft, and arthrogrypotic-like deformities of the lower extremities consisting of atrophy, flexed abducted hips, webbed knees, and a narrow pelvis (Fig. 5-1). Frequently the absence of the sacrum is palpable. The anal wink is absent, the lower limbs are flaccid, and the deep tendon reflexes are absent. Often there will be preservation of the perineal sensation and dorsal column afferents from the lower extremities, which is disproportionate to the motor loss. Since it has been suggested that all patients with agenesis of two or more segments will have neurogenic bladder, the presence of perineal sensation cannot be relied upon to indicate sphincter function.[4,13] Some of the multisystem abnormalities reported to be associated with sacral agenesis are listed in Table 5-1.

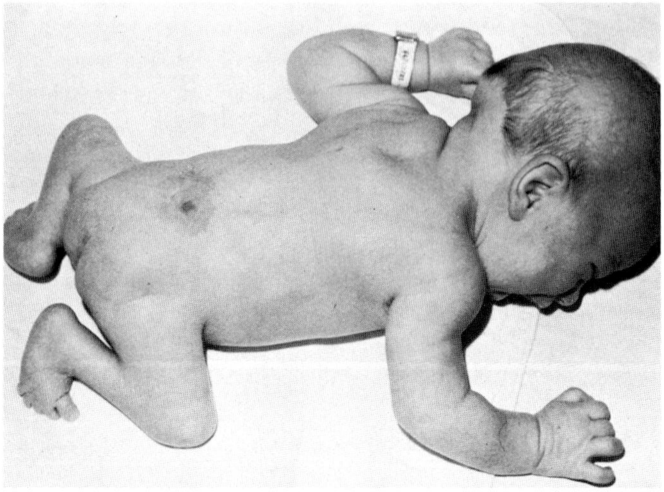

Figure 5-1. Infant with lumbar and sacral agenesis. Note popliteal webbing, gluteal dimple, and associated myelomeningocele.

Table 5-1
Abnormalities Associated with Sacral Agenesis[1-15]

Neurologic	Cardiopulmonary	Gastrointestinal	Orthopedic	Urologic
Paraparesis	Agenesis	Inperforate anus	Spinal curvature and fusion	Neurogenic bladder
Paraplegia	Tracheo-esophageal (T-E) fistula	Hernia	Hemisacrum	Horseshoe kidney
Neurogenic bladder	Dextrocardia	Fistula	Hip dislocation	Duplication
Spina bifida	Atresia	Situs inversus	Pelvic deformity	Hypospadias
Myelomeningocele	Congenital heart defects	Reduplication	Knee dislocation	Extrophy
Microcephaly	Rib anomalies		Talipes equinovarus	
Hydrocephalus			Talipes calcaneovalgus	
Lipoma and dermoid cyst				
Microophthalmia				

The diagnosis may be established by lumbosacral spine x-rays (Fig. 5-2). The possibility of exaggerated lumbosacral angle may result in nonvisualization of the sacrum in the anteroposterior (AP) view, and therefore a lateral film is required to identify true sacral agenesis.[4,8] Since presacral and intraspinal tumors, diastematomyelia, and hydromyelia have been reported, we have also recommended myelography.[11,13] We have now studied 6 patients with sacral agenesis without finding occult spinal lesions. Diagnostic delay has been reported in patients with minor expressions of sacral agenesis and occurs most frequently in patients with only symptomatic neurogenic bladder. For these patients we

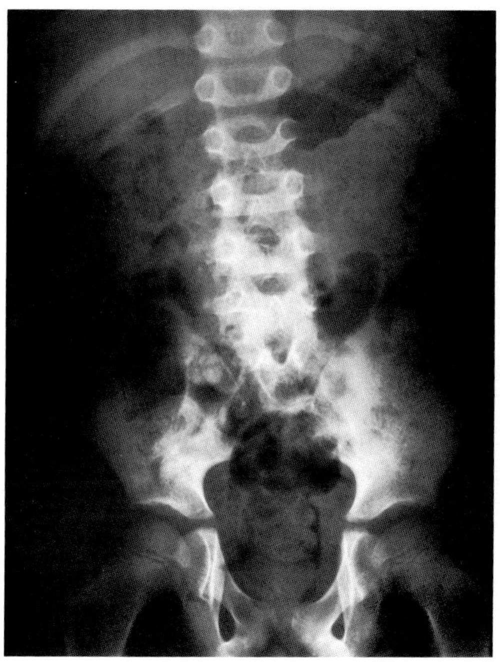

Figure 5-2. Anterior–posterior x-ray demonstrating complete absence of sacrum and pelvic changes.

REFERENCES

1. Andrish J, Kalamchi A, MacEwen GD: Sacral agenesis: A clinical evaluation of its management, heredity, and associated anomalies. Clin Orthoped Rel Res 139:52–57, 1979
2. Dounis E: Sacrococcygeal agenesis. Acta Orthop Scand 49:475–480, 1978
3. Hohl AF: Zur Pathologie des Beckens: I. Das Schrag-Ovale Becken. Leipzig, Wilhelm Engelmann, 1852
4. Mariani AJ, Stern J, Khan AU, et al: Sacral agenesis: An analysis of 11 cases and review of the literature. J Urol 122:684–686, 1979
5. Price DL, Dooling EC, Richardson EP Jr: Caudal dysplasia (caudal regression syndrome). Arch Neurol 23:212–220, 1970
6. Braren V, Jones WB: Sacral agenesis: Diagnosis, treatment and followup of urological complications. J Urology 121:543–544, 1979
7. Sarnat HB, Case ME, Graviss R: Sacral agenesis: Neurologic and neuropathologic features. Neurology 26:1124–1129, 1976
8. White RI, Klauber GT: Sacral agenesis: Analysis of 22 cases. Urology 8:521–525, 1976
9. Streeter GL: Factor involved in the formation of the filum terminale. Am J Anat 25:1–11, 1919
10. Ignelzi RJ, Lehman RAW: Lumbosacral agenesis: Management and embryological implications. J Neurol Neurosurg Psychiat 37:1273–1776, 1974
11. Kenefick JS: Hereditary sacral agenesis associated with presacral tumours. Br J Surg 60:271–274, 1973
12. Rosenthal RK: Congenital absence of the coccyx, sacrum, lumbar vertebrae and the lower two thoracic vertebrae: Report of a case. Bull Hosp Joint Dis 29:287–292, 1978
13. Williams DI, Nixon HH: Agenesis of the sacrum. Surg Gynecol Obstet 105:64–88, 1957
14. Banta JV, Nichols O: Sacral agenesis J Bone Joint Surg 51-A:693–703, 1969
15. Olliver CP: Traite des Maladies de la Moelle Epiniere (ed 3), vol I. Paris, Mequignon-Marvis, 1837
16. Sheptak PE: Diastematomyelia—Diplomyelia, in Handbook of Clinical Neurology, vol 32, 1978, pp 239–254
17. Herren RY, Edwards JE: Diplomyelia (duplication of the spinal cord). Arch Path 30:1203–1214, 1940
18. Lichtenstein BW: "Spinal dysraphism"; spina bifida and myelodysplasia. Arch Neurol Psychiat 44:792–810, 1940
19. James CCM, Lassman LP: Diastematomyelia and the tight filum terminale. J Neurol Sci 10:193–196, 1970
20. Hendrick EB: Progress in Neurological Surgery. Amsterdam, Excerpta Medica, 1974, pp 60–66
21. James CCM, Lassman LP: Spinal dysraphism (Spina Bifida Occulta). London, Butterworths, 1972
22. Vani PM, Seetharam W, Dinakar I: Diastematomyelia (a case report). Ind Pediatr 16:541–544, 1979
23. Matson DD; Neurosurgery of Infancy and Childhood (ed 2). Springfield, Charles C Thomas, 1969, pp 84–89
24. Sedzimir CB, Roberts JR, Occleshaw JV: Massive diastematomyelia without cutaneous dysraphism. Arch Dis Child 48:400–402, 1973
25. Milhorat TH: Pediatric Neurosurgery. Philadelphia, FA Davis, 1978, pp 155–157
26. Agnoli AL, Schonmayr R, Popovic M, et al: The value of neuroradiological investigations in intraspinal malformations of the lumbosacral spine in childhood. Neuroradiology 16:91–92, 1978
27. Barson AJ: The vertebral level of termination of the spinal cord during normal and abnormal development. J Anat 106:489–497, 1970
28. Kennedy PR: New data on diastematomyelia. J Neurosurg 51:355–361, 1979
29. Ritchie GW, Flanagan MN: Diastematomyelia. Can Med Assoc J 100:428–433, 1978

30. Von Bazan UB: The association between congenital elevation of the scapula and diastematomyelia. J Bone Joint Surg 61:59–61, 1979
31. Winter RB, Haven JJ, Moe JH, et al: Diastematomyelia and congenital spine deformities. J Bone Joint Surg 56:27–39, 1974
32. Gilmor RL, Batnitzky S: Diastematomyelia—Rare and unusual features. Neuroradiology 16:87–88, 1978
33. Hilal SK, Marton D, Pollack E: Diastematomyelia in children. Radiology 112:609–621, 1974
34. Scatliff JH, Till K, Hoare RD: Incomplete, false and true diastematomyelia. Radiology 116:349–354, 1975
35. Till K: Paediatric Neurosurgery, London, Blackwell, 1975, pp 293–296
36. Claussen CD, Lohkamp FW, Von Basan UL: The diagnosis of congenital spinal disorders in computed tomography (CT). Neuropadiatrie 8:405–417, 1977
37. Reigel DH, Scarff TB, Woodford J: Surgery for tethered spinal cord in myelomeningocele patients. Dev Med Child Neurol 18(Suppl 37):165, 1977
38. Guthkelch AN: Diastematomyelia with median septum. Brain 97:729–744, 1974
39. James CCM, Lassman LP: Diastematomyelia with median septum in spina bifida occulta: Indications for surgery: Kinder Chir 22:460–464, 1977
40. Basauri L, Palma A, Suleta A, et al: Diastematomyelia report of 10 cases. Acta Neurochir 51:91–96, 1979
41. Shaw JF: Diastematomyelia. Dev Med Child Neurol 17:361, 1975
42. Till K: Recent Progress in Neurological Surgery. Amsterdam, Excerpta Medica, 1974, pp 60–66
43. James HE, McLaurin RL, Watkins WT: Remission of pes cavus in surgically treated spinal dysraphism. J Bone Joint Surg 61:1096–1098, 1979
44. Reigel DH: Kyphectomy and myelomeningocele repair. Mod Tech Surg: Neurosurg 13:1–9, 1979

6. Dermal Sinus

A. B. Eisenbrey

Deceptively innocent, whether buried in the hair of the scalp at the occiput or near the lumbosacral junction at the midline, the tiny dermal sinus may be of devastating importance. Rare lesions, when not associated with an obvious lipomatous mass or neurologic deficit present from birth, have been overlooked or disregarded as insignificant until local infection, meningitis, or paraplegia develops.

Certainly related to neural tube development and closure,[1] both cephalic and caudal, precise or unified ontogenetic explanations for its presence are lacking. These are in some cases persistent segmental residua of the posterior neuropore or of the neurenteric canal (yolk sac) origin. The extension intraspinally and the location at the upper lumbar levels of an attached dermoid are explained by the relative ascent of the spinal cord secondary to continued longitudinal and caudal growth of spinal segments.

The dermal sinus can be differentiated in most cases from pilonidal sinuses originating immediately above the anus. The term pilonidal sinus does not refer to time of origin or location, but to the nidus of hair with it. A prospective study of craniospinal axis congenital abnormalities[2] revealed a 3 percent incidence in a total of 1977 neonates, about half of which had a dimple and the others a presumed sinus. Only 5 patients were explored; one had a sinus extending to the dura and the others a fibrous band ending at the coccyx. The considerable number of pilonidal sinuses manifest in adolescence or later become so as the result of chronic irritation and inflammation.[3]

At the lumbosacral level only a dimple may be present, or a true sinus tract 1 to 3 mm in diameter communicating through subcutaneous tissue and containing hair and secretory epithelium (sweat and sebaceous glands) of histologically well-developed dermal structure can be found (Figures 6-1 and 6-2). The tract may lead between, or sometimes through, altered spinous processes to epidural and dural coverings. It may end here or continue clearly into the subarachnoid space attaching to filum terminale and conus medullaris. The tract, if a well-developed tube, may contain the debris characteristic of

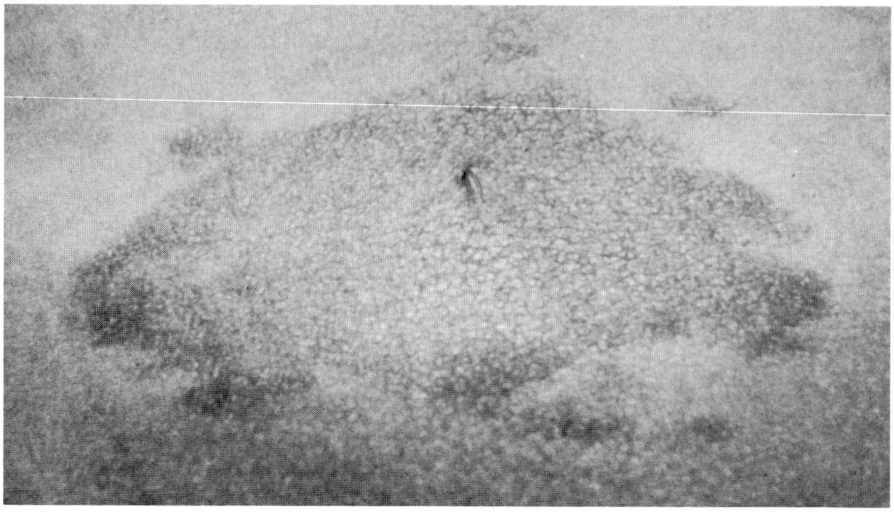

Figure 6-1. Dermal sinus at the lumbosacral junction with protruding hair and surrounding angiomatous changes.

dermoid or epidermoid cysts, loculated as pearly nodules of various sizes and acting as an expanding tumor with its secondary effects of compression and traction. Most important, whether or not evident communication with the surface is noted (discharge or inflammation), the sinus and its contents serve as a nidus for infection descending downward from the skin and subsequent bacterial meningitis and intra- or extramedullary abscess.[4] The uninfected content of these tracts, cheesy and high in cholesterol, is an infrequent though definite cause of sterile meningitis. Bacterial meningitis has been produced by *Escherichia coli* and *Staphylococcus aureus,* and occasionally other organisms. Discharge from these tracts requires immediate attention, antiobiotic therapy, and planning for surgery.

Identification of patients with these lesions, whether tiny or large, depends less on neurologic surgeons than on obstetricians, pediatricians, and parents. Despite the relative sophistication of physicians and the public, a surprising number of these lesions are discovered only after infection or neurologic deficit is present.

The discussion thus far has been restricted to the tiny sinus tract surrounded by normal or slightly angiomatous skin. More obvious lipomatous masses spreading beneath otherwise normal skin may be present. More than one dimple or tract may be seen. Patches of hair, palpably abnormal spinal processes, and alteration in the lumbar curvature are associated. The degree of neurologic involvement and deficit will give some clue to the complexity of the underlying lesion. Discussed elsewhere is this text in detail, both lipomatous meningocoel and diastematomyelia may have significant dermal sinus tracts. Those lesions at midlumbar, thoracic, and cervical levels do not fit readily into the class of embryologic dysgenetic accidents related to the posterior neuropore. The dermal sinus is almost incidental to the more obvious lesions unless infected, but should not be disregarded. The sinuses located in cervical and thoracic areas present the hazards of spinal cord compression or compromise during surgery. When infected, however, the rapid and castastrophic development of transverse myelitis is a rule.

Neurologic evaluation must include careful inspection of the extremities and a view of the palmar and plantar surfaces where developmental asymmetry is readily visualized. Narrow or shortened feet, high arch, and of course a small

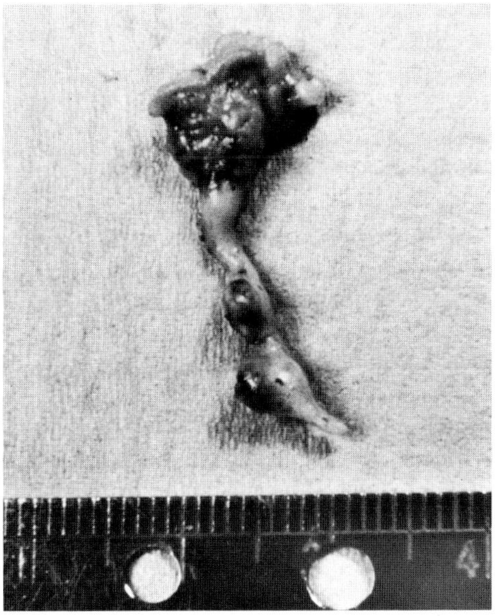

Figure 6-2. Surgical specimen: a small dermal sinus and tract that terminated on the dura.

extremity, should warn of spinal cord or cauda equina involvement. Awkward children, as they begin to walk and play, may be seen first by orthopedic surgeons; in those patients with disturbance of bowel or bladder control urologic studies may have been done.

Experience justifies an emphatic recommendation that all dermal sinuses be excised to their full extent. A qualified elective delay is not contraindicated when no infection has been present. The surgical technique is straightforward. Injection of the tract or probing should not be done. At surgery some magnification is helpful. Preparation for full laminectomy of several segments is advisable. Elliptical incision about the surface lesion and careful dissection downward with exposure by removal of spinal process and lamina are undertaken. Preoperative x-rays, particularly if normal, will not identify the pathway of the tract. Adequate access to the dural attachment is needed and the dura is opened to assure definition of the limits of penetration. All too frequently the band or tract will extend through the dura cephalad, requiring laminectomy as high as the conus medullaris. Removal of an intramedullary mass may result in significant neurologic deficit despite the use of magnification. The presence or history of infection will make the procedure difficult and increase risk because of adhesions or abscess. There will be circumstances that necessitate following a portion of the capsule wall to remain after its contents and lining have been removed. This is particularly true in the presence of infection. Closure of the dura and deeper layers of muscle and fascia despite the presence of infection has been the author's preference, thus avoiding postoperative fistulae established with the use of open drainage.

We do not believe that each of these patients must have preoperative myelography, but experience with one case in which a presumably thorough intradural exploration at the site of dural penetration had revealed no continuation of the tract subsequently was found to have a dermoid attached to the conus. The expanding availability of computerized axial tomography for whole-body scan recommends its use as an adjunct in preoperative evaluation of patients with suspected lesions of this type, as well as the use of amipaque contrast myelography in some cases.

The appropriate selection of antiobiotics is most important and their administration is indicated where infection is or has been present.

INTRACRANIAL DERMAL SINUS

The infrequent dermal sinus of the scalp that extends intracranially must receive the same respect as those of the spine. Located near the midline from nasion to occiput, but more often the latter, they present in most reported instances as a tumor of the posterior fossa. Over 80 percent of these present before the age of 4.[5] The opening of the tract at the skin may overlay a small subcutaneous mass narrowing to a stalk, caudally penetrating the skull through a defect not always seen on x-ray. Intracranially the mass can be large, interhemispheric or intraventricular. The hazards of meningitis (sterile or bacterial) or abscess exist in these patients and are serious enough to justify shaving the head for better inspection. Patients who have recurrent meningitis especially deserve such care. Computerized tomography is of great value in such lesions and it must be remembered that the fatty cholesterol content of dermoids is low density in most cases. The venous phases of cerebral arteriography have been valuable in assessing these lesions. Obstructive hydrocephalus has been a presenting feature with associated increasing head size, headache, nausea, vomiting, and ataxia.

Once again, these are surgical lesions that require careful dissection through a generous suboccipital craniectomy and complete removal if there is evidence of a tract with penetration of the bone. Simple excision of the lesion where no intracranial extension exists will suffice.

REFERENCES

1. Gerlach J: Congenital malformation of the spinal cord, in Handbook of Clinical Neurology, vol. 32. Amsterdam North Holland Publishing Company, 1978, pp 449–463
2. Powell KR, Cherry JD, Horigan TJ, et al: A prospective search for congenital dermal abnormalities of craniospinal axis. J Pediat 87:744–750, 1975
3. Haworth JG, Zachary RB: Congenital Dermal Sinuses in Children. Lancet, 2:10–14, 1955
4. DiTullio MV Jr: Intramedullary spinal abscess, a case report with a review of 33 previously described cases. Surg Neurol 7:351–354, 1977.
5. Giuffrè R, Curatolo P: Cranial Dermal Sinuses in Childhood and Adolescence. Neurochirugia 21:72–75, 1978.

BIBLIOGRAPHY

Angevine JB: Clinically relevant embryology of the vertebral column and spinal cord. Clin Neurosurg 20:95–113, 1973

Blechschmidt E: Stages of Human Development Before Birth. Philadelphia, WB Saunders, 1961

James CCM, Lassman LP: Spinal Dysrhaphism. London, Butterworths, 1972

Matson D: Neurosurgery of Infancy and Childhood (ed 2). Springfield, Charles C Thomas, 1969

7. Congenital Malformations of the Brain

David G. McLone

Congenital cerebral malformations are an important part of a text on pediatric neurosurgery not because they are surgical lesions, but because they are for the most part, nonsurgical lesions. Early diagnosis and differentiation from diseases that have a more optimistic outlook are essential. The heartbreak of the family unprepared for the child's lack of development and needless surgical procedures can be prevented by an awareness on the part of the physician of the signs of these anomalies and the utilization of appropriate diagnostic procedures to rule out treatable conditions.

DEVELOPMENT

Many of the congenital anomalies described here represent insults to the fetal nervous system leading to arrested development or to the loss of fetal tissues. A brief outline of the developmental sequence gives some insight into the timing of the arrested development. In 1908 Mall[1] pointed out that whatever the noxious stimulus to the developing ovum might be, the stage of development reached at the time of the experiment was the decisive factor in determining the final malformation.

Prechordal mesoderm is responsible for induction of rostral neural ectoderm and determines not only the differentiation of the ectoderm as nervous tissue, but also its morphology. This same prechordal mesoderm is also responsible for the median facial bones.[2] Defective prechordal mesoderm, because of mechanical, genetic, or environmental teratogens, is reflected in abnormal development of the midface as well as the abnormal form of the cerebral hemispheres.

Following closure of the rostral neural tube, the prosencephalon gives rise to the telencephalon and the diencephalon. From the telencephalon the cerebral hemispheres develop as lateral diverticula that bud from either side and expand rapidly. The corpus callosum begins as a small bundle near the anterior commissure, then enlarges, expanding superiorly and then posteriorly as the cerebral hemispheres balloon in size.

By the 14th gestational week the sylvian fissure begins to form. The smoothed surface insula starts as a conical structure and is outlined by the circular sulcus at 18 weeks. The frontal, temporal, and parietal opercula fold over the insula at 28 to 29 weeks. By 30 weeks numerous gyri have formed and are well defined.

As the human brain develops in utero, it gains neurons at the rate of hundreds of thousands a minute. Neurogenesis is at its greatest during the 12th through the 20th weeks, during which time almost all of the cerebral cortical neurons are formed. Cerebral cortical neurons arise in the periventricular germinal matrix and migrate to their place in the cortex.

Arrested Development of the Cerebral Hemispheres

Microcephaly

Microcephaly is a condition common to most of the anomalies in this section. A small brain is enclosed within a small skull. Because the small skull is the result of the lack of growth of the brain,[3] the term "microencephaly" is actually more accurate. The normal brain-to-body-weight ratio is 1 to 30, whereas in microcephaly it may be 1 to 100. Adult microcephalic brains weigh less than 900 grams and may be as small as 300 grams. Individuals are classified as microcephalic if their head circumference is less than three standard deviations below the mean for age and sex.[4]

Based on Darwin's theory of evolution, microcephaly was thought to be an "atavism," or relapse to earlier stages of phylogenic development. Studies have shown the microcephalic brain to be more human than apelike, however, and more probably represents arrest of development at various fetal stages.

Microcephaly is not an entity with a single etiology, but is reduced brain growth from a variety of causes,[5] some of which are unknown. From a neurosurgical point of view, the important factor to establish is that the small cranial cavity is not the result of premature closure of the cranial sutures. Some of the known causes are genetic, such as autosomal recessive, chromosomal deletions, and trisomies. Inflammatory causes include rubella, toxoplasmosis, and cytomegalic inclusion disease.[6] Material intoxication with poisons and metabolic disorders, such as phenylketonuria,[7] have also been implicated in microcephaly. The mechanism is thought to be an insult to the developing cerebrum at a time just prior to or during neurogenesis. This insult interferes with the development and migration of the periventricular matrix cells, which leads to diminution of cerebral cortical volume and heterotopia.

In a typical microcephalic child, the frontal bone recedes over a much reduced anterior fossa. The small brain usually does not cover the cerebellum and the cortical gyral pattern is abnormal. Cortical architecture shows few large cells and a predominance of primitive cells. The ventricular system is often large. Porencephaly, lissencephaly, absence of the corpus callosum, and heterotopias are common.

The development of microcephalic children varies over a wide range. Some will die shortly after birth while others will grow to adulthood. Many are profoundly retarded, but some will reach borderline intelligence and be capable of simple tasks.

Lissencephaly

Lissencephaly is an uncommon congenital anomaly and one of several conditions characterized by maldevelopment of the cerebral convolutions.[8] Like many of the other microcephalic conditions, it probably represents an arrest in cortical development at an early fetal stage. Agyria denotes a completely smooth surface (true lissencephaly) while pachygyria (macrogyria) is the term used when a few broad gyri with shallow sulci are present.[9] This anomaly results from an interruption of neuronal migration from the ventricular germinal matrix. Pachgyria and agyria differ only in degree. This condition can be lobar in distribution but more commonly involves the entire hemisphere.

Clinically, the "lissencephalic sydrome" includes microcephaly, decerebrate posture, severe psychomotor retardation, seizures, unresponsiveness to visual and auditory stimuli, failure to thrive, and death before two years of life.

Computerized tomography (CT) scanning shows wide sylvian fissures, absence of the operculum, wide subarachnoid spaces, large ventricles, and a smooth cortical surface (Fig. 7-1). Angiography reveals absence of the sylvian point, straight ascension of the middle cerebral arteries, and poor definition of the sylvian triangle.

Micropolygyria

An excessive formation of secondary sulci complicating an otherwise normal convolutional pattern leading to the formation of multiple small convolutions (Fig. 7-2) is termed micropolygyria. It is quite different from ulegyria, which is the result of a destructive process. Micropolygyria[10] on section reveals an increase in cells in abnormal architectural patterns that produce small plications in the cortical surface.

Micropolygyria varies greatly from brain to brain. It often is patchy and unilateral, and may have been of no clinical significance. Conversely, it may be extensive and involve major portions of the hemisphere, causing a hemiparesis. Frequently it is associated with other brain anomalies such as the Arnold–Chiari Type II malformation.

Ulegyria (Sclerotic Microgyria)

Inflammatory processes or anoxic episodes occurring in the perinatal period can lead to ulegyria. Inflammatory arterites or anoxia cause the death of cortical neurons, laminar necrosis, and atrophy of previously formed cerebral cortical gyri. The gyri appear small (microgyria), and the sulci are open. Histologic

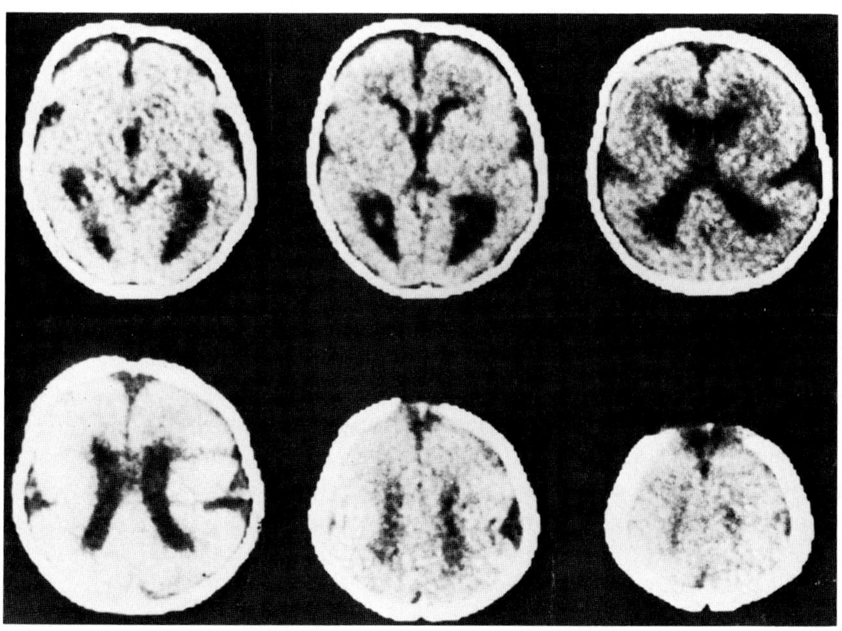

Figure 7-1. A CT scan of a child with lissencephaly. The cerebral cortical surface is smooth without identifiable gyri or sulci. The sylvian fissures are deep grooves, and the insular opercularization is not well formed. There is moderate ventricular enlargement.

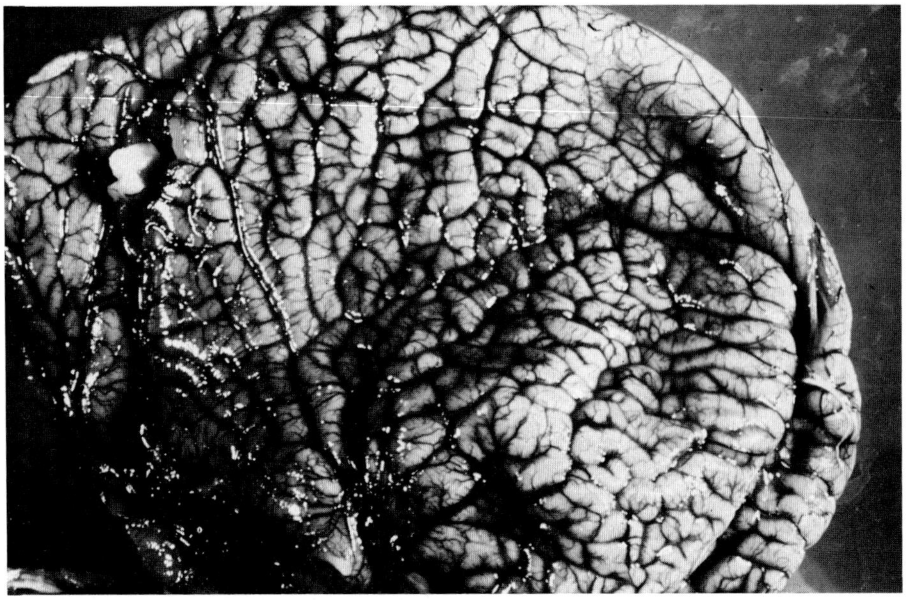

Figure 7-2. An extreme case of micropolygyria. Not the innumerable small plications superimposed on the gyral pattern. The process involves the entire cerebral cortical surface.

sections reveal the destructive process and often show calcification of the cortical vasculature. This process is often lobar in distribution and is probably the result of involvement of the metabolically most active, and therefore most susceptible, portion of the cortex. When this process is widespread, microcephaly is present.

Agenesis of the Corpus Callosum

Phylogenically and ontogenically the corpus callosum is a relatively new structure. Development of the corpus callosum[11] begins in the lamina terminalis and remains limited to the rostral brain until the fourth fetal month. From the fifth month it grows rapidly. Agenesis may be complete (Fig. 7-3) or partial, with the more caudal portions absent in partial cases. Such malformations as holoprosencephally and the Dandy–Walker malformation are often associated with agenesis of the corpus callosum.

The etiology is varied. Familial[12] cases occur and trisomy[13] is a frequent cause. X-ray[14] and other teratogens have produced this lesion in animal models.

No typical clinical syndrome can be identified. Many individuals appear normal, even with sophisticated neurologic testing. On the other hand, this malformation can accompany a more extensive brain anomaly associated with mental retardation, seizures, cranial nerve involvement, spasticity, and paralysis.

Angiography[15] shows, in the anteroposterior projection (Fig. 7-4), that the anterior cerebral artery at the genu loops laterally and curves back onto itself, but never reaches the midline. In the lateral projection (Fig. 7-5) the anterior cerebral artery meanders superiorly. The pneumographic picture in the anterior-posterior projection (Fig. 7-6) has the appearance of a "butterfly." This results in the unimpeded third ventricle ascending between the two lateral ventricles. Here CT scanning demonstrates the large third ventricle at cuts above the divergent lateral ventricles. The anterior horns of the lateral ventricles diverge and the dome of the third ventricle can be seen between them (Fig. 7-7).

Only symptomatic treatment is necessary and the prognosis depends on associated anomalies.

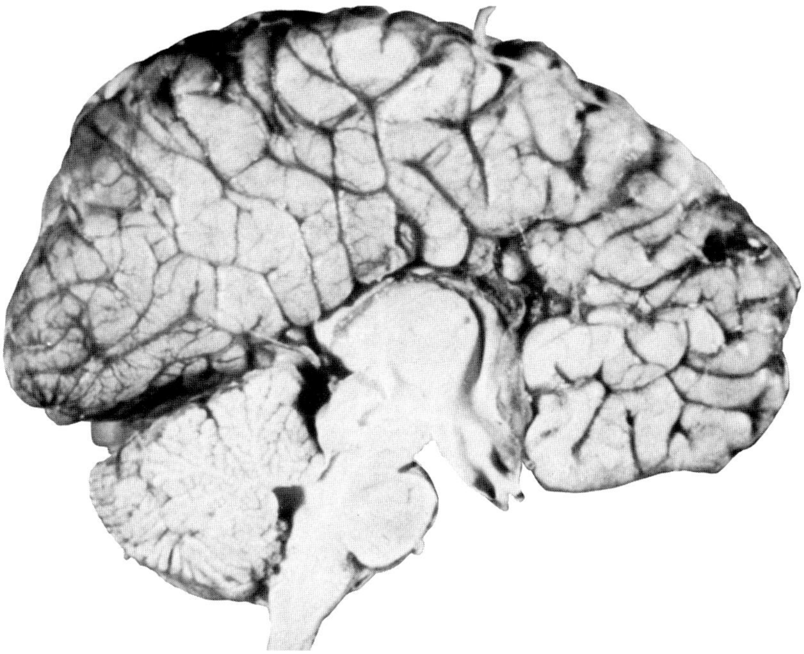

Figure 7-3. A gross sagittal section of the brain demonstrates agenesis of the corpus callosum. The columns of the fornix ride high over the dome of the third ventricle. No septum pellucidum is seen.

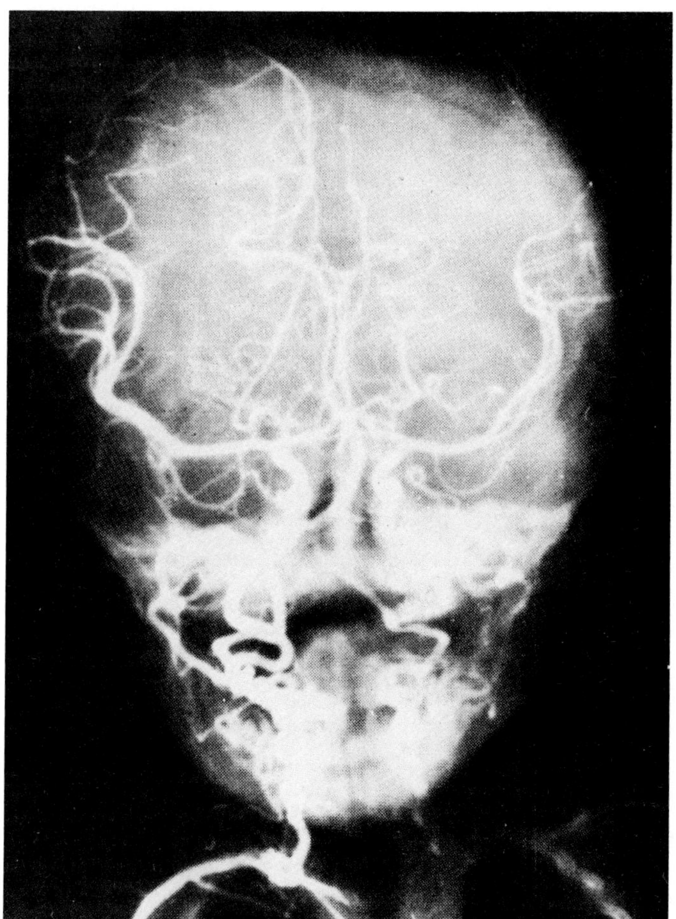

Figure 7-4. An anteroposterior projection of a cerebral angiogram demonstrates the wandering course of the anterior cerebral artery. The artery curves laterally at the genu, never to return to the midline.

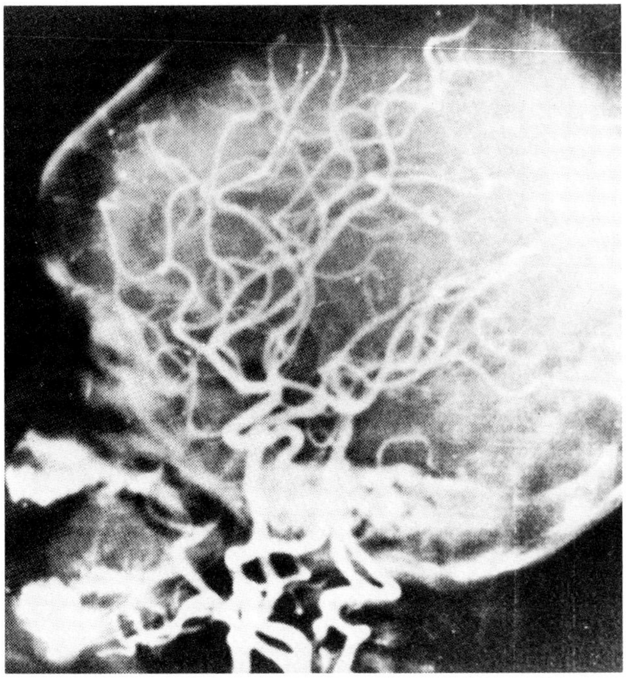

Figure 7-5. A cerebral angiogram in the lateral projection shows the meandering course of the anterior cerebral artery roughly parallel to the ascending frontoparietal arteries.

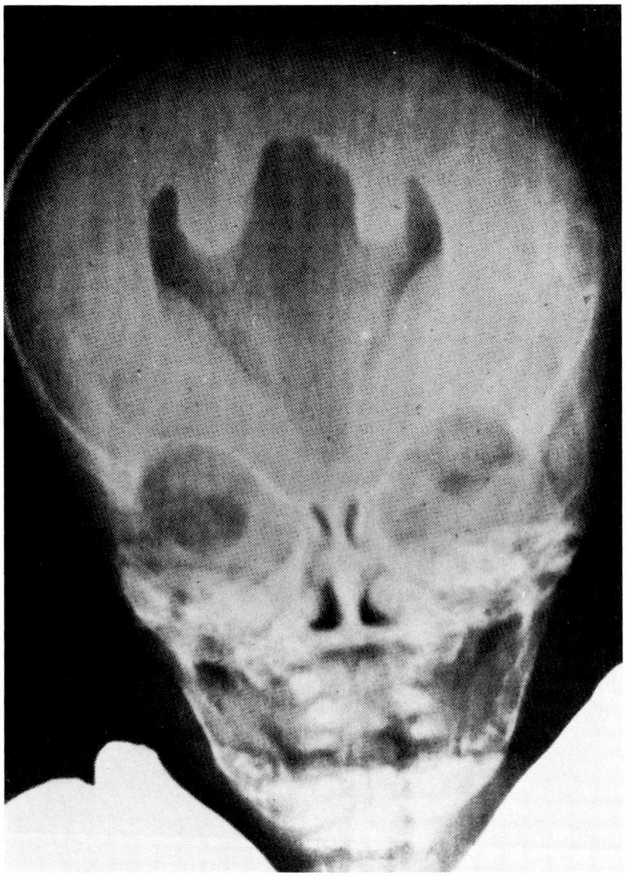

Figure 7-6. An anteroposterior pneumoencephalogram illustrates the upward expansion of the third ventricle between the two lateral ventricles, giving the appearance of a butterfly.

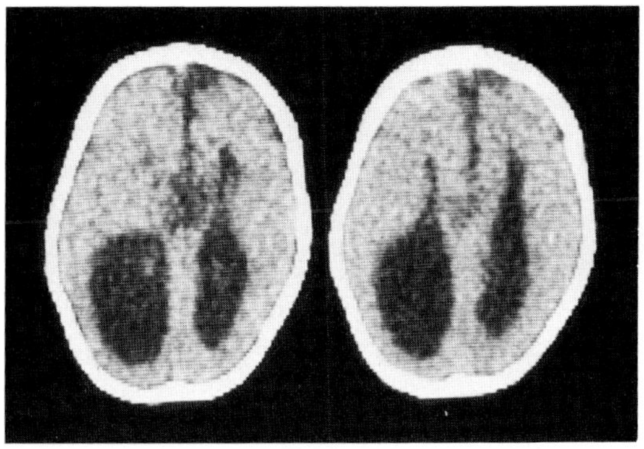

Figure 7-7. A CT scan demonstrates the divergence of the anterior portions of the lateral ventricles and a portion of the third ventricle between the lateral ventricles.

Cerebral Mantle Defects

This group of anomalies blends one into the other, sometimes imperceptibly, and they probably differ only in terms of the extent of the defect. While porencephaly is usually a unilateral defect, schizencephaly and hydranencephaly are usually symmetrical. Schizencephaly refers to clefting of the hemisphere; however, if the cleft represents almost the entire hemisphere, it is hydranencephaly.

Hydranencephaly

Cruveilhier[16] first used the terms anencephalie, hydrocephalique, hydrocephalic anencephaly, and hydroanencephalie to describe this congenital condition. Cruveilhier believed it to be a combination of anencephaly and hydrocephalus. Other terms used in recent literature include "ox bladder brain," "Rh indenblasen-porencephalie," and "hydromicrocephaly." Some cases of hydranencephaly are included in the literature under hydrocephalus, porencephaly, and schizencephaly.

Hydranencephaly is usually incompatible with survival beyond early infancy. A few cases have survived, but none have developed functional intellectual capacities.

The cerebral hemispheres are wholly or partially reduced to sacs of cerebrospinal fluid (Fig. 7-8) covered by thin layers of pia-arachnoid with remnants of cerebral tissue and vessels. This membrane often contains hemorrhagic area, hemosiderin, and phagocytic cells. Progressive hydrocephalus may be present or the child may have a frankly microcephalic head. The fluid in the cyst is usually crystal clear but ventricular taps and birth trauma can produce hemorrhagic fluid.

The pathogenesis of hydranencephaly remains controversial although most agree that the anlage of the neopallium reaches a level of development only to be destroyed and reabsorbed prior to birth. Yakovlev,[17] and Yakovlev and Wadsworth,[18,19] however, describe a series of congenital brain anomalies that they feel represent various stages of arrested development of the cerebral hemispheres or alar plate of the rostral neural tube. Schizencephaly or bilateral clefting of the cerebral hemispheres could range from small opercullar clefts through total absence of the hemispheres. Most of the cortical clefts are in the distribution of the middle cerebral artery (Figs. 7-9 and 7-10).

The predominant theory favors ischemia as the mechanism.[20] At some point following development of the cerebral hemispheres, vascular occlusion, principally in the distribution of the carotid arteries, leads to infarction, necrosis, and absorption of the cerebral mantle and usually portions of the deep gray matter fed by the lenticulostriate arteries. The vascular occlusion is thought to be either mechanical, umbilical cord, or amniotic bands, or inflammatory secondary to syphilis, toxoplasmosis, or other meningo-encephalities.

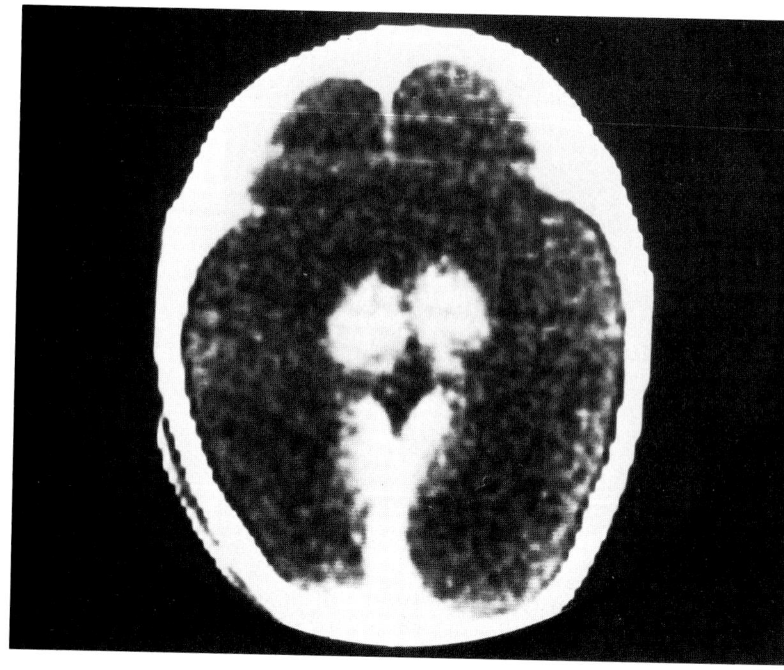

Figure 7-11. A CT scan demonstrates the normal cranial form containing cerebrospinal fluid, the egglike thalami, and the remnants of the medial occipital cortex.

Early diagnosis is important for prognostic reasons in order to spare the family prolonged mental anguish and needless expenses. A ventricular shunt is often indicated to control the expanding head for nursing purposes.

Porencephaly

Asymmetrical cerebral defects or porencephaly may affect any of the cerebral lobes. True porencephaly should communicate with the ventricular system as a passageway or pore.[23] Porencephaly has been used, however, to describe cerebral cavitation or cysts within cerebral substance whether they communicate with the ventricular system or the subarachnoid pathways, or have no communication. It is probably appropriate to confine this term to cysts within

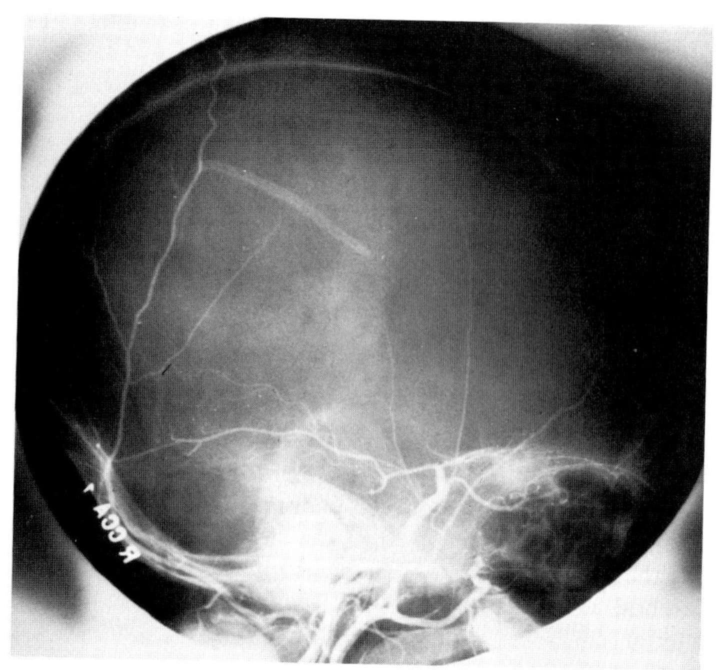

Figure 7-12. A cerebral angiogram demonstrates that the internal carotid artery terminates in the ophthalmic artery, posterior communicating artery, one lenticulostriate artery, and a whisp of an anterior cerebral artery. Note that the posterior cerebral artery is present but very attenuated.

cerebral substance and to exclude cysts within the pia-arachnoid. It is difficult to classify some of the cysts at the cerebral surface because, although they are partially within cerebral substance, the majority of the cyst is within the pia-arachnoid. This is especially true of some of the middle fossa cysts, which may represent absence of temporal lobe, a cerebral defect, or an arachnoid cyst.

Choux[24] has classified the supratentorial cysts by their location and communication as follows: (1) internal cyst (noncommunicating—intracerebral cyst, and communicating—cerebroventricular cyst); (2) external cyst (extracerebral and cerebral—noncommunicating and communicating), and (3) ventriculoperipheral cyst (porencephalic cyst of Heschl).

From a therapeutic standpoint, the porencephalies are quite different from the previously mentioned cerebral defects. Although this anomaly in our and other's experience has a high incidence of mental retardation, it can be compatible with normal intelligence.[25] It also is often a progressive lesion, thus making early diagnosis important to preserve the child's intellect.

The majority of porencephalic cysts appear to be congenital lesions, possibly unilateral intrauterine vascular accidents. Acquired forms have been described as a result of trauma, strokes, and iatrogenic porencephaly following tapping of a hypertensive ventricular system.

A classical sign of porencephaly is an asymmetrical head. This sign is not common in our experience, although there is usually asymmetry of the intracranial contents with displacement of the sagittal sinus in the congenital forms. Psychomotor retardation, seizures, and endocrine abnormalities are common. In Choux's series half of the children had a hemiparesis. About half of the children will have progressive head enlargement beyond the normal growth curve.

Computerized tomographic scanning has been very useful in localizing these cysts. Pneumo or other contrast encephalography is helpful in establishing paths of communication with the cyst. Cerebral angiography assists in localizing the cyst and may give some insight into the origin of the cavity.

We have tended to approach those lesions that verge on the subarachnoid space directly in an attempt to communicate them with the cerebrospinal fluid pathways. Deep lesions that communicate with the ventricular system are better managed by cerebrospinal fluid diversion through a shunt.

Abnormal Lobar Patterns

Holoprosencephaly

With the division of the prosencephalon into telencephalon and diencephalon, the single telencephalic vesicle at the cephalic tip of the neural tube gives rise to the two lateral hemispheres. Induction of the rostral neural ectoderm is by the prechordal mesoderm. This ties these two primitive tissues together developmentally. The prechordal mesoderm also gives rise to the median facial bones. Defects in one leads to abnormalities in the other. If this vesicle does not cleave or incompletely cleaves into two lateral hemispheres, the cerebral mantle develops as a single structure (Fig. 7-13). The term holoprosencephaly has been used to describe this malformation. This is probably not a good term because "holo" implies whole in the sense of complete, which certainly is not the case. Arhinencephaly is often used to describe this lesion, although the olfactory lobes are affected, they are usually present.

In addition to the lack of cleavage into cerebral hemispheres, other structures are either absent or dysplastic. Often the olfactory bulbs are small and the cingulate gyrus remains fused.

The degree to which the cerebrum remains undivided varies from total to

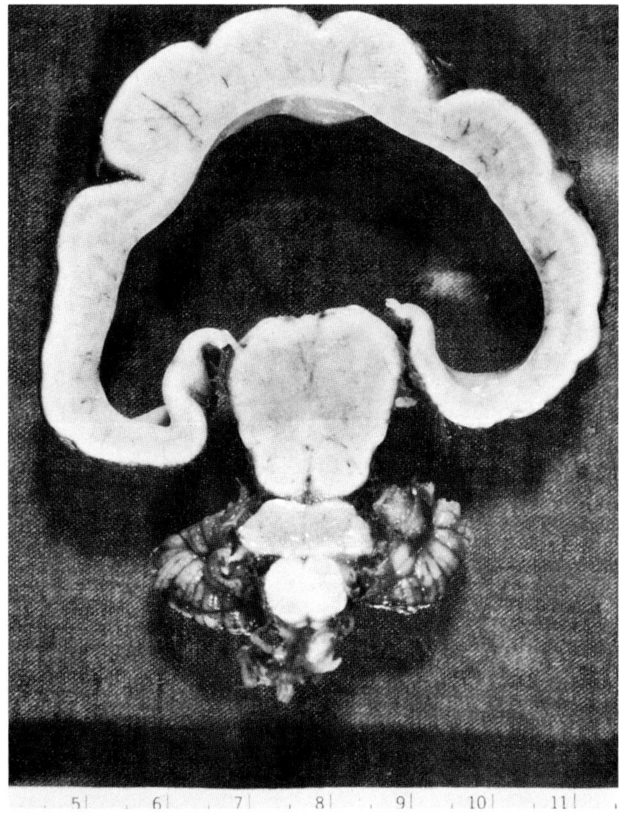

Figure 7-13. A gross specimen of a child with trisomy and holoprosencephaly. The interhemispheric fissure is absent, and the cerebral cortical surface is almost lissencephalic in appearance. The large monoventricle is typical of the alobar type.

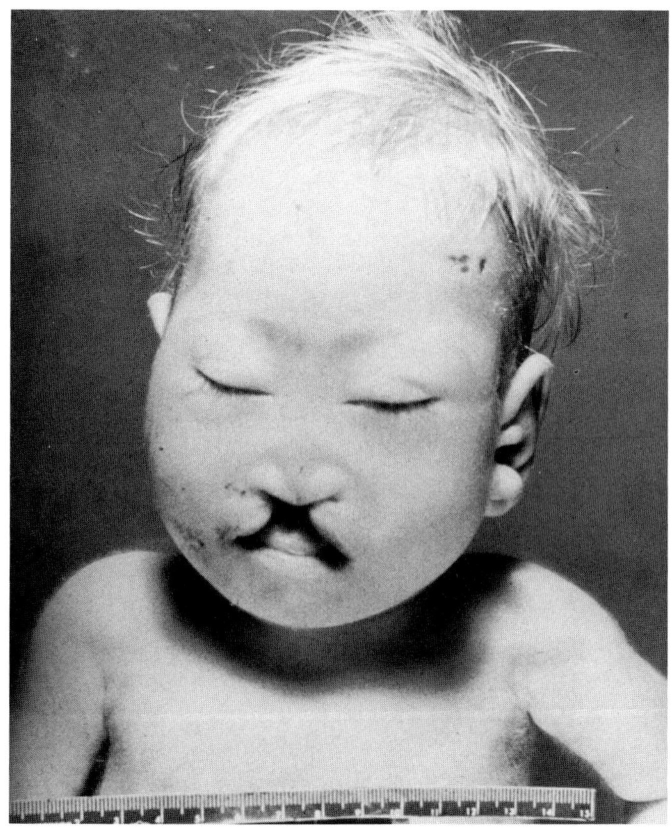

Figure 7-14. A child born with a midline cleft, flat nose, and hypotelorism. This midfacial cleft predicts the holoprosencephaly malformation.

partial. The malformation thus has been classified by degree of cleavage.[26–28] Alobar indicates a monoventricle with no interhemispheric fissure and semilobar and lobar describe lesser malformations.

This brain malformation is usually reflected in the development of the face and forms a class of teratologic anomalies characterized by median faciocerebral dysplasia.[2,29] A spectrum of malformations results. At one end is cyclopia with a proboscis-like nose and at the other is orbital hypotelorism with cleft lip (Fig. 7-14). In the middle are ethmocephaly and cebocephaly (Fig. 7-15) with hypotelorism and a single nasal aperture. The more severe the facial involvement, the more likely the holoprocephaly is to be severe. The child with cyclopia thus has an alobar cerebrum and the child with hypotelorism will have a semi- or lobar malformation. These facial features are pathognomonic of the underlying brain malformation.

Clinically, the infants are easily recognized by the characteristic facial features. Most are poikilothermic, spastic, and hyperreflexic, and show periodic apnea and seizures. Growth and psychomotor development are almost totally lacking.

Survival beyond infancy is unusual.[30] Those who survive are severely retarded, except for an occasional child with lobar holoprosencephaly who may develop sufficient intelligence to function in society.

Trisomy[30,31] often is the cause of this malformation, but normal 46-chromosome karyotypes are common. If an affected child is born to a couple, the risk of a second affected child is increased on subsequent pregnancies.

Alobar holoprosencephaly has a dorsal (Fig. 7-16) sac or fluid-filled space posterior to the pallium in the prepineal area. In the semi and lobar forms the sac persists as an interhemispheric cyst. It may protrude extracranially as an encephalocele that is continuous with the ventricular system.

Although the facial anomalies bespeak the cerebral malformation, further diagnostic studies may be indicated. Osaka, Handa, Matsumoto, et al.[28] have

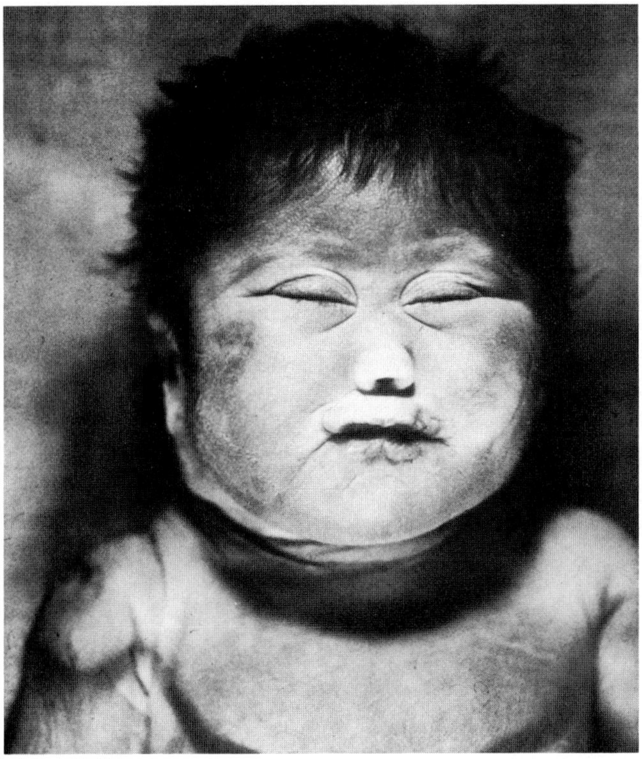

Figure 7-15. A child born with cebocephaly. Note the small nose with a single nostral and the marked hypotelorism. This child had alobar holoprosencephaly at postmortem examination.

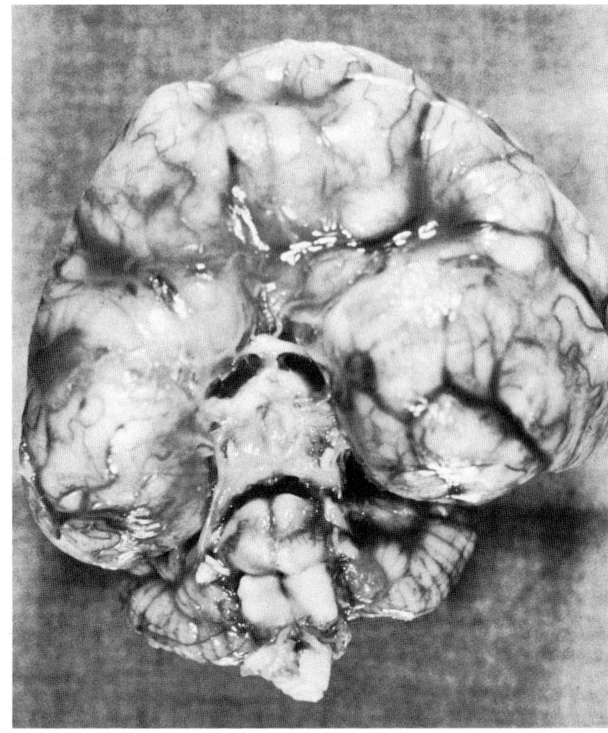

Figure 7-16. The brain of a child with cebocephaly viewed posteriorly. The interhemispheric fissue is absent. The cavity above the quadrigeminal plate is surrounded by the holoprosencephalic cerebrum forming the dorsal sac.

described the angiographic finding in these malformations. The azygous anterior cerebral artery is a most obvious feature. The single artery courses just below the inner table of the skull. The sylvian triangle of the middle cerebral artery is also absent, which suggests the maldevelopment of the temporal lobe. The venous phases show absence or deficiencies in the internal cerebral veins and deep venous system.

The single or monoventricle and the dorsal sac are revealed by CT scanning (Fig. 7-17). In the lesser forms the partial interhemispheric fissure can be seen.

Hydrocephalus develops in some of these children and may require ventricular shunting. This has been especially true in the lobar form with an encephalocele.

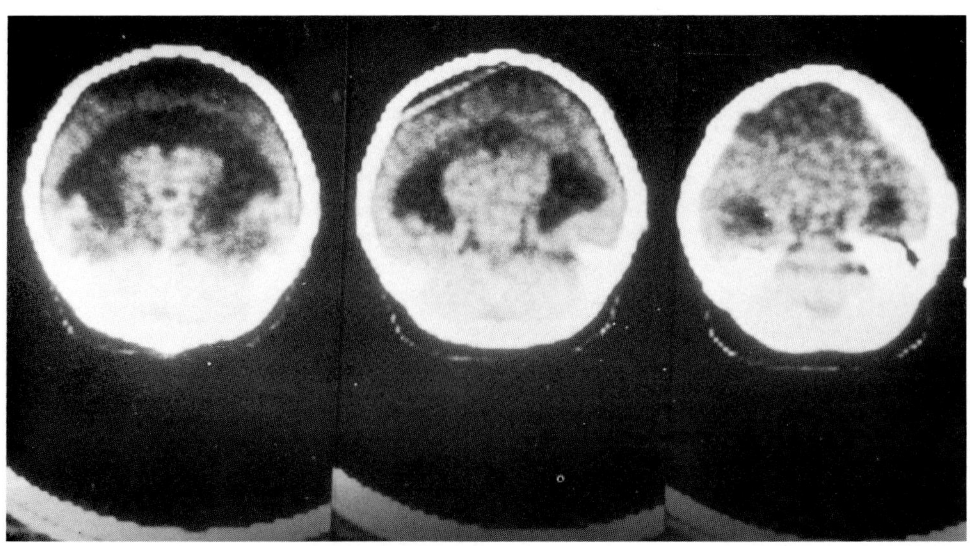

Figure 7-17. A CT scan of a child with holoprosencephaly. There is a large monoventricle with no interhemispheric fissure.

Megalencephaly (Macrencephaly)

Abnormally large brains weighing 1600–2850 grams have been found in normal, exceptional, and mentally defective individuals.[32]

Megalencephaly is not a clinical or etiologic entity since few of the cases resemble one another. The brain is always large but the gray and white matter are enlarged in some cases whereas in others only the gray matter is hypertrophied. Usually the spinal cord is also larger than normal. In some brains the nerve cells are large and the distance between them is increased. The glia may be the hypertrophic factor and occasionally giant cells are found.

Pathologists prefer to reserve this term for brains that large because of the presence of additional structures.[9] The first type would be the diffuse overgrowth of glia or diffuse gliomas.[33] The second type of abnormally large brain would be a generalized increase not associated with neuroglia, and the third type is a heterogeneous group that would include massive heterotopias and storage diseases.

Megalencephaly may be evident at birth or noted in the postnatal period. The head grows rapidly and the fontanelles remain open and sunken. The head circumference is usually 4–7 cm above average. Craniofacial disproportion is noted and hydrocephalus or chronic subdural effusions are suspected. Frontal bossing, parietal bone prominence, "setting sun," and cutaneous venous engorgement usually are not present, and CT scanning shows normal ventricles and no evidence of an extracerebral fluid collection.

Developmental delays, retardation, spasticity, and hypotonia may be present, and therefore the prognosis is not always good. Convulsions and sudden death occur in megalencephalic children but many have lived into the seventh decade.

REFERENCES

1. Mall FP: A study of the causes underlying the origin of human monsters. J Morphol 19:3, 1908
2. DeMyer W: Zeman W, Palmer CG: The face predicts the brain: Diagnostic significance of median facial anomalies for holoprosencephaly (arhinencephaly). Pediatrics 34:256, 1974
3. Moss ML: Functional anatomy of cranial synostosis. Child's Brain 1:22, 1975
4. Westropp CK, Barber CR: Growth of the skull in young children. Part 1. Standards of head circumference. J Neurol Neurosurg Psychiat 19:52, 1956
5. Hicks SP: Some effects of ionizing radiation and metabolic inhibition on the developing mammalian nervous system. J Pediat 40:489, 1952
6. Baron J, Youngblood L, Siewers CMF, Medeatis D Jr: Incidence of cytomegalovirus, herpessimplex, rubella, and toxoplasma antibodies in microcephalic, mentally retarded and normocephalic children. Pediatrics 44:932, 1969
7. Stevenson RE, Huntley CC: Congenital malformations in offspring of phenylketonuric mothers. Pediatrics 40:33, 1967
8. Walker AE: Lissencephaly. Arch Neurol Psychiat 48:13, 1942
9. Norman RM: Malformations of the nervous system, in Greenfield's Neuropathology. Baltimore, Williams & Wilkins, 1963, pp 324–440
10. Warner F: The histogenetic principle of microgyria and related cerebral malformations. J Nerv Ment Dis 118:1, 1953
11. Rakic P, Yakovlev PI: Development of the corpus callosum and cavum septi in man. J Comp Neurol 132:45, 1968
12. Menkes JH, Philippart M, Clark DB: Hereditary partial agenesis of corpus callosum. Arch Neurol 11:198, 1964
13. Warkany J, Passarge E, Smith LB: Congenital malformations in autosomal trisomy syndromes. Am J Dis Child 112:502, 1966

14. Hicks SP: Developmental malformations produced by radiation. Am J Roentgenol 69:272, 1953
15. Raimondi AJ: Pediatric Neuroradiology. Philadelphia, WB Saunders, 1972
16. Cruveilhier J: Anatomie pathologique du corps humain. p 1. Paris. Traite d'anatomie pathologique generale. Paris, vol 4, p 75, 1829
17. Yakovlev PI: Pathoarchitectonic studies of cerebral malformations. J Neuropath Exp Neurol 18:22, 1959
18. Yakovlev PI, Wadsworth RC: Schizencephalies: A study of the congenital clefts in the cerebral mantle: I. Clefts with fused lips. J Neuropath Exp Neurol 5:116, 130, 1946
19. Yakovlev PI, Wadsworth RC: Schizencephalies: A study of the congenital clefts in the cerebral mantle: II. Clefts with hydrocephalus and lips separated. J Neuropath Exp Neurol 5:169, 1946
20. Marburg O, Casamajor L: Phlebostasis and phlebothrombosis in newborn and in early childhood. Arch Neurol Psychiat 52:170, 1944
21. Hamby WB, Krauss RF, Beswick WF: Hydranencephaly: Clinical diagnosis. Pediatrics 6:371, 1950
22. Alexander E Jr, Davis CH Jr, Kitahata LM: Hydranencephaly: observations on transillumination of the head of infants. AMA Arch Neurol Psychiat 76:578, 1956
23. Heschl R: Gehirndefekt und hydrocephalus, Vierlelysharschr. pnakt. Heilkunde Prag 61:59, 1859
24. Choux M, Raybaud C, Pinsard N, et al: Intracranial supratentorial cysts in children excluding tumor and parasitic cysts. Child's Brain 4:15, 1978
25. Cohn R, Neumann MA: Porencephaly: Clinicopathologic study. J Neuropath Exp Neurol 5:257, 1946
26. Osaka K, Sato N, Yamasaki S, et al: Dysgenesis of the deep venous system as a diagnostic criterion for holoprosencephaly. Neuroradiology 13:231, 1977
27. Osaka K, Tanimura T, Yamasaki S, et al: Holoprosencephaly. Neurol Med Chir (Tokyo) 18:33, 1978
28. Osaka K, Handa H, Matsumoto S, et al: Development of the cerebrospinal fluid pathway in the normal and abnormal human embryos. Childs Brain 6(1):26, 1980
29. DeMyer W, Zeman W, Palmer DG: Familial alobar holoprosencephaly (arhinencephaly) with median cleft lip and palate. Report of patient with 46 chromosomes. Neurology 13:913, 1963
30. Miller JQ, Picard EH, Alkan MD, et al: Neurological manifestations of 13–15 trisomy (A chromosome abnormality in arhinencephaly). Trans Am Neurol Assoc 62:51, 1962
31. Buhler E, Bodis L, Rossier H, et al: Trisomie 13–15 mit cebocephalie. Ann Paediat (Basel) 199:198, 1962
32. Jakob A: Normale und Pathologische Anatomie und Histologie des Grosshirns. Leipzig, F. Deuticke, 1927
33. Weil A: Megalencephaly with diffuse glioblastomatosis of the brain stem and the cerebellum. Arch Neurol 30:795, 1933

8. Intracranial Arachnoid Cysts

Frank M. Anderson
Hervey D. Segall

Arachnoid cysts apparently can develop in any area of the intracranial spaces where arachnoid membrane is present. The fundamental nature and origin of these cysts remain obscure, but probably most evolve between layers of embryonic arachnoid when the primitive mesenchyme is developing.[1–4] They may progressively enlarge from small and variable channels, particularly if prenatal intracystic bleeding occurs,[5,6] or from the forces of venous or arterial pulsation within these tissues.[7]

The cysts contain liquid that closely resembles cerebrospinal fluid (CSF), but the histology of their membranous walls differs; Jakubiak, Dunsmore, and Beckett[2] reported four supratentorial cysts that all appeared grossly to be arachnoidal, but microscopic study showed that two of these contained complex ependymal, choroidal, or glial elements and could therefore secrete fluid. Others have reported similar findings.[2,8–10] Many anatomic and functional mechanisms may account for cyst behavior in various locations; occasionally they cause no symptoms during life or are quiescent for many years before producing serious problems.[4]

We will consider the diagnosis and management of various cysts with respect to their locations, using the common categories—supratentorial, suprasellar, quadrigeminal or collicular, and posterior fossa.

SUPRATENTORIAL CYSTS

Supratentorial cysts range from about 4 cm in diameter to huge cystic masses occupying one half of the calvarium. They tend to lie in the middle fossa and sylvian fissure, over the convexity of one hemisphere, or parasagitally, between hemispheres (Fig. 8-1). They cause severe distortion and compression of the brain, but the cortex is not penetrated and communication is usually not

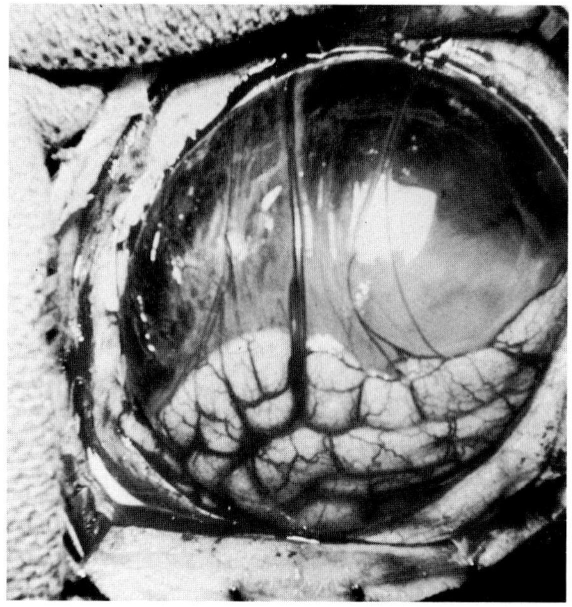

Figure 8-1. A very large supratentorial arachnoid cyst as exposed by temporoparietal craniotomy. There is severe displacement and identation of the temporal lobe. Superficial cerebral veins are clearly shown in cyst wall. (Reprinted with permission from Smith JL: Neuro-ophthalmology Focus 1980:388, 1979. Copyright © by Masson Publishing USA, Inc., New York.)

present between cyst and ventricular or subarachnoid spaces. The longitudinal sinus and falx may be markedly displaced.

Symptoms and findings produced by this type of cyst arise principally from elevated intracranial pressure secondary to mass effect and the displacement and obstruction of ventricles. Infants usually have periodic vomiting and show lethargy and irritability; limb weakness and convulsions are uncommon. Older children and adults describe headaches and on occasion develop abrupt pressure symptoms due to traumatic or spontaneous bleeding into the cyst or subdural space.[6] In some patients the head is enlarged at birth or grows more rapidly than average in early life, and patients with long-standing cysts tend to have rather large heads. Infants usually show fullness of fontanels, perhaps suture widening, and asymmetric head enlargement with smooth protrusion over one parietal or temporal region. Hemiparesis, visual loss, and retardation may be observed. Transillumination of the head in infants almost invariably shows a large lucent area over the cyst.

Radiologic Features

Plain x-rays of the skull often show asymmetry of the vault and protrusion of bone over the lesion. Pneumoencephalography is apt to be of limited value because in almost all cases it discloses only a non-air-filled mass. Angiography may be useful, indicating a large avascular cystic structure and wide displacement of one or both cerebral hemispheres. We have also shown that superficial cerebral veins lie on the outer convex cyst surface next to the dura, whereas arterial branches remain on the cortical surface, displaced and distorted by the cyst (Fig. 8-2A, B).[11] Angiography may also reveal or exclude an isodense subdural hematoma in a traumatized patient whose computerized tomography (CT) scan has shown bloody cyst fluid.[12]

Computerized tomography offers very valuable aid in identifying supratentorial cysts. These typically appear as large, smoothly demarcated, water-density masses between the dura and distorted brain (Fig. 8-2C); the displaced ventricles may show only mild enlargement. Cysts in the sylvian fissure often appear square due to compression of the adjacent temporal lobe and insula[13] (Fig. 8-2D).[13] They may be much more extensive than the scan suggests.

Differentiation from tumors is normally not difficult because neoplasms

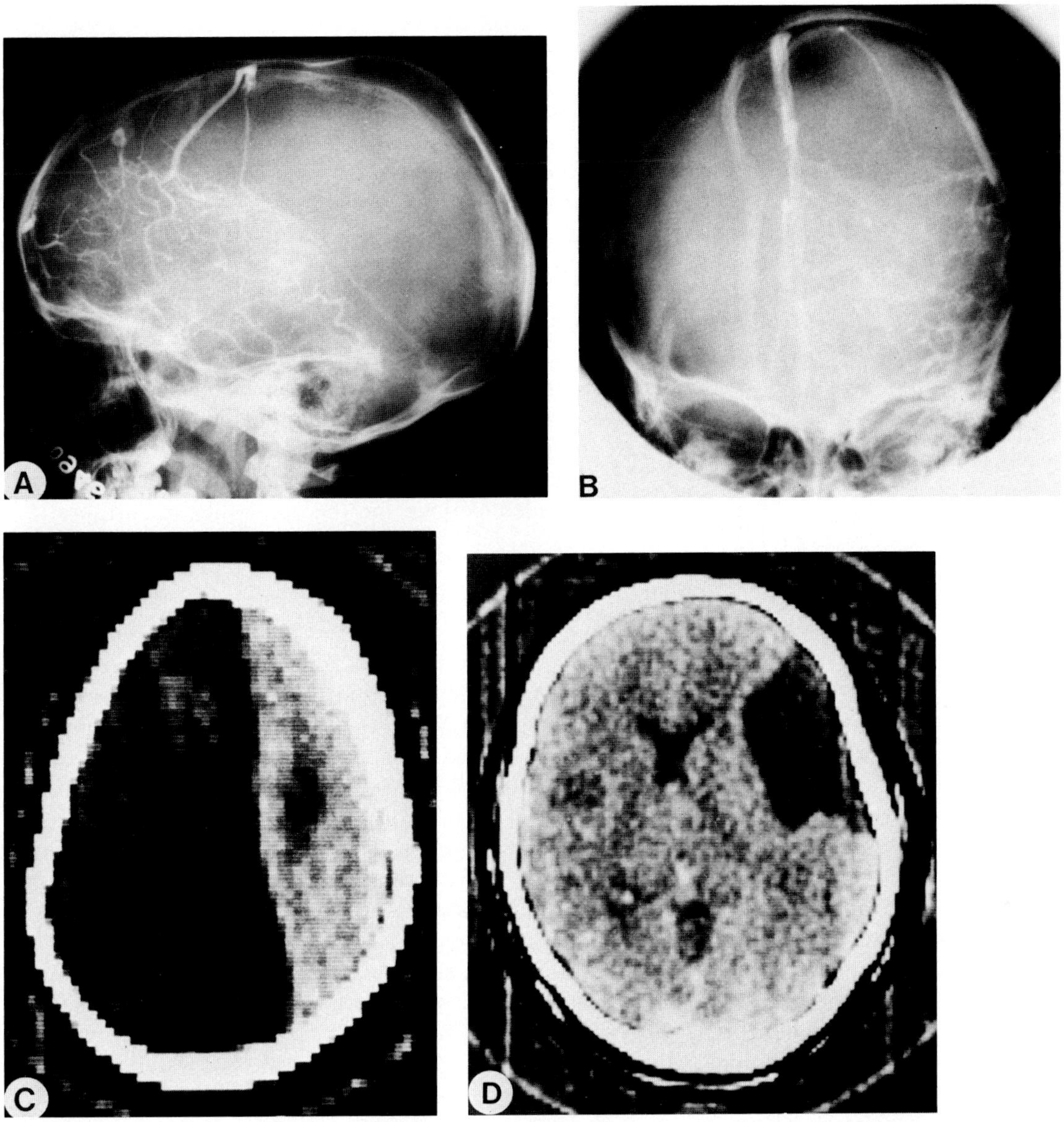

Figure 8-2. A, B. Lateral and anteroposterior angiograms in a 5-year-old mildly retarded girl with a large parasagittal cyst. The hemisphere is outlined by arterial vessels, whereas superficial veins remain within the outer cyst wall. This arrangement is diagnostic.[23] Note also asymmetry of skull. C. A CT scan in the same patient shows a hugh supratentorial cyst and marked distortion and displacement of cerebrum. D. Cyst in right sylvian fissure. Note flattened cortical markings on frontal and temporal opercula and insula. (Reprinted with permission from Anderson FM, Seigel HD, Caton WL: Use of CT-scanning in supratentorial arachnoid cysts. J Neurosurg 50:333–338, 1979.)

show enhancing tissues and their cysts are much smaller than the arachnoid variety; chronic subdural hematomas are less globular, contain denser fluid, and are encapsulated. Dysplastic lesions such as porencephaly are irregularly contoured and usually show communication with ventricles or subarachnoid space; also their walls are uneven, lacking a regular gyral pattern. Identification of these hypoplastic deformities is very important because they are basically untreatable, and quite unlike potentially curable cysts. In infants cysts must be differentiated from hydrocephalus, chronic subdural hematomas, and intracranial tumors; in older children other space-taking lesions such as cerebral abscesses and arteriovenous anomalies are also to be considered.

Supratentorial cysts have been treated with craniotomy and removal of accessible portions of the membranes,[1,2,14,15] by a small diagnostic bone flap and cystoperitoneal shunt,[16] or by primary cyst shunt alone.[17,18] Close observation without surgery has also been proposed in patients with no threatening pressure signs.[12,19,20] Our experience in 24 cases leads us to feel that craniotomy and subtotal removal of cyst wall is to be preferred, with cystoperitoneal shunt later if required; ventriculostomy from cyst to lateral ventricle is not worthwhile.[21] We hesitate to advise shunting from the cyst as a primary procedure in young children, but in adults, particularly the elderly, this may be wiser initially, with craniotomy later if needed.

Following operation, CT scans should be obtained in two or three months and periodically thereafter to observe for persistence of a significant cyst space; if this continues longer than about six months, a shunt is recommended. Delayed hydrocephalus may also develop from meningeal or aqueduct adhesions, requiring ventriculoperitoneal or cardiac shunt. Some patients treated for large cysts show a tendency to bleed into the residual space, especially with trauma, and should be observed for extended periods for the possibility of intracystic or subdural hemorrhage.[15,19–21]

SUPRASELLAR CYSTS

The sites of origin of suprasellar cysts and their relations to surrounding structures are often difficult to establish. For instance, some of these lesions may arise by upward ballooning of arachnoid from the sella,[22] whereas others have no direct contact with sellar structures. They may or may not communicate with the third ventricle or subarachnoid spaces. Sansregret, Ledoux, Duplantis, et al.[23] believed that cysts that do communicate are actually outpouchings from the third ventricle caused by sarcoid, tuberculosis, or other inflammations; they presented autopsy material demonstrating sarcoid in one case. Other concluded that such acquired lesions differed from arachnoid cysts, and were not comparable.[5]

Symptoms of these cysts include headache, diminished vision, mental dullness, pituitary disorders (including diabetes insipidus),[5] sexual precocity,[24,25] and nodding movements of the head. These are produced by upward compression and distortion of the third ventricle, aqueduct, and pituitary stalk, as well as encroachment on the chasm, and may of course arise from other types of space-taking lesions such as craniopharyngiomas and hypothalamic gliomas. Findings comprise evidence of raised intracranial pressure, visual field and acuity defects, endocrine difficulties, and, rarely, the peculiar intermittent movements of the head described by Benton, Nellhaus, Huttenlocher, et al.[26] as "the bobble-head doll syndrome."

Roentgenograms of the skull usually reveal some change in the sella, such as enlargement or erosion of clinoids with perhaps loss of the upper portion of the dorsum. Angiograms show the changes caused by an avascular suprasellar mass, perhaps posterior displacement of the basilar artery, and signs of hydrocephalus. If pneumoencephalography shows a non-air-filled lesion, but the third ventricle is elevated and indented, cyst must be considered.[39] It has been shown that the hanging head position is important in these studies because some "noncommunicating" cysts fill only in this posture.[25,27] Kasdon, Douglas, and Broughham[28] reported that CT scans clearly showed a smooth, oval, water-density suprasellar structure, and differentiated cyst from an enlarged third ventricle when pneumoencephalogram was also done. Lee[29] confirmed this and also demonstrated that ventriculoperitoneal shunt diminished ventricular size but did not alter the size or contour of the cyst in his case (Fig. 8-3A, B, C). Leo, Pinto, Hulvot, et al.[30]

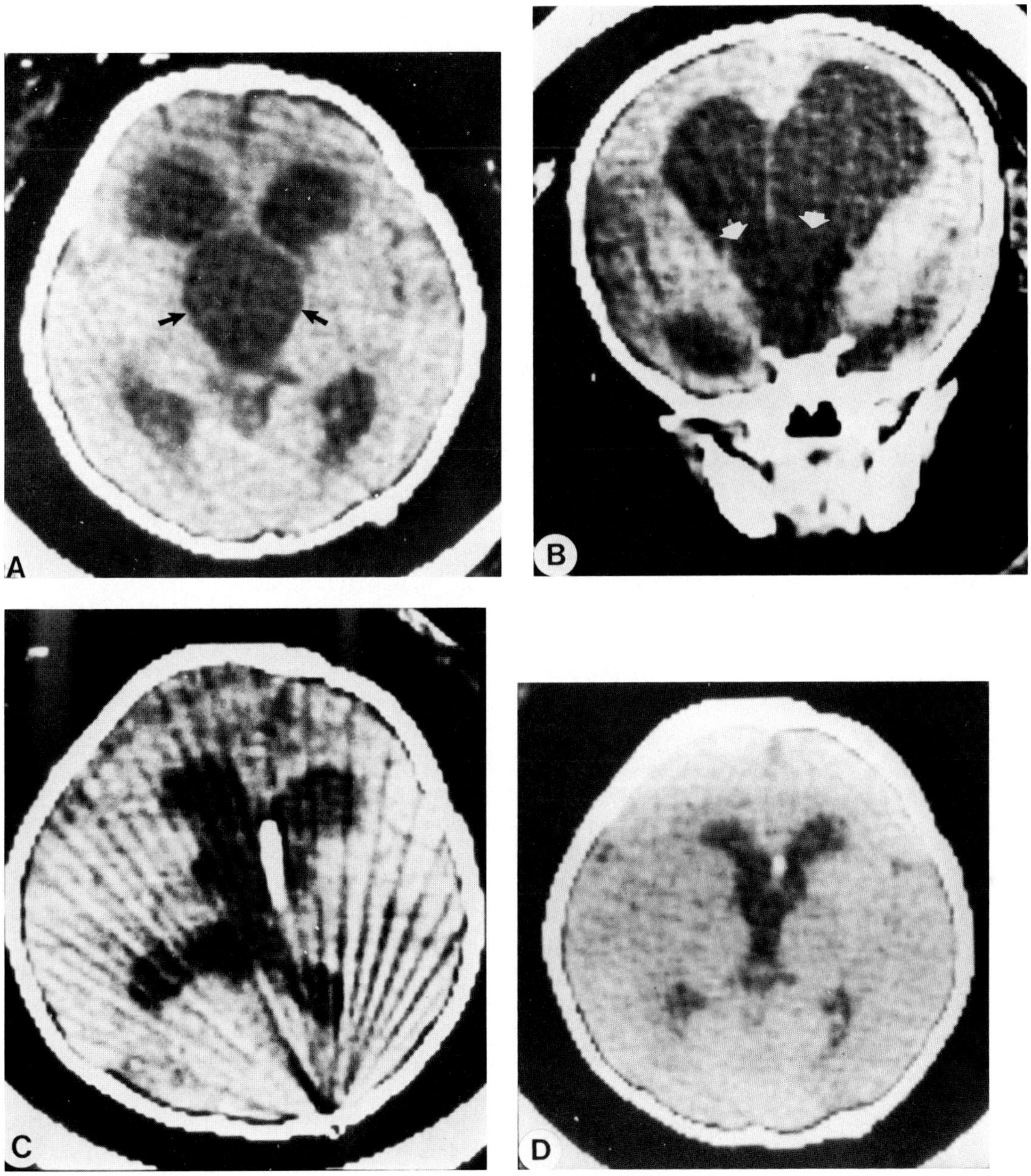

Figure 8-3. Female, 14 months, with enlargement of head and slowed development. A, B. CT scans show suprasellar cyst (arrows), which apparently causes obstruction of outflow from lateral ventricles. Earlier air injection by needle had determined that the midline space was possibly a cyst rather than third ventricle. C. After ventriculoperitoneal shunt, cyst was unchanged. Following transcallosal exposure, partial resection of cyst and relocation of shunt tube to cyst bed. Cyst and ventricles are now much smaller (case of Dr. F. L. Johnson).

injected Conray into a lateral ventricle, then repeated the CT scan; the opaque solution did not enter the cyst, which blocked the foramina of Monro.

Treatment

An ideal method of treatment for cysts in the suprasellar region has not been established. Aspiration is ineffective, and craniotomy with partial resection of the cyst wall has often been followed by refilling of the lesion.[5,25,28] A ventriculoperitoneal or cystoperitoneal shunt seems not to be dependable. The following plan of management, drawn from many sources, has been reasonably successful. Ventriculoperitoneal shunt is established, followed by frontotemporal craniotomy and resection of as much cyst wall as possible. A segment of shunt tubing is placed in the cyst bed and the other end inserted into one lateral ventricle. This tube may be attached instead to the existing peritoneal shunt.[5,28]

In the future it may prove more satisfactory to visualize and resect such cysts by a transcallosal approach.[31]

QUADRIGEMINAL CYSTS

Quadrigeminal cysts, also described as "collicular" or "incisural," are situated between the collicular plate and the incisural notch of the tentorium, and originate within or closely applied to the quadrigeminal cistern. Probably these cystic dilations of meninges develop because adjacent outflow channels, such as the ambient cistern, become occluded.[26,27] As with cysts in other intracranial areas, these are usually arachnoidal but may be more complex, the membranes being lined with well-organized ependymal or glial elements.[14,32] Even small cysts in this region may create serious neurologic difficulties because space is restricted and the adjacent structures have complex functions.[5,26] When a quadrigeminal cyst enlarges, it pushes backward above as well as beneath the tentorium, indenting the anterior cerebellar lobe. Simultaneous forward growth compresses the colliculi, fourth ventricle, and posterior part of the third ventricle, and may displace nearby cranial nerves (Fig. 8-4A).

Symptoms and findings include hydrocephalus, with undue head growth and suture widening in infants, and headache, nausea, lethargy, and papilledema in older patients. Impairment of pupillary reactions and eye movements, facial pain, limb weakness, and ataxia have been noted, and hearing defects occur occasionally.[32]

Although it is relatively easy to judge the general location of lesions that might cause the above symptoms, exact localization and identification of these cysts may be difficult. Diagnostic problems resemble those encountered with the suprasellar cysts. Pineal and third ventricle tumors, gliomas of the brain stem, tentorial meningiomas, and arteriovenous malformations all produce a clinical picture very similar to that caused by quadrigeminal cysts, and these must be differentiated before operation, if possible. Careful air contrast studies can provide important diagnostic help.[27,29] Kruyff[27] performed detailed ventriculography and pneumonencephalography in six infants, accurately localized and tentatively identified quadrigeminal cysts in all, and suggested that these are not uncommon. In the case of Huckman, Davis, and Coxe[39] a pneumoencephalogram showed a nonfilling defect in the pineal area, but diagnosis of the cyst was not considered seriously until an angiogram showed that the nonvascular mass caused posterior bowing of the precentral cerebellar vein, indicating an extracerebellar lesion. Computerized tomography is a very important investigative aid and may define these cysts clearly (Fig. 8-4B). It is logical to assume that this method will prove to be the most important, but not the only, diagnostic test required for such lesions.

It may be difficult in some situations to determine whether surgical treatment of a quadrigeminal cyst can be better carried out from above or below the tentorium. Alexander[33] reported a case successfully treated subtentorially with incision of the cerebellum, partial cyst resection, and creation of a fistula through posterior wall of the third ventricle. Huckman et al.[39] explored their patient via a low occipital flap, and provided a communicating pathway from the cyst through the anterior medullary velum into the fourth ventricle (Fig. 8-4A);

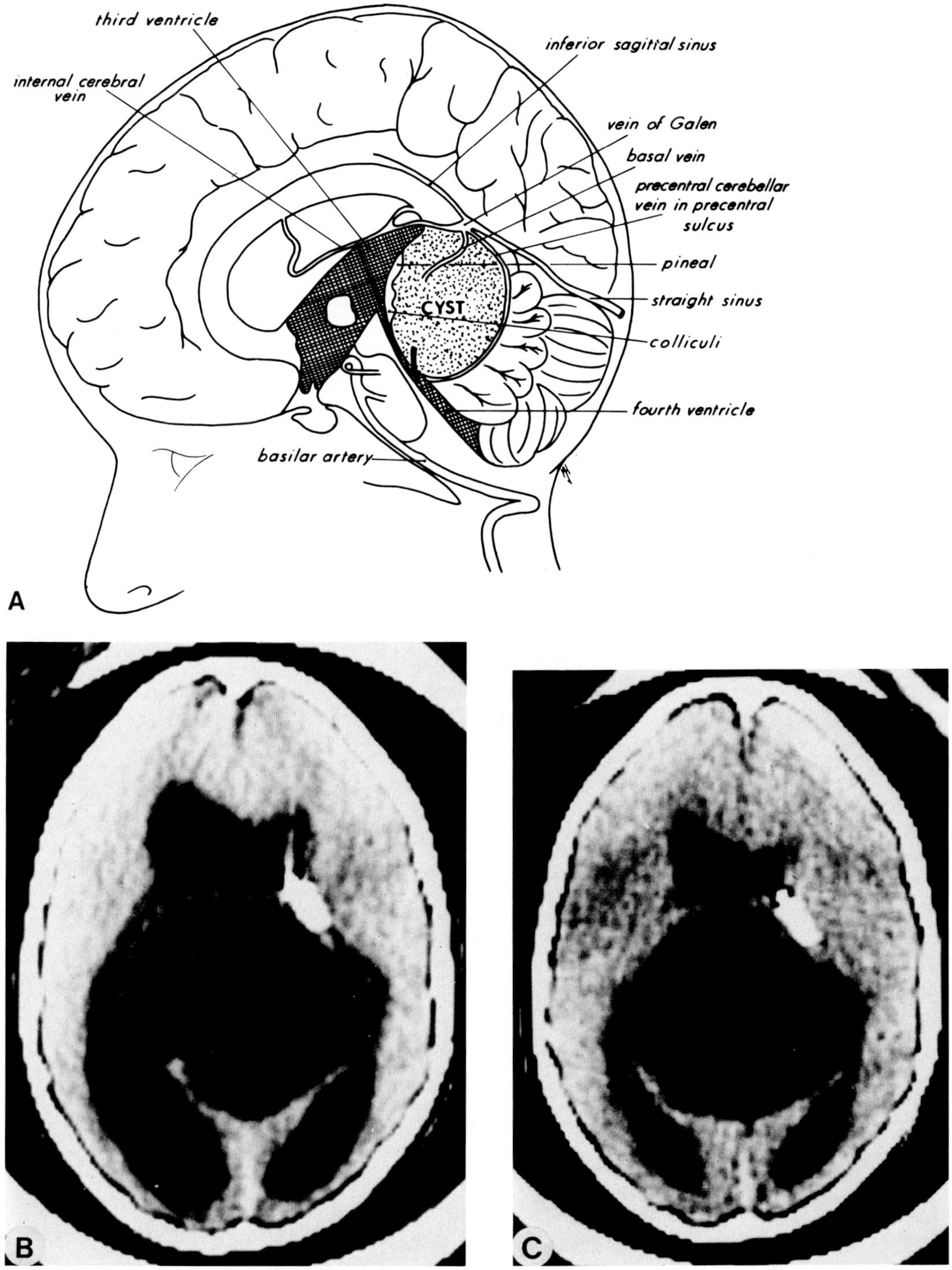

Figure 8-4. A. Diagram illustrating relation of a quadrigeminal cyst to surrounding structures. The sylvian aqueduct, upper brain stem, vein of Galen, and precentral cerebellar vein are distorted and functionally threatened. Arrow indicates surgical opening from cyst into fourth ventricle. B. A CT scan in a 9-year-old girl with myelomeningocele and hydrocephalus. Ventriculoperitoneal shunt was nonfunctional. A large quadrigeminal cyst is well shown; the ventricular system is dilated. C. Following revision of shunt, ventricles are smaller but cyst remains unchanged. (Diagram reprinted with permission from Huckman MS, Davis DO, Coxe WS: Arachnoid cyst of the quadrigeminal plate. J Neurosurg 32:367–370, 1970.)

shortness of the tentorium was an important advantage in this case. Others have established communication between the cyst and a lateral ventricle by means of a direct opening[34] or shunt tube.[5] Lee[29] treated three patients by cardiac shunt from cyst or lateral ventricle but two of these were not improved; this method is not generally recommended because of its high failure rate (Fig. 8-4C). It seems clear that cysts in the quadrigeminal region have a strong tendency to refill and produce recurring symptoms, unless a permanent fistula can be established between the cyst and ventricular or subarachnoid compartments.

CEREBELLAR CYSTS

Arachnoid cysts confined to the posterior fossa usually lie posteriorly, partly encased in the vermis or one cerebellar hemisphere, or are extra-axial and lateral, displacing the brain stem and adjacent hemisphere and extending toward the cerebellopontine angle (Fig. 8-5). Several reports[8,9,35] describe histologic evidence of the potential for CSF secretion within these cysts, namely, a tuft of choroid plexus, or an ependymal or hyperplastic cyst lining. The fact that spinal fluid can penetrate cyst walls was shown by Drayer, Rosenbaum, Maroon, et al.[36] in one case; after metrizamide was injected intraspinally, it was found to be present in an extra-axial cyst within a few hours. This also indicates to us, however, that fluid can pass outward into subarachnoid channels, thus lowering intracystic pressure and perhaps accounting for variations in clinical symptoms.

The location of posterior fossa cysts is such that the flow of spinal fluid through the fourth ventricle and aqueduct is eventually threatened, leading to elevated pressure and hydrocephalus. With extra-axial cysts, distortion and malfunction of the brain stem and cranial nerves are probably inevitable but may be long delayed.

Symptoms and signs caused by cysts in a cerebellar hemisphere or the vermis are basically those of fourth ventricle obstruction, including headache, lethargy, nausea, and ataxia, all of which may develop slowly and intermittently.[10,15] Extra-axial lesions produce complex difficulties, which include hearing loss, facial pain,[22] ataxia, brain-stem disturbances, and elevated pressure.[10] These are sometimes precipitated by sudden changes in head posture, and vary in severity.

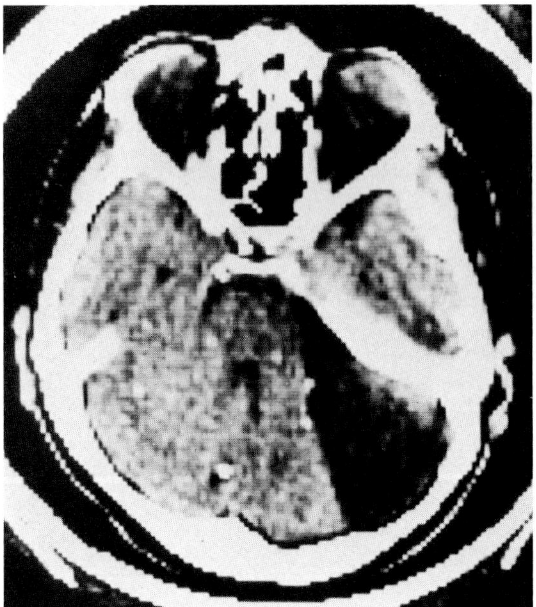

Figure 8-5. A CT scan shows arachnoid cyst of posterior fossa displacing right cerebellar hemisphere. This cyst extended forward and to the left, anterior to the brain stem. Surgical resection relieved all symptoms of raised intracranial pressure (case of Dr. V. T. Petersons).

Because the patient's clinical course may be quite similar to that caused by other space-taking lesions, careful diagnostic investigation is required. Gliomas and epidermoid tumors of the cerebellum, acoustic neuromas, vascular anomalies, and the Dandy–Walker malformation all must be considered.

Roentgenograms of the skull may show protrusion and thinning of occipital squama over a cerebellar cyst,[14] and other signs of chronic elevated pressure. If judiciously used, ventriculography and pneumoencephalography may be helpful in clarifying diagnosis, but vertebral angiography is generally safer and more useful in this situation;[37] a clear filling defect excludes vascular neoplasma and arteriovenous malformations, and other angiographic signs identify anomalies of the Dandy–Walker type. To distinguish a cyst from a large cisterna magna, hematoma, or cholesteatoma, CT scans are essential, perhaps with sagittal reconstruction or an intraspinal injection of air.[30,38] As noted, metrizamide injection with delayed scan is also a very useful supplemental aid.[36]

Treatment

Most writers have advised that cysts in this region be treated by operation, but it is stressed that preoperative diagnosis and surgical planning should be as accurate as possible. Thorough exploration is required to make certain that the cyst is fully visualized, widely resected, and perhaps opened into the subarachnoid space when possible.[14] Also, search should be made for a second cyst if there is any suspicion of this from preoperative investigation.[10,37]

Ventriculoperitoneal shunt or external ventriculostomy is recommended before craniotomy if the patient has high intracranial pressure, and some writers have felt that a shunt alone is sufficient for definitive treatment in certain cases.[38] Because there is a tendency for postoperative adhesions to cause obstruction of spinal fluid flow and hydrocephalus, these patients should be regularly observed for an extended period after surgery.[14] Computerized tomographic scans should be obtained within a month or less, and periodically for at least one year; if the cyst does not return but hydrocephalus develops, a shunt is recommended rather than reoperation.

REFERENCES

1. Ghatak NR, Mushrush GJ: Supratentorial intra-arachnoid cyst: Case report. J Neurosurg 35:477–482, 1971
2. Jakubiak P, Dunsmore RH, Beckett RS: Supratentorial brain cysts. J Neurosurg 28:129–136, 1968
3. Rengachary SS, Watanabe I, Brackett CE: Pathogenesis of intracranial cysts. Surg Neurol 9:139–144, 1978
4. Starkman SP, Brown TC, Linell EA: Cerebral arachnoid cysts. J Neuropathol Exp Neurol 17:484–500, 1958
5. Grollmus J, Wilson CB, Newton TH: Paramesencephalic arachnoid cysts. Neurology 26:128–134, 1976
6. Tiberin P, Gruszkiewicz J: Chronic arachnoidal cysts of the middle cranial fossa and their relation to trauma. J Neurol Neurosurg Psychiat 24:86–91, 1961
7. Williams B, Guthkelch AN: Why do cerebral arachnoid pouches expand? J Neurol Neurosurg Psychiat 37:1085–1092, 1974
8. Handa H, Bucy PC: Benign cysts of the brain simulating brain tumor. J Neurosurg 13:489–499, 1956
9. Harrison MJE: Cerebral arachnoid cysts in children. J Neurol Neurosurg Psychiat 34:316–323, 1971
10. Little JL, Gomez MR, MacCarty CS: Infratentorial arachnoid cysts. J Neurosurg 39:380–387, 1973

The poor prognosis for intellectual ability in children with severe craniofacial dysostosis has now been ascribed to the combination of craniosynostosis and hydrocephalus. Recognition of these factors had led to the early treatment of both of these conditions, with consequent excellent cosmetic as well as intellectual results.

Even a single synostotic suture may cause neurologic problems. Anderson and Johnson[10] documented 19 cases in which ocular deficits due to raised intracranial pressure could be ascribed to an isolated sagittal suture fusion. Recently, Hirsch, Renier, and Saint-Rose[11] continuously recorded intracranial pressure in patients with craniosynostosis, and again documented raised intracranial pressure in patients with fusion of a single suture.

In the past some individuals were skeptical about the value of craniectomy in the management of craniosynostosis.[12,13] Shillito and Matson[14] accounted for this skepticism by pointing out that it "stems in part from failure to achieve cosmetic improvement when surgery is carried out too late and in part from the use of surgical procedures which either never free the involved bones from one another adequately, or do not maintain this separation for an adequate period."

Simmons and Peyton[15] first attempted to inhibit early refusion of an artificial suture with the use of tantalum foil applied to the edge of the artificial suture. Since then various techniques have been used to prevent early refusion, including polyethylene film,[16] rubber,[17] methyl methacrylate,[18] Zenker's solution,[11] the outer layer of dura, and most recently silastic sheeting, which now is the most popular method in use. It is absolutely imperative that this interposition substance be inserted whenever a linear craniectomy is done if patency of that artificial suture is to be maintained. We initially confined the use of silastic to infants, but experience soon demonstrated that early and undesirable refusion may occur in children up to 2 years of age without the insertion of silastic interposition substance.

PATHOLOGY

The cranial sutures allow for the rapid expansion of brain mass during infancy and childhood. The human brain grows more rapidly during the first six months of life than it does during the remainder of life. Brain weight at birth is 335 grams and by age 1 year it is 925 grams. Since brain growth determines growth and shape of the overlying skull vault, expansion of the cranial vault is uneven when a suture is synostosed. Compensatory growth following Virchow's law occurs in the opposite direction of that of the closed suture, because the force of cerebral expansion is exaggerated wherever there is no resistance. Since most grain growth is complete by age 2 years, the sutures begin fibrous union at that time. By age 8 years the sutures are largely ossified.

The cause of premature synostosis remains unclear. Virchow[1] initially suggested meningitis as a possible cause, and over the years theories implicating intrauterine infection, birth trauma, endocrine dysfunction, syphilis, radiation during pregnancy, intrauterine constraint,[19] and metabolic disorders such as rickets and hypophosphatasia have all been mentioned as causes of premature craniosynostosis.

Reilly, Leeming, and Fraser[20] showed that craniosynostosis could be secondary to any metabolic derangement that caused the histologic changes of rickets. They found that two thirds of patients with hypophosphatasia, one quarter of those with azotemic osteodystrophy, one half with hypophosphatemic aminoacidura, one third with simple hypophosphatemic vitamin D refractory rickets, and one quarter with ordinary vitamin D deficiency rickets developed craniosynostosis.

Table 9-1
Characteristics of Craniofacial Dysmorphism

Syndrome	Genetics: Sporadic	Genetics: Autosomal Dominant	Genetics: Autosomal Recessive	Craniofacial Findings	Associated Findings
Crouzon	Yes (25%)	Yes	No	Craniosynostosis involving coronal sutures, basal skull sutures frequently associated with maxillary hypoplasia, shallow orbits, proptosis	Hydrocephalus rare
Saethre-Chotzen	No	Yes	No	Same	Ptosis, brachydactyly; soft-tissue syndactyly; often asymmetric; hydrocephalus rare
Apert	Yes (95%)	Yes	No	Same	Osseous & soft tissue, syndactyly of digits 2, 3, 4, of hands & soft-tissue syndactyly of digits 2, 3, 4, of feet; shortened upper extremities; hydrocephalus common
Carpenter	No	No	Yes	Same	Polysyndactyly of feet, soft-tissue syndactyly of hands; hydrocephalus rare
Pfeifer (Noack)	Yes (occasional)	Yes	No	Same	Partial soft-tissue syndactyly of hands & feet; broad thumbs & great toes; hydrocephalus rare
Summitt	No	No	Yes	Same	Variable syndactyly, obesity, gynecomastia
Baller-Gerold	No	No	Yes	Same	Radial aplasia
Lowry	No	No	Yes	Same	Fibial aplasia
Gorlin-Chaudry-Moss	No	No	Yes	Same	Hypertrichosis; anomalies of eyes, teeth, heart and external genitalia
Herrmann-Opitz	Yes	Yes	No	Same	Brachysyndactyly of hands, absent toes; soft-tissue syndactyly of 2, 3, 4, fingers
Herrmann-Pallister-Opitz	Yes	Yes	No	Same	Severe symmetrically malformed limbs, cleft lip and palate; radial aplasia; microcephaly

(*continued*)

Table 9-1
(*continued*)

Syndrome	Genetics: Sporadic	Genetics: Autosomal Dominant	Genetics: Autosomal Recessive	Craniofacial Findings	Associated Findings
Sakati-Nyhan-Tisdale	Yes	Yes	No	Same	Polysyndactyly, short limbs, congenital heart disease, ear anomalies
7P-	Yes	Yes	No	Same	Deletion of band P21 on chromosome 7; simian crease; hypogenitalism; nevus flammus on forehead
Weiss	No	No	Yes	Same	Medially deviated great toes; occasional mild syndactyly
Fairbanks	Yes	Yes	No	Same	Short legs; failure of tooth eruption
Craniotelencephalic dysplasia	Yes	Yes	?*	Craniosynostosis with protruding frontal region (? variant of Crouzon)	Isolated or may be associated with Apert's syndrome, encephalocele; hydrocephalus
Kleebattscahdel	Yes	Yes	No	Craniosynostosis with trilobular-shaped skull (? variant of Crouzon)	Isolated or may be associated with thanatrophic dwarfism or Apert's syndrome; hydrocephalus

Reprinted with permission from Hoffman HJ: Early neurosurgical repair in craniofacial dysmorphism. J. Neurosurg 51:796–803, 1979.
*Two personal cases in two siblings.

Moss[21] postulated that craniosynostosis is secondary to a primary malformation of the cranial base. The abnormal development of the cranial base creates alteration in the tensile force transmitted through dural fiber tracts to the calvarium, resulting in synostosis of the calvarial sutures. As evidence for this, Moss pointed out that surgical removal of a normal calvarial suture area is consistently followed by restoration of normal sutural margins. In the case of craniosynostosis, creation of an artificial suture is rapidly followed by reformation of synostotic ossification unless an interposition substance is used.

Craniosynostosis is typically an intrauterine event, with the child presenting at birth with a characteristic deformity. Postnatal synostosis can occur, however, and may be related to the lack of brain growth in primary microcephaly, to shunted hydrocephalus, to sutural trauma, to metabolic derangement, or to the progressive synostosis found in some patients with Crouzon's disease. Norwood, Alexander, Davis, et al.[22] drew attention to this entity when they reported a group of patients who developed recurrent multiple suture closures after craniectomy for craniosynostosis.

Any or all of the cranial sutures can be prematurely closed. When the synostosis is accompanied by abnormalities of the facial skeleton, the term craniofacial dysmorphism is used. In the past many of these patients were socially ostracized and only reluctantly were brought for treatment; accordingly,

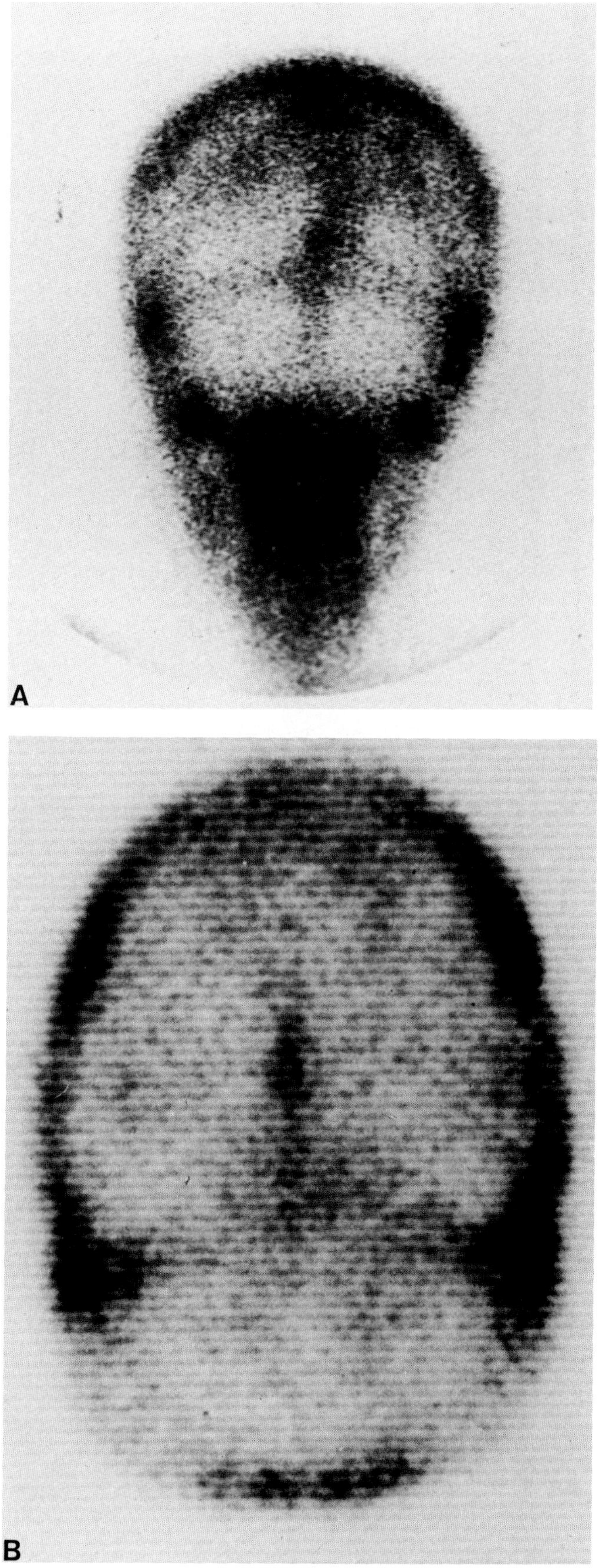

Figure 9-1. A. Bone scan in infant showing normal activity in sagittal, coronal and metopic sutures. B. Bone scan showing area of hyperactivity in closing sagittal suture.

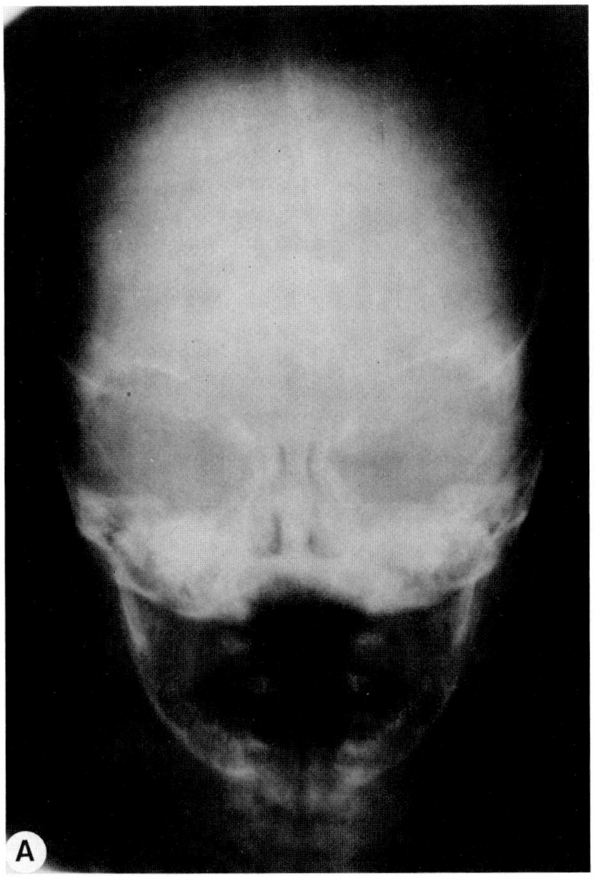

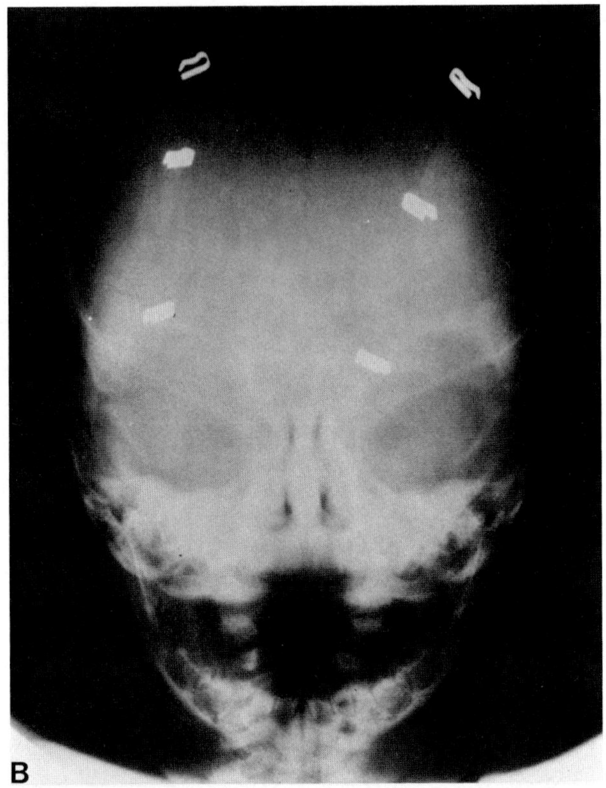

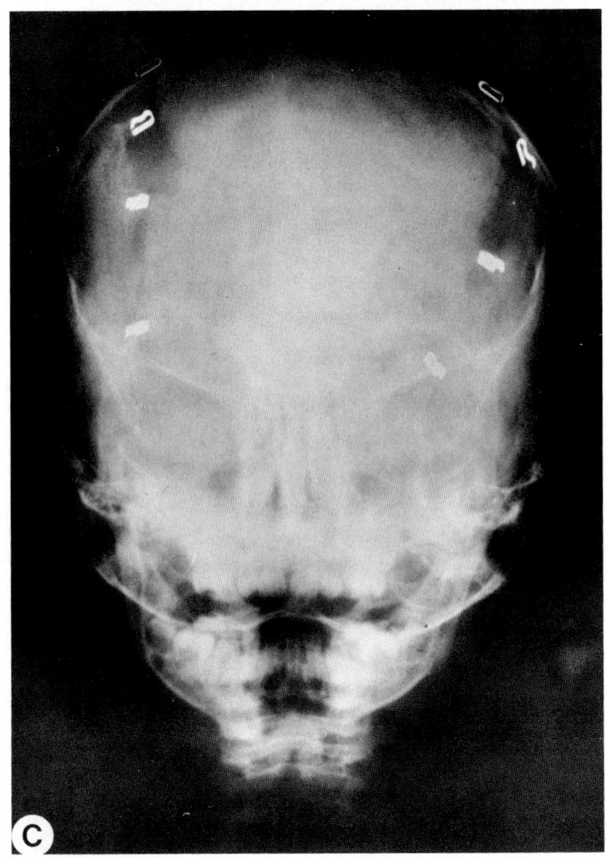

Figure 9-2. A. Anteroposterior (AP) x-ray of skull of neonate with sagittal synostosis. B. AP x-ray of same neonate immediately after sagittal craniectomy showing bony gap and tantalum clips holding silastic in place. C. AP x-ray of same infant at age 1 year showing filling in with bone of craniectomy site, maintenance of artificial suture by silastic, and tremendous growth in width with release of closed sagittal suture. D. Lateral view of skull of same neonate prior to repair. E. Lateral view immediately after repair. F. Lateral view of same infant at age 1 year showing correction of scaphocephaly.

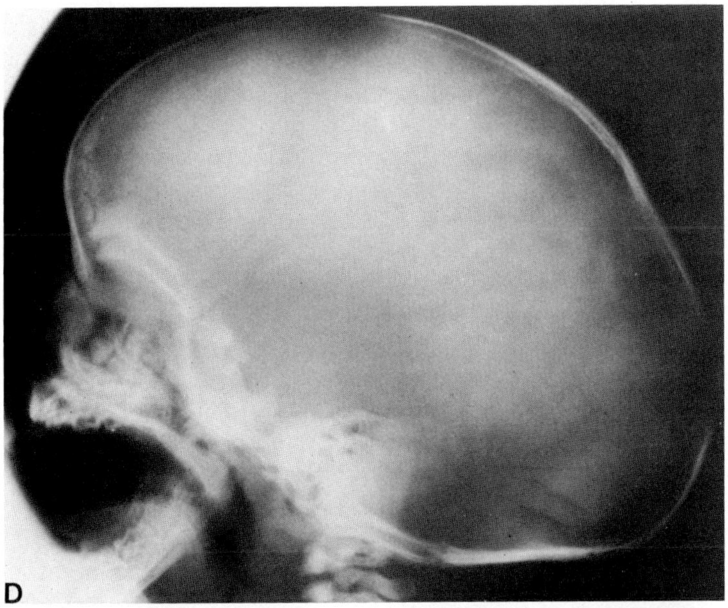

D

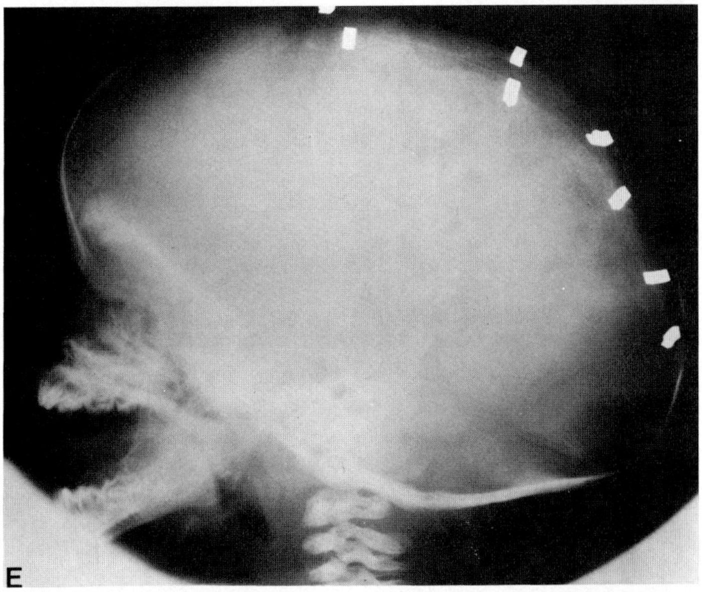

E

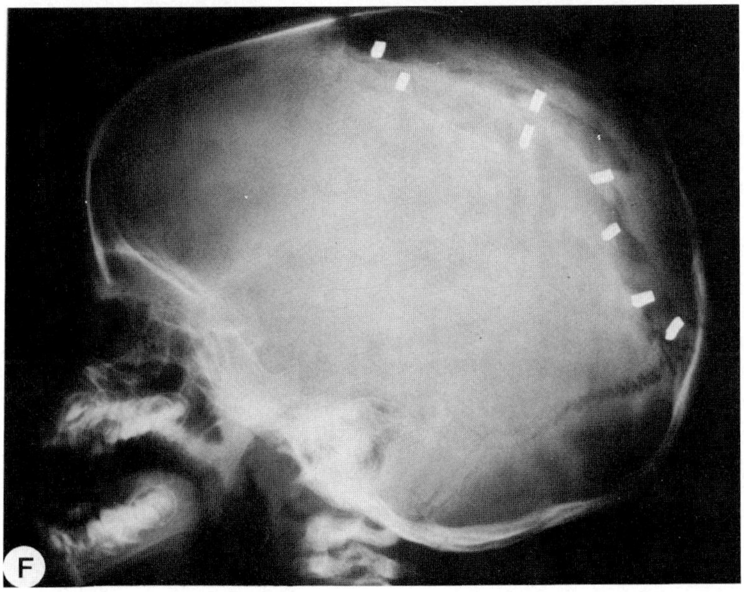

F

the percentage of patients with various types of craniosynostosis varies greatly depending on when the series was sampled. The craniofacial dysmorphic states number 17 in type and are detailed in Table 9-1.[23–27]

INVESTIGATION

Standard skull x-rays not only will show the closed suture, but will document the cranial vault shape. The computerized tomography (CT) scan will reveal any cerebral anomalies, including hydrocephalus, and will document head shape in another modality. Radioisotope bone scanning with technetium (^{99m}Tc) methylene diphosphonate given intravenously will confirm synostosis that might be questionable on skull x-ray alone (Fig. 9-1). Clinical acumen remains the most reliable guideline in assessing craniosynostosis.

SAGITTAL SYNOSTOSIS

Sagittal synostosis is the most common type of synostosis affecting a single suture. Eighty percent of the patients are males. The condition is rarely associated with other congenital anomalies. Although familial cases are rare, they occasionally occur.[28]

Premature fusion of the sagittal suture produces a characteristic scaphocephalic or boat-shaped appearance of the head. Since the two parietal bones are fused at the vertex, brain growth occurs predominantly at the coronal and lamboid sutures, producing enormous frontal bossing and a prominent occiput. The biparietal diameter remains narrow, and there is a prominent ridge along the sagittal suture. The head thus appears long and narrow with a keel-like configuration over the closed suture.

Surgical Repair

The original standard treatment for sagittal synostosis was bilateral parasagittal craniectomies 1 cm in width on either side of the midline. In 1973 Shillito[29] indicated the advantage of a single midline sagittal craniectomy. We have been using this craniectomy for the past 15 years and have never encountered undue bleeding from the sagittal sinus. More radical procedures for the treatment of sagittal synostosis have been recommended in recent years, but they are justifiable only in cases in which surgery has been delayed beyond early infancy, or in which primary surgery is performed without the benefit of a silastic interposition substance.[30–33] These more radical techniques all rely on extensive removal of bone and thus result in a more rapid correction of the abnormal head shape. We have found that a simple linear craniectomy, if performed within the first few months of life, will lead to complete correction of the abnormal head shape by age 6 months, providing that the craniectomy is kept patent with the use of interposition substance (Figs. 9-2, 9-3, and 9-4).

The surgical repair procedure is shown in Figure 9-5. To proceed, the patient's head is positioned prone with the neck extended. The midline scalp incision begins immediately anterior to the normally closed fontanelle and extends just behind the lambda. Scalp clips are applied to the skin edges to prevent bleeding. Burr holes are placed on either side of the midline just behind the coronal suture, and just in front of the lambdoid suture. The craniotome is then used to make cuts between the anterior and posterior burr holes, and bone is

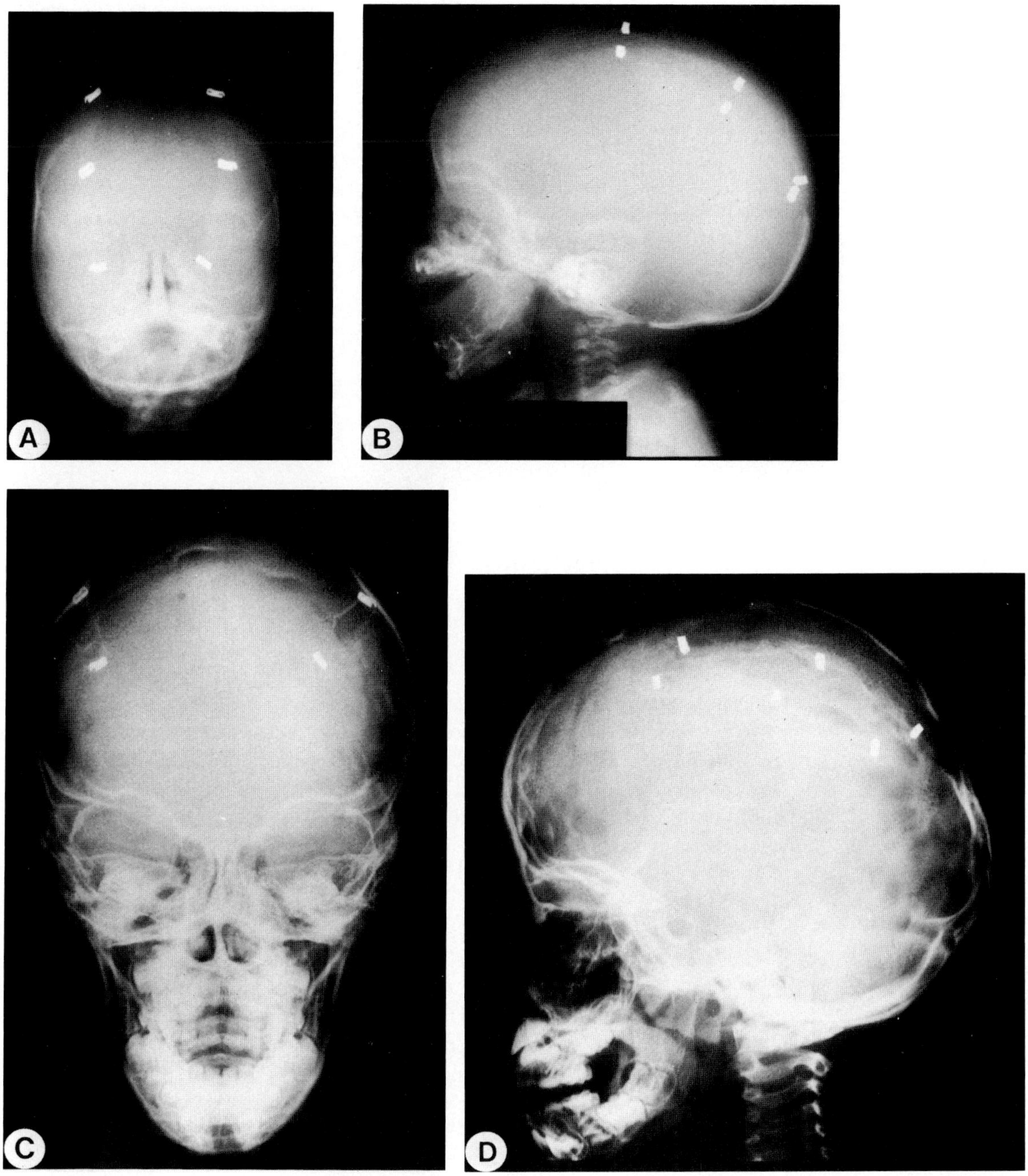

Figure 9-3. A, B. AP and lateral views of skull of neonate immediately after correction of sagittal synostosis. C, D. AP and lateral views of skull in same patient at age 5 years showing maintenance of correction due to persistence of suture provided by interposition substance.

rongeured across the midline between the two anterior and two posterior burr holes. The midline strut of bone, measuring some 3 cm in width and including the center keel, is stripped off the underlying sagittal sinus with ease. The artificial suture is then extended across the coronal suture anteriorly, and across the lambdoid suture posteriorly. When this is done, one can see the two parietal bones separating with each beat of the brain (Fig. 9-6). Molded silastic sheeting is then applied to the edge of the parietal bone on either side, and held in place with Ingram tantalum clips (Codman, Randolph, Mass.). The scalp is closed in two layers without drainage and a tight elastoplast dressing is applied.

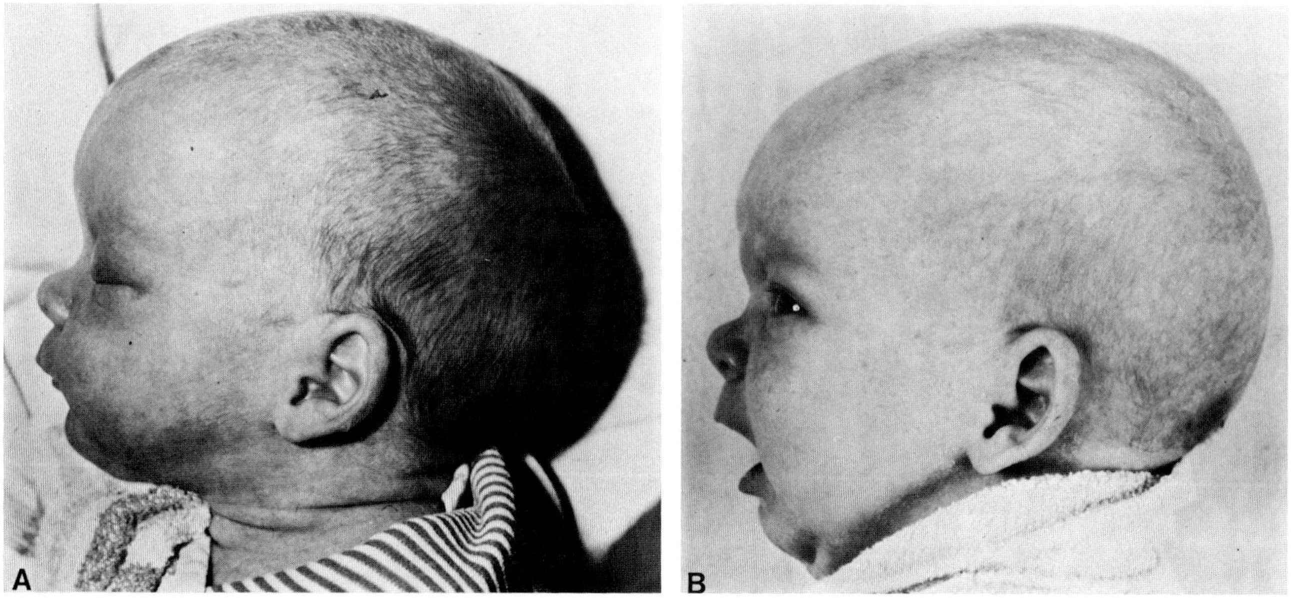

Figure 9-4. A. Newborn with scaphocephalic head characteristic of sagittal synostosis. B. Same child at age 5 months showing complete correction of head shape after simple linear craniectomy.

CORONAL SYNOSTOSIS

Coronal synostosis accounts for some 18 percent of patients with craniosynostosis. Premature closure of both coronal sutures is commonly seen in conjunction with craniofacial dysmorphism or multiple suture synostosis. All of the craniofacial dysmorphic states were considered rare prior to the development of modern craniofacial surgery, a field ushered in by Tessier[34] 15 years ago. Now that such patients are being made reasonably attractive by proper treatment, and since so many of the craniofacial dysmorphic states are autosomal dominant (Table 9-1), many of the offspring will have the same disorder. We are thus beginning to see patients whose parents were treated for some form of craniofacial dysmorphism in infancy. Modern techniques will make these patients even more attractive than in the past, particularly if the surgery is carried out in the neonatal period, so the actual incidence of these anomalies will probably increase dramatically. Apert's syndrome is said to occur in 1:160,000 births.[23] The number of surviving patients with this disorder is said to be reduced to 1:2,000,000 population because of the high incidence of morbidity and mortality in the disorder. This is certainly not true now that these children are being treated aggressively in the neonatal period. With their hydrocephalus adequately managed, not only do they have an acceptable appearance, but their brain functions well. Rather than dying, they will survive and produce more offspring with Apert's syndrome, so that the reported incidence of 1:160,000 will rise.

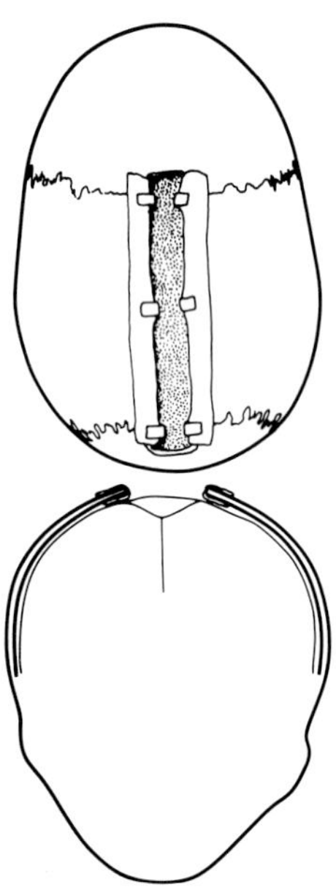

Figure 9-5. Surgical technique for repair of sagittal synostosis.

The inherent pathology of coronal synostosis and the craniofacial dysmorphic states involves premature fusion of the frontosphenoidal and frontoethmoidal sutures (Fig. 9-7).[35] These sutures, together with the coronal sutures, form a complete ring around the anterior end of the skull (Fig. 9-8). With closure of these sutures, the anterior fossa is foreshortened, so that the middle fossa can extend in front of the anterior fossa. Because the midportion of the face is attached to the anterior fossa. Because the midportion of the face is attached to the anterior fossa, it fails to grow, resulting in a hypoplastic maxilla. The

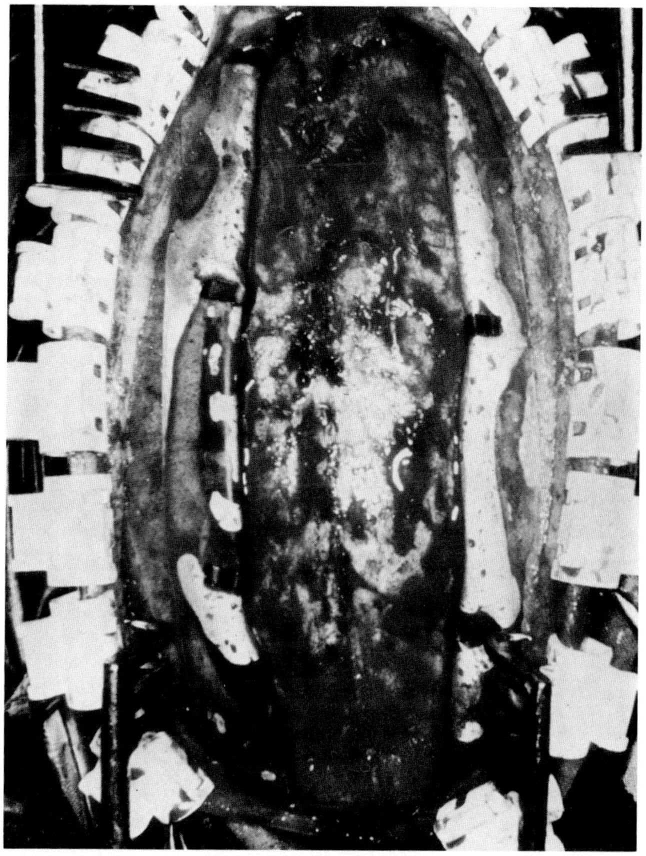

Figure 9-6. View of operation showing removal of sagittal suture and application of interposition substance.

retropositioning of the frontal bone in conjunction with the hypoplastic maxilla produces shallow orbits and results in progressive proptosis (Fig. 9-9).

Patients with synostosis of only one coronal suture present with a characteristic plagiocephaly. The forehead on the involved side has a flattened or concave appearance above the eye, and the eye on the involved side is higher than its contralateral mate. Without prompt and proper treatment in infancy, the ipsilateral cheek becomes flattened, and the nose tends to deviate toward the opposite normal side (Fig. 9-10). With premature fusion of both coronal sutures, both frontal bones are flattened and concave above the supraorbital margin, the

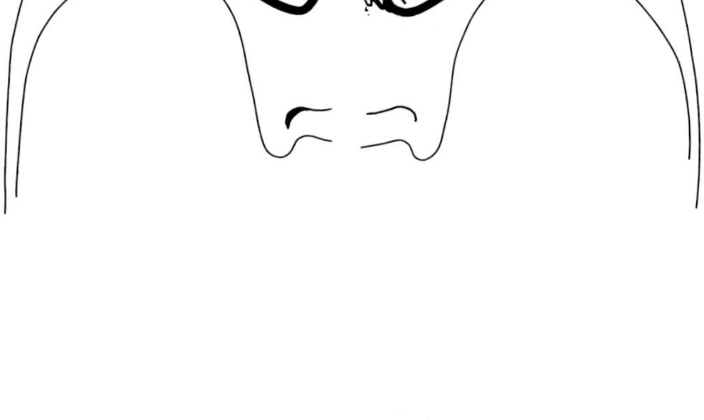

Figure 9-7. Diagram of closed frontoethmoidal and frontosphenoidal sutures.

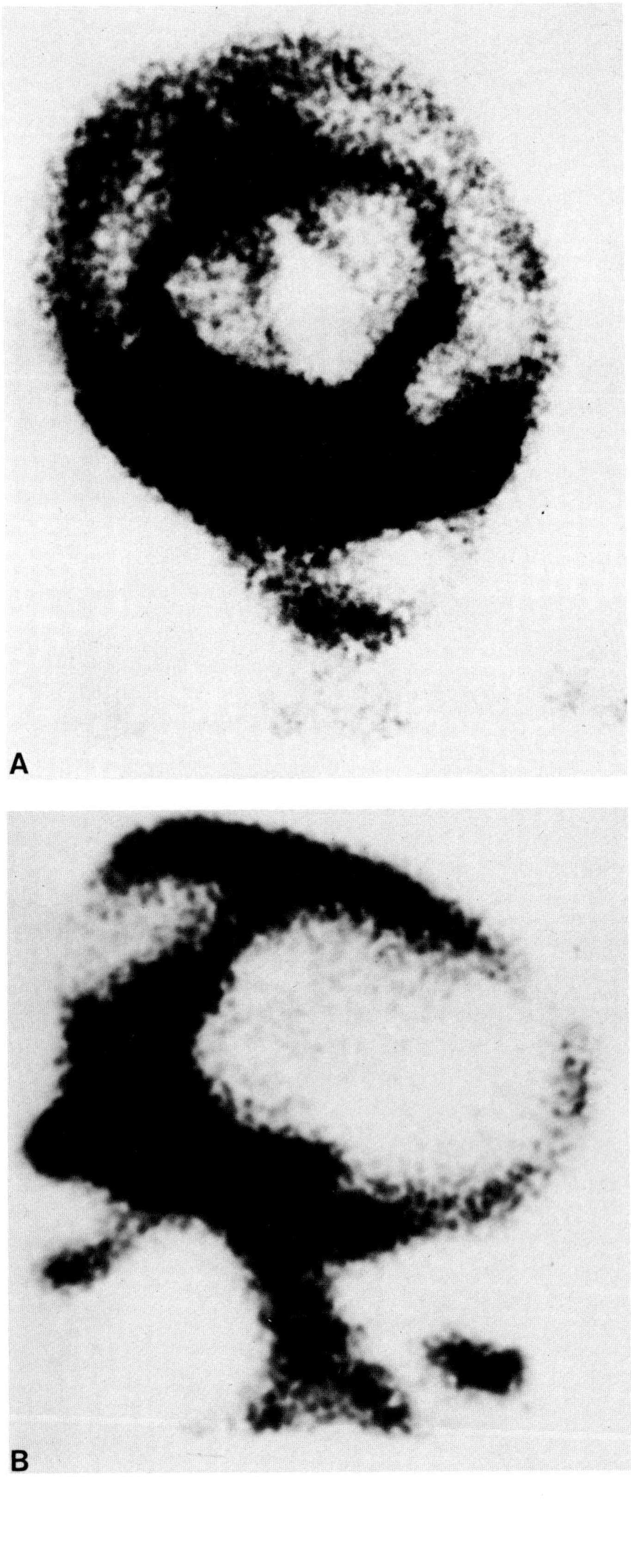

A

B

Figure 9-8. Bone scan of neonate with Crouzon's disease showing pathologic uptake of isotope in closing coronal, frontosphenoidal, and frontoethmoidal sutures, which together form a ring at the front end of the skull. (Reprinted with permission from Hoffman HJ: Craniofacial anomalies, in Wilson, Hoff (eds): Current Surgical Management of Neurologic Disease, New York, Churchill Livingstone, 1980.)

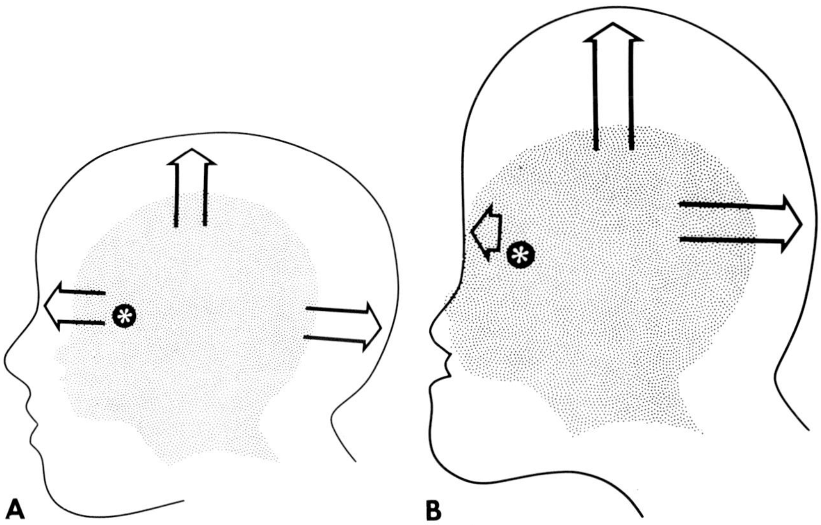

Figure 9-9. A. Normal growth of anterior cranial fossa. B. Lack of growth of anterior cranial fossa due to premature fusion of coronal frontoethmoidal and frontosphenoidal sutures results in characteristic deformity of craniofacial dysmorphism.

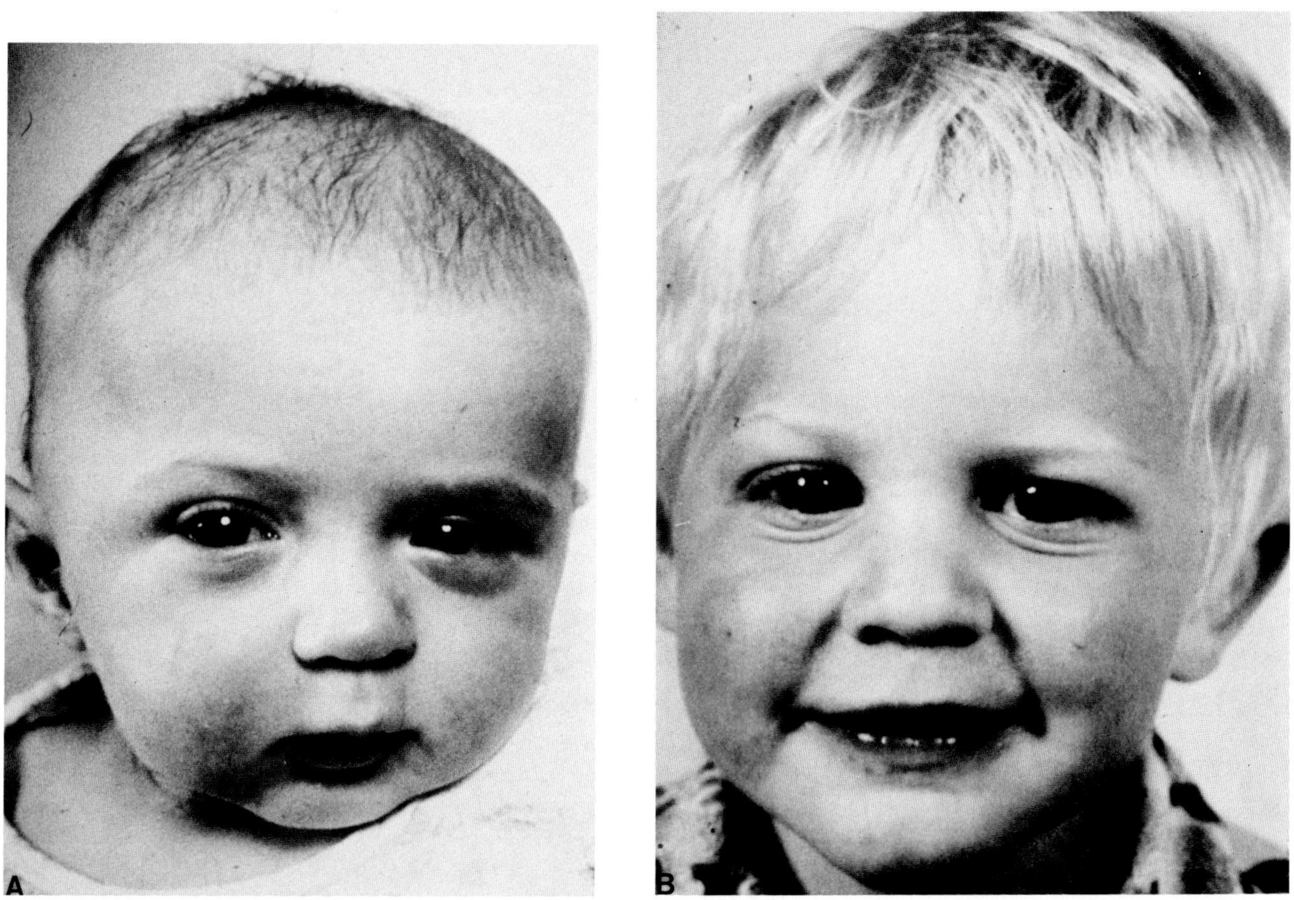

Figure 9-10. A. Infant with unilateral coronal synostosis showing characteristic facies. Note higher eye on right, deviation of nose to left, and concavity of forehead about right eye. B. Same child at age 4 years having undergone lateral canthal advancement at 4 weeks. Note complete correction of anomaly.

anterior fossa is foreshortened, and the attached face maxilla becomes progressively hypoplastic, resulting in proptosis. These patients exhibit the characteristic facies of craniofacial dysmorphism.

Surgical Repair

Early in infancy the procedure of lateral canthal advancement[36] adequately deals with both unilateral and bilateral coronal synostosis (Figs. 9-11, 9-12). This procedure begins with a frontal craniotomy. An osteotomy through the floor of the anterior fossa just behind the supraorbital margin frees the supraorbital margin from adjacent structures. One can thus advance the lateral extent of the supraorbital margin to a normal position, and secure it in this position with a strut of bone that is fastened to the silastic-edged parietal bone posteriorly. It is essential that the pterion be rongeured away, and the open artificial basal skull suture thus made continuous with the artificial coronal suture. The growing frontal lobe will then move the forehead and the attached face into a normal position (Fig. 9-13).

In the older child with unilateral coronal synostosis, the same operative procedure can be used, and we have indeed used lateral canthal advancement on children as old as 3 years of age with perfectly satisfactory results. The minor cosmetic nuisance of having the nose point away from the side of the closed suture remains in these older children, even though the eye and the forehead assume a normal appearance.

When bilateral coronal synostosis occurs without involvement of the basal skull sutures, however, the face grows in normal fashion, and so a bilateral lateral canthal advancement can be carried out until 18 months of age. Beyond that age, the entire supraorbital bar must be moved forward in one piece in order adequately to advance the anterior fossa since brain growth is largely over by then.

In the older child with craniofacial dysmorphism who has not had an adequate repair of the craniosynostosis in infancy, a radical craniofacial repair must be undertaken. The procedure begins with a tracheotomy. If there is some degree of hydrocephalus, it is useful to insert a lumbar drain to allow escape of cerebrospinal fluid (CSF). When the ventricles in such cases are normal in size or when the patient has an indwelling diversionary CSF shunt, this is obviously not

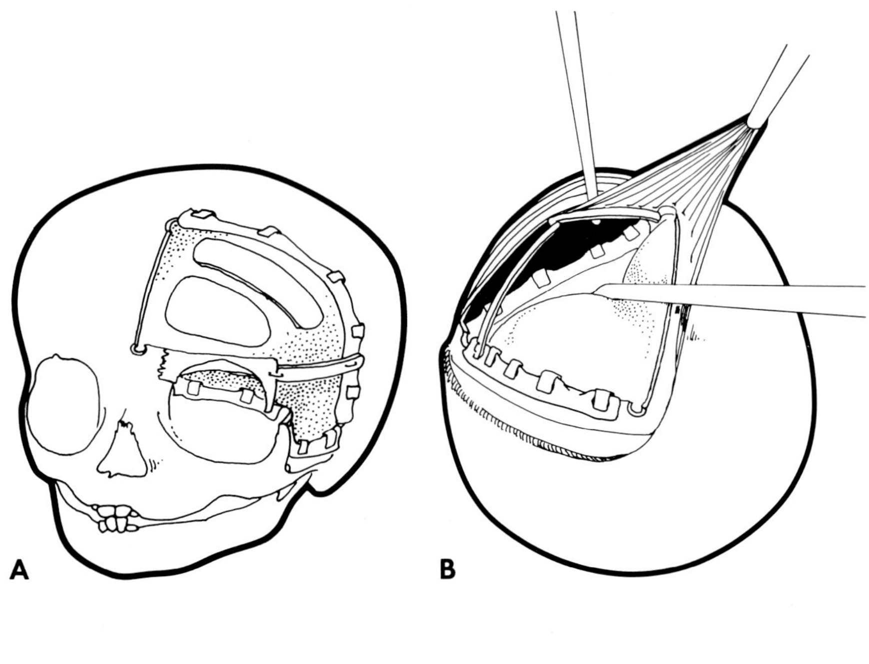

Figure 9-11. A, B. Operative diagram of unilateral lateral canthal advancement.

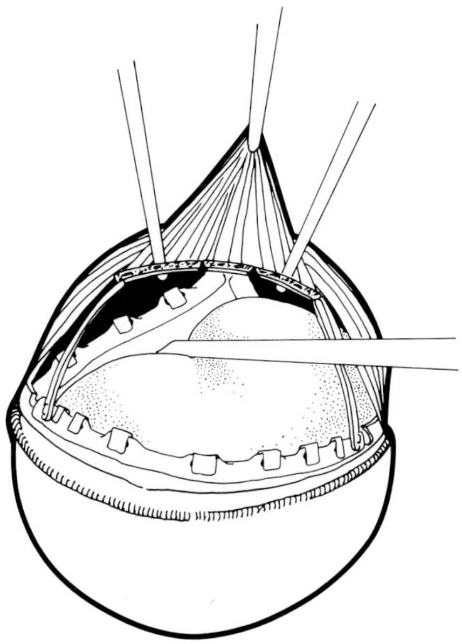

Figure 9-12. Operative diagram of bilateral lateral canthal advancement.

necessary. Mannitol, 20 percent in a dose of 2 g/kg, is given to provide adequate brain shrinkage. Blood and fluid loss are carefully monitored during the procedure, with adequate replacement being carried out.

A bicoronal scalp incision well behind the coronal suture and extending down to the ears bilaterally is used. The periosteum is incised and carried down into the orbits with the scalp flap. The lacrimal sac is identified and dissected free from the orbital wall. The periosteum is then elevated from the lateral orbital wall, and inferior orbital rim, as well as from the zygoma.

The entire frontal bone back to the coronal suture is removed to one segment. The inferior frontal osteotomy is then extended horizontally to include the temporal bone and is continued in a stepwise fashion inferiorly toward the base of the skull. This outlines a poserior slot in the temporal bone, which guides the subsequent advancement of the supraorbital margin and allows maintenance of bony contact (Fig. 9-14).

Horizontally, the osteotomy extends into the lateral orbital wall, then continues through the orbital roof and across the nasion. Once this is done bilaterally, it is possible to remove the supraorbital bar in one piece.

At this point one has an excellent view of the dura long the floor of the anterior fossa and so any dural leaks incurred during the removal of bone can be easily repaired. Frequently, with craniofacial dysostosis there are numerous stalactites of bone protruding up from the floor of the anterior fossa, and many of these patients have had previous attempts at surgical correction as well. Consequently, dural lacerations are common during craniofacial repair. It is absolutely imperative that all of these dural tears be adequately sealed to avoid postoperative rhinorrhea, which is a dreaded complication.

The maxilla is advanced with a Lefort 3 osteotomy. The root of the nose is sectioned horizontally into the medial orbital wall; the osteotomy is then continued along the medial wall behind the lacrimal sac to the inner third of the orbital floor. The lateral wall of the orbit is split in a sagittal plane, and the osteotomy continued into the orbital floor. The osteotomy is then extended to the malar bone, and the maxilla is advanced and fixed in position by interdental wiring. Consequently, the patient must be old enought to have primary dentition. If there are any abnormalities of the nasal structure, a rhinoplasty can be done. The advancement of the forehead can be as much as 20–30 mm in these children,

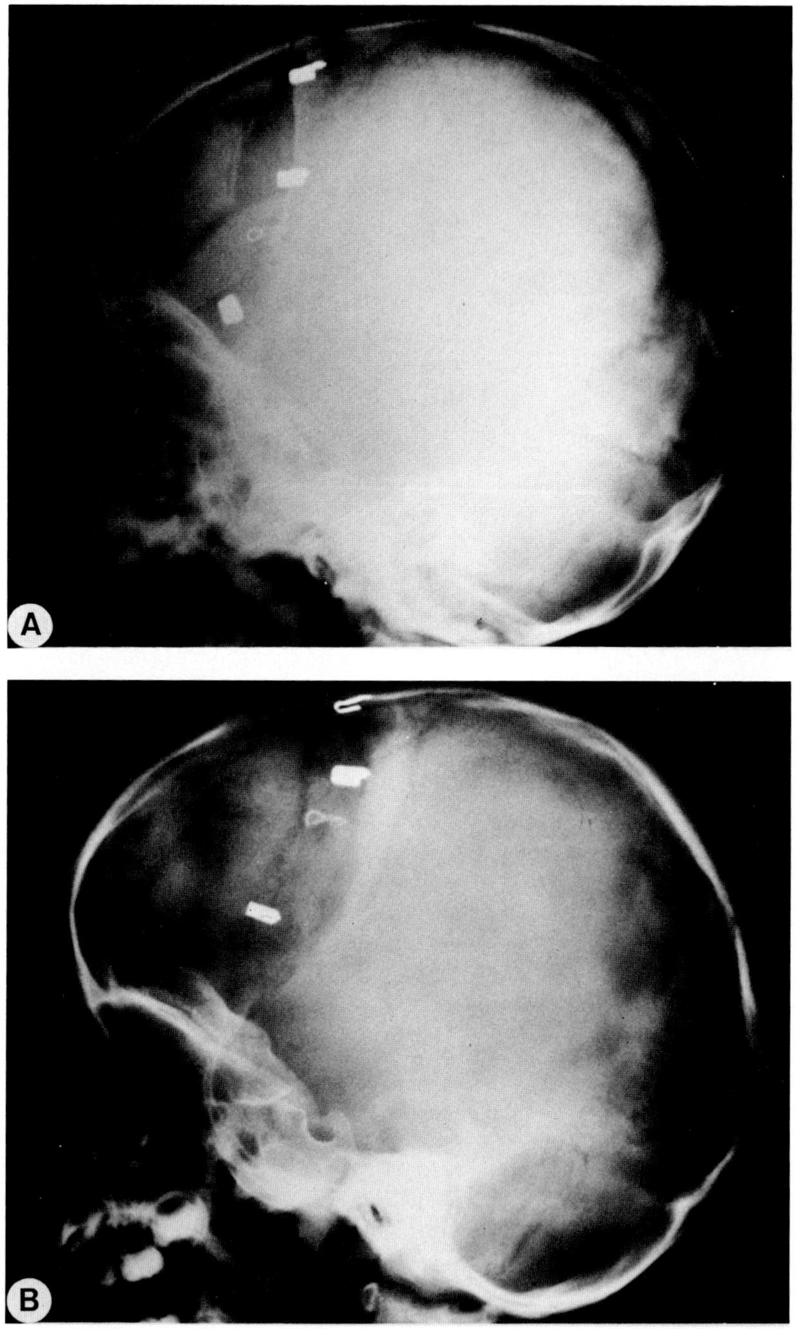

Figure 9-13. A. Lateral skull x-ray of infant with unilateral coronal synostosis immediately after unilateral lateral canthal advancement. B. Same patient at age 3 years. Note tremendous growth of anterior fossa and spreading apart of wires that initially secured bony strut.

and consequently bone grafts (split ribs) must be taken to fill in the defects created by the advancement. The frontal bone flap is then replaced.

Since this procedure allows free communication between cranial cavity, face, and mouth, there is very significant risk of infection; prophylactic antibiotics are used and the wound is profusely irrigated with Betadine. (Betadine solution—10% povidone-iodine—is manufactured by Purdue, Frederide Co., 123 Sunrise Avenue, Toronto, Canada.)

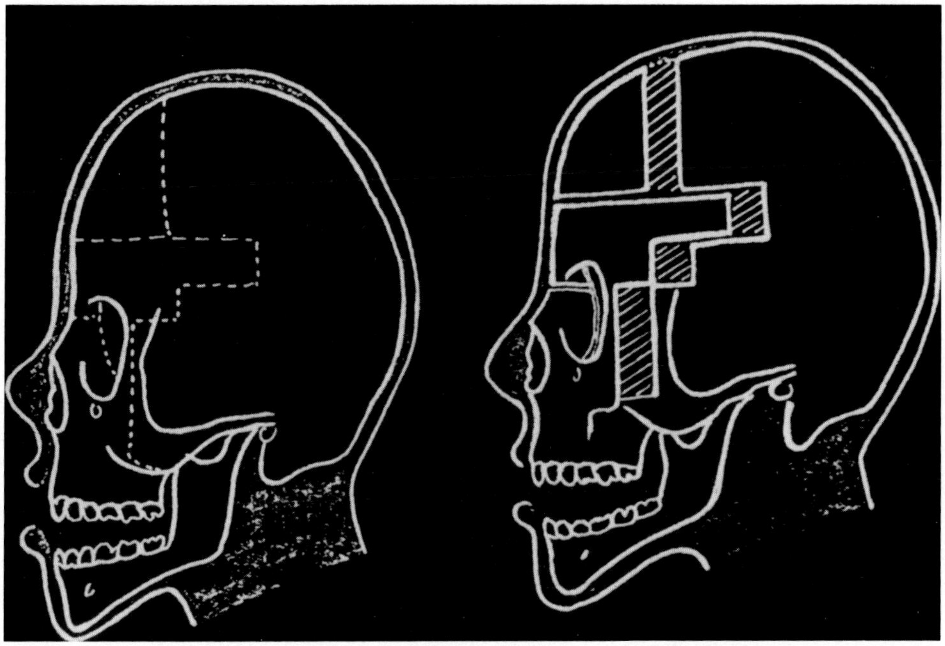

Figure 9-14. Operative diagram of technique of advancement of forehead and face in older patient with craniofacial dysmorphism.

The child with craniofacial dysmorphism or coronal synostosis treated with a bilateral lateral canthal advancement during infancy can develop a perfectly normal face and head shape, and thus grow up with dignity, free from the taunts that inevitably beset the strange-looking child (Figs. 9-15, 9-16).

In the past the older child with craniofacial dysmorphism could obtain some improvement from the on-lay grafts of Longacre.[37] Modern treatment, however, initially described by Tessier,[34] has finally brought relief to all patients with craniofacial dysmorphism, and remains the treatment of choice for those who have not been treated effectively in infancy. With proper repair, these children can be rendered normal in appearance no matter how severe their deformity (Fig. 9-17).

TRIGONOCEPHALY

Trigonocephaly is created by premature closure of the metopic suture. In our institution it accounts for some 16 percent of the cases of craniosynostosis. The metopic suture is one of the first sutures to close, with closure beginning late in the first year of life, and finishing by the age of 8 years. Normally, the metopic suture accounts for the rounding and broadening of the frontal bone. Should the metopic suture close early, particularly during intrauterine life, the forehead remains pointed and angular, and a ridge develops along the closed metopic suture (Fig. 9-18). The orbits tend to angulate inwardly, and there is marked hypotelorism. When the metopic suture closes after birth, the ridging is usually present only along the posterior aspect of the suture, and the forehead frequently has a normal contour and there are no ocular abnormalities. This type of synostosis of the metopic suture has no clinical significance and frequently is familiar in nature.

Unlike the other forms of craniosynostosis, trigonocephaly is commonly seen in association with a variety of underlying anomalies of the brain, the most

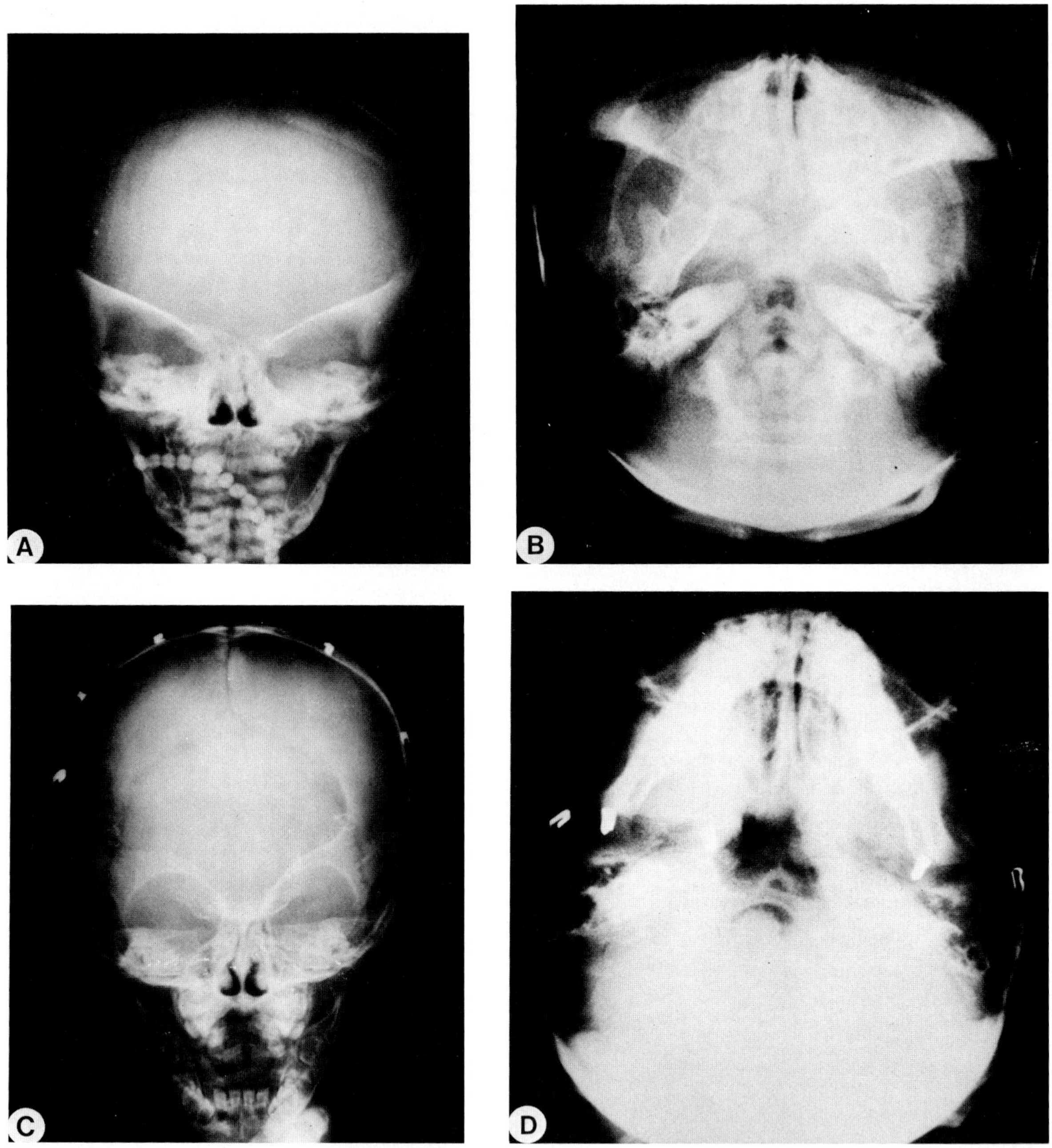

Figure 9-15. A, B. Anteroposterior (AP) and basal views of skull in infant with Crouzon's disease. Note halequin orbits, thickened pterion bilaterally, and obtuse angle of sphenoid wings. C, D. AP and basal views of same infant at age 3 years. Child underwent bilateral lateral canthal advancement at age 2 weeks. E, F. AP and lateral views of face of same infant immediately prior to surgery. G, H. AP and lateral views of same child at age 5 years showing normal appearance. This child had only one operative correction (bilateral lateral canthal advancement) as neonate. (Reprinted with permission from Hoffman HJ: Early neurosurgical repair in craniofacial dysmorphism. J Neurosurg 51:796–803, 1979.)

severe of which is holoprosencephaly.[38] For this reason, many of these patients with trigonocephaly show significant degrees of retardation. In the series described by Anderson, Gwinn, and Todt[39] 30 percent were retarded, a fact that the authors attributed to the gradual constriction of the frontal lobes by the narrow anterior cranium. The need for early diagnosis and treatment is therefore obvious when the condition is severe.

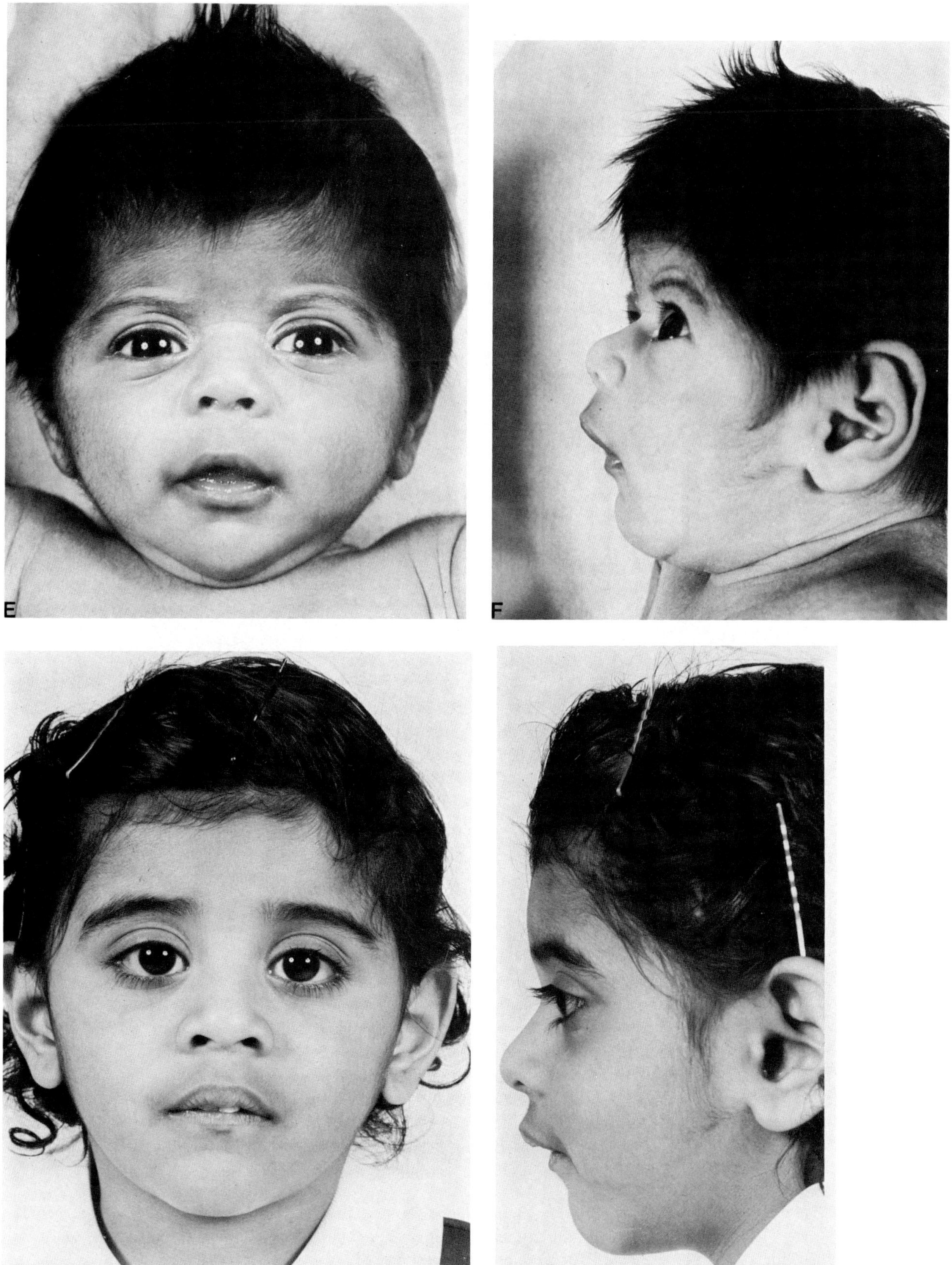

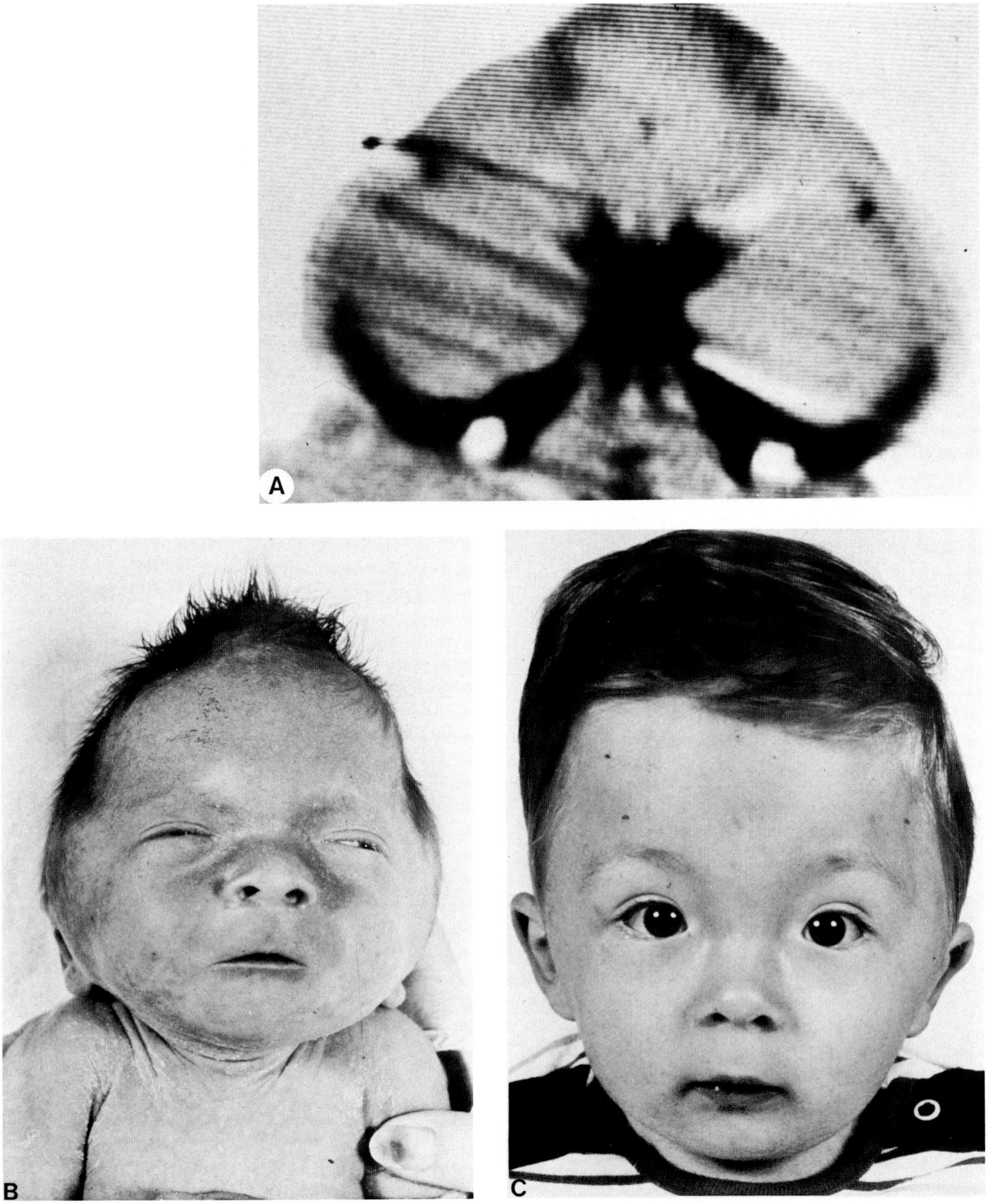

Figure 9-16. A. A CT scan of neonate with characteristic trilobed skull of Kleeblattschadel. B. Photograph of same infant. C. Same child at age 2 years having undergone bilateral canthal advancement and morcellation craniotomy at age 2 weeks. Not only does this child appear normal, but he is functioning with a normal IQ.

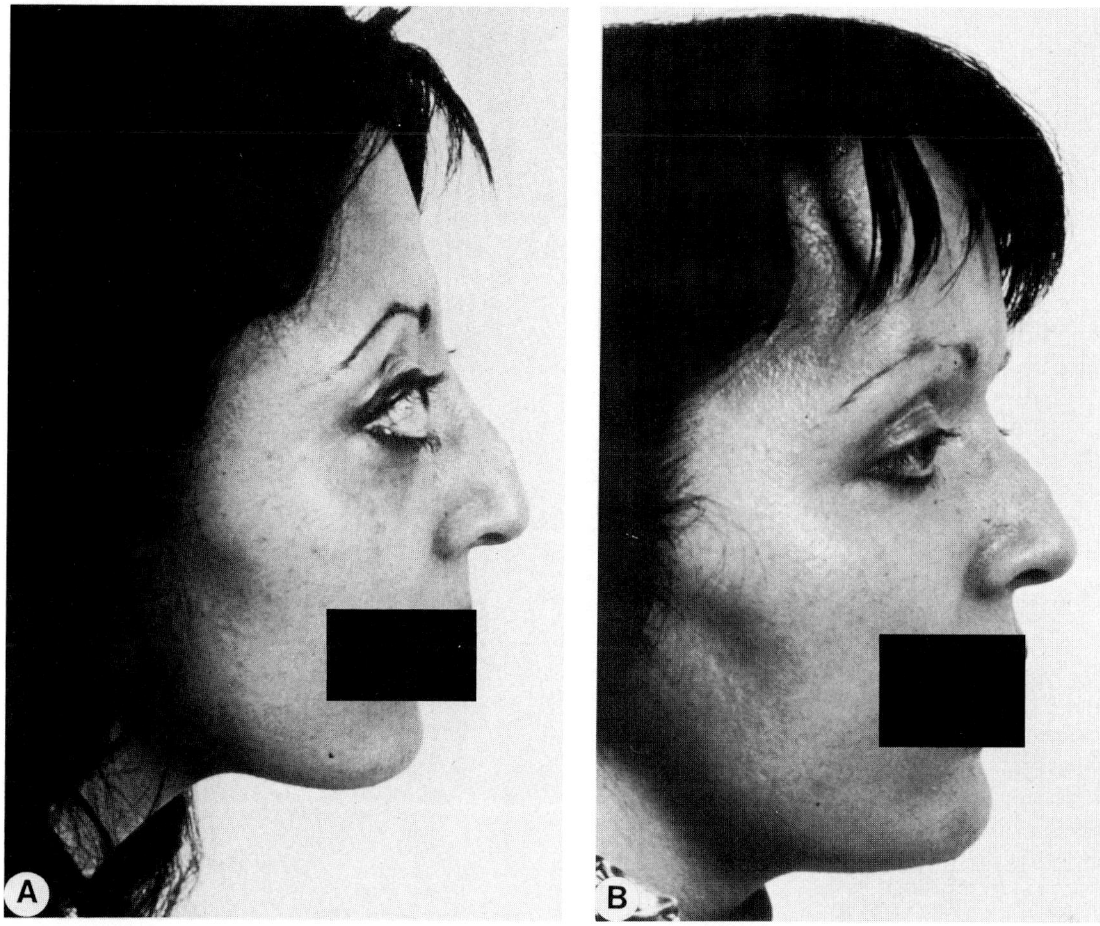

Figure 9-17. A. Young woman with untreated Crouzon's disease showing exorbitism and oxycephaly. B. Same young woman after Tessier repair, she now has a normal appearance.

Although trigonocephaly was initially described in 1862, surgical management was initially mentioned by Matson in 1960.[40] In 1962 Anderson et al.[39] reviewed the literature and presented what is now the accepted therapeutic approach to trigonocephaly.

Surgical Repair

In the surgical repair procedure, shown in Figure 9-19, the entire frontal bone is removed from just above the supraorbital margin to just in front of the coronal suture. The midline ridge extends down onto the nasion and must be chiseled or burred away. The bone fragments of the removed frontal bone are then loosely applied to the dura and held there by the preserved sheet of frontal periosteum. Since the metopic suture closes early, interposition substance is not used in this condition. Following this procedure the forehead achieves a normal contour almost immediately, and with the passage of time the orbits move out into normal position, and have a normal radiologic appearance. In the severe forms of trigonocephaly, in which the forehead is markedly "depressed" above the orbits, a bilateral lateral canthal advancement is of value. This procedure is also used when trigonocephaly occurs in conjunction with bilateral coronal synostosis.

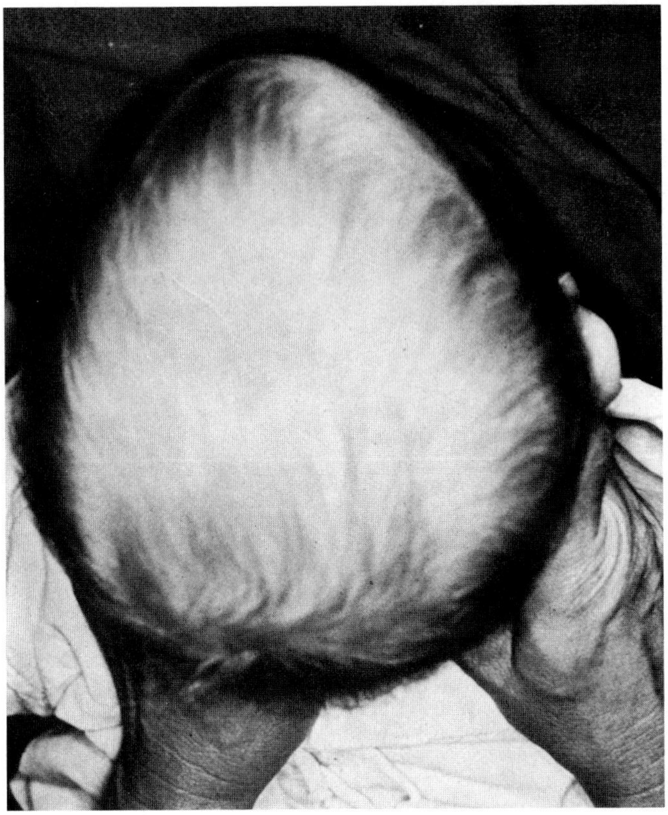

Figure 9-18. Triangular forehead of trigonocephaly.

LAMBDOIDAL SYNOSTOSIS

Lambdoid synostosis is unusual; in our series at the Hospital for Sick Children it accounts for only 9 percent of all cases of craniosynostosis. Left untreated, this form of synostosis produces flattening of the back of the head on the involved side, with the ear on this side being higher and more anteriorly placed (Fig. 9-20). The differentiation between lambdoidal synostosis and positional flattening of the head frequently presents difficulties. Radiologically, a closed lambdoid suture may appear open, but typically there is a sclerotic margin along one edge of the suture (Fig. 9-21). The bone scan in such cases becomes

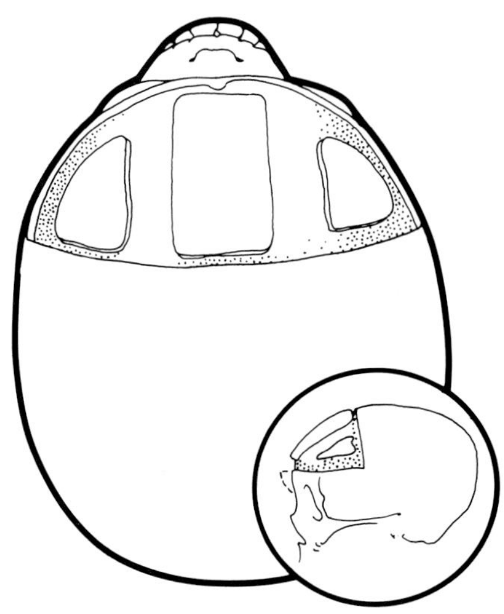

Figure 9-19. Operative technique for repair of trigonocephaly.

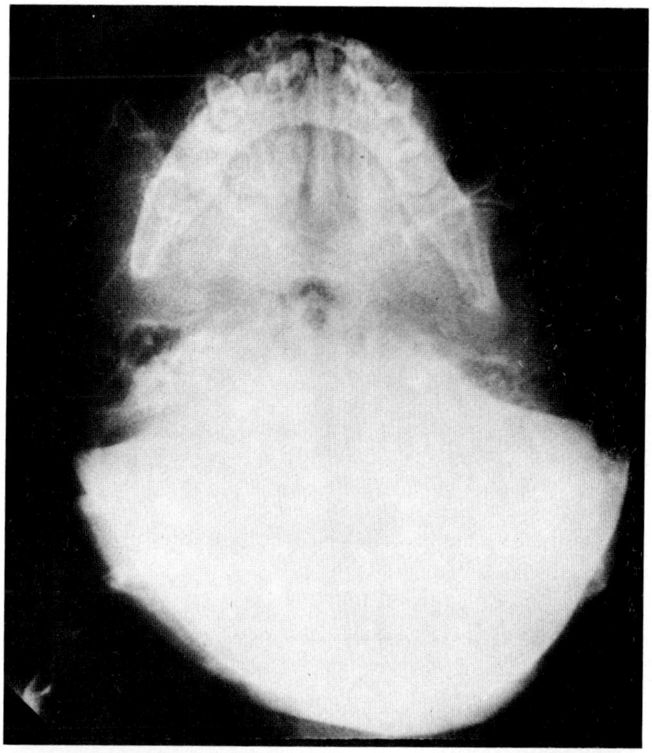

Figure 9-20. Basal view of skull showing flattening of occiput and bulging of ipsilateral frontal region in child with unilateral lambdoid synostosis.

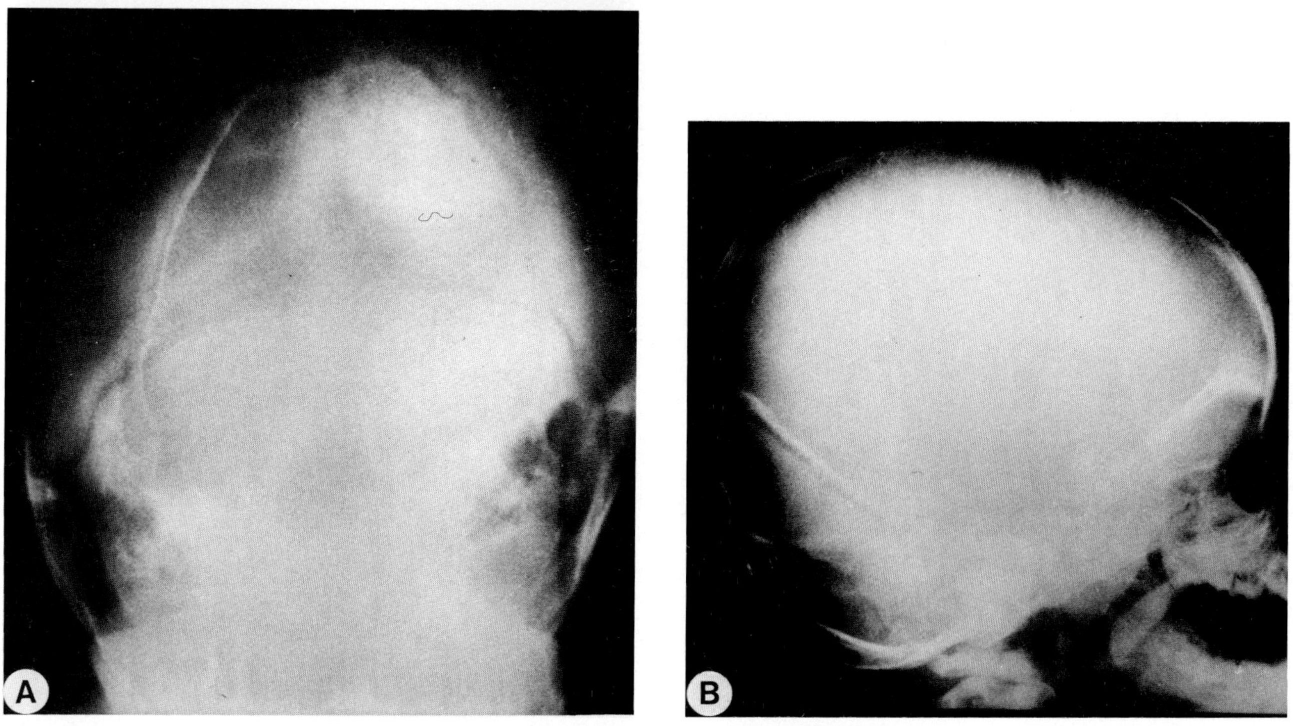

Figure 9-21. A. Towne's view of infant with unilateral lambdoid synostosis showing sclerosis along edge of lambdoid suture. B. Lateral view.

invaluable in that a closed suture will show no activity as compared with the contralateral lambdoid suture, and a suture in the process of closing will show hyperactivity compared with the normal open contralateral suture.

Surgical Repair

Lambdoid synostosis responds very nicely to a simple linear craniectomy extending from the sagittal suture medially to the asterion laterally. Silastic sheeting is used to cover the bony edges. If the disease is bilateral, the linear craniectomy is carried out bilaterally. The removed abnormal lambdoid suture shows a characteristic appearance. In those cases in which the suture appears radiologically open, the external appearance of the suture indeed looks normal, but the inner aspect of the closed suture shows a remarkable hyperostosis and bony ridging, which accounts for the sclerotic edge one so commonly sees on x-ray in lambdoid synostosis (Fig. 9-22).

MULTIPLE SUTURE SYNOSTOSIS

Multiple suture synostosis unassociated with craniofacial dysmorphism accounts for some 7.6 percent of cases of craniosynostosis in the authors' series. The head shape varies according to the sutures involved. A not infrequent combination is that a sagittal and both lambdoid sutures (Fig. 9-23). Marked frontal bossing, ridging over the sagittal suture, and a very narrow head from posterior to the coronal suture are the result.

Surgical Repair

Multiple suture synostosis in the past was frequently treated in several stages. With the modern techniques of pediatric neuroanesthesia, it is possible to open all sutures simultaneously. The head is supported by a special crutch head rest applied to the occipital prominences, and a *meisterschnitt* incision is used so

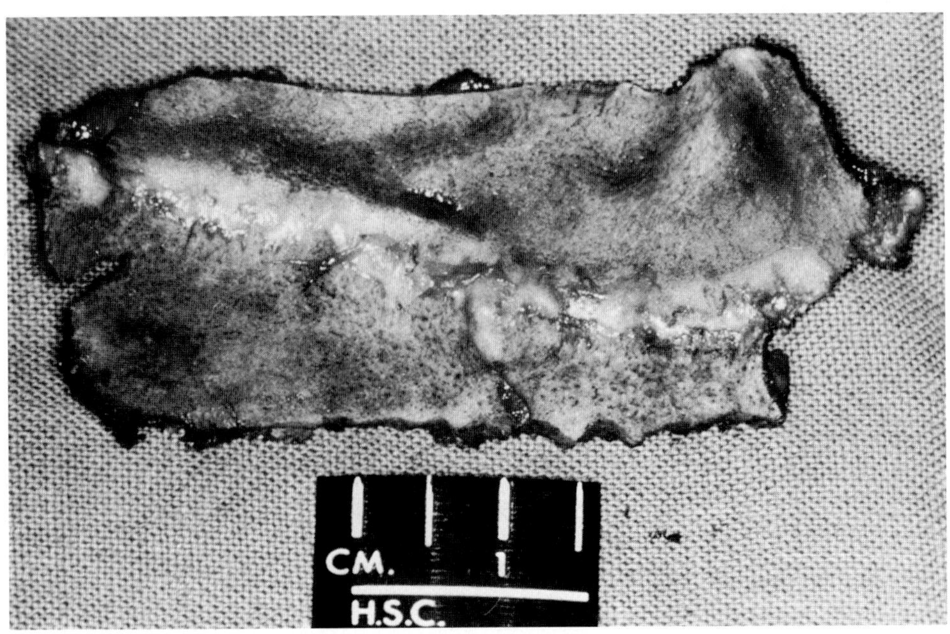

Figure 9-22. Inner aspect lambdoid suture showing hyperostosis along suture line.

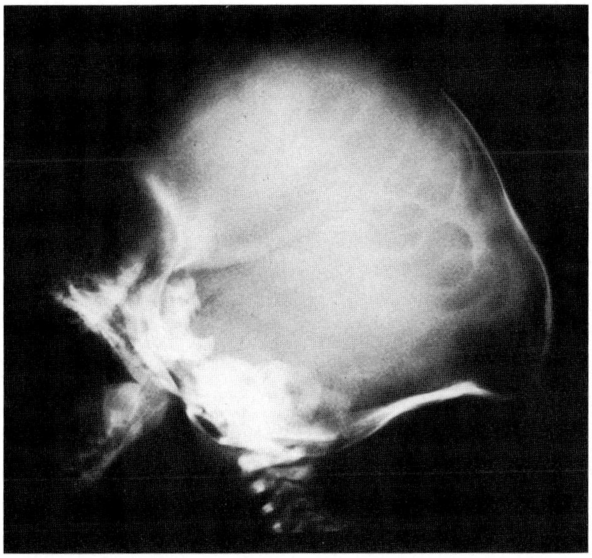

Figure 9-23. Lateral view of skull of infant with closure of sagittal and both lambdoid sutures.

that the scalp can be reflected both anteriorly and posteriorly. It is thus possible to perform multiple linear craniectomies and, if necessary, a bilateral lateral canthal advancement, all at the same time (Fig. 9-24).

HYPOPHOSPHATASIA

Rathbun[41] in 1948 coined the term hypophosphatasia and used it to describe a genetically determined metabolic disorder characterized by abnormal mineralization of bone, diminished alkaline phosphatase activity, and increased urinary excretion of phosphoryethanolamine. Hypophosphatasia was divided into three groups by Fraser.[42] Group 1 included the most severely affected patients in whom

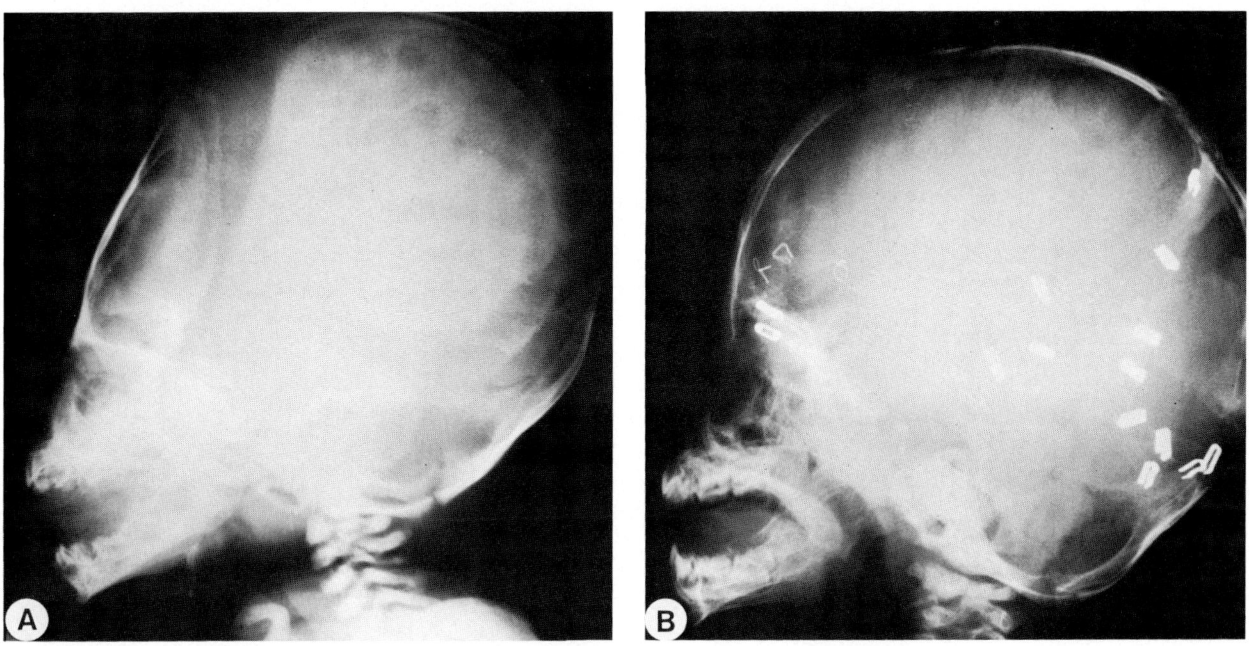

Figure 9-24. A. Lateral skull x-ray of neonate with closure of all sutures. B. Same child at age 18 months after correction at age 1 week. Note normal head shape.

lesions were present at birth or within the first six months of life. These patients typically presented with fibrous synostosis of the cranial sutures, a nonossified calvarium, a small head, and signs of raised intracranial pressure. Release of the constricting fibrous calvarium frequently improved the patient's cerebral state, but the majority of these infants also have respiratory problems related to a constrictive rib cage and so die in infancy because of respiratory insufficiency.

Group 2 became symptomatic beyond the age of 6 months, and only a minority presented with typical multiple suture craniosynostosis. These patients responded well to multiple linear craniectomies.

Group 3 consisted of those patients who developed minimal problems that did not manifest themselves until adult life, and that did not require treatment.

Hypophosphatasia is an autosomal dominant disease and can be detected early in pregnancy; thus many of the cases of hypophosphatasia of the severe type are being aborted in high-risk pregnancies and so are not presenting for treatment.

HYPERTELORISM

Hypertolorism is a rare abnormality consisting of an increased breadth between the eyes. It occurs in a ratio of 1:60,000 population. Normally, during embryonic development, the eyes initially separate from the diencephalon as diverticula and migrate to a lateral position on the head as in lower animals. As the face matures, the eyes rotate forward, reducing the orbital angle from 180 degrees to 71 degrees by birth, and to 68 degrees by maturity. Hypertelorism therefore may result not only from failure of this forward migration, but also

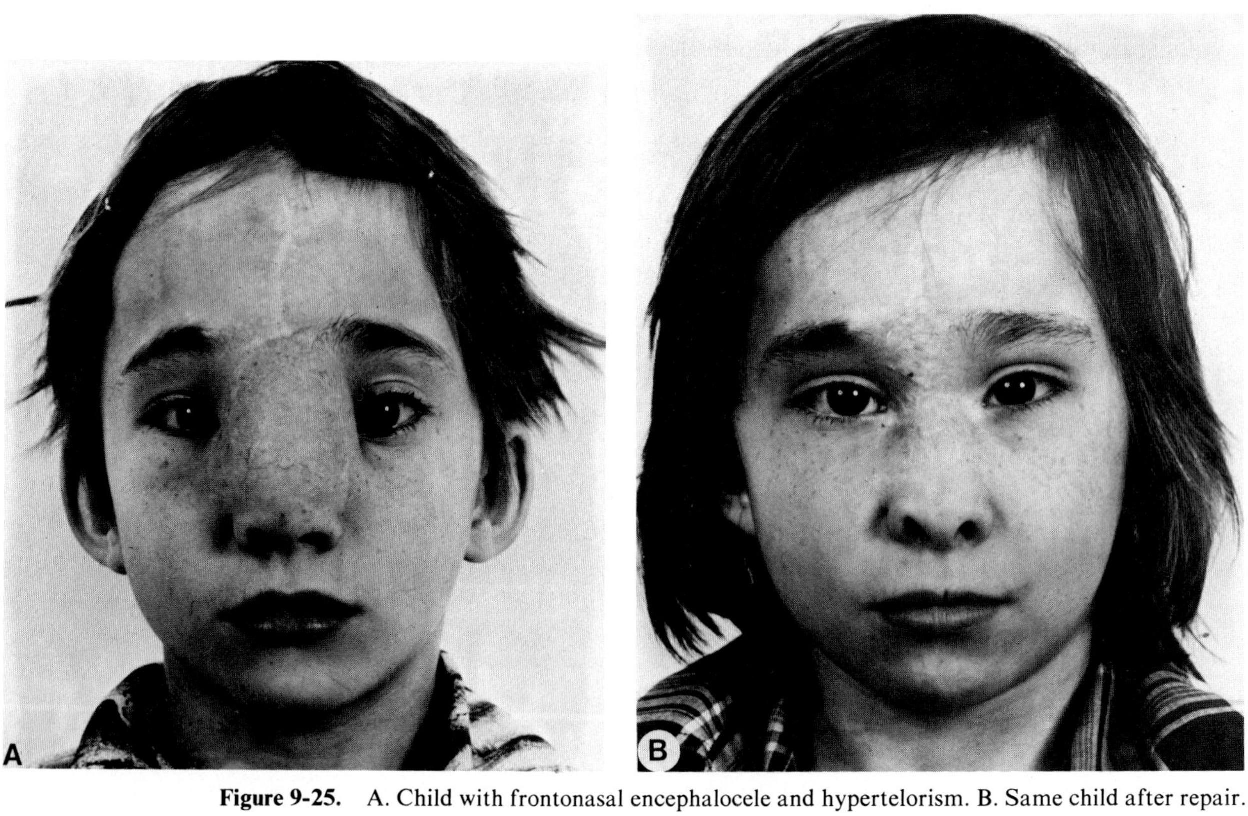

Figure 9-25. A. Child with frontonasal encephalocele and hypertelorism. B. Same child after repair.

from its obstruction by congenital malformation such as encephaloceles (Fig. 9-25).

In the median cleft face syndrome[43] hypertelorism occurs in conjunction with one or more facial malformations, which include a V-shaped frontal hairline (widow's peak), cranium bifidum occultum, median cleft nose, and cleft lip and palate. Hypertelorism can also occur in association with the craniofacial dysmorphic states. Occasionally, hypertelorism is seen as a completely isolated event. In such instances brain development and intellect are always normal (Fig. 9-26).

Tessier[44] described hypertelorism according to the measured distance between the anterior lacrimal crests as seen on skull x-rays. This distance was called the intraorbital distance (IOD). The normal IOD ranges from 18.5 to 29.5 mm in women and from 19.5 to 30.7 mm in men. In first-degree hypertelorism, the IOD is between 30 and 34 mm; in second-degree hypertelorism it is between 34 and 40 mm; and in third-degree cases it is greater than 40 mm.

Earlier attempts at treating hypertelorism consisted only of altering soft-tissue structure. Schmid[45] in 1966 described his experience with shifting the bony medial walls of the orbit. Tessier[46] in 1967 described the now classic procedure for moving both orbits medially, and allowing total correction of hypertelorism.

Unlike most cranial anomalies, hypertelorism is best corrected in the older child or adult. When it coexists with a frontonasal encephalocele, however, a combined repair can be done early in childhood. We have carried this out as early as 10 months of age. In most cases of sincipital encephalocele, however, the

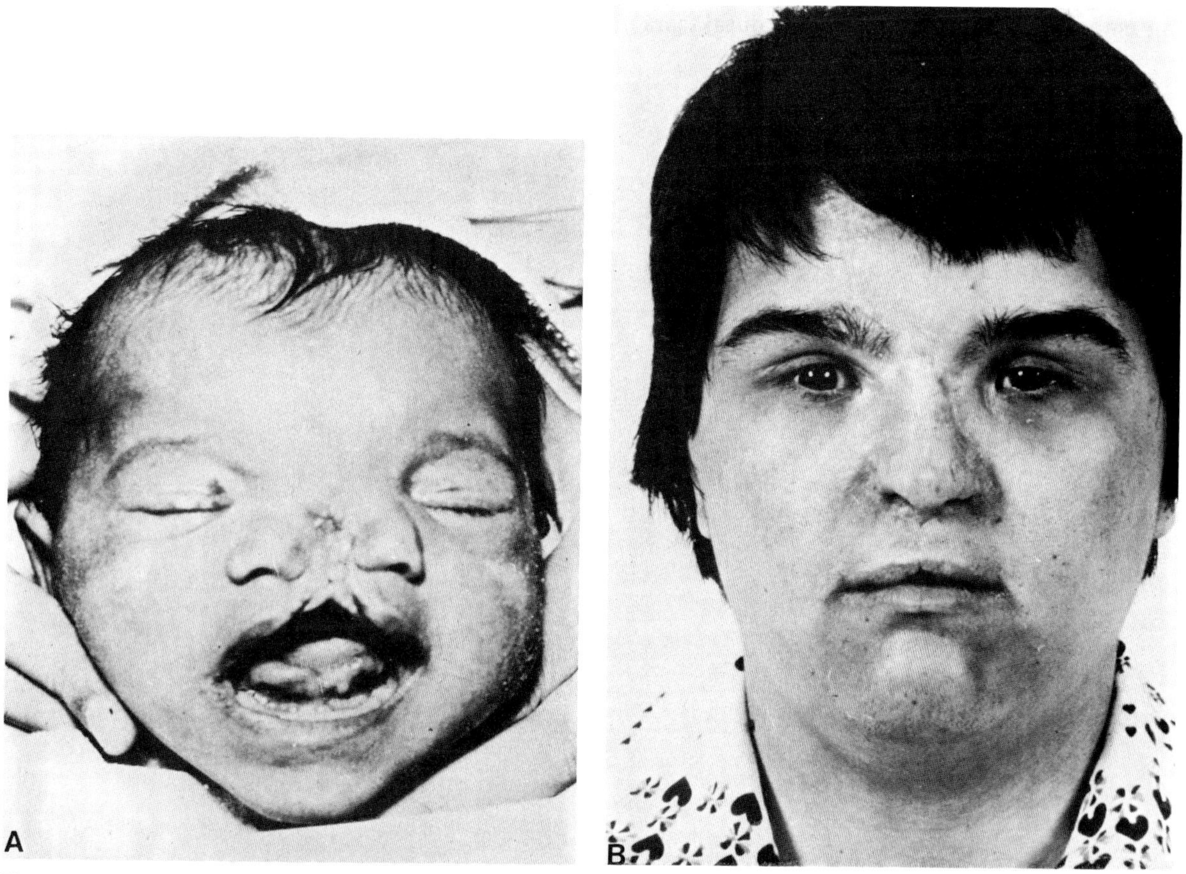

Figure 9-26. A. Infant with median cleft and hypertelorism. B. Same patient after repair of hypertelorism.

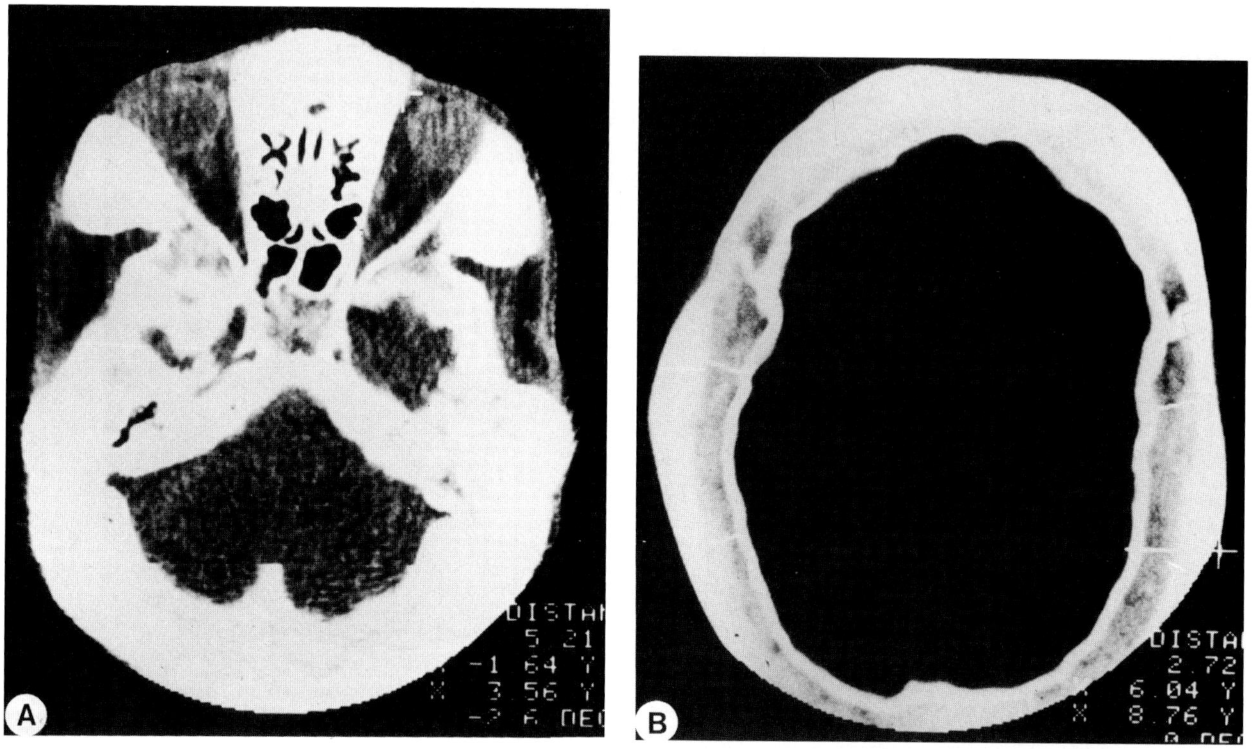

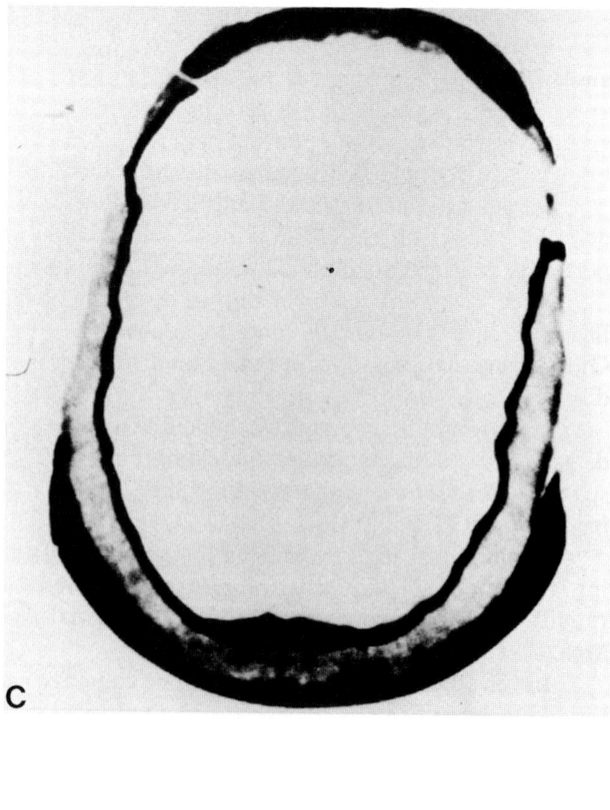

Figure 9-30. A. A CT scan of skull of patient with craniometaphyseal dysplasia showing thickened skull and hypertelorism. B. A CT scan of same patient showing tremendous thickening of cranial vault. C. A. CT scan, same patient, showing reduction in size of vault.

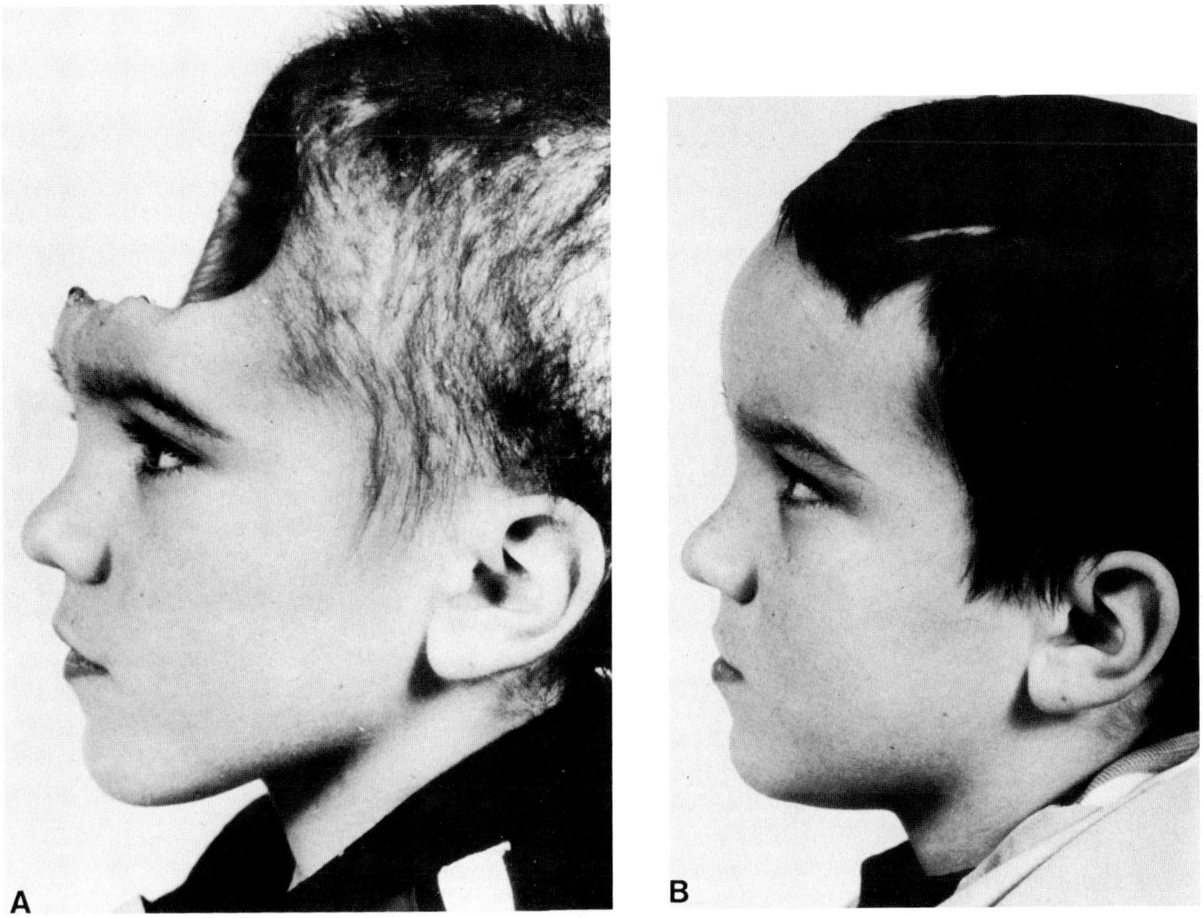

Figure 9-31. A. Young boy with large skull defect after cranial trauma. B. Same child six months after repair of defect with split rib grafts.

In craniometaphyseal dysplasia there is tremendous growth of dense bone in the skull and long bones, resulting in a tremendously enlarged and distorted skull. By using high-speed instruments and the principles of craniofacial surgery, these patients can be given a normal appearance (Fig. 9-30).

Split rib grafts have proved of invaluable use for the repair of large skull defects, particularly when they occur in cosmetically important areas (Fig. 9-31).

Tumors in and about the skull base can be resected, with the resulting defects repaired with rib grafts (Fig. 9-32).

Cranial vault size and shape can be radically altered in a wide variety of disorders, including those cases of gross macrocrania that are the result of inadequate management of infantile hydrocephalus.

CONCLUSIONS

Craniofacial anomalies have become a focus of attention in recent years. Reasonable treatment is being provided at last to patients with these disorders. In the past such patients were objects of ridicule, frequently housed in circuses and amusement parks to be gawked at by idle crowds. Modern surgical techniques have made it possible for these patients to achieve a normal appearance and to lead a normal life.

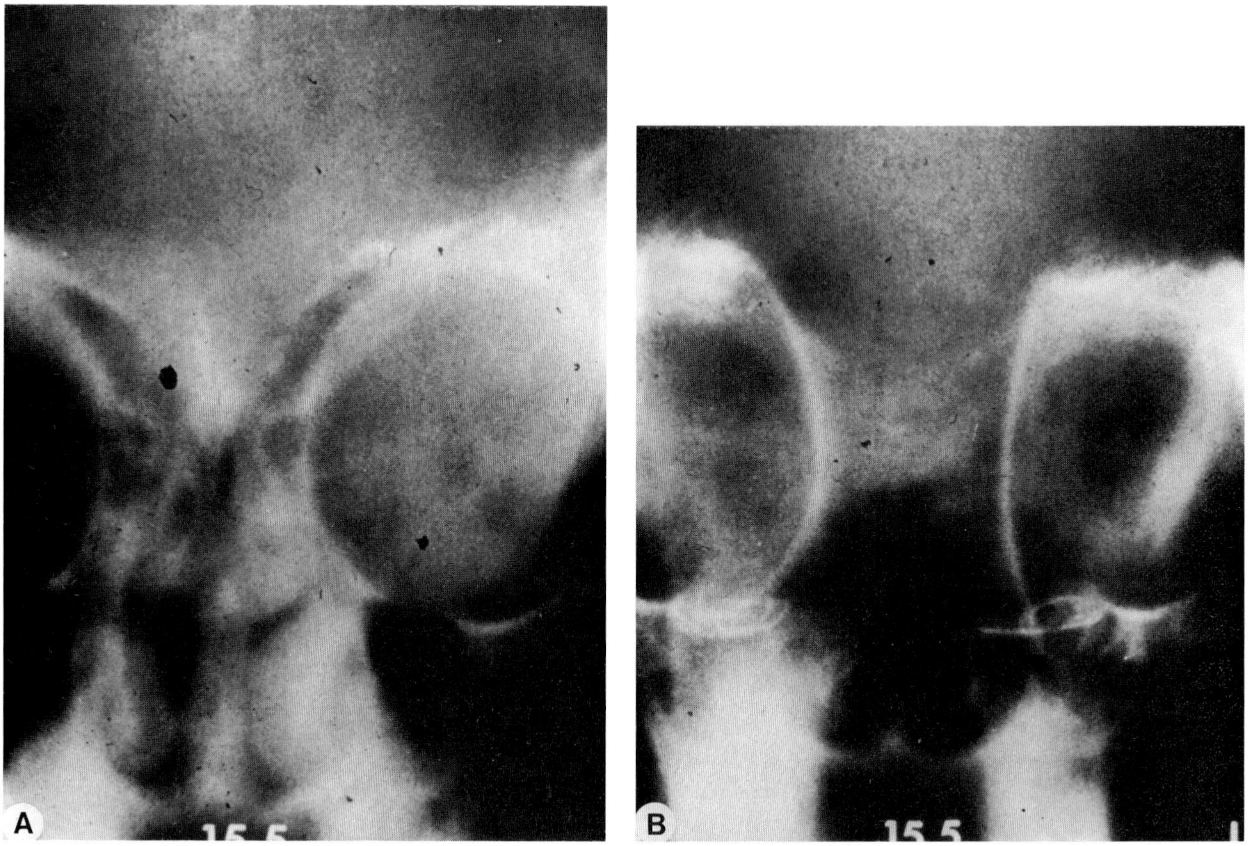

Figure 9-32. A. Facial x-ray of child with recurrent Ewing's sarcoma involving ethmoid air cells. B. Following block resection of ethmoid air cells, the orbital walls have been reconstructed of split rib grafts.

REFERENCES

1. Virchow R: Uber den Cretinismus, Namentlich in Franken und uber pathologische Schadelformen. Verh Phys-Med Ges Wurzburg 2:230, 1851
2. Greig DM: Oxycephaly. Edinburgh Med J 33:189–218, 1926
3. Apert E: De l'acrocephalosyndactylie. Bull Meme Soc Med Hop Paris 23:1310, 1906
4. Crouzon O: Dysostose cranio-faciale hereditaire. Bull Meme Soc Med Hop Paris 33:545, 1912
5. Vincken PJ, Bruyn GW: Handbook of Clinical Neurology, vol 30, Part 1, Congenital Malformations of the Brain and Skull. Amsterdam; Elsevier North-Holland, 1977, pp 219–255
6. Lannelongue M: De la craniectomie dans la microcephalie. CR Acad Sci Paris 110:1382, 1890
7. Faber HK, Towne EB: Early craniectomy as a preventive measure in oxycephaly and allied conditions: With special reference to the prevention of blindness. Am J Med Sci 173:701, 1927
8. Larsen H: Die Schadeldeformat mit Augensymptomen. Klin Monatsbl Augenheilkd 51:145, 1913
9. Bertelsen TI: The premature synostosis of the cranial sutures. Acta Ophthalmol suppl 51:63, 97–113, 1958
10. Anderson FM, Johnson FI: Craniosynostosis: A modification in surgical treatment. Surgery 40:961, 1956
11. Hirsch J, Renier D, Saint-Rose C: Intracranial pressure in craniostenosis. Ninth Meeting, International Society for Pediatric Neurosurgery, Budapest, Hungary, July 20–22, 1981

12. Hemple DJ, Harris LE, Svien HJ, et al: Craniosynostosis involving the sagittal suture only: Guilt by association? J Pediat 58:342, 1961
13. Freeman JM, Berkowf S: Craniostenosis review of the literature and report of thirty-four cases. Pediatrics 30:57, 1962
14. Shillito J, Matson DD: Craniosynostosis: A review of 519 surgical patients. Pediatrics 41:829, 1968
15. Simmons DR, Peyton WT: Premature closure of the cranial sutures. J Pediat 31:528, 1947
16. Ingraham FD, Matson DD, Alexander E Jr: Experimental observations in the treatment of craniosynostosis. Surgery 23:252, 1948
17. Keener EB: Experimental observations on the use of rubber in the treatment of craniosynostosis. J Neurosurg 15:642, 1958
18. Foltz EL, Loeser JD: Craniosynostosis. J Neurosurg 43:48 1975
19. Higginbottom MC, Jones KL, James HE: Intrauterine constraint and craniosynostosis. Neurosurgery 6:39–44, 1980
20. Reilly BJ, Leeming JM, Fraser D: Craniosynostosis in the rachitic spectrum. J Pediat 64:396, 1964
21. Moss ML: The pathogenesis of premature cranial synostosis in man. Acta Anat (Basel), 37:351, 1959
22. Norwood CW, Alexander E Jr, Davis CH, et al: Recurrent and multiple suture closures after craniectomy for craniosynostosis. J Neurosurg 41:715, 1974
23. Bergsma D: Birth Defects and Atlas and Compendium. Baltimore, Williams & Wilkins, 1973
24. Cohen MM: Genetic perspectives on craniosynostosis and syndromes with craniosynostosis. J Neurosurg 47:886, 1977
25. Holtermuller K, Wiedemann HR: Kleeblattschadel syndrom Med Wochenschr 14:439, 1960
26. Jabour JT, Taybi H: Craniotelencephalic dysplasia. Am J Dis Child 108:627, 1964
27. McPherson E, Hall JG, Hickman R: Chromosome 7 short arm deletion and craniosynostosis: A 7P-syndrome. Genetics 35:117, 1976
28. Bell HS, Clare FB, Wentworth AF: Familial scaphocephaly. J Neurosurg 18:239, 1962
29. Shillito J: A new cranial suture appearing in the site of craniectomy for synostosis. Radiology 107:83, 1973
30. Rougerie J, Derome P, Anquez L: Craniostenosis et dysmorphies cranio-faciales: Principles d'une nouvelle technique de traitment et ses resultats. Neurochirurgie 18:429, 1972
31. Stein SC, Schut L: Management of scaphocephaly. Surg Neurol 7:153, 1977
32. Venes J, Sayers MP: Sagittal synostectomy: Technical note. J Neurosurg 44:390, 1976
33. Jane L, Edgerton MT, Futrell W, et al: Immediate correction of sagittal synostosis. J Neurosurg 49:705, 1978
34. Tessier P: Osteotomies totales de la face, syndrome de Crouzon, syndrome d'Apert, oxycephalies, scaphocephalies, turricephalies. Ann Chir Plast 12:273–286, 1967
35. Seeger JF, Gabrielson TO: Premature closure of the frontosphenoidal suture in synostosis of the coronal suture. Radiology 101:631, 1971
36. Hoffman HJ, Mohr G: Lateral canthal advancement of the supraorbital margin: A new corrective technique in the treatment of coronal synostosis. J Neurosurg 45:376–381, 1976
37. Longacre JJ: The early reconstruction of congenital hypoplasia of the facial skeleton and skull surgical management of facial deformation secondary to craniosynostosis, in Longacre JJ (ed): Craniofacial Anomalies. Pathogenesis and Repair. Philadelphia, Lippincott, 1968, pp 151–161
38. Osaka K, Matsumoto S: Holoprosencephaly in neurosurgical practice. J Neurosurg 48:787, 1978
39. Anderson FM, Gwinn JL, Todt JC: Trigonocephaly: Identity and surgical treatment. J Neurosurg 19:723, 1962
40. Matson DD: Surgical treatment of congenital anomalies of the coronal and metopic sutures. J Neurosurg 17:413, 1960

41. Rathbun JC: Hypophosphatasia, a new developmental anomaly. J Dis Child 75:822, 1948
42. Fraser D: Hypophosphatasia. Am J Med 22:730, 1957
43. Demyer W: The median cleft face syndrome: Differential diagnosis of cranium bifidum occultum; hypertelorism and median cleft nose, lip, and palate. Neurology 17:961, 1967
44. Tessier P: Experiences in the treatment of orbital hypertelorism. Plast Reconstruct Surg 53:1, 1974
45. Schmid E: Surgical management of hypertelorism, in Longacre JJ (ed): Craniofacial Anomalies, Pathogenesis and Repair. Philadelphia, Lippincott, 1968, pp 155–161
46. Tessier P, Guiot G, Rougerie J, et al: Osteotomies cranio-naso-orbito-faciales hypertelorisma. Ann Chir Plast 12:103, 1967

10. Anomalies of the Craniocervical Junction

Steven L. Wald
Robert L. McLaurin

Anomalies of the craniovertebral junction have been a source of confusion to the clinician since the first description of deformity of the skull base by Ackermann in 1790.[60] The extent of involvement of bony, neural, or meningeal elements, the relationship to clinical symptomatology, and the pattern of association with other skeletal or neural structures are diverse and complicated. Multiple classifications have been proposed based on presumed etiology, functional presentation, radiologic findings, and dynamic pathophysiology. While each of these offer particular advantages, a basic understanding of the embryologic development[43] in this area is required and aids in the understanding and classification of the various bony anomalies of the craniocervical junction.

EMBRYOLOGY

The skull base (chondrocranium) and occipital bone develop by the process of membrane formation, chondrification, and ossification. Ossification is either of the membranous or endochondral type. Endochondral ossification involves the passage from a stage of mesodermal differentiation to cartilage and then bone. Membranous ossification proceeds from the stage of mesenchymal differentiation to a prebone stage and does not involve a cartilaginous phase. The skull base is formed entirely by endochondral ossification whereas the occipital squama is formed by both processes.

Condensation of the mesoderm around the notochord forms two masses of tissues, referred to as the prechordal and parachordal cartilages. As chondrification proceeds the parachordal cartilage or basal plate fuses with the rostral four occipital sclerotomes and forms an unsegmented cartilage that extends from the sella turcica to the anterior lip of the foramen magnum (Fig. 10-1). Four ossification centers then develop around the foramen magnum (Fig. 10-2). The basioccipital bone gives rise to the central part of the skull base or clivus. The

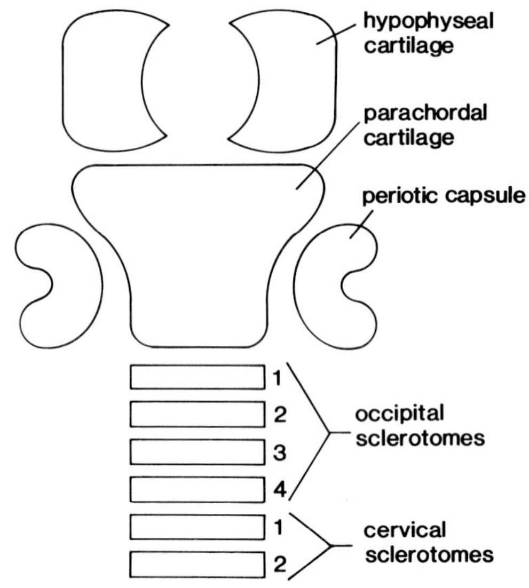

Figure 10-1. Chondrification of craniocervical junction.

paired exoccipital bones develop on either side of the foramen magnum, eventually forming its lateral boundaries as well as the hypoglossal canals and the occipital condyles. The squamosal portion of the occipital bone develops from supraoccipital and interparietal centers. The interparietal portion, located above the mendosal suture, is the only part of the occipital bone to undergo membranous ossification. These two centers are fused at birth; fusion between the other centers occurs postnatally. Ossification between the sphenoid and basioccipital bone begins at age 12 with closure completed between 16 and 20 years of age.[67]

The atlas is formed by the fusion of the caudal half of the last occipital sclerotome and the cranial and caudal halves of the first cervical sclerotome. The first cervical sclerotome also gives rise to the odontoid process. The tip of the odontoid is probably derived from the most caudal occipital sclerotome, although disagreement persists on this point.

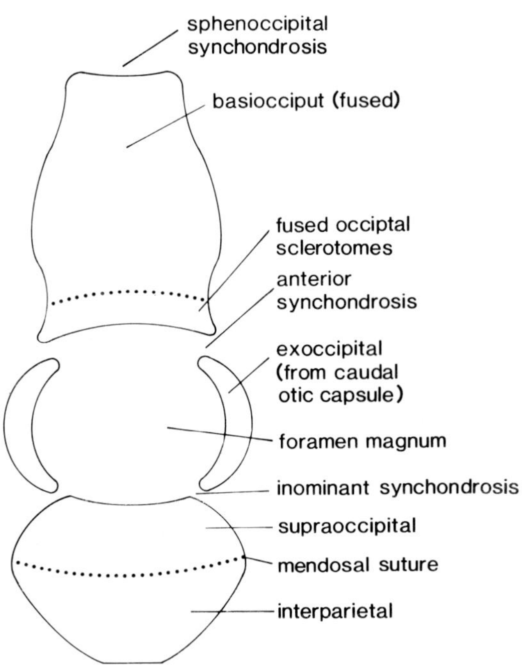

Figure 10-2. Ossification of craniocervical junction.

RADIOLOGIC ANATOMY AND MEASUREMENTS

Multiple roentgenologic methods and measurements have been devised for evaluation of the craniocervical junction. While each is valuable for determining certain aspects of anatomic relationships, differences in technique, lack of specificity, dependence on facial structures, and variance during flexion or extension require that multiple views and positions be obtained. Standard views are usually suggestive of an abnormality of the craniovertebral region, but tomography is often required to clarify pathologic relationships and is particularly valuable for demonstrating normal and pathologic sutures and synchondroses.

Standard radiologic measurements include the basilar angle, Bull's angle,[6] Chamberlain's line,[10] McGregor's line,[50] the digastric line of Fischgold and Metzger,[25] the bimastoid line,[25] the height index,[38] and the anterior–posterior dimension of the foramen magnum.[52] The basilar angle is drawn from the nasion to the tuberculum sella to the anterior lip of the foramen magnum. (Fig. 10-3). This angle should not exceed 140 degrees. Chamberlain's line extends from the posterior aspect of the hard palate to the posterior rim of the foramen magnum (Fig. 10-3). McGregor's line joins the posterior end of the hard palate to the lowest point of the occipital bone. The digastric line joins the digastric notches. The bimastoid line connects the mastoid tips and should be within 2 mm of the odontoid tip. Klaus' height index is determined by drawing a line from the tuberculum sella to the internal occipital protuberance and measuring the distance from this line to the tip of the odontoid. The normal anterior–posterior diameter of the foramen magnum, as described by McRae and Barnum,[52] should exceed 19 mm.

In many instances myelography is required to elucidate the relationships of bony abnormalities to neural structures. Supine myelography is considered a necessary part of the procedure by some authors.[80] Dynamic testing may be done and is useful in planning surgical therapy. Vertebral angiography has been studied,[3] but its usefulness is questioned. Computerized tomography (CT) of basal structures has been recently employed to visualize abnormal bony relation-

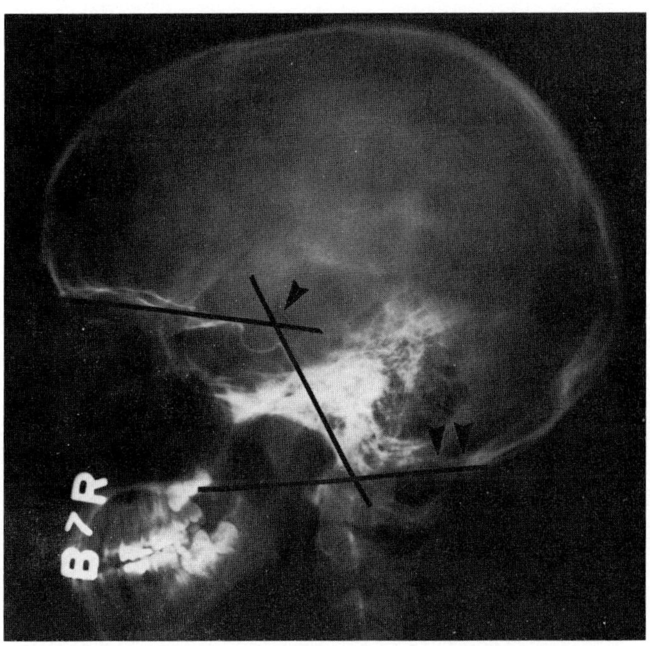

Figure 10-3. Chamberlain's line (double arrow) and basilar angle (single arrow).

ships about the foramen magnum.[58] This procedure, combined with contrast augmentation and myelography, may provide valuable information as further experience with the technique is gained.

ANOMALIES OF THE CRANIOVERTEBRAL JUNCTION

As shown in Tables 10-1, 10-2, and 10-3, numerous bony abnormalities have been reported about the craniocervical junction. Many of these anomalies are found in combination with other skeletal dysplasias and combinations of anomalies involving the cranial base and cervical spine are common. Furthermore many of these are asymptomatic and only called to attention during incidental radiographic procedures. Discussion of the various craniovertebral anomalies will concentrate on those lesions with symptomatic manifestations and their surgical management.

MALFORMATIONS OF THE BASIOCCIPUT AND FORAMEN MAGNUM

Basilar Impression

The literature is replete with examples of basilar impression and platybasia. As pointed out by O'Connell and Turner,[60] Rokitansky in 1844 clearly described indentation of the skull by the cervical spine, followed by a more detailed report by Berg and Retzius in 1855.[2] These two terms have been used synonymously, although they represent different processes. Platybasia implies an abnormal basilar angle (more than 140 degrees) such that the basiocciput or clivus assumes a more horizontal course with respect to the axis of the spine. This is of primary interest to anatomists and anthropologists, but has had little use in clinical medicine.

Basilar impression or invagination represents the upward displacement of the margins of the foramen magnum into the posterior fossa (Fig. 10-4). The elevation is most prominent medially such that the rim of the foramen magnum curves upward while the lateral parts of the posterior fossa angle downward.[80] There is reduction of volume in the posterior fossa and an irregular contour to the foramen magnum. The cerebellar tonsils may be situated below the rim of the foramen magnum as in an Arnold–Chiari deformity. The abnormal tonsillar herniation, however, is not usually representative of a true Arnold–Chiari malformation as the cervical roots will pass in the usual rostral-caudal direction and associated anomalies are not present. The clivus is reduced in length.[65]

Etiology

The causes of basilar impression can be divided into primary or congenital and secondary or acquired (Table 10-1). Although considerable areas of overlap exist and combinations of abnormalities are common, primary causes represent a true congenital malformation while secondary basilar impression is associated with a disease process leading to structural change in the skull base. Acquired basilar impression is relatively rare, being found in only 3 to 8 percent of all cases.[65] Paget's disease is the most frequently mentioned secondary cause.[64] Abnormalities of bone and calcium metabolism are rarely reported to produce basilar impression. Traumatic basilar impression is extremely rare, although trauma of varying intensity has been reported as a precipitating event.[60]

While many instances of presumed congenital etiology can be found in the

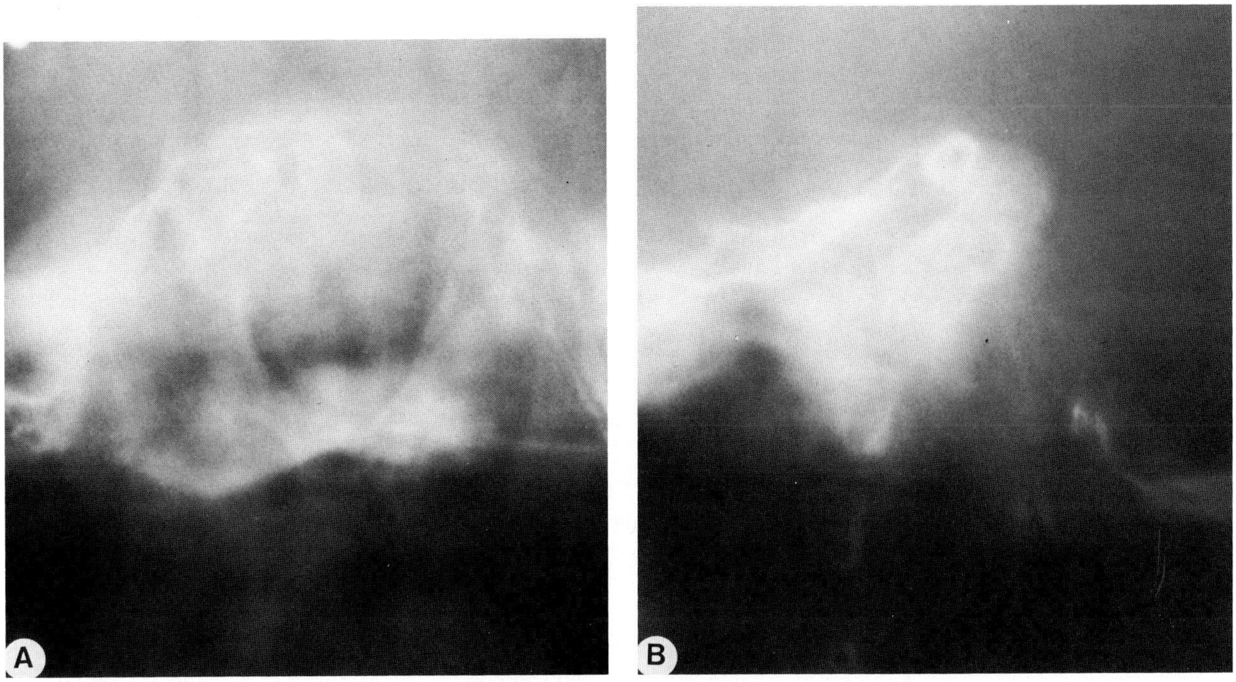

Figure 10-4. Tomograms of severe basilar impression due to osteogenesis imperfecta. A. Anteroposterior. B. Lateral.

Table 10-1
Malformations of the Basiocciput and Foramen Magnum

- Basilar Impression[33,53,60]
  - Primary or congenital
    - Down's syndrome[56]
    - Achondroplasia[47,70,78]
    - Mucopolysaccharidosis
    - Arnold–Chiari malformation[15,16,27]
    - Cleidocranial dysplasia[37,49]
    - Osteogenesis imperfecta[34,49,60]
  - Secondary or acquired
    - Osteomalacia[9,35]
    - Paget's disease[73]
    - Fibrous dysplasia[38]
    - Rickets
    - Hypothyroidism[22]
    - Hyperparathyroidism[44]
    - Neoplastic[18]
    - Infectious
    - Traumatic
- Basioccipital Clefts[36,40,46,65,75]
- Hypoplasia of the Clivus[17]
- Occipital Condylar Hyperplasia[18,39,68]
- Third Occipital Condyle[46,54,68]
- Occipital Vertebra[46,54]
- Paracondylar Processes[65,68]
- Basilar Processes[13,65,68]
- Bone Masses on the Anterior Rim of the Foramen Magnum[13,65]
- Persistent Mendosal Suture
- Premature Closure of the Occipital Synchondroses[11,39]

literature, the paucity of clinical reports in infants and younger children is striking. Gardner[28] and Lindgren[44] felt that the invagination could be explained by the transition from a recumbent posture to an upright stature. The weight of the relatively heavy skull and brain presumably exerts more pressure than the craniocervical junction can support. While the disease is congenital, the bony abnormality is developmental. In addition constant radiographic landmarks required for measurements are obscured in the infant by incomplete ossification and calcification of the chondrocranium and cervical spine.

Congenital causes of basilar impression are represented by a group of diseases characterized by both biochemical and structural bony abnormalities of a genetic origin. Achondroplasia is inherited as an autosomal dominant. Inadequate endochondral bone formation leads to retardation of growth of the skull base. The clivus is shortened and assumes a more vertical orientation. The posterior fossa is deformed, but recent studies indicate that its volume is preserved by a compensatory elevation of the tentorium.[63] The odontoid is high, although Pierre-Kahn, Hirsch, Renier, et al.[63] found true basilar impression in only one of 10 patients. The atlas lies in close proximity to the occiput. Atlantoccipital assimilation has not been reported, although fibrous fusion between the posterior arch and occiput is implied[12] and may account for the radiographic appearance of basilar impression. Significant deformation and stenosis of the foramen magnum are characteristic.[47,63,78]

Down's syndrome also involves the skull base and foramen magnum. Michejda and Menolascino,[56] in reviewing this topic, suggested multiple factors that might be responsible or play a role in the abnormal development of the basiocciput. Delayed fusion of basal synchondroses coupled with endocrinologic factors and abnormal mucopolysaccaride metabolism are areas requiring further research.

Associated Conditions

Herniation of the cerebellar tonsils has often been reported with basilar impression.[15,16,27,71] While these two entities are seen in association and as isolated malformations, supporting a primary congenital etiology, tonsillar herniation has also been described in secondary basilar impression.[23] Debate continues regarding the etiology of the Arnold–Chiari complex and the exact interplay of basilar impression and tonsillar herniation remains to be elucidated.

Although less frequent the association of basilar impression and syringomyelia is reported.[32,51,64] Again it is very difficult to determine whether the syrinx is primary or secondary, as symptomatology may be related to either lesion.

Other skeletal malformations have been reported in association with basilar impression.[65] Associated anomalies include a high arched palate, poly- and syndactyly, pes cavus, iris heterochromia, Sprengel's deformity, scoliosis, torticollis, and skull abnormalities.

Symptoms

Basilar impression is a radiologic abnormality and as such may or may not be associated with clinical symptomatology. In infants developmental abnormalities in the region of the craniocervical junction are often accompanied by hydrocephalus, whereas in the symptomatic adult or adolescent ventricular dilatation is much less frequent. The onset of symptoms is insidious and usually progressive. Diffuse, bilateral headache and occipital pain, often precipitated by head movement, are the most common complaints. The pain is often most severe in the morning and may be unilateral, resembling occipital neuralgia. Weakness of one or both legs or arms, paresthesias, and dysesthesias are less frequently reported. Complaints referrable to cranial nerve dysfunction include diplopia, facial pain, dysphagia, and hearing disturbances. Symptoms attributed to disruption of the vertebrobasilar circulation are drop attacks, transient paralysis, and amaurosis fugax.[72]

Signs

A characteristic physical feature, although infrequently noted, is a stocky, short neck with restriction of passive movements of the head. Facial asymmetry may accompany this finding.

Neurologic signs can be grouped into those causing disturbances of the cerebellum, of the pyramidal tracts, and of the cranial nerves. Rarely do these signs occur in isolation. Nystagmus is the most common sign of basilar impression but is nonspecific. It may be in any direction and is reported to be supravestibular in origin.[65] Ataxia and dysmetria are less frequently found.

Spastic paraparesis is the most common initial sign pointing to the pyramidal tract. Upper extremity paresis rarely occurs as the only or predominant sign. Sensory changes are usually not striking, although pain of a sharp, shooting nature may be elicited (Lhermitte sign). Bladder disturbance is rare.

Hypoglossal paresis may be the only neurologic sign.[65] Accessory nerve palsy is more common than it is reported. Vocal cord paresis and dysarthria point to the vagus or its branches. Facial paresis and trigeminal involvement have been recorded.[1,61]

Radiographic Investigation

As previously noted a complete skull series and cervical spine survey are always indicated. Careful determination of relationships of structures to constructed lines is required and will often lead to the diagnosis as well as suggest the need for tomography. The odontoid tip should not be greater than 5 mm above Chamberlain's line or 7 mm above McGregor's line.[33] The normal distance of the digastric line is 10 mm and is reduced in the presence of invagination. The digastric line is the upper limit in position of the odontoid tip.[18] Klaus' height index should not be less than 30 mm. McRae's line, the anteroposterior diameter of the foramen magnum, should be greater than 19 mm.

Additional Investigation

Electroencephalogram abnormalities have been reported in 45 percent of 50 patients.[65] Cerebrospinal fluid studies are nonspecific, with protein elevations observed in a substantial number of patients.

Differential Diagnosis

Basilar impression must be differentiated from other lesions of the posterior fossa and foramen magnum. Tumors of the brain stem, cerebellum, and fourth ventricle rarely produce the characteristic bone changes and are often associated with hydrocephalus, which is not common in uncomplicated basilar impression. McRae has presented 68 patients, noting their referring diagnosis at the time of admission.[54] These include multiple sclerosis, cervical fracture or dislocation, degenerative spinal disease, spinocerebellar degenerative disease, and hysteria. To this can be added myelitis, amyotrophic lateral sclerosis, and variants of bulbar and pseudobulbar palsy.

Treatment

In the presence of significant and particularly progressive symptomatology, treatment is directed to providing adequate space. While conservative measures, including head and neck immobilization, may offer temporary relief, surgical decompression is eventually required.

Standard neurosurgical treatment has consisted of occipital craniectomy to include excision of the posterior rim of the foramen magnum and bilateral cervical decompressive laminectomy. The dura is opened and arachnoid adhesions, if present, are lysed. The dura is left open or, preferably, a graft is employed. Prior to 1960 the operative mortality was as high as 36 percent, but recent operative experience indicates a mortality of 5 percent.[20,62] Nearly two thirds of patients are either improved or demonstrate cessation of their progressive disease.[19]

Menezes, VanGilder, Graf, et al.[55] have formulated a physiologic approach to the cervicomedullary region based on the mechanism of compression and the ability to achieve reduction at the craniocervical junction. Myelography with pluridirectional tomography demonstrated the direction of compression and dictated the surgical approach. Patients with anterior compression underwent resection of the offending structure—odontoid, clivus, or atlas—by a transoral approach.[30] Instability required posterior or posterolateral fusion. Dorsal impingement on neural structures was treated by suboccipital craniectomy and cervical decompression. All patients were improved or recovered and morbidity was minimal.

BASIOCCIPITAL CLEFTS

Retention of sclerotomal segmentation results in complete or partial clefts or fissures in the basiocciput. They are best visualized using a modified Water's projection and tomography. The clefts are similar to the normal synchondroses, being smooth, often paired, and 3–5 mm in depth.[36] They may be associated with additional fetal malformations or be entirely asymptomatic.

OCCIPITAL CONDYLAR HYPOPLASIA

Hypoplasia of the occipital condyles is most commonly asymptomatic. Because of the relatively elevated position of the atlas, the foramen magnum may be compromised, producing neurologic dysfunction. Roentgenograms demonstrate the odontoid to be high in relation to Chamberlain's and McGregor's lines. Anteroposterior tomography reveals elevation of the dens above the digastric line and allows for an estimation of the height of the occipital condyles. Occipital condylar hypoplasia has been described in Morquio's disease, spondyloepiphyseal dysplasia, and Conradi's syndrome.[18,29,35,76]

THIRD OCCIPITAL CONDYLE, OCCIPITAL VERTEBRA, AND OCCIPITALIZATION OF THE ATLAS

Anomalous bony formations around the foramen magnum are difficult to classify because of their diversity. A third condyle is located in the midline above the anterior arch of the atlas, but is separated from the atlas. While it may be a type of occipital vertebra,[46] it should not be misdiagnosed as an occipitalized axis.

Often the lateral condyles are hypoplastic, the atlas is high, and the clivus is short. It is usually asymptomatic, but it may restrict head and neck movements.

Differentiation between an occipital vertebra and an occipitalized atlas is often difficult. McRae[54] has reviewed and established criteria to differentiate these lesions. The lack of a foramen for the passage of the vertebral artery or suboccipital nerve supports a diagnosis of occipital vertebra. Both lesions are usually asymptomatic.

PARACONDYLAR PROCESS

This accessory bony structure extends from the paracondylar surface of the occipital bone toward the transverse process of the atlas. In its pure form, it is asymptomatic, but it is usually found in conjunction with other anomalies of the craniocervical region. The epitransverse process of the atlas is its mirror image projecting from the transverse process of the atlas toward the occiput.

PREMATURE CLOSURE OF THE OCCIPITAL SYNCHONDROSES

As development of the chondrocranium proceeds, sutures between the two exoccipital centers and the basioccipital bone anteriorly (anterior synchondrosis) and the supraoccipital bone posteriorly (innominate synchondrosis) can be seen.

They are easily visualized at 1 year of age and persist until nearly 4 years of age. Premature synostosis of these sutures has been documented by Kruyff.[39] Anterior synostosis results in improper migration and formation of the occipital condyles and asymmetry of the foramen magnum. Of the eight infants reported by Kruyff, all were neurologically intact, although he speculated that problems might develop as the children grew. Careful observation was suggested.

CONGENITAL SKULL DYSPLASIAS

The skeletal dysplasias (Table 10-2) are a diverse group of inherited disorders. Many of these disorders are characterized by prominent changes in the calvarium and others produce pronounced thickening or sclerosis of the skull base and foramen magnum.

Osteopetrosis is a rare disorder characterized by dense, compact, homogeneous bone. Encroachment of the skull base foramina may result in cranial nerve deficits, especially affecting the optic nerve.[42,77]

Pyknodysostosis combines the features of cleidocranial dysostosis and osteopetrosis.[21] The disease is characterized by multiple long bone fractures and a thickened skull base.

Table 10-2
Congenital Skull Dysplasias

Osteopetrosis (Albers–Schonberg disease)[42,77,79]
Pyknodysosteogenesis[21]
Progressive Diaphyseal Dysplasia (Engelmann–Camurati Disease)[69,77]
VanBuchem's Disease[74]
Endemic Fluorosis
Craniometaphyseal Dysplasia (Pyle's Disease)[8,57]
Achondroplasia[47,70,78]

more than a 50 percent reduction of CSF production, a finding that has been used to support the existence of an extrachoroidal source of CSF.[46]

As depicted by Figure 11-3, there are many sites within the CSF–blood–brain compartment in which solvent and solute changes can occur, making it difficult to isolate any portion of the system. The extracellular fluid of the brain is in continuity with and identical in composition to CSF,[3] with the ependyma between these compartments offering no barrier to free exchange.[10]

It is possible that a substantial source of nonchoroidal CSF is the extracellular fluid since it can drain unimpeded into the ventricles. Support for this idea has been given substance by Cserr, Cooper, and Milhorat,[14] who reported that 20 percent of an extracellular marker injected into the brain flowed into the CSF. These findings would not be at variance with Rall,[60] who calculated that it would require an extracellular fluid flow of greater than 25 percent of CSF formation to produce a distortion in the profile of an extracellular marker and he could find no evidence for such a profile distortion. Available evidence indicates that about 80 percent of CSF is derived from the choroid plexus with the remaining 20 percent originating from another source.

Formation Rate

Open drainage techniques were the first methods used to estimate CSF formation and consisted of either measuring the amount of fluid drained per unit of time or removing a known volume of fluid and recording the time it took to restore the opening CSF pressure. More recently Potts[57] has described a radiologic method whereby the rate of ascent of fluid in the lateral ventricles, whose cross-sectional area has been measured, is used to calculate CSF production. The most accurate method of measuring CSF formation is that of ventricular perfusion, a technique introduced by Papenheimer, Heisey, Held, et al.[30,53] and his associates. This method has been used extensively in animals but has been limited in clinical use as it is invasive. In this technique artificial CSF containing a known concentration of a nondiffusible reference material, such as albumin tagged with an isotope of iodine, which moves only by bulk flow, is infused into the ventricles while CSF is removed from the cisterna magna or lumbar subarachnoid space at a constant low pressure. By quantitating the

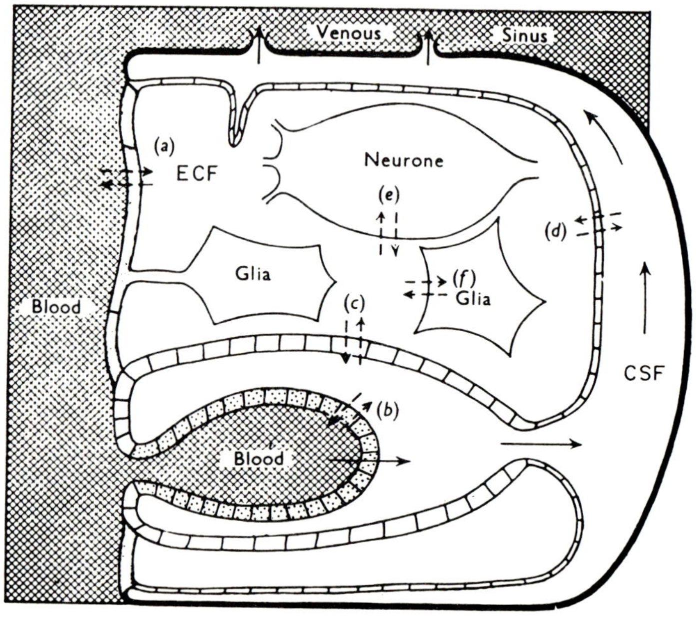

Figure 11-3. Diagrammatic representation of the blood–brain–CSF system. Solid arrows indicate bulk flow of CSF. Broken arrows show sites of possible exchange of CSF and its constituents across the (a) blood–brain barrier, (b) choroidal epithelium, (c) ependyma, (d) pia, and (e), (f) cell membranes of neurons and glia. The thick line is that of the arachnoid–dural boundary. (Reprinted with permission from Davson H, Bradbury MWB: The fluid exchange of the central nervous system. Symposia of the Society for Experimental Biology 19:349, 1965.)

volumes of fluid into and out of the system and measuring the concentration difference of the reference marker in the two fluids, it is possible to calculate the rate of CSF formation. Clinical studies have indicated CSF formation rates of about 20 ml/hr or 500 ml/day.[15,39,61] As the volume of CSF in the ventricles and subarachnoid space averages 150 ml, there is a threefold turnover of CSF daily.

Formation Rate Alterations

Most physical and chemical alterations tend to reduce CSF formation with the one notable exception being that of cholera toxin, which is reported to double CSF output.[24] Drugs that decrease CSF formation do so by interfering with cellular respiration (dinitrophenol) and inhibiting carbonic anhydrase (acetazolamide or furosemide) or Na-K-ATPase (cardiac glycosides).[54] It is not clear as to whether glucocorticoids alter CSF formation as some studies show no change[41,71] while others have shown a diminished production rate.[65,75] Unfortunately, the reduced CSF formation rates have only a transient effect on pressure within the ventricles and the various drugs that diminish CSF production have not been found to be at all useful clinically in the control of hydrocephalus.[15,61]

Welch[78] has reviewed the studies investigating the role of pressure in decreasing CSF production and reports that although the process is pressure responsive, the effect is only slight until high pressures are reached. It is most likely that the effect of pressure occurs at the first stage in CSF production, that of filtration, a concept supported by a recent study.[76]

Clinical and experimental studies on the changes produced by choroid plexectomy have been reported by Milhorat.[46] He noted that the removal of the choroid plexus from the lateral ventricles in hydrocephalic patients rarely results in ventricular diminution, and in most cases the ventricles continue to enlarge. This work also refutes the previous assumption that the pulsations of the choroid plexus are necessary to produce ventricular enlargement.[5] This surgical technique to reduce CSF formation has little to offer for the control of hydrocephalus and has been virtually abandoned.

It has long been suggested that the hydrocephalus associated with a choroid plexus papilloma results from the tumor tissue secreting fluid in excess of the reserve absorptive capacity of the patient since the hydrocephalus can be cured following the removal of the papilloma.[42] Unequivocal evidence of CSF oversecretion by a choroid plexus papilloma has been documented by ventriculolumbar perfusion studies on two occasions.[21,49]

To summarize, in general the means to control hydrocephalus by reducing CSF production do not currently exist; the one exception is the removal of a choroid plexus papilloma.

CEREBROSPINAL FLUID ABSORPTION

Absorption Forces

That CSF drains in response to a pressure gradient has been well demonstrated as the rate of absorption is related to infusion pressure[15,30,35,52,58] and under normal conditions the CSF pressure in the SAS exceeds that of the superior sagittal sinus.[69,74] In addition to this hydrostatic force, Weed[73] proposed an additive colloid osmotic force similar to that promulgated by Starling for the distal end of a capillary. Such a pressure by necessity would require the presence of a semipermeable membrane. This concept was called into question by Davson,[16] who argued that as the brain had no lymphatic system, there must exist a way to remove substances as large as plasma proteins and the presence of a semipermeable membrane would preclude this. Subsequent physiologic studies[18,79] have confirmed the lack of a colloid osmotic force. Although studies have shown that pinocytosis by endothelial cells is influenced by pressure,[2,28] this process may not be metabolically dependent because the absorptive process is reported to be unaltered by the death of the animal.[84] The only proven force responsible for CSF absorption thus is that of a hydrostatic gradient from the SAS to the venous sinuses.

Absorption at the Arachnoid Villus

The arachnoid villi are clusters of cells that project from the SAS through the dura into the adjacent venous structures. Electron micrographic studies[1,68] have shown that the villi are covered by a layer of endothelium continuous with that of the inner surface of the venous sinuses. Those villi that are grossly visible are called arachnoid granulations or pacchionian bodies.

Key and Retzius[36] in 1875 were the first to propose that the CSF drains into the venous system via the arachnoid villi through open channels. Weed[72] confirmed their observation as to the site of drainage but was convinced that the process was one of filtration through an intact (i.e., semipermeable) membrane. This concept was seriously challenged by Welch, Pollay, and Friedman,[56,79,80] who observed the presence of pressure-responsive open channels that permitted the one-way passage of particulate matter as large as intact erythrocytes from the SAS into the venous sinuses.

Initial light and electron micrographic studies indicated open communication between the SAS and the venous sinuses.[33,34,79] Subsequent reports took issue with this finding and characterized the endothelial covering of the villus as having tight junctions, continuous, and without openings.[1,2,68] Additional work on the subject by Gomez, Potts, Deonarine, et al.[27,28,59] have validated the original views of open communications from the SAS to the venous sinuses with endothelial-lined tubules (Fig. 11-4). The discrepancy in anatomic findings may relate to the pressure at which the villus is fixed since when the fixation is at a zero pressure gradient, it is collapsed and the channels are not evident.

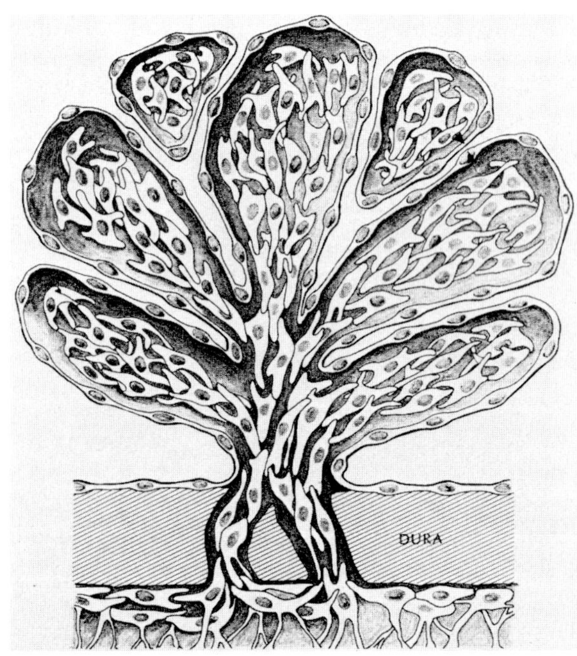

Figure 11-4. Diagrammatic representation of an arachnoid granulation projecting through the dura into a venous sinus. Arachnoid cells from the SAS extend into the granulation to become its stroma. Endothelium lining the venous sinus covers the surface of the granulation and extends into its fissures and tubules. On a single micrographic section it is not possible to demonstrate continuity of the endothelial-lined tubules from the SAS to the venous sinus, a fact that has led some observers to disclaim the presence of open channels. Physiologic studies, however, give strong support for these openings. (Reprinted with permission from Potts DG, Reilly KF, Deonarine V: Morphology of the arachnoid villi and granulations. Radiology 105:333–341, 1972.)

Another hypothetical mechanism that could bridge the gap between the open and closed theories of CSF drainage was proposed by Tripathi,[70] who has reported the presence of a dynamic transendothelial vacuolization process during which temporary openings would allow passage of particles and CSF (Fig. 11-5). This concept has been questioned by Welch[78] but, if accepted, it seems more convincing as an additional pathway rather than as the only mechanism by which drainge occurs.

Absorption at Sites Other than the Arachnoid Villus

Other than the arachnoid villus, possible sites for CSF absorption would be the SAS, lymphatics, brain, and choroid plexus. Arachnoid villi have been shown to be present along the spinal nerves[58,81,85] so it is likely that they are the drainage route for studies reporting CSF absorption from the spinal SAS.[12,38] It has thus far been impossible to isolate a portion of the SAS in mammals that lacks arachnoid villi, and hence there are no reliable studies indicating CSF absorption directly from the SAS.[43]

A number of animal studies have shown that substances injected into the ventricles or SAS can be found in the lymphatics of the cervical and spinal nerves, nasal mucosa, and cervical lymph nodes.[7,9,11,25,31,66] Recent experiments in our laboratory have shown that isotopically labeled albumin infused under elevated pressure into the ventricles of rabbits resulted in a high concentration of the tracer in the olfactory bulbs, optic nerves, episcleral tissue, and cervical lymph nodes; there was, however, no evidence of transventricular absorption of CSF.[44]

Usually the brain is not thought to be the site for CSF absorption and, in fact, there is evidence to suggest that it may contribute to the total volume of CSF.[14,45,55] That the hydrocephalic brain might absorb CSF was proposed in 1921 by Wislocki and Putnam.[83] Reports from several laboratories purport to show transventricular absorption in animals made hydrocephalic by the injection

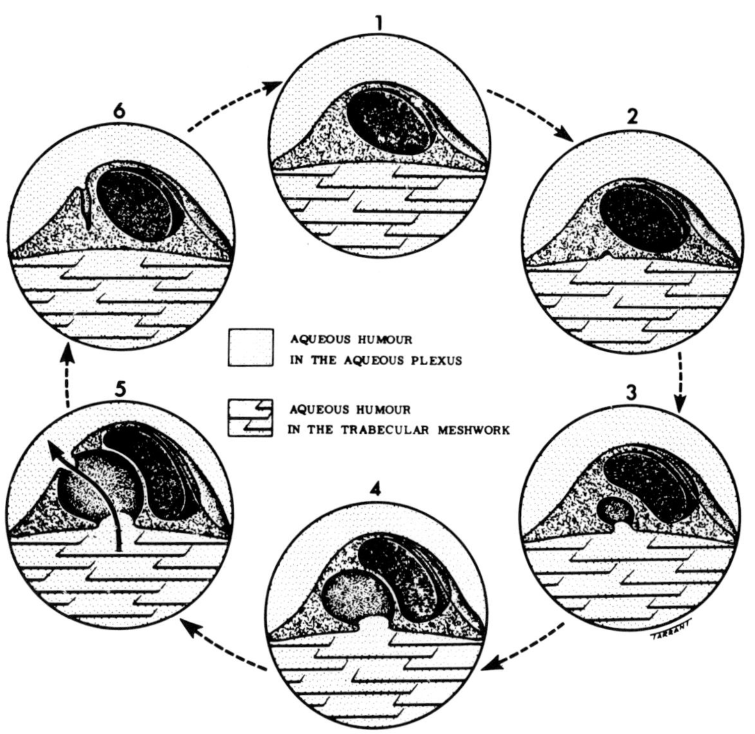

Figure 11-5. Diagrammatic representation of a hypothetical dynamic transendothelial vacuolization process originally described for drainage of aqueous humor and subsequently for CSF absorption. A basal infolding progresses to become a giant vacuole, which in turn becomes a transcellular pore that would permit the bulk flow of fluid and particulate mater. (Reprinted with permission from Tripathi, RC: Mechanisms of aqueous outflow across the trabecular wall of Schlemm's canal. Exp Eye Res 11:116–121, 1971.)

of kaolin into the cisterna magna.[6,64] These studies have subsequently been shown to be invalid because the kaolin model results in CSF being diverted into the dilated central canal of the spinal cord to exit from the filum termanile into the spinal SAS, where it is presumably absorbed by villi.[22,23] The presence of isotopes in the periventricular white matter in the hydrocephalic state as well as edema in the same region detected by computerized tomographic scans has also served as evidence for transventricular absorption.[32,48] This effect, however, can be explained on the basis of molecular movement in response to a concentration or pressure gradient and does not necessarily signify net transfer of CSF. Welch[78] has pointed out that the brain capillaries are impermeable to the reference substances used to indicate net transfer, and since CSF absorption occurs in response to a pressure drop, ventricular pressure would have to be greater than capillary pressure, a condition that would collapse the capillaries and prevent CSF absorption. It is unlikely, therefore, that the hydrocephalic brain absorbs CSF, unless this occurs by an as-yet-unidentified metabolic process.

Studies do suggest that the choroid plexus absorbs approximately one tenth of the total volume of CSF secreted.[63,82] Although there are definite anatomic changes in the choroid plexus that are associated with hydrocephalus,[20] they cannot be equated with CSF absorption. Contrary to one report,[50] experimental evidence indicates little bulk CSF absorption by the choroid plexus in hydrocephalus.[22]

Absorption in Hydrocephalus

Hydrocephalus, with the single exception of oversecretion of CSF by a choroid plexus papilloma,[21,49] results from impairment of CSF absorption.[37,39,47,62] The rate of CSF production in hydrocephalic patients is either normal or near normal,[14,39,61] and unless the CSF continues to accumulate, the rate of absorption must equal the rate of formation. If CSF absorption totally ceased with no decrease in production, the contents of the cranial cavity would be replaced by CSF in approximately three days. As the quantity of CSF retained in the noncompensated state is only a small fraction of the total secretion, the overwhelming majority of CSF output must be absorbed. It is likely that the arachnoid villi are still the site for most CSF absorption in communicating as well as in noncommunicating hydrocephalus since in the latter the obstruction within the ventricular system is usually not complete[29,35] and dilatation of the central canal of the spinal cord, rupture of the lamina terminalis of the third ventricle, and other pathways would allow for the passage of ventricular CSF into the SAS.[4,8,22,23,62]

In summary, the arachnoid villi probably absorb most of the draining CSF in both types of hydrocephalus. Compensatory CSF absorption in hydrocephalus may occur via the lymphatics but it is doubtful that the same is true of the brain or choroid plexus.

REFERENCES

1. Alksne JF, Lovings ET: Functional ultrastructure of the arachnoid villus. Arch Neurol 27:371–377, 1972
2. Alksne JF, White LE Jr: Electron-microscope study of the effect of increased intracranial pressure on the arachnoid villus. J. Neurosurg 22:481–488, 1965
3. Ames A III, Sakanoue M, Endo S: Na, K, Ca, Mg, and Cl concentrations in choroid plexus fluid and cisternal fluid compared with plasma ultrafiltrate. J Neurophysiol 27:672–681, 1964

4. Becker DP, Wilson JA, Watson GW: The spinal cord central canal: Response to experimental hydrocephalus and canal occlusion. J Neurosurg 36:416–424, 1972
5. Bering EA Jr: Circulation of the cerebrospinal fluid. Demonstration of the choroid plexuses as the generator of the force for flow of fluid and ventricular enlargement. J Neurosurg 19:405–413, 1962
6. Bering EA Jr, Sato O: Hydrocephalus: Changes in formation and absorption of cerebrospinal fluid within the cerebral ventricles. J Neurosurg 20:1050–1063, 1963
7. Bradbury MWB: Proportion of cerebrospinal fluid draining into jugular lymphatic trunk of the cat. J Physiol (London) 276:67–68, 1977
8. Bradbury MWB, Lathem W: A flow of cerebrospinal fluid along the central canal of the spinal cord of the rabbit and communications between this canal and the sacral subarachnoid space. J Physiol (London) 181:785–800, 1965
9. Brierley JB, Field EJ: The connexions of the spinal subarachnoid space with the lymphatic system. J Anat 82:153–166, 1948
10. Brightman MW: The intracerebral movement of proteins injected into blood and cerebrospinal fluid of mice. Progr Brain Res 29:19–40, 1968
11. Casley-Smith JR, Foldi-Borcsok E, Foldi M: The prelymphatic pathways of the brain as revealed by cervical lymphatic obstruction and the passage of particles. Br J Exp Path 57:179–188, 1976
12. Coben LA, Smith KR: Iodide transfer at four cerebrospinal fluid sites in the dog: Evidence for spinal iodide carrier transport. Exp Neurol 23:76–90, 1969
13. Cserr HF: Physiology of the choroid plexus. Physiol Rev 51:273–311, 1971
14. Cserr HF, Cooper DN, Milhorat TH: Flow of cerebral interstitial fluid as indicated by the removal of extracellular markers from rats caudate nucleus. Exp Eye Res 25(suppl):461–473, 1977
15. Cutler RWP, Page L, Galicich J, et al: Formation and absorption of cerebrospinal fluid in man. Brain 91:707–720, 1968
16. Davson H: Physiology of the Ocular and Cerebrospinal Fluids. London, Churchill Livingstone, 1956
17. Davson H: Physiology of the Cerebrospinal Fluid, London, Churchill, 1967, 445 pp
18. Davson H, Hollingsworth G, Segal MD: The mechanism of drainage of the cerebrospinal fluid. Brain 93:665–678, 1970
19. Dohrmann GJ: The choroid plexus: A historical review. Brain Res 18:197–218, 1970
20. Dohrmann GJ: The choroid plexus in experimental hydrocephalus. A light and electron microscopic study in normal, hydrocephalic, and shunted hydrocephalic dogs. J Neurosurg 34:56–69, 1971
21. Eisenberg HM, McComb JG, Lorenzo AV: Cerebrospinal fluid overproduction and hydrocephalus associated with choroid plexus papilloma. J Neurosurg 40:381–385, 1974
22. Eisenberg HM, McLennan JE, Welch K: Ventricular perfusion in cats with kaolin induced hydrocephalus. J Neurosurg 41:20–28, 1974
23. Eisenberg HM, McLennan JE, Welch K, et al: Radioisotope ventriculography in cats with kaolin-induced hydrocephalus. Radiology 110:399–402, 1973
24. Epstein MH, Feldman AM, Brusilow SW: Cerebrospinal fluid production: Stimulation by cholera toxin. Science 196:1012–1013, 1977
25. Faber FW: The nasal mucosa and the subarachnoid space. Am J Anat 62:121–148, 1937
26. Gomez DG, Chambers AA, Dibenedetto AT, et al: The spinal cerebrospinal fluid absorptive pathways. Neuroradiology 8:61–66, 1974
27. Gomez DG, Potts DG: Arachnoid villi: Plasticity of the endothelium. J Cell Biol 55:89a, 1972
28. Gomez DG, Potts DG, Deonarine V, et al: Effect of pressure gradient changes on the morphology of arachnoid villi and granulations of the monkey. Lab Invest 26:648–657, 1973
29. Hammock MK, Milhorat TH, Davis DA: Isotope cisternography and ventriculography in the diagnosis of hydrocephalus. Dev Med Child Neurol 16(supp 32):58–71, 1974
30. Heisey SR, Held D, Pappenheimer JR: Bulk flow and diffusion in the cerebrospinal fluid system of the goat. Am J Physiol 203:775–781, 1962

84. Wolfson LI, Katzman R: Infusion manometric test in experimental subarachnoid hemorrhage in cats. Neurology (Minneapolis) 22:856–862, 1972
85. Woollam DHM, Millen JW: Observations on the production and circulation of the cerebrospinal fluid, in Wolstenholme GEW, O'Connor CM (eds): Ciba Foundation Symposium on Production, Circulation and Absorption of the Cerebrospinal Fluid. Boston, Little, Brown, 1958, pp 124–146

12. Circulation of the Cerebrospinal Fluid

Thomas H. Milhorat

Although the discovery of the cerebrospinal fluid (CSF) can be attributed to Cotugno (1764), who proved against all Galenic authority that a watery medium and not a vapor was present within the cerebral ventricles, the circulatory character of this unique body fluid was scarcely recognized until the beginning of the 20th century. In 1914, following a series of ingenious experiments on hydrocephalus, Dandy and Blackfan[1] demonstrated that when the aqueduct of Sylvius was occluded in dogs, the cerebral ventricles proximal to the block would become greatly enlarged and distended with fluid. This important finding was soon confirmed by others and could hardly have left doubt that a significant volume of the CSF was formed continuously within the cerebral ventricles, and that the direction of flow was downward toward the subarachnoid space. Somewhat later, Dandy reported that enlargement of all four ventricles would occur as a consequence of inflammatory scarring of the basilar cisterns,[2] providing additional evidence that, following drainage out of the cerebral ventricles, the route of circulation was upward through the subarachnoid space toward the cerebral convexities.

In recent years the study of the CSF and its disorders has taken on new dimensions. The development of the electron microscope and the introduction of radiopharmaceuticals into clinical and experimental medicine have greatly increased our ability to examine fundamental brain processes, and we can now discuss in a manner unknown to our predecessors the structural basis of the blood–brain barrier, the fine anatomy of the CSF spaces, and molecular transport within the central nervous system.

THE CSF SYSTEM

The CSF system in humans and other higher vertebrates consists of two distinct but continuous compartments: (1) the macroscopic CSF cavities, which encircle the brain and spinal cord in a series of interconnecting channels; and (2) the interstitial space of the brain and spinal cord, which surround individual cellular elements. These two compartments are in direct anatomic continuity, so that the extraparenchymal cavities may be regarded as expanded lacunae of the brain interspaces.[3]

Macroscopic Cavities

The macroscopic CSF cavities consist of three cerebral ventricles, the aqueduct of Sylvius, the fourth (cerebellar) ventricle, the central canal of the spinal cord, and the subarachnoid space (Fig. 12-1). Each cavity is continuous with the next through one or more well-defined openings and the system terminates at the level of the dural sinuses where expansions of the subarachnoid space, the arachnoid villi, protrude into the venous circulation.

The surface of the ventriculo-subarachnoid pathway is lined by a single layer of cells that constitutes a semipermeable membrane. A ciliated, low columnar epithelium, the ependyma, lines the three cerebral ventricles, the aqueduct of Sylvius, the fourth ventricle, and the central canal of the spinal cord. This is an "open" epithelium and lacks tight junctions, except for an investment covering the choroid plexuses. The cisterns and channels of the subarachnoid space, on the other hand, are formed by an inner membrane of pial cells and an outer membrane of arachnoid cells.

Interstitial Space

The interspaces of the brain and spinal cord, in contrast to those in other organs, are comparatively narrow channels that are separated from the vascular compartment by a highly impermeable capillary membrane. This membrane, which forms the structural basis for the blood–brain barrier, is actually a double layer of cells composed of the capillary endothelium and a perivascular investment of astrocytes. In most areas of the brain the cells of the capillary endothelium are joined by pentalaminar tight junctions (zonulae occludentas), which are capable of restricting the intercellular movement of molecules having the diameter of 20 angstroms or more.[5–7] Beyond the blood–brain barrier the brain interspaces form a maze of interconnecting and patent channels that are

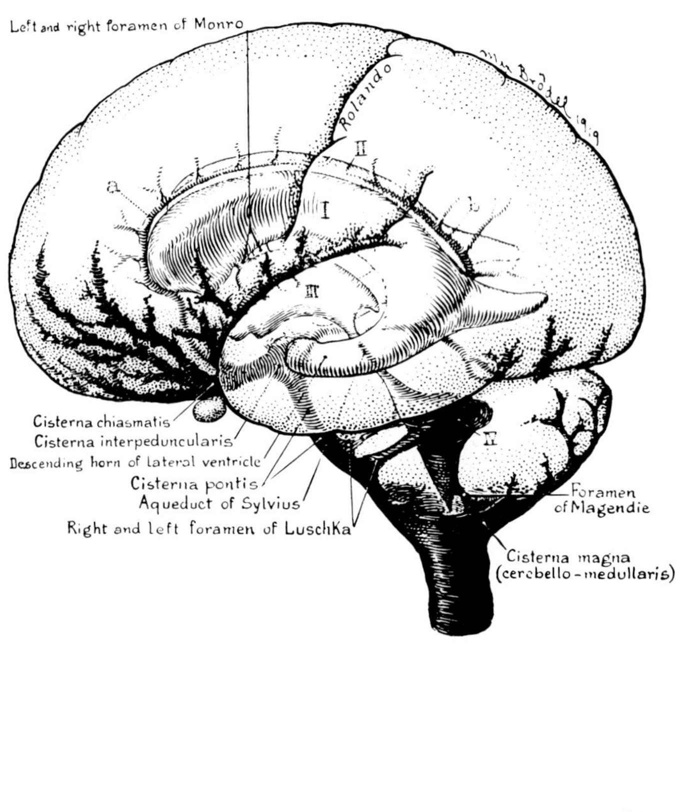

Figure 12-1. The macroscopic CSF spaces. Max Brödel drawing. (Reprinted with permission from Dandy WE: The brain, in Lewis D (ed): Practice of Surgery, vol 12. Hagerstown, WF Prior, 1932.)

anatomically continuous with the adjacent CSF cavities. Brightman[8-10] has demonstrated that when proteins such as ferritin and horseradish peroxidase are injected into the CSF, these large markers move with relative ease between ependymal and pial cells to distribute widely throughout the brain extracellular space. Ventricular perfusion studies, employing a variety of substances including inulin, sulfate, and dextran,[11-13] have shown a similar extracellular distribution. From these and other data it is estimated that the extracellular channels of the brain and spinal cord have an average width of about 150 angstroms.

CSF CIRCULATION

Major Pathways of Flow

On the basis of extensive data concerning the migration of dyes, radioisotopes, and other tracers injected into the CSF, it now is firmly established that the CSF flows in bulk from sites of origin to sites of absorption (Fig. 12-2). The fluid that is formed in the lateral ventricles passes out through the paired interventricular foramina of Monro to reach the third ventricle. The CSF then flows caudally through the aqueduct of Sylvius and fourth ventricle where it passes into the subarachnoid space by one of three exits. It may exit through the paired lateral foramina of Luschka, which direct fluid around the brain stem into the cerebellopontine angle and prepontine cisterns, or through the midline foramen of Magendie, which directs fluid through the vallecula into the cisterna magna. A small volume of fluid may also exit through the central canal of the spinal cord.[15] From the cisterna magna, fluid then flows in several directions: (1) superiorly into the subarachnoid space investing the cerebellar hemispheres; (2) caudally into the spinal subarachnoid space; and (3) cephalad, into the premedullary, prepontine, and interpeduncular cisterns.

From the basilar cisterns the bulk flow of fluid continues cephalad along two major routes: (1) a ventral route through the interpeduncular cistern, from which fluid passes, mainly through the sylvian fissure and prechiasmatic cisterns, to the subarachnoid space investing the lateral and frontal aspects of the cerebral hemispheres; and (2) a dorsomedial route through the ambient cisterns and cisterna venae magnae cerebri, from which fluid passes to the subarachnoid space investing the medial and posterior aspects of the cerebral hemispheres. In the spinal subarachnoid space the bulk flow of fluid appears to follow a

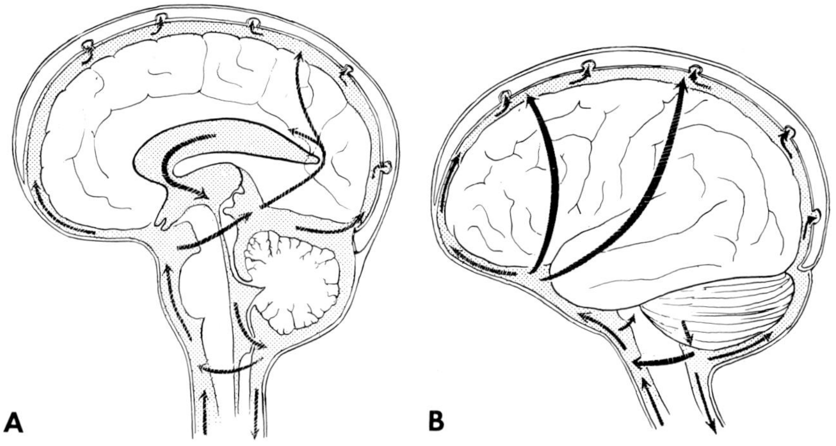

A B

Figure 12-2. Pathways of CSF bulk flow. (Reprinted with permission from Milhorat TH: Hydrocephalus and the Cerebrospinal Fluid. Baltimore, Williams & Wilkins, 1972.)

downward route behind the cord (posterior to the dentate ligaments) to the lumbar theca, and then upward in front of the cord to the basilar cisterns.[15] The circulation of the CSF within the macroscopic cavities terminates at the level of the dural sinuses where absorption takes place across the arachnoid villi.

Mechanics of Flow

The manner in which fluid circulates within the CSF cavities has been a controversial subject. For many years it was held that a true circulatory current did not exist and that the CSF traveled by simple ebb and flow movements resulting from the arterial pulse, as modified by respiration, body position, coughing, and so on.[16–18] With the advent of isotope cisternography, however, the existence of a consistent flow pattern toward the cerebral convexities has been established (Fig. 12-3). Di Chiro[19,20] has demonstrated that body position and physical activity of the patient do not affect the pattern of spreading, and although an ebb and flow component is probably present, the CSF moves in a true circulatory current.[15]

Although the exact mechanism for propelling the CSF along its circulatory route is incompletely understood, the following factors are involved to some extent: (1) the continuous outpouring of newly formed CSF; (2) the ciliary action of the ventricular ependyma; (3) the ventricular pulsations, representing the combined effects of respiratory variations and the pulsations emanating from the choroid plexuses and cerebral arteries; and (4) the pressure gradient across the arachnoid villi. Of these, the last factor is probably the most important. As Shulman, Yarnell, and Ransohoff[21] have shown, the mean CSF pressure in humans (150 mm saline) is considerably higher than the pressure in the superior sagittal sinus (90 mm saline). This differential is required to promote drainage and absorption across the arachnoid villi, and doubtless contributes to the cephalic movement of the CSF.[3] Recently, Bradley[22] emphasized the "suction pump" action of the dural sinuses. This action, which depends upon the high velocity of the central blood flow through the fixed diameter of the sinuses, and the low intraluminal pressure that develops at the circumference of the sinus wall

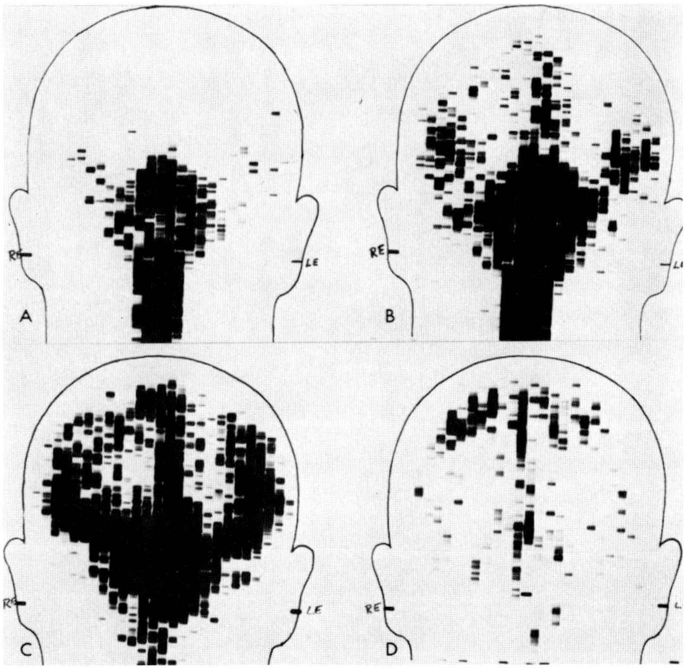

Figure 12-3. RISA cisternogram in a normal human. A. At one hour. B. At three hours. C. At six hours. D. At 24 hours. (Reprinted with permission from Di Chiro G: Movement of the cerebrospinal fluid in human beings. Nature (London) 204:209, 1964.)

where the arachnoid villi enter, may explain how the circulation of CSF continues through a wide range of postural pressures.

It is likely that in certain areas of the CSF system the circulation stagnates. A notable example of this is in the lumbosacral cul-de-sac where intrathecal drugs, blood, and purulent material may be retained for prolonged intervals.[14] Zulch,[23] in discussing neoplasms that seed the CSF pathways, pointed out that the location of tumor implants often coincides with areas in which the circulation "sludges down." The frequent spread of pinealomas to the anterior recesses of the third ventricle, and of medulloblastomas to the cauda equina, thus may indicate areas of circulatory stagnation.

Lesser Pathways of Flow

Lesser pathways of flow, along extracellular channels, are present across all surfaces lining the CSF cavities (Fig. 12-4). Long regarded as little more than diffusional pathways, these delicate channels are nonetheless responsible for some bulk transport of CSF and have the following functions under normal conditions.

Transependymal and Transpial Flow

Evidence exists that the CSF is constantly formed by two mechanisms: secretion by the choroid plexuses, and "lymphatic-like" drainage of the brain extracellular fluid.[3] Although the exact contributions from choroidal and extrachoroidal sites remain to be determined, the latter are probably significant since the maximum reduction in the rate of CSF formation that can be achieved by choroid plexectomy is only about 40 percent.[24] Recently Cserr with Ostrach[25] and with Cooper and Milhorat[26] have provided convincing evidence of bulk flow pathways within the brain parenchyma, supporting the view that the interstitial fluid of the central nervous system drains to the adjacent CSF cavities through extracellular channels. On the basis of these and other data,[27-30] it is likely that a steady, net addition of new fluid occurs at all points along the ependymal and pial surfaces until the major sites of CSF absorption are reached.[14]

Transarachnoid Flow

The major route by which constitutents of the CSF are returned to the blood is across the arachnoid villi. In addition, subsidiary routes of absorption probably exist across the proximal leptomeninges, with drainage into the extradural

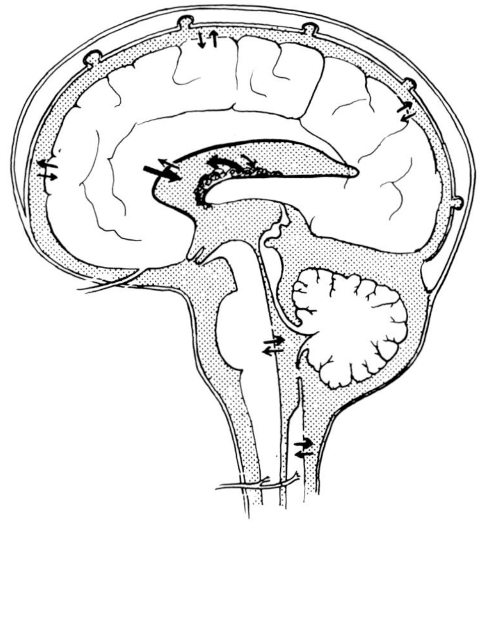

Figure 12-4. Lesser pathways of CSF flow. (Reprinted with permission from Milhorat TH: Hydrocephalus and the Cerebrospinal Fluid. Baltimore, Williams & Wilkins, 1972.)

lymphatics of the cranial and spinal nerves.[4] These lesser pathways of flow, like those across the pia and ependyma, may assume added importance in hydrocephalus, and are potential routes for removing fluid from the macroscopic CSF cavities (see "CSF Circulation in Hydrocephalus").

FUNCTIONS OF THE CSF

Modern interest in the CSF has been more concerned with the origin, circulation, and absorption of the brain fluids than with their functions. Nevertheless, there is growing evidence that the medium is far more than a "cushion for the brain" and that its flowing character and biologic functions justify its description as "the third circulation." Granted that many questions remain unanswered, the following may be cited as specific functions of the CSF.

Protection and Support

An obvious function of the CSF is to surround, support, and protect nervous tissue. The CSF system is hydrostatically precise and responds to a wide variety of physiologic influences.[14] In this manner the delicate neural tissue is cushioned from external forces applied to the rigid skull and spinal column.

Internal Milieu

Another obvious role of the CSF is to provide a specialized watery environment for nervous tissue. Within limits, the chemical composition of the CSF is closely regulated by the blood–brain barrier, and large or polar molecules, many of which have toxic or potentially toxic properties, are almost totally excluded from the brain interspaces. The ability of the blood–brain barrier to restrict the movement of blood products into and out of the brain serves, in addition, to maintain the interstitial fluid as a protein-poor product of the plasma.[3] This milieu is clearly necessary for the proper functioning of nervous tissue, which requires a watery environment for the generation and conduction of electrical impulses.

Lymphatic-like Role

An especially important function of the CSF is to serve as a modified lymphatic system. This 'lymphatic-like' role was particularly emphasized by Cushing,[31] who observed that the CSF, like the lymph, "proves to be in continual movement in a definite direction through a highly specialized pathway that cuts across the blood circle to envelop an organ in which a lymphatic apparatus of the usual type does not exist." Cushing was also aware that the anatomic arrangement of the brain interspaces and cavities was not unlike that of the lactiferous channels and ducts, and that both systems ultimately drain to the venous circulation.

The most clinically apparent lymphatic-like role of the CSF is to remove products of cerebral metabolism. Although there are few quantitative data, evidence is accumulating that a number of substances metabolized by the brain, as well as a number of substances that cross the blood–brain barrier, are cleared by net transport into the CSF. These include the following lipid-insoluble substances: inulin,[32] mannitol,[32] sulfanilic acid,[32] urea,[33] albumin,[34] globulin,[35] dopamine,[36–38] homovanillic acid,[37] serotonin,[36] and norepinephrine.[39] From a clinical standpoint the laboratory analysis of CSF for enzymes and other type-specific proteins is often helpful in the diagnosis of various neurologic disorders.[14]

Finally, when the brain is damaged by disease, the lymphatic-like role of the CSF takes on added importance. Because of the blood–brain barrier, large or polar molecules cannot be removed transcerebrally (across cerebral capillaries), and the capacity of pinocytotic systems within the cerebral parenchyma is limited. It thus remains for the CSF, which irrigates the brain and spinal cord as it flows in bulk toward the arachnoid villi, to remove products as varied as erythrocytes, bacteria, and necrotic and purulent material.[3]

Intracerebral Transport

Since the CSF is a circulating medium that irrigates regions of the brain known to participate in neuroendocrine activity, it is not surprising that from time to time the suggestion has been made that the medium serves as a vehicle for intracerebral transport. As early as 1910, Cushing and Goetsch[40] suggested that the active principle of the posterior lobe of the hypophysis might be released into the third ventricle for distribution within the nervous system, and a similar route of transport was proposed for the hormones of the hypothalamus and pineal gland.

Among the more intriguing pieces of evidence that have recently come to light is the observation that when biogenic amines are injected into the cerebral ventricles, they have a precise and predictable effect on pituitary function.[41,42] Porter, Kamberi, and Ondo[43] have shown that the injection of dopamine directly into the hypophyseal portal system has no effect on neuroendocrine function but that the administration of equivalent doses into the third ventricle is followed within 20 minutes by the release of luteinizing hormone and follicle-stimulating hormone from the pituitary gland. These and other comparable data[44] provide strong evidence that the intraventricular administration of biogenic amines stimulates the letdown of pituitary-releasing factors from cellular elements in contact with the CSF. Although much work remains to be done, there is accumulating evidence that the specialized ependymal cell of the third ventricle, the tanycyte, which projects from the ventricular surface into the infundibular recess, may form an essential link in the control of pituitary function by responding as a sensor to substances circulating in the CSF.[45]

CSF CIRCULATION IN HYDROCEPHALUS

Obstruction of the CSF pathways, from whatever cause, leads inevitably to an altered flow of CSF within the intracranial cavities. Although the abnormal patterns of circulation vary with the location and completeness of the block, there is, in almost every case, an attempt to establish compensatory pathways of absorption.

Communicating Hydrocephalus

With lesions obstructing the subarachnoid space, there is a free flow of CSF out of the cerebral ventricles up to the level of the block. Since the circulatory route beyond this point is blocked, however, there is a net accumulation of fluid within the trapped chambers, and the forward circulation of the CSF is slowed, or even totally arrested. As a consequence of the continuous ventricular pulsations, fluid proximal to the block undergoes “mixing.” This “mixing effect” is important and accounts for the fact that when tracers are injected into the lumbar theca they will distribute throughout the obstructed system, and will migrate upward into the lateral ventricles. In patients undergoing isotope cisternography, retrograde filling of the ventricular system is a characteristic sign of communicating hydrocephalus (Fig. 12-5).

Noncommunicating Hydrocephalus

In cases of hydrocephalus in which the cerebral ventricles are separated from the distal CSF pathways by an obstruction within the ventricular system, the fluid proximal to the block is subjected to the mixing forces cited above. Distal to the block, the flow of fluid may or may not be altered. Frequently, the subarachnoid fluid flows normally toward the cerebral convexities. This can occur even when the ventricular obstruction is comparatively complete (e.g., aqueductal stenosis), and indicates that the circulation of fluid in the subarachnoid space is not dependent upon the pulsations emanating from the choroid plexuses or upon the flow of fluid out of the cerebral ventricles.[14] In many cases, however, the convexity subarachnoid space and/or basilar cisterns are mechani-

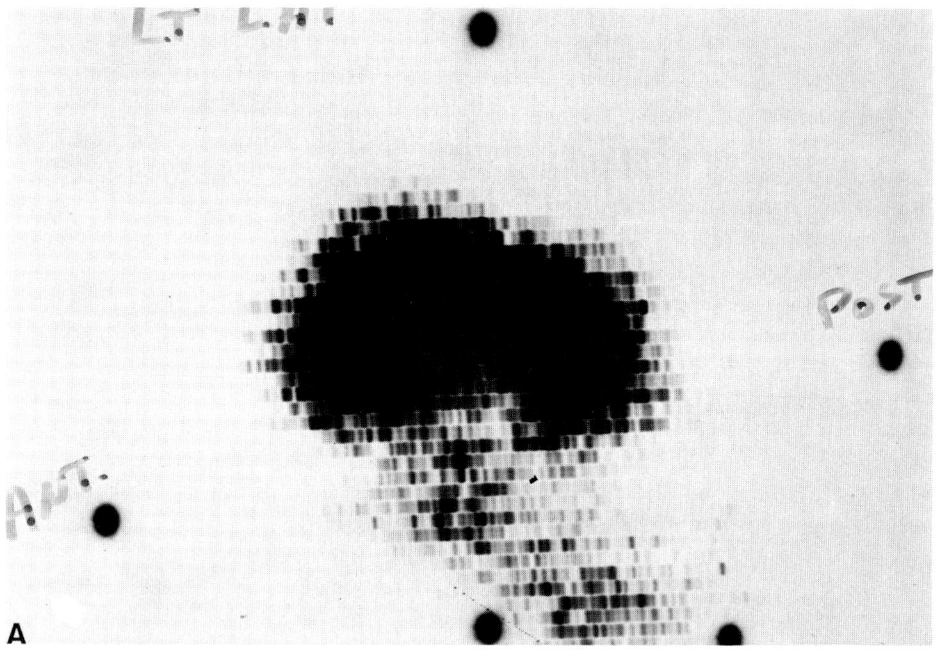

A

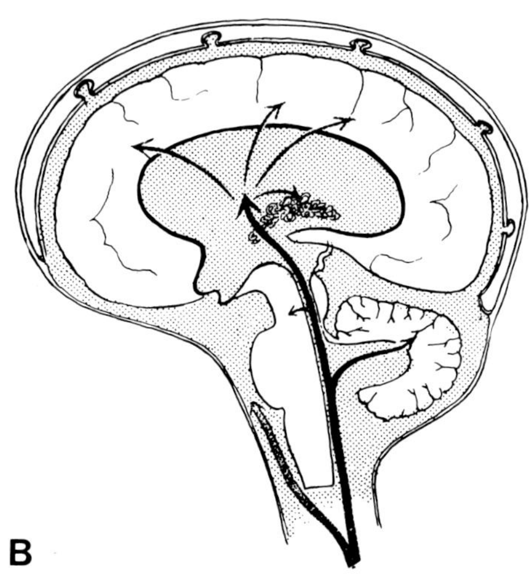

B

Figure 12-5. Retrograde circulation of CSF in communicating hydrocephalus. A. RISA cisternogram of patient with hydrocephalus secondary to subarachnoid hemorrhage. A 24-hour scan shows reflux of radiotracer into the lateral ventricles and nonfilling of the basilar cisterns and subarachnoid space. The halo or "double-density" pattern around the lateral ventricles suggests migration of the tracer into the periventricular tissue. B. Diagram of CSF circulation in communicating hydrocephalus. (Reprinted with permission from Milhorat TH: Hydrocephalus and the Cerebrospinal Fluid. Baltimore, Williams & Wilkins, 1972.)

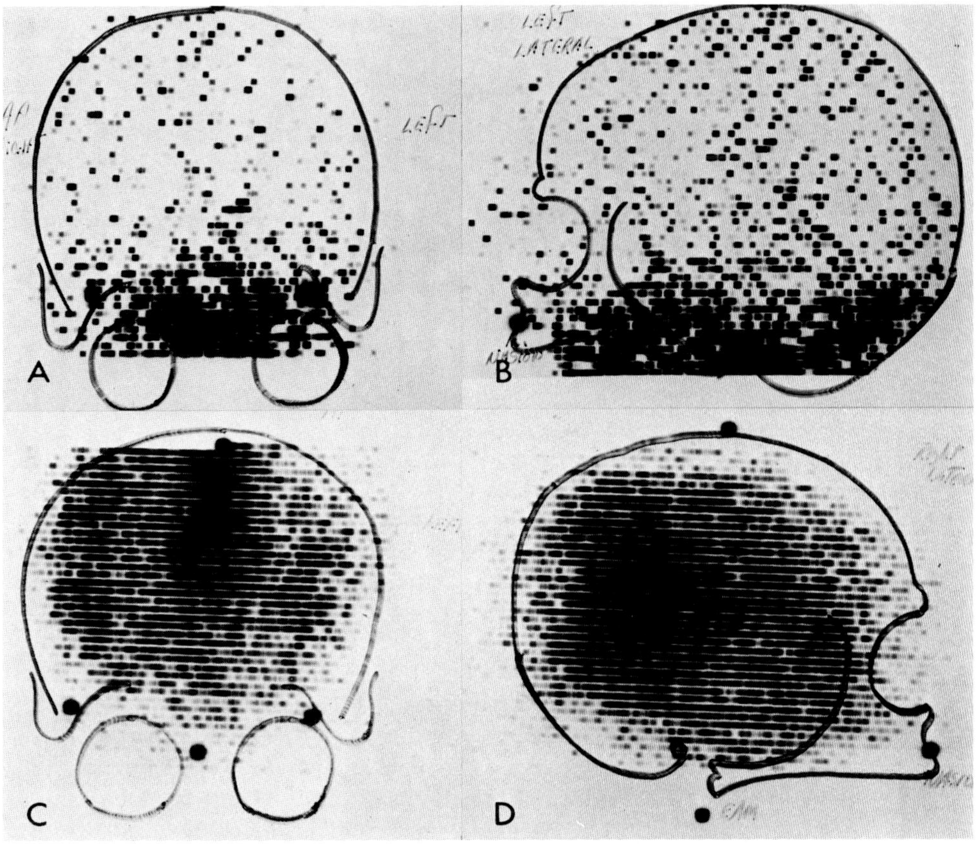

Figure 12-6. Flow of subarachnoid fluid in noncommunicating hydrocephalus. A, B. RISA cisternogram in patient with congenital aqueductal stenosis and massive ventricular enlargement. On 48-hour scan little or no tracer has passed above the level of the cisterna magna. C, D. A 48-hour RISA scan, same patient, following ventricular shunt. The convexity subarachnoid space has reexpanded. (Reprinted with permission from Milhorat TH: Hydrocephalus and the Cerebrospinal Fluid. Baltimore, Williams & Wilkins, 1972.)

cally obstructed by the enlarged ventricular system (Fig 12-6).[46,47] This phenomenon probably accounts for the frequent failure of internal shunts such as third ventriculostomy or ventriculocisternostomy (Torkildsen shunt) in the treatment of noncommunicating hydrocephalus.[14]

Compensatory Pathways of Flow

A characteristic finding in hydrocephalus, regardless of its type, is an increased permeability of the surfaces lining the obstructed system. When dyes or radioisotopes are injected into the CSF, the tracers can be demonstrated to migrate rapidly and in increased amounts into structures such as the septum pellucidum, the choroid plexuses, the periventricular zone of the brain, and the leptomeninges proximal to the block (Fig. 12-7).[14,48,49] The easy penetrability of the periventricular boundaries can sometimes be shown graphically during human isotope ventriculography, and results in a "double-density" pattern: a dense inner area of uptake, corresponding to the radiotracer in the cerebral ventricles; and a less dense outer area of uptake, corresponding to the radiotracer in the brain surrounding the ventricles (see Fig. 12-6).[50] The presence of periventricular white matter edema was recently demonstrated by computerized contract tomography (CCT) and may become a useful criterion for helping to distinguish normal pressure hydrocephalus from cerebral atrophy (Fig. 12-8).

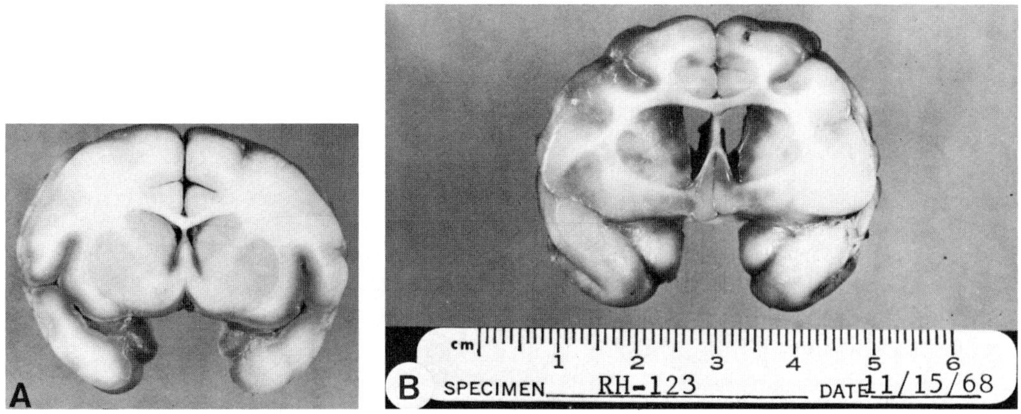

Figure 12-7. Increased permeability of ventricular surface in experimental hydrocephalus. A. Distribution of intraventricularly injected phenolsulfonphthalein (PSP) in normal rhesus monkey. After 45 minutes the dye has migrated across the ependyma to a depth of 1–2 mm. B. Distribution of intraventricularly injected PSP in rhesus monkey with obstruction of fourth ventricle (inflatable balloon). After 45 minutes the dye has migrated deeply into the periventricular grey and white matter. (Reprinted with permission from Milhorat TH, Clark RG: Some observations on the circulation of phenosulfonphthalein in cerebrospinal fluid: Normal flow and flow in hydrocephalus. J Neurosurg 35:522, 1970.)

The fate of fluid once within the cerebral parenchyma is not known. There is growing evidence that at least some of this fluid is absorbed, and Levin, Milhorat, Fenstermacher, et al.[51] have reported an apparent increase in cerebral capillary permeability in experimental hydrocephalus. More recently, McLone[52] has presented evidence that when lanthanum colloid is injected into the lateral ventricles of hydrocephalic mice, the tracer moves transcerebrally by extracellular routes to enter cerebral vessels in the subarachnoid space. Before transependymal absorption can be accepted unequivocally as a major compensatory mechanism in hydrocephalus, however, it is obvious that more work needs to be done.

Despite the foregoing uncertainties, it is evident that a major adjustment in the dynamics and circulation of the CSF must take place in almost every case of

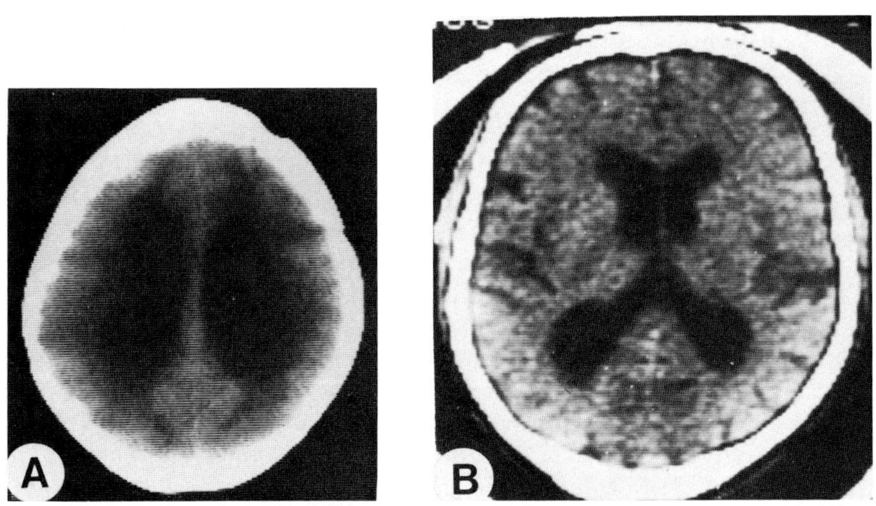

Figure 12-8. A. CCT scan of patient with normal pressure hydrocephalus. B. CCT scan of patient with presenile dementia. In hydrocephalus CCT scan may demonstrate a halo of periventricular white matter edema, whereas scans of patients with cerebral atrophy never do.

chronic hydrocephalus. Were this not to occur, then in patients with complete blocks the ventricles would be forced to enlarge by several hundred cubic centimeters a day. In this regard it is appropriate to point out that Hammock, Milhorat, and Davis[53] have recently shown that in most cases of "complete" ventricular obstruction radioisotopes invariably bypass the block, albeit at a delayed rate. This suggests that a considerable volume of fluid may actually circulate along normal pathways. Overall, it is likely that within any obstructed CSF system fluid will flow along the route or routes of least structural resistance. This probably explains the phenomenon of transventricular absorption as well as the development of ventricular diverticula and hydromyelia in certain types of hydrocephalus.

REFERENCES

1. Dandy WE, Blackfan KD: Internal hydrocephalus: An experimental, clinical and pathological study. Am J Dis Child 8:406, 1914
2. Dandy WE: Experimental hydrocephalus. Ann Surg 70:129, 1919
3. Milhorat TH: The third circulation revisited. J Neurosurg 42:628, 1975
4. Dandy WE: The brain, in Lewis D (ed): Practice of Surgery, vol 12. Hagerstown, WF Prior, 1932
5. Bodenheimer TS, Brightman MW: A blood–brain barrier to peroxidase in capillaries surrounded by perivascular spaces. Am J Anat 122:244, 1968
6. Fenstermacher JD, Johnson JA: Filtration and reflection coefficients of the rabbit blood–brain barrier. Am J Physiol 211:341, 1966
7. Reese TS, Karnovsky MJ: Fine structural localization of a blood–brain barrier to exogenous peroxidase. J Cell Biol 34:207, 1967
8. Brightman MW: The distribution within the brain of ferritin injected into cerebrospinal fluid compartments. 1. Ependymal distribution. J Cell Biol 26:99, 1965
9. Brightman MW: The distribution within the brain of ferritin injected into cerebrospinal fluid compartments. 2. Parenchymal distribution. Am J Anat 117:193, 1965
10. Brightman MW: The intracerebral movement of proteins injected into blood and cerebrospinal fluid of mice. Prog Brain Res 29:19, 1968.
11. Levin VA, Fenstermacher JD: Cortical ECS and diffusion profiles in the cat, dog, and monkey perfused through the subarachnoid space. Fed Proc 28:578, 1969 (abstract)
12. Rall DP, Oppelt WW, Patlak CS: Extracellular space of brain as determined by diffusion of inulin from the ventricular system. Life Sci 1:43, 1962
13. Levin VA, Fenstermacher JD, Patlak CS: Sucrose and inulin space measurements of cerebral cortex in four mammalian species. Am J Physiol 219:1528, 1970
14. Milhorat TH: Hydrocephalus and the Cerebrospinal Fluid. Baltimore, Williams & Wilkins, 1972
15. Di Chiro G: Observations on the circulation of the cerebrospinal fluid. Acta Radiol (Diagn) (Stockholm) 5:988, 1966
16. Sachs E, Wilkins H, Sams CF: Studies on cerebrospinal circulation by a new method. Arch Neurol Psychiat 23:130, 1930
17. Grundy HF: Circulation of cerebrospinal fluid in the spinal region of the cat. J Physiol (London) 163:457, 1962
18. Davson H: Physiology of the Cerebrospinal Fluid. London, Churchill, 1967
19. Di Chiro G: Movement of the cerebrospinal fluid in human beings. Nature (London) 204:209, 1964
20. Di Chiro G: New radiographic and isotopic procedures in neurological diagnosis. JAMA 188:524, 1964
21. Shulman K, Yarnell P, Ransohoff J: Dural sinus pressure in normal and hydrocephalic drugs. Arch Neurol 10:575, 1964
22. Bradley KC: Cerebrospinal fluid pressure. J Neurol Neurosurg Psychiat 33:387, 1970
23. Zulch KJ: In Olwercrona H, Tönnis W (eds): Handbucher Neurochirugie, vol 3. Berlin, Springer, 1956

24. Milhorat TH, Hammock MK, Fenstermacher JD, et al: Cerebrospinal fluid production by the choroid plexus and brain. Science 173:330, 1971
25. Cserr HF, Ostrach LH: Bulk flow of interstitial fluid following intracranial injection of Blue Dextran 2000. Exp Neurol 45:50, 1974
26. Cserr HF, Cooper DN, Milhorat TH: Flow of cerebral interstitial fluid as indicated by the removal of extracellular markers from rat caudate nucleus. Exp Eye Res suppl:467–473, 1977
27. Milhorat TH: Choroid plexus and cerebrospinal fluid production. Science 166:1514, 1969
28. Pollay M, Curl F: Secretion of cerebrospinal fluid by the ventricular ependyma of the rabbit. Am J Physiol 213:103, 1967
29. Sato O, Bering EA: Extra-ventricular formation of cerebrospinal fluid. Brain Nerve (Tokyo) 19:883, 1967
30. Cserr HF: Physiology of the choroid plexus. Physiol Rev 51:273, 1971
31. Cushing H: The Third Circulation. London, Oxford University Press, 1926
32. Cserr HF, Rall DP, Fenstermacher JD, et al: Studies relating to the function of cerebrospinal fluid in Squalus acanthias. Bull Mt Desert Island Biol Lab 7:16, 1967
33. Cserr HF, Fenstermacher JD, Rall DP: Permeabilities of the choroid plexus and blood–brain barrier to urea, in Schmidt-Nelson B (ed): International Colloquy on Urea and the Kidney, International Congress Series No. 195. Amsterdam, Excerpta Medica, 1970
34. Hochwald GM, Wallenstein MC: Exchange of alpha-globulin between blood, cerebrospinal fluid, and brain in the cat. Am J Physiol 212:1199, 1967
35. Hochwald GM, Wallenstein MC: Exchange of alpha-globulin between blood, cerebrospinal fluid, and brain in the cat. Exp Neurol 19:115, 1967
36. Guldberg HC, Yates CM: Some studies of the effects of chlorpromazine, reserpine and dihydroxyphenylalanine on the concentrations of homovanillic acid, 3, 4-dihydroxyphenylacetic acid and 5-hydroxyindol-3-ylacetic acid in ventricular cerebrospinal fluid of the dog using the technique of serial sampling of the cerebrospinal fluid. Br J Pharmacol 33:457, 1968
37. Portig PJ, Sharman DF, Vogt M: Release by tubocurarine of dopamine and homovanillic acid from the perfused caudate nucleus. J Physiol (London) 194:565, 1968
38. Portig PJ, Vogt M: Activation of a dopaminergic nigro-striatal pathway. J Physiol (London) 197:20, 1968
39. Schanberg SM, Breese GR, Schildkraut JJ, et al: 3-methoxy-4-hydroxyphenylglycol sulfate in brain and cerebrospinal fluid. Biochem Pharmacol 17:2006, 1968
40. Cushing H, Goetsch E: Concerning the secretion of infundibular lobe of the pituitary body and its presence in the cerebrospinal fluid. Am J Physiol 27:60, 1910
41. McCann SM, Kalra PS, Donoso AO, et al: The role of monoamines in the control of gonadotropin and prolactin secretion, in Knigge KM, Scott DE, Weidl A (eds): Brain–Endocrine Interaction, Median Eminence: Structure and Function. Berlin, S Karger, 1972
42. Weiner RI, Gorski RA, Sawyer CH: Hypothalamic catecholamines and pituitary gonadotropin function, in Knigge KM, Scott DE, Weidl A (eds): Brain–Endocrine Interaction, Median Eminence: Structure and Function. Berlin, S Karger, 1972
43. Porter JC, Kamberi IA, Ondo JG: Role of biogenic amines and cerebrospinal fluid in the neurovascular transmittal of hypophysiotropic substances, in Knigge KM, Scott DE, Weidl A (eds): Brain–Endocrine Interaction, Median Eminence: Structure and Function. Berlin, S Karger, 1972
44. Knigge KM, Scott DE, Weidl A (eds): Brain–Endocrine Interaction, Median Eminence: Structure and Function. Berlin, S Karger, 1972
45. Kendall JW, Jacobs JJ, Kramer RM: Studies on the transport of hormones from the cerebrospinal fluid to hypothalamus and pituitary, in Knigge KM, Scott DE, Weidl A (eds): Brain–Endocrine Interaction, Median Eminence: Structure and Function. Berlin, S Karger, 1972
46. Milhorat TH, Hammock MK, Di Chiro G: The subarachnoid space in congenital hydrocephalus. Part I. Cisternographic findings. J Neurosurg 35:1, 1971

47. Milhorat TH, Hammock MK, Chandra RS: The subarachnoid space in congenital obstructive hydrocephalus. Part II. Microscopic findings. J Neurosurg 35:7, 1971
48. Milhorat TH, Clark RG: Some observations on the circulation of phenosulfonphthalein in cerebrospinal fluid: Normal flow and flow in hydrocephalus. J Neurosurg 35:522, 1970
49. Milhorat TH, Clark RG, Hammock MK, et al: Structural, ultrastructural, and permeability changes in the ependyma and surrounding brain favoring equilibration in progressive hydrocephalus. Arch Neurol (Chicago) 22:397, 1970
50. Milhorat TH, Hammock MK: Isotope ventriculography. Interpretation of ventricular size and configuration in hydrocephalus. Arch Neurol (Chicago) 25:1, 1971
51. Levin VA, Milhorat TH, Fenstermacher JD, et al: Physiological studies on the development of obstructive hydrocephalus in the monkey. Neurology (Minneapolis) 21:238, 1971
52. McLone DG: Development of brain extracellular space in hydrocephalic (Hy-3) mice. J Neurol Neurosurg Psychiat 36:155, 1972
53. Hammock MK, Milhorat TH, Davis DA: Isotope cisternography and ventriculography in the diagnosis of hydrocephalus. Dev Med Child Neurol 16:58, 1974

13. Hydrocephalus: Historical Notes, Etiology, and Clinical Diagnosis

Thomas H. Milhorat

HISTORICAL NOTES

The large head, attributable to "water on the brain," has long attracted interest and speculation. Hippocrates cited examples, and Galen, in his instructions to his students, emphasized how meager the symptoms might be despite great enlargement of the skull and its integuments.[1] Although ancient descriptions abound, there is little evidence that early physicians had more than a vague understanding of hydrocephalus. A common belief was that the condition was due to an accumulation of fluid around the surface of the brain.[2] This view, advanced by Galen, and perpetuated by the designation "water on the brain," led to many errors in diagnosis and treatment. It thus remained for Vesalius,[3] who was responsible for the clarification of so many ill-conceived anatomic matters, to give the first accurate description of the pathology of hydrocephalus. In his celebrated account of a 2-year-old girl with congenital hydrocephalus, Vesalius noted that "the water had not collected between the skull and its outer surrounding membrane, but within the ventricles of the brain." He also discussed the gross changes accompanying ventriculomegaly, and provided sufficient information to conclude that his patient probably had aqueductal stenosis ("the cerebellum and entire base of the brain were in their natural state"). As if to convince disbelievers how extraordinary the condition could be, Vesalius proclaimed that the ventricles in this case contained "nine pounds of water or three Augsburg wine measures, so help me God!"

Much of the confusion concerning these early accounts of hydrocephalus was the result of an erroneous understanding of the cerebrospinal fluid (CSF). According to Galen, a vaporous substance, the "spiritus animalis," was manufactured within the cerebral ventricles, and to this he ascribed the functions of energy and motion for all parts of the body. So influential was Galenic dogma that it survived for 1000 years, and as late as the 16th century, Vesalius, the first anatomist of the Renaissance, was able to hold this view. Some authorities such as Thomas Willis (1664) came to the conclusion that the pineal gland or choroid plexuses pumped fluid into the cerebral ventricles,[4] but most continued to teach, as Von Haller (1760) did, that the ventricles contained a vapor during life that condensed after injury or death as water and gravitated to the spaces surrounding the brain and spinal cord.[5] And so it was left for Cotugno (1774) to prove beyond question that the cavities of the brain contained a fluid during life, and that recovery of this fluid could be accomplished reliably by percutaneous tap.[6]

Following Cotugno's discovery of the CSF (or "Liquor Cotunni" as he preferred to call it), observations concerning the pathology of hydrocephalus soon multiplied. Morgagni,[7] expanding upon earlier findings of Vesalius, confirmed the fact that the hydrocephalic brain was often reduced "to the thinness of a membrane" and noted that the physician who taps such brains may conclude mistakenly that the skull and dura have merely been perforated. Morgagni also observed that hydrocephalus could occur in adult patients as an acquired disorder without visible enlargement of the head. Almost simultaneously, Robert Whytt,[8] a contemporary of Morgagni's, described the pathologic features of communicating hydrocephalus in patients dying of tuberculous meningitis. This paved the way for Cheyne (1808),[9] and later for West (1848),[10] to provide a rough classification of hydrocephalus that included acute and chronic types, congenital examples resulting from malformations of the brain, and acquired cases due to tumors, hemorrhage, and infections of the meninges.

During the 19th century the understanding of the CSF advanced in bits and pieces. Magendie (1825)[11] discovered the foramen that bears his name, and subsequently produced a series of important papers in which he described the movement of the CSF. This epoch-making contribution was at least 100 years ahead of its time,[12] and marked a radical departure from the contemporary view that the CSF was merely a stagnant pool having no purpose but to suspend and buffer the brain. In 1859 Luschka confirmed the presence of the foramen of Magendie and described two additional openings, situated laterally, for which he is known.[13] A complete description of the CSF pathways, however, was not available until 1875 when Key and Retziüs[14] published their classic atlas on the anatomy of the central nervous system. This provided an accurate description of the subarachnoid space, and included beautiful and detailed drawings, based on dye injection studies at necropsy, of the ventricles, the meninges, the cisterns, and the arachnoid villi.

Despite the foregoing advances, the management of hydrocephalus remained an enigma until the beginning of the 20th century. To be sure, early physicians had employed blood-letting, head wrapping, and percutaneous taps in the care of hydrocephalic patients, but there were few serious attempts to treat the disorder by surgical means until the specialty of neurosurgery was pioneered by Cushing and his followers. Cushing was quick to recognize the importance of developing new knowledge in his chosen field of surgery, and it is often remarked that his establishment of "The Old Hunterian," a laboratory for experimental surgery at the Johns Hopkins Hospital, was among his most lasting contributions. With this modest beginning, and without precise goals other than to understand hydrocephalus better, Cushing and his associates—among them S. J. Crowe, James Bordley, Jr., Emil Goetsch, Walter E. Dandy, and Lewis Weed—ventured into the backwaters of CSF physiology. In 1914 Dandy, in conjunction with a pediatrician, Kenneth Blackfan,[15] hit upon an ingenious technique for producing experimental hydrocephalus in dogs. By slipping a pledget of cotton into the aqueduct of Sylvius, Dandy showed that the cerebral ventricles proximal to the block would become greatly enlarged and distended with fluid. This finding was soon confirmed by others and could hardly have left doubt that a considerable volume of CSF was formed continuously within the cerebral ventricles and that the route of circulation was toward the subarachnoid space. Somewhat later Dandy[16] reported that if the choroid plexus of one lateral ventricle were removed, and if the foramina of Monro of both lateral ventricles were obstructed, the ventricle containing a choroid plexus would dilate and the ventricle lacking a choroid plexus would collapse. This observation, made in a single dog experiment without a histologic study, led Dandy to conclude that the choroid plexuses were the sole source of the CSF, a view that was accepted without serious criticism for many years.

On the basis of such experimental observations, it is not surprising that surgical operations for hydrocephalus were soon devised. In 1918 Dandy[17] introduced the technique of choroid plexectomy as a means for decreasing the rate of CSF formation. This imaginative procedure consisted of excising the choroid plexuses from both lateral ventricles and, despite its technical difficulty, was for many years the most commonly performed operation for infantile hydrocephalus in the United States. The historic importance of choroid plexectomy and the notable contributions of Scarff in the subsequent development of endoscopic cauterization techniques were recently summarized in a delightful review article.[18] Unfortunately, as experience with bilateral extirpation and/or cauterization of the choroid plexuses increased, it became clear that these procedures invariably failed to benefit patients with noncommunicating hydrocephalus, and were only occasionally successful in cases of communicating hydrocephalus, most often when the condition was arrested or nearly so.[1] Most perplexing was the observation that, in the majority of patients with progressive hydrocephalus, the cerebral ventricles continued to enlarge at a rate equal to or sometimes greater than that recorded preoperatively.[19] In the 1950s, because of generally poor results, choroid plexectomy was abandoned by most neurosurgeons as a treatment for hydrocephalus.

With the experience gained by the many unsuccessful efforts to treat hydrocephalus by reducing the rate of CSF formation, it is only natural that the attention of surgeons turned increasingly to means of enhancing drainage and absorption. By trial and error, a variety of techniques were evolved for directly removing intracranial mass lesions, for fenestrating Dandy–Walker cysts and septae occluding the aqueduct of Sylvius, for decompressing anomalies of the craniospinal junction (e.g., Arnold–Chiari malformation), and for bypassing ventricular blocks by intracranial shunts or fistulas. In all this there was great energy and invention, and it is hardly possible adequately to acknowledge the monumental contribution of Torkildsen in the development of ventriculocisternostomy[30] or of Dandy[21] and Stookey and Scarff[22] in the development of third ventriculostomy.

Efforts to treat hydrocephalus by diverting CSF to remote body cavities also advanced apace. In 1908 Kausch[23] described a technique for shunting CSF to the peritoneum, but the procedure did not catch on, or at least did not meet with immediate success in the hands of others. Recognizing the potential merits of such shunts, however, neurosurgeons doggedly pursued the possibilities of extracranial diversion of the CSF. In time almost every conceivable operation was attempted, including shunts to the heart, the jugular vein, the ureter, the pleural space, the fallopian tube, the mastoid air cells, the sagittal sinus, the intestinal tract, the gallbladder, the spinal epidural space, the thoracic duct, the bladder, and even Stensen's duct.[1] Experience has shown that two sites are especially well suited for accepting and removing CSF: the right atrium of the heart, and the peritoneal cavity. Somewhat less effective are the pleural space and ureter.

A major development, which can be said to mark the modern era of hydrocephalus surgery, came in 1952 with the introduction of valve-regulated shunts. Nulsen and Spitz,[24] and almost simultaneously Holter,[25] produced a one-way flow device that for the first time made shunts to the bloodstream feasible, and avoided many of the complications of uncontrolled CSF drainage. Following this breakthrough new interest was focused on hydrocephalus surgery, which, in some quarters, was still regarded as a futile exercise. In the period of just a decade, a whole new technology arrived and today, 30 years later, one has only to look in the surgical trade journals to appreciate the staggering number of valves, reservoirs, and catheters that are constantly being designed.

Without question the development of simple and effective extracranial shunts stands today as the single most important advance in the surgical treatment of hydrocephalus. So greatly have these ingenious devices improved the outlook for patients with hydrocephalus that the results of early operations (e.g., choroid plexectomy) seem as dismal in comparison as the results of 19th century surgery must have appeared to Cushing and Dandy. Extracranial shunting procedures are now employed as the treatment of choice for patients with communicating hydrocephalus, and for most cases of noncommunicating hydrocephalus that are not amenable to direct operations or intracranial shunts. As surgical experience has grown, the mortality of first operations has been reduced almost to zero and the five-year survival rate, including patients with all types of hydrocephalus, now approaches 90 percent.[26]

How far we may go, and how much we will be able to improve upon these promising results, only time and experience will tell. What is clear is that the introduction of catheters and valves into the body cavities has inherent disadvantages and that it is with such matters that neurosurgeons must concern themselves in the years to come. Among the more significant problems that still confront us are the following.

1. Extracranial shunts, regardless of design, are associated with a high incidence of complications. Obstruction and infection are the most common shunting problems, and thromboembolism and septicemia are of added concern in patients with ventriculoatrial shunts.
2. In growing patients a single shunting operation is rarely definitive. To accommodate somatic growth, a minimum of three, and sometimes more, shunting operations are required from infancy through adolescence.
3. Since we know little about the biophysics of hydrocephalus, it is far from clear which of the many valve-regulated systems are most effective under the given conditions of intracranial pressure, ventricular size, type of hydrocephalus, and so on.

EPIDEMIOLOGY

The overall incidence of hydrocephalus in the general population is not known. Since the condition occurs in association with a large number of childhood and adult intracranial diseases, it is obvious that the reported incidence of infantile hydrocephalus—namely, 3 per 1000 live births[26]—is grossly understated.[27] The incidence of hydrocephalus occurring as a single congenital disorder is given as 0.9 to 1.5 per 1000 births, and that of hydrocephalus occurring with spina bifida and myelomeningocele varies from 1.3 to 2.9 per 1000 births.[28]

Whereas the causes of acquired hydrocephalus are often apparent, the etiologic factors responsible for congenital hydrocephalus are for the most part obscure. In a small number of cases, maternal malnutrition, toxins, cytomegalic inclusion virus, or toxoplasmosis can be shown to play a role.[1] An inheritable form of aqueductal stenosis has also been described[29] that occurs only in males and is transmitted from one generation to the next by a female carrier (X-linked hydrocephalus). This is an extremely rare condition and probably accounts for less than 1 percent of all cases of congenital hydrocephalus. In patients with acquired hydrocephalus, the most important etiologic factors include trauma, intracranial bleeding, meningitis, and tumors.

ETIOLOGY

Current knowledge concerning the etiology of hydrocephalus was put on firm ground in 1949 with the publication of *Observations on the Pathology of Hydrocephalus* by Dorothy Russell.[30] One of the most important conclusions of this study, and one that has been upheld to date, is that in almost every case of hydrocephalus there is a pathologic obstruction at some point along the pathways of CSF circulation. This can usually be demonstrated even in cases of choroid plexus papilloma, so that with few exceptions hydrocephalus may be regarded as a disturbance of CSF *absorption.*

For clinical purposes it is useful to divide defects of CSF absorption into two types: (1) lesions that obstruct the ventricular system, and (2) lesions that obstruct the subarachnoid space. The former, by preventing the free circulation of fluid out of the cerebral ventricles, produces a "noncommunicating" type of hydrocephalus, although in such cases the extraventricular pathways may be secondarily obstructed by expansion of the brain against the undersurface of the skull.[31,32] With lesions primarily obstructing the subarachnoid space, there is a free flow of fluid out of the ventricles up to the point of the block and the hydrocephalus is therefore termed "communicating." Table 13-1 classifies the more common lesions causing hydrocephalus.

Congenital Obstructions

The vast majority of lesions causing congenital hydrocephalus occur proximal to the outlets of the fourth ventricle. This produces a noncommunicating type of hydrocephalus, and in approximately 70 percent of cases a lesion obstructing the aqueduct of Sylvius can be demonstrated.[1] Though imprecise, the term "aqueductal stenosis" is used to denote any intrinsic narrowing of the iter. Of the four main types (see Table 13-1), aqueductal gliosis or forking will be found in all but a few cases. The former usually occurs as an isolated finding and is characterized by narrowing or obliteration of the aqueductal lumen by a proliferation of subependymal astrocytes. In contrast, aqueductal forking is almost always associated with other congenital anomalies (e.g., spina bifida and myelomeningocele) and consists of two greatly narrowed channels, one behind the other, which are separated by normal intervening nervous tissue. There is increasing evidence that at least some cases of aqueductal stenosis are the result, and not the cause, of hydrocephalus.[33,34] Such occlusions apparently occur as a consequence of compression and angulation of the upper brain stem by the enlarged lateral ventricles, converting a primary communicating hydrocephalus into a secondary type of noncommunicating hydrocephalus.

Aside from aqueductal stenosis, the most common lesions causing congenital hydrocephalus are the Arnold–Chiari malformation, congenital atresia of the

Table 13-1
Classification of Hydrocephalus

Noncommunicating Hydrocephalus	Communicating Hydrocephalus
Congenital lesions Aqueductual obstruction (stenosis) Gliosis Forking True narrowing Septum Atresia of the foramina of Luschka and Magendie (Dandy–Walker cyst) Masses Benign intracranial cysts Vascular malformations Tumors Acquired lesions Aqueductual stenosis (gliosis) Ventricular inflammation and scars Masses Tumors Nonneoplastic masses	Congenital lesions Arnold–Chiari malformation Encephalocele Leptomeningeal inflammations Lissencephaly Congenital absence of arachnoid granulations Acquired lesions Leptomeningeal inflammations Infections Hemorrhage Particulate matter Masses Tumors Nonneoplastic masses Platybasis Oversecretion of CSF (choroid plexus papilloma)

foramina of Luschka and Magnedie, and intracranial masses such as vascular malformations, arachnoid cysts, and congenital tumors (Table 13-1).

Acquired Obstructions

A variety of acquired intracranial lesions can obstruct the CSF pathways and lead to hydrocephalus. During the first year of life, the most common of these by far is fibrosis of the leptomeninges. This lesion usually results from either meningitis or intraventricular hemorrhage and produces a communicating type of hydrocephalus. After the first year of life, the incidence of intracranial tumors increases significantly, so that in adult life neoplastic lesions rank second only to subarachnoid hemorrhage as the leading cause of hydrocephalus.[1]

CSF Oversecretion

The principal exception to the rule that hydrocephalus results from obstruction of the CSF pathways concerns the rare case of CSF oversecretion by choroid plexus papillomas. This mechanism, long suggested on the basis of indirect clinical evidence,[35–37] has been confirmed by ventriculolumbar perfusion studies in infants with communicating hydrocephalus and papillary tumors of the lateral ventricle.[38,39]

It is important to point out that despite the ability of choroid plexus papillomas to elaborate excessive amounts of CSF, hydrocephalus associated with these tumors may have other causes. Papillomas arising in the third and fourth ventricles, for example, usually produce hydrocephalus by directly obstructing the ventricular system. With papillomas of the lateral ventricles, furthermore, Russell,[30] and subsequently Hoytema,[40] have suggested that obstruction of the distal subarachnoid pathways may be a more important pathogenetic mechanism than generally appreciated. Supporting this view are the following facts: (1) Occult subarachnoid bleeding is a recognized complication of these tumors.[41] (2) At the time of clinical presentation, approximately 50 percent of patients will have xanthochromic CSF and elevation of the CSF protein.[42,43] (3) Pneumoencephalography and isotope cisternography frequently demonstrate obstruction of the distal subarachnoid pathways.[44] (4) Chronic arachnoiditis is a common finding at autopsy.[30,42] (5) Hydrocephalus may persist following the complete removal of tumors from the lateral ventricles.[44,45] These observations, taken together with evidence that choroid plexus papillomas may arise in the absence of hydrocephalus,[1] have raised the possibility that oversecretion of the CSF alone may be insufficient to produce hydrocephalus when the mechanisms for CSF drainage and absorption are normal.[1] Since a permanent cure of hydrocephalus is sometimes achieved by the removal of papillary tumors from the lateral ventricles, however, it is likely that, in these cases at least, oversecretion of the CSF is the most important pathogenetic mechanism.[26]

Impaired Cerebrovenous Drainage

It has been long argued, mainly on theoretical grounds, that if the cephalic venous pressure is markedly increased, the resulting back pressure on the arachnoid villi might cause hydrocephalus.[30,46,47] To date experimental efforts to confirm this proposition have been unimpressive. Whereas Bering and Salibi[46] reported a moderate degree of hydrocephalus in dogs following ligation of the major veins of the neck, other authors have reported no evidence of ventricular enlargement following experimental occlusion of the sagittal sinus,[48] the torcular Herophili,[49] or the vein of Galen.[50] From a clinical standpoint, it is well established that radical neck dissection, superior vena cava syndrome, and dural sinus thrombosis are rarely associated with ventricular enlargement in adults despite temporary or sustained elevations of intracranial pressure.[51–53] Kalbag and Woolf[54] have shown that cerebral atrophy may be a late complication of cerebrovenous occlusions, and, overall, this is probably the best explanation for occasional examples of mild to moderate ventriculomegaly occurring in association with dural sinus thrombosis, unless the lesion has been complicated by subarachnoid bleeding.[1]

The effects of cerebrovenous occlusions in infants are not so well understood. Some authorities have cited a venous link with hydrocephalus based on the distensibility of the immature skull,[47,55,56] and it is my opinion, but by no means an established fact, that the syndrome of "external hydrocephalus" characterized in infants by the triad of macrocrania, capacious subarachnoid space, and normal to slightly enlarged ventricles is often due to increased cerebrovenous pressure resulting from an obstruction of venous return at any point from the dural sinuses to the right atrium of the heart.[57]

CLINICAL DIAGNOSIS

Infantile Hydrocephalus

An excessive rate of cranial enlargement is usually the first and most consistent finding in patients under the age of 2 years with hydrocephalus.[26] Since this is a compensatory phenomenon that tends to dissipate the rise in intracranial tension, overt symptoms are delayed and papilledema is rarely encountered. More important than any single measurement indicating absolute enlargement of the head are serial measurements demonstrating an *excessive rate* of growth. By conventional usage the term *macrocrania* has been adopted to describe a head whose maximum circumference is in or above the 98th percentile.

includes all cases of arrested or compensated hydrocephalus, constitutional ventriculomegaly, and cerebral atrophy. Although the last condition rarely poses a diagnostic problem in young patients, since the head tends to be small rather than enlarged, hydrocephalus and cerebral atrophy frequently coexist, so that a normal or small-sized head does not automatically exclude some element of hydrocephalus.

The definitive diagnosis of normal pressure hydrocephalus in children invariably requires special tests. Evidence of progressive ventricular enlargement on serial CCT scans is obviously diagnostic, but when ventricular size is stable, difficulties arise. In the past considerable weight was given to pneumoencephalographic findings such as obliteration of the cerebral sulci (in cases of hydrocephalus) and the presence of a capacious subarachnoid space (in cases of cerebral atrophy). Such criteria unfortunately are far from reliable, and in some instances hydrocephalus and cerebral atrophy coexist. In most clinics today, the standard workup of patients with suspected normal pressure hydrocephalus includes a complete neurologic examination, CCT, isotope or metrizamide cisternography, and neuropsychologic testing. In doubtful cases continuous intraventricular pressure recordings or a lumbar spinal infusion test can be carried out. Although the literature is filled with claims that one test or another is the most helpful in predicting surgical outcome, the diagnosis of normal pressure hydrocephalus is still made most accurately on the basis of clinical findings supplemented by appropriate laboratory tests.[26]

Arrested Hydrocephalus

Arrested hydrocephalus may be defined as a state of chronic hydrocephalus in which the CSF pressure has returned to normal and in which the pressure gradient between the cerebral ventricles and brain parenchyma has been dissipated.[1] Under these conditions, the size of the cerebral ventricles remains stable or decreases, new neurologic signs do not appear, and there is evidence of continuing psychomotor development with increasing age. This definition is consistent with the findings in patients with surgically treated hydrocephalus.

Spontaneous arrest of hydrocephalus is most likely to occur when the CSF obstruction is incomplete and when the block is distal (subarachnoid space) rather than proximal (intraventricular). Patients with this diagnosis should be followed for at least a year with periodic neurologic examinations, IQ tests, and CCT to rule out the insidious development of normal pressure hydrocephalus. It is important to point out that if the hydrocephalic process is truly arrested, continuing damage to the brain ceases, and normal developmental processes such as myelinization and neuronal maturation resume. This is manifested clinically by a steady development of psychomotor function, albeit at a subnormal level. It is my opinion that spontaneously arrested hydrocephalus is rarely an optimal physiologic state if the cerebral ventricles are significantly enlarged, and if it can be established on the basis of clinical and neuroradiologic evidence that this is not the result of cerebral atrophy. Under such circumstances consideration should be given to a ventricular shunting procedure.

REFERENCES

1. Milhorat TH: Hydrocephalus and the Cerebrospinal Fluid, Baltimore, Williams & Wilkins, 1972
2. Milhorat TH: Structural function of the choroid plexus and other sites of cerebrospinal fluid formation. Int Rev Cytol 47:225, 1976
3. Vesalius A: De Corporis Humani Fabrica. Basileau, Joannis Oporini, 1543
4. Willis T: De Cerebri Anatomie. Londini, T Roycroft, 1664

5. von Haller A: Elementa Physiologiae, IV. Lausanne, 1760
6. Cotugno D: De Ischiade Nervosa Commentarius. Naples, Apud Fratres Simonios, 1764
7. Morgagni GB: The Seats and Causes of Diseases Investigated by Anatomy. London, A. Millar & T. Cadell, 1761
8. Whytt, R: Observations on the Dropsy of the Brain. Edinburgh, Balfour, Auld, & Smellie, 1768
9. Cheyne J (1808), cited in Milhorat TH: Hydrocephalus and the Cerebrospinal Fluid Baltimore, Williams & Wilkins, 1972
10. West C: Lectures on the Diseases of Infancy and Childhood. London, Longman, 1848.
11. Magendie F: Memoire sur le liquide qui se trouve dans le crane et l'epine de l'homme and des animaux. J Physiol Exp Path 5:27–37, 1825
12. Cushing H: The Third Circulation. London, Oxford University Press, 1926
13. Luschka H von (1859) as cited in Russell DS: Observations on the Pathology of Hydrocephalus. London, Her Majesty's Stationery Office, 1949
14. Key EAH, and Retzuis G: Studien in der Anatomie des Nervensystems und des Bindegewebes. Stockholm, Samson & Wallin, 1875
15. Dandy WE, Blackfan KD: Internal hydrocephalus: An experimental, clinical and pathological study. Am J Des Child 8:406, 1914
16. Dandy WE: Experimental hydrocephalus. Ann Surg. 70:129, 1919
17. Dandy WE: Extirpation of the choroid plexus of the lateral ventricules in communicating hydrocephalus. Ann Surg 68:569, 1918
18. Scarff JW: The treatment of nonobstructive (communicating) hydrocephalus by endoscopic cauterization of the choroid plexus. J Neurosurg 33:1, 1970
19. Milhorat TH: Failure of choroid plexectomy as treatment for hydrocephalus. Surg Gynec Obstet 139:505, 1974
20. Torkildsen A: A new palliative operation in cases of inoperable occlusion of the Sylvian aqueduct. Acta Chir Scand 82:117, 1939
21. Dandy WE: An operative procedure for hydrocephalus. Bull Johns Hopkins Hosp 33:189, 1922
22. Stookey B, Scarff JE: Occlusion of the aqueduct of Sylvius by neoplastic and non-neoplastic processes with a rational surgical treatment for relief of the resultant obstructive hydrocephalus. Bull Neurol Inst NY 5:348, 1936
23. Kausch W: Die behandlung des hydrocephalus der kleinen kinder. Arch Klin Chir 87:709, 1908
24. Nulsen, FE, Spitz EB: Treatment of hydrocephalus by direct heart shunt from ventricle to jugular vein. Surg Forum 2:399, 1952
25. Holter J: Personal communication
26. Milhorat TH: Pediatric Neurosurgery. Philadelphia, FA Davis, 1978
27. Milhorat TH: Congenital hydrocephalus, in Sano K, Ishii S, LeVay S (eds): Recent Progress in Neurological Surgery. Amsterdam, Excerpta Medica, 1973
28. Myrianthopoulos, NC, Kurland LT: Present concepts of the epidemiology and genetics of hydrocephalus, in Fields WS, Desmond MM (eds): Disorders of the Developing Nervous System. Springfield, Charles C Thomas, 1961
29. Bickers DS, Adams RD: Hereditary stenosis of the aqueduct of Sylvius as a cause of congenital hydrocephalus. Brain 72:246, 1949
30. Russell DS: Observations on the Pathology of Hydrocephalus. London, Her Majesty's Stationery Office (Spec. Rep. Ser. Med. Res. Coun. No. 265), 1949
31. Milhorat TH, Hammock MK, Chandra RS: The subarachnoid space in congenital hydrocephalus: II. Microscopic findings. J Neurosurg 35:7, 1971
32. Milhorat TH, Hammock MK, Di Chiro G: The subarachnoid space in congenital hydrocephalus I. Cisterographic findings. J Neurosurg 35:1, 1971
33. Williams B: Is aqueductal stenosis a result of hydrocephalus? Brain 96:399, 1973
34. Raimondi AJ, Clark SJ, and McLone DG: Pathogenesis of aqueductal occlusion in congenital murine hydrocephalus. J Neurosurg 45:66, 1976
35. Ray BS, Peck FC: Papilloma of the choroid plexus of the lateral ventricles causing hydrocephalus in an infant. J Neurosurg 13:405, 1956
36. Fairburn B: Choroid plexus papilloma and its relation to hydrocephalus. J Neurosurg 17:166, 1960

37. Matson DC, Crofton ED: Papilloma of the choroid plexus in childhood. J Neurosurg 17:1002, 1960
38. Milhorat TH, Hammock MK, Davis DA, et al: Choroid plexus papilloma: I. Proof of cerebrospinal fluid overproduction. Child's Brain 5:273, 1977
39. Eisenberg HM, McComb JG, Lorenzo AV: Cerebrospinal fluid overproduction and hydrocephalus associated with choroid plexus papilloma. J Neurosurg 40:381, 1974
40. Hoytema GJ van: Thesis, University of Amsterdam, 1956
41. Russell DS, Rubenstein LJ: Pathology of Tumours of the Nervous System. London, Arnold, 1959
42. Laurence KM, Hoare RD, Till K: The diagnosis of the choroid plexus papilloma of the lateral ventricle. Brain 84:628, 1961
43. Matson DD: Neurosurgery of Infancy and Childhood. Springfield, Charles C Thomas, 1969
44. McDonald JV: Persistent hydrocephalus following the removal of papillomas of the choroid plexus of the lateral ventricles: Report of two cases. J Neurosurg 30:736, 1969
45. Raimondi AJ, Gutierrez FA: Diagnosis and surgical treatment of choroid plexus papillomas. Child's Brain 1:81, 1975
46. Bering EA, Salibi B: Production of hydrocephalus by increased cephalic-venous pressure. Arch Neurol Psychiat 81:693, 1959
47. Shapiro K, Shulman K: Facial nevi associated with anomalous return and hydrocephalus. J Neurosurg 45:20, 1976
48. Woolf AL: Experimentally produced cerebral venous obstruction. J Pathol Bacteriol 67:1, 1954
49. Guthrie TC, Dunbar HS, Karpell B: Ventricular size and chronic increased intracranial venous pressure in the dog. J Neurosurg 33:407, 1970
50. Hammock MK, Milhorat TH, Earle K, et al: Vein of Galen ligation in the primate: Angiographic, gross, and light microscopic evaluation. J Neurosurg 34:77, 1971
51. Bradshaw P: Benign intracranial hypertension. J Neurol Neurosurg Psychiatry 19:28, 1956
52. Fitz-Hugh GS, Robins RB, Craddock WD: Increased intracranial pressure complicating unilateral neck dissection. Laryngoscope 76:893, 1966
53. Gardner WJ: Ortitic sinus thrombosis causing intracranial hypertension. Arch Otolaryngol 30:253, 1939
54. Kalbag RM, Woolf JT: Cerebral Venous Thrombosis. London, Oxford University Press, 1967
55. Hooper R: Hydrocephalus and obstruction of the superior vena cava in infancy: Clinical study of the relationship between cerebrospinal fluid pressure and venous pressure. Pediatrics 28:792, 1961
56. Norrell H, Wilson C, Howieson J, et al: Venous factors in infantile hydrocephalus. J Neurosurg 31:561, 1969
57. Milhorat TH: Hydrocephalus, in Hoff (ed): Harry S. Goldsmith's Practice of Surgery. Hagerstown, Harper & Row, 1980, Chap 7
58. Raimondi AJ: Pediatric Neuroradiology. Philadelphia, WB Saunders, 1972
59. Milhorat TH: Acute hydrocephalus. N Eng J Med 283:857, 1970
60. Yakovlev PI: Paraplegias of hydrocephalus (a clinical note and interpretation). Am J Ment Defic 51:561, 1947
61. Bourneville JN: Hydrocephalic. Prog Med (Paris) 12:17, 1900
62. Doriff BG, Shapiro LM: A clinicopathologic study of sexual precocity with hydrocephalus: Report of two cases occurring in females, with postmortem observations in one. Am J Dis Child 53:481, 1937
63. Hammock MK, Milhorat TH, Baron IS: Normal pressure hydrocephalus in patients with myelomeningocele. Dev Med Child Neurol 37(suppl):55, 1976
64. Laurence KM: The natural history of hydrocephalus. Lancet 2:1152, 1958
65. Laurence KM, Coates S: The natural history of hydrocephalus: Detailed analysis of 182 unoperated cases. Arch Dis Child 37:345, 1962
66. Hagberg G: The sequelae of spontaneously arrested infantile hydrocephalus. Dev Med Child Neurol 4:583, 1962
67. Schick RW, Matson DD: What is arrested hydrocephalus? J Pediat 58:791, 1961
68. Milhorat TH, Hammock MK: "Arrested" versus normal pressure hydrocephalus in children. Clin Proc Child Hosp Nat Med Cent 28:168, 1972

14. Treatment of Hydrocephalus

Harold D. Portnoy

Modern therapy for the treatment of hydrocephalus began with the introduction of the valve-regulated shunt in 1952, by Nulsen and Spitz,[71] and in 1957 by Pudenz, Russell, Hurd, et al.[84] Other forms of treatment for hydrocephalus will be reviewed, but the main thrust of this chapter is to thoroughly acquaint the reader with the use of the various types of shunts and, in particular, with ways to avoid complications.

NONOPERATIVE TREATMENT

Many attempts have been made to control hydrocephalus by reducing cerebrospinal fluid (CSF) formation. Acetazolamide reduces the formation rate in animals to as much as 30 percent of control values,[73,75] but it is ineffective in controlling hydrocephalus in humans. It has been demonstrated, in humans, that the effect of large intravenous doses of acetazolamide lasts but 30 seconds, and chronic acetazolamide therapy has not been of significant help in the treatment of infantile hydrocephalus.[9,61,91] Oral isosorbide also has been utilized but has been found unsatisfactory for long-term use because hypernatremic dehydration occurs after 72 hours of continuous administration.[41] This agent appears to reduce CSF formation and produce an osmotic removal of CSF from the ventricles.

Reduction in CSF formation has been accomplished experimentally in animals by necrosing the choroid plexus using radioactive gold.[88,92,96] This technique produces almost a one-third decrease in the CSF formation rate in dogs with kaolin-induced hydrocephalus[92]—about the same decrease found by Bering[7] following surgical resection of the choroid plexus. Cryosurgery of the choroid plexus has also been reported to reduce the CSF formation rate in dogs by approximately one third.[10] These techniques have not been tried in humans. Since the CSF absorption rate in infants with hydrocephalus may be very low,[56,80] obliteration of the choroid plexus by any means is likely to be of insignificant value except in the mildest cases.[63]

OPERATIVE TREATMENT

Direct Intervention

Direct attack on an aqueduct stenosis, Dandy–Walker cyst, Arnold–Chiari malformation, or similar lesion has resulted in a relatively high mortality. A percutaneous stereotactic third ventriculostomy therefore is the only surgical procedure that may obviate, in select situations, the necessity for a permanent shunt.[1,4,11,12,26,54,83,102]

Choroid Plexectomy

Choroid plexectomy, whether by the original technique devised by Dandy,[19] by the technique of endoscopic cauterization,[97,98] or by craniotomy,[63] has not proved effective in the treatment of hydrocephalus. This hazardous procedure can be carried out only in children with marked hydrocephalus, and the formation of CSF continues from extrachoroidal sources.[14,62–66,97,98]

Intracranial Shunts

Intracranial shunts are used in the treatment of noncommunicating hydrocephalus to channel CSF from the ventricles to the subarachnoid space. The technique is successful only if the subarachnoid space and basilar cisterns are patent. The patency of the subarachnoid space thus must be ascertained prior to surgery.

Many techniques have been described, but the two that have continuing usefulness are third ventriculostomy and the Torkildsen procedure (ventriculocisternostomy).

Third ventriculostomy was first advocated by Dandy in 1922,[17] via a subfrontal approach. It required section of a normal optic nerve, and there was a mortality of 10–15 percent. The procedure was subsequently simplified and revised to preserve sight, but the high mortality of a craniotomy persisted.[18,24] A reduction in mortality was accomplished by the introduction of a percutaneous technique by McNickle in 1947.[58] A blunt needle introduced through the anterior fontanel was used to puncture the floor of the third ventricle. Guiot, Derome, Hertzog, et al.[34] further refined the operation by using the Bertrand leukotome to fenestrate the floor of the third ventricle. An endoscopic technique has also been described.[86] Sayers,[93] Sayers and Kosnils,[94] and later Hoffman,[43] improved on the result of this procedure by first allowing the subarachnoid space to reopen by using a preoperative extracranial shunt. More recently Hoffman[42] has avoided the preoperative shunt by subjecting the child to preoperative ventricular taps.

The Hoffman technique is described because of its relative simplicity.[43] The child is placed in a stereotaxic unit, and a needle is inserted through the fontanel into the ventricle. One-half milliliter iodophendylate (Pantopaque®—Lafayette Pharmaceuticals, Division of Alcon Laboratories, Inc. Lafayette, Indiana, 47904) is introduced into the third ventricle (Fig. 14-1). A Bertrand leukotome is then aligned under radiographic control so as to penetrate the floor of the third ventricle just behind the tip of the dorsum sella. The leukotome is introduced through the same skin puncture as the initial needle, the thrust through the thin floor of the third ventricle. The cutting loop is opened, rotated full circle, and retracted into the leukotome, which is then withdrawn. The Pantopaque will then flow into the interpeduncular cistern.

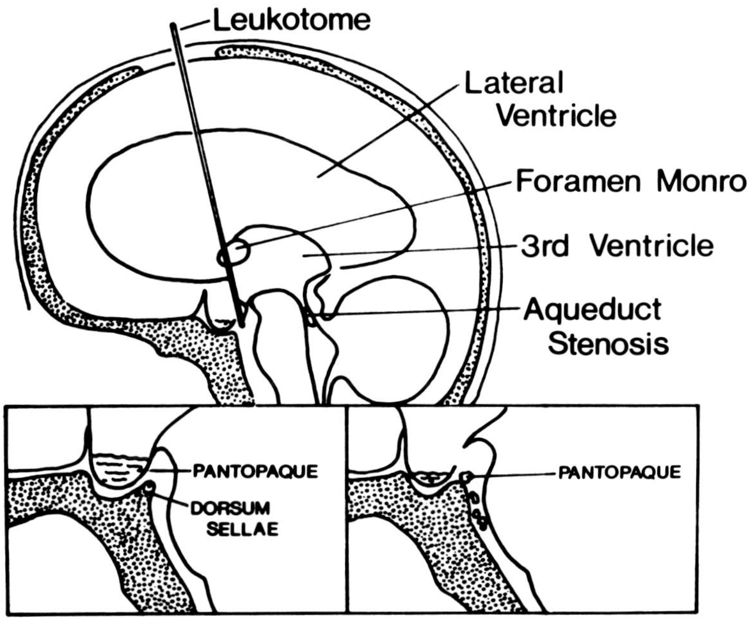

Figure 14-1. Third ventriculostomy. Lower left insert: Pantopaque layered in floor of third ventricle. Lower right insert: Pantopaque flowing into interpeduncular cistern after fenestration by the leukotome.

Ventriculocisternostomy was introduced by Torkildsen in 1939,[68] primarily for the treatment of tumors obstructing the third ventricle, aqueduct of Sylvius, or fourth ventricle, or aqueductal stenosis in children and adults. In a review of the literature, Scarff[98] noted an operative mortality rate of 30 percent, and an initial success rate of only 58 percent. Because of these high mortality and low success rates, the operation is seldom used as a primary procedure. Its major use is for bypassing an unresectable tumor at posterior fossa exploration. Failure is usually the result of continued obstruction of the basilar cisterns and collapse of the subarachnoid space. The shunt should provide a means of temporarily reducing intraventricular pressure to foster expansion of the subarachnoid space, for testing the patency of the shunt and subarachnoid space, and for readily converting the ventriculocisternosotomy into an extracranial shunt.

A trephine is placed in the right posterior parietal region, and a ventricular catheter is inserted, if possible, into the frontal horn, so as to minimize contact with the choroid plexus, and attached to a reservoir. After a suboccipital incision is made, a silicone rubber catheter is passed subgaleally between the two incisions and connected to the outlet of the reservoir, which is then placed in a subgaleal pocket between the two incisions. The distal catheter is clamped until the end of the suboccipital exploration.

A small perforation for the distal catheter is made in the dura at the level of the cerebellar tonsil. The catheter is cut to length so that the tip will reside at the level of the second or third cervical vertebra. Care is taken to pass the distal catheter tip into the subarachnoid space anterior to the spinal cord. This last maneuver, described by Matson,[60] positions the catheter tip away from the main operative site and obliterated cisterna magna (Fig. 14-2).

If the postoperative clinical status of the patient is satisfactory, and a computerized tomographic (CT) scan demonstrates a reduction in ventricular size, no further manipulations are necessary. When the clinical status suggests persistent hydrocephalus, the reservoir is tapped daily, for four to seven days, to relieve the intraventricular pressure and foster reexpansion of the subarachnoid space. Patency of the subarachnoid space may be confirmed by injecting a radioisotope into the reservoir and following the course of the isotope over the next 48 hours.[50] If the subarachnoid space is not patent, the system is converted to a standard extracranial shunt.

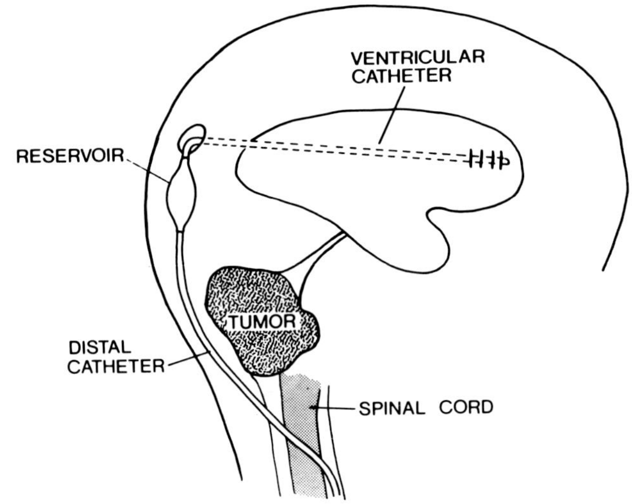

Figure 14-2. Ventriculocisternostomy. A reservoir is placed between the ventricular and cervical subarachnoid space catheters.

Extracranial Shunts

Ventriculoatrial (VA), ventriculoperitoneal (VP), and lumboperitoneal (LP) shunts are mainstays in the modern treatment of hydrocephalus. The common essential features of these shunts is that they are manufactured from, or encased in, medical-grade silicone rubber, a material that is well tolerated by the body and causes little tissue reaction or intravascular thrombosis[8,48,59] and that they are valve-regulated, which prevents excess drainage of CSF and reflux of blood into the cerebral ventricles.[5,71,84]

An ideal shunt will drain excess CSF, maintain a normal intracranial pressure, and produce no complications. To attain this ideal, the surgeon should have a good working knowledge of (1) normal cerebrospinal fluid hydrodynamics (see Chapters 11 and 12), (2) the mechanics of shunt drainage of CSF and how it differs from normal absorption, (3) the types of shunt-related complications, and (4) the operative procedure for inserting the desired type of shunt. These factors are reviewed in the following sections.

Because many shunts are manufactured, the discussion is presented in a general sense, rather than related to a specific brand. The surgeon should have no difficulty relating the concepts presented to a given brand of shunt.

Mechanics of Shunt Drainage of CSF

A shunt is a mechanical device usually composed of one or more tubes and valves. Flow (F) through the shunt is governed by the differential pressure across the shunt (ΔP), and the resistance of the shunt (R) according to the equation[38,82]

$$F = \frac{\Delta P}{R}$$

In comparison with the valve, the resistance of the tubing is neglible; thus the valve defines the resistive qualities of the shunt.[77]

All commercial valves available are simple differential pressure valves (DPV). This means that the valve opens and closes at a certain difference in pressure between the inlet and outlet. Once the valve is open, flow through the DPV is governed by the difference between the inlet and outlet pressures and the resistance of the valve. The various DPVs have been tested by several investigators,[25,31,38,82,87] and while individual brands of valves have slightly different pressure–flow characteristics, there are basically two types of DPV: low-resistance valves (LRV) and high-resistance valves (HRV).[82] The springball and diaphragm valves comprise the LRV, while most of the HRVs are slit valves. (The pressure–flow characteristics of the LRV are illustrated in Figure 14-3.) Only the springball valve (Hakim–Cordis) and the silicone rubber diaphragm valve (Pudenz) fall into this category.[77,82] When the LRV value opens, valve resistance drops rapidly, that is, the valve no longer effectively obstructs the flow of fluid, and the resistance to flow through the shunt approximates that of the shunt tubing. From Figure 14-3 it can be seen that even if the normal production of CSF were doubled, inlet pressure (intraventricular pressure) would not significantly increase above the inlet pressure at zero flow (i.e., the closing pressure of the valve). With an LRV, intraventricular pressure thus is maintained essentially just above the rated closing pressure of the valve. As discussed later, *this statement is true only if the outlet of the valve is at atmospheric pressure.*

In contrast to the LRV, the HRV does not open widely once the opening pressure is exceeded. All of the silicone rubber slit valves fall into this category and, to a lesser extent, so do the miter valves. As a slit valve undergoes increasing pressure, the lips of the valve separate, which presents a gradually increasing cross-sectional orifice to the flow of fluid.[82] This relationship between pressure and cross-section orifice results in a nonlinear increase in flow with increasing pressure, as depicted in Figure 14-4 for a "medium-pressure" valve. The LRV regulates inlet (intraventricular) pressure by attempting to match inflow (CSF formation) with some point on the pressure–flow curve. Variations in flow through the valve within the normal range of CSF formation result in a wide range of inlet pressures; thus it is much more difficult to maintain a specific intraventricular pressure using an HRV than an LRV. This variation in inlet pressure is amplified if the outlet of the valve is not maintained at atmospheric pressure.

A significant problem with silicone rubber slit valves is a varying pressure–flow curve which depends on the pretreatment of the valve (Figure 14-4).[25] In our laboratory it was found that the valve must soak without disturbance for at least 24 hours after filling in order to obtain repeatable results. When utilizing this calibration technique, a slit valve will have the same pressure–flow curve when tested several months apart or after removal as an implant.[80] A slit valve irrigated

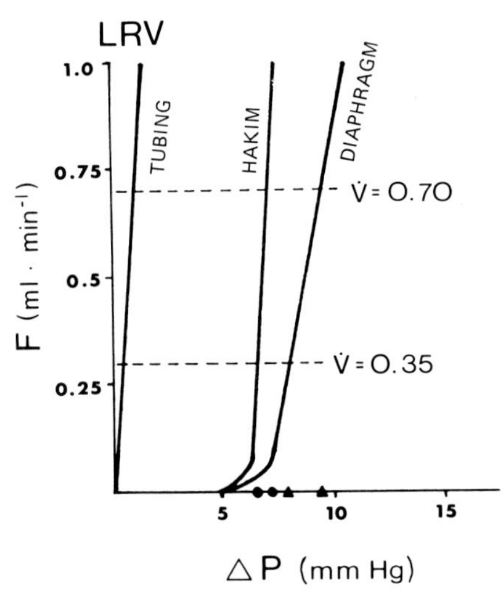

Figure 14-3. Pressure–flow characteristics of low-resistance valves. Note that doubling of the formation rate (V) minimally affects the differential pressure (ΔP) across the valve [Hakim springball valve (●) Pudenz silicone rubber diaphragm valve (▲)].

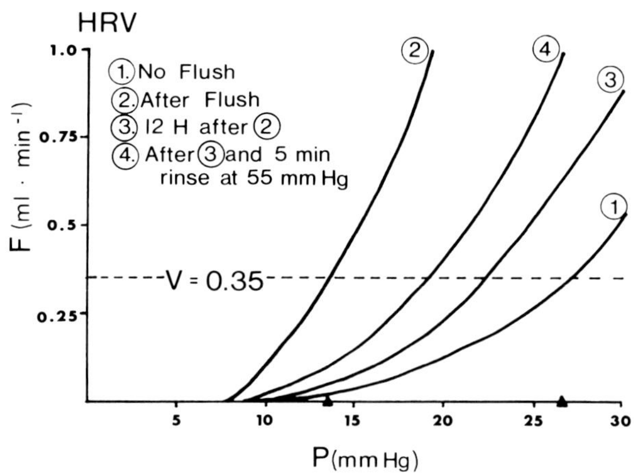

Figure 14-4. Pressure–flow characteristics of a medium-pressure silicone rubber slit valve (from data supplied by J. Ekstedt[25]). When the valve has not been flushed (curve 1), inlet pressure (P) is markedly affected by formation rate ($\dot{V}$). At a formation rate of 0.35 ml · min^{-1}, inlet pressure for this medium-pressure valve is quite high (▲). Testing at time of surgery would result in a curve similar to curve 2, and the apparent inlet pressure at 0.35 ml · min^{-1} would be much lower.

and tested at surgery will have an excessive flow when compared to the above method of calibration.

A DPV can only maintain the desired inlet pressure if the outlet pressure is at atmospheric pressure, the condition that exists when the valve is bench-tested. Should the outlet pressure vary in any direction, the inlet pressure will vary in exactly the same manner. Variations in valve outlet pressure can arise from several causes. As Yamada, Tajima, and Nagaya[99] have demonstrated, right auricular pressure (RAP) and intraperitoneal pressure (IPP) vary considerably during infant activities, especially crying. They found that when infants were quiet, RAP was usually slightly negative (−10–0 mm H_2O) while IPP was usually positive (10–50 mm H_2O). When crying RAP varied from −100 to −200 mm H_2O during inspiration to 400–800 mm H_2O during expiration, and IPP varied from 30–150 mm H_2O during inspiration to 400–750 mm H_2O during expiration.

A more constant alteration in outlet pressure is produced by the siphoning effect of the vertical distal catheter when the patient is upright.[13,32,81,82,100] Any water-filled vertical tube produces a hydrostatic pressure (HP) equal in millimeters H_2O to the vertical height between the two ends of the tube (not the length of the tube). The vertical distal catheter of the shunt, whether going to the auricle or peritoneal cavity, produces such an HP at the outlet of the valve (Fig. 14-5). In a lumboperitoneal shunt, the vertical height of the spine must also be calculated as part of the HP of the system.

The pressure that drives CSF through a shunt can be expressed by the

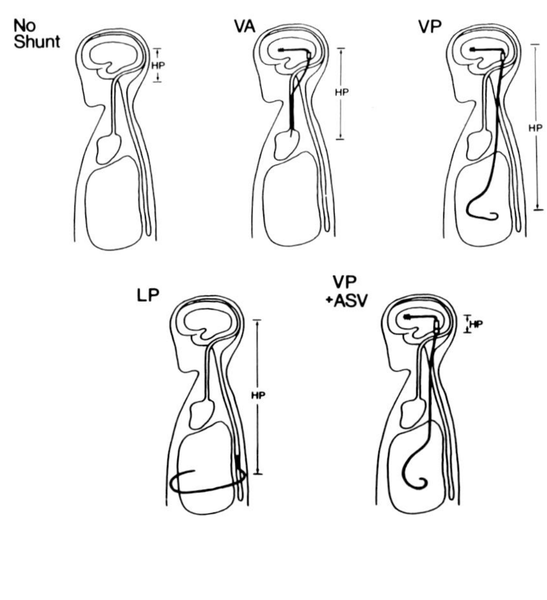

Figure 14-5. The hydrostatic pressure (HP) in the normal and shunted individual with various types of shunt. In each instance the HP is governed by the vertical height between the ventricle and the point of equilibration with atmospheric pressure.

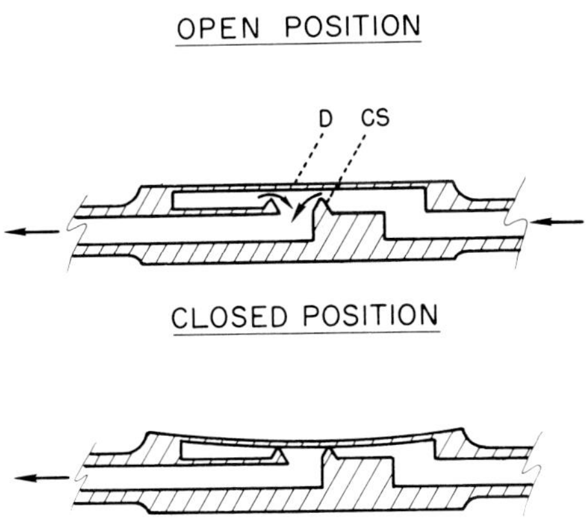

Figure 14-6. The antisiphon valve: D, diaphragm; CS, crown seat. (Reprinted with permission from Portnoy HD Schulte RR, Fox JL, et al: Antisiphon and reversible occlusion valves for shunting in hydrocephalus and preventing post-shunt subdural hematomas. J Neurosurg 38:729–739, 1973.)

following equation: PP = IVP + HP − (DCP + CP), where PP is shunt perfusion pressure, IVP is intraventricular pressure, HP is hydrostatic pressure (positive in head-up position, negative in head-down position), DCP is distal cavity pressure (peritoneal or auricular), and CP is the closing pressure of the DPV.[32,81] Cerebrospinal fluid will continue to flow through the shunt until PP equals zero. In the supine position, HP is zero, and the valve will close when the IVP equals DCP + CP. When the patient is erect, the HP becomes significant. If HP exceeds DCP + CP, IVP will drop below atmospheric pressure before the shunt ceases to flow, and may drop as low as −400 mm H_2O.[32,81] The shunt has bypassed the natural antisiphon effect of the internal jugular veins.[35]

From the foregoing discussion, it can be seen that in the supine position IVP is governed primarily by the pressure–flow characteristics of the valve, whereas in the upright position IVP is determined primarily by the hydrostatic pressure, although the rate of drainage will be governed by the pressure–flow characteristics of the valve. A shunt with an LRV will drain rapidly, and acutely produce a negative IVP. With an HRV the drainage is slower.

The siphon effect can be eliminated in vivo by equilibrating the outlet of the DPV with atmospheric pressure.[79,82] This will restore the pressure–flow characteristics of the valve to those measured at the time of calibration when the valve outlet was at atmospheric pressure. In vivo equilibration has been accomplished in two ways. Hakim[37] has developed a complex valve that opens and closes in response to a balloon sensor within the valve, and is linked to a balloon beneath the scalp (essentially at atmospheric pressure). Portnoy, Schulte, Fox, et al.[81] devised the antisiphon valve (ASV), which, when placed just distal to any DPV, does not allow the DPV outlet pressure to drop significantly below atmospheric pressure. Of these valves only the ASV is commercially available (Fig. 14-6).

The ASV works in the following manner. Implanted beneath the scalp, the diaphragm of the valve and the overlying scalp act as a single unit in equilibrium with atmospheric pressure. If the pressure within the valve exceeds atmospheric pressure, the diaphragm (D) is displaced away from the valve crown seat (CS) and CSF flows through the valve; if the pressure within the valve drops below atmospheric pressure, then the diaphragm seats and the valve closes.*

---

*If the area beneath the inlet and outlet portions of the diaphragm were the same size, a negative pressure exerted at the outlet would require a similar positive pressure at the inlet to pop open the valve. A strong negative pressure created by a long distal catheter could theoretically require a high CSF pressure to open the valve. To prevent this problem the areas of the diaphragm under the inlet and outlet have an 8:1 ratio. Thus, even with a 800 mm distal catheter, a CSF pressure of 100 mm H_2O will open the valve. To prevent the overlying scalp from exerting enough pressure to occlude the ASV, there is a 0.125 mm offset between diaphragm and crown seat. Full closure of the valve, therefore, does not occur unless at least −100 mm H_2O is exerted at the outlet.

While the in vivo effectiveness of the ASV has been demonstrated,[79,81] it is important to realize that it cannot be used with every DPV. The ASV can only be used with a proximal valve and must be placed immediately following the outlet of the valve. It will have minimal effect on a distally placed slit valve.[82]

The ASV performs most ideally with an LRV and should not be used with a medium or high pressure HRV. If an LRV having a closing pressure of 90 mm H_2O (6.6 mm Hg) is implanted, IVP will be held at slightly above this pressure when the patient is supine (Figure 14-7).

If the patient stands and the vertical length of the distal catheter is 300 mm, the differential pressure across the valve will increase by an HP of 300 mm H_2O (22 mm Hg). The valve opens and CSF flows rapidly through the shunt until the PP equals zero. This will occur when the IVP is −15 mm Hg. The addition of an ASV eliminates the siphon effect, and IVP again approximates 7 mm Hg.

In a supine patient, a typical medium-pressure HRV usually maintains a much higher IVP (Fig. 14-4, curve 1). If all CSF formed left through the shunt illustrated, the IVP would be 27 mm Hg. On the patient's standing, the same 300 mm H_2O (22 mm Hg) hydrostatic pressure increases the perfusion pressure across the valve, CSF flow increases, and IVP decreases to −15 mm Hg, but at a much slower rate than with an LRV. When the patient lies down, the IVP again slowly increases. Ideally an HRV is selected that underdrains when the patient is supine, and overdrains to the same degree when the patient is standing. The addition of an ASV to an HRV eliminates the balancing overdrainage and the shunt becomes inadequate.

Since an infant usually remains supine, it is generally necessary when using an HRV to select one with a "low-pressure" rating. When the infant begins to walk, such a low-pressure slit valve will act much like an LRV and begin to overdrain. This has led some neurosurgeons to increase the pressure rating of the shunt valve prophylactically when the child reaches 1 year of age. An alternative

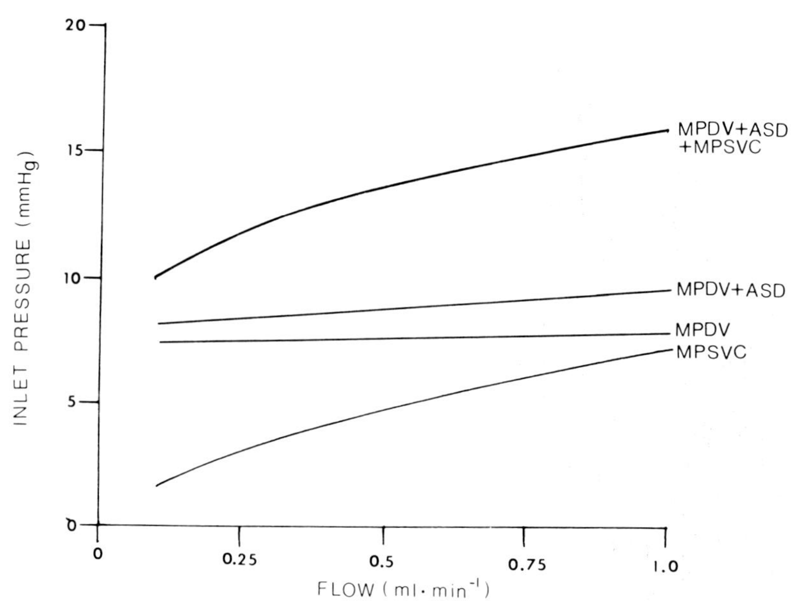

Figure 14-7. Demonstration of the additive resistive effects of shunt components in series. Note the additive effects of MPDV and MPSVC resulting in a high pressure shunt. MPDV, medium-pressure diaphragm valve; MPSCV, medium-pressure slit valve catheter; ASD, antisiphon device.

is to install a medium-pressure LRV coupled with an ASV that maintains approximately the same IVP regardless of the position of the child.

Two valves in series can cause a hidden problem. Usually only one of the two valves is looked upon as the control valve, and the existence of the other virtually is ignored. The resistances of valves in series are additive. As demonstrated in Figure 14-7, when a medium-pressure distal slit valve is added to a medium-pressure proximal diaphragm valve, the result is a high-pressure shunt with pressure–flow characteristics most resembling those of the slit valve. If pressure control is desired at the proximal valve, then the distal slit valve catheter should be a low-pressure type. It should have almost no resistance to flow. The combination of a medium-pressure proximal valve and medium-pressure distal slit valve may work adequately without an ASV, but fail with the ASV. The neurosurgeon usually condemns the ASV, not realizing that the complex valve system is a high-pressure shunt that should not contain an ASV.

If the object of a shunt is to maintain a relatively constant specific intracranial pressure, then the best valve system is an LRV with an ASV. Second best is an HRV without an ASV. An LRV without an ASV will work, but frequently will result in a low intraventricular pressure. A medium- or high-pressure HRV should not be used with an ASV because the child may not be adequately shunted.

Types of Shunts and Related Complications

The ability to maintain a viable shunt depends on knowing what complications can develop and then selecting the shunt components and operation to avoid these complications. Although many types of shunt procedures have been devised, only the ventriculoatrial (VA), ventriculoperitoneal (VP), and lumboperitoneal (LP) shunts have had success in the hands of a wide variety of neurosurgeons. The first two shunts may be used for all forms of hydrocephalus while the last is limited to communicating hydrocephalus.

The VA shunt was the first to be generally successful in the treatment of hydrocephalus.[3,15,22,27,47,49,71,72,74,84] Since the venous catheter must be repeatedly lengthened in the growing child, the VA shunt poses a major problem in shunt maintenance.[5,78] An infant shunted shortly after birth may require two, three, or more revisions for this reason alone. In addition septicemia and venous thrombosis are significant complications.[30,51,70]

For these reasons the VP shunt has become increasingly popular in the treatment of hydrocephalus, particularly in the growing child.[2,23,39,46,52,89,101] The simple expedient of placing 25–30 cm of tubing within the peritoneal cavity allows the shunt to lengthen as the child grows. A shunt inserted in a newborn frequently lasts 3 to 4 years before revision is required. If infected, the VP shunt rarely leads to a generalized infection. Because of the antimicrobial activity of peritoneal fluid,[6] the tip of the infected peritoneal catheter usually is walled off much like a ruptured appendix. More often the walling off occurs simply as a reaction to the catheter (or adherent powder from surgical gloves). Whether due to infection or not, the result is an obstructed shunt and sometimes abdominal cyst formation.[20,29,33,55]

In addition to the above, there are a variety of complications seen in nearly all series of patients that result in revisions, such as disconnection of shunt components, fracture of a catheter, erosion of the shunt through the skin, loss of the ventricular catheter into the ventricle, kinking of a proximal or distal catheter, particulate matter within the shunt, an erroneously placed catheter, over- and undershunting, and the formation of a subdural hematoma.[30,32,39,44,46,47,49,52,74,79,81,82]

Operative Procedures

In the infant a VP or LP shunt avoids the problem of multiple revisions for lengthening a distal catheter. The components should be selected to minimize complications, or to help in localizing a complication, if one should develop. The VA and VP shunts should include a reservoir. The components should be radiopaque so that any separation of the shunt can be readily detected on a plain skull, chest, or abdomen radiograph.

The reservoir allows easy percutaneous access to the shunt. If a shunt infection is suspected, CSF can be readily obtained from the reservoir for culture, a positive bacterial culture can be obtained even when cultures of ventricular and spinal fluids are negative.[69] The reservoir is also helpful in localizing a block. If, after the reservoir is depressed, it readily expands, the block is distal. A slowly expanding reservoir suggests a ventricular catheter obstruction, although in the presence of a small ventricle the reservoir may take 30 to 60 seconds to expand. Definitive localization of the block can be obtained by injecting either an isotope or contrast medium into the reservoir and following its course.[28,40,67,95]

The necessity for selecting an appropriate DPV has already been reviewed. Whenever craniocerebral disproportion (or, as in the adult, normal pressure hydrocephalus) exists, it may be advisable to include an on–off valve to attempt to prevent the formation of a postoperative subdural hematoma.[81] Closure of the shunt for three to four days postoperatively by utilizing an on–off valve may prevent formation of the subdural hematoma by temporarily expanding the brain and sealing the subdural space.

Ventricular catheter obstruction can be virtually eliminated by the use of a flanged ventricular catheter[36,76] and placing the tip of the catheter in the frontal horn away from the choroid plexus.[5] In the last 12 years during which this catheter has been used, the revision rate for occluded ventricular catheters has been 4 percent. Removal of the catheter is easily accomplished by rotating the catheter as it is extracted. This sweeps the choroid plexus from the flanges.

A shunt should never be inserted in the presence of infection. Any infection should be cleared completely, whether it be meningitis or a simple skin infection in the operative field.

The surgical procedure should be simple. General endotracheal anesthesia is preferred, although local anesthesia can be used. There should be only a few short incisions and revisions should be through the same scars, or placed completely away from the old surgical site. Large and crisscrossing incisions invite tissue breakdown and shunt infection.

VP shunt. The following technique is simple and avoids complications by planning ahead. The child should urinate just before surgery or, in the infant, the Crede maneuver can be carried out after the infant is anesthetized. If there is any question of a full urinary bladder, the bladder should be catheterized.

Presoaking the shunt components in a closed container with 50,000 units of bacitracin and 0.5 gram of neomycin added to 250 ml of saline may reduce infections.

The infant is placed with the head rotated to the left (Fig. 14-8). A small, slightly curved incision is made over the parietal boss and the skull trephined (Fig. 14-8B). With the use of a hemostat, a subgaleal pocket is formed inferior to the incision to accept the valve (Fig. 14-8A). A flat-bottomed valve is preferred. Next a tunneling device is passed from the scalp incision subgaleally (through the pocket) and subcutaneously to a small incision over the lateral aspect of the rectus abdominis muscle just above the level of the umbilicus (Fig. 14-8C). The catheter is drawn up from the abdominal to the scalp incision. Occasionally a

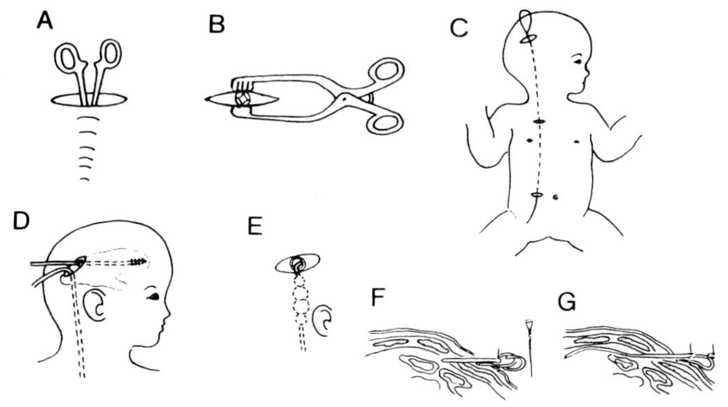

Figure 14-8. Technique for insertion of a ventriculoperitoneal shunt.

subclavicular incision is also needed. The peritoneal catheter is cut to length and attached to the distal end of the valve with a connector. Separation of the catheter from the valve is minimized if the two sutures holding the valve and catheter to the connector are tied together.

The dura and brain surface are coagulated and incised. The incision in the dura should just allow insertion of a ventricular cannula. If the cerebral mantle is thin, the catheter should be inserted directly into the ventricle. If the mantle is thick, the catheter is inserted through a ventricular cannula (Fig. 14-8D). The catheter is cut long, attached to the valve, and the valve and extra length of catheter pulled down into the subgaleal pocket as illustrated in Figure 14-8E. If a wire-reinforced catheter is used, it will not kink as it passes over the trephine edge. Should the catheter loosen from the valve, it will not fall into the ventricle since the catheter is slightly long. This method is preferrable to the use of a valve that fits into the trephine, or the use of an angled connector as a disconnection will result in the catheter falling into the ventricle.

The peritoneal end of the peritoneal catheter is then inserted into the abdominal cavity. Though many neurosurgeons prefer insertion by laparotomy, the procedure is simplified by using a trochar (Fig. 14-8F).[85] The trochar is aimed toward the lower quadrant, and care is taken not to impinge bowel between the trochar tip and the spine. The catheter is then fed through the trochar into the abdomen (Fig. 14-8G). At each stage of the procedure, the shunt is tested to be sure there is free flow and no kink in the tubing. Insertion of the catheter by trochar not only quickens the procedure, but probably produces less scar tissue at the entrance of the catheter into the peritoneal cavity. Scar tissue at this site will bind the catheter, resulting in a catheter that stretches rather than one that pulls out of the cavity. A stretched catheter will eventually snap, requiring a premature revision. At completion of the procedure, the wounds are closed in layers.

When the peritoneal catheter requires lengthening, a new catheter should not be added to the end of the old one. The connector between the two segments cannot migrate up the subcutaneous channel. This will result in a fractured catheter, or disconnection. A completely new catheter should be inserted.

VA shunt. Insertion of the proximal catheter and valve of a ventriculoatrial shunt is similar to that for a VP shunt (Fig. 14-9). A low-pressure atrial slit valve catheter, or open-end catheter, is chosen so as not significantly to alter the characteristics of the shunt as determined by the proximal valve.

In addition to the incision over the right parietal boss, a second incision is made over the lower end of the valve as it lies in the subgaleal pocket, and a third transverse incision is made over the medial aspect of the sternomastoid muscle

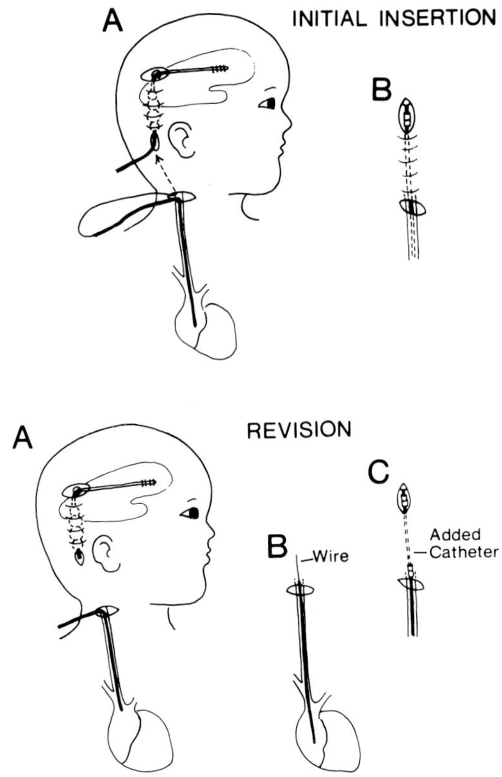

Figure 14-9. Technique for insertion and revision of a ventriculo-atrial shunt.

about halfway between the ear and midclavicle (upper Fig. 14-9A). The ventricular catheter and valve are inserted in the same manner as described for a VP shunt, except that a small piece of silicone rubber tubing attached to the valve outlet is used to pull the valve down into the subgaleal pocket.

The cervical incision is carried down to the junction of the jugular and facial veins. An estimation of the appropriate length of distal catheter is determined by measuring the clavicular to T6 vertebral body distance on a chest radiograph. When possible the atrial catheter is inserted through a small nick in the facial vein, into the jugular vein. In infants this may not be possible, and the catheter is introduced directly into the jugular vein. The appropriate length of atrial catheter may be determined electrocardiographically by inserting a needle into the proximal end of the catheter and filling the catheter with saline. The catheter thus becomes an intracardiac electrode when attached to the appropriate lead of the electrocardiogram EKG. As the tip of the catheter passes into the atrium, the P-wave, which is initially downward, becomes biphasic. If advanced to the triscupid valve, the P-wave becomes deflected upward and the catheter should be withdrawn.[57,90] The length as determined by the EKG method should be within 1 cm of the length previously determined from the chest radiograph.

Keeping in mind the concept of planning ahead for a revision, the proximal end of the atrial catheter is tunneled subcutaneously to the incision at the lower end of the valve (upper Fig. 14-9B). A connector is not placed at the jugular vein. The temporary piece of tubing attached to the valve outlet is discarded and the atrial catheter cut to length and connected to the valve outlet. The facial or jugular vein need not be ligated about the catheter. Venous ooze from the opening in the vein is readily stopped with a little absorbable gelatin sponge.

When lengthening is contemplated, the two distal incisions are reopened (lower Fig. 14-9A). The atrial catheter is disconnected from the valve and pulled down into the cervical incision. A 0.035-inch-diameter Seldinger guide wire is then inserted into the catheter after being lubricated with a drop of sterile iodophendylate (Pantopaque) (lower Fig. 14-9B). The catheter, supported by the guide wire, is advanced to the new position as determined by an intraoperative radiograph or EKG. A short segment of new catheter is then attached to the atrial catheter and retunneled to the incision at the lower end of the valve (lower Fig. 14-9C). There it is cut to size and connected to the valve outlet.[45,104] The atrial catheter thus may be advanced several times. A new atrial catheter must be inserted only when the proximal end of the atrial catheter reaches the opening in the jugular vein.

LP shunt. The LP shunt is useful in cases of communicating hydrocephalus because it avoids the problem of proximal catheter occlusion by the choroid plexus and minimizes the problem of shunt lengthening with growth. A significant drawback is that there is no practical way to eliminate overdrainage attributable to the siphon effect. Siphoning can be minimized by increasing the resistance of the shunt through the use of small tubing and a high-resistance slit valve.

For the infant the method described by Hoffman, Hendrick, and Humphreys can be used.[44] The shunt is composed of a T-shaped silastic catheter with a distal slit-valve tip. The operation is performed with the infant on its side, with the abdomen, flank, and midline of the back exposed. A small incision is made over the T12 and L1 spinous processes, and a portion of these adjacent lamina removed. A small dural and arachnoid incision is made. The dura is closed over the catheter. The distal tip of the catheter is tunneled beneath the skin to the flank, and then to the abdomen over the rectus muslce. The peritoneal catheter is then inserted into the peritoneal cavity by means of a trochar.

For the older child and adult, the LP shunt procedure described by Spetzler with Wilson and Grollmus[16] and with Wilson and Schulte[21] may be preferred since a laminectomy is not necessary. The shunt itself consists of a thin spring-reinforced silastic tubing with multiple holes at the proximal end and a slit valve at the distal end. The patient lies in the lateral decubitus position with knees flexed. The operating table is tilted up slightly to expand the lumber subarachnoid space. A small skin incision is placed over the L3 and L4 spinous processes. Through the incision a 14 g Touhey spinal needle is introduced into the subarachnoid space in a cephalad direction. The proximal end of the catheter is inserted for 4 to 8 cm, and the needle withdrawn over the catheter, leaving the catheter in the lumbar subarachnoid space. If the catheter is properly placed, CSF flows from the distal end. A tunneling instrument is used to form a subcutaneous tunnel to a small incision in the flank and then to a small incision over the ipsilateral rectus muscle. By applying gentle suction to the tunneling instrument, the catheter is drawn first between the lumbar and flank incisions, and then between the flank and abdominal incisions. With a peritoneal trochar, the distal end of the catheter is placed into the abdominal cavity. A sleeve supplied with the catheter allows it to be secured to the tissues to prevent catheter migration.

Because the LP shunt does not usually contain a reservoir, patency of the shunt is best determined by introducing a radioisotope into the subarachnoid space and determining whether the isotope flows into the peritoneal cavity.

REFERENCES

1. Amacher AL, Page LK: Hydrocephalus due to membranous obstruction of the fourth ventricles. J Neurosurg 35:672–676, 1971
2. Ames RH: Ventriculo-peritoneal shunts in the management of hydrocephalus. J Neurosurg 27:525–529, 1967

3. Anderson FM: Ventriculo-auriculostomy in treatment of hydrocephalus. J Neurosurg 16:551–557, 1959
4. Balakrishnan V, Dinning TAR: Non-neoplastic stenosis of the aqueduct presenting in adolescence and adult life. Surg Neurol 7:333–338, 1977
5. Becker DP, Nulsen FE: Control of hydrocephalus by valve regulated venous shunt: Avoidance of complications in prolonged shunt maintenance. J Neurosurg 28:215–226, 1968
6. Bercovici B, Michel J, Miller J, et al: Antimicrobial activity of human peritoneal fluid. Surg Gynec Obstet 141:885–887, 1975
7. Bering EA Jr: Problems of the dynamics of the cerebrospinal fluid with particular reference to the formation of cerebrospinal fluid and its relationship to cerebral metabolism. Clin Neurosurg 5:77–89, 1958
8. Braley S: The silicones as subdural engineering materials. Ann NY Acad Sci 146:148–157, 1968
9. Schain, RJ: Carbonic anhydrase inhibitors in chronic infantile hydrocephalus. Am J Dis Child 117:621, 1969
10. Bryan N, Coe JE: Experimental alteration in cerebrospinal fluid production following cryosurgery of the choroid plexus. J Neurosurg 62–64, 1969
11. Crosby RMN, Henderson CM, Paul RL. Catheterization of the cerebral aqueduct for obstructive hydrocephalus in infants. J Neurosurg 38:596–601, 1973
12. Crosby RMN, Paul RL: Treatment of Hydrocephalus: Direct attack on the obstruction. Am Surg 35:701–704, 1969
13. Shucart WA, Connolly R: Experimental negative intraventricular pressures. J Surg Res 19:43–46, 1975
14. Cserr HF: Physiology of the choroid plexus. Physiol Rev 51:273–311, 1971
15. Shurtleff DB, Foltz EL: Clinical observations on twenty hydrocephalic children subjected to ventriculoatrial shunt: A preliminary report. J Dis Child 98:467–468, 1959
16. Spetzler RF, Wilson CB, Grollmus JM: Percutaneous lumboperitoneal shunt. Technical note. J Neurosurg 43:770–773, 1975
17. Dandy WE: An operative procedure for hydrocephalus. Bull Johns Hopkins Hosp. 33:189–190, 1922
18. Dandy WE: Diagnosis and treatment of strictures of the aqueduct of Sylvius (causing hydrocephalus). Arch Surg 51:1-14, 1945
19. Dandy WE: Exterpation of the choroid plexus of the lateral ventricles in communicating hydrocephalus. Ann Surg 68:569–579, 1918
20. Davidson RI: Peritoneal bypass in the treatment of hydrocephalus, historical review and abdominal complications. J Neurol Neurosurg Psychiatr 39:640–646, 1976
21. Spetzler R, Wilson CB, Schulte R: Simplified percutaneous lumboperitoneal shunting. Surg Neurol 7:25–29, 1977
22. Spitz EB: Neurosurgery in the prevention of exogenous mental retardation. Pediatr Clin N Am 6:1215–1235, 1959
23. Stark GD, Drummond MB, Poneprasert S, et al: Primary ventriculo-peritoneal shunts in the treatment of hydrocephalus associated with myelomeningocele. Arch Dis Child 49:112–117, 1974
24. Stookey B, Scarff J: Occlusion of the aqueduct of Sylvius by neoplastic and non-neoplastic processes with a rational surgical treatment for relief of the resultant obstructive hydrocephalus. Bull Neurol Inst NY 5:348–377, 1936
25. Ekstedt J, Friden H: Hydrodynamic properties of CSF shunt systems, in Shulman K, Marmarou A, Millek JD (eds): Intracranial Pressure IV. Berlin, New York, Springer-Verlag, 1980, pp 483–488
26. Elvidge AR: Treatment of obstructive lesions of the aqueduct of Sylvius and the fourth ventricle by interventriculostomy. J Neurosurg 24:11–23, 1966
27. Emery JL: Intracranial effects of long-standing decompression of the brain in children with hydrocephalus and meningomyelocele. Dev Med Child Neurol 7:302–309, 1965
28. Evans RC, Thomas MD, Williams LA: The use of the valvogram for the detection of shunt blockage in hydrocephalic children. Dev Med Child Neurol 17(suppl 35):94–98, 1975

29. Fischer EG, Shillito J Jr: Large abdominal cysts: A complication of peritoneal shunts. Report of three cases. J Neurosurg 31:441–444, 1969
30. Forrest DM, Cooper DGW: Complications of ventriculo-atrial shunts. A review of 455 cases. J Neurosurg 29:506–512, 1968
31. Fox JL, McCullough DC, Green RC: Cerebrospinal fluid shunts: An experimental comparison of flow rates and pressure valves in various commercial systems. J Neurosurg 37:700–705, 1972
32. Fox JC, McCullough DC, Green RD: Effect of cerebrospinal fluid shunts on intracranial pressure and on cerebrospinal fluid dynamics. 2. A new technique of pressure measurements: Results and concepts. 3. A concept of hydrocephalus. J Neurol Neurosurg Psychiatr 36:302–312, 1973
33. Grosfeld JL, Cooney DR, Smith J, et al: Intra-abdominal complications following ventriculoperitoneal shunt procedures. Pediatrics 54:791–796, 1974
34. Guiot G, Derome P, Hertzog E, et al: Ventriculo-cisternostomie sous controle radioscopique pour hydrocephalie obstructive. Presse Med 76:1923–1926, 1968
35. Guyton AC: Textbook of Medical Physiology (ed 4). Philadelphia, WB Saunders 1971, pp 224–226
36. Hakim S: Contribution al estudio de la fisopatologia del pulso del liquido cefalo-raquideo. Prevencion de la obstruccion del cateter ventricular en las ventriculo-atriostomios. Ciencias Neurol 3:3–16, 1969
37. Hakim S: Hydraulic and mechanical mis-matching of valve shunts used in the treatment of hydrocephalus. The need for a servo-valve shunt. Dev Med Child Neurol 15:646–653, 1973
38. Hakim S, de la Roche D, Burton JD: A critical analysis of valve shunts used in the treatment of hydrocephalus. Dev Med Child Neurol 15:230–255, 1973
39. Hammon WM: Evaluation and use of the ventriculoperitoneal shunt in hydrocephalus. J Neurosurg 34:792–795, 1971
40. Harbert J, Haddad D, McCullough D. Quantitation of cerebrospinal fluid shunt flow. Nucl Med 112:379–387, 1974
41. Hayden PW, Foltz EL, Shurtleff DB: Effect of an oral osmotic agent on ventricular fluid pressure of hydrocephalic children. Pediatrics 41:955–967, 1968
42. Hoffman HJ: Personal communication, 1980
43. Hoffman HJ: The advantages of percutaneous third ventriculostomy over other forms of surgical treatment for infantile obstructive hydrocephalus, in Morley T (ed): Current controversies in Neurosurgery. Philadelphia, WB Saunders, 1974, pp 691–703
44. Hoffman HJ, Hendrick EB, Humphreys RF: New luboperitoneal shunt for communicating hydrocephalus. Technical note. J Neurosurg 44:258–261, 1976
45. Hooper R: A lengthening procedure for ventriculo-atrial shunts. Technical note. J Neurosurg 30:93–96. 1969
46. Ignelzi RJ, Kirsch WM: Follow-up analysis of ventriculoperitoneal and ventriculo-atrial shunts for hydrocephalus. J Neurosurg 42:679–682, 1975
47. Illingsworth RD, Logue V, Symon L. et al: The ventriculocaval shunt in the treatment of adult hydrocephalus. Results and complications in 101 patients. J Neurosurg 35:681–685, 1971
48. Irving IM, Castilla P, Hall EG, et al: Tissue reaction to pure and impregnated Silastic. J Pediatr Surg 6:724–729, 1971
49. Ivan LP, Stratford JG, Gerrard JW et al: Surgical treatment of infantile hydrocephalus: Ten years' experience in the use of ventriculoatrial shunts with the Holter valve. Can Med Assoc J 98:337–343, 1968
50. James AE, Mathews ES, Dorst JP: Technique of cerebrospinal imaging, in James AE, Wagner HN, Cooke RE (eds): Pediatric Nuclear Medicine. Philadelphia, WB Saunders, 1974, pp 144–157
51. Strenger L: Complications of ventriculovenous shunts. J Neurosurg 20:219–224, 1963
52. Keucher TR, Mealey J: Long-term results after ventriculoatrial and ventriculoperitoneal shunting for infantile hydrocepahlus. J Neurosurg 50:179–186, 1979
53. Kushner J, Alexander E Jr., Davis CH Jr., et al: Kyphoscoliosis following lumbar subarachnoid shunts. J Neurosurg 34:783–791, 1971

54. Little JR, Houser OW, MacCarty CS: Clinical manifestations of aqueductal stenosis in adults. J Neurosurg 43:546–552, 1975
55. Llewellyn RC: Abdominal pseudocysts and ascites formation after ventriculoperitoneal shunt procedures. Report of four cases. J Neurosurg 43:476–480, 1975
56. Lorenzo AC, Page LK, Walter GV: Relationship between CSF formation, absorption and pressure in human hydrocephalus. Brain 93:679–692, 1970
57. McLaurin RL, Glass IH, Kaplan S: Ventriculoatrial shunt for hydrocephalus. Electrocardiographic control for accurate placement. Am J Dis Child 105:216–218, 1963
58. McNickle HF: The surgical treatment of hydrocephalus. A simple method of performing third ventriculostomy. Br J Surg 34:302–307, 1947
59. Marzoni FA, Upchurch SE, Lambert CJ: An experimental study of silicone as soft tissue substitute. Plas Reconstr Plas 24:600–608, 1959
60. Matson DD: Neurosurgery of Infancy and Childhood (ed 2). Springfield, Charles C Thomas, 1969
61. Mealey J Jr, Barker DT: Failure of oral acetazalamide to avert hydrocephalus in infants with myelomeningocele. J Pediatr 72:257–259, 1968
62. Milhorat TH: Choroid plexus and cerebrospinal fluid production. Science 166:1514–1516, 1969
63. Milhorat TH: Failure of choroid plexectomy as treatment for hydrocephalus. Surg Gynec Obstet 139:505–508, 1974
64. Milhorat TH: The third circulation revisited. J Neurosurg 628–645, 1975
65. Milhorat TH, Hammock MK, Chien T, et al: Normal rate of cerebrospinal fluid formation five years after bilateral choroid plexectomy. Case report. J Neurosurg 44:735–739, 1976
66. Milhorat TH, Hammock MK, Fenstermacher JD, et al: Cerebrospinal fluid production by the choroid plexus and brain. Science 173:330–332, 1971
67. Sty JR, D'Souza BJ, Daniels D: Nuclear anatomy of diversionary control nervous system shunts in children. Clin Nucl Med 3:271–275, 1978
68. Torkildsen A: New palliative operation in cases of inoperable occlusion of sylvian aqueduct. Acta Chir Scand 82:117–123, 1939
69. Myers MG, Schoenbaum SC: Shunt fluid aspiration. An adjunct in the diagnosis of cerebrospinal fluid shunt infection. Am J Dis Child 129:220–222, 1975
70. Nugent GR, Lucas R, Judy M, et al: Thromboembolic complications of ventriculo-atrial shunts. Angiocardiographic and pathologic correlations. J Neurosurg 24:34–42, 1966
71. Nulsen FE, Spitz EB: Treatment of hydrocephalus by direct shunt from ventricles to jugular vein. Forum 2:399–403, 1952
72. Ojemann RG: Initial experience with the Hakim valve for ventriculovenous shunt. J Neurosurg 28:283–287, 1968
73. Oppelt WW, Paclak CS, Rall DP: Effect of certain drugs on cerebrospinal fluid production in the dog. Am J Physiol 206:247–250, 1964
74. Overton MC III, Snodgrass SR: Ventriculovenous shunts for infantile hydrocephalus. A review of five years experience with this method. J Neurosurg 23:517–521, 1965
75. Tschirgi RD, Frost RW, Taylor JL: Inhibition of cerebrospinal fluid formation by a carbonic anhydrase inhibitor, 2-acetylamino -1, 3, 4-thiadiazole -5- sulfonamide (Diamox). Proc Soc Exp Biol Med 87:373–376, 1954
76. Portnoy HD: New ventricular catheter for hydrocephalic shunts. J Neurosurg 34:702–703, 1971
77. Portnoy HD: Unpublished data
78. Tsingoglou S, Forrest DM: Therapeutic and prophylactic lengthening of distal catheter of the Holter ventriculo-atrial shunt.
79. Portnoy HD, Croissant PD: New devices for shunting hydrocephalics. Neurocir Mex 3:55–66, 1973
80. Portnoy HD, Croissant PD: Pre- and postoperative cerebrospinal fluid absorption studies in patients with myelomeningocele shunted for hydrocephalus. Child's Brain 4:47–64, 1978
81. Portnoy HD, Shulte RR, Fox JL, et al: Antisiphon and reversible occlusion valves for

for shunting in hydrocephalus and preventing post-shunt subdural hematomas. J Neurosurg 38:729–738, 1973

82. Portnoy HD, Tripp L, Croissant PD: Hydrodynamics of shunt valves. Child's Brain 2:242–256, 1976
83. Turnbull IM, Drake CG: Membranous occlusion of the aqueduct of Sylvius. J Neurosurg 24:24–33, 1966
84. Pudenz RH, Russell FE, Hurd AH, et al: Ventriculoauriculostomy. A technique for shunting cerebrospinal fluid into the right auricle. Preliminary report. J Neurosurg 14:171–179, 1957
85. Raimondi AJ, Matsumoto S. A simplified technique for performing the ventriculo-peritoneal shunt. Technical note. J Neurosurg 26:357–360, 1967
86. Vries JK: An endoscopic technique for third ventriculostomy. Surg Neurol 9:165–168, 1978
87. Rayport M, Reiss J: Hydrodynamic properties of certain shunt assemblies available for the treatment of hydrocephalus. Part 1: Report of a case of communicating hydrocephalus with increased cerebrospinal fluid production treated by duplication of shunting device. Part 2: Pressure–flow characteristics of the Spitz–Holter, Pudenz–Heyer, and Cordis–Hakim shunt systems. J Neurosurg 30:455–467, 1969
88. Rish BL, Meacham WF: Experimental study of intraventricular instillation of radioactive gold. J Neurosurg 27:15–20, 1967
89. Robertson JS, Maraga MI, Jennett B: Ventriculoperitoneal shunting for hydrocephalus. Br Med J 1:289–292, 1971
90. Robertson JT, Schick RW, Morgan F, et al: Accurate placement of ventriculo-atrial shunt for hydrocephalus under electrocardiograph control. J Neurosurg 18:255–257, 1961
91. Rubin RC, Henderson ES, Walker MD, et al: The production of cerebrospinal fluid in man and its modification by acetazolamide. J Neurosurg 25:430–436, 1966
92. Weiss MW, Nulsen FE, Kaufman B: Selective radionecrosis of the choroid plexus for control of experimental hydrocephalus. J Neurosurg 36:270–275, 1972
93. Sayers MP: Surgery for obstructive hydrocephalus. Acta Neurol Lat Am 1 (suppl):245–254, 1971
94. Sayers MP, Kosnik J: Percutaneous third ventriculostomy, experience and technique. Child's Brain 2:24–30, 1976
95. Savoiardo M, Solero CL, Passerini A, et al: Determination of cerebrospinal fluid shunt function with water soluble contrast medium. J Neurosurg 49:398–407, 1978
96. Weiss MH, Roessman U: Radioactive tissue changes induced to control experimental hydrocephalus. J Neurosurg 36:266–269, 1972
97. Scarff JE: The treatment of nonobstructive (communicating) hydrocephalus by endoscopic cauterization of the choroid plexuses. J Neurosurg 33:1–18, 1970
98. Scarff JE: The treatment of hydrocephalus: A historical and critical review of methods and results. J Neurol Neurosurg Psychol 26:1–26, 1963
99. Yamada H, Tajima M, Nagaya M: Effect of respiratory movement on cerebrospinal fluid dynamics in hydrocephalic infant with shunts. J Neurosurg 42:194–200, 1975
100. Yamada S, Ducker TB, Perot PL: Dynamic changes of cerebrospinal fluid in upright and recumbent shunted experimental animals. Child's Brain 1:187–192, 1975
101. Weiss SR, Raskind R: Twenty-two cases of hydrocephalus treated with a silastic ventriculoperitoneal shunt. Internat Surg 51:13–19, 1969
102. Wilkinson HA, LeMay M, Dre JH: Adult aqueductal stenosis. Arch Neurol 15:643–648, 1966
103. Yamada H, Tajima M: A method for lengthening the distal catheter of a Pudenz ventriculoatrial shunt. J Neurosurg 40:663–664, 1974

15. Results of Treatment for Hydrocephalus as a Guide to Future Management

Frank E. Nulsen
Harold L. Rekate

This discussion will be confined to hydrocephalus developing either in infancy (both genetic and acquired) or in later life, when a congenital defect in cerebrospinal fluid (CSF) pathways becomes operable. Hydrocephalus secondary to neoplasm is not included. We are considering 405 such cases treated by shunting from 1956 to 1976.

Prior to 1956 we lacked the mechanical ability adequately to control excessive CSF accumulation in the head. In our hands bypass procedures to provide ventricular CSF access to cisterns around a blocked aqueduct, for example, did not result in adequate absorption of CSF (as does a Torkildsen procedure[1] in the child who *acquires* a blocked aqueduct or third ventricle from tumor). Choroid plexectomy[2] did not arrest the process. Cerebrospinal fluid diversion to other body areas was only rarely effective, although certain of Cone's peritoneal shunts[3] and most of Matson's ureteral shunts[4] proved highly effective in their hands.

We had introduced a valve-checked venous shunt that proved highly effective in one case in 1949,[5]* but had to be abandoned because of the frequent complication of subdural fluid collections secondary to ventricular overdrainage. (The reported success occurred in a patient whose neonatal subdural hematomas caused both marked hydrocephalus and obliterated subdural spaces.) In 1956 Spitz and Holter supplied us with valve-regulated shunt equipment that combined the simple check valve function we had found inadequate, with a positive valve resistance to forward flow so that CSF diversion would cease when intracranial pressure became lowered to a specific level. Spitz had wisely required radiopacification of the equipment so that later ventricular catheter and venous catheter obstruction could be related to anatomic position. Spitz presented his results with use of this shunt at annual meetings of The Harvey Cushing Society in 1958, 1959, and 1963, but no publications are available. Multiple revisions were necessary for shunt dysfunction in these early patients

*Although this was titled "a shunt from ventricular to jugular vein," the article and diagram describe placement into superior vena cava *via* jugular vein.

before guidelines for shunt maintenance could be learned, and case infection rate became significant with multiple procedures. By 1962 it was evident that good intelligence quotient (IQ) development was best correlated with the multiplicity of revisions the growing child had undergone. This reflected the needed alertness of family and surgeons in striving to idealize shunt regulation for these patients. (Space does not permit discussion of a similar, equally effective valve-regulated shunt designed by Pudenz, in collaboration with Heyer and Schulte, also introduced in 1956. Comparisons of methodology and results, with such workers as Foltz, assisted development of our guidelines for shunt management. In a 1981 review,[6] Pudenz provides an excellent perspective for viewing this account of our experience.)

CASE SELECTION

It early became evident that as a final referral center we would be forced to treat every nutritionally healthy child destined for monstrous head growth. This would apply even to cases of hydranencephaly with no brain above the thalamic level, if either the parents or a long-term nursing facility were to be faced with a head growing week by week to huge proportions.

Preoperative study always included limited pneumoventriculography sufficient to rule out mass lesion, to define the degree and nature of the hydrocephalus, and to assure that the CSF was free of infection and high protein or blood content so as to be suitable for shunting. In addition a Blackfan test would be done to determine whether indigo-carmine dye placed in ventricles could be recovered from lumbar subarachnoid CSF. Mild hydrocephalus would not be treated unless there developed clear evidence for continued progression of ventricular enlargement.

RESULTS

Of 340 children shunted between July 1956 and July 1976, we have 271 survivors with adequate studies on 243. Sixty-one of these deaths occurred mercifully in infancy where "social shunts" were undertaken in problems of severe myelodysplasia, extreme hydrocephalus at birth, or hydrocephalus following severe brain damage from neonatal hemorrhage or meningitis. The other eight deaths in older children were tragic. Those from overt shunt dysfunction, four in number, occurred prior to 1973 (two were venous catheter obstruction and two were coapted ventricles not responding to redrainage of tiny ventricles plus massive bony decompression). The remaining four were children with myelodysplasia and Arnold–Chiari malformations who seemed totally well despite proven shunt dysfunction, only to die abruptly at home from presumed respiratory arrest after up to three years of apparent shunt independence.

Although our ongoing analysis of results includes evaluation of performance in schooling, vocation, and social relationships, we here discuss results purely in terms of recent IQ determinations in patients aged 5 to 29 years. Older patients rarely showed downgrading from the original estimate unless an insult from shunt dysfunction occurred. This limited index of brain function correlates reasonably with other areas of performance in life, and neurologic defects attributable to hydrocephalus occurred only in the low IQ groups.

These IQ levels, as in our 1973 publication,[7] have been correlated with the widths of frontal cerebral mantle existing within the last year. This measurement is defined through pneumography in a lateral brow-up x-ray as the distance from the roof of the lateral ventricles (averaged when asymmetric) to the inner table of the skull in the axis of the coronal suture. Past correlation of ventriculogram measurements with computerized tomographic (CT) scan permits us now to estimate frontal mantle from CT scan alone. Cerebral volume measurements would be more quantitative, but attention to frontal mantle does answer the question: What is adequate control of hydrocephalus?

To evaluate the effects upon brain of hydrocephalus alone, we must exclude from our analysis of the 243 cases 81 patients who either at birth presented brain configurations reflecting maldevelopment not explainable by hydrocephalus alone, or who had severe brain insults developing hydrocephalus. These include cases of anoxic insults, bacterial meningitis, cerebral trauma, and intracranial bleeding, frequently in relation to respiratory distress. Hydrocephalus followed from impairment of CSF absorption. These patients were shunted either because they might become educable if an additional insult from progressive hydrocephalus were prevented, or because a social shunt was needed to avoid monstrous head growth.

In addition to this group of 81 brain-damaged patients, we further separated 82 children requiring shunts for hydrocephalus who had myelomeningoceles and presumed Arnold–Chiari malformations. This leaves us with 80 cases of "pure" hydrocephalus not complicated by primary brain damage or by myelodysplasia. Forty-three of these patients had blockade at the aqueduct that sometimes was responsible for a large head at birth but occasionally did not give symptoms until early adolescence. Thirteen cases (including eight Dandy–Walker malformations) showed fourth ventricle enlargement with block at the fourth ventricle outlets. The balance (24 cases) were shown to have communicating hydrocephalus. We assumed that the CSF absorption problem developed in utero. The behavior of all of these types of pure hydrocephalus appeared similar in showing significant correlation between IQ levels and control of ventriculomegaly, *except* for unpredictably good and poor outcomes in Dandy–Walker cases.

In Figure 15-1 the 80 cases are displayed in relation to IQ score in the *y*-axis and *final* frontal cerebral mantle width in the *x*-axis. Dandy–Walker malforma-

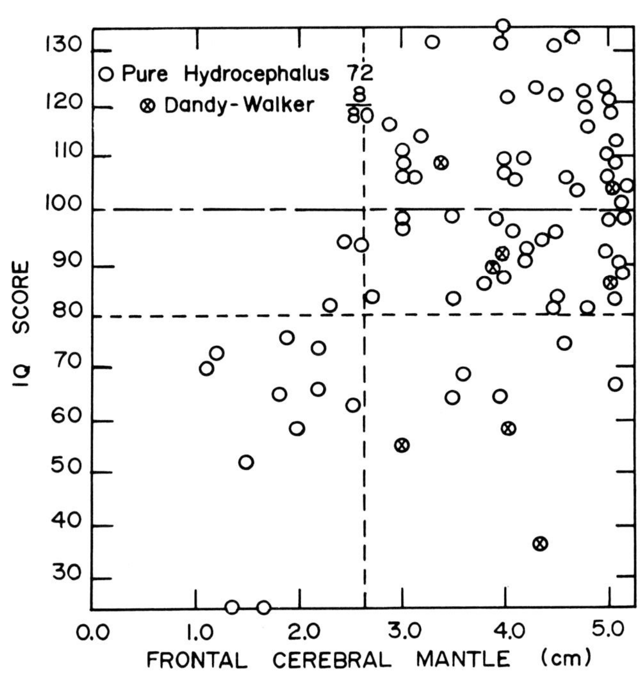

Figure 15-1. Current frontal mantle width in relation to IQ scores for 80 patients (ages 5–29) treated for "pure" hydrocephalus. Eight cases of Dandy–Walker malformation are included but with separate designation.

tions are designated separately. It is apparent that for any mantle under 2.0 cm the results will be just educable to dismal. There is a zone between 2.0 and slightly less than 3.0 cm where, in this small number, normal IQs of 100 are not reached. The surprising finding is that once we achieve a final mantle of 3.0, the IQ distribution, approaching normal, is much the same as it is at 3.5 or 4.0 or 5.0 cm. The important implication for management of hydrocephalus by shunt is that successful development does *not* depend upon shunting ventricles to a normal size reflected by a frontal mantle of 5.0 to 5.5 cm.

The reasons for failure to develop adequate frontal mantle in treated hydrocephalus relate in part both to severity of ventricular dilatation and to the age at which treatment was begun. All 8 patients failing to grow mantles of 2.0 cm (best IQ 76; mean IQ 45) were not adequately shunted until after age 6 months. Initial mantles varied from 0.6 to 1.5 cm. Six cases with a final mantle of over 2.0 cm but less than 3.0 cm (IQ range 63–95) were all first adequately shunted after age 5 months with initial mantle of 2.0 cm or more. All cases shunted before age 5 months grew adequate mantles, including nine with initial mantles of 1.0 cm or less. Four cases shunted after 6 months did grow adequate mantles. No growth in mantle, however, occurred in any of 5 patients first shunted after age 18 months.

A significant conclusion can be drawn from these data. If infantile hydrocephalus is severe with frontal mantle of less than 2.0 cm, the opportunity for a good developmental result from treatment diminishes with time. By 4 or 5 months of age, the progressive reduction in cerebral mantle no longer shows reversibility with shunting.

Patients with myelodysplasia and Arnold–Chiari malformation are considered separately just as they were in 1973[7] because the relationship between late frontal cerebral mantle thickness and IQ is highly variable (or unpredictable) as compared with the correlations existing in pure hydrocephalus. Since these cases were in the hands of neurosurgeons from birth, a failure to develop the 3.0-cm width of cerebral mantle (judged adequate in pure hydrocephalus) was quite rare. But the IQ distribution disappointingly was much lower than for the corresponding adequate mantle cases of pure hydrocephalus. Over 50 percent fell below IQ 80 (versus 15 percent) and only 15 percent were above IQ 100 (versus 51 percent). Further analysis is needed to define the role of neonatal brain insults, infections, and both the morbidity and deprivations of the paraplegic state in this downgrading. It may become possible to define whether variable intrinsic cerebral and stem malformations contribute to random lowering of mental capacities in myelodysplasia. These findings by no means diminish the indications for treatment by shunt when significant hydrocephalus develops. Further downgrade of even a marginal IQ by uncontrolled hydrocephalus would be a cruelty to the patient, family, and society. But we cannot prognosticate in myelodysplasia that shunting can minimize the threat of reduced mental capacity, as it does in pure hydrocephalus.

This review of late results correlates intelligence with adequacy of control of ventriculomegaly, as defined by width of frontal cerebral mantle. Severely thinned mantles will expand (with good IQ result) only if shunting is begun by 4 or 5 months of age. A near normal IQ distribution is found in patients with "pure" hydrocephalus who develop mantles of 3.0 cm or more. Shunt regulation therefore should aim to maintain mild ventriculomegaly so as to avoid the occurrence of coapted or slit ventricles that can disrupt shunt function.

It is meaningless to discuss the results of palliation of hydrocephalus by shunt without considering how prolonged shunt maintenance has been achieved, as well as the problems that continue to plague us and our patients.

METHODS AND PROBLEMS IN SHUNT MAINTENANCE

Retrospectively a cause has been assigned to each case of shunt dysfunction as we try to improve guidelines for the proper maintenance of each shunt component. Elective revisions have greatly reduced the incidence of overt shunt dysfunction requiring emergency intervention. But these still occur, and the avoidance of catastrophes has related to continuous availability of our "shunt service" to patients, alongside enforced follow-up visits and parent–doctor education.

Up to age 18 to 24 months, inadequate shunting can permit the infant to thrive without symptoms despite insidious reenlargement of ventricles. (Six low IQ cases first treated by us for thin mantles after age 6 months had been shunted early elsewhere with no concern when rapid head growth resumed. One of our own cases was similarly damaged by failure to enforce follow-up.) The still-elastic skull jacket yields enough to prevent an increase in intracranial pressure (ICP) sufficient to cause symptoms and the potential for ultimate brain function becomes downgraded. Head growth is abnormal with full fontanel; and ventricular reenlargement is defined by CT or ultrasound scans (formerly by pneumography via Rickham reservoir).

After there is sufficient rigidity of skull to prevent its quick expansion, significant enlargement of ventricles does not occur without major somatic symptoms. The child now signals the beginning of dysfunction with complaints of headache before anorexia or vomiting and irritability or lethargy present a textbook picture of ICP increase. Changes in behavior, including worsening school performance, demand investigation, almost invariably to reaffirm that, in the absence of somatic symptoms, ventricular reenlargement has not occurred.

Following is a brief discussion of our complications with prolonged shunt maintenance, and what has been learned on how best to guarantee continued function of each shunt component and to cope with sepsis.[8–10]

Distal catheter obstruction has been the most frequent cause of shunt dysfunction. Up to 1968 these were placed in the venous system. By 1972 peritoneal shunts were placed initially with the expectancy of ultimate conversion to a more definitive venous shunt. We claimed in 1968 that venous obstruction would not occur until body growth caused this radiopaque catheter tip to migrate above the T_5 vertebral body level, and there have been only four exceptions to this. Since catheter placement below T_7 (level of tricuspid valve in infancy) often led to endocarditis and pulmonary embolic phenomena, a prophylactic maintenance schedule involved keeping the tip between T_7 and T_4 in the growing child. Elective revisions could be needed at ages 1, 3, 7, and 14 years as prescribed by x-ray delineation of the catheter's ascent with growth. Roughly twice-per-year venous catheter obstruction is still encountered, usually from failure to anticipate its ascent above T_5 in a new body growth spurt. Signs of ICP increase can occur abruptly. Reservoir needling reveals ICP of over 500 mm H_2O with no reduction by pumping the valve. Drainage of CSF by needle will yield transient improvement. The needed major shunt revision under general anesthesia can be postponed by externalizing the shunt into a collecting bottle. Our incidence of shunt sepsis was high when the patient was "carried" by repeated reservoir needling before delayed surgery.

The definitive revision involves preparing the surgical field for the alternative of intraperitoneal shunting, should atrial venous entry not be feasible. Before 1974, 12 atrial replacements were done by thorocotomy because peritoneal shunts failed and no venous channel for re-entry could be discovered. At present, femoral venous catheterization has guided over 20 atrial placements (in cases with thrombosed internal jugular veins from previous shunting) by directing the catheter tip through the atrium to a point in the external jugular system close to the existing shunt system in the neck. A new venous catheter can then be pulled down to the atrium under fluoroscopy as the femoral catheter is withdrawn. It must be stressed that *elective* venous catheter lengthening does not involve the technical problems of venous channel occlusion.

Peritoneal placement of the distal catheter, at first doomed to early occlusion, is now yielding years of adequate function owing to improvements in silastic catheter properties. When catheter block was explainable by migration that left only a short length within the abdomen, prolonged function of a newly placed peritoneal catheter occurred. But replacement of a long intraabdominal coil unexplainably blocked has carried a high probability of early reblock, probably related to a previous peritoneal inflammatory process. It appears that lifetime adequacy of distal drainage will always be afforded by a venous catheter in proper position after full body growth, and may be afforded by an increasing proportion of peritoneal catheters.

Ventricular catheter occlusions have been reduced by placement of the tip in frontal horn (under x-ray control with air introduction) so as to avoid enmeshment in choroid. But the development of slit ventricles with low ICP regulation (CSF overdrainage) has not been as easily reversible by a change to higher resistance valve regulation as originally assumed. Before the ventricular catheter tip was modified to contain multiple small openings, sudden blockades resulted in death in two instances. Now the symptoms appear always to begin as mild, intermittent headaches. The shunt usually reopens with only a moderate rise in ICP, and only three major morbidities have occurred. With symptoms of shunt dysfunction, percutaneous insertion of a no. 25 needle into the reservoir did not reveal the expected high pressure found in the usual distal blockage; rather, either no CSF flow was obtained or it flowed poorly without pulse into the manometer. Saline and air introduction would usually open the block temporarily and define either a poor position of a ventricular catheter or a correct position in a slit-like ventricle. Often a new ventricular catheter had to be placed in the still generous frontal horn of the contralateral ventricle. The valve runoff pressure would be found low and a higher resistance valve system would be substituted (occasionally the valves were blocked by particulate matter).

It thus became evident that *valve changes* were a necessary part of shunt maintenance, just as much as repositioning of distal and proximal catheter tips. That level of valve pressure regulation that would arrest abnormal head growth in the small infant and permit adequate growth of cerebral mantle would be so low as to permit ventricular coaptation in an older child.

The slit ventricle syndrome from CSF overdrainage has become the most frequent shunt dysfunction problem in our long-term shunt-dependent patients and will be discussed further. Since the use of a multipored catheter tip, abrupt total occlusion has occurred in only one instance with serious morbidity. In this case massive temporal decompression permitted recovery and gradual ventricular regrowth with valve change.

Shunt dysfunction can arise from disconnection of shunt components when there is insufficient slack in tubing between fixation points near a burr hole and at a cervical site of entry into the venous system. Routine x-rays to show the position of shunt elements will always reveal the separation and a palpable CSF accumulation will usually overlie the site.

Infections have related to external contamination of a shunt element, manifest as surgical wound infections, or as more subtle internal shunt infection (CSF bacterial sepsis) involving no subcutaneous reaction to the prosthesis. The former have become relatively rare, including the external contamination occurring when a shunt element becomes exposed by skin breakdown. Infants with precariously thin scalps, especially when large-headed, must be shunted with miniaturized reservoir buttons and valve units, or the valve assembly can be placed under more generous skin along the chest wall.

Internal shunt sepsis usually has included involvement of CSF in ventricles (and meningitis in communicating hydrocephalus). The bacteria are usually skin-dwelling organisms of low virulence (*Staphylococcus epidermidis*, diphtheroids).[11] The symptoms arise from the drainage into the venous system or the peritoneum. Skin organisms are introduced either by surgical incision or by needling of the Rickham reservoir. Signs of sepsis can follow the shunt invasion as much as six months later.

The usual symptoms of infected CSF drainage into the bloodstream via a catheter properly placed above the tricuspid valve at first are insidiously benign. Sweats and chills finally develop in a child who has probably carried intermittent low-grade fever for weeks. Frequent blood cultures at the time of fever with prompt implant into anaerobic media have been necessary, often to grow diphtheroid organisms. The CSF shows similar growth. Occasionally, the symptoms of bacteremia from "nonpathogens" that grow only within the shunt-contained CSF have been so minimal that in four instances patients presented with hypertension and edema secondary to "shunt nephropathy."[12,13] Long-standing low-grade fever without symptoms had been disregarded. These experiences demand routine urinalysis for venous shunt patients as part of follow-up for one year after the last shunt invasion, as well as temperature charting as home for one month postoperatively.

Drainage of infected CSF into the peritoneal cavity has resulted either in low-grade signs of increased ICP from reduced CSF absorption (often with a palpable abdominal fluid encystment) or in abdominal signs and symptoms varying from intermittent low-grade focal pain and tenderness to a full-blown picture of acute abdomen and peritonitis.[14]

The treatment of the shunt-dependent patient seriously ill from bacteremia, nephropathy, or peritoneal reaction has involved prompt externalization of the shunt with removal of the distal catheter when the CSF showed organisms on Gram stain or cellular reaction. After obtaining blood and CSF cultures, wide-spectrum CSF penetration antibiotics are begun intravenously and an intraventricular antibiotic is introduced via the reservoir. If the ventricular fluid cultures positive, a new shunt is placed in a new locus only after several days of antibiotic therapy. Occasionally the infection can be cured without shunt removal.[15] Despite the long hospitalization and outpatient treatment often involved, death from sepsis occurred in only three "social shunts" where aggressive treatment was not pursued in the face of existing brain damage or a high level of paraplegia. Two highly shunt-dependent children suffered serious brain insults affecting higher functions, especially memory, from failure properly to control ICP with shunt replacements. (Sepsis may play a major role in the "unpredictable" downgrading of myelodysplastics where CSF contamination via an open sac was thought to have been cured without brain insult.)

Present prophylaxis against infection with shunt placement or revision[16] includes the usual measures at surgery to minimize contact of shunt elements with skin, irrigation of wounds with bacitracin, use of IV antibiotics just prior to surgery and for 24 hours postoperatively, and injection of gentamycin solution into the ventricular reservoir at the close of the procedure. Although possibilities for surgical field contamination are increased by x-ray monitoring of both ventricular and distal catheter positions, the operation infection rate has been reduced to under 5 percent since 1976. Needling of the shunt reservoir, frequently done for shunt assessment and determination of brain mantle growth before CT exam availability, carried retrospectively an infection rate of 1.5 percent. Since 1976, 10 mg of gentamycin have been injected before needle removal and no infections have resulted. These results suggest that CSF loading with gentamycin at surgery has been a major deterrent against internal shunt infection.

An earlier complication of shunting was subdural hematoma, often developing remote to the procedure after trivial trauma from a fall. This has been preventable by selection of a valve that avoids CSF overdrainage and low ICP. Before 1974 hemiparesis was incurred in 4 patients with residuals in 2 patients, always when small ventricles were catheterized by the occipital–parietal route. Small ventricles are now reached through a coronal burr hole under x-ray guidance. Focal seizures with electroencephalogram findings relating to the cortical site of catheter penetration have occurred in 2 patients currently no longer requiring anticonvulsants. Early postoperative seizures in an infant usually are related to sepsis. All of our chronic seizure problems relate to a brain-damaging etiology before shunting.

A final complication has been far more difficult to recognize—a growing CSF collection not in communication with the shunted lateral ventricle. These include Dandy–Walker fourth ventricle cysts not remaining in communication via aqueduct, extraarachnoid cysts in the suprasellar region, and porencephalic cysts in cerebrum losing their communication with shunted ventricles. Correct diagnosis and proper contrivance of a shunt, often two-headed, are clearly afforded by initial and follow-up CT examinations.

ARRESTED HYDROCEPHALUS AND SHUNT INDEPENDENCE

The dictum of "once a shunt, always a shunt" was disproved by 1963.[17] At a time when revisions were not done electively, certain patients showed no signs of shunt dysfunction after more than five years of growth without revision. Ultimately these shunts were proved to be blocked distally by surgical exposure, and removed. Later open shunts requiring elective lengthening distally after several years were managed with the incorporation of an on–off valve.[18] The shunt was occluded at the bedside two or three days postoperatively when the child was fully active and painfree. Any symptoms from ICP increase would begin by four hours and become maximal by 24 hours. Mild headache or nausea led to further observation if ICP by reservoir tap was less than 250 mm H_2O. A second trial of closure was planned if the first attempt was almost tolerated.

It was found early that shunt occlusion was never tolerated in obstructive or noncommunicating hydrocephalus. Hence occlusion trials or permissive gradual occlusion of a peritoneal shunt with growth have been limited to cases where either contrast studies or the Blackfan test proved communication of lateral ventricle with cisterna magna or lumbar CSF. This determination was unclear in the myelomeningocele cases and occlusion trials were rarely undertaken. Four myelodysplastics, however, chanced to develop shunt occlusion without symptoms, mostly patients whose original hydrocephalus was not severely progressive. But a grave unpredictability has been found in patients seemingly shunt independent who carry Arnold–Chiari malformation. Three patients, rushed in as emergencies, suffered abrupt respiratory compromise, with one death and one permanent cerebral insult from anoxia. Retrospectively, the death at home of 3 patients, carried as shunt independent for one month to three years, probably resulted from respiratory arrest at the time of stress from a febrile illness, usually upper respiratory infection, without prodromal symptoms of headache. These occurrences raise serious questions. We feel that children with Arnold–Chiari malformation should be presumed to be shunt dependent for life, unless chance shunt occlusion has caused absolutely no symptom, past or present.

By contrast the experience with both fortuitous and planned shunt blockade in communicating hydrocephalus allows clear conclusions:[19] (1) None of these patients became critically ill with shunt blocks and none suffered a measurable brain insult (ICP never exceeded 200 mm while pressures in excess of 500 mm were found in noncommunicating cases). (2) Once the patient was asymptomatic with shunt independence, there were no late sequellae. (3) None of these patients, in the absence of somatic symptoms, showed either insidious reenlargement of ventricles, or neurologic alterations, or reduction of intellectual functions. Abrupt shunt block is not tolerated with smaller than normal ventricular size. Two cases have been "weaned" to shunt independence in stages by achieving ventricular regrowth through increasing valve resistance. In five others a permanent shunt addiction may relate to earlier pressure regulation that permitted a degree of ventricular coaptation.

THE FUTURE FOR SHUNT MANAGEMENT WITHOUT COMPLICATIONS

Unfortunately experience with the present state of the shunting art belies the simplistic goal of a single shunt placement for palliation of infantile hydrocephalus. At best an experienced and concerned shunt team can manage these patients with planned revisions directed by a compulsive follow-up program that prevents the emergencies of shunt dysfunctions. Even this limited goal has not been fully achievable so that "hot-line" access to the team must be kept available to parents educated to the importance of system recognition.

The review of our past problems in shunt maintenance suggests that the greatest continuing question is how to avoid the slit ventricles that develop, especially in patients with high brain performance. In the majority of cases presently destined for lifetime shunt dependency, this occurrence can involve

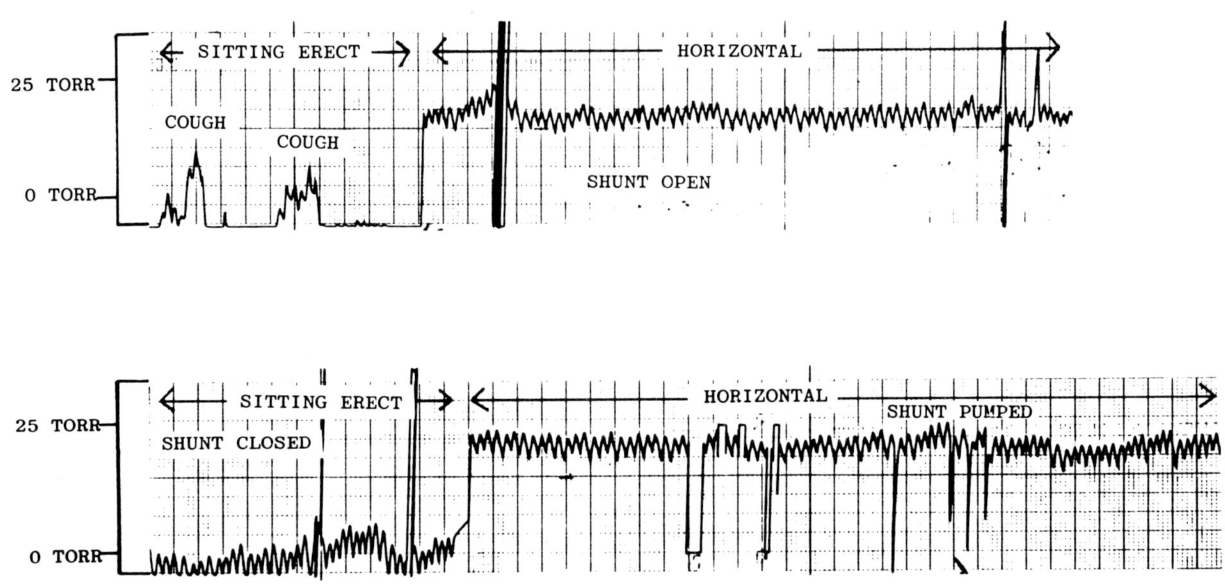

Figure 15-2. Telemetry ICP recording with shunt open and with shunt closed showing effect of sitting and recumbent posture. With shunt closed there was no threat to life or function but mild symptoms prevented tolerance. The large pulse wave, seen with tiny ventricles, may be a factor in symptoms despite minimal ICP elevation. (Reprinted with permission from Nulsen FE, Leung A, Fleming DG, et al: Chronic intracranial pressure monitoring by telemetry: Clinical experience. Ann Biomed Eng 8:505–513, 1980.)

multiple revisions to reestablish stable CSF drainage, involving both ventricular catheter repositioning and valve replacement. The latter must sometimes be done in stages because the ICP increase that can first be tolerated is still too low to yield sufficient ventricular regrowth. In communicating hydrocephalus, where ultimate shunt independence is a reasonable possibility, continued dependence is often associated with slit ventricles. It is reasonable to assume that a number of potential independents have become permanently shunt addicted by a low level of ICP control that permitted this artificial ventricular configuration. As an example Figure 15-2 shows the telemetrically recorded ICP[20] in L. M., a potentially shunt-independent patient, who has acquired slit ventricles. As a result total shunt closure, while producing only mild ICP elevation, is associated with mild headaches and vomiting sufficient to prevent long-term tolerance. An antisiphon device was used as an intermediate step toward "weaning" L. M. from her shunt addiction.

Retrospectively, this difficult problem should have been arrestable in its earlier stages. Serial CT examinations can establish when huge ventricles are reduced to a moderate size that permits more than adequate cerebral mantle thickness. In theory this would be the time to provide a changed valve control, sufficiently precise to maintain ventricles at this ideal size. There are two difficulties: (1) The psychologic trauma and the admitted infection risk of a revision are difficult to accept in an asymptomatic patient still not positively faced with shunt dysfunction. (2) We presently lack the expertise to guarantee that the new valve assembly will operate as intended. In other words, new problems may be created for the patient when one could have left well enough alone.

Not only are the dynamics of ICP regulation via CSF flow through shunt clearly variable for each individual, but also there are major variations of ICP in normals, with changes in position and levels of activity, including sleep, that are accentuated by positional effects upon CSF flow through shunts.

The concept of the antisiphon device, as developed by Portnoy, Schulte, Fox, et al.,[18] is attractive as a means of avoiding severe lows in ICP that with shunts can exceed the negativity that normals develop when upright. Our still limited experience with incorporating this device in shunts has occasionally led to ventricular reenlargement in infants and to ICP levels not tolerated in patients already showing slit ventricles.

Certain patients require ICP control within extremely narrow limits, so as to demand repeated valve changes before a proper set is found by trial and error. Such a situation existed in T. M., age 15. He harbored an atrio-venous malformation (AVM) in the upper brain stem that caused total aqueduct occlusion. When lateral and third ventricles became large, extreme ataxia prevented independent walking. But if ventricles became too small, increased drowsiness, left hemiparesis, and right cerebellar signs developed. Many valve changes by trial and error established brief intervals of near normal ventricular size consistent with independent function and good school performance. Figure 15-3 shows the placement of two shunts in parallel, each controlled by an on–off switch. Initially when CSF flow was permitted only through shunt A (high-resistance antisiphon shunt), ICP transmitted by a telemetric device exceeded 200 mm H_2O with a marked increase in ataxia and headache. A switch to permit CSF flow through low-resistance shunt B gave ICP below 100 mm H_2O when recumbent with markedly negative ICP when erect. Clinically the patient passed through an interval of excellent function for him, before ventricular coaptation occurred in association with stupor and left hemiplegia. Ultimately the patient came to tolerate shunt A regulation of ICP with shunt B closed off. Figure 15-4 compares telemetric ICP behavior with an antisiphon device (shunt A) and

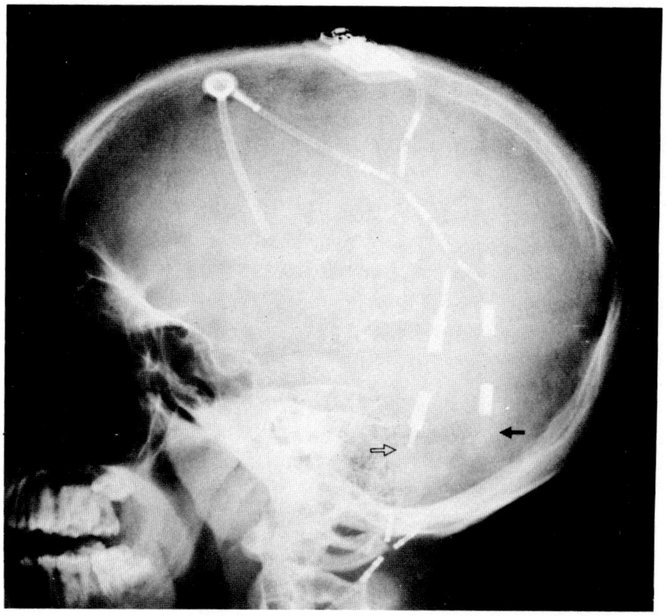

Figure 15-3. Lateral skull x-ray shows placement of intraventricular catheter connected to two shunt systems in parallel that rejoin a single distal venous catheter. The posterior shunt incorporates a high-resistance Hakim valve with an antisiphon device (opposite closed arrow). The anterior shunt contains a medium resistance Holter valve with an on–off switch (opposite open arrow). Telemetric ICP sensor is placed under scalp to connect with ventricular catheter and reservoir proximal to valve regulators.

without a device (shunt B). By good luck T. M. has continued within these levels of ICP and with good clinical performance for eight points with ventricles at near normal size.[20]

Clearly, for highly pressure-sensitive patients such as T. M., a "dial-a-valve" device would be ideal along with telemetric ICP monitoring so as to vary shunt resistance and flow in order to reach the ideal set. It should be possible theoretically finally to develop closed-loop control of ICP in which ICP feedback would direct the valve set correct for that hour.[21]

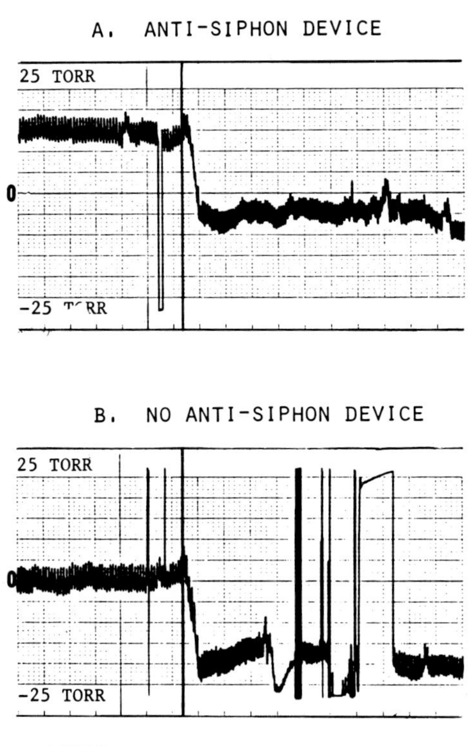

Figure 15-4. Telemetric ICP recording which compares the pressure regulation when only shunt A with antisiphon device is open with the pressure when shunt B permits CSF flow at lower pressures. A marked siphon effect occurs when erect (lower tracing).

CONCLUSIONS

Children with hydrocephalus uncomplicated by gross malformations of the brain or birth injury have an excellent chance for normal intellectual, social, and vocational development as long as they are treated early and adequately to obtain a frontal brain mantle of at least 3.0 cm. Serious complications such as crises of ICP increase from shunt block and ventriculitis can result in downgrading of this rather optimistic picture. With compulsive attention to procedures for the avoidance of shunt complications and ready access to the "shunt team," these serious complications can be minimized.

Ideal management of certain highly pressure-sensitive patients with hydrocephalus, as well as avoidance of slit ventricles and of unnecessary permanent shunt dependency, involves the development of a variable resistance valve (possibly in combination with ICP telemetry) so as to avoid the multiple operations often needed to achieve satisfactory ICP regulation.

REFERENCES

1. Torkildsen A: A follow-up study 14 to 20 years after ventriculocisternostomy. Acta Psychiatr Neurol Scand 35:114–121, 1960
2. Scarff JE: Non-obstructive hydrocephalus. Treatment by endoscopic cauterization of the choroid plexuses. Am J Dis Child 63:297–334, 1942
3. Cone WV, Lewis RD, Jackson IJ: Shunting of cerebrospinal fluid into the peritoneal cavity. Meeting, American College of Physicians, Montreal, 1949
4. Matson DD: Ventriculoureterostomy. J Neurosurg 8:398–404, 1951
5. Nulsen FE, Spitz EB: Treatment of hydrocephalus by direct shunt from ventricle to jugular vein. Surg Forum 2:399–403, 1952
6. Pudenz RH: The surgical treatment of hydrocephalus—An historical review. Surg Neurol 15:15–26, 1981
7. Young HF, Nulsen FE, Weiss MH, et al: The relationship of intelligence and cerebral mantle in treated infantile hydrocephalus. J Pediatr 52:38–44, 1973
8. Nulsen FE, Becker DP: Control of hydrocephalus by valve-regulated shunt, surgical technique. J Neurosurg 26:362–374, 1967
9. Becker DP, Nulsen FE: Control of hydrocephalus by valve-regulated venous shunt: Avoidance of complications in prolonged shunt maintenance. J Neurosurg 28:215–226, 1968
10. Nulsen FE, Becker DP: Control of hydrocephalus by valve-regulated shunt: Infections and their prevention, in Clinical Neurosurgery. Vol. 14, Baltimore, Williams & Wilkins, 1967, pp. 256–273
11. Rekate HL, Ruch T, Nulsen FE: Diphtheroid infections of cerebrospinal fluid shunts: The changing pattern of shunt infection in Cleveland. J Neurosurg 52:553–556, 1980
12. Beeler BA, Crowder JG, Smith JW, et al: Propionibacterium acnes: Pathogen in central nervous system shunt infection. Report of three cases including immune complex glomerulonephritis. Am J Med 61:935–938, 1976
13. Bolton WK, Sande MA, Normansell DE, et al: Ventriculo-jugular shunt nephritis with corynebacterium bovis. Successful therapy with antibiotics. Am J Med 59:417–423, 1975
14. Rekate HL, Yonas H, White RJ, et al: The acute abdomen in patients with ventriculoperitoneal shunts. Surg Neurol 11:442–445, 1979
15. McLaurin RL: Treatment of infected ventricular shunts. Child's Brain 1:306–310, 1975
16. Venes JL: Control of shunt infection. Report of 150 consecutive cases. J Neurosurg 45:311–314, 1976
17. Nulsen FE: The control of progressive hydrocephalus in infancy by valve-regulated venous shunt, in K. Shulman (ed): Workshop in Hydrocephalus. Philadelphia, University of Pennsylvania, 1965, pp 256–273

18. Portnoy HD, Schulte RR, Fox JL, et al: Anti-siphon and reversible occlusion valves for shunting in hydrocephalus and preventing postshunt subdural hematomas. J Neurosurg 38:729–738, 1973
19. Rekate HL, Nulsen FE, Mack HL, et al: Establishing the diagnosis of shunt independence. Monogr Neur Sci (in press)
20. Nulsen FE, Leung A, Fleming DG, et al: Chronic intracranial pressure monitoring by telemetry: Clinical experience. Ann Biomed Eng 8:505–513, 1980
21. Rekate HL: Closed-loop control of intracranial pressure. Ann Biomed Eng 8:515–522, 1980

16. Shunt Complications

Robert L. McLaurin

The history of the evolution of ventricular shunting for hydrocephalus is largely a history of efforts to prevent the complications of shunting. Until such time as pharmacologic control of cerebrospinal fluid (CSF) production is achieved, the treatment of hydrocephalus will necessarily rely mainly on the establishment of artificial conduits for the venting of CSF from the ventricular system. Such devices have been fraught with mechanical and biologic complications. This chapter attempts to summarize these untoward occurrences.

COMMON TO ALL TYPES OF SHUNTS

Malfunction

The most common complication of a ventricular shunt, regardless of the terminus, is mechanical malfunction of the shunt system. Malfunction may be the result of either obstruction or disconnection of the component parts of a shunt system. Obstruction may occur at the proximal (ventricular) end, within the pumping device or valve, or at the distal end.

There have been several reviews of the complications occurring in sizable series of shunts. The largest series reported to data is that of Forrest and Cooper, which included 455 cases of ventriculoatrial shunts in which 520 revisions were performed.[8] Complications involving the proximal catheter were the most frequent, and this has been true in nearly all reported series.

Malfunction at the proximal end of the shunt may be due to disconnection with separation of the ventricular catheter from the rest of the shunt system. This complication has become less frequent in recent years as a result of the use of a one-piece ventricular catheter reservoir. Prior to utilization of this particular device, it was not uncommon for ventricular catheters to become disconnected and to lie free within the ventricle. There has been no report to indicate that a free catheter within the ventricle causes any harm. It may be noted, however,

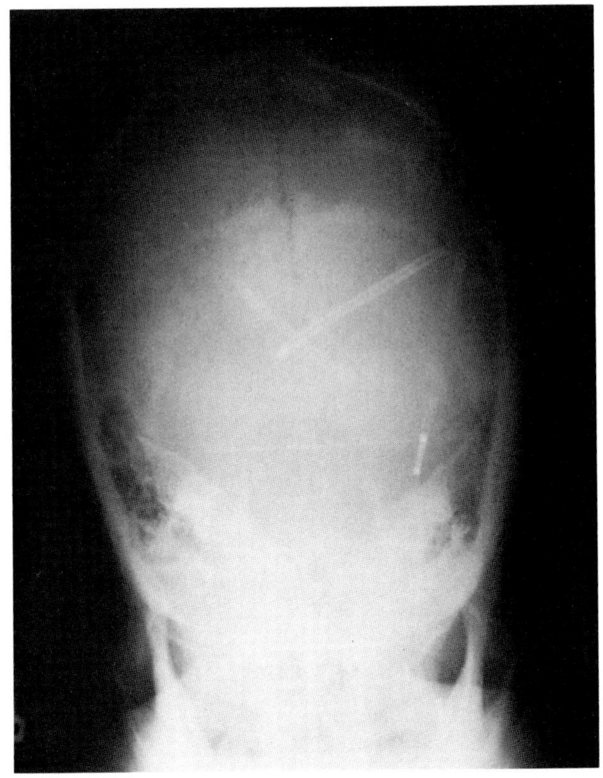

Figure 16-1. A free-floating catheter within the shunted ventricular system of a patient with shunt infection. It was essential to remove the catheter in order to cure the infection.

that it is not possible to cure ventricular or shunt infections in the presence of a free-floating ventricular catheter (Fig. 16-1).

A second cause of malfunction at the ventricular end is blockage of the ventricular catheter by choroid plexus and glial tissue growing into the lumen of the ventricular catheter (Fig. 16-2). This complication can be minimized by proper placement of the ventricular catheter; the tip of the catheter should be placed sufficiently far anteriorly in the lateral ventricle so that it is beyond the anterior extent of the choroid plexus. Ideally the tip of the ventricular catheter, therefore, should be anterior to the foramen of Monro.

A third cause of ventricular catheter failure has been contraction of the ventricle, resulting in the catheter becoming embedded in the wall of the

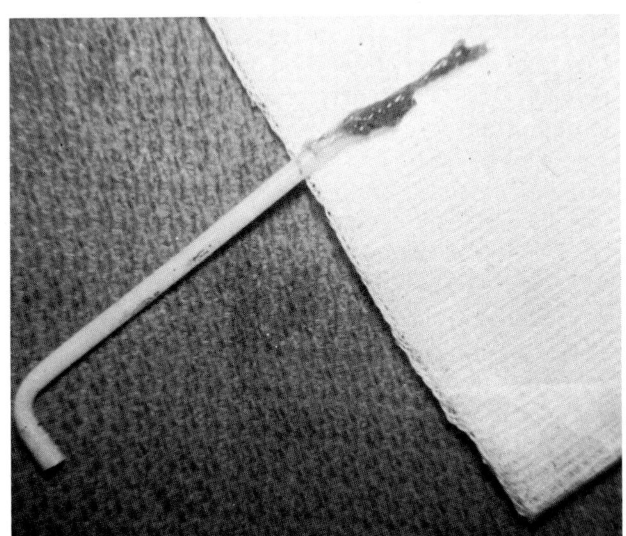

Figure 16-2. Ventricular catheter removed because of malfunction with adherent choroid plexus that had grown through the multiple openings into the lumen.

ventricle or piercing the wall and entering the white matter. This has been the mechanism of development of the "slit ventricle" syndrome in which the patient has symptoms and signs of intracranial hypertension in the presence of a small ventricular system. This complication has been one of the most difficult to resolve. The use of a high-pressure valve in the system may be of very significant benefit. Epstein, Fleischer, Hochwald, et al. have described the procedure of subtemporal craniectomy for recurrent shunt obstruction due to small ventricles.[5] These authors advocate the use of this procedure in such cases for the following reasons: It vents the acutely increased intracranial pressure; it allows some degree of dilatation of the ipsilateral ventricle, providing a greater likelihood of restoration of patency of the ventricular catheter; and it also allows access to palpation to determine the presence of intracranial hypertension.

Malfunctions involving the valve and pumping device have been quite few in nearly all reported series. Incompetence of a valve may allow retrograde blood flow, with clotting and occlusion in a vascular shunt. Such valve incompetence fortunately is quite rare and generally can be detected prior to insertion of the valve by meticulous testing at the time of surgery. The hazard of retrograde incompetence is considerably less in the presence of peritoneal shunting than it was previously when vascular shunts were used more commonly.

Although there has been concern generally about the effect of high protein content of the spinal fluid on valve function, it is noteworthy that no definite relationship has been substantiated. This writer has seen several instances of spinal fluid protein in excess of 1000 mg% with no apparent effect on the functional integrity of the shunt system.

Malfunction relating to the distal part of the shunt also may be attributed to disconnection, to migration, or to blockage at the distal end. Obstruction at the distal end within the vascular system or the peritoneal cavity is considered in more detail in subsequent sections of this chapter. Disconnection may occur at the site of attachment of the distal catheter to the lower end of the pumping device or at the site of a more distal connection. Raimondi, Robinson, and Kuwamura, et al. have advocated the use of a one-piece shunt and reported the complications occurring in 357 patients having peritoneal shunts.[22] Of these, 161 had a one-piece shunt and 196 a three-piece shunt. The complications were fewer in those with the one-piece shunt and this difference was partially attributable to the lack of problems caused by disconnection. A distal shunt tubing can migrate from the peritoneal cavity or vascular compartment and the direction of migration is generally toward the ventricular end of the shunt system (Fig. 16-3).

Several diagnostic procedures have been advocated to determine the functional status of a shunt system. Evans, Thomas, and Williams describe the use of valvography employing a water-soluble contrast medium instilled directly into the shunt system.[6] With this method patency of the distal end of the shunt could be seen directly on injection, and reflux into the ventricular system also could be visualized. The authors noted that no instances of false-positive valvograms were encountered but occasional false-negative results were obtained. A similar type of shuntogram has been described using radionuclides injected directly into the shunt system and followed by scintillation scanners in its passage distally in the shunt system.[23]

Infection

Infection constitutes the second most frequent type of shunt complication. Two types of shunt infection can be delineated. The first is an infection occurring primarily on the external surface of the shunt involving the subcutaneous soft

ties.[16] Lateralization of the abnormality was to the right hemisphere in 11 patients. In a comparative group of infants with hydrocephalus and no shunting, there was a high incidence of normal traces and no significant lateralization. The matter was pursued further by Graebner and Celesia, who also compared a group of shunted hydrocephalics with a nonshunted group.[10] There was a higher incidence of abnormal records in the shunted group and focal paroxysmal discharges were seen much more frequently in the shunted patients. In addition there was an incidence of clinical seizures in 48 percent of the shunted group and 20 percent of the nonshunted group. Ines and Markund later evaluated a large series of hydrocephalics for EEG abnormalities and seizures; in 65 patients with right-sided shunts there were 22 with grand mal seizures, 16 with left focal seizures, 4 with right-sided seizures, and 6 with other minor seizures.[14] The authors noted that the majority of seizures begin within four years after placement of the shunt.

Another recent report was that of Varfis, Berney, and Beaumanoir, who noted that 19 of 29 shunted hydrocephalic patients developed an epileptogenic focus and that during a follow-up period of four years 17 of the 19 experienced clinical seizures.[28] By observing serial EEGs it was found that the irritative abnormalities occurred usually during the second year after operation and that a slow wave pattern usually preceded the occurrence of the irritative abnormality. It was further noted that myelomeningocele patients had the lowest incidence of epilepsy while the highest incidence occurred in patients with hydrocephalus due to cerebral hemorrhage. The authors also concluded that the younger the patient at the data of operation, the greater the chance of development of an epileptogenic scar.

It must be concluded that the incidence of EEG abnormality and seizure activity is sufficiently high after shunting to indicate some routine evaluation of this potential complication. Routine use of anticonvulsant therapy is probably not necessary, except in the high-risk groups (e.g., cerebral hemorrhage, porencephalic cyst) but serial observation of EEGs during the first few years after shunting is indicated so that anticonvulsant therapy can be used if an irritative focus occurs.

Subdural Accumulations

Subdural hematomas and effusions have been a recognized complication of successful shunting of hydrocephalics but it is significant that this complication only rarely causes clinical manifestations of its presence. Unilateral subdural accumulations may cause focal neurologic deficit due to shift of the intracranial structures (Fig. 16-4). More often, however, bilateral and rather symmetric effusions may be present without clinical evidence. The existence of such accumulations has become increasingly more apparent since the advent of CT

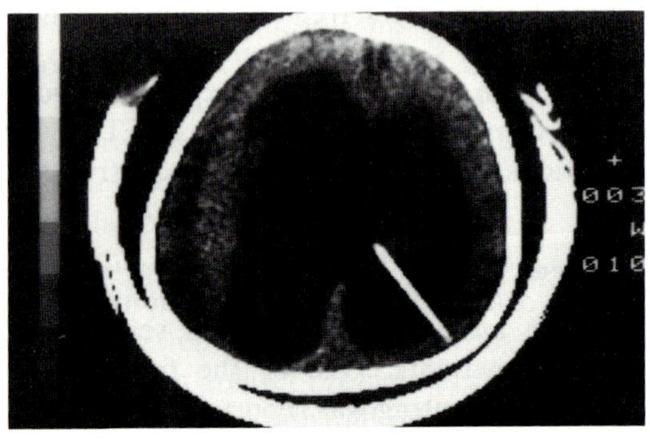

Figure 16-4. A CT scan of shunted hydrocephalus with a left subdural accumulation.

scanning. It appears likely that subdural effusions are frequently a manifestation of the existence of a craniocephalic disproportion and that no specific treatment is necessary in most instances.

Craniosynostosis

Craniosynostosis has been reported as a complication of shunting. Andersson reported three such instances, two of which occurred in patients with associated myelomeningocele and the third in a patient treated for aqueduct stenosis.[1] In addition to premature closure of the sutures, there was marked increase in the thickness of the skull bones. The author recommended that low-pressure valves not be used because of this particular complication. It should be noted that while this complication may have some cosmetic effect, there has been no definite indication that it restricts brain growth in the treated hydrocephalic patient.

A rare complication of shunting has been described by Hoffman and Tucker as "cephalocranial disproportion" in which there occurred cerebellar and brain-stem herniation into the upper spinal canal.[13] Six of the eight reported cases had communicating hydrocephalus treated by lumboperitoneal shunts. The symptoms included signs of lower brain-stem dysfunction and myelography or air study demonstrated tonsillar herniation. Posterior fossa decompression was carried out with significant improvement in all patients. The authors speculate that the basic problem is that secondary craniosynostosis results from overshunting of the patients. Further normal growth of the brain then leads to a cephalocranial disproportion, and this in turn leads to herniation downward as the brain volume exceeds the available space.

UNIQUE TO VASCULAR SHUNTS

The complications that are unique to ventriculovascular shunts fall into two principal groups cardiac and pulmonary. Although the incidence of such complications is difficult to determine, their severity has led to preference, in most instances, for the use of peritoneal shunting.

The following cardiac complications have been reported: (1) mural thrombosis occurring in the right atrium or extending into the atrium from the superior or inferior vena cava; (2) bacterial endocarditis; (3) cardiac arrhythmias, which have been attributed to irritation by the distal catheter; (4) cardiac tamponade resulting from perforation of the right atrium by the distal shunt catheter; and (5) detachment of a distal shunt tubing remaining in the heart or embolization to the pulmonary arteries.

Emery and Hilton reported the necropsy findings on 15 patients with vascular shunts.[4] In every instance the catheter entering the heart was surrounded by fibrinous material extending for various distances into the auricle. Attached to the end of the fibrinous collar were masses of fibrinous clot. On one occasion the tricuspid valve was obstructed by such a clot. In 6 of the 15 cases, the wall of the right atrium contained vegetation that was probably the result of trauma.

The existence of clots within the atrium may not produce any specific manifestations until emboli occur in the pulmonary vascular system. The first indication of the existence of such a problem therefore may be either a malfunction of the distal end of the shunt or irreversible secondary changes due to pulmonary hypertension. The presence of a detached catheter lying within the cardiac chambers may be correctable by retrieval, under radiographic control, through the inferior venous drainage system (Fig. 16-5).[27]

Obstruction of the vena system above the heart is another vascular complication that only rarely proceeds to a symptomatic state. Obstruction of the superior vena cava has occurred infrequently but results in the characteristic evidence of blockage of the venous drainage from the head and neck. It may be noted that the distal shunt catheter introduced into the jugular vein may become misdirected into the subclavian vein rather than progressing toward the atrium. Again, it is possible in many instances to redirect the catheter under radiographic control by manipulation performed via the inferior venus system.[27]

The most consistent vascular complication consists of emboli in the pulmo-

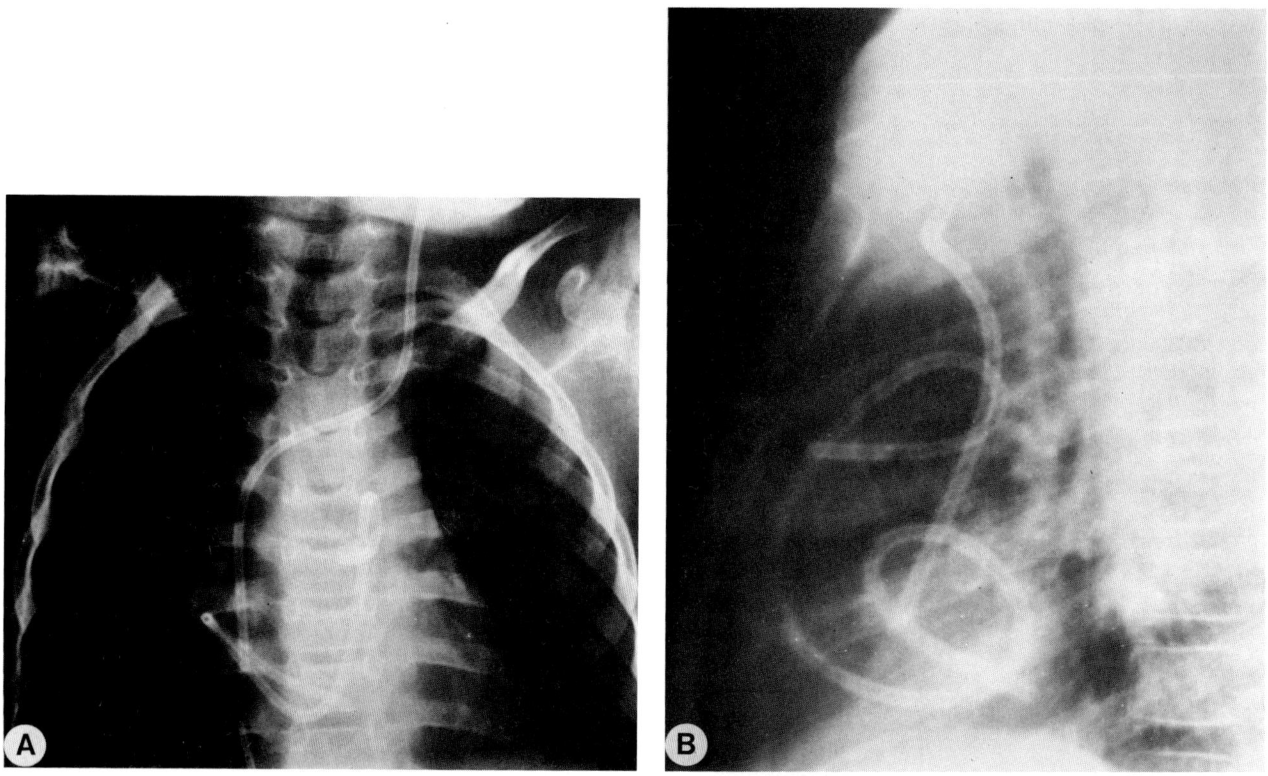

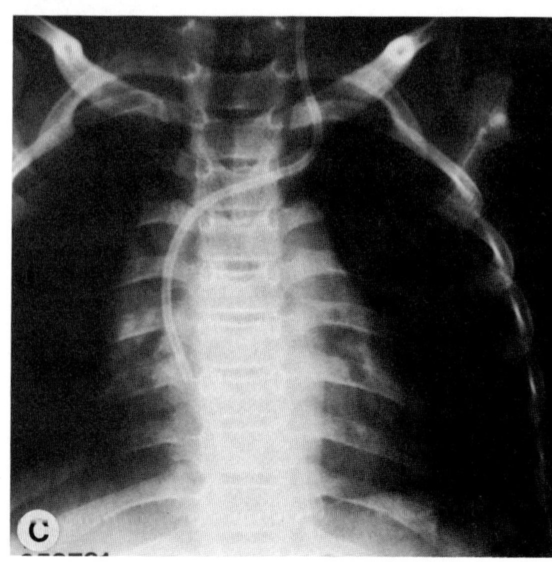

Figure 16-5. A. Left ventriculoatrial shunt in proper position. Embolized right VA shunt is coiled in the heart with the distal end in the main pulmonary artery. B. Lateral view of same. C. Following removal of embolized shunt tubing by transvenous retrieval.

nary system. Emery and Hilton found pulmonary emboli in all but 1 of 15 patients studied at necropsy.[4] The emboli varied markedly in size but in the majority of instances had completely occupied and obstructed small arteries. In many instances there was no edema or cellular infiltration of the vessel walls around the embolized vessel. Friedman, Zitta-Gozum, and Chatten, in reviewing the pulmonary vascular histology in 65 patients who had died following ventriculojugular shunting, found that approximately half of the patients had pulmonary vascular lesions.[9] They noted that the age of the patient, composition of the tubing, location of the distal tubing, and the nature of coexisting disease did not seem to influence the incidence of pulmonary thromboembolism. This is at some variance with the opinion of Nugent, Lucas, Judy, et al., who concluded that infection played a major role in the occurrence of thrombosis in their patients.[19] They reported that most of the patients who had thromboembolic phenomena were myelomeningocele patients and had experienced repeated septicemia. Emery and Hilton also noted mycotic aneurysms, periarteritis, and intimal degeneration in several of their patients.[4]

The signs of pulmonary thromboembolism are the result of pulmonary hypertension. This includes accentuation of the second heart sound and disappearance of physiologic "splitting" of the second heart sound. The most serious consequence of pulmonary hypertension is the development of right heart failure (copulmonale). Although this is a rare complication of vascular shunting, it appears to represent an end state that is irreversible.

UNIQUE TO PERITONEAL SHUNTS

Intraabdominal complications of peritoneal shunts include (1) inguinal hernia and/or hydrocele, (2) ascites and cyst formation, (3) intestinal volvulus and obstruction, (4) perforation of a viscus or to the outside, and (5) spread of neoplasm or infection to the peritoneal cavity. An extensive review of intraabdominal complications was made by Davidson in 1976, and included a very complete bibliography up to that time.[3]

A frequent complication of peritoneal shunts is the occurrence of inguinal hernia. Grosfeld, Cooney, Smith, et al. noted an incidence of 16.8 percent in a series of 185 peritoneal shunts.[11] All of the patients underwent hernia repair, and bilateral hernias or patent processus vaginalis occurred in 75 percent. The authors attribute this high incidence to the fact that shunting is performed in most instances while the processus vaginalis is still patent. The superimposed CSF in the peritoneal cavity then converts itself into a clinical hernia. Prompt operation of the inguinal hernia is recommended and bilateral exploration seems advisable. A less common complication has been described by Scherzer.[25]

Abdominal cysts and ascites have been discussed by several authors. Fischer and Shillito, on the basis of the character of the cyst wall, speculate that infection of previous abdominal procedures contributes to the occurrence of a cyst.[7] Parry, Schumacher, and Llewellyn, on the other hand, describe cysts that were formed solely by intestinal serosal surfaces but no fibrous cyst wall.[21] Although most authors believe that the occurrence of an abdominal cyst precludes reestablishment of a functioning shunt, Parry et al. report instances of subsequent use of the peritoneal cavity with no sign of cyst recurrence or shunt malfunction.[21] In this writer's experience, abdominal cyst formation has invariably led to the need for vascular shunting.

Surprisingly, the occurrence of intestinal volvulus and obstruction has been a rare complication. Sakoda, Maxwell, and Brackett reported the first such case in 1971, in which a single adhesive band was found in the region of the tubing about which the volvulus had occurred.[24]

Perforation may occur into the bowel, bladder, or vagina. Grosfeld et al. reported seven instances of perforation of a viscus in 185 cases.[11] Schulhof, Worth, and Kalsbeck, in 1975, reviewed the literature concerning bowel perforation and found descriptions of only 12 patients.[26] In almost all instances, the shunt had continued to function despite the perforation. Only 2 of the 12 patients had evidence of peritonitis, although 6 patients had ventriculitis due to gram negative bacilli. Grosfeld et al. noted that 4 or 5 patients with colon perforation were asymptomatic and were treated conservatively without formal laparotomy or attempts at colon repair, and all survived.[11]

Perforation of the vagina has been reported in several instances and umbilical perforation and fistulae have also been noted.[2]

Peritoneal spread of infection is part of the sequellae of an infected shunt. Management of the infection is covered in Chapter 52, and the possible consequent of peritoneal cyst formation has been noted (vide supra).

The peritoneal shunt also may act as a conduit for the spread of neoplasm when the shunt is performed as a part of the management of intracranial tumors. Hoffman, Hendrick, and Humphreys have reported an incidence of approximately 10 percent of peritoneal metastases when shunting is performed in the presence of medulloblastoma. As a result of this experience, the authors have recommended the use of a milipore filter encased in the shunt system.[12]

COMPARISON OF VA AND VP SHUNT COMPLICATIONS

In recent years there has been a definite trend toward peritoneal rather than vascular shunting. The principal reason for this has been that while the incidence of complications may not be significantly different in the two groups, the severity and consequences of the complications have been greater in the vascular shunts. A recent review by Keucher and Mealey analyzed the relative incidence of complications in the two types of shunt.[15] The series included 119 patients who had initial vascular shunts and 72 with initial peritoneal shunts. Children who survived until 5 years of age with uninfected vascular shunts required an average of 1.46 revisions whereas those with uninfected peritoneal shunts averaged 1.02 revisions. Distal obstructions and prophylactic lengthening accounted for more than half of the revisions in vascular shunts. Proximal revisions were more common in peritoneal systems while distal revisions were more common in vascular systems. Twice as many children with peritoneal shunts did not need revision as did those with vascular shunts. The authors also noted that although the infection rate was the same in vascular and peritoneal shunts, the consequences of infection were much more serious in the vascular systems. It was concluded, therfore, that peritoneal shunts required fewer revisions and the patients suffered from fewer and less serious complications. On the basis of this review and the experience of other observers, it seems reasonable to conclude that at present peritoneal shunts should be used, if possible, whenever shunting is necessary in the treatment of hydrocephalus.

REFERENCES

1. Anderson H: Craniosynostosis as a complication after operation for hydrocephalus. Acta Paediatr Scand 55:192–196, 1966
2. Antunes ACM, Ribeiro TR: Spontaneous umbilication fistula from ventriculoperitoneal shunt drainage. J Neurosurg 43:481–482, 1975
3. Davidson RI: Peritoneal bypass in the treatment of hydrocephalus. Historical review and abdominal complications. J Neurol Neurosurg Psychiatr 39:640–646, 1976

4. Emery JL, Hilton HB: Lung and heart complications of the treatment of hydrocephalus by ventriculoauriculostomy. Surgery 50:309–313, 1966
5. Epstein FJ, Fleischer AS, Hochwald GM, et al: Subtemporal craniectomy for recurrent shunt obstruction secondary to small ventricles. J Neurosurg 41:29–31, 1974
6. Evans RC, Thomas MD, Williams LA: Shunt blockage on hydrocephalic children: The use of the valvogram. Clin Radiol 27:489–495, 1976
7. Fischer EG, Shillito J Jr: Large abdominal cysts: A complication of peritoneal shunts. J Neurosurg 31:441–444, 1969
8. Forrest DM, Cooper DGW: Complications of ventriculo-atrial shunts. A review of 455 cases. J Neurosurg 29:506–512, 1968
9. Friedman S, Zita-Gozum C, Chatten J: Pulmonary vascular changes complicating ventriculovascular shunting for hydrocephalus. J Pediatr 64:305–314, 1964
10. Graebner RW, Celesia GG: EEG findings in hydrocephalus and their relation to shunting procedures. Electroenceph Clin Neurophysiol 35:517–521, 1973
11. Grosfeld JL, Cooney DR, Smith J, et al: Intra-abdominal complications following ventriculoperitoneal shunt procedures. Pediatrics 54:791–796, 1974
12. Hoffman NJ, Hendrick EB, Humphreys RP: Metastasis via ventriculoperitoneal shunt in patients with medulloblastoma. J Neurosurg 44:562–566, 1976
13. Hoffman HJ, Tucker HJ: Cephalocranial disproportion. A complication of the treatment of hydrocephalus in children. Child's Brain 2:167–176, 1976
14. Ines DF, Markand ON: Epileptic seizures and abnormal electroencephalographic findings in hydrocephalus and their relation to the shunting procedures. Electroenceph Clin Neurophysiol 42:761–768, 1977
15. Keucher TR, Mealey J: Long-term results after ventriculoatrial and ventriculoperitoneal shunting for infantile hydrocephalus. J Neurosurg 50:179–186, 1979
16. Laws ER Jr, Niedermeyer E: EEG findings in hydrocephalic patients with shunt procedures. Electroenceph Clin Neurophysiol 29:325, 1970
17. Little JR, Rhoton AL Jr, Mellinger JF: Comparison of ventriculoperitoneal and ventriculoatrial shunts for hydrocephalus in children. Mayo Clin Proc 47:396–401, 1972
18. McLaurin RL: Infected cerebrospinal fluid shunts. Surg Neurol 1:191–195, 1973
19. Nugent GR, Lucas R, Judy M, et al: Thrombo-embolic complications of ventriculoatrial shunts. Angiocardiographic and pathologic correlations. J Neurosurg 24:34–42, 1966
20. Nulsen FE, Becker DP: Control of hydrocephalus of valve-regulated shunt. J Neurosurg 26:362–374, 1967
21. Parry SW, Schumacher JF, Llewellyn RC: Abdominal pseudocysts and ascites formation after ventriculoperitoneal shunt procedures. Report of four cases. J Neurosurg 43:476–480
22. Raimondi AJ, Robinson JS, Kuwamura K: Complications of ventriculoperitoneal shunting and a critical comparison of the three-piece and one-piece systems. Child's Brain 3:321–342, 1977
23. Rudd TG, Shirtleff DB, Loeser JD, et al: Radionuclide assessment of cerebro-spinal fluid shunt function in children. J Nucl Med 14:683–686, 1973
24. Sakoda TH, Maxwell JA, Brackett CE Jr: Intestinal volvulus secondary to a ventriculoperitoneal shunt. Case report. J Neurosurg 35:95–96, 1971
25. Scherzer AL: Hydrocele following placement of a ventriculoperitoneal shunt. J Pediatr 86:811, 1975
26. Schulhof LA, Worth RM, Kalsbeck JE: Bowel perforation due to peritoneal shunt. A report of seven cases and a review of the literature. Surg Neurol 3:265–269, 1975
27. Schwartz DC, McSweeney WJ: Intravascular manipulation of ventriculoatrial shunt catheters, in McLaurin R (ed): Myelomeningocele. Proceedings of a Multidisciplinary Symposium. New York, Grune & Stratton, 1976
28. Varfis G, Berney J, Beaumanoir A: Electro-clinical follow-up of shunted hydrocephalic children. Child's Brain 3:129–139, 1977
29. Venes JL: Control of shunt infection. Report of 150 consecutive cases. J Neurosurg 45:311–314, 1976
30. Wald SL, McLaurin RL: Shunt-associated glomerulonephritis. Neurosurgery 3(2):146–150, 1978

17. Mechanisms of Intracranial Hypertension in Children

Kenneth Shapiro
Anthony Marmarou

"The control of intracranial pressure is perhaps the principal task in the neurosurgical care of infants."[16] This statement may be extended to the wider range of ages encountered in pediatric neurosurgery, as many of the medical and surgical diseases encountered in children are accompanied by intracranial hypertension. Widely differing disease processes, including neoplasms, congenital lesions, and metabolic and infectious syndromes, such as Reye's syndrome, will require evaluation and treatment for elevated intracranial pressure. If intracranial hypertension is a common accompaniment of the disease processes of children, then an understanding of the mechanisms leading to intracranial hypertension is of paramount importance to the neurosurgeon. The neurosurgeon involved in the care of children, however, must be cautious in applying to children the concepts of intracranial hypertension derived from experience with adults. Although many of its clinical manifestations are similar in both age groups, distinct differences exist. Children may harbor an intracranial mass lesion for some time without showing definite signs of intracranial hypertension, only to deteriorate rapidly and dramatically to an unsalvageable state. Often intracranial masses may be accompanied by subtle signs of failure to accomplish developmental milestones and an increase in head circumference—phenomena not seen in the adult. Further, unique properties of the immature brain and its container affect the brain's response to changes in intracranial pressure. These differences include the water content of the immature brain, the level of arterial blood pressure that perfuses the immature brain, and the "plasticity" of the immature nervous system. The following discussion addresses the mechanisms that lead to raised intracranial pressure and attempts to integrate the unique properties of the immature nervous system in discussing these mechanisms.

NORMAL INTRACRANIAL PRESSURE

The upper limit of normal intracranial pressure (ICP) in adults and older children is usually given at 15 mm Hg. Transient changes due to coughing, sneezing, or straining will often lead to pressures exceeding 30–50 mm Hg, but ICP returns rapidly to baseline levels. Efforts to measure ICP in younger children and infants by spinal puncture using manometers are open to criticism because of the lack of cooperation from the child and the displacement of fluid into the manometric measuring device. In spite of these difficulties, published norms for children range from 3 to 7.4 mm Hg and for infants from 1.5 to 5.9 mm Hg.[10,12,16] Using visual estimates of fontanel configuration, Welch reported normal ICP of 3–4 mm Hg from the first hours of life to 7 months of age.[16] By applying a noninvasive applanation transducer to the fontanel, Salmon, Hajjar, and Bada found that the normal ICP of infancy is approximately 8 mm Hg.[12]

All reported values for the ICP of younger children are lower than those reported for adults, but are probably reasonable approximations of the actual level of ICP. A teleologic explanation might account for this relatively low normal ICP in children. In adults the ability to effectively perfuse the brain depends on maintenance of an adequate cerebral perfusion pressure (CPP). The CPP is simply the difference between mean arterial blood pressure and ICP. Usually a CPP exceeding 50 mm Hg is needed to maintain adequate cerebral perfusion in adults.[4] The critical CPP of the immature brain has not been determined. Since the mean arterial blood pressure of infants and children is considerably lower than that of adults, a lower normal ICP may be a mechanism of maintaining adequate cerebral perfusion for the brains of younger children if their CPP approximates that found in adults.

Measurements of ICP using closed system, low-volume-displacement electrical transducers to interface with the CSF pathways yield considerably more information than a pressure that exceeds atmospheric pressure by 4–8 mm Hg. A strip chart recorder can be used to display the pulsatile ICP waveform that can be divided into three major components (Fig. 17-1). The *baseline* or diastolic level is commonly referred to as the intracranial pressure (ICP), while the rhythmic components are associated with *cardiac* and *respiratory* activity. To describe

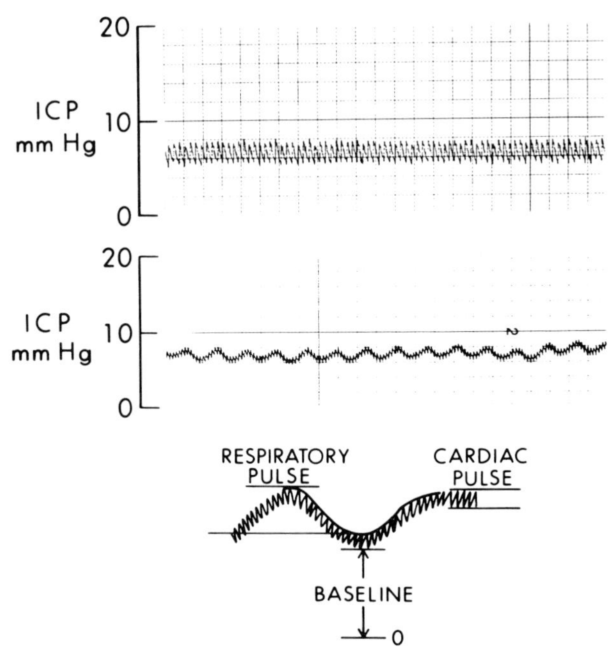

Figure 17-1. The intracranial pressure waveform consists of a respiratory and cardiac pulse superimposed upon a steady-state level that is above atmosphere. The upper panel displays the ICP at fast paper speed to accent the cardiac pulsation. Specification of ICP should include a measure of both baseline level and amplitude of pulsatile components.

ICP completely, one should specify the magnitude of the baseline or "steady-state" level and the amplitude and periodicity of the pulsatile components. At present there is no standardization of nomenclature, so that the pulsatile components are usually excluded and disastolic pressure is specific as the ICP. Although some workers report ICP as a mean pressure, paralleling the convention used in systemic blood pressure, this has not been universally adopted.

STEADY-STATE DYNAMICS

In the condition of physiologic equilibrium, both the baseline ICP and the amplitude of the pulsatile components of ICP remain constant. This implies that the net intracranial volume is also in a state of dynamic equilibrium or steady state. If volume is removed or added to the system, the net seepage of fluid into or out of the cerebrospinal fluid (CSF) spaces will be in a direction that returns pressure to its steady-state level. This dynamic equilibrium is found in a system where volume changes induced by the heartbeat and CSF formation occur continuously, so that it is logical to ask what factors govern volume interchange in the steady state and how these changes affect baseline ICP. These questions were addressed by using a mathematical model of the CSF system that subdivided the physical mechanisms into three major categories: mechanisms associated with CSF formation, the mechanisms for volume storage or compliance, and mechanisms dealing with fluid absorption (Fig. 17-2).[6] Conceptually the formation of CSF was depicted as a fluid pump that continuously introduces fluid into the CSF spaces of the neural axis. The rate of formation of fluid (I_f) was considered constant and independent of the pressure head seen by the pump mechanism, in accordance with observations that the rate of CSF formation is minimally, if at all, affected by changes in the ICP.

According to this model, the newly formed fluid entered a compliant storage space that could expand to accommodate the added volume or proceed via outflow pathways to be absorbed across the arachnoid villi into the dural venous sinuses. The compliance mechanism was represented by an element (C), which decreased its contractibility with increasing volume, much like the impedance offered by a rubber balloon a maximum inflation. Both the resistance of the CSF channels leading to the arachnoid villi and the resistance of the villi to fluid flow were combined into a single resistance element (R_o). This component represented the total resistance to the outflow of CSF, which, under normal conditions, was considered to remain fixed and independent of intracranial pressure. The final element of this model is the dural sinus pressure (P_d). Fluid crossing the arachnoid villi must overcome the P_d, so that the exit pressure of CSF is determined by P_d.

From this conceptual framework a theory was developed to describe the interaction of the formation, storage, and absorptive elements in the steady state.

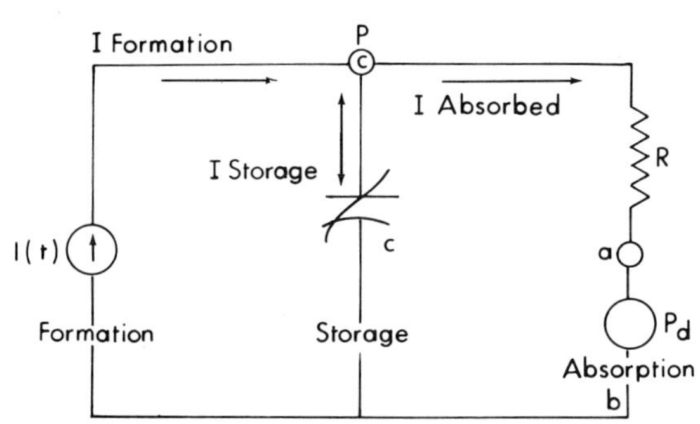

Figure 17-2. The CSF system was depicted by an equivalent electrical circuit that distributed the CSF parameters among three fundamental mechanisms: formation, represented by a constant-current generator; storage, represented by a nonlinear capacitance (C); and absorption, represented by resistance element (R). The venous outflow site (dural sinus) was represented by a constant pressure source P_d. The system equations were derived from this configuration.

First, both pressure and volume are in equilibrium and there can be no net increase or decrease in the total volume of the CSF space. The CSF formed must pass through the absorptive elements, so that no net fluid is stored and the total volume within the CSF spaces remains constant.

Since all fluid formed passes through the resistive element (R_o), a pressure gradient will be developed across the absorptive element that is equal to the product of fluid flow (I_f) and the fluidic resistance (R_o). The greater the magnitude of flow or resistance, the greater the pressure gradient ($I_f \times R_o$). As long as a condition of equilibrium is imposed upon the system, the pressure of the CSF space must be of sufficient magnitude to continuously force all newly formed fluid through the arachnoid villi and to overcome the exit pressure. This requires that the CSF pressure (ICP) be equal to the sum of the pressure gradient developed by the absorptive element ($I_f \times R_o$) and the exit pressure: ICP = ($I_f \times R_o$) + P_d.[1]

The steady-state intracranial pressure thus is proportional to three parameters: the rate of CSF formation, the resistance to CSF absorption, and the dural sinus pressure. When these parameters remain constant, the ICP level remains unchanged and the compliance element does not participate actively.

How is this dynamic equilibrium altered in cases of raised ICP? According to the model, a sustained elevation of pressure can develop with an increase in CSF formation, an increase in outflow resistance, or an increase in the venous pressure at the site of fluid absorption. Our computer studies show that the contribution of the product of outflow resistance and formation rate ($I_f \times R_o$) is approximately 10 percent of total ICP.[9] The remainder is attributed to the magnitude of dural sinus pressure (P_d). With this distribution the outflow resistance would have to increase markedly to effect a significant rise in the ICP. In contrast elevations of sagittal sinus pressure by venous sinus obstruction would be transmitted directly to the CSF system, resulting in an increase in the resting ICP level. Since the increase in P_d equals the change in ICP, the gradient across the arachnoid villi is not altered, CSF absorption remains constant, and the equilibrium shift to a higher ICP level is sustained. This concept is supported by the work of Johnston, who demonstrated normal CSF resistance in the presence of raised ICP induced by venous obstruction and by use in children with anomalies of venous return.[3,14] In both of these conditions, there is no net storage of volume and presumably no change in the compliant element. When the latter two events occur, neural axis dynamics are no longer in a steady state and new concepts must be invoked.

NONSTEADY-STATE DYNAMICS

As implied in the preceding paragraph, steady-state pressure dynamics cannot be transposed directly to pathologic conditions. In contrast to the physiologic steady state where net volume storage does not occur, pathologic settings are often associated with net changes in volume within the neural axis. To understand the interaction between pressure and volume changes, additional concepts and parameters are required.

The cornerstone for analyzing these volume–pressure interactions is the Monro–Kellie doctrine. This states that, after fontanel and suture closure, the container of the neural axis forms a rigid box with the craniospinal, intradural volume being *nearly* constant. Since the components of neural axis volume, neural parenchyma, CSF, and blood are essentially incompressible, any change in one of these components must be accompanied by reciprocal changes in one or both of the others in order to preserve the constancy of neural axis volume. When an additional component is introduced, such as a hematoma, the same principle applies. Exchanges of volume must also be analyzed in terms of rate, as changing properties of tissue may allow volume exchanges to occur over time, which may not be possible acutely. In children with open fontanels or unfused sutures, the container is not rigid, thereby modifying the Monro–Kellie hypothesis.

The interaction among the three components of neural axis volume depends on the ease of egress and the amount of each component that is available for exchange with the other components. The largest constituent of neural axis volume is the brain, comprising approximately 80 percent of total volume. The brain can respond to volume additions to the neural axis by undergoing compression, dislocation, or shift. The effectiveness of the brain as a buffer to added volume depends on the rate of volume addition. A slowly growing brain tumor, for example, is more likely to cause compression and deformation than a rapidly enlarging epidural hematoma that will shift the brain through the tentorial hiatus. The ability of the brain to accommodate mass also depends upon the brain's viscoelastic properties. Theoretically cerebral edema might alter the elasticity of the brain, rendering it less capable of accommodating volume additions to the neural axis.

The second volume component of the neural axis is the CSF, constituting approximately 10 percent of total neural axis volume. Since CSF absorption can increase with increasing pressure gradients across the valve at the arachnoid villi, significant compensatory reserves are available for volume exchange.[17] Estimates of between 30 and 70 percent of total compensatory reserves for volume exchange or buffering are enabled through the mechanism of increased absorption or displacement of CSF into the spinal subarachnoid spaces.[5,7] Since the capacity to increase CSF absorption is not infinite, the rapidity of volume interchange required to preserve the relative constancy of total neural axis volume is important.

The final component of intracranial volume is blood, which normally constitutes the remaining 8–10 percent of total neural axis volume. Since most blood is contained on the venous or capacitance side of the vasculature, many view the cerebrovascular volume as the mechanism for the rapid interchange of volume. Although it is attractive, this mechanism has not been well documented.

Clearly this mechanism must play some role in young children, as scalp veins supplied via the emissary system characteristically become engorged in children with intracranial hypertension and must represent a mechanism to dissipate ICP.

If changes in volume occur within the neural axis, the rapidity with which reciprocal shifts in volume occur to a large part determines the change of ICP within the neural axis. Other factors include the elastic properties of the components within the closed box. Many inanimate containers have "ideal" elastic properties. Such properties include a coefficient of deformation that does not vary with time and is constant for all degrees of expansion of that container. In such an "ideal" container pressure varies directly with volume so that a pressure–volume relationship can be described that is linear with the compliance or rate of volume–pressure change (dV/dP) being constant. The containers of the neural axis and neural parenchyma, however, do not have ideal elastic properties. This results in a nonlinear relationship between ICP and volume added to the neural axis. For equal volume increments, the dV/dP ratio, or compliance, decreases as pressure increases. This was first demonstrated by Ryder, Epsey, Kimbell, et al. in 1953, who described the general form of the curve as "hyperbolic."[11]

The relationship between neural axis volume and ICP is hyperbolic or exponential up to an ICP of 50 mm Hg (Fig. 17-3A). When pressure exceeds

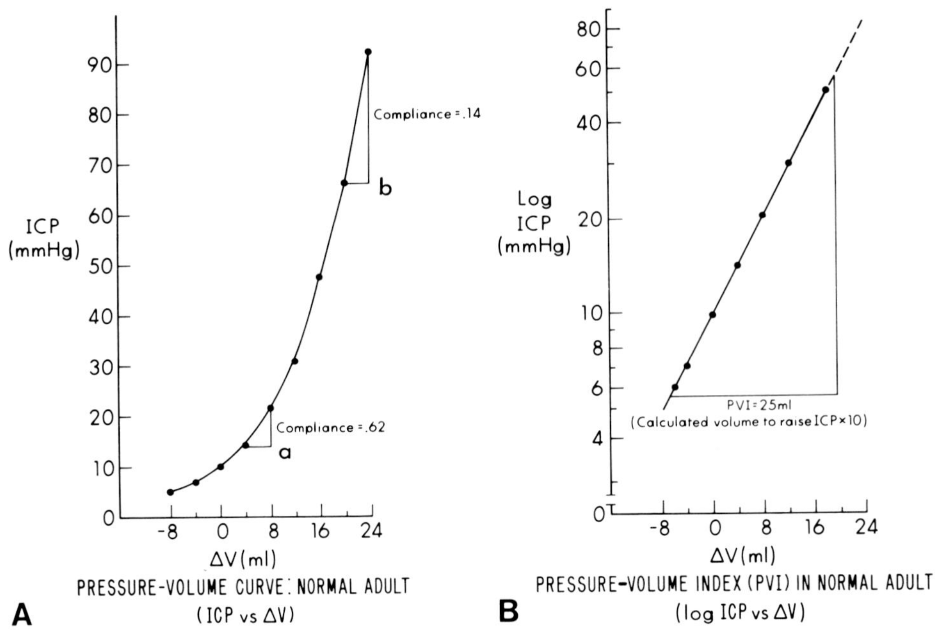

Figure 17-3. A. Neural axis pressure–volume curve obtained by measuring the immediate cerebrospinal fluid pressure response to successive bolus injections ($+ \Delta V$) or withdrawals ($- \Delta V$) of CSF in a normal adult. Compliance ($\Delta V/\Delta P$) is measured at two places on this curve: at point *a* compliance is greater than at point *b*. The differences in compliance at these points are a normal function of CSF pressure. B. The same pressure–volume curve has been transformed to a linear function by plotting the response of CSF pressure on a logarithmic scale. Only two points are needed to define this linear function. The pressure volume index (PVI) is the calculated volume (milliliters) needed to raise CSF pressure by a factor of 10.

50 mm Hg, the curve tends to flatten as the arterial blood pressure is approached. Over the entire range of ICP, the pressure–volume curve thus may be described by a sigmoid-shaped curve. The pressure–volume is measured by rapidly inserting known volumes of fluid into the CSF pathways and recording the magnitude of ICP change. Compliance, according to physical definition, is given by the ratio of volume change (ΔV), which is graphically equivalent to the slope of the pressure–volume curve. Elastance, the reciprocal of compliance, can be extracted from the curves or computer by similar bolus techniques. Since the slope of this curve reflects the ability of the neural axis to accommodate or buffer additional increments of volume, steeper curves identify dynamic settings that have limited compensatory reserves. Inasmuch as compliance changes with pressure, we have however, found little use for the numerical determinations of compliance by this definition.

When pressure–volume data are plotted on a logarithmic pressure axis against volume, the exponential curve is transformed into a straight line (Fig. 17-3B). The slope of this straight-line transformation is the pressure volume index (PVI) and is the calculated volume (in millileters) needed to raise ICP by a factor of 10.[7] A *steep* exponential curve is associated with a *reduced* buffering capacity, and is characterized by a low PVI. An exponential curve with a more gradual increase in slope describes a *more* compliant system and is characterized by a higher PVI value.

In adult humans the normal PVI is approximately 25 ml. This level of PVI can be expressed in more physical terms and indicates that 25 ml of fluid must be added to the CSF compartment in order to raise baseline ICP by a factor of 10.[13] The PVI is directly proportioned to the available buffering capacity. A 50 percent reduction in PVI is equivalent to a 50 percent reduction in volume

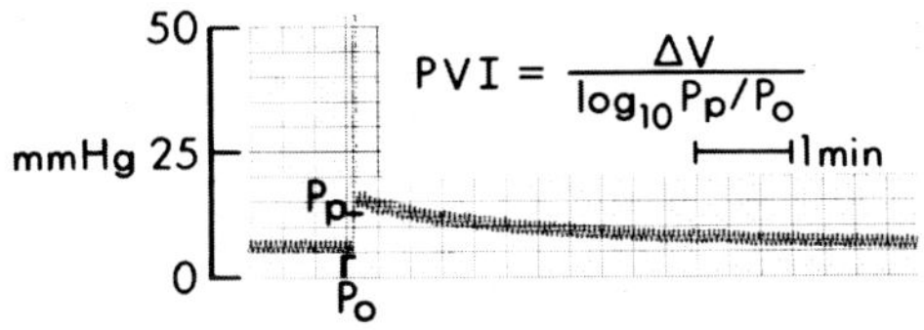

Figure 17-4. This strip chart recording shows the ICP response to a bolus injection of CSF into the cisterna magna of a child. Following injection the baseline pressure P_o is immediately raised to P_P, the peak pressure response to the injection. Pressure then begins to return toward P_o as CSF is absorbed. The PVI can be calculated from the formula, using data derived from the bolus injection.

buffering capacity at all points along the exponential portion of the pressure–volume curve.

In clinical settings the PVI can be determined by adding a known volume (ΔV) to the CSF space at initial pressure (P_o) and recording the peak pressure (P_p) measured immediately after the bolus addition. Both pressures must be measured on the same relative portion of the respiratory and cardiac ICP pulse wave to avoid error. The PVI can be calculated using the formula PVI = $\Delta V/\log_{10}(P_p/P_o)$ (Fig. 17-4). In normal children ranging from infancy to 14 years of age, we have found that PVI varies in proportion to estimated neural axis volume.[13] Normal infants will have PVIs of 8 ml while the adult PVI of 25 ml is reached at around 14 years of age. These studies provide important reference data for assessing pressure–volume relationships in pathologic settings. But even more important, we have found that the slope of a normal infant's or young child's pressure–volume curve is greater than that of a normal teenager (Fig. 17-5). A 10-ml volume added to the neural axis of the teenage child may produce modest elevations of ICP, but the same bolus increment may be lethal in an infant. The factors responsible for volume buffering represent the combined storage ability of both intracranial and spinal compartments. Most workers agree that, theoretically, the venous capacitance system is at least partly responsible for volume buffering, so that as added volume accumulates within the neural axis, venous blood is expressed from these capacitance vessels. Additional buffering capacity may be gained by the relative ease of distending the spinal dural tube at the expense of epidural venous blood volume. We have estimated that 48 percent of this "pool" of compensatory reserve is derived from the supratentorial compartment, 20 percent infratentorial, and 32 percent spinal.[8]

The expression of these nonsteady-state dynamics depends on many factors. Conceptually the simplest situation exists when neural axis pressure–volume relationships describe a stable pressure–volume curve. As volume is added to this system, ICP rises along this curve and the pressure response to each increment of added volume is predicted by the curve. This situation often fails to materialize in many clinical settings, as most disease processes are dynamic, with shift from one pressure–volume curve to another. This dynamic shift may be caused by increases in cerebral blood volume, cerebral edema, and the like,

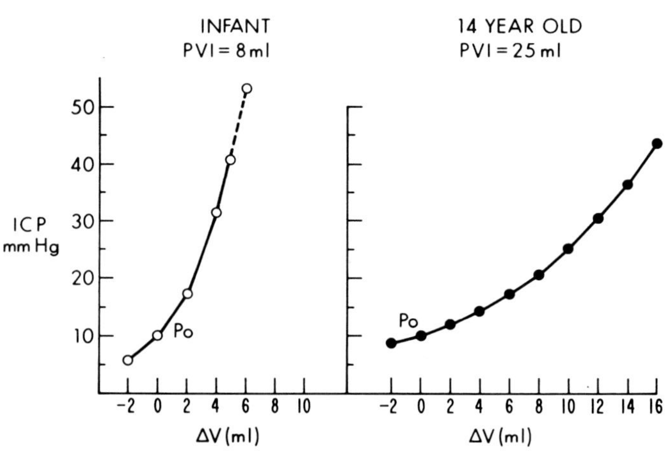

Figure 17-5. The pressure–volume curves shown were generated by injecting and withdrawing CSF from a normal infant (left) and a teenager (right). The slope of the infant's pressure–volume curve is steeper than that of the teenager, resulting in less ability to buffer equal increments of volume.

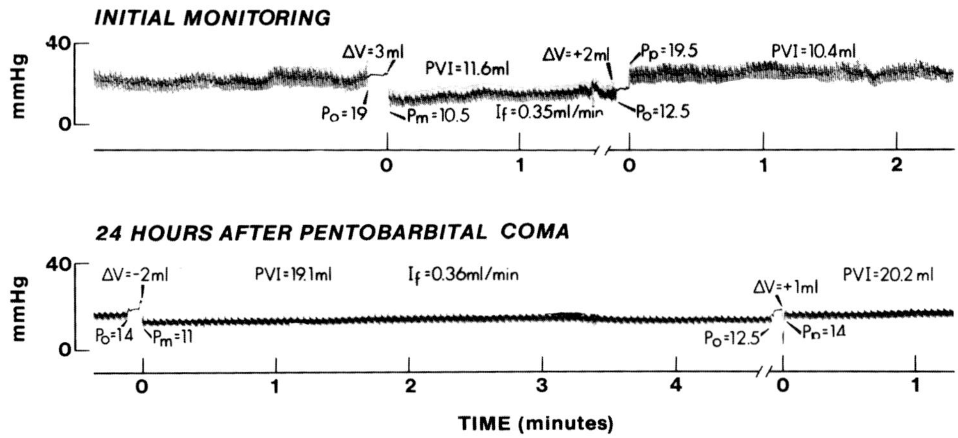

Figure 17-6. The strip chart recordings shown were obtained through a ventricular catheter placed in a child with severe closed-head injury. (GCS=8). The upper tracing shows that PVI was markedly reduced from the predicted normal (23 ml) for this child and was manifest by dramatic elevations of intracranial pressure. The lower tracing shows a PVI determination performed after barbiturate coma was induced in this child. The PVI of 19 ml represents an improvement in the slope of this child's pressure–volume curve and was associated with normalization of intracranial pressure.

exhausting the compensatory reserve bent on preserving normal ICP. We have observed this shifting of pressure–volume curves without significant changes in ICP in a variety of neurosurgical conditions, and also as a response to treating these conditions (Fig. 17-6). This concept of varying pressure–volume curves as opposed to movement along a single curve is reasonable intuitively, as there are not only redistributions of volume, but there probably also are changes in the biomechanical properties of the brain in response to a variety of insults.

NONSTEADY-STATE DYNAMICS IN YOUNGER CHILDREN

The conceptual model and analysis discussed in the preceding sections are based on the "rigid box" container of the neural axis implicit in the Monro–Kellie hypothesis. Weed observed that this does not hold for infants because the skull has not acquired the rigid container property found in the adult.[15] Clinicians caring for infants with hydrocephalus have repeatedly observed that the immature brain with open sutures accommodates added intracranial volumes by skull expansion, often with little elevation of intracranial pressure. The response of the infant to osmotic dehydration by reducing total neural axis volume as evidenced by a sunken fontanel is yet another exception to the Monro–Kellie hypothesis found in young children.[15]

In the preceding section, we stated that the pressure–volume relationship in infants described curves similar to, but steeper than, those found in older children and adults. At first glance this evidence appears to contradict the work of Weed. This conflict can be resolved, however, by realizing that the clinical phenomena seen in children with open sutures usually occur over time. Infants with acute changes in intracranial volume will often have experienced a period of intracranial hypertension that is secondarily accompanied by partial dissipation of ICP elevation as the head enlarges. Our studies in infants were not carried to extreme ICP levels. With the rapid absorption of the added CSF, it is unlikely that the generation of a pressure–volume curve stretched the container of the brain in these infants.

Theoretic models have shown that the bulk intracranial compliance is governed by the spring properties of the meninges and the compressible nature of the vasculature, particularly the more compliant venous bed. Few studies, however, have been conducted to isolate and clearly identify the exact contribution of each of these components to the total compliance. Pressure–volume studies in craniectomized animals have shown that below a pressure range of 50 mm Hg removal of both dura and bone did not affect the shape of the pressure–volume curve. From these experiments it was concluded that in the acute stage the elastic properties of the arachnoid layers, combined with the venous bed, determine the overall compliance.[6]

In these experiments, conducted in the normal physiologic range of pressure and volume, the tensile properties of both arachnoid and dura were not affected. Clinically, in cases where there is prolonged tissue stress, such as is seen with infantile hydrocephalus, the meninges are stretched beyond the normal physiologic range, changing the elastic properties of the dural envelope. Bench tests of the viscoelastic properties of human dura performed by conventional mechanical methods have shown that dura is quite stiff.[2] Clinicians must infer from their own observations that dynamic changes in the mechanical properties of the container must occur in order to accommodate growth of the brain and to allow the brain to expand in children with rising ICP.

The preceding discussion of the factors responsible for steady-state ICP and the mechanism of its change form the foundation for analyzing ICP dynamics in clinical settings. Many of the principles detailed here require modification when applied to the pediatric patient. In addition to the Monro–Kellie hypothesis, other basic concepts of ICP physiopathology may not be directly applicable to the immature nervous system. The notion of a critical cerebral perfusion pressure, well described in adults, has yet to be investigated in young children. The effect of raised ICP on the immature brain with its high water content and changing myelin content has not been systematically investigated. These issues, while beyond the scope of this chapter, may influence the response of the immature brain to raised ICP.

REFERENCES

1. Davson H: Physiology of the cerebrospinal fluid. London, Churchill Livingstone, 1967, p 445
2. Galford JE, McElahany JH: A viscoelastic study of the scalp, brain and dura. J Biomech 3:211–221, 1969
3. Johnston I: Reduced CSF absorption syndrome. Reappraisal of benign intracranial hypertension and related conditions. Lancet 2:418–421, 1973
4. Johnson IH, Rowen JO, Harper AM, et al: Raised intracranial pressure and cerebral blood flow. I Cisterna magna infusion in primates. J Neurol Neurosurg Psychiatr 35:285–296, 1972
5. Lofgren J, Zwetnow NN: Cranial and spinal components of the cerebrospinal fluid pressure-volume curve. Acta Neurol Scand 49:575–585, 1973
6. Marmarou A: A theoretical and experimental evaluation of the cerebrospinal fluid system. Ph.D. thesis, Drexel University, Philadelphia, 1973
7. Marmarou A, Shulman K: Pressure–volume relationships—basic aspects, in McLaurin RL (ed): Head Injuries. New York, Grune & Stratton, 1976, pp 230–236
8. Marmarou A, Shulman K, LaMorgese J: Compartmental analysis of compliance and outflow resistance of the cerebrospinal fluid system. J Neurosurg 43:523–534, 1976
9. Marmarou A, Shulman K, Rosende R: A nonlinear analysis of the cerebrospinal fluid system and intracranial pressure dynamics. J Neurosurg 48:332–344, 1978
10. Munro D: Cerebrospinal fluid pressure in the newborn. JAMA 90:1688–1689, 1928
11. Ryder HW, Epsey FP, Kimbell FD, et al: The mechanism of the change in

cerebrospinal fluid pressure following an induced change in the volume of the fluid space. J Lab Clin Med 41:428–435, 1953
12. Salmon JH, Hajjar W, Bada HS: The fontogram: A noninvasive intracranial pressure monitor. Pediatrics 60:721–725, 1977
13. Shapiro K, Marmarou A, Shulman K: Characterization of clinical CSF dynamics and neural axis compliance using the pressure volume index: I. The normal pressure volume index. Ann Neurol 7(6):508–514, 1980
14. Shapiro K, Shulman K: Facial nevi associated with anomalous venous return and hydrocephalus. J Neurosurg 45:20–25, 1976
15. Weed LH: Some limitations of Monro–Kellie hypothesis. Arch Surg 18:1049–1068, 1929
16. Welch K: The intracranial pressure in infants. J Neurosurg 52:693–699, 1980
17. Welch K, Friedman V: The cerebrospinal fluid valves. Brain 83:454–469, 1961

18. Treatment of Intracranial Hypertension

Derek A. Bruce

In Chapter 17 the mechanisms that function to maintain a normal intracranial pressure-to-volume relationship were discussed. This chapter reviews the therapeutic means available to treat increased intracranial pressure. The fact that the pressure is altered suggests that some resetting of the homeostatic mechanisms or some dysfunction thereof has occurred. Increased intracranial pressure (ICP) is not a disease but a symptom of some underlying pathologic process in the intracranial cavity. It is rare that events external to the cranium can produce intracranial hypertension, although bilateral acute obstruction of the internal jugular veins can produce transient intracranial hypertension, as can prolonged CO_2 retention and severe systemic hypertension. The normal intracranial cavity is exposed to intermittently high pressures (e.g., in coughing, sneezing, straining, etc.). As long as mechanisms such as vascular pressure autoregulation are functioning and the period of increased pressure is short, no ill effects from intracranial hypertension occur. The deleterious effects of increased ICP appear to be those of secondary brain ischemia and displacement and herniation of brain substance—cingulate, uncal, and tonsilar.[1] The ICP that produces deterioration of neurologic function thus will vary depending upon the course of the intracranial hypertension and the state of the various homeostatic mechanisms within the cranium. It appears that diffuse increases in ICP (hydrocephalus, pseudotumor cerebri) are better tolerated than focal lesions since the latter are more likely to produce herniation syndromes.

There is no single therapy for intracranial hypertension since elevated ICP is not a disease but merely a symptom of a variety of pathologic events that can occur within the cranium. Therapy must be directed toward correction of the underlying pathologic factors, if possible. The intracranial space contains blood, cerebrospinal fluid (CSF), brain, and any other pathologic lesion (e.g., hematoma or tumor) that may be added. An increase in any one compartment, if large enough or rapid enough, can lead to increased ICP. Correction of the increased ICP may be directed against a primary event as in hydrocephalus or designed to decrease some nonpathologic compartment in an effort simply to decrease overall volume, as in the use of mannitol to lower ICP in the face of a mass lesion. With the multiplicity of therapy available, selection of the best method of treatment of elevated ICP has to be based on an accurate diagnosis of the underlying pathology. This is important not only in selecting the most effective initial therapy, but also in planning later therapy. Hyperventilation, for example, may be very effective in lowering the ICP following head trauma or in Reye's syndrome in the initial stages of disease, but after several days increased cerebral edema may be present or a hematoma may have formed and now a different type of therapy will be required. The physician must not be restricted to the use of one or two modalities of therapy since, in the patient with severe intracranial hypertension, a whole gamut of therapy for physiologic manipulation to surgical decompression may be necessary to prevent secondary brain ischemia resulting from intracranial hypertension.

When considering the causes of increased ICP, the following equation is helpful in visualizing the various compartments of the cranium:

$$V_{CSF} + V_{blood} + V_{brain} + V_{other} = V_{intracranial\ space}$$

Each of these compartments will be discussed separately, to examine what diseases affect each compartment and what methods are available for treatment (Table 18-1).

V_{OTHER}

Under this heading are all the lesions that add a new component to the intracranial space (tumor, abscess, hematoma, etc.). When one of these lesions is the cause of intracranial hypertension, the best therapy is surgical removal of the mass. This may be definitive therapy and, therefore, such a treatable cause of increased ICP must always be sought. The other various methods of treatment to be discussed below and shown in Table 18-1 may well be applicable, particularly when the added intracranial mass lesion is not readily removable or has been present for a long period and is associated with significant cerebral edema.

Surgery is the ideal therapy when the cause of increased intracranial volume is an increased V_{other}. Tumor, abscess, hemorrhage, giant aneurysms, arteriovenous malformations (AVMs), etc., thus all lend themselves to surgical removal and reestablishment of the normal intracranial volume. There are situations in which a mass lesion may be present (e.g., infection and metastatic disease) yet surgery may not be indicated. The intracranial hypertension must then be treated by some other method, such as corticosteroids, antibiotics, chemotherapy, or radiation. In patients with rapid neurologic deterioration secondary to a rapidly expanding mass lesion (e.g., epidural hematoma), there is a need to apply general therapy to lower ICP until a diagnosis is made. These therapies include head-up position, hyperventilation, and endotracheal intubation, *if done with full anesthetic precautions for rapid sequence induction and osmotic therapy.* The dangers of some increase in size of the hematoma are offset by reversal of any

Table 18-1
Treatments Available to Lower ICP or Improve Intracranial Compliance

Blood Volume	CSF	Brain Bulk
Head-up position	Diamox®	Steroids
Midline head position	Furosemide	Osmotic diuretics
Controlled intrathoracic pressure	Ethacrynic acid	Tubular diuretics
Decrease $PaCO_2$	CSF drainage	Barbiturates (?)
Barbiturates (?)	Steroids	Controlled blood pressure

associated herniation and improvement in cerebral perfusion. The danger of the therapy comes in seeing an improvement in the patient's neurologic examination and then not continuing to make a definitive diagnosis of the underlying pathophysiology. If an expanding mass is present, the sequence of increased ICP and herniation will repeat itself. This is not "rebound" but a manifestation of the progressive nature of the primary lesion, which must be diagnosed and treated. When a difficult-to-approach mass lesion is present (e.g., deep hematoma secondary to ruptured AVM), ICP monitoring can be very useful in helping to decide whether immediate surgery is advisable or necessary. If the ICP is easily controlled below 20 torr and there are no signs of progressive herniation, then surgery can be postponed until the patient is in a more favorable condition for a complex operation and the brain swelling and increased ICP have subsided. The use of ICP monitoring can also be helpful when multiple lesions are present and surgery is deemed inadvisable or impossible (e.g., multiple abscesses or mycotic aneurysm). The knowledge of the level of ICP permits rational selection of therapy and allows the physician to measure the response to therapy, thereby helping to define when further therapy or a different type of therapy is necessary. It is our firm belief that severe intracranial hypertension associated with coma can only be adequately treated with the help of intracranial pressure monitoring.

Besides the role of surgery in the definitive removal of an intracranial mass lesion, there are two other situations in which surgical intervention may be helpful: the performance of internal and of external decompressions. Internal decompression is the surgical excision of a portion of the brain to decrease intracranial volume, at least temporarily. This is a technique that has little role in the treatment of children with brain disease. It has been particularly applicable to traumatic injuries in adults when relatively silent polar areas are involved with hemorrhagic contusion and edema. Because these lesions act as a focal mass, surgical removal of the frontal or temporal pole has been advocated. In adults ICP monitoring can be used in a predictive fashion; that is, those with an ICP over 20 torr despite therapy require surgery, whereas those in whom the ICP remains below 20 torr are likely to recover without surgical intervention.[2] Whenever therapy involves the removal of potentially viable brain, the treatment must be questioned, and in children this type of destructive surgery is rarely necessary or justifiable.

The final role of surgery is in the treatment of intracranial hypertension by external decompression. This, as the name implies, is the removal of portions of the cranium to enlarge the intracranial volume. This type of therapy can be rationalized when an ultimately self-limiting process that does not produce primary brain damage is present, the ICP cannot be kept below 20–25 mm Hg with intensive medical therapy, and the chances of good recovery are good, if secondary ischemia and herniation can be avoided. In trauma the results have been discouraging, probably because the traumatically damaged brain does not fulfill these criteria. Hoffman has suggested a role for decompressive craniectomy in children with Reye's syndrome and has reported encouraging results. The role for this type of therapy is very limited and careful judgment is required before such an operation is performed. The potential benefit of bifrontal craniectomy with opening of the dura is that transtentorial herniation is less likely to occur because the brain can now decompress anteriorly. Cerebral perfusion pressure also may be improved. In the author's experience, craniectomy in Reye's syndrome is rarely associated with a significant lowering of the ICP and the beneficial results obtained are probably due to decreased tentorial herniation. Residual brain damage may be very severe (Fig. 18-1).

When the increase in intracranial volume is due to an increased V_{other}, the most satisfactory treatment is the surgical removal of the offending mass lesion,

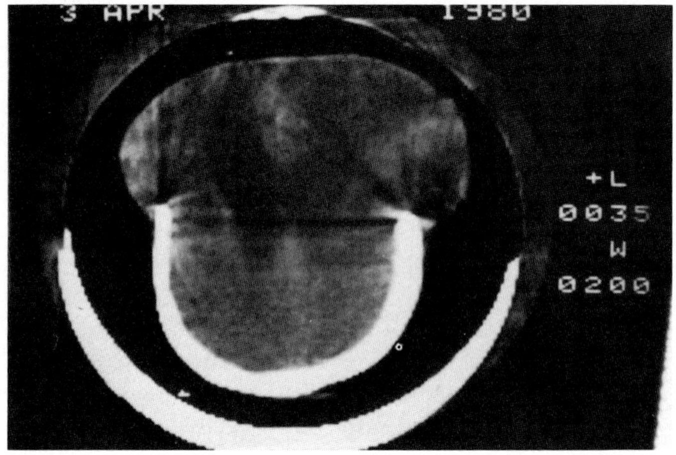

Figure 18-1. CT scan two weeks following decompressive craniotomy in patient with Reye's syndrome. Note enlarged ventricular system and marked decreased density of both frontal lobes.

when possible. When this is impossible, other ancillary methods to decrease intracranial volume by removing CSF, brain, water, or blood may all be applicable. These treatments are discussed in the following.

V_{CSF}

Ventricular shunting or ventricular drainage is the treatment of choice when increased CSF is the cause of the increase in intracranial volume, or hydrocephalus. The treatment of hydrocephalus is discussed in Chapter 14 and will not be elaborated on here. Other situations, however, lend themselves in CSF drainage as an ancillary measure to control intracranial hypertension. These may be divided into acute and subacute cases. Many units still use an intraventricular catheter to monitor the ICP, even when ventriculomegaly is not present. One of the advantages of this technique is that it gives access to the CSF and removal of small amounts of CSF can terminate waves of intracranial pressure. The second theoretic reason for the use of CSF drainage is to create a gradient of pressure from the edematous brain to the ventricles, thereby encouraging movement of water from the brain into the ventricles and aiding in the resolution of cerebral edema.[3,4] Practically, this does not seem to be effective as a continuous therapy since, when the ventricles are small, the removal of CSF leads to collapse of the ventricle around the catheter, loss of drainage capability, and frequently loss of ICP recording. In the face of a swollen brain (i.e., small ventricles), therefore, while intermittent removal of small amounts of ventricular CSF may be an effective ancillary measure to maintain the ICP below 20 mm Hg, it cannot be done continuously and is of limited value. The subacute instances where CSF drainage may be effective are during the resolution of an episode of cerebral edema. There are a number of situations during which the ventricular size enlarges abnormally during the course of treatment for increased ICP. This is especially true following trauma in children but may occur during recovery from Reye's syndrome, meningitis, or subarachnoid or ventricular hemorrhage. In the child with severe closed-head injury, subarachnoid hemorrhage, and diffuse brain swelling, the ICP can usually be controlled in the first 3–10 days by a combination of position, hyperventilation, and medications. It is not uncommon that after a period of 24–48 hours of a stable, normal ICP, the pressure again rises between the third and 15th day. At this time a repeat computerized tomographic (CT) scan will show either enlarged subarachnoid spaces, especially frontally, or ventricular dilation, or both (Fig. 18-2).[5] At this time therapy to

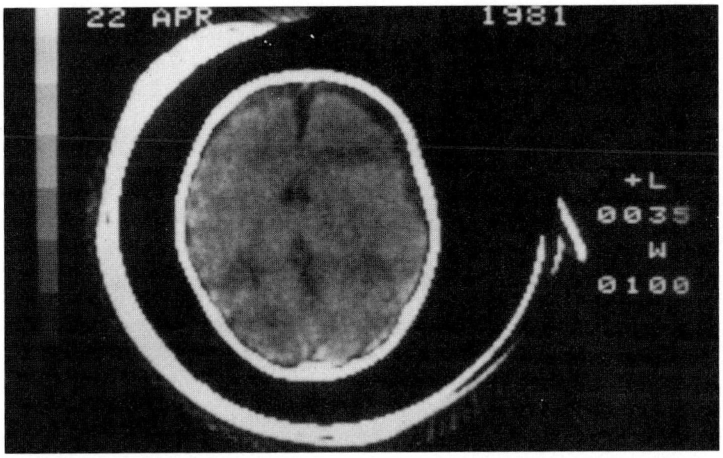

Figure 18-2. CT scan in 2-year-old suffering head trauma taken two weeks following trauma. Note increased subarachnoid spaces over frontal lobes.

maintain a normal pressure is primarily removal of the excess CSF via lumbar or ventricular drainage. A permanent ventricular shunt usually is not necessary in these children as this is a transient phase. The cause of the increased CSF is believed to be an increase in outflow resistence. This change from the swollen brain with little *extracerebral* CSF to excess CSF emphasizes that disturbances of the intracranial homeostatic mechanisms are dynamic events and a constant review of the underlying pathology is required to govern the sensible choice of specific therapy. Changes in therapy based on changes in the underlying pathology are frequently necessary. The formation of CSF, which also contributes to intracranial volume, can be decreased by a variety of drugs and, in children with acute hydrocephalus, ICP may be transiently controlled by the use of such medications. Diamox® Sequel tablets (Lederle Laboratories, Pearl River, New Jersey, 10965),[6] furosemide (Lasix®—Elkins-Sim, 2 Esterbrook Lane, Cherry Hill, New Jersey, 08034),[7] and corticosteroids[8] all may transiently decrease CSF production. There is good evidence[9] that the use of corticosteroids very rapidly decreases pressure waves and, ultimately, lowers the ICP in patients with posterior fossa tumors and hydrocephalus. Except in the sickest children, we routinely use steroids rather than ventricular drainage or shunting in children with posterior fossa lesions, especially those that are malignant, in an effort to avoid peritoneal metastases. Unfortunately none of the methods of decreasing CSF production have been shown to have any long-term benefit in the treatment of intracranial hypertension and all are associated with side effects. One other medication, isosorbide,[10] has been used chronically in the treatment of borderline hydrocephalus in childhood and seems to have some minor role to play.

Whether or not the increase in ICP is due to an increase in CSF, a variety of therapies that reduce the volume of CSF are available. These range from the use of drugs that decrease CSF formation to withdrawal and removal of CSF from the lumbar space or the ventricles, and they can help maintain a normal ICP.

V_{BLOOD}

Most intracranial blood volume is in the venous sinuses and pial blood vessels. Only quite small amounts, 5 ml/100 g of grey matter and 3.5 ml/100 g of white matter, are present within the brain parenchyma.[11] Theoretically the displacement of pial venous blood is one of the factors responsible for acute compensation for volume changes in the cranium. There is good evidence, however, that intracerebral blood volume increases with increasing ICP,[12] and this is believed to be due to vasodilatation in response to lowered cerebral perfusion pressure (CPP), or pressure autoregulation. As the ICP is elevated, there is, in fact, a shift of blood volume from the pial vessels at the venous end of the system to the arterial end because of arterial dilatation. Two separate events may occur in response to elevation of ICP. The intracerebral blood volume may increase while the total intracranial blood volume, at least in the early stages of increasing ICP, may decrease as blood is squeezed from the pial circulation to the sinuses. The net effect on the intracranial blood volume thus is not a simple one and remains to be completely clarified.

It is possible to have a primary increase in cerebral blood volume that can produce swelling of the brain, increased ICP, and, depending on the location of the blood, a change in the elastic properties of the brain itself. In this situation the compliance in the cranium could be either increased or decreased depending on whether the increased blood volume was in the pial circulation, and therefore readily expressible into the venous sinuses, or within the cerebral substance itself. Increased $PaCO_2$ leads to an increase in cerebral blood flow (CBF) and cerebral blood volume (CBV); increased ICP, and papilledema, and, in the face of acute infarction, it can produce vasodilatation and acute hemorrhage as a result of the increased CBF.[13]

Can an increase in CBV alone be adequate to raise the ICP and, if so, under what conditions? Carbon dioxide intoxication has already been mentioned. Raichle, Grubb, Phelps, et al.[14] have demonstrated an increased CBV in patients with pseudotumor cerebri but concluded that the increase in CBV was insufficient to account for the increase in ICP. Cerebrovascular dilatation occurs following experimental head injury[15] and there is a suggestion that this vasodilatation may be blocked by prostaglandin inhibitors.[16] Following certain types of head injury in children, acute swelling of the brain is seen. Bruce, Bilaniuk, Dolinskas, et al.[17] have suggested that in children the swelling is most likely due to increased intracranial blood volume. As yet studies on rCBV have not conclusively proved that all the swelling is due to blood volume, although CT scan density measurements suggest that the increased brain bulk is not the result of edema but more likely of increased blood volume.[18] In the acute encephalopathy of Reye's syndrome, increased CBF is present, and this must also be accompanied by an increase in CBV. We believe that there is adequate evidence that in many acute brain insults in childhood increased blood volume is at least one factor contributing to the decrease in intracranial compliance and the increase in ICP.

The simplest way to decrease intracranial blood volume is to place the patient in a 30-degree head-up tilt. This will decrease the venous pressure in intracranial dural sinuses and permit collapse of the upper cervical extradural veins, and thus allow a decrease in ICP. Proper ventilator settings, if the patient is on mechanical ventilation, are important since too long an inspiratory phase will produce prolonged increased intrathoracic pressure—increased venous pressure reflecting back to the head with increased venous sinus pressure. Similarly, too high levels of positive end respiratory pressure (PEEP) theoretically produce increases in central venous pressure that could also be reflected back to the intracranial space. In practice we have not found the use of PEEP to be associated with elevated ICP. The best explanation for this is that when large amounts of PEEP are required, there is usually markedly reduced pulmonary compliance and the intrapulmonary pressure is not transmitted directly to the central veins. Significant rises in central venous pressure therefore do not occur. While lowering of systemic arterial pressure might be expected to decrease intracranial blood volume, the reverse is true. This is so because the decrease in systemic arterial pressure (SAP) produces a fall in CPP that results in vasodilatation at the arterial end of the tree. There is evidence, however, that lowered

SAP does have some beneficial effect in lowering brain compliance, and this is discussed in the following.[19]

The single most effective therapy to decrease rCBV is to reduce the arterial CO_2. This results in decreased vascular caliber and reduction of CBF and CBV.[20,21] The response of the cerebral vessels to changes in $PaCO_2$ is preserved in most disease states until the point of impending brain death, and therefore a good response to hyperventilation can usually be expected. Acutely, hyperventilation can almost always be performed adequately in the child with the use of an oral airway, bag, and mask. While adult studies suggest that lowering the $PaCO_2$ below 20 torr has little further effect on CBF,[21] this does not appear to hold true for children. Clinically we have found that a favorable decrease in ICP occurs with lowering of the $PaCO_2$ from 20 to 17 torr. When severe hyperventilation to this degree is used, it is advisable to have a jugular venous bulb catheter in place to monitor the cerebrovenous AVD O_2 and the venous PaO_2 since a fall in cerebrovenous PaO_2 below 20 torr may be a sign of too large a decrease in CBF. The jugular bulb catheter can also be used to monitor the match between cerebral blood flow and metabolism.[22] It is unlikely that true cerebral ischemia can be produced by hyperventilation since, as CBF decreases due to elevated $PaCO_2$, the local increase in metabolites will produce vascular dilatation and prevent a severe decrease in CBF. Metabolic studies by MacMillan and Seisjo[23] showed no evidence of changes in energy charge potential until the CO_2 was decreased below 10 torr.

It seems likely that one of the beneficial effects of barbiturates on intracranial hypertension is due to vasoconstriction with an acute decrease in cerebral blood volume inside the brain. Whether this is a secondary effect of decreased metabolism or a prime effect on the cerebral vessels remains unclear. The barbiturates are discussed in greater detail below.

V_{BRAIN}

The final intracranial component that can expand is the brain tissue itself. The processes underlying expansion of the brain can be tumor, in which case the definitive therapy is to remove the lesion if possible; infection; or, most frequently, brain edema. Brain edema is an increase in the water content of the brain and occurs as a result of either disturbances of cellular function interfering with cell pumping mechanisms, disruption of the blood–brain barrier, disturbances of transcapillary pressures or in association with disturbance of CSF circulation, or hydrocephalus. The last has been discussed under CSF increases and will not be considered here. When brain edema is believed to be the pathologic process responsible for the increased ICP, therapeutic considerations have to be based on the location and cause of the cerebral edema. The approach to therapy can be divided into three phases: (1) decreasing the formation of the edema, (2) improving neuronal or axonal function in the presence of edema, and (3) increasing the rate of removal of the edema fluid.

The edema fluid may be intracellular—neurons, glial, or both; in the extracellular space; or occasionally between the lamellae of the myelin. While removal of fluid from the brain may not depend upon the location of the fluid, the effect of other drugs that influence edema is dependent upon the location of the edema fluid. When the excess water is intracellular, this is the result of some disturbance of cellular metabolism, usually interference with energy production (e.g., following anoxia or ischemia) and the edema is secondary to the cellular dysfunction. The ideal therapy in these instances is to correct the disordered cell function. At present few, if any, agents are available for this purpose. When anoxia or ischemia is of limited duration, reestablishment of oxygen delivery will correct the metabolic defect, and therefore maintenance of adequate cerebral circulation and oxygen and glucose delivery are primary considerations in all types of cellular edema.

The most common type of edema requiring therapy is extracellular edema, so-called vasogenic, which occurs as a result of disturbances of the blood–brain barrier, or a combination of extra- and intracellular edema, as occurs in the later stages of infarction. At present the way in which this type of extracellular edema influences cerebral function is unclear. There appear to be three major detrimental effects: (1) interference with local neuronal/axonal function (mechanism not yet known); (2) local expansion of brain with distortion and displacement of brain leading to cerebral herniation, subfalcine, transtentorial, or cerebellar tonsillar; and (3) diffuse increase in ICP producing pressure waves, decreased CBV, and focal or global ischemia as a result of lowered cerebral perfusion pressure. Experimental studies on vasogenic edema have demonstrated that removal of the area of damaged blood–brain barrier can limit and stop the progressive accumulation of edema fluid.[24] While it is very rare to use resection of brain as a treatment for brain edema, the removal of severely contused brain (e.g., temporal tip lobectomy) following trauma is occasionally performed to control the ICP and this has the additional benefit of removing the source of the edema fluid. The concept of removing the source of the edema is more pertinent when the edema source is not normal or damaged brain but a separate pathophysiologic lesions (e.g., brain tumor, abscess, or hematoma). Here removal of the source will stop edema formation. When large mass lesions are removed, the decompression of the brain may be followed by a period of increased swelling and edema and therefore other methods of therapy to control brain edema may have to be continued for several days following removal of mass lesions. The factors involved in edema formation are the state of the hydraulic conductance of the cerebral capillaries, the compliance of brain tissue, the intravascular hydrostatic pressure, the intravascular oncotic pressure, the cerebral tissue hydrostatic pressure, and the cerebral oncotic pressure. Although most of these factors cannot be manipulated, the systemic arterial pressure, the intravascular oncotic pressure, and possibly the hydraulic conductance of the capillaries can be effected. Experimental studies show that if the SAP is lowered sufficiently, little or no cerebral edema will occur following a cold lesion of the cortex.[25] In practice the use of this information should lead at least to preventing cerebrovascular hypertension (age-appropriate) in children with brain edema. To lower the blood pressure below the normal mean can be safely performed only if both blood pressure and ICP are continuously monitored to ensure that adequate CPP is preserved. When there is severe brain edema with coma and difficult-to-control ICP, modest lowering of the SAP can occasionally be a useful ancillary measure. This is discussed again under barbiturates.

Increasing the intravascular osmolality, thus speeding removal of edema fluid, is probably the most widely used method of treating cerebral edema and intracranial hypertension. The three commonly used agents are urea, mannitol, and glycerol. Mannitol is the one most frequently used. The theory behind the use of these agents is that by increasing serum osmolality, fluid, mostly free water, will move from the brain tissue into the blood down an osmotic gradient. It has been demonstrated that the maximum water removal is from the normal brain rather than from the edematous brain.[26,27] This remains a poorly explained phenomenon and cannot be the result of disturbances of the blood–brain barrier since it has been shown that the barrier is intact in all but the area of edema formation. Urea has been shown to enter the brain through an intact barrier. This knowledge led to the theoretic concern that urea might leak into the brain and end up reversing the osmotic gradient, thus producing a rebound in intracranial pressure. There is little or no hard evidence that rebound is a clinically significant phenomenon and urea has one advantage over the other drugs mentioned. It is a smaller molecule and less volume has to be given to obtain the same osmotic effect. Over the past two or three years, the initial doses of both urea and mannitol have decreased from the more standard doses of 1–2 g/kg to small doses of 0.25–0.5 g/kg. The ideal mode of delivery is to give the smallest amount that will effectively lower the ICP. The complications associated with osmotic therapy are electrolyte imbalance, dehydration, and possibly renal failure. Repeat measurements of serum electrolytes and osmolality are necessary with repeated use of osmotic therapy. Fluid replacement is performed to preserve vascular volume and the ideal situation is to preserve isovolemia with increased serum osmolality. With both urea and mannitol, as the serum osmolality rises about 320–330 mOsm there is increasing concern for effects on the renal tubules and it is advised that another agent be used at this time. Glycerol has been used IV and PO to lower ICP and shows promise as a valuable agent for control of increased ICP. The most obvious benefit is that glycerol is not excreted via the kidneys, but is metabolized in the body. The concentration gradients in the renal tubules therefore are not disturbed and tubular failure has not been reported. Very high levels of serum osmolality can be obtained, over 400 mOsm, with apparent safety. This is a drug that is likely to see increasing use.

Hyperosmotic therapy should be valuable in lowering the ICP and reducing edema in both cellular and extracellular edema. The amount of water removed will depend upon the tissue perfusion, the osmotic gradient, but also upon the site and state of the brain water. Little is known about the state of brain water (i.e., bound or unbound). The major contraindication to the use of osmotic agents is when hyperemia and an increased cerebral blood volume are present. The use of hyperosmotic agents increases CBF[28] independently of its effect on ICP, and therefore should be used with caution in the early treatment of head injuries or Reye's syndrome.

DMSO is gain being investigated as an agent to reduce ICP. At present there is no good information on either the efficacy of the drug or the best methods and dose of administration or complications. While there is an osmotic effect, this does not seem to be the prime mechanism whereby ICP is decreased and studies are underway to investigate the usefulness and complications associated with this drug. It is not recommended as an agent for intracranial hypertension control at the present time and is not available for general use.

In discussing the factors responsible for edema formation, alterations of blood–brain barrier and increased capillary hydraulic conductance were mentioned. In vasogenic edema in particular, therapy to restore the integrity of the blood–brain barrier should be useful. Corticosteroids, especially methylprednisolone and dexamethasone, have been demonstrated to have a clinically beneficial effect on certain patients with cerebral edema. The best clinical responses are seen in patients with brain tumors or abscesses. A beneficial role of steroids on the outcome of patients with brain trauma or infarction remains unproved. The effect of corticosteroids is not clear. A simple decrease in tissue water content does not occur, yet clinical and experimental improvement in neurologic function, the electroencephalogram (EEG), and intracranial compliance are all seen early after administration.[29,30] Crocker, Zimmerman, Phelps, et al.[31] demonstrated that steroids appear to decrease the area and amount of blood–brain barrier leakage and may be beneficial by decreasing edema formation or by some direct membrane effect in the area of edema. Methylprednisolone has been shown to facilitate the release of oxygen from hemoglobin and it is possible that some systemic effect facilitating substrate delivery to the brain underlies the beneficial actions of these drugs. Whatever the mechanism involved, corticosteroids have a firm place in the therapy of brain edema secondary to tumor or infection. In other lesions (e.g., trauma or infarction), the use of steroids is very much the decision of the individual physician. When used to control symptomatic cerebral edema, large doses are employed (1 mg/kg/day divided into four doses). Once the reason for the edema has resolved, the dosage is cut rapidly and every effort made to stop the steroids within the shortest possible time.

Work by Bourke[32] and with his co-workers, Kimelberg, Daze, et al.,[33] has shown that swelling of the glial cells accompanies trauma and hypoxia and that this swelling appears to be related to a chloride-mediated transport system within the glial cell membrane. These investigators have demonstrated that ethacrynic acid decreases this glial cell swelling and, in animal models, improves mortality statistics. They have also tested ethacrynic acid derivatives that have little or no diuretic effect but appear to be even more potent against the glial swelling. This field of research seems to hold promise for the development of a whole new group of specific agents with which to treat brain edema, particularly that associated with glial swelling.

Diuretic agents, such as furosemide and ethacrynic acid, also decrease CSF production and may lower ICP by removing water from the body or by effects on sodium pumping at the membrane. In children furosemide is most effective in lowering ICP when there is evidence of fluid overload. When a rapid decrease in ICP is desired, a combination of a tubular diuretic plus a hyperosmolar agent may produce a better response than either drug alone. When tubular diuretics are employed to treat edema and ICP, careful management of fluid status is necessary with close monitoring of intake and output, electrolytes, and serum osmolarity.

The final group of drugs that have received clinical and experimental support as agents to control brain swelling, edema, and increased ICP are the barbiturates. Three barbiturates have been used: sodium pentothal, pentobarbital, and phenobarbital. The mechanism of action of these drugs is unknown. They do decrease CBF and cerebral metabolism, however. The decrease in CBF tends to limit formation of edema by lowering end-capillary pressure. The decrease in cerebral metabolism may permit the cells to tolerate a degree of ischemia or anoxia that would otherwise be detrimental. While experimental studies of focal ischemia, particularly, have shown some protective effect of barbiturates, this has yet to be demonstrated in the clinic. The use of barbiturate therapy, then, is mainly to lower the ICP. The use of high doses of barbiturates is a major undertaking and requires a pediatric intensive care unit. Of the three drugs, phenobarbital appears to have the fewest cardiovascular side effects but also appears to have the least effect on the EEG and, at present, appears to be less capable of controlling intracranial hypertension. Pentobarbitol has been the most commonly used agent, but when levels above 3 mg% are obtained in children, hypotension is common. This drop in SAP is due to decreasing peripheral resistance, not to altered cardiac output, and can be controlled with volume and dopamine, if necessary.

Significant dangers from hypotension and infection exist when barbiturates are used and their use should be restricted to areas where continuous supervision of therapy can be maintained. There seems to be a definite value in the use of barbiturates following head trauma in children and in Reye's syndrome. In both of these states there is significant cerebral hyperemia and it may be that the barbiturates have a maximum effect in those situations where flow is greater than metabolism. In patients with severe brain swelling post anoxia or ischemia, we have not found the use of barbiturates to lead to an improved outcome.[35] While it has proved possible to control the ICP, no patient recovered beyond the vegetative state, whereas in those patients who did not develop intracranial hypertension, 30 percent recovered to a moderately disabled or better state.

SUMMARY

Intracranial hypertension is not a disease but a reflection of some imbalance between volume and pressure in the cranium. The clinical signs and symptoms of intracranial hypertension may be difficult to recognize in children. This is absolutely true in the unconscious child and before instituting treatment of intracranial hypertension, it is necessary to establish what is producing the imbalance in the cranium and that the ICP is indeed elevated. This requires special neuroradiologic studies and measurement of the ICP. The various compartments of the intracranial space may contribute in different degrees to the cause of the raised ICP and the selection of therapy has to be based on an understanding of the role of each compartment. The deleterious effects of ICP appear to be due to cerebral distortion and focal or global ischemia. While the normal brain can resist significantly elevated ISP, the damaged brain may not, and therapy is directed toward maintaining a normal ICP below 20 torr, if possible. Except in rare circumstances, it is possible with modern techniques to control the ICP in children. The benefit to the patient in terms of improved recovery, however, will depend upon the underlying pathologic processes. When there is a reversible underlying disease, the control of ICP can lead to dramatic recovery (e.g., head injury), whereas when the underlying disease leads to irreversible loss of neurons (e.g., anoxia, ischemia), control of ICP and preservation of life at a vegetative level may be a disservice to the patient and family.

There is no single therapy for increased ICP and it is important constantly to review the various pathophysiologic mechanisms that may be active within the cranium to select the most appropriate therapy. This therapy may be quite different from day to day in any one patient, depending upon the cause and course of the disease process. In the unconscious patient, the use of ICP monitoring is an invaluable aid—and, we feel, a necessity if therapy is to be given in a safe and controlled fashion.

REFERENCES

1. Bruce DA: CSF pressure dynamics and brain metabolism, in Wood JH (ed): Neurobiology of Cerebrospinal Fluid. New York, Plenum Press, 1980
2. Teasdale G, Galbraith S, Jennett B: Operate or observe? ICP and the management of the "silent" traumatic intracranial hematoma, in Shulman K, Marmarou A, Miller JD, et al (eds): Intracranial Pressure IV. New York, Springer Verlag, 1980, pp 36–38
3. Reulen HJ, Tsuyumie H, Tach A, et al: Clearance of edema fluid into cerebrospinal fluid. J Neurosurg 48:754, 1978
4. Bruce DA, ter Weeme C, Kaiser G, et al: Mechanisms and time course for clearance of vasogenic cerebral edema, in Popp AJ, Bourke FJ, Nelson LR, et al (eds): Neural Trauma. New York, Raven Press, 1979, pp 155–171
5. Bruce DA, Raphaely RC, Goldberg AI, et al: The pathophysiology, treatment and outcome following severe head injury in children. Child's Brain, 5:174, 1979
6. Pollay M: Formation of CSF: Relation of studies of isolated choroid plexus to the standing gradient hypothesis. J Neurosurg 42:666–673, 1975
7. Cottrell JF, Robustelli A, Post K: Furosemide and mannitol induced-changes in intracranial pressure and serum osmolality and electrolytes. Anesthesiology 47:28–30, 1977
8. Weis MH, Nulsen FE: The effect of glucocorticoids on CSF flow in dogs. J Neurosurg 32:452–458, 1970
9. Brock M, Zillig C, Weigand H, et al: The effects of dexamethasone on ICP in cases of posterior fossa tumors, in Beks JWF, Bosch DA, Brock M (eds): Intracranial Pressure III. Berlin/Heidelberg/New York, Springer-Verlag, 1976, pp 236–246

10. Lorber J: Isosorbide in medical treatment of infantile hydrocephalus. J Neurosurg 49:702–711, 1973
11. Kuhl DE, Alavi A, Hoffman EJ, et al: Local cerebral blood volume in head-injured patients. Determination by emission computed tomography of ^{99}mTc-labeled red cells. J Neurosurg 52:309–320, 1980
12. Grubb RZ Jr, Raichle ME, Phelps ME, et al: Effects of increased intracranial pressure on cerebral blood volume, blood flow and oxygen utilization in monkeys. J Neurosurg 43:385–398, 1975
13. Laurent JP, Molinari GF, Oakley JC: Experimental model of cerebral hematoma. J Neuropathol Exp Neurol 35:560–568, 1976
14. Raichle ME, Grubb RZ Jr, Phelps ME, et al: Cerebral hemodynamics and metabolism in pseudotumor cerebri. Ann Neurol 4:104–111, 1978
15. Saunders ML, Miller JD, Stablain D, et al: The effects of graded experimental trauma on cerebral blood flow and responsiveness to CO_2. J Neurosurg 52:18, 1979
16. Wei EP, Dietrich D, Povlishock JT, et al: Functional, morphological, and metabolic abnormalities of the cerebral microcirculation after concussive brain injury in cats. Circ Res 46:37–47, 1980
17. Bruce DA, Bilaniuk LT, Dolinskas C, et al: Diffuse cerebral swelling following head injuries in children: The syndrome of "malignant brain edema." J Neurosurg 54(2):170–178, 1981
18. Zimmerman RA, Bilaniuk LT, Bruce DA, et al: Computed tomography of pediatric head trauma: Acute general cerebral swelling. J Radiol 126:403, 1978
19. Lofgren J: Effects of variations in arterial pressure and arterial CO_2 tension on the cerebrospinal fluid pressure volume relationships. Acta Neurol Scand, 49:586–598, 1973
20. Kuhl DE, Reivich M, Alavi A, et al: Local cerebral blood volume determined by three dimensional reconstruction of radionucleide scan data. Circ Res 36:610, 1978
21. Reivich M: Arterial PCO_2 and cerebral hemodynamics. Am J Physiol 206:25, 1964
22. Swedlow D, Lewis L: Measurement of cerebral blood flow in children. Anesthesiology 53, 1980
23. McMillan V, Seisjo BK: The influence of hypocapnia upon intracellular pH and upon some carbohydrate substrates, amino acids and organic phosphates in the brain. J Neurochem 21:1283, 1973
24. Aarabi B, Long DM: Dynamics of cerebral edema. The role of an intact vascular bed in the production and propagation of vasogenic edema. J Neurosurg 51:779, 1979
25. Bakay L: Radio-isotope studies in brain edema, in Klatzo I, Seitelberger F (eds): Brain Edema. New York, Springer-Verlag, 1967, pp 517–529
26. Pappius HM, McCann WP: Effects of steroids on cerebral edema in cats. Arch Neurol 10:207, 1969
27. Millson C, James HE, Shapiro HM, et al: Intracranial hypertension and brain edema in albino rabbits. Part II. Effects of acute therapy with diuretics. Acta Neurochirug 56:167–181, 1981
28. Bruce DA, Langfitt TW, Miller JD, et al: Regional cerebral blood flow, intracranial pressure and brain metabolism in comatose patients. J Neurosurg 38:131, 1973
29. James HE, Bruce DA, Welsh F: Cytotoxic edema produced by 6 aminonicotinamide and its response to therapy. Neurosurgery 3:196–200, 1978
30. Miller JD, Sakalas R, Ward JD, et al: Methyl prednisolone treatment in patients with brain tumors. Neurosurgery 1:114, 1977
31. Crocker EF, Zimmerman RA, Phelps ME, et al: The effects of steroids on the extravascular distribution of radiographic contrast material and technetium pertechnetate in brain tumors as determined by computer tomography. Radiology 199:471, 1976
32. Bourke RS: Evidence for mediated transport of chloride in cat cerebral cortex in vitro. Exp Brain Res 8:219–231, 1969
33. Bourke RS, Kimelberg HK, Daze MA, et al: Studies on the formation of astroglian swelling and its inhibition by clinically useful agents, in Popp AJ, Bourke RS, Nelson LR, et al (eds): Neural Trauma. New York, Raven Press, 1979, pp 95–113

III TRAUMA

19. Scalp Injuries

C. Dennis Bucko
Glenn W. Kindt

The scalp exhibits unique qualities and also shares many characteristics common to other areas of the body. The anatomy is unique; the biologic processes of wound healing are common.

ANATOMY

The scalp is composed of five distinct tissue layers: (1) skin, (2) subcutaneous tissue, (3) musculoaponeurotic layer, (4) areolar layer, and (5) periosteum.

The outer layer of *skin* is basically a protective layer because of its thickness (3–8 mm) and hair coverage. Obviously the scalp hair is unique and adequate reconstruction is difficult or impossible when large segments of scalp are lost. Indeed, scalp avulsion would probably almost never occur were it not for long hair.

The *subcutaneous* layer is also quite thick and forms a cushion to insulate the underlying skull from injury. The major vessels that supply the overlying skin with a rich vascular network are located in this layer (Fig. 19-1) and may give rise to serious blood loss from relatively minor wounds. On the other hand, this uniquely rich blood supply may often save crushed soft tissue in long, narrow-based, random flaps that would be lost in other areas of the body with poorer blood supply. In addition this rich blood supply also protects the superficial scalp against infection.

The *galea aponeurotica* is a condensation of the fascia of the frontalis and occipitalis muscles and covers the major area of the skull. This tough, strong fibrous layer is connected to the skin by fibrous septae that run through the subcutaneous layer. It is therefore often difficult to close scalp defects by

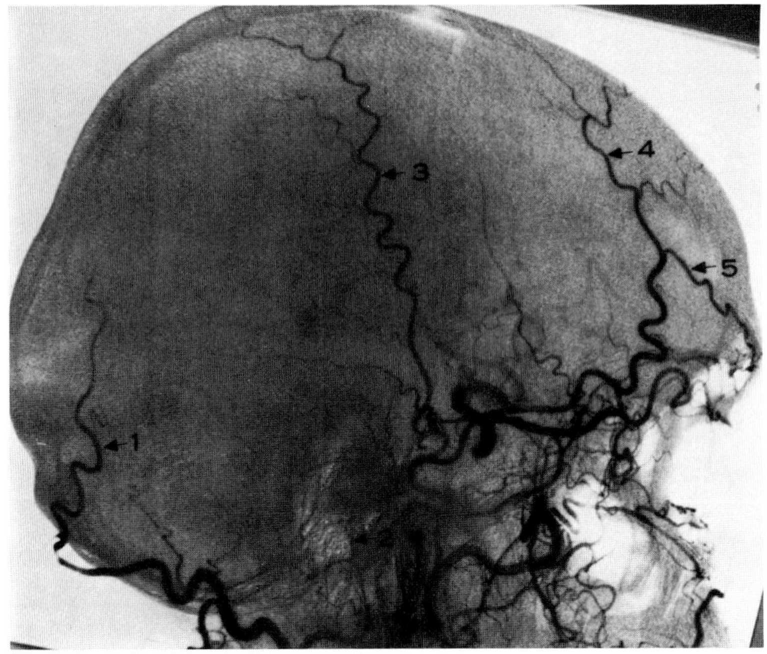

Figure 19-1. A common carotid angiogram in a patient with internal carotid occlusion, which demonstrates the scalp arteries clearly. (1) Occipital artery. (2) Posterior auricular artery. (3) Parietal branch of superficial temporal artery. (4) Frontal branch of superficial temporal artery. (5) Supraorbital artery showing anastomosis with superficial temporal artery.

stretching adjacent tissue because of this unique arrangement of skin connected to inelastic galea.

The *areolar layer* deep to the galea is really an avascular plane, which separates from the underlying pericranium quite easily. This allows scalp mobility and is also a convenient surgical plane. On the other hand, infection[1] and bleeding from emissary veins in this layer may spread widely. Direct intracranial extension of infection may also occur through these veins.

The *periosteum* is the final protection for the skull from outside invasion. Fortunately it has a good blood supply and will support skin grafts, and can even be used as a flap for covering denuded bone.

BASIC PRINCIPLES OF WOUND CARE

Scalp wounds are like any wound in that all tissues heal by the same basic processes; these processes can be affected by the manner in which the wounds are treated. This treatment may make the difference between a successfully primarily healed wound and an infected painfully disfiguring wound requiring secondary treatment, as pointed out by Cushing during World War I.[2] Even minor scalp wounds have been responsible for severe infection such as tetanus[3] and sepsis.[4,5] The following basic principles of wound care are directed at achieving a closed, healed wound.

1. Gentle cleansing with mild agents such as betadine or soap should be performed as soon after wounding as possible since the incidence of wound infection increases significantly with delay in treatment.[6]
2. Hemostasis must be obtained to avoid hematoma formation.
3. Devitalized tissue should be conservatively debrided.
4. All foreign bodies must be removed.
5. The tissues must be handled gently to promote successful healing.

EVALUATION OF PATIENT

The initial evaluation of any patient with a scalp injury should include at least a short neurologic examination since even minimal lacerations or contusions may be associated with intracerebral injury. Further central nervous system evaluation may include skull x-rays, computerized axial tomography (CAT) scans, and angiography.

Tetanus prophylaxis must be considered and immunization should follow the guidelines suggested by the American College of Surgeons.[7] Children up to the age of 10 are usually protected by the initial series of diphtheria, pertussis, tetanus immunizations.

Adequate anesthesia is essential to successful evaluation and treatment of most scalp wounds. Usually a few cubic centimeters of 1 percent xylocaine with adrenalin injected into the wound edges in the subcutaneous plane are adequate for small lacerations. The entire scalp can be easily anesthetized by selective nerve blocks of the supraorbital, occipital, and greater auricular nerves in a circumferential pattern for treatment of major scalp injuries; thus it is rarely necessary or desirable to use general anesthesia for treatment of even major scalp lacerations in a cooperative child.

Following adequate evaluation, and after achieving satisfactory anesthesia, we prefer gentle cleansing of the wound with betadine scrub. It is usually not necessary to shave the hair as it can be adequately cleansed and then kept away from the wound edges with soap, vaseline, or K-Y jelly. It also camouflages the wound during healing.

Hemostasis of the wound edges is usually adequate within 5 to 10 minutes following the injection of xylocaine with adrenalin, although some larger arterioles may need clamping and ligation with 4–0 or 5–0 chromic catgut suture. Electrocautery is usually adequate and faster, however. Orticochea has described a tourniquet for the scalp that may be used for temporary hemostasis in adults.[8]

If uncontrolled bleeding in the subgaleal plane gives rise to a hematoma following blunt injury, it is usually not aspirated or treated other than to advise 24–48-hour application of cold compresses. The blood dissipates very rapidly, does not usually cause significant inflammation, and overlying skin necrosis is very unusual. Cephalhematoma of the newborn and subgaleal hematoma due to vacuum extraction are also treated conservatively, although subgaleal abscess can occur if lacerations of the scalp are present.[9]

Usually debridement of scalp wounds is unnecessary as previously noted since the ability of severely contused scalp flaps to survive is amazing, and primary closure of scalp wounds with traumatic tissue loss is particularly difficult because of inelasticity of the underlying galea. If the blood supply to any portion of the scalp is in doubt, the fluorescein test may be used:[10] this test consists of injection of two ampules (10 cc) of 5 percent fluorescein intravenously (adult dose), waiting 20 minutes for the capillary circulation to pick up the dye, and then visualizing perfused areas with an ultraviolet light. Nonfluorescing areas should be debrided since it is unlikely that these poorly perfused areas will survive. The use of fluorescein in neonates, however, has not been approved by the Federal Drug Administration.

Foreign bodies such as glass, dirt, stones, and avulsed hair must be carefully removed mechanically with small forceps or hemostat. Frequently it is necessary to elevate flaps and search carefully for imbedded materials. Blind probing with hemostats or forceps in puncture wounds may reveal the gritty feel of buried glass or gravel. Tangential x-rays of the scalp soft tissues may occasionally be helpful in locating imbedded radiopaque material.

Systemic antibiotics are rarely indicated in simple scalp lacerations since the risks associated with their use outweigh any possible benefits (human bites and fetal lacerations may be exceptions). Indeed, when the initial dose is given more than two or three hours after injury, the rate of infection may actually increase, and resistant strains of bacteria may be seen.[11] Although scalp infections (cellulitis and subgaleal abscess) can occur, proper wound care as previously described should keep the incidence below 1 percent.

TREATMENT OF LACERATIONS

Simple or complex burst lacerations seen in the emergency room can be closed by aligning the wound edges, as in putting a jigsaw puzzle together, if no tissue has been lost. Either 4–0 or 5–0 monofilament nylon sutures should be used to effect a single layer closure. Although the scalp is relatively inelastic, defects up to 3 cm in an older child can usually be closed by the technique of wide undermining of the adjacent scalp and performing multiple incisions in the galea parallel with the wound edges without injuring the subcutaneous vessels.

Scalp lacerations following the use of fetal monitoring electrodes during labor usually heal without treatment;[12] however, infection with abscess, sepsis, and death following such minor injuries have been reported.[13] Plavdal and Werch,[14] who reported 31 cases of fetal scalp abscess (0.4 percent of monitored labors), advise surgical drainage, local wound care, and systemic antibiotics (10 of 29 cultures revealed staphylococci). Laceration of the vagina and postpartum sepsis may also predispose to abscess, and systemic antibiotics should probably be used in such cases.[15]

Small abscesses of the scalp may also be seen following fetal blood sampling and usually heal after drainage.[16]

Small sloughs of scalp occasionally seen in neonates receiving intravenous infusions (hyperalimentation, antibiotics, or chemotherapy) can usually be treated conservatively with topical antibiotics.[17] Grafts or flaps are rarely needed although up to 10 weeks may be required for spontaneous wound healing.

Although primary closure of wounds is ideal, in some cases delayed closure is preferred. These could include grossly infected wounds or wounds that are suspected of being infected because of heavy bacterial contamination, such as human bites. If the degree of bacterial contamination is uncertain, quantitation may be obtained on a biopsy of the wound followed by culture[18] or by standardized dilutional techniques with Gram stain[19] to determine if a critical level of bacteria (10^5 bacteria per gram of tissue) is present. If the concentration of bacteria is less than this number, (excluding *streptococcus* or *Proteus*),[20] the wound can be closed or grafted with a better than 90 percent chance of primary healing.[21] If the bacterial count is greater than 10^5 bacteria per gram of tissue, or if a single organism is seen on the Gram stained slide after appropriate dilutions, the wound should not be closed. The open wound should be treated with frequent wet dressing changes, skin allografts (homograft), or amniotic allografts, or xenografts (pigskin) until one of the grafts takes, or until the bacterial concentration drops below 10^5 bacteria per gram of tissue.[22]

TREATMENT OF WOUNDS WITH TISSUE LOSS

Defects of scalp larger than 3 or 4 cm can rarely be closed primarily in children and the use of grafts and/or flaps must be considered. The choice must be based on factors such as the size and location of the defect, the age of the patient, the depth of the wound, the vascular status of the bed, and the skill and experience of the surgeon. The management of larger scalp defects has been reviewed by Thompson, Spivak and Bennett;[23] Dingman and Johnson;[24] Paletta;[25] and Khanna.[26]

Skin Grafts

Grafts may be taken from the patient (autografts), from another person or cadaver (allograft or homograft), or from an animal of another species (xenograft or heterograft). Reliably permanent coverage can be obtained only with autografts. Although allografts may become vascularized ("take"), immunologic rejection usually occurs within two weeks. Xenografts do not become vascularized. Allografts and xenografts thus are useful only as temporary biologic dressings that may decrease wound pain, decrease the bacterial count in the wound tissues, and prepare a bed for a later autograft.[27] These functions may also be served by human amniotic membrane.[28]

Autogenous skin grafts can be cut full thickness or split thickness. Although full-thickness grafts contract less and are more durable, split grafts usually take better and the size of the graft is not limited, as it is with a full-thickness skin graft, by the available donor sites. Full-thickness grafts therefore are more suitable for small defects (up to 6–8 cm in an older child). These small hairless areas may be excised later and closed primarily or covered with hair-bearing punch autografts.[29]

Split-thickness skin grafts can be used in any size defect if the periosteum is intact to serve as a vascular bed. A thick split-thickness skin graft (15 thousandths of an inch) can be taken from the buttock at the time of injury for primary closure, or it may be taken a few days later if temporary coverage with allografts or xenografts has been employed.[30] Thinner grafts are used in infants because of the thinner donor skin. Skin grafts can even be placed on dura, although this is usually not recommended since later removal for definitive reconstruction with cranioplasty and flap coverage is very difficult. Skin grafts can even be used in patients in traction, with Crunchfield tongs.[31]

Although skin grafts may take over small areas of nonvascularized bed by the "bridging phenomenon,"[32] and skin grafting on bare bone using "reverse dermal grafts"[33] has been reported, whenever significant areas of bare bone are exposed (greater than 1 cm), flaps are necessary. Of course it may be possible to graft skin onto skull if the outer cortex has been previously removed and the wound allowed to granulate,[34] however, this is time consuming and rarely supplies a durable cover (see "Total Scalp Avulsion").

Skin Flaps

Local flaps of skin, subcutaneous tissue, and galea are used whenever a more durable, hair-bearing cover is needed or when the bed of the wound is unsuitable for a graft because of poor blood supply. Many such flaps have been described.[35–37] The design of these flaps must take into consideration the size and location of the defect, the scalp tension in the donor area, and the anatomy of the vascular pattern in the flap base. One should always attempt to raise an arterial (axial pattern) flap rather than a random (musculocutaneous) flap because of the increased margin of vascular safety with the former, which includes a large artery and its venae comitantes along the axis of the flap.[38] Fluorescein can be used to predict areas of vascular insufficiency in the flap as previously described.

If small areas of periosteum are absent following a subtotal scalp loss, the

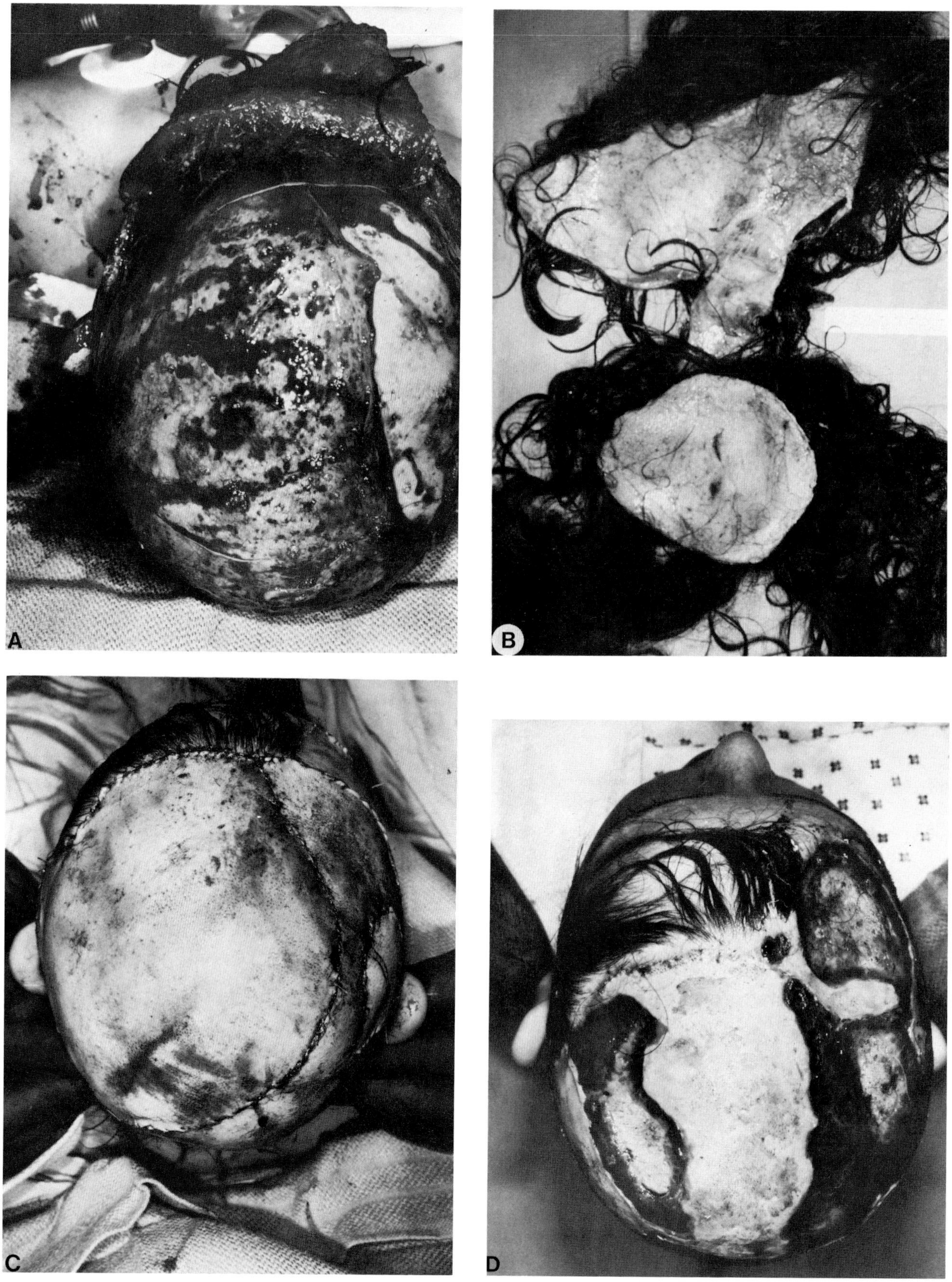

Figure 19-2. A. A 12-year-old girl with avulsion of 90 percent of scalp (anterior forehead flap spared). B. Avulsed scalp—two separate pieces. C. Split-thickness scalp grafts taken from avulsed scalp with Padgett dermatome and sutured over periosteum. D. Partial failure of scalp grafts requiring second grafting with split-thickness skin grafts from buttock. E. Twelve months after injury with some fine hair growth from split-thickness scalp grafts. F. Twelve months after injury showing inadequate hair coverage requiring hairpiece.

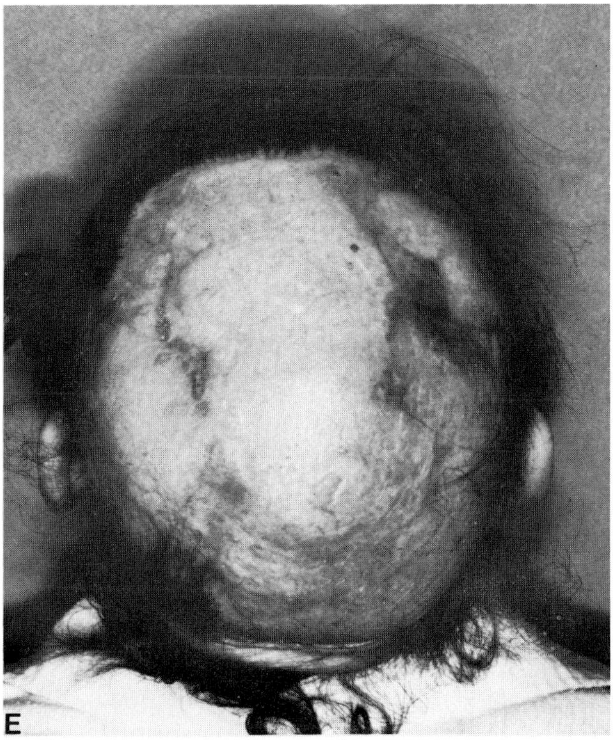

E

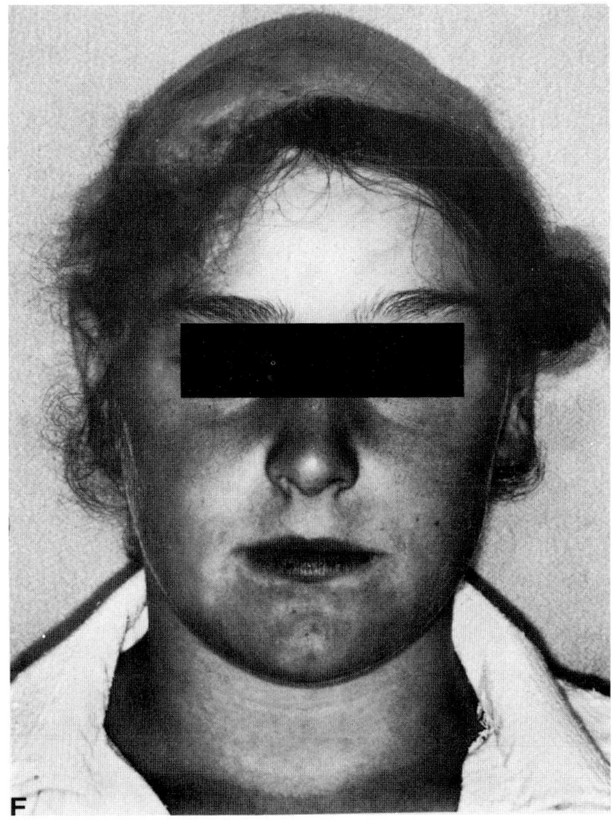

F

denuded bone can be covered with local scalp flaps, leaving the donor area periosteum intact. Skin grafts can then be used to cover the donor area. Alternatively a periosteal flap may be raised from beneath an intact scalp and rotated to cover denuded bone. Split-thickness skin grafts are then applied to the periosteal flap.

If more than one third of the scalp is lost, the wound is unsuitable for grafting, local flaps will not be large enough for adequate coverage and other techniques must be used. The oldest technique is multiple-staged pedicle transfers from the neck, chest, or back.[39,40] Alternatively free microvascular flaps from the groin,[41–43] latissimus dorsi,[44] thorocodorsal area,[45,46] or omentum[47] can be used for single-staged coverage of these defects. These flaps are particularly useful when larger areas need coverage; when brain is exposed, necessitating cranioplasty; and when patients have received previous irradiation.

TOTAL SCALP AVULSION

Total scalp avulsion usually occurs in young women as a result of long hair catching in a rapidly rotating shaft such as a tractor power take-off or lathe. The scalp is usually torn free in the subgaleal areolar plane at the level of the nuchal ridge, ears, and eyebrows. Occasionally ears and brows are included in the avulsed segment. Fortunately periosteum is often left intact, although some denuded bone may be present.

The surgical treatment is aimed primarily at achieving a covered wound. The temptation to replace the avulsed scalp as a composite graft should be resisted since this predictably will be unsuccessful; only one successful case has been reported in the English literature in an 80 percent scalp avulsion.[48] The avulsed scalp should be saved and cooled, however, because it can be replaced as a free microvascular flap if microsurgical expertise is available and if the vessels are suitable for repair or vein grafting. Seven cases[49–54] have now been reported, and whenever possible this is the method of choice for treatment of total or subtotal scalp avulsion.

If the periosteum is intact, and the avulsed scalp is not suitable for microvascular replantation, the scalp can still be used as a donor site for split-thickness skin grafts (Fig. 19-2).[55–57] The hair is shaved and thick grafts can be taken with a Padgett dermatome. Occasionally these grafts will even grow hair, although it is rarely thick enough to be effective, and these patients usually require a hairpiece. Supplemental skin grafts also frequently will be necessary as total take of these grafts from the avulsed scalp is rare.

The use of the avulsed scalp as a full-thickness skin graft after defatting the undersurface occasionally has been partially successful,[58] but revascularization is unreliable and necrosis usually destroys the graft.[59–61] We therefore do not recommend this method of treatment.

If the avulsed scalp is not available or is badly damaged, then split-thickness skin grafts from elsewhere on the body are used for coverage if the periosteum is intact.[62] Grafting may be performed at the time of injury or a few days later after temporary coverage with biologic dressings. These grafts may also be unstable, however, and replacement will full-thickness grafts or even an abdominal flap may be necessary.[63]

In all or most of the periosteum is lost and microvascular replantation of the avulsed scalp is not feasible, removal of the outer cortex with a chisel and split-thickness skin grafting one week later has been the only reasonable treatment available.[64,65] This process may take many weeks because of difficulty in providing a satisfactory bed for the grafts, and often the results may be cosmetically and functionally unacceptable because of repeated breakdown of scar and skin adherent to skull. Replacement with full-thickness skin grafts or dermal overgrafting[66] is often necessary. Microvascular transfer of free flaps now makes such treatment obsolete in most cases since a greater omentum free flap can be used to cover the entire skull and provide a vascular bed for split-thickness skin grafts.[67-70]

BURNS

Burns of the scalp are treated like burns of other parts of the body; this subject has been reviewed by Boswick[71] and by Stuckey.[72] Superficial burns (dermis is viable) need only cleansing, shaving, topical antibiotics, and observation. Full-thickness skin losses larger than 1–2 cm usually need coverage. The depth of the burn is usually obvious by one or two weeks after the burn, and grafting can be performed if needed. Often the initial split-thickness skin graft is adequate for permanent coverage, however, occasionally later reconstruction by replacement with full-thickness skin grafting, serial excision and closure, or overgrafting is needed to produce stable scalp coverage. An obvious full-thickness skin injury can be excised immediately and grafted within two or four days after the burn or closed primarily if less than 3 or 4 cm wide.

Electrical burns of the scalp frequently involve bone. Standard treatment would include frequent dressing changes until the depth of the wound is obvious, removal of the outer cortex of bone, and coverage with flaps or grafts. The graft may be taken at the time of recortication, and the wound covered with a biologic dressing for 48 hours; then the graft can be laid on the wound, which should have an adequate vascular bed. In more severe burns, where bone necrosis becomes obvious and brain may be involved, excision of full-thickness necrotic bone is usually indicated. Luce and Hoopes,[73] however, have reported early coverage of burned bone with local rotation flaps with reconstitution of the skull using the devitalized bone as a "bone graft" before necrosis ensued as an alternative to the more conservative delayed treatment. Worthen[74] has shown biopsy proof of bone regeneration in a similar case. Burned brain is indistinguishable from inflamed brain, and therefore Ranev and Shidarsky[75] advocate avoiding brain debridement and watching for abscess formation. Two out of 4 patients treated in this manner died, however.

The subject of burn alopecia has been reviewed by Huang, Larson, and Lewis.[76] If less than 15 percent of the scalp hair is lost, series excision of hairless scalp over many months is successful. If up to 50 percent is lost, local hair-bearing flaps may be used; however, greater losses can only be covered with a hairpiece.

REFERENCES

1. Goodman SJ, Cahan L, Chow AW: Subgaleal abscess. West J Med 127:169, 1977
2. Cushing HA: A study of a series of wounds involving the brain and its enveloping structures. Br J Surg 15:555, 1918
3. Nourmand H: Clinical studies on tetanus: Notes on 42 cases in Southern Iran with special emphasis on portal of entry. Clin Pediatr 12:62, 1973
4. Limogelli W, Ogle O, Clark M, et al: Fatal massive edema of the head and neck secondary to scalp laceration. J Oral Surg 35:215, 1977
5. Hanson PG, Standridge J, Jarrett F, et al: Freshwater wound infection secondary to *Aeromonas hydrophilia*. JAMA 238:1053, 1977
6. Robson MC, Duke WF, Krizek TJ: Rapid bacterial screening in the treatment of civilian wounds. J Surg Res 14:426, 1973
7. Committee on Trauma of the American College of Surgeons: Report. Bull Am Coll Surg 64(7):20, 1979
8. Orticochea M: A pneumatic tourniquet to control haemorrhage during operations on the scalp. Br J Plast Surg 30:223, 1972
9. Plauche WC: Vacuum extraction–Use in a community hospital setting. Obstet Gynec J 52(3):289, 1978
10. Dibbell D, Hedberg JR, McCraw JB, et al: A quantitative examination of the use of fluorescein in predicting viability of skin flaps. Ann Plast Surg 3:101, 1979
11. Burke JF: The effective period of preventative antibiotic action in experimental incisions and dermal lesions. Surgery 50:161, 1961
12. Cordero L, Hon E: Scalp abscess: A rare complication of fetal monitoring. J Pediatr 78:533, 1971
13. Tuberville DF, Heath R, Bowen F, et al: Complications of fetal scalp electrodes: A case report. Am J Obstet Gynec 122:530, 1975
14. Plavidal F, Werch A: Fetal scalp abscess secondary to intrauterine monitoring. Am J Obstet Gynec 125:65, 1976
15. Winkel C, Snyder D, Schlaerth J: Scalp abscess: A complication of the spiral fetal electrode. Am J Obstet Gynec 126:720, 1976
16. Balfour HH, Block SH, Bowe ET, et al: Complications of fetal blood sampling. Am J Obstet Gynec 107(2):288, 1970
17. Brown AS, Hoelzer DJ, Piercy SD: Skin necrosis from extravasation of IV fluids in children. Plast Reconstr Surg 64:145, 1979
18. Robson MC, Heggers JP: Bacterial quantification of open wounds. Mil Med 134:19, 1969
19. Heggers JP, Robson MC, Ristroph JD: A rapid method of performing quantitative wound cultures. Mil Med 134:666, 1969
20. Robson MC, Heggers JP: Surgical infection. II. The β-hemolytic streptococcus. J Surg. Res. 9:289, 1969

21. Robson MC, Krizek TJ: Predicting skin graft survival. J Trauma 13:213, 1973
22. Robson MC, Heggers JP: Delayed wound closure based on bacterial counts. J Surg Oncol 2:379, 1970
23. Thompson LW, Spivak J, Bennett JC: Management of large scalp defects. J Trauma 10(2):153, 1970
24. Dingman RO, Johnson HA: Surgery of the scalp. Surg Clin N Am 57(5):1011, 1977
25. Paletta FX: Soft tissue injuries of the face and scalp. Clin Plast Surg 4:479, 1977
26. Khanna NN: Management of scalp defects. Am Surg 37(6):363, 1971
27. Krizek TJ: Biologic dressing, in Kuzek TJ, Hoopes JE (eds): Symposium on Basic Science in Plastic Surgery. St. Louis, CV Mosby 1976, p 63
28. Koss N, Robson M, Krizek TJ: Scalping injuries. Plast Reconstr Surg 55:439, 1975
29. Cronin TD: Use of hairbearing punch grafts for partial traumatic losses of the scalp. Plast Reconstr Surg 42:446, 1968
30. Oneill J, Grossfeld J, Boles E: The extended use of skin homografts. Arch Surg 99:263, 1969
31. Rus J: Open treatment of avulsion of scalp using a Crutchfield skull caliper. Acta Chir Plast 18:80, 1976
32. Gingrass P, Grabb WC, Gringrass RP: Skin graft survival on avascular defects. Plast Reconstr Surg 55:65, 1975
33. Stallings JO, Huffman WC, Bernstein L: Skin grafts on bare bone. Plast Reconstr Surg 43:152, 1969
34. Kazanjian VH, Webster RC: The treatment of extensive losses of the scalp. Plast Reconstr Surg 1:360, 1946
35. Orticochea M: Four flap scalp reconstruction technique. Br J Plast Surg 20:159, 1967
36. Orticochea M: New 3-flap scalp reconstruction technique. Br J Plast Surg 24:184, 1971
37. Vecchione IR, Griffith L: Closure of scalp defects by using multiple flaps in pin wheel design. Plast Reconstr Surg 62:74, 1978
38. McGregor IA, Morgan G: Axial and random pattern flaps. Br J Plast Surg 26:202, 1973
39. Horashima T, Nakajima T, Maruyama Y: Deltovertebral flap to cover a large scalp defect. Plast Reconstr Surg 59:951, 1977
40. Brown G: The indirect deltopectoral flap. Br J Plast Surg 29:122, 1976
41. Kaplan H, Wexler MR, Fiensod M: Free groin flap for the reconstruction of the scalp following tumor resection. Ann Plast Surg 2:445, 1979
42. Buncke HJ, Alpert B, Shah K: Microvascular grafting. Clin Plast Surg 5(2):185, 1978
43. Biemer E, Duspira W: Free transfer of a groin flap to the skull following scalp avulsion. Chir Plast 3:277, 1976
44. Maxwell GP, Steuber K, Hoopes JE: A free latissimus dorsi myocutaneous flap. Case Report. Plast Reconstr Surg 62:462, 1978
45. Harii K, Torri S, Sekiguchi J: The free lateral thoracic flap. Plast Reconstr Surg 62:212, 1978
46. Baudet J, Guimberteau J, Nascemento E: Successful clinical transfer of two free thoraco-dorsal axillary flaps. Plast Reconstr Surg 58:680, 1976
47. Harii K, Ohmori S: Use of the gastroepiploic vessels as recipient or donor vessels in the free transfer of composite flaps by microvascular anastomosis. Plast Reconstr Surg 52:541, 1973
48. Lu MM: Successful replacement of avulsed scalp. Plast Reconstr Surg 43:231, 1969
49. Muller GDE, Rustee EJ, Snell JA: Successful replantation of an avulsed scalp by microvascular anastomosis. Plast Reconstr Surg 58:133, 1976
50. Van Beek AC, Zook EG: Scalp replantation by microvascular revascularization. Plast Reconstr Surg 61:774, 1978
51. Buncke HJ, Rose EH, Brownstein MJ, et al: Successful replantation of two avulsed scalps by microvascular anastomosis. Plast Reconstr Surg 61:666, 1978
52. Biermer E, Stock W, Wolfensberger C, et al: Successful replantation of a totally avulsed scalp. Br J Plast Surg 32:19, 1979

53. Spira M, Daniel RK, Agris J: Successful replantation of totally avulsed scalp with profuse regrowth of hair. Plast Reconstr Surg 62:447, 1978
54. Nahai F, Hurteau J, Vasconez L: Replantation of an entire scalp and ear by microvascular anastomosis of only one artery and one vein. Br J Plast Surg 31:339, 1978
55. Dalak Z: Successful replacement of completely avulsed scalp. Br J Plast Surg 8:55, 1956
56. Jakubik J, Barinka L: Scalping injury of the head and its treatment. Acta Chir Orthop Trauma Cech 34:527, 1967
57. Nummi P, Aippe A: Replacement of the avulsed scalp. Scand J Plast Reconstr Surg 5:67, 1971
58. Delak Z, Zelinka A: Successful replacement of the completely avulsed scalp J Plast Surg 7:55, 1955
59. McWilliams CA: Principles of the four types of skin grafting with an improved method of treating total avulsion of the scalp. JAMA 83:183, 1924
60. Straith CL, McEvitt WG: Total avulsion of the scalp. Occup Med 1:451, 1946
61. Robinson F: Complete avulsion of the scalp. Br J Plast Surg 5:37, 1952
62. Caldwell E: Complete scalp avulsion. Arch Surg 111:159, 1976
63. Curtin JW, Latham WD, Greeley PW, et al: Catastrophic loss of the scalp and contiguous structures. Plast Reconstr Surg 32:1, 1963
64. Rylander C, Kisner W: Avulsion of the scalp. Am J Surg 58:150, 1942
65. Jensen F, Petersen N: Repair of denuded cranial bone by bone splitting and free skin grafting. J Neurosurg 44:728, 1976
66. Thompson N, Ell P: Dermal overgrafting in the treatment of venous stasis ulcers: A substitute for skin flap repair in some injuries of the extremities. Plast Reconstr Surg 54:290, 1974
67. Harii K: Clinical application of free omental flap transfer. Clin Plast Surg 5:273, 1978
68. McLean DH, Buncke HJ: Autotransplantation of omentum to a large scalp defect with microsurgical revascularization. Plast Reconstr Surg 49:268, 1972
69. Browning FS, Cartwood DS, Price DJ, et al: Scalp and cranial substitution with autotransplanted greater omentum using microvascular anastomosis. Br J Plast Surg 66(3):152, 1979
70. Ikuta Y: Autotransplantation of omentum to cover large denudation of the scalp. Plast Reconstr Surg 55:490, 1975
71. Boswick JA: Burns of the head and neck. Surg Clin N Am 53:97, 1973
72. Stuckey JG: The surgical management of massive electrical burns of the scalp. Plast Reconstr Surg 54:359, 1974
73. Luce EA, Hoopes JE: Electrical burns of the scalp and skulls. Plast Reconstr Surg 54:359, 1974
74. Worthen EF: Regeneration of skull following a deep electrical burn. Plast Reconstr Surg 48:1, 1971
75. Ranev D, Shindarsky B: Operative treatment of deep burns of the scalp. Br J Plast Surg 22:309, 1969
76. Huang TT, Larson DL, Lewis SR: Burn alopecia. Plast Reconstr Surg 60:763, 1977

20. Skull Fractures

John Mealey, Jr.

The nature and physical forces of injury and the skull contour, thickness, and buttressing determine the occurrence and type of fractures in infancy and childhood. Experimental data on fractures are lacking in this age group,[1] but compared with the adult greater skull deformation is believed necessary to produce tensile failure in children.

LINEAR FRACTURES

Some 90 percent of fractures found in children are linear and involve the vault. Fracture lines may extend from suture to suture or buttress or follow no predictable pattern. In young children they are characteristically more separated or diastatic. Diagnosis on x-rays is difficult at times due to the variable developmental sutural patterns and synchondroses that may be found.[2] Computed tomography (CT) would be advisable when there is a clinical question of associated intracranial pathology.

The majority of children with head injuries of sufficient magnitude to result in linear fracture of the calvarium are symptomatic and should be admitted to the hospital. Children with uncomplicated linear skull fractures generally resume normal activities within a few days. Most fractures will heal by bony union and will no longer be evident roentgenographically after six months. An epicranial cerebrospinal fluid (CSF) collection may sometimes develop acutely when the dura is lacerated at a linear fracture site. These lesions usually are transient and resolve spontaneously.[3] Early operative intervention will occasionally be indicated when the scalp swelling is persistent or progressive (Fig. 20-1).

DEPRESSED SKULL FRACTURES

Depressed fractures in newborns are quite rare in relation to the frequency of births. Ordinarily they are closed, incomplete, and frontal or parietal in location. These depressions have long been associated with difficult births and

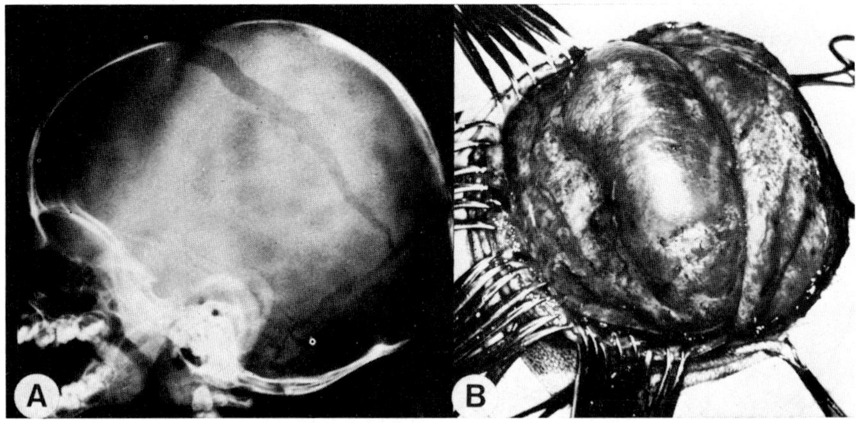

Figure 20-1. A. Widely separated linear left parietal skull fracture in a 17-month-old infant with a large scalp swelling two days after closed-head injury. B. Appearance of the pseudoencapsulated persistent epicranial fluid collection over the fracture after the scalp was reflected at operation for duraplasty three weeks later.

forceps deliveries. Most often the infant appears well otherwise. An intrauterine etiology has also been documented with or without prior trauma to the maternal pelvis, notably from pressure on the fetal skull by the sacral promontory.[4] Conventional treatment of skull depressions in newborns has been surgical elevation. Spontaneous elevations have been reported within 24 hours and after several months without any intervention.[5] Skull indentations in newborns have also been elevated nonsurgically.[6]

Depressed skull fractures in children account for about half of all the skull fractures of this type seen in the population at large.[7,8] Fractures are considered depressed when the inner table is displaced by more than the thickness of the skull. These injuries are most apt to be found in the frontal region, followed, in order, by parietal, temporal, and occipital locations. Roughly a third of the depressed skull fractures in the pediatric age group are simple or closed. The most severe compound craniocerebral nonmissile wounds are found in victims of motor vehicle accidents. Neurologic deficits are usually secondary to localized brain damage, notably hemiparesis, and are noted in less than half of the cases. Prolonged unconsciousness is exceptional. X-ray diagnosis of depressed fractures may be furthered by tangential views and the use of an image intensifier (Fig. 20-2). Cranial computed tomography (CCT) is generally advisable. This study

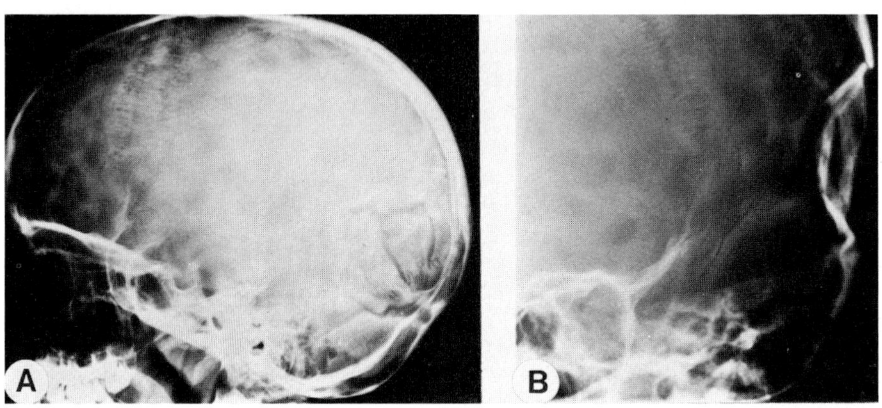

Figure 20-2. A. Depressed left parietooccipital fracture. B. Oblique view demonstrates the extent of depression and comminution resulting in dural, transverse sinus, and cerebral lacerations. The intracranial soft tissue trauma was not indicated by CT done with and without injection of contrast medium.

provides an additional dimension of the degree of the cranial depression, an indication of the extent of any underlying fluid collection, hemorrhage, and/or regional edema, and is a valuable adjunct for surgical treatment and follow-up (Fig. 20-3). Computed tomography, however, may not reliably delineate dural and dural sinus tears, small hematomas, or brain lacerations subjacent to the fracture.

Essentially all compound depressed skull fractures should be debrided and elevated as soon as feasible. The occasional one at the vertex overlying the longitudinal sinus in a neurologically normal patient may be exceptional. The principal goal of such treatment is prevention of infection, which makes operation within the first 24 hours after injury advisable. Restoration of the cranial contour follows as a secondary aim. Operation may not be advised for some simple fractures with only slight skull indentations or which are cosmetically concealed within the hairline. Surgical elevation should be considered in the majority of closed injuries where the fragments are depressed by more than 0.5–1.0 cm, however, since conventional x-rays tend to underestimate the degree of depression and comminution, dural lacerations occur in at least a third of closed depressed skull fractures, in young people and brain lacerations in nearly a quarter,[8] and the prognosis, if they are left untreated, is not well known.

At operation on compound wounds, the scalp laceration may be extended or in some cases incorporated in a scalp flap to gain adequate exposure. A conventional scalp flap, preferably behind the hairline, is appropriate for closed injuries. In young children with simple indentations, a burr hole or craniectomy at the margin of the depression may be used to lever the fragments into satisfactory position. In most cases, however, a craniectomy is advisable, encircling to a greater or lesser extent the periphery of the fracture, extracting the more central fragments, and elevating the margins of the defect. Elective subdural exploration is generally not indicated when CT is otherwise nonrevealing. When there is concomitant cerebral laceration, the dural defect should be

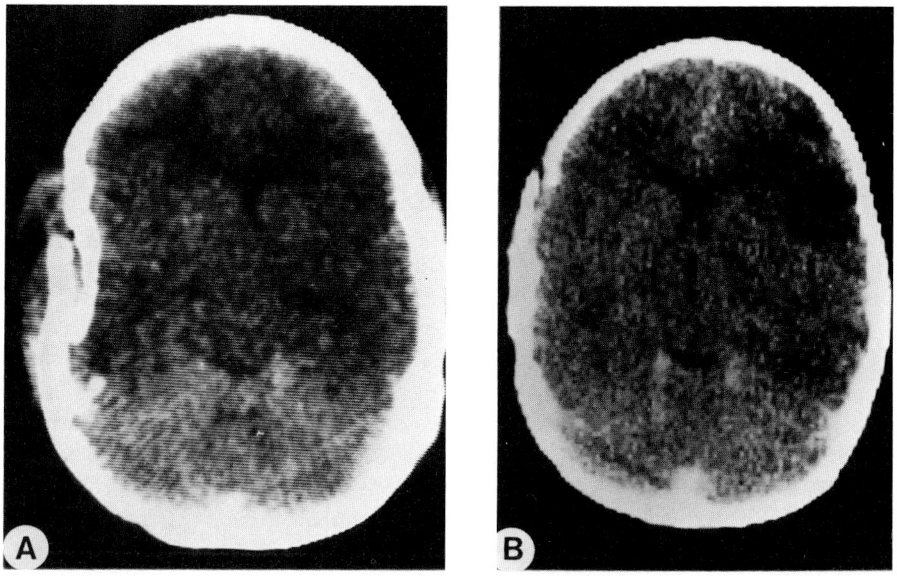

Figure 20-3. A. Cranial computed tomography of a 4-year-old child with a closed depressed left parietal skull fracture demonstrating the extent of the depression and associated diffuse brain edema. The dura was found intact at operation. B. Postoperative study five days later shows a satisfactory elevation and decreased attenuation in the right cerebral hemisphere due to contrecoup contusion and edema responsible for a left-sided hemiparesis of delayed onset.

extended for adequate hemostasis and debridement. Dural closure is desirable, using free pericranial grafts where necessary. If the frontal sinus is exposed, the mucous membrane is stripped away, the bone decorticated by curettement, and the cavity packed with muscle or fat. The bone fragments are replaced as a primary mosaic cranioplasty to reconstitute the desired skull contour prior to scalp closure. Skull x-rays should be repeated to confirm the completeness of the debridement and elevation.

Replacement of the bone fragments after a definitive surgical repair has become an accepted practice.[9] Replacement of bone has been advocated even when it is not possible to close the dura.[10] Established infection in the wound would appear the only absolute contraindication. In most of the cases, there is a solid bone union that obviates the need for cranioplasty. The incidence of serious postoperative wound infections following definitive treatment of compound depressed skull fractures where the bone fragments have been replaced is under 5 percent.

The value of prophylactic antibiotics in the perioperative management of compound depressed skull fracture has become more debatable, with a trend away from routine use. Antibiotic coverage would be considered when there is gross contamination or infection, when there is extension into the paranasal sinuses, and when methyl methacrylate has been inserted. Most of the children with blunt injuries resulting in depressed skull fractures recover without disabling neurologic and mental deficits and the mortality observed is generally under 10 percent.

PENETRATING CRANIOCEREBRAL TRAUMA

The principles of treatment of craniocerebral missile wounds have been well established from military experiences.[11,12] Early definitive operation is advisable for optimal wound healing and prevention of infection. Complicating hematomas, in-driven bone, and retained metal fragments can be localized from CCT, upon which surgery should be based (Fig. 20-4). Devitalized tissue, clot, bone clusters, and accessible metal fragments should be removed. Primary dural and scalp closures are ordinarily indicated. Antibiotics, while no substitute for adequate wound debridement, are customarily administered. Retained bone fragments have been implicated as the major cause of infection and brain abscess and reoperation has been considered mandatory. Recent data from Vietnam[13] and from experimental studies[14] indicate that an isolated peripheral bone fragment remaining after an otherwise adequate debridement in a well patient is best left undisturbed. Penetrating craniocerebral wounds range from the inconspicuous or obscure to gross impalement of the head.[15,16] In transorbital penetrations the globe may be spared with vision preserved. Skull x-rays may not reveal the puncture. The compound craniocerebral nature of head wounds of this type and their potential for early or late infections and vascular complications should be recognized.[17,18] With an obvious impalement, preparations for craniotomy should be complete or the debridement in progress prior to extraction of the foreign body. Orbital and intracranial penetration may be demonstrated by CT and direct early surgical treatment.[19]

BASAL SKULL FRACTURES

Fractures of the base of the skull have been diagnosed in 6 to 14 percent of head injuries collated in children.[15,20,21] Conventional skull x-rays were diagnostic in less than 10 percent of children with convincing clinical signs.[21] Multidirec-

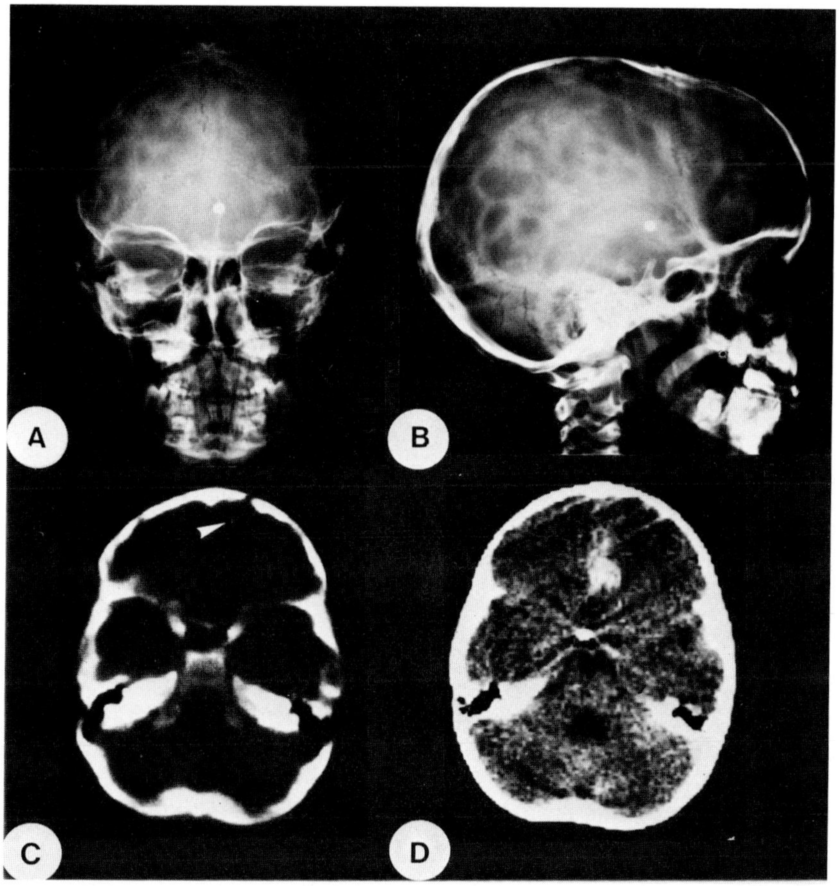

Figure 20-4. A, B. Frontal craniocerebral pellet gun injury in a neurologically intact child with the missile lodged above the dorsum sellae. C. Cranial computed tomography with bone window settings show the right inferior frontal skull penetration and an in-driven bone fragment (arrow). D. Higher transverse tomogram demonstrates hemorrhage and air along the missile tract and the retained metal fragment. Craniocerebral debridement and dural closure were done without any attempt at removal of the metal pellet. Recovery was complicated by transient diabetes insipidus but thereafter was complete.

tional tomography with hypocycloidal blurring has greatly improved the detection of basal skull fractures. Cranial computed tomography provides a further dimension for radiographic delineation of these fractures.[22]

Cerebrospinal Fluid Rhinorrhea

Frontal skull fractures that tear the meninges and extend into the paranasal sinus cavities or cribriform plate are the usual cause of cranionasal fistulas. This complication has been diagnosed in 1 to 3 percent of civilian head injuries[23–25] and documented in less than 1 percent of head injuries reported in children.[15,20,21] Traumatic cerebrospinal fluid rhinorrhea has been described in children as young as 2 years[26] but is seldom encountered in the first decade of life.[27,28]

Cerebrospinal fluid rhinorrhea develops within 48 hours or by the end of the first week in 60 to 70 percent of the cases.[24,29] The onset may be more delayed in the remainder, but within one month after injury over 90 percent of such cases will have occurred, and the condition is seldom first encountered beyond three months. Diagnostic determinations from glucose oxidase test tapes must be interpreted with caution since positive results in nasal secretions and tears may occur in a majority of normal children.[30]

Since rhinorrhea will cease spontaneously in 80 percent or more of the cases within a week or so after injury,[25,31] initial management has been expectant. Bed rest in semi-Fowler's position and repeated lumbar punctures have been recommended,[32] and have also been considered as potentially deleterious.[25] Bacterial meningitis has been observed in 3 to 25 percent of frontobasal skull fractures with CSF rhinorrhea, generally early, and under conditions where some form of antimicrobial therapy had been administered.[24,33] The natural risk of meningitis in unselected patients with posttraumatic rhinorrhea may be under 10 percent.[34] The risk of remote meningitis is probably very low.[32] The case mortality with this form of bacterial meningitis is comparatively small—6 percent in one study in adults.[35]

In both retrospective[36] and prospective[34] studies of acute traumatic CSF fistulas, a significant effectiveness of prophylactic antibiotics in preventing meningitis could not be demonstrated. Prophylactic antibiotic therapy does not prevent meningitis due to organisms supposedly sensitive to the antimicrobial drugs being administered.[31] The avoidance of antibiotic prophylaxis would also eliminate inherent drug complications and reduce the opportunity for more virulent supervening infections with resistant organisms. The trend away from prophylactic antimicrobial therapy in acute traumatic CSF fistulas has been extended to the pediatric age group.[37]

Surgical repair of traumatic cranionasal fistulas remains controversial in terms of selection of appropriate patients, localization of a causal dural defect, and timing of the operation. Operative repair has been advocated in virtually every case where traumatic CSF rhinorrhea has ever been documented,[24] and this same policy of routine anterior fossa exploration has been advised in children.[26] The contrary and probably more widely followed practice has been to reserve surgical treatment for children with persistent or recurrent leaks beyond the acute phase of injury or where meningitis has supervened early or late. Rhinorrhea and/or intracranial air associated with middle face fractures are ordinarily transient and resolve after facial fixation is done without neurosurgical intervention.[28,33]

Special diagnostic procedures have been used to confirm and localize CSF leaks before surgical repair is undertaken. Colorimetric dye and fluorescein studies have generally been unsuccessful or frankly contraindicated because of neurotoxicity.[38,39] Pantopaque has been helpful in some cases.[40] When the leak is copious, radionuclide cisternography may be helpful,[41] but when it is scanty or transitory, this study is frequently nondiagnostic. At present the best means of defining the anatomic site of the fistula is by thin, multisection complex motion tomography. High-resolution CT and edge-enhancement programs promise an even better definition of traumatic defects in the skull base (Fig. 20-5).

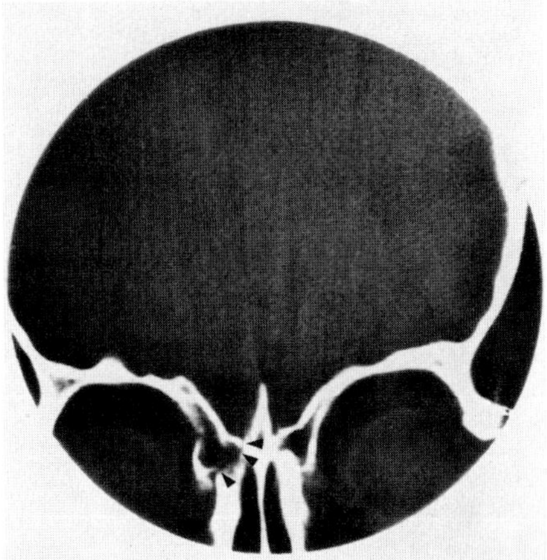

Figure 20-5. High-resolution CT with 5-mm collimation showing fracture line through right cribriform plate and frontoethmoidal sinus (arrowheads) in a youth with head and maxillofacial injuries, CSF rhinorrhea, and pneumocephalus. (Courtesy of Dr. Richard L. Gilmor, Department of Radiology, Indiana University School of Medicine, Indianapolis.)

Radiologic localization of leaks may be feasible by CCT after subarachnoid instillation of metrizamide.[42]

Operation is usually done electively when traumatic brain swelling has largely subsided. An intradural approach is generally advisable, initially through a unilateral or bifrontal bone flap, if necessary, according to the laterality of the rhinorrhea, the radiology, and operative findings.[24,28,43] Magnification is helpful. Muscle, fat, flaps of dura and falx, pericranium, temporalis fascia, fascia lata, homologous dura,[25] and freeze-dried dura[37,44] have all been used in the repair of dural defects and are superior to grafts of synthetic materials. The graft is laid on intradurally with a generous overlap and secured by several anchoring sutures. Tissue adhesives seem potentially useful and isobutyl 2-cyanoacrylate is reportedly safe for this purpose.[45,46] For some parasellar fistulas, transcranial packing of the sphenoid sinus through the tuberculum sella has proved successful.[43] Surgical repair by conventional craniotomy techniques obliterates most of the CSF leaks. Obliteration of the leak, however, does not invariably prevent recurrent bouts of bacterial meningitis in children as well as in the adult population. Ventriculoperitoneal or lumboperitoneal shunts and transsphenoidal packing have also been done to resolve recalcitrant CSF rhinorrhea in patients with fistulas originating in the middle and posterior cranial fossas and after craniotomies had failed.[47]

Cerebrospinal Fluid Otorrhea

This dural fistula is usually located in the middle cranial fossa through the thin tegmen typani of the petrous bone, from longitudinal extensions of fractures of the temporal squama or parietal bone. A posterior fossa origin of cranioaural fistulas may be suspected in exceptional cases. Cerebrospinal fluid otorrhea has been diagnosed in 0.5 to 6 percent of pediatric head injuries.[15,20,21] Bleeding in the middle ear from a lacerated drum and hemotympanum without ensuing CSF otorrhea are observed more often. Cranioaural fistulas are unusual prior to 5 years of age due to the underdevelopment of the mastoid air cells. Cerebrospinal fluid otorrhea is initially bloody and may be delayed in onset for several days by a blood clot. When the eardrum is not ruptured, the CSF may be channeled into the nasopharynx via the eustachian tube and be difficult to recognize. In most cases CSF otorrhea ceases spontaneously within a week[33] and meningitis occurring early or late is uncommon.[32] The treatment is ordinarily expectant.

Prophylactic antibiotics are not routinely advisable for patients with basal skull fractures and blood in the middle ear or obvious CSF otorrhea. The reported incidence of meningitis complicating acute traumatic CSF otorrhea is 4.5 percent.[36] *Pneumococcus, Staphylococcus aureus,* and *Hemophilus influenza,* which are frequently present in the nasopharynx and among the usual causes of posttraumatic bacterial meningitis, are not ordinarily found in the normal bacterial flora of the external auditory canal. In a prospective study of basal skull fractures in 50 patients, mostly with blood in the middle ear or CSF otorrhea, antibiotics were not administered and meningitis was not observed over a 3- to 24-month follow-up.[48]

Surgical repairs have been reported in 1 to 5 percent of cases when the otorrhea has been persistent, chronic, and intermittent, or associated with meningeal infection,[25,49] and advocated for such sporadic cases in childhood.[26] Operation was done in 9 of 24 cases in children when the otorrhea seemed persistent.[50] Radiography is especially important when surgical exploration is considered and hypocycloidal tomography is usually diagnostic. Computed tomography of the temporal bone can provide additional diagnostic information.[22,51] Although endaural surgery and mastoidectomy have been employed to obliterate cranioaural fistulas, a transcranial intradural operation seems more appropriate for localization and grafting of the defect, particularly when there is useful hearing. A subtemporal approach generally done first can be extended to inspect the posterior aspect of the petrous bone by division of the tentorium if indicated. Magnification aids in the definition of the more elusive lesions.

Cranial Nerve Injuries

Olfactory Nerve

Parital, unilateral, or complete loss of the sense of smell has been described in 3 to 10 percent of head injuries.[23,49] This deficit would be difficult to ascertain in young children even if regularly attempted. Natural recovery may occur by the end of one year, but traumatic anosmia when complete tends to be permanent in most cases.

Optic and Extraocular Nerves

Blunt head trauma may cause indirect optic nerve injury with instantaneous blindness of one eye, as a rule, due to contusion or ischemia of the nerve in its intracranial and intracanalicular course.[52] Some spontaneous recovery of vision may be expected in up to 50 percent of patients, usually within days or weeks, but rarely is it complete.[53,54] This condition is rare in children.[55,56] Surgical treatment is ordinarily considered only in the isolated case where it can be ascertained that some vision is preserved initially, that further loss has since developed, usually over several days, and that light perception at least is retained. Under these circumstances the orbit and optic canal can be explored transcranially or transethmoidally to decompress the optic nerve. Good visual recovery following surgical treatment is generally unusual.[57] The large Japanese experience is exceptional; less than 15 percent of these cases, however, were operated on during the first week after head injury.[58]

Fractures of the base of the skull and/or orbit may cause immediate primary palsies of the extraocular nerves. Blowout fractures of the orbits involving the floor or medial aspect may mimic a third nerve palsy.[52] Injury to the extraocular nerves has been reported in 1 to 9 percent of head injuries among the general population,[49,54] and in decreasing order of frequency to the sixth, third, and fourth cranial nerves.[59] Multiple partial injuries are observed more frequently than complete ophthalmoplegia. The sixth nerve is most apt to be involved bilaterally. Over 75 percent of the third and sixth nerve palsies recover spontaneously. The prognosis is poorer for the isolated trochlear nerve contusional injuries due to blows to the vertex of the head.[52]

Facial Nerve

Facial paralysis is the most common cranial nerve injury that occurs at birth and tends to recover promptly. Extracranial anastomosis of the facial nerve at the stylomastoid foramen to other cranial or phrenic nerves may fail to restore facial function in young children with persisting paralysis. This observation probably reflects an intracanalicular causal etiology rather than the more conventional view of an extracranial origin of the nerve damage.[60]

Peripheral facial nerve palsies in general occur in about 1 percent of head injuries studied in children.[15,21] The onset of the paralysis may be delayed in about 12 percent of the cases for several days and then gradually becomes more complete over two or three more days.[49,61] Hypocycloidal tomography delineated a fracture in 75 percent of children with peripheral facial palsies associated with acute head injury.[50]

Satisfactory natural recovery may be expected in up to 90 percent of the facial palsies resulting from basal skull fractures.[23,62] The outlook is especially favorable with expectant treatment when facial paralysis is incomplete or delayed in onset. Signs of spontaneous recovery are usually detected clinically and from electrical testing within one to three months after injury. Beyond this time exploration of the nerve should be considered if the paralysis remains complete.

Acoustic Nerve

Dizziness, hearing loss, and tinnitus have been noted in a third or more of the cases after head injury.[23,63] These symptoms are recognized in older children, but easily may be overlooked in the very young. Conductive hearing deficits usually associated with longitudinal fractures of the petrous bone and middle ear damage generally tend to improve. Significant partial or complete sensorineural deafness has been described in 1.5 percent of head injuries, occurring after either longitudinal or transverse fractures of the petrous bone in most instances, but also where there are no signs of fracture.[49] The actual incidence of this problem in children is unknown but probably is very low.[21]

Trigeminal and Lower Cranial Nerves

Intracranial damage to the trigeminal complex after head trauma in children is very rare, is associated with extensive basal skull fractures and penetrating injuries, and may be partial or complete,[64] Injuries to the ninth through 12th cranial nerves are not ordinarily observed in patients who survive after trauma to the head. Unilateral paralysis of these four nerves due to penetrating wounds around the jugular foramen is well documented.[65]

REFERENCES

1. Gurdjian ES: Recent advances in the study of the mechanisms of impact injury of the head—A summary. Clin Neurosurg 19:355–370, 1972
2. Allen WE II, Kier EL, Rothman SLG: Pitfalls in the evaluation of skull trauma. A review. Radiol Clin N Am II: 479–503, 1973
3. Epstein JA, Epstein BA, Small M: Subepicranial hydroma. A complication of head injuries in infants and children. J Pediatr 59:562–566, 1961
4. Alexander E, Davis CH Jr: Intra-uterine fracture of the infant's skull. J Neurosurg 30:446–454, 1969
5. Loeser JD, Kilburn HL, Jolley T: Management of depressed skull fracture in the newborn. J Neurosurg 44:62–64, 1976
6. Saunders BS, Lazoritz S, McArtor RD, et al: Depressed skull fracture in the neonate. J Neurosurg 50:512–514, 1979
7. Jennett B, Miller JD, Braakman R: Epilepsy after nonmissile depressed skull fracture. J Neurosurg 41:208–216, 1974
8. Jamieson KG, Yelland JDN: Depressed skull fractures in Australia. J Neurosurg 37:150–155, 1972
9. Kriss FC, Taren JA, Kahn EA: Primary repair of compound skull fractures by replacement of bone fragments. J Neurosurg 30:698–702, 1969
10. Jennett B, Miller JD: Infection after depressed fracture of skull. Implications for management of nonmissile injuries. J Neurosurg 36:333–339, 1972
11. Meirowsky AM: Penetrating craniocerebral trauma. Clin Neurosurg 12:253–265, 1966
12. Hammon WH: Analysis of 2187 consecutive penetrating wounds of the brain from Vietnam. J Neurosurg 34:127–131, 1971
13. Carey ME, Young HF, Rish BL, et al: Followup study of 103 American soldiers who sustained a brain wound in Vietnam. J Neurosurg 41:542–549, 1974

14. Pitlyk PJ, Tolchin S, Steward W: The experimental significance of retained intracranial bone fragments. J Neurosurg 33:19–24, 1970
15. Mealey J Jr: Pediatric Head Injuries. Springfield, Charles C Thomas, 1968
16. Reeves DL: Penetrating craniocerebral injuries. Report of two unusual cases. J Neurosurg 23:204–205, 1965
17. Duffy GP, Bhandari YS: Intracranial complications following transorbital penetrating injuries. Br J Surg 56:685–688, 1969
18. Bulluck MH, Baker GS, Henderson JW: Injuries of the brain caused by penetration of the orbit. Minn Med 42:1408–1413, 1959
19. Lunsford LD, Woodford J, Drayer BP: Cranial computed tomographic demonstration of intracranial penetration by an orbital foreign body. Neurosurgery 1:57–59, 1977
20. Dugger GS: Head injury, in Farmer TW (ed): Pediatric Neurology. New York, Harper, 1964, pp 392–442
21. Hendrick EB, Harwood-Nash DCF, Hudson AR: Head injuries in children: A survey of 4465 consecutive cases at the Hospital for Sick Children, Toronto, Canada. Clin Neurosurg II:46–65, 1964
22. Claussen CD, Lohkamp FW, Krastel A: Computed tomography of trauma involving brain and facial skull (craniofacial injuries). J Comput Assist Tomogr 1:472–481, 1977
23. Gurdjian ES, Webster JE: Head Injuries. Mechanisms, Diagnosis and Management. Boston, Little Brown, 1958
24. Lewin W: Cerebrospinal fluid rhinorrhea in non-missile head injuries Clin Neurosurg 12:237–252, 1966
25. Raaf J: Posttraumatic cerebrospinal fluid leaks. Arch Surg 95:648–651, 1967
26. Caldicott WJH, North JB, Simpson DA: Traumatic cerebrospinal fluid fistulas in children. J Neurosurg 38:1–9, 1973
27. Jamieson KG, Yelland JDN: Surgical repair of the anterior fossa because of rhinorrhea, aerocele, or meningitis. J Neurosurg 39:328–331, 1973
28. Jefferson A, Reilly G: Fractures of the floor of the anterior cranial fossa. The selection of patients for dural repair. Br J Surg 59:585–592, 1972
29. Robinson RG: Cerebrospinal fluid rhinorrhea, meningitis and pneumocephalus due to non-missile injuries. Aust NZ J Surg 39:328–334, 1970
30. Hull HF, Morrow G III: Glucorrhea revisited. Prolonged promulgation of another plastic pearl. JAMA 234:1052–1053, 1975
31. Mincy JE: Posttraumatic cerebrospinal fluid fistula of the frontal fossa. J Trauma 6:618–622, 1966
32. Brawley BW, Kelly WA: Treatment of basal skull fractures with and without cerebrospinal fluid fistulae. J Neurosurg 26:56–61, 1967
33. Leech PJ, Paterson A: Conservative and operative management for cerebrospinal-fluid leakage after closed head injury. Lancet 1:1013–1016, 1973
34. Klastersky J, Sadeghi M, Brihaye J: Antimicrobial prophylaxis in patients with rhinorrhea or otorrhea: A double-blind study. Surg Neurol 6:111–114, 1976
35. Hand WL, Sanford JP: Posttraumatic bacterial meningitis. Ann Intern Med 72:869–874, 1970
36. MacGee EE, Cauthen JC, Brackett CE: Meningitis following acute traumatic cerebrospinal fluid fistula. J Neurosurg 33:312–316, 1970
37. Shulman K: Late complications of head injuries in children. Clin Neurosurg 19:371–380, 1972
38. Evans JP, Keegan HR: Danger in the use of intrathecal methylene blue. JAMA 174:856–859, 1960
39. Mahaley MS, Odom GL: Complication following intrathecal injection of fluorescein. J Neurosurg 25:298–299, 1966
40. Allen MB, Gammal TE, Ihnen M, et al: Fistula detection in cerebrospinal fluid leakage. J Neurol Neurosurg Psychiatr 35:664–668, 1972
41. DiChiro G, Ommaya AK, Ashburn WL, et al: Isotope cisternography in the diagnosis and follow-up of cerebrospinal fluid rhinorrhea. J Neurosurg 28:522–529, 1968
42. Naidich TP, Moran CJ: Precise anatomic localization of atraumatic sphenoethmoidal

cerebrospinal fluid rhinorrhea by metrizamide cisternography. J Neurosurg 53:222–228, 1980
43. Ray BS, Bergland RM: Cerebrospinal fluid fistula: Clinical aspects, techniques of localization, and methods of closure. J Neurosurg 30:399–405, 1969
44. Rosomoff HL: Ethylene oxide sterilized, freeze-dried dura mater for the repair of pachymeningeal defects. J Neurosurg 16:197–208, 1959
45. VanderArk GD, Pitkethly DT, Ducker TB, et al: Repair of cerebrospinal fluid fistulas using a tissue adhesive. J Neurosurg 33:151–155, 1970
46. Maxwell JA, Goldware SI: Use of tissue adhesive in the surgical treatment of cerebrospinal fluid leaks. Experience with isobutyl 2-cyanoacrylate in 12 cases. J Neurosurg 39:332–336, 1973
47. Spetzler RF, Wilson CB: Management of recurrent CSF rhinorrhea of the middle and posterior fossa. J Neurosurg 49:393–397, 1978
48. Ignelzi RJ, VanderArk GD: Analysis of the treatment of basilar skull fractures with and without antibiotics. J Neurosurg 43:721–726, 1975
49. Hughes BJ: The results of injury to special parts of the brain and skull, in Rowbotham GF (ed): Acute Injuries of the Head. Their Diagnosis, Treatment, Complications and Sequels (ed 4). Baltimore, Williams & Wilkins, 1964, pp 408–433
50. Harwood-Nash DC: Fractures of the petrous and tympanic parts of the temporal bone in children: A tomographic study of 35 cases. Am J Roent Rad Ther Nucl Med 110:598–607, 1970
51. Hammerschlag SB, Wolpert SM, Carter BL: Computed tomography of the skull base. J Comput Assist Tomogr 1:75–80, 1977
52. Walsh FB, Hoyt WF. Craniocerebral trauma, hypoxia and injuries by other physical agents, in Clinical Neuro-ophthalmology, vol. 3. Baltimore, Williams & Wilkins, 1960, chap 14, pp 2331–2537
53. Hooper RS: Orbital complications of head injuries. Br J Surg 39:126–138, 1951
54. Turner JWA: Indirect injuries of the optic nerve. Brain 66:140–151, 1943
55. Hooper R: Head injuries in childhood. Aust NZ J Surg 32:11–22, 1962
56. Schneider P: Perte de vision par traumatisme crânien fermé. Ophthalmologica 156:377–384, 1968
57. Kennerdell JS, Amsbaugh GA, Myers EN: Transantral-ethmoidal decompression of optic canal fracture. Arch Ophthalmol 94:1040–1043, 1976
58. Fukado Y: Results in 400 cases of surgical decompression of the optic nerve. Mod Prob Ophthalmol 14:474–481, 1975
59. Rucker CW: The causes of paralysis of the third, fourth and sixth nerves. Am J Ophthalmol 61:1293–1298, 1966
60. McHugh HE: Facial paralysis in birth injury and skull fractures. Arch Otolaryng 78:443–455, 1963
61. Jongkees LBW: Facial paralysis complicating skull trauma. Arch Otolaryng 81:518–522, 1965
62. Miehlke A: Surgery of the Facial Nerve. Philadelphia, WB Saunders, 1973, pp 74–80
63. Barber HO: The diagnosis and treatment of auditory and vestibular disorders after head injury. Clin Neurosurg 19:355–370, 1972
64. Jefferson G, Schorstein J: Injuries of the trigeminal nerve, its ganglion and its divisions. Br J Surg 42:561–581, 1955
65. Mohanty SK, Barrios M, Fishbone H, et al: Irreversible injury of cranial nerves 9 through 12 (Collet-Sicard syndrome). Case report. J Neurosurg 38:86–88, 1973

21. Concussion and Contusion following Pediatric Head Trauma

Derek A. Bruce
Luis Schut

Concussion has been defined in its simplest, most restrictive sense either as "a temporary state of unconsciousness produced by trauma to the head"[1] or "the loss of consciousness and associated traumatic amnesia which occurs as the consequence of head trauma in the absence of physical damage to the brain."[2] These definitions imply: (1) that concussion is transient, yet no time period is defined; and (2) that structural damage does not occur. In animal experiments neuronal cell change in the brain-stem reticular formation has been described following traumatic unconsciousness with recovery,[3,4] suggesting that structural damage may indeed be part of the concussive process. A broader, less restrictive definition is that concussion is a clinical syndrome characterized by immediate and transient impairment of neuronal function, such as alterations of consciousness or disturbance of vision, due to mechanical forces (Committee to Study Head Injury Nomenclature, 1966). Again, the time period of the disturbance is not defined and we know that posttraumatic disturbances, such as deficits in short-term memory, may last for weeks following even minor trauma.[5] Symonds[6] proposed that concussion could not be restricted to transient states of unconsciousness since the etiology was diffuse neuronal and axonal injury, and that a spread of injury must occur from mild and completely reversible to severe and irreversible. This hypothesis was expanded by Hooper,[7] and most recently by Ommaya and Gennarelli,[8] who proposed the following hypothesis for concussion.

> Concussion represents a graded set of clinical syndromes following head injury wherein increasing severity of disturbance in level and content of consciousness is caused by mechanically-induced strains affecting the brain in a centripetal sequence of disruptive effect on function and structure. The effects of this sequence always begin at the surface of the brain in the mild cases and extend inwards to affect the diencephalic, mesencephalic core at the more severe levels of trauma.*

---

*Reprinted with permission from Ommaya AK, Gennarelli TA: Cerebral concussion and traumatic unconsciousness: Correlation of experimental and clinical observations on blunt head injuries. Brain 97:633–654, 1974.

This concept of radial injury helps explain many of the clinical disturbances that occur, yet that are not associated with traumatic unconsciousness (e.g., amnesia). Further it suggests that there may be a continuum of degree of injury that goes from mild amnesia to continued deep coma. The mechanism of concussion is believed to be due to shearing stresses set up within the brain substance.[9,10] Linear acceleration alone does not appear to produce concussion, whereas rotational acceleration does.[9]

When consciousness is lost, the disruptive force has been sufficient to affect not only cortex and subcortical white matter function, but also the brain-stem reticular formation and the deep midthalamic nuclei. The loss of function may be due to physiologic blockade at the neuronal body, synapse, dendrite, axons, or some combination of these, that is associated with, as yet, unidentifiable pathologic damage or may be due to disruption of myelin sheaths and axons with concomitant, irreversible structural damage. When the patient is seen, it may be impossible to decide how much underlying irreversible injury has occurred. This is particularly true if the patient is seen immediately following head injury. In human adult head injury autopsy material, major contusions or lacerations are present in 75 percent of patients[11] and there is almost always evidence of structural damage to the brain. When primary brain-stem hemorrhages are seen, there are usually accompanying changes in the supratentorial portion of the brain,[12] thus supporting the radial concept of injury. In children, however, no microscopic lesion may be found at autopsy, only severe, diffuse swelling of the brain,[13] suggesting that in this age group concussion itself may cause death (e.g., by prolonged apnea) or may precipitate changes that cause death without producing identifiable structural change in the brain (e.g., acute swelling and vasodilatation). We shall discuss the clinical aspects of concussion in children on the basis of the hypothesis of Ommaya and Gennarelli as we feel that this is the best functional definition of concussion.

CLINICAL ASPECTS OF CONCUSSION

Any injury to the head that is associated with transient amnesia fulfulls the criteria of concussion. In younger children a history of amnesia may be very difficult to obtain, and in those under 2 years of age, concussion may be impossible to diagnose unless a period of traumatic unconsciousness has occurred. In older children and adults, there is good evidence[14] that the length of posttraumatic anmesia is a good measure of the severity of the concussive injury. The clinical syndrome of concussion is different at different ages in infancy and childhood and we consider the syndromes separately.

Traumatic unconsciousness is uncommon in children under 1 year of age. Many injuries to the head in this age group are the result of short falls (e.g., from the bed or changing table) and skull fractures are very frequently seen, but loss of consciousness is rarely reported. Occasionally a history is obtained of a period of limpness with the eyes rolled up, but this is infrequent. The usual history is that of a child who is crying immediately after the fall and seems to be awake and alert without any identifiable traumatic unconsciousness. Minutes to hours after the injury, the child becomes irritable, pale, often cold and clammy, and begins to vomit. The vomiting may be quite intractable for a period of hours. The child's level of consciousness may also change, with increasing somnolence and general listlessness. This history in an adult would most likely be associated with an expanding mass lesion. This is rarely the case in infancy.

The physical examination shows a pale, somnolent child with rather floppy extremities. The fontanel is generally soft, and the fundi clear. Plantar responses will generally be extensive, which is normal to the end of the first year of life, and abdominal reflexes are usually absent. A localized subgaleal hematoma may be felt and the remainder of the general physical examination is usually normal. We feel that skull x-rays should be obtained in this group of children, since the frequency of linear skull fractures is high. A computerized axial tomography (CAT) scan has generally been normal with the occasional appearance of subarachnoid hemorrhage. If the child is rousable to painful stimuli and the fontanel soft, we do not routinely perform a CAT scan. If a full fontanel is found or the sutures are split suggesting elevated intracranial pressure (ICP), a CAT scan is necessary since the rare epidural hematoma will be found. Occasionally the deterioration in consciousness can be pinned down to a clear history of a seizure, but this is infrequent.

The majority of children requires no special therapy. The vomiting in the milder cases may have stopped by the time the children present to the emergency room. Those with a fracture or continued vomiting we do admit, at least for overnight, and occasionally intravenous therapy is necessary to prevent dehydration. Prolonged somnolence or vomiting, the onset of seizures, the development of a full fontanel, or bradycardia suggest the need for a CAT scan. We have not found that an electroencephalogram (EEG) or nucleid scanning are helpful in this group of children. Seizures occurring at the time of injury, which do not recur, do not require therapy. Seizures that occur later (i.e., more than one hour posttrauma) do, and we use phenobarbital. Phenobarbital is usually continued for a period of two years before it is stopped. There are no proven long-term effects on the brain of this type of trauma.

This pattern of delayed vomiting and somnolence is referred to as "the pediatric concussion syndrome,"[15,16] but it does not fit in with our theory of concussion as a sudden neurophysiologic malfunctioning. The injury that is usually sustained is low velocity and would not be expected to set up great shearing stresses within the brain. Experimentally Foltz, Jenkner, and Ward[17] showed that the reticular formation activity, which is absent following a concussive blow, could return and then disappear secondarily without any new trauma being delivered. It is possible that this delayed dysfunction in the reticular formation occurs in childhood and infancy and is responsible for the above-described clinical pattern. Frequently there is no initial loss of consciousness, however, suggesting that this explanation is less than adequate. It is possible that subclinical seizures are occurring and producing the deteriorating pattern, but in this group of children, the EEG is usually normal. As we discuss later, sudden increases in intracranial blood volume might produce an increase in ICP with a similar symptomatology. That the ICP is high seems quite unlikely since, in general, the fonanel is not full. This is a completely reversible process with no obvious pathology following a traumatic insult and, therefore, fulfills the criteria for concussion. The symptoms are similar to vagal stimulation and could be precipitated by chemical stimulation of the floor of the fourth ventricle as a result of neuroactive chemicals (e.g., histamine), which have been demonstrated in cerebrospinal fluid following trauma. The delay between injury and the onset of symptoms may be due to the diffusion time taken for the chemicals to exist from the lateral and third ventricles and reach the floor of the fourth ventricle. The excellent recovery suggests that little or no pathologic damage is done to the brain and it is clear that, as yet, we have no explanation for the delayed onset of symptoms.

Traumatic unconsciousness in the child less than 1 year old is most commonly seen in the shaken child in whom diffuse white matter injury, acute subarachnoid hemorrhage and/or subdural bleeding, and acute brain swelling occur. The rarity of posttraumatic unconsciousness in the infant may be related to the immaturity of the brain, the poor myelination, or, more likely, the fact that the mechanisms of injury and the input forces are quite different in this age group. Whether or not the "pediatric concussion syndrome" is an aspect of concussion remains questionable.

In children older than 1 year, the various degrees of concussion to the brain can be more easily identified. The pattern of a minor injury without loss of consciousness that is later followed by pallor, nausea, vomiting, and lethargy (pediatric concussion syndrome) is less common as age increases. Our own experience is that this syndrome occurs most commonly with polar injuries after minor falls (e.g., from a swing or roller skates) and most frequently follows blows to the occiput. With such injuries transient cortical blindness may occur, and this is especially difficult to diagnose in the prespeech child. This blindness may be a cause of great anxiety, fear, and agitation, but no clear explanation for it can be found. Fortunately traumatic blindness almost always resolves and is believed to represent some local concussive phenomenon. The CAT scan in these children is normal.

Minor episodes of concussion and brief periods of traumatic unconsciousness come to the attention of the physician less as age increases, and in the teenager many episodes of concussion occur on the sports field that pass unnoticed or are considered too minor to warrant medical attention. In the group of children more than 7 years of age, the most common pattern of behavior associated with concussion that requires hospitalization is one of marked fluctuation in the level of consciousness. Typically this state is produced by a significant injury of the acceleration/deceleration type, usually in a pedestrian struck by an automobile. Consciousness usually is lost for less than an hour and often the loss is only transient. There then follows a period of some recovery of consciousness, which is followed by marked waxing and waning of consciousness. The level of consciousness varies from talking and answering questions, or at least obeying commands, to deep stupor without any withdrawal to pain. Skull fracture may or may not be present and the CAT scan is frequently normal with the most common pathologic lesion being subarachnoid hemorrhage in approximately 20 percent of patients. We believe it is valuable to obtain a CAT scan in these patients, especially if there is evidence of local trauma and skull fracture, as epidural hematomas may present in a similar fashion. The EEG is usually diffusely abnormal but without evidence of seizure discharges. Recovery occurs and it is rare that any treatment other than IV fluids and supportive therapy is required. Because of the benign course of this syndrome, there is little information on the state of the ICP or other physiologic parameters. We have occasionally monitored the ICP in these children and have generally found it to be normal.

Recovery proceeds more slowly than would be expected from the admission state of the children and 7–10 days is the average hospital stay. The period of posttraumatic amnesia, which is a measure of the severity of the concussion, usually lasts for much of the hospital stay and is frequently greater than a week. These children commonly have minor personality changes, irritability, increased aggressiveness, and generally less controlled behavior for a period of weeks to months following injury. Further they frequently experience minor difficulties in school and complain of difficulties with concentration and learning new information. Studies on short-term memory in children who have sustained head injuries have clearly demonstrated that these complaints have identifiable neuropsychologic correlates.[5] It is therefore important that all children sustaining this severity of concussion be followed for at least one year, and that parents and teachers be properly alerted to the possible difficulties they may encounter. Follow-up CAT scans in this group of patients are usually entirely normal and show no evidence of focal or diffuse atrophy.

Another commonly seen clinical pattern of concussion follows more severe head injury in children. The children became unconscious immediately but fairly rapidly show signs of an improving neurologic state. While talking is rare, purposeful movements and occasional obeying of commands and spontaneous eye opening may occur. This is followed within minutes to hours by the sudden deterioration of consciousness, with pallor, bradycardia, loss of purposeful pain responses, and spontaneous eye opening. In about 25 percent of these children, unilateral decerebrate posturing, alternating pupillary dilatation, and episodes of apnea will occur. While this history and course are consistent with an expanding mass lesion, especially an epidural hematoma, and this must always be ruled out, we find that such a lesion is rare. These children rarely have skull fractures and the CAT scan usually shows evidence of diffuse swelling of the brain with loss of cerebrospinal fluid spaces and no other specific focal lesion. The mechanism of this swelling appears to be mainly an increase in blood volume and not true cerebral edema.[18,19] These children frequently require endotracheal intubation and mechanical hyperventilation to prevent the continued deterioration. With intensive supportive care, recovery recurs rapidly within two to three days with little or no focal neurologic deficit. The period of posttraumatic amnesia tends to be shorter and the delayed memory defects less in this group of children than in those who present with a waxing and waning level of consciousness.

How does this pattern fit our hypothesis for concussion? The lack of structural lesion on the CAT scan and the rapid, usually complete, recovery fulfill the criteria for concussive injury. It would appear that the acute brain swelling that occurs in this group either causes the secondary deterioration by causing increased ICP or is an accompaniment of a similar IV ventricular stimulation, as was hypothesized to occur in the younger infants. In favor of the first hypothesis are the autopsy findings, in children, of severely swollen brains with minimal microscopic evidence of tissue injury and increased venous volume.[13,20] If inadequately treated, this clinical pattern thus can result in death. Neither seizures nor shock appear to be responsible for the acute brain swelling.[21] Concentration and short-term memory appear to be less impaired in this group than in the previous group. This characteristic requires more intensive study, but might be explained by a mechanism of injury that produces less shearing within the white matter but precipitates acute brain swelling.

The final pattern seen in children without identifiable mass lesions following trauma is that of the immediate onset of deep coma with alteration of pupillary responses and decorticate or decerebrate posturing or flaccidity. These children do not have a lucid period and represent a severe degree of shearing injury. The CAT scan most often shows diffuse swelling, but occasionally deep white matter, corpus callosum, or brain-stem hemorrhages are also seen, thus confirming the shearing injury.[22] With intensive care and rehabilitation, the majority of these patients will recover, although 50 percent will be left with neurologic or intellectual deficits. Although the severity of the injury implies that it is clearly associated with some irreversible structural lesions, we believe that this represents the most severe form, and transient amnesia the least severe form, of cerebral concussion.

It appears that the most useful clinical approach to the problem of concussion is to consider it as a spectrum of functional and pathologic changes in the brain produced by shear stress. The most minor result may be brief amnesia, and the most severe may be prolonged coma. In children it appears that there are some delayed effects of the concussion that produce secondary nausea and vomiting, pallor, and occasionally deterioration in the level of consciousness some time following injury. At present the mechanism of these changes is unclear and an epidural mass lesion must always be considered. Further, with more severe degrees of concussion, a pattern of acute swelling of the brain can occur that appears to be due to acute suffusion of the brain with blood. Whether the increase in blood volume is responsible for an increase in ICP that produces secondary deterioration, or whether it is an accompaniment of some chemical or neuronally mediated brain stem or pontine irritation that produces deterioration and cerebral hyperemia at one time, is not yet clear. What is clear is that children may die from head injury as a result of acute brain swelling with little or no evidence of pathologic changes within the brain, and that therapy to support ventilation, decreased cerebral blood flow (CBF), and decreased cerebral blood volume (CBV) can prevent this. In children death, then, may result from concussion, if the above hypothesis is correct. But we have shown that even when diffuse shearing injury of the white matter has occurred, recovery may take place. Death from concussion thus should always be preventable, unless the severe swelling is produced by prolonged apnea and anoxia such that there has been too much secondary injury to the brain for a recovery to occur.

It is clear that concussion of the brain no longer can be equated to a lack of pathologic damage, but must be considered as a spectrum of injury. The postconcussive syndrome, while uncommon in children in its full-blown fashion, is seen associated with difficulties in short-term memory, learning, and behavior. As a result concussion in its various degrees up to and including traumatic unconsciousness should not be taken lightly in the infant or child population, and the parents should be made cognizant of the potential for future problems.

CONTUSION

Contusion implies bruising or microscopic hemorrhage within the cerebral substance and it occurs as a result of two separate mechanisms. Local trauma to the static head may produce inbending and local depressed skull fracture, the impact being transferred to the underlying brain and thus resulting in bruising and contusion. In adults contrecoup contusions in the area contralateral to the impact are quite common. In children we have found such contusions to be a rare occurrence. The second mechanism is associated with acceleration/deceleration injuries to the freely movable head. The inferior surfaces of the frontal lobes and the anterior surfaces of the temporal lobes are contused and sometimes lacerated by back-and-forth motion over the bony prominences of the orbital roof and sphenoid wing respectively. This latter mechanism is uncommon in children (10 percent of a series of 76 severe head injuries[20] and the majority of contusions that we encounter are associated with local trauma to the scalp, bone, and underlying brain.

The CAT scan can readily identify hemorrhagic contusion and separate this from true intracerebral hemorrhage. The course of these lesions is one of progressive local cerebral edema and frequently progressive displacement of intracranial structures over several days (Fig. 21-1). There then follows slow resolution, usually with good recovery of function. Often local areas of encephalomalacia are seen on follow-up CAT scan (Fig. 21-1). We have seen in a number of patients, especially shaken babies, areas of focally decreased density on the CAT scan early after injury. Over time these lesions behave like contusions with an increase in local swelling and spreading edema, and are followed by resolution and residual encephalomalacia. While some of these local decreased density areas probably represent infarction, some appear to represent contusions but with minimal hemorrhage.

Contusions may be present clinically and produce no symptoms at all. More frequently there is gradual deterioration of local neurologic function over several

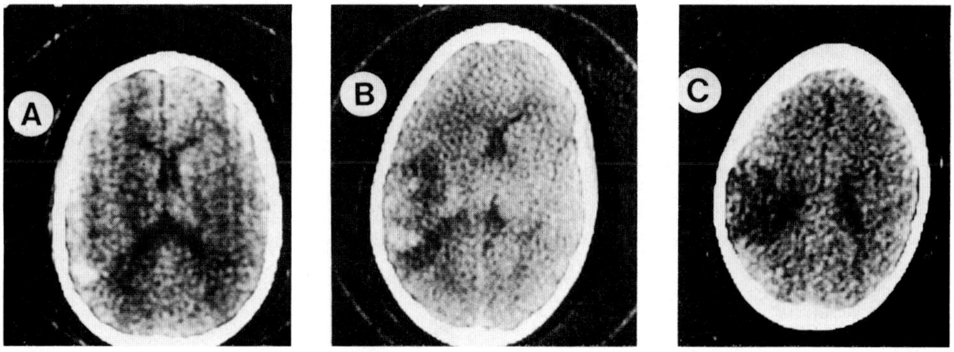

Figure 21-1. Serial CAT scans following left parietal contusion. A. Immediate postinjury CAT scan showing left parietal hemispheric contusion. B. Repeat CAT scan seven days posttrauma showing spreading edema and midline displacement. C. Follow-up CAT scan one month later showing residual encephalomalacia.

days with deterioration of level of consciousness. This is related to swelling and spreading edema from the focus (Fig. 21-1). There is then a period of slow resolution with improving level of consciousness, and then later improvement in local neurologic dysfunction. We do not feel that these lesions, even when polar, should be surgically treated as much of the involved brain may recover. If the swelling is severe, then intracranial pressure monitoring with control of the ICP to less than 20 mm Hg may be required to prevent herniation and to promote recovery. Occasionally, when a large hematoma accompanies the contusion, surgical evacuation may be required. Surgical intervention may be required more frequently when the lesions are in the temporal tip, but we believe that surgery should be postponed and medical therapy used whenever possible since this regimen will avoid the removal of any potentially viable brain. We treat the patients with steroids—dexamethasone, 1.5 mg/kg, or prednisolone, 5–10 mg/kg per 24 hours—immediately after the CAT scan diagnosis is made. There is no evidence, however, that steroids have a significant effect on the outcome or time course of these lesions.

Pathologically 75 percent of adults dying of head injury have evidence of contusion at autopsy. In children under 4 years of age, this percentage is very low, with an increase to almost the adult level by age 5. In our own experience, the incidence of contusions in those children who die primary deaths following head injury has been only about 40 percent.

The responses of the child's brain to trauma are clearly different from those of the adult. The infant rarely is rendered unconscious unless severely shaken, and contusion is rarely present. The older child is easily rendered unconscious, with usually rapid recovery. At both these ages, a delayed onset of lethargy, nausea, and vomiting frequently occurs. In the milder cases, this seems to be unassociated with elevated ICP and the CAT scan is usually normal or shows mild swelling. The process is generally self-limiting and therapy is supportive. In more severe cases, an increased CBV with diffuse brain swelling is often seen, and in these children the deterioration may be to deep coma. Recovery almost always occurs, but an increased level of intensive care support, including hyperventilation, may be necessary. This postconcussive brain swelling, however, can be fatal and must always be taken seriously. Finally, even when evidence of early physical disruption of the white matter (shearing injury) has occurred, good functional recovery can be seen if early intensive care and late physiotherapy and rehabilitation are maximized.

Cerebral contusion in children is most frequently associated with direct trauma to the head and usually occurs under the site of a traumatic fracture.

Contrecoup injuries are uncommon. Similarly, multiple contusions as a result of movement of the frontal and temporal lobes over the bony prominences of the orbital roof and temporal fossa are infrequent in children. We do not recommend surgical evacuation or removal of potentially viable brain unless other nonsurgical therapies have failed to control intracranial pressure. When a deteriorating level of consciousness or a significant midline shift is present, intracranial pressure monitoring is recommended as the only way to judge the need for decompressive medical therapy.

REFERENCES

1. Tomlison BE: Pathology, in Rowbotham GF (ed): Acute Injuries of the Head. Baltimore, Williams & Wilkins, 1964, p 99
2. Ward AA Jr: The physiology of concussion. Clin Neurosurg 12:95–111, 1966
3. Windle WF, Groat RA: Disappearance of nerve cells after concussion. Anat Rec 93:201–209, 1945
4. Windle WF, Groat RA, Fox CA: Experimental structural alterations in brain during and after concussion. Surg Gynec Obstet 79:561–572, 1944
5. Levin HS, Eisenberg HM: Neuropsychological outcome of closed head injury in children and adolescents. Child's Brain 5(3):281–292, 1979
6. Symonds CP: Concussion and its sequelae. Lancet 1:5, 1962
7. Hooper R: Patterns of Acute Head Injury. London, Edward Arnold, 1969
8. Ommaya AK, Gennarelli TA: Cerebral concussion and traumatic unconsciousness: Correlation of experimental and clinical observations on blunt head injuries. Brain 97:633–654, 1974
9. Ommaya AK, Gennarelli TA: Experimental head injury, in Vinken PJ, Bruyn GW (eds): Handbook of Clinical Neurology, vol. 23. New York, American Elsevier, 1975, pp 67–87
10. Holbourn AHS: Mechanics of head injury. Lancet 2:438, 1943
11. Courville CB: Contrecoup injuries of the brain in infancy. Arch Surg 90:157–165, 1965
12. Budzilovich GN: On pathogenesis of primary lesions in blunt head trauma with special reference to the brain stem injuries, in McLaurin RL (ed): Head Injuries New York, Grune & Stratton, 1976, pp 39–43
13. Lindenberg R, Fisher RS, Durlacher S, et al: The pathology of the brain in blunt head injuries of infants and children, in Proceedings of the Second International Congress of Neuropathology, vol. 1. Amsterdam, Excerpta Medica, 1955, pp 477–479
14. Russell WR, Smith A: Post-traumatic amnesia in closed head injury. Arch Neurol 5:4–17, 1961
15. Schnitker MT: A syndrome of cerebral concussion in children. J Pediatr 35:557–561, 1949
16. Pickles W: Acute general edema of the brain in children with head injuries. N Engl J Med 242:607–611, 1950
17. Foltz EL, Jenkner FL, Ward AA: Experimental cerebral concussion. J Neurosurg 10:342–352, 1953
18. Zimmerman RA, Bilaniuk LT, Bruce DA, et al: Computed tomography of pediatric head trauma: Acute general cerebral swelling. Radiology 126:403–408, 1978
19. Lewis AJ: Mechanisms of Neurological Disease. Boston, Little Brown, 1976
20. Bruce DA, Raphaely RD, Goldberg AI, et al: The pathoiphysiology, treatment and outcome following severe head injury in children. Child's Brain 5(3):174–191, 1979
21. Bruce DA, Alavi A, Bilaniuk LT et al: Diffuse cerebral swelling following head injuries in children. The syndrome of malignant brain edema. J Neurosurg 54(2):170–178, 1981
22. Zimmerman RA, Bilaniuk LT, Gennarelli T: Computed tomography of shearing injuries of the cerebral white matter. Radiology 127:393–396, 1978
23. Bruce DA, Schut L, Bruno L, et al: Outcome following severe head injuries in children. J Neurosurg 48:679–688, 1978

22. Posttraumatic Hematomas

Robert L. McLaurin

Posttraumatic intracranial hemorrhage is generally a surgically correctable lesion that must be recognized early and treated cautiously but with dispatch. A minority of children admitted following head injury will be candidates for surgical treatment but it must be constantly recognized that failure to recognize a hematoma may transform an otherwise mild injury into a fatal or permanently disabling entity. The advent of the computerized tomographic (CT) scan has markedly simplified the process of recognition of a hematoma, and also of monitoring its progress if it is elected to treat the patient without surgery.

EXTRADURAL HEMORRHAGE

Extradural hemorrhage is probably the most favorable type of traumatic intracranial bleeding that occurs in childhood, provided it is recognized and treated expeditiously. Fortunately, because of its moderately predictable clinical presentation and its characteristic appearance by computerized tomography, it is usually rather easily detected.

The incidence of extradural hemorrhage in the pediatric age group has varied among reports by differing authors. The occurrence of such bleeding in the neonatal period associated with head trauma during birth is extremely low.[1] The statement has been made that extradural hemorrhage is rare in the extremes of life. This, however, is not borne out by those who are specifically involved in pediatric care. Jamieson and Yelland noted that approximately 25 percent of all traumatic hematomas in the age range 0 to 20 years were extradural alone and another 10 percent were combined extradural and intradural in location.[2] Matson reported 44 extradural hematomas[3] and Choux, Grisoli, and Peragut summarized experiences with 104 cases in children.[4]

The reason generally provided for the presumed low incidence in infancy is the adherence of dura to the overlying skull at the suture lines at this age. Choux et al., nevertheless, discredited this concept by demonstrating the richness of diploic and dural vascularization during infancy.[4] Moreover, they found no indication, by injections into the extradural space, of attachment of the dura to suture lines, with the exception of the coronal suture. Seventeen of the 104 patients reported were less than 2 years of age.

The mechanism of the development of extradural hematomas has been the subject of much speculation and some investigation. Of historical interest is the demonstration by Bell in 1816 that a hammer blow delivered to a cadaver skull was capable of separating the dura from the skull without fracturing the skull.[5] He concluded that without such mechanical separation, the force of bleeding from the middle meningeal artery was incapable of causing hematoma accumulation. Subsequent experiments on dogs confirmed that some separation is indeed essential to allow initiation of extradural bleeding.[6] The truth of Bell's observations regarding the lack of need for fracture has been substantiated by many subsequent observers. Galbraith, reporting a series of 46 cases of extradural hemorrhage without skull fracture, found that 91 percent were below the age of 30 years and 28 percent were less than 10 years old.[7]

The respective roles of arterial versus venous bleeding as a cause for extradural hemorrhage has been debated in the literature. There is little question that the classical hematoma, occurring in the temporal fossa, associated with fracture over the middle meningeal artery, and accompanied by a rapidly progressive neurologic deterioration, is arterial in origin. Conversely there is no doubt that extradural bleeding occurring from direct injury to a major dural sinus—for example, depressed fracture over the sagittal sinus—is of venous origin (Fig. 22-1). The unsettled issue is the origin of those hematomas that are atypical in location or those in which there is a protracted clinical course.

The classical clinical presentation of the child with extradural hematoma includes an initial injury of rather minor significance. It should not be inferred, however, that extradural hemorrhage may not follow more severe trauma. The characteristic history involves a blow to the head, usually temporal, which causes either no disturbance of consciousness or, at most, a brief lapse of contact. This is followed by the classic "lucid interval," during which the child seems relatively normal prior to inevitable deterioration. Choux et al. reported that 57 percent of patients had no disturbance of consciousness at the time of injury, and this rose to 85 percent in infants.[4] The lucid interval was present in 68 percent and lasted from a few minutes to 30 days; in 60 percent of cases it lasted longer than 24 hours, thus refuting the frequent teaching that the typical extradural hematoma is lethal in 6 to 12 hours.

The characteristically rapid course of deterioration is due not only to the arterial force of the bleeding point, but also to the location in relation to the brain stem. A hematoma developing in the low temporal fossa causes herniation of the

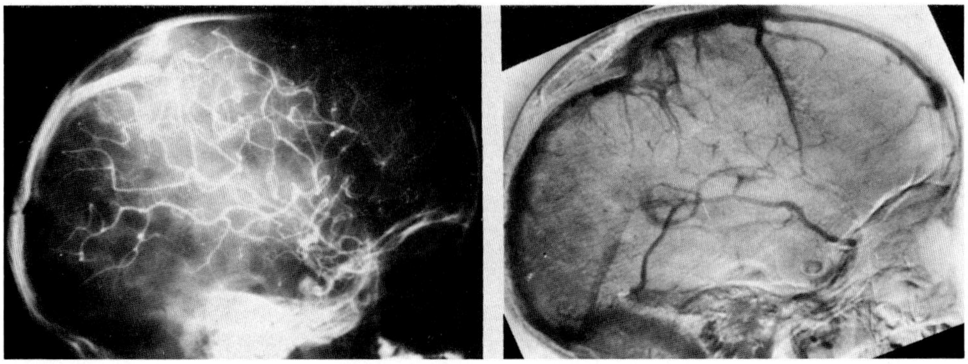

Figure 22-1. Depressed fracture over sagittal sinus. Venogram shows depression of the sinus that was due partly to extradural hematoma beneath the fracture.

medial temporal lobe and displacement and compromise of the brain stem occur fairly rapidly. A similar hematoma occurring over the upper convexity of the cerebral hemisphere causes brain-stem signs only later, since a greater degree of brain molding is necessary before the brain stem is affected.

The neurologic deterioration contains all the elements of an expanding mass lesion: headache, vomiting, nuchal stiffness, weakness of opposite extremities progressing to decerebrate extension and accompanied by a Babinski response, anisocoria with dilatation and loss of light reactivity on the hematoma side, and finally decline of consciousness, which may proceed to coma and death. Several aspects of the clinical manifestations should be noted specifically. The existence of soft tissue swelling in the temporal area, when accompanied by neurologic deterioration, must be considered to indicate extradural hematoma until proven otherwise. Changes in vital signs should not be relied on to indicate need for intracranial investigation; such changes are late developments.[8] Seizures are an infrequent sign of extradural hemorrhage. They occurred in none of the 44 cases reported by Matson[3] and in 10 percent of those in the series of Choux et al.[4]

Radiologic diagnostic investigation is primarily based on computer tomography at present. As noted above the absence of skull fracture by no means excludes the diagnosis and therefore is unnecessary in the face of neurologic deterioration. Angiography was performed prior to CT scan but has very limited

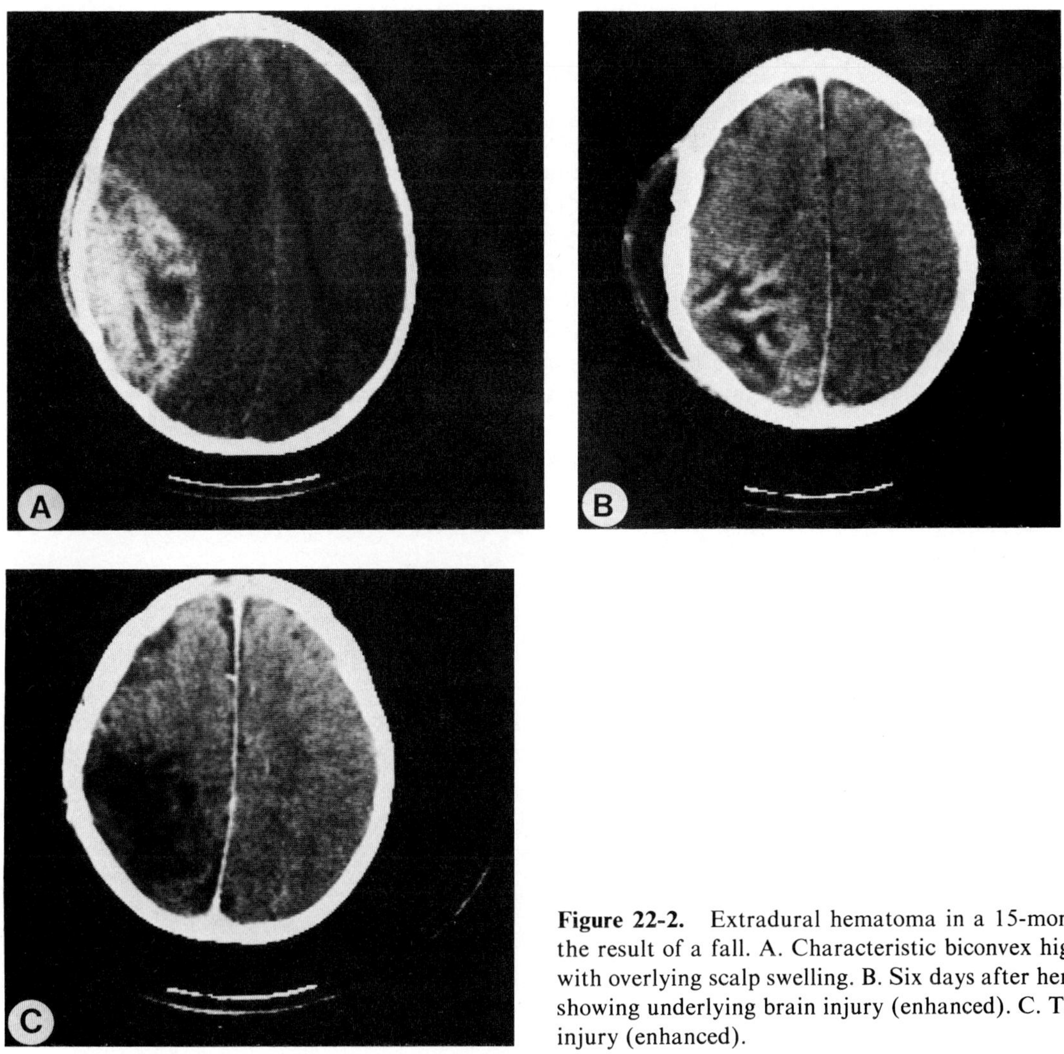

Figure 22-2. Extradural hematoma in a 15-month-old infant as the result of a fall. A. Characteristic biconvex high-density lesion with overlying scalp swelling. B. Six days after hematoma removal showing underlying brain injury (enhanced). C. Three weeks after injury (enhanced).

application now. The CT scan appearance of an extradural hematoma is usually very easily distinguished, consisting of a well-localized, biconvex, high-density lesion subjacent to the inner skull table, usually temporoparietal, and accompanied by appropriate mass effect and anatomic shift (Fig. 22-2).

The child should be treated by hyperventilation and administration of mannitol if neurologic decline is occurring during diagnostic evaluation and surgical preparation. Such measures to retard intracranial decompensation may provide one or more hours of safety and the difference between ultimate complete recovery and persistent neurologic deficit.

The definitive treatment of extradural hemorrhage should always be surgical removal, and delay of such treatment is unacceptable when the diagnosis has been established. The surgical procedure includes an appropriately placed craniotomy (usually temporal), evacuation of the hematoma, identification and control of the dural bleeding points, and finally suturing of the dura to the overlying extracranial soft tissues to prevent postoperative reaccumulation.

The results of treatment of arterial extradural hematomas in infancy and childhood have been difficult to evaluate because statistics in many instances have included patients with associated intracranial hematomas. In general, however, it is appropriate to conclude that (1) the results of treatment of extradural hemorrhage are better than those relating to intradural hemorrhage, and (2) the result depends principally on the speed of recognition and evacuation of the blood clot. Choux et al. reported a mortality of 17 percent and two thirds of those were comatose from the beginning with associated brain lesions.[4] Occasional cases of residual motor or ocular impairment following recovery otherwise were also reported.

The rare occurrence of extradural hemorrhage in the posterior fossa in childhood should be described briefly. The clinical manifestations and three case reports were summarized by Arkins, McLennan, Winston, et al.[9] These authors note that the posterior fossa location is unique to children and the mechanism is direct occipital trauma. As with supratentorial hematomas, however, skull fracture is not necessary. The clinical picture usually includes a lucid period followed by decreasing consciousness and manifestations of brain-stem impairment. The lateralized motor signs and anisocoria are missing. In emergency situations the authors suggest ventricular tap, which confirms the presence of acute hydrocephalus. As with temporal hematomas, the definite diagnostic test is usually the CT scan and treatment consists of immediate craniotomy and clot removal.

SUBDURAL HEMORRHAGE

Subdural hematoma may present acutely or as a chronic lesion; the difference is related principally to whether there is an accompanying cerebral contusion. As was noted in relation to extradural hemorrhage, bleeding into the subdural space may also be either arterial or venous in origin. If it originates from arterial sources, usually cortical arteries, the clinical presentation will be rapid and usually within the first 12 hours. If bleeding occurs from the venous structures, usually the bridging veins between cortex and sinuses, the clinical presentation probably is dependent on the severity of associated brain injury rather than on the bleeding itself. If there is significant neural damage, the clinical deterioration thus will be rapid (acute), while if there is little or no brain damage initially, the presentation will be protracted and delayed (chronic).

Acute Subdural Hemorrhage

According to the above pathophysiologic considerations, acute subdurals may be of either arterial or venous origin. They are seen occasionally as a result of birth damage or later as a consequence of external impact, usually from vehicular accidents or falls.

In the newborn distress occurs within 12 hours of delivery, frequently with dilation of the ipsilateral pupil and with respiratory difficulty. The fontanel is usually full or tight and subhyaloid hemorrhages may be seen in the fundi. Abroms, McLennan, and Mandell recently reviewed the literature on acute subdural hematomas neonatally and reported two cases following breech delivery.[10] The Apgar scores were lowered and vasomotor collapse, hypotonia, seizures, and signs of transtentorial herniation occurred.

In the older child, acute subdural hemorrhage is usually, but not invariably, accompanied by cerebral contusion of at least moderate severity. The entity is not commonly seen, and occurred in only 8 percent of 85 children with severe head injury reported by Bruce, Raphaely, Goldberg, et al.[11] The presence of cerebral contusion enhances the neurologic deterioration by providing an additional factor leading to cerebral edema, increased intracranial pressure, and shift of midline structures. The same galaxy of signs (e.g., motor, pupillary, consciousness) as were described with extradural hemorrhage may be seen. Although the occurrence of a lucid interval is rare in the presence of acute subdural bleeding, it may be seen rarely. Indeed, in a review of 66 patients who experienced a lucid period and then died after head injury (not limited to children), Reilly, Adams, Graham, et al. found 41 intradural hematomas.[12]

The diagnosis of acute subdural hematoma today is usually made definitively by CT scan (Fig. 22-3). The characteristic appearance is a high-density crescentic lesion overlying one or both hemispheres. It is most often unilateral and accompanied by compression of the ipsilateral ventricle. There is often evidence of contusion of the underlying brain tissue and a shift of midline structures to the opposite side to an extent that exceeds that attributable to the hematoma.

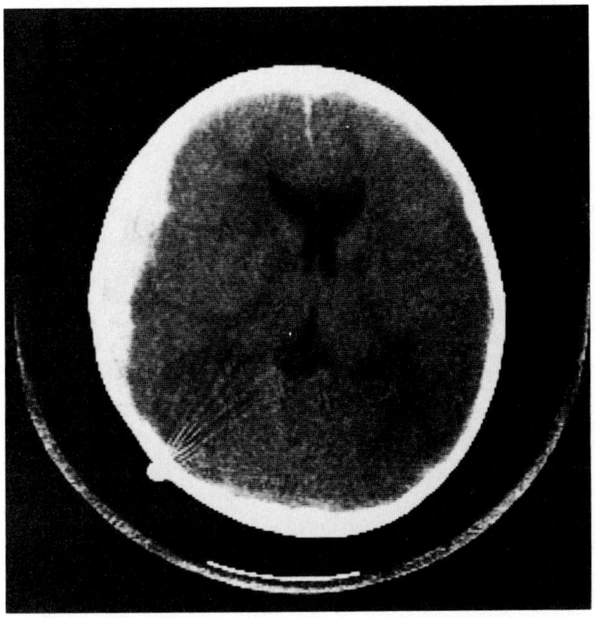

Figure 22-3. Acute subdural hematoma in a child following a vehicular accident. The crescentic surface hematoma is accompanied by a midline shift to the opposite side.

To the best of our knowledge, there are no reports in the literature dealing with the treatment and results of treatment of acute subdural hemorrhage in the pediatric age group. The general policy in our institution has been to evacuate subdural hematomas that exceed 5 mm in thickness. Although some observers believe that acute lesions can be removed by needle in the newborn period, it has been our experience that more extensive cranial opening is required. In the older child, the associated cerebral swelling should be treated with hyperventilation and osmotherapy. The cranial opening should be at least 3 inches in diameter, to permit adequate visualization of the cortex to allow control of bleeding points. Vigorous use of osmotic agents at the time of surgery also minimizes the risk of brain herniation following hematoma evacuation. The dura and skull should be closed and replaced after removal of the clot. Finally, most children with acute subdural hemorrhage will be candidates for intracranial pressure monitoring and this may be inserted at the same operation.

The results of treatment of children with acute subdural hematomas are generally considerably less favorable than for those with extradural bleeding. The residual deficit is more dependent on the severity of brain contusion than on the compressive effect of the surface lesion.

Brief mention should be made of acute subdural hematomas occurring in the posterior fossa of newborns. These have been reported rarely and usually result from a tear of the tentorium. The clinical presentation is characterized by developments during the first week of life that include changes in the cry, poor suck and vomiting, hypotonia, and intracranial hypertension due to hydrocephalus. Early recognition and evacuation are mandatory for survival.

Chronic Subdural Hemorrhage

Chronic subdural hematoma seems to occur rather rarely in the pediatric ages beyond 2 years except as a complication of ventricular shunting. During infancy, however, it is seen frequently, presumably on the basis of trauma, and presents some unique considerations. It should be noted that there is no concensus with regard to correct treatment and the following remarks will reflect the bias of the author.

The term "hematoma" is used somewhat loosely in describing this disease entity since the content of the accumulation may be quite thin and thereby resemble hydroma fluid rather than the breakdown of a blood clot. Although subdural effusions may occur also as a consequence of meningitis, and rarely as a complication of blood disorders such as leukemia and hemophilia, the majority are considered to be the result of trauma. In many instances the trauma has not been recognized. It is noteworthy that chronic subdural hematoma rarely occurs as a result of birth trauma and is not a complication of prematurity. The frequency of "battering" is difficult to assess, but probably the hematoma that results from abuse is more likely to be acute. For reasons that are totally unclear, most reported series of infantile chronic subdural hematomas show a preponderance of male infants.

The principal features of clinical presentation are due to intracranial hypertension and to cortical irritation. The former result in enlargement of the cranial vault, abnormal width and tension of the fontanel, irritability, and vomiting. "Sunset" appearance of the eyes is seen only rarely and papilledema has never been present in our experience. Signs of intracranial hypertension are the presenting features in approximately 60 percent of cases, while the remaining 40 percent with seizures that may be localized or generalized. Any infant with onset seizures after 3 months of age, in the absence of fever or disturbances of calcium or carbohydrate metabolism, must be considered as possibly harboring a subdural hematoma.

Examination of the infant may reveal macocrania but this is rarely greater than 2 cm above the 90th percentile limit, in contrast to more severe enlargement due to hydrocephalus. It has also been stated that biparietal enlargement characterizes subdural accumulations whereas hydrocephalus is more likely to cause fronto-occipital expansion.[3]

Retinal or subhyaloid hemorrhages are not uncommonly seen, although these may imply a more acute or recent process. The incidence of this finding has varied up to nearly 50 percent in various reported series, but during the past decade it has been noted in only about 10 percent in our experience. Anemia may also be found in infants with subdural hematoma; in Matson's series is was noted in about one third,[3] whereas Till found a 40 percent incidence of hemoglobin less than 10 grams.[13] The cause of anemia is related partially to the nutritional deficit that may be present from poor feeding and partially to the loss of a significant component of the total blood volume within the intracranial space.

The most frequent clinical presentation is difficult to define. It consists of a hyperirritable infant who has been eating poorly. Lateralizing neurologic signs are rarely present.

Transillumination of the head may provide supportive information about the presence of subdural effusion but it must be interpreted with extreme caution. Although excessive light transmission is not definitive diagnostically, it may be supportive of a presumptive diagnosis if it is seen bilaterally in the frontal areas.

X-ray examination of the skull may be of diagnostic assistance by demonstrating signs of mild or moderate intracranial hypertension, that is, suture separation and macrocrania, and rather rarely the presence of skull fracture. It should be emphasized that in all cases of unexplained subdural hemorrhage x-rays of the long bones and thoracic cage should be made for evidence of possible widespread injury.

The most definitive noninvasive diagnostic method is computerized tomography. The characteristic picture is the presence of symmetric hypodense surface accumulations over the frontal lobes and extending variable distances backward. Generally there is no shift or enlargement of the ventricular system. The surface accumulations are crescentic in shape, in contrast to the lenticular configuration of chronic subdural hematomas in adults. In contrast also to adult subdural hematomas are widened cerebral sulci, suggesting atrophy, large sylvian cisterns, and wide interhemispheric fissures. The depth of the effusion is variable and may be a few millimeters to as much as 3–4 cm. In the latter circumstance there is a strong likelihood of craniocerebral disproportion.

A more recently developed noninvasive diagnostic technique is gray-scale B-mode ultrasonography. Although this is not universally available at this time, it has advantages over CT scan in being less expensive, utilizing mobile equipment, and avoiding exposure to x-radiation. Sonography has proved to have quite adequate resolution to determine the presence and size of surface accumulations, and offers a relatively easy method of following the size of subdural accumulations during treatment (Fig. 22-4).

Prior to the advent of CT scan and ultrasonography, the definitive method of diagnosis was by subdural tap, and this may still have some application at present. This procedure should be carried out only with meticulous attention to scalp preparation and sterile technique as a precaution against introduction of infection into a subdural effusion. Tapping is usually done through the lateral border of the anterior fontanel or the coronal suture. A short 20- or no. 21-gage

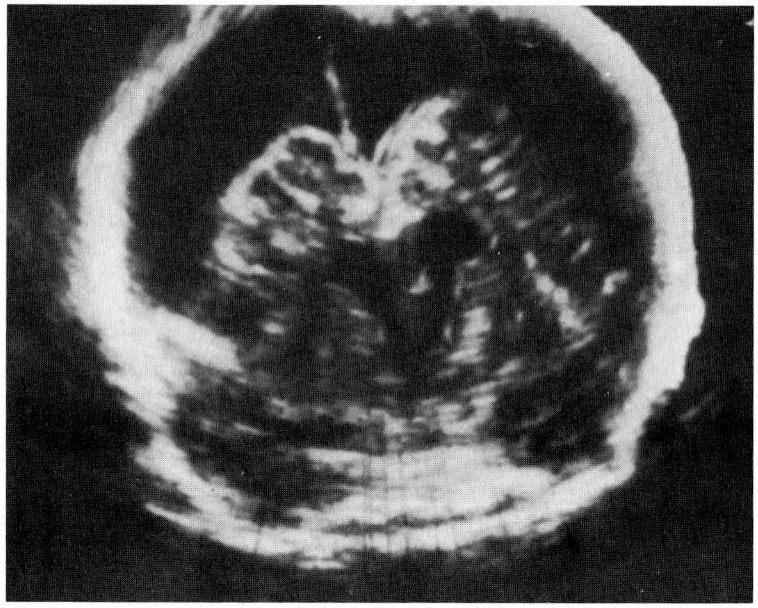

Figure 22-4. B-mode ultrasonogram showing large bilateral subdural hematomas compressing the underlying brain of an infant.

spinal needle is introduced at least 2 cm lateral to the midline to avoid the midline sinus and its draining veins. Bilateral taps should always be done since the incidence of bilaterality of subdural hematomas in this age group is extremely high.

Treatment of infantile subdural hematomas continues to be a controversial matter. There is not complete agreement regarding the proper management of either the liquid contents of the hematoma or the membranes that envelop those contents. It is generally accepted that the membranes, growing from the inner dural layer, begin to develop within one week of the subdural bleed and increase in thickness over a period of several weeks. The membranes are known to contain delicate blood vessels and these may contribute to the subdural accumulation.

The specific methods of treatment have included (1) tapping only,[14] (2) tapping followed by shunting of the subdural affusion,[15,16] and (3) tapping followed by craniotomy for membrane stripping and possibly accompanied by shunting.

This writer has generally favored treatment by tapping only and it is believed that this is effective in the majority of patients. Tapping of the subdural space is performed only in response to the presence of intracranial hypertension, manifested either by clinical features (e.g., irritability, vomiting) or by increased tension of the fontanel Fig. 22-5. Seizures are not an indication of intracranical hypertension. Tapping is done by the method described above and fluid is allowed to drain from the subdural space as long as it flows spontaneously; it should never be aspirated. It must be recognized, however, that cessation of flow of the subdural fluid does not indicate that the subdural space has been emptied; it means only that the intracranial and ambient pressures have equilibrated.

In our experience repeated tapping has been successful in most cases.[14] Characteristically the interval between taps is progressively increased as the fluid becomes less bloody. The total number of taps necessary may vary from one to about 10, but if it exceeds that number, shunting should be considered.

An alternative method of treatment, advocated by many experienced neurosurgeons, is early shunting after the diagnosis has been established. Shunting has been done into the pleural space,[15] but more often into the peritoneal space.[16] Shunting has the advantage of avoiding repeated taps and

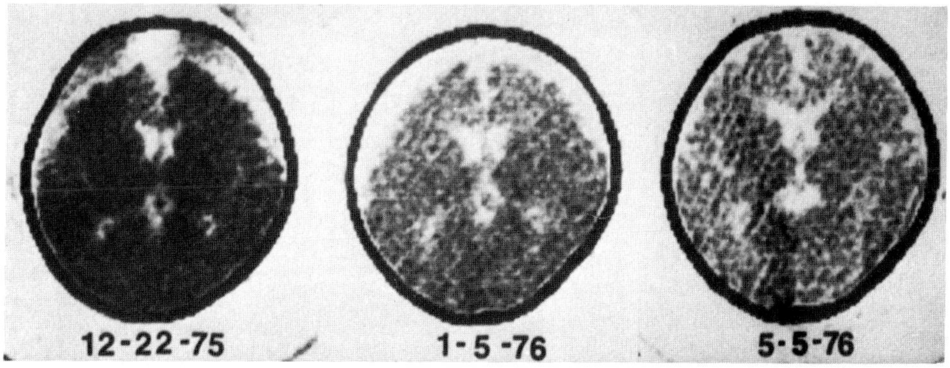

Figure 22-5. Chronic subdural hematoma in an infant showing gradual reexpansion of the brain and obliteration of the surface accumulation. No treatment was done during this period.

may shorten hospitalization; it has the disadvantage of subjecting the infant to a major surgical procedure and then either permanent retention of the foreign body or a second procedure for its removal.

While craniotomy for membrane removal is not generally performed at present, it still has its advocates. It is based on the belief that membranes may contribute to the persistence of subdural effusion and also may cause some constriction of the growing brain. Opponents of membrane removal note that subdural membranes can hardly restrict brain growth, which normally overcomes restraints imposed by dura, skull, and scalp. They also point out that it has been demonstrated that membranes spontaneously disappear after subdural effusion has been effectively evacuated by shunting.[17]

The results of treatment of chronic subdural hematomas in infants have shown remarkable consistency regardless of the method used. Most series have shown that approximately 75 percent of infants have normal development while 25 percent have shown greater or lesser psychomotor retardation. What cannot be determined is whether the developmental delay is due to presence of the subdural effusion causing cerebral compression or to an associated parenchymal damage from the initial injury.

Intracerebral Hemorrhage

Intracerebral hemorrhage is an infrequent complication of trauma in infancy and childhood but does occur rarely. It is recognized that intraparenchymal hematomas do occur in the tissue adjacent to the third ventricle in newborn premature infants, but these are not properly termed traumatic in the sense of being due to mechanical forces. The exact cause for such hemorrhages from the germinal matrix is not understood but probably is related to hypoxia or to alternations of intravascular or intraventricular pressures at birth. In any event, there is no surgical implication other than the possible secondary development of hydrocephalus.

True traumatic intracerebral hematoma, neverthelss, does rarely occur from the birth process.[1] It is located in the subcortical area and leads to significant damage to the developing brain. Such hematomas are distinctly less common than surface hemorrhages but may be demonstrated by ultrasonography or CT scan. To the best of our knowledge, surgical evacuation has never been advocated.

In older children intracerebral hemorrhage is clearly seen as a consequence of trauma, which may be rather mild or very severe. In the case of mild trauma, it

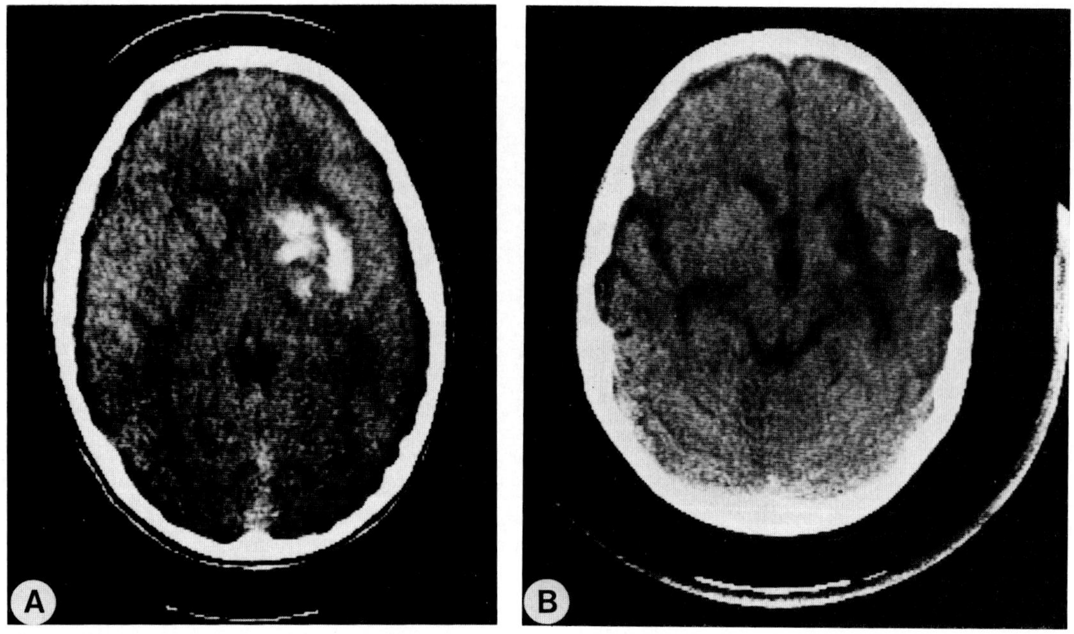

Figure 22-6. Intracerebral hematoma in a child following a blow to the head. A. Hematoma in left subcortical structures with compression of ventricle and shift of midline to right. B. Six months later showing area of atrophic change at site of hematoma.

is likely that they would never have been recognized except for CT scan. The child may show progressive symptoms over a period of several days, probably due to actual delay in hematoma formation or to the occurrence of perihematoma edema. The existence of delayed traumatic intracerebral hematoma has been clearly documented by Brown, Mullen, and Duda.[18]

Intracerebral hemorrhage may occur alone as a consequence of more severe injury or may be associated with cerebral contusion or concomitant surface hemorrhage. The CT scan is crucial for diagnosis and for decision-making with regard to evacuation (Fig. 22-6). Deeper clots, particularly those accompanied by contusion, should be managed nonoperatively if possible by monitoring and control of intracranial pressure and by CT scan observation. Removal should be considered only if the hematoma is easily accessible and is responsible for regional shift and neurologic deterioration. The relative rarity of this indication is illustrated by the absence of any surgically removed hematomas in the series of 85 severely injured children recently analyzed by Bruce and associates.[11] Although four intracerebral hematomas were recognized, none were considered operable.

The late effects of intracerebral hematomas include residual porencephalic cystic areas, which frequently communicate with the adjacent ventricle. There is apparently a rather high incidence of seizures in these patients although they may not be a direct result of the intraparenchymal hemorrhage.

REFERENCES

1. Natelson SE, Sayers MP: The fate of children sustaining severe head trauma during birth. Pediatrics 51:169–174, 1973
2. Jamieson KG, Yelland JDN: Extradural hematoma: Report of 167 cases. J Neurosurg 29:13–23, 1968

3. Matson DD: Neurosurgery of Infancy and Childhood (ed 2). Springfield, CC Thomas, 1969, p 934
4. Choux M, Grisoli F, Peragut J: Extradural hematomas in children. 104 cases. Child's Brain 1:337–347, 1975
5. Bell C, cited by Jacobson WHA: On middle meningeal hemorrhage. Guy's Hosp Rep 43:147–308, 1886
6. Ford LE, McLaurin RL: Mechanisms of extradural hematomas. J Neurosurg 20:760–769, 1963
7. Galbraith S: Age-distribution of extradural hemorrhage without skull fracture. Lancet 1:1217–1218, 1973
8. McLaurin RL, Ford LE: Extradural hematoma. Statistical survey of 47 cases. J Neurosurg 21:364–371, 1964
9. Arkins TJ, McLennan JE, Winston KR, et al: Acute posterior fossa epidural hematomas in children. Am J Dis Child 131:690–692, 1977
10. Abroms IF, McLennan JE, Mandell F: Acute neonatal subdural hematoma following breech delivery. Am J Dis Child 131:192–194, 1977
11. Bruce DA, Raphaely RC, Goldberg AI, et al: Pathophysiology, treatment and outcome following severe head injury in children. Child's Brian 5:174–191, 1979
12. Reilly PL, Adama JH, Graham DI, et al: Patients with head injury who talk and die. Lancet 2:375–377, 1975
13. Till K: Subdural hematoma and effusion in infancy. Br Med J 3:400–402, 1968
14. McLaurin RL, Isaacs E, Lewis HP: Results of nonoperative treatment in 15 cases of infantile subdural hematoma. J Neurosurg 34:753–759, 1971
15. Ransohoff J: Chronic subdural hematoma treated by subdural-pleural shunt. Pediatrics 20:561–563, 1957
16. Collins WF, Pucci GL: Peritoneal drainage of subdural hematoma in infants. J Pediat 58:482–485, 1961
17. Shulman K, Ransohoff J: Subdural hematoma in children: The fate of children with retained membranes. J Neurosurg 18:175–181, 1961
18. Brown FD, Mullan S, Duda EE: Delayed traumatic intracerebral hematomas. J Neurosurg 48:1019–1022, 1978

23. Late Complications of Head Injury

Howard M. Eisenberg

Recently there has been renewed interest in the acute management of severe head injury. Improvements in care have been shown to increase the chance of survival.[1] In many cases, however, the ability of a child to reach full potential after injury depends on the management of late or chronic complications. The complications discussed in this chapter include cranial defects, growing skull fracture, carotid-cavernous sinus fistula, seizure disorder, and persistent neuropsychologic dysfunction. Other important late complications such as hydrocephalus and cerebrospinal fluid rhinorrhea and otorrhea are reviewed in other chapters.

CRANIAL DEFECTS

Cranial defects are most often caused by operative removal of bone fragments after compound depressed fractures. Less commonly they occur when a bone flap cannot be replaced because of severe brain swelling. The latter is less frequent now than in the past because of the more effective use of controlled respiration, osmotic diuretics, and other drugs to control brain swelling. Similarly there now seems to be less enthusiasm for treating severe brain swelling by removing large portions of the skull.

The most common reasons to treat these defects are protection of the brain and improvement of the appearance of the patient. Other indications for operation are the occasional presence of annoying symptoms attributed to these defects, including headache, throbbing sensations, and feelings of dizziness. Distortion of the brain by migration of the ventricles toward the bony defect has been observed in association with these skull defects;[2,3] however, these changes are more likely the result of direct injury to the underlying brain and disruption of the dura than of the skull defect itself. Defects below the temporal or occipital muscles or small defects less than 2–3 cm in diameter often can be left untreated.

The important considerations in the management of skull defects relate to the age of the patient, the time between the injury and reconstruction, and the choice of materials used to reconstruct the defect.

Cranioplasty can frequently be delayed in children under the age of 3 years. Large defects, particularly in children younger than 2 years, often close spontaneously. The newly formed bone generally conforms to the shape of the skull, providing a satisfactory cosmetic result. Another reason for delay of repair in young children is that the use of synthetic materials for reconstruction is unsatisfactory because of the rapid head growth that occurs during this period. This necessitates the use of autogenous bone, making the operation somewhat more difficult. Compound injuries should be considered contaminated, and when a synthetic graft is planned, a period of 6 to 12 months is recommended before repair of the defect. In these cases an x-ray of the skull should be made before reconstruction to rule out the presence of osteomyelitis.

The preference for different materials used for reconstruction varies among neurosurgeons. When reconstruction is done in children under the age of 3 years, autogenous bone is the best material. Rib, the most commonly used graft, is split so that bony plates with one cortical surface can be placed edge to edge to cover the defect (Figure 23-1).[4] Other sources of bone such as iliac crest can also be used. The autogenous bone graft, once in place, becomes infiltrated with osteoblasts and acts as a scaffold for new bone formation. The graft can then compensate for growth of the skull. The disadvantages of autogenous grafts are the possibility of resorption before bone growth has closed the defect and the added difficulty of acquiring bone for grafting. In children older than 3 years, synthetic materials are generally satisfactory. Alloplastic grafts can be fashioned at the time of operation when the skull defect is exposed, assuring a good fit. Common complications of synthetic grafts are dislodgement and those complications associated with insertion of any foreign body, infection and breakdown of the overlying skin.

Repair of defects of the low forehead, particularly those that require reconstruction of an orbital rim or nasion, represent more difficult problems. Silastic prostheses are suitable for repair of these types of deficit. Silastic can be

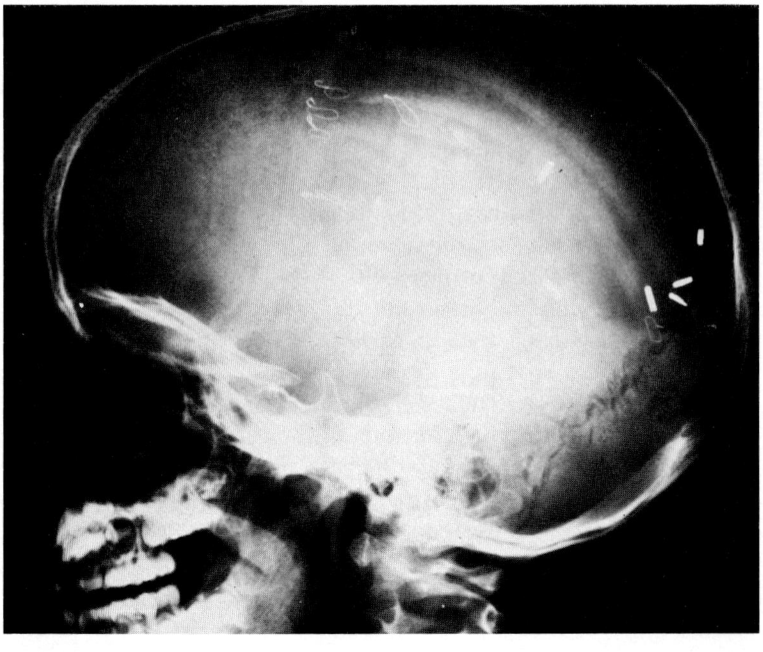

Figure 23-1. Cranioplasty using rib graft in a 3-year-old boy.

premolded over mesh into the complex curves that are required for a good cosmetic result. Although these grafts are not as rigid as other synthetic grafts, the protection provided is adequate. Other materials used to repair low forehead deficits with good cosmetic results are autogenous bone[5] and, more recently, a combination of a polyurethane mesh and autogenous bone.[6]

GROWING SKULL FRACTURE

An infrequent complication of head injury is the formation of a skull defect at the site of a fracture. The defect most often detected by visible or palpable swelling of the overlying scalp may also be associated with signs of brain injury such as hemiparesis or seizures. Although the condition was reported in the early 1800s,[7] the anatomy of the lesion, its pathogenesis, and even its natural history are still debated. The condition has been considered under other rubrics; traumatic leptomeningeal cyst is the most common.

Dyke[8] first used the term leptomeningeal cyst, and although this terminology has been perpetuated it may be a misnomer, adding to the confusion about the anatomy of the lesion and its pathogenesis. It is agreed that the basic substrate for development of the condition is a skull fracture and an underlying dural tear. This has been repeatedly shown clinically and in animal experiments.[9,10] A popular concept of the pathogenesis was first stated by Taveras and Ransohoff.[11] They hypothesized that the condition developed initially as an outpouching of arachnoid through the lacerated dura. This arachnoid protrusion may increase in size because fluid that enters it is partially prevented from leaving by surrounding adhesions acting as one-way valves. The enlarging arachnoid cyst, aided by normal pulsations of the brain, gradually erodes the edges of the fracture and causes progressive enlargement of the skull defect. This popular concept, although appealing, has been questioned. Lende and Erickson[7] did not see an arachnoid or leptomeningeal cyst in any of their five cases. At their operations they found fibrotic scar and gliotic brain between the edges of the bone. In one case a cyst was seen within this scar tissue, which they considered a porencephalic cyst. Similar operative findings have been described by Stein and Tenner.[12] They assumed that the leptomeningeal cysts seen in other reported cases were actually superficial porencephalic cysts covered by gliotic brain. Of ten cases treated at the Hospital for Sick Children in London,[13] seven were found at operation to have cysts. Six of these cysts were clearly porencephalic; four communicated with the ipsilateral lateral ventricle. A leptomeningeal cyst was not seen in any of these cases. A true leptomeningeal cyst in the setting of trauma must then be considered a rare finding. The pathology found most frequently at operation is a fibrotic and gliotic scar insinuated between the edges of the bony defect.

A growing skull fracture occurs only in infants and children. In a review of the world literature up to 1960,[7] the initial injury in half of the cases occurred before 12 months of age and in 90 percent of cases before 3 years of age. Matson's[2] oldest patient was 12 years of age at the time of injury but the next oldest in his series was less than 4 years old. Excluding the oldest case, the mean age of the remaining 16 cases in his series was 10½ months. All other reports also emphasize the early age at the time of the initial injury. In another series of cases,[14] the oldest child was 2 years of age at time of injury. The remaining eight were injured at 1 year of age or less. Similarly in 10 other cases seven were injured under 1 year of age.[13] The occurrence of this lesion in virtually only infants and young children has been explained by two features of early childhood: the dura and skull are firmly attached and the head grows at a rapid rate.

The most common presenting symptom is a scalp mass. Other symptoms are those that can be attributed to an associated brain injury, the most common being seizures and focal weakness. The condition is almost always first noticed by finding scalp swelling or a palpable skull defect after a head injury. X-rays show a characteristic bony defect lying in the course of a skull fracture (Figure 23-2). Frequently the preexisting fracture is diastatic. The bony defect is irregular, with saucerized margins. Sometimes the edges are everted and the inner table frequently appears eroded, although erosion of the outer table has also been described. The bony defect has been noted to cross the suture lines.[13] An almost universal finding is dilatation of the ipsilateral lateral ventricle. This has been found in almost every instance in which the lateral ventricles were studied.[2,13,14] The cause of the ventricular dilatation is not certain. It has been hypothesized

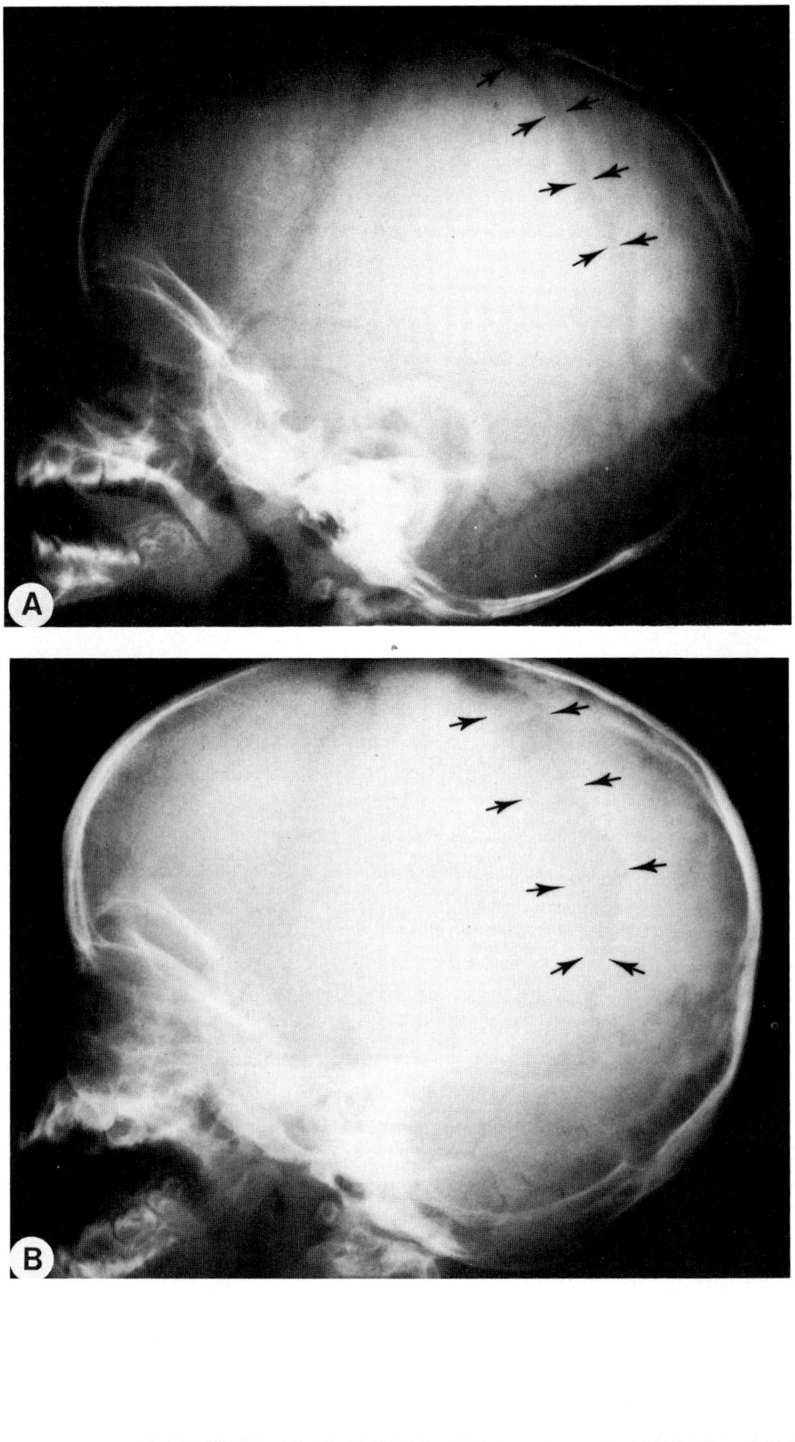

Figure 23-2. Evolution of a growing skull fracture. A. Diastatic parietal skull fracture in an 8-month-old girl. B. Widening of the fracture demonstrated five months later.

that it may be related to pressure in the ventricle unopposed by the resistance of a normally intact dura.[15] A more likely explanation is that it is caused by atrophy. The frequent finding that the midline is shifted toward the side of the dilated lateral ventricle supports this latter idea. In many cases there is an obvious porencephalic cyst, which not infrequently communicates with the lateral ventricle.[2,13]

Although there is clinical and anatomic evidence that a severe brain injury has taken place in many of these cases, the relationship between the cerebral injury and the skull defect is not clear. It is not known whether the cerebral injuries progress as a result of the defect or injury to the underlying brain aggravates the bony changes. Experiments made in young dogs and cats have shown that discontinuity of the bone and dura was required to cause progressive skull defects but adding an injury to the underlying brain did not appear to increase their incidence or size.[9,10]

The natural history of the condition has not been clearly defined. There is probably a period of early rapid progression. Some defects reach a very large size in relatively short periods of time, one or two months. This rapid progression is probably followed by a period of slower change or even stability. It is, however, unlikely that the condition ever spontaneously improves with resolution of the swelling and new bone formation. Occasionally a skull defect in a fracture line is found in an adult with a history of head injury in childhood.[16] Several untreated cases have been described. In most of these,[16–18] the defect once found did not appear to progress; no new neurologic findings occurred and change in the skull defect was not apparent in serial x-rays. In one reported untreated case,[18] however, the skull defect increased in size over a year and a neurologic deficit progressed from a monoparesis to a hemiparesis. In view of this potential for change after detection, these defects should be repaired when they are discovered in early childhood. When they are found in adults or adolescents as an incidental finding, and when small, the necessity for operation may be questioned.

The operative repair of these lesions can be more difficult than imagined by those who are inexperienced. The dural defect may be considerably larger than the bony defect. This features should be kept in mind when planning a scalp flap. When the bony defect is uncovered, a fibrotic and gliotic scar is frequently seen between the bone edges. Occasionally there are visible or palpable cysts in the scar or below the scar. The scar is dissected from the bone edges and bone removed until the dura is visible circumferentially. Occasionally 3–4 cm of bone on each side must be removed to visualize the dural edges. Usually it is not necessary to remove the scar. Occasionally a superficial cyst may be encountered and removed or fenestrated. The most important part of the repair is closure of the dura. The dural repair should be made using pericranium or fascia. Although a cranioplasty is generally done at the time of dural repair, it may be postponed without jeopardizing the repair.[2]

CAROTID-CAVERNOUS SINUS FISTULA

This is a rare complication of head injury in adults and there is little doubt that it is even less common in children. Even in large series, the number of patients less than 20 years old are few. The details of three cases occurring in childhood have been reported. The youngest was 2½ years old[19] and the other two were 7 years of age.[20,21] Considering these cases it is likely that the lesion and its effects are similar in adults and children.

The fistula develops when a basal fracture or penetrating injury results in a tear of the internal carotid artery or one of its small branches as it passes through the cavernous sinus. The time from injury to recognition of the fistula varies. In one series slightly less than half of the cases were recognized as early as 24 hours after injury.[22] Occasionally the fistula does not become apparent for several months. The signs and symptoms that are most characteristic include pulsating exophthalmus, visual failure, and chemosis. Occasionally, as a result of communication between the sinuses, both eyes may be affected, even though the fistula is demonstrated only on one side. True bilateral-carotid cavernous sinus fistulas occur but are very rare. Of the signs and symptoms, proptosis is the most common, occurring in virtually all cases. Cranial nerve deficits are common; in addition to visual loss, the most common are deficits of extraocular movement. Decreased facial sensation is not infrequent. Visual failure may be due to ischemia of the retina,[23] or to the development of cataracts, vitreous opacities, or glaucoma. The lesion can be easily diagnosed when pulsating exophthalmus occurs after head injury. The pulsation and bruit, when present, can be decreased by compression of the ipsilateral common carotid artery. The definitive diagnosis is made by angiography. Flow through the fistula may be so rapid that even when a rapid film-changing sequence is used, the anatomy of the fistula may not be seen by injection of the ipsilateral carotid artery. In some cases injection of a vertebral or contralateral carotid artery may show the site of the leak more precisely. The differential diagnosis includes all other causes of proptosis in children, particularly orbital encephalocele, intraorbital tumor, orbital pseudotumor, cavernous sinus thrombosis, and other orbital vascular anomalies.

Death or neurologic deficit associated with untreated fistulas is rare. Hamby[24] reviewed 322 cases reported by Sattler. In this large series, there were nine deaths due to hemorrhage. Six were from fatal epistaxis and three from intracranial bleeding. Spontaneous resolution of the lesion has been reported but probably is not common. Dandy and Follis[25] estimated that approximately 10 percent of cases resolved spontaneously. Because of progressive visual loss, cranial nerve palsies, and disfigurement, treatment is almost always recommended. Visual loss can occur, however, following operative occlusion of the fistula.

An operation commonly used to occlude the fistual involves a combination of trapping and embolization.[24] The intracranial carotid artery is occluded above the cavernous sinus at the point at which the artery becomes intradural. If possible, this occlusion is made proximal to the ophthalmic artery; if not, the ophthalmic artery is separately occluded. A muscle embolus is then introduced into the internal carotid artery through an arterotomy made in the external carotid artery. Blood flow through the common carotid carries the embolus to the site of the fistula and occludes the intracavernous branches of the carotid artery. The operation is completed by ligation of the common, external, and internal carotid arteries. Before an occlusive operation is done, it must be established that there will be adequate perfusion of the ipsilateral hemisphere. In some recent cases, an anastomosis between an extracranial artery and a branch of the middle cerebral artery has been made, to assure flow to the ipsilateral hemisphere after occlusion. The carotid artery should not be permanently occluded in the neck before the internal carotid artery above the fistula is occluded. If this is done, blood may be shunted from the brain into the fistula, causing cerebral ischemia. Although the trapping embolization operation is generally successful, it does result in loss of a carotid artery.

Other treatments aimed at preserving the carotid artery have been developed. Direct occlusion of the fistula has been described by Parkinson.[26] This operation entails opening the cavernous sinus and repairing the fistula while leaving the carotid artery intact, however, profound hyperthermia and cardiac arrest are required. A less complicated operation that spares the carotid artery has been proposed by Mullan.[27] This operation entails packing the cavernous sinus. The anterior portion of the sinus can be packed by passing gelfoam or similar material through an opening in the junction of the superior and inferior ophthalmic veins. The material is then advanced into the cavernous sinus (Fig. 23-3). The posterior portion of the sinus can be similarly packed through an

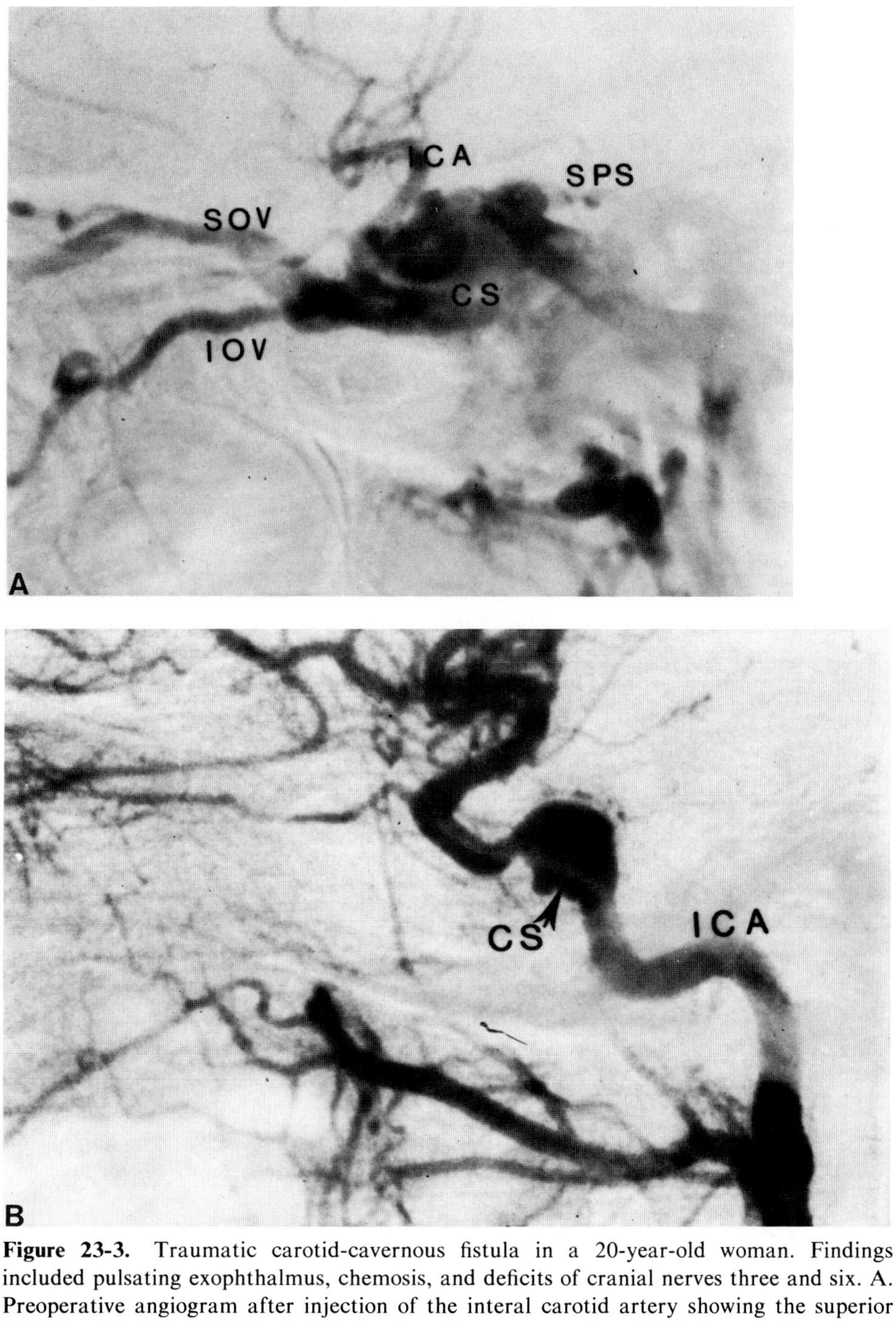

Figure 23-3. Traumatic carotid-cavernous fistula in a 20-year-old woman. Findings included pulsating exophthalmus, chemosis, and deficits of cranial nerves three and six. A. Preoperative angiogram after injection of the interal carotid artery showing the superior (SOV) and inferior (IOV) ophthalmic veins, the cavernous sinus (CS), the superior petrosal sinus (SPS), and the internal carotid artery (ICA). B. Angiogram after anterior packing of the cavernous sinus. A small portion of the sinus still opacifies but there is no anterior or posterior venous drainage. The signs and symptoms have resolved.

opening in the superior petrosal sinus. The middle portion of the cavernous sinus can be occluded by passing long lengths of a fine phosphor bronze wire (0.005 mm in diameter) directly into the sinus through a fine (33-gage) cannula. The type of occlusion required depends on the site of the leak. Arteriography and a Doppler apparatus placed on the affected eye assist in determining the flow through the fistula during the operation. When wire is inserted directly into the sinus, intraoperative arteriograms aid in locating the intracavernous portion of the artery so that it can be avoided during insertion of the wire. More recently these fistulas have been occluded with detachable balloons introduced by catheter, into the fistula via the carotid artery in the neck.[41,42]

POSTTRAUMATIC SEIZURES

A review of a series of over 4000 consecutive cases of head injury admitted to a pediatric hospital showed that 7.4 percent of these children had at least one seizure sometime after the injury.[28] This incidence is similar to those found in other studies, and when groups of patients seen at different clinics in different countries were compared, the incidence was surprisingly constant.[29] It is generally agreed that approximately half of the children who have seizures following a head injury have a seizure within the first 24 hours.[28,29] The effect of age on the occurrence of posttraumatic seizures is not certain. Seizures appear to be more common following birth injuries.[28] But while some studies showed little difference among young children, older children, and adults,[29,30] other studies showed more definite effects of age.[28,31] In one study it was found that in children below 5 years of age the incidence fell as the age increased but that after the age of 5 there was no apparent relationship between age and the occurrence of seizures.[28]

The most extensive recent studies of posttraumatic epilepsy in children have been made by Jennett[29,32] and by Jennett with Miller and Braakman[30] and with Teather and Bennie.[33] In these studies seizures were divided into early (occurring during the first week) and late (occurring at any time thereafter).[32] The basis for this distinction is related primarily to the frequency of seizures, their type, and the prognostic value of early seizures. Jennett found that seizures in children occurred 30 times more often in the first week after the injury than in any succeeding week and that a much higher percentage of the early seizures were focal, or at least started with focal features, than did late seizures. Early seizures correlated strongly with the event of late seizures. In these studies approximately 20 percent of children with an early seizure developed a late seizure, and of those children who developed a late seizure, approximately 70 percent developed recurrent attacks. The estimated instance of early seizures and of late seizures was each approximately 5 percent. In children with early seizures, the severity of injury per se did not appear significantly to influence the appearance of late seizures—that is, children with apparently trivial injuries followed by an early seizure were at as high a risk of developing late seizures as children who had more severe injuries followed by early seizure. In addition prevention of early seizures seemed unlikely to decrease the risk of late seizures. Late seizures were equally common in children who had a single seizure, status, or repeat seizures in the first week. The specific features of the head injury that appear to increase the incidence of seizures include depressed fracture, particularly with penetration of the dura, hematomas, especially subdural, and posttraumatic amnesia lasting more than 24 hours.[28,29]

A question of concern is which children to treat with prophylactic anticonvulsants and how long to continue these medications. Children particularly prone to developing seizures as characterized above should benefit from prophylactic anticonvulsants. The question of when to discontinue this medication is not answered by the data. It has been shown that those children who develop posttraumatic epilepsy may not have their first seizure until one or more years after injury.[33,34] Only approximately half of the children who developed seizures did so in the first 12 months. The rest developed seizures later, sometimes several years after the injury. Changes found by electroencephalography probably have only limited predictive value for the occurrence of seizures. When children with epilepsy due to all causes were studied after their medication was discontinued, those with severe electroencephalogram (EEG) abnormalities relapsed at a higher rate than those who had no or only mild abnormalities. Patients with severe EEG abnormalities, however, made up a small fraction of the total group at risk.[35] No similar study has been made of head-injured children who never had a seizure or who only had a seizure in the first week after injury but were given prophylactic anticonvulsants. A definite rule therefore cannot be formulated with regard to how long to continue prophylactic anticonvulsants in these children. Those patients who have had seizures and in whom control has been achieved should be continued on medication for at least two to three years. It is probable that approximately 25 percent of these children will relapse when the medication is stopped.[35] This risk may be acceptable to many of these patients and their parents.

NEUROPSYCHOLOGIC DEFICITS

A serious and pervasive complication of head injury is neuropsychologic deficit. Although not only a late complication, these deficits may persist and present problems in long-term management. Residual psychologic impairment has been found in children with even brief periods of coma, sometimes after only momentary loss of consciousness.[36] When a group of children and adolescents were assessed after head injury by testing multiple indices,[37] impairment of memory was the most commonly found abnormality, exceeding linguistic deficits or visuospatial impairment. When these memory deficits were more closely analyzed, retrieval of information was found to be more severly affected than storage. The occurrence of retrieval deficits has been emphasized in the memory disorders associated with Korsakoff's syndrome.[38] In view of the importance of temporal lobe structures for memory and their vulnerability in head injury,[39] it may be inferred that involvement of these regions is partially responsible for impaired retrieval in head-injured patients. When the memory deficits were related to specific areas of injuries, it was found that patients with left temporal lobe lesions had impairment of verbal memory that was not found in patients with right temporal lobe lesions, while those patients with a right temporal lobe lesion had impairment of visual memory.[40]

The degree of neuropsychologic impairment generally correlated well with the duration of coma and the severity of acute neurologic impairment.[37] General intelligence assessed by measuring intelligence quotient showed that global intelligence was generally in the normal range in all but the most severly injured patients.[37] When postinjury measurements were compared with premorbid ability, however, it was found that only partial intellectual recovery was generally achieved.

A neuropsychologic assessment should be part of the follow-up of any child who has sustained a head injury, particularly one associated with loss of consciousness. The capacity of a child merely to attend school does not necessarily imply a good recovery since learning problems may be overlooked. A neuropsychologic profile can assist in planning the resumption of schooling and determining the need for special education and rehabilitative services.

REFERENCES

1. Bruce DA, Schut L, Bruno LA, et al: Outcome following severe head injuries in children. J Neurosurg 48:679–688, 1978
2. Matson DD: Neurosurgery of Infancy and Childhood (ed 2). Springfield, Charles C. Thomas, 1969
3. Milhorat TH: Pediatric Neurosurgery. Philadelphia, FA Davis, 1978
4. Longacre JJ, DeStefano GA: Further observations of the behavior of autogenous split-rib grafts in reconstruction of extensive defects of the cranium and face. Plat Reconstruct Surg 20:281–296, 1957
5. Longacre JJ, Kahl JB, Wood RW: Reconstruction of extensive defects in and about the orbit. Am J Ophthalmol 61:763–768, 1966
6. Maniscalco JE, Leake D, Habal MB: Cranioplasty use of a combination graft. J Fla Med Assoc 63:869–871, 1976
7. Lende RA, Erickson RC: Growing skull fractures of childhood. J Neurosurg 18:479–489, 1961
8. Dyke CG: The roentgen-ray diagnosis of the skull and intracranial contents, in Golden R (ed): Diagnostic Roentgenology. New York, T Nelson and Sons, 1938, p 7
9. Lende RA: Enlarging skull fractures of childhood. Neuroradiology 7:119–124, 1974
10. Goldstein F, Sakoda T, Kepes JJ, et al: Enlarging skull fractures: An experimental study. J Neruosurg 27:541–550, 1967
11. Taveras JM, Ransohoff J: Leptomeningeal cysts of the brain following trauma with erosion of the skull. A study of seven cases treated by surgery. J Neurosurg 10:233–241, 1953
12. Stein, BM, Tenner MS: Enlargement of skull fracture in childhood due to cerebral herniation. Arch Neurol 26:137–143, 1972
13. Kingsley D, Till K, Hoare R: Growing fractures of the skull. J Neurol Neurosurg Psychiatr 41:312–318, 1978
14. Ito H, Miwa T, Onodra Y: Growing skull fracture of childhood with reference to the importance of the brain injury and its pathogenetic consideration. Child's Brain 3:116–126, 1977
15. Sato O, Tsugane R, Kageyama N: Growing skull fractures of childhood possible mechanism of its focal ventricular dilatation. Child's Brain 1:148–157, 1975
16. Vas CJ, Winn JM: Growing skull fractures. Dev Med Child Neurol 8:735–740, 1966
17. Addy DP: Expanding skull fracture of childhood. Br Med J 4:338–339, 1973
18. Ramamurthi B, Kalyanaraman S: Rationale for surgery in growing fractures of the skull. J Neurosurg 32:427–430, 1970
19. Broughton WL, Gee W, Doppman J, et al: Nonpulsatile exophthalmos in carotid-cavernous sinus fistula. J Pediat Ophthalmol 14:221–224, 1977
20. Arseni C, Horvath L, Caurea V, et al: Carotid-cavernous fistula in the child. Rev Roum Med Neurol Psych 16:29–32, 1978
21. Agnetti V, Pav A, Pinna L, et al: Cerebral pseudo-angiomatous pattern in a case of carotid-cavernous fistula. J Neurosurg Sci 18:75–79, 1974
22. Henderson JW, Schneider RC: The ocular findings in carotid-cavernous fistula in a series of 17 cases. Trans Am Ophthalmol Soc 56:123–141, 1958
23. Sanders MD, Hoyt WF: Hypoxic ocular sequelae of carotid-cavernous fistulae. Study of the causes of visual failure before and after neurosurgical treatment in a series of 25 cases. Br J Ophthalmol 53:82–97, 1969
24. Hamby WB: Carotid-Cavernous Fistula. Springfield, Charles C Thomas, 1966
25. Dandy WE, Follis RH: On the pathology of carotid-cavernous aneurysms (pulsating exophthalmos). Am J Ophthalmol 24:365–385, 1941
26. Parkinson D: A surgical approach to the cavernous portion of the carotid artery. Anatomical studies and case report. J Neurosurg 23:474–483, 1965

27. Mullan JF: Technique of thrombosis of carotid cavernous fistulae, in Schmidek HH, Sweet WH (Eds): Current Techniques in Operative Neurosurgery. New York, Grune & Stratton, 1976, pp 25–30
28. Hendrick EB, Harwood-Nash DC, Hudson AR: Head injuries in children: A survey of 4465 consecutive cases at the Hospital for Sick Children, Toronto, Canada. Clin Neurosurg 11:46–65, 1964
29. Jennett WB: Trauma as a cause of epilepsy in childhood. Dev Med Child Neurol 15:56–62, 1973
30. Jennett WB, Miller JD, Braakman R: Epilepsy after nonmissle depressed skull fracture. J Neurosurg 41:208–216, 1974
31. Kollevold T: Immediate and early cerebral seizures after head injuries. J Oslo City Hosp 28:77–86, 1978
32. Jennett WB: Early traumatic epilepsy. Lancet 1:1023–1025, 1969
33. Jennett WB, Teather D, Bennie S: Epilepsy after head injury. Residual risk after varying fit-free intervals since injury. Lancet 2:652–653, 1973
34. Weiss GH, Caverness WF: Prognostic factors in the persistence of posttraumatic epilepsy. J Neurosurg 37:164–169, 1972
35. Holowach J, Thurston DL, O'Leary J: Prognosis in childhood epilepsy follow-up study of 148 cases in which therapy had been suspended after prolonged anticonvulsant control. N Engl J Med 286:169–174, 1972
36. Klonoff H, Low MD, Clark C: Head injuries in children with a prospective five year follow-up. J Neurol Neurosurg Psychiatr 40:1211–1219, 1977
37. Levin HS, Eisenberg HM: Neuropsychological outcome of closed head injury in children and adolescents. Child's Brain 5:281–292, 1979
38. Warrington EK, Weiskrantz L: Amnesic syndrome. Consolidation or retrieval? Nature (London) 228:628–630, 1970
39. Jennett WB: Head injuries and the temporal lobe, in Herrington (ed). Current Problems in Neuropsychiatry. Br J Psychiatr special publ, no 4, Asford, Headley Bros Ltd, 1969
40. Levin HS, Eisenberg HM: Neuropsychological impairment after closed head injury in children and adolescents. J Pediatr Psychol (in press)
41. Debrun G, Lacour P, Caron JP, et al: Detachable balloon and calibrated-leak balloon techniques in the treatment of cerebral vascular lesions. J Neurosurg 49:635–649, 1978
42. Barrow DL, Fleischer AS, HOffman JC: Complications of detachable balloon catheter technique in the treatment of traumatic intracranial arteriovenous fistulas. J Neurosurg 56:396–403, 1982

24. Spinal Cord Injury

Joan L. Venes

Injury to the spine and spinal cord is an infrequent occurrence in the pediatric age group[21] and is often accompanied by lack of radiologic evidence of fracture or dislocation. A high index of suspicion is required for the diagnosis of spinal cord injury in the acutely injured child.

Vertebral or spinal cord injury should be suspected in the unconscious child, the conscious child who complains of neck or back pain, or the child in whom there is asymmetry or lack of response to stimulation. A careful history may indicate the possibility that significant flexion, extension, or rotational distortion forces have been applied to the spinal column. Examination of the unconscious patient may suggest spine injury; for example, contusion to the forehead indicates possible hyperextension of the cervical spine, a palpable gap suggests disruption of spinous processes, and bruising, particularly over the thoracic spine, may indicate significant underlying cord trauma. The elasticity of the cartilaginous spine and supporting ligamentous structures allows severe cord damage to occur in the absence of radiologic evidence of fracture or dislocation.[4] It is also not unusual for the level of spinal cord injury to be at variance with the level of vertebral injury in those children in whom radiographic evidence of spine injury is seen. A longitudinal traction force caused by the difference between the inherent elasticity of the spinal column and the lesser elasticity of the dura and meninges may cause disruption of neural tissue over several cord segments. In the cervical spine, loss of normal lordosis or the presence of prevertebral swelling may be the only diagnostic finding on plain x-ray. Associated soft tissue injury is less easily appreciated in thoracolumbar injuries.

CASE ILLUSTRATION

A 2½-year-old child fell from the second story of a building and was found unconscious with ecchymoses over the upper back. Nonpurposeful withdrawal of pain could be elicited in the upper extremities, but no response was noted in the

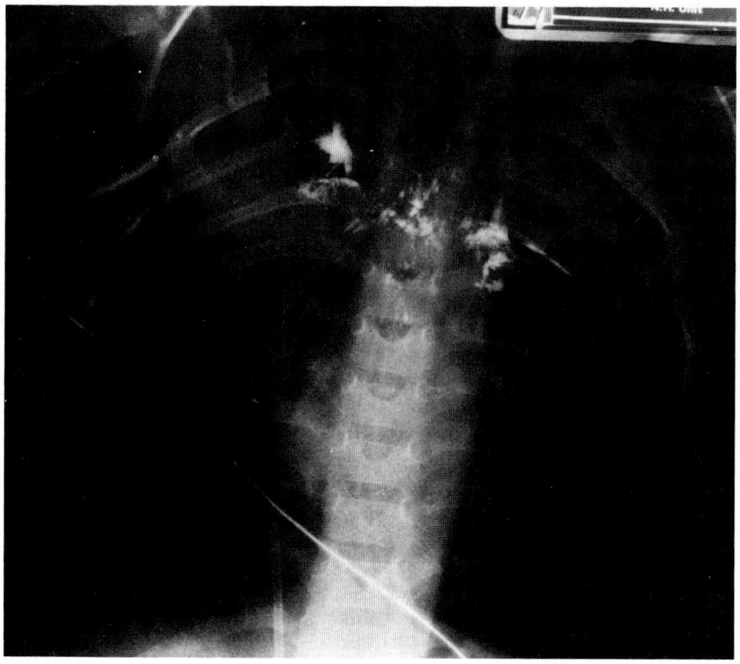

Figure 24-1. Pantopaque myelography in child with normal plain spine x-ray and total transverse loss of function below T4. Note extravasation of contrast material into mediastinum.

lower extremities. Respirations were shallow and the patient was intubated and placed on ventilatory assistance. Chest and cervicodorsal spine films showed no evidence of fracture or dislocation. This initial impression was confirmed by polytomography at a later date. A C1–2 myelogram demonstrated extravasation of Pantopaque into the mediastinum, indicating dural and probable cord disruption in the upper thoracic area (Fig. 24-1). The child remains without function below the upper thoracic level 18 months after injury.

CLINICAL DIAGNOSIS

Spinal cord concussion may be seen occasionally in cases of blunt trauma to the spine unassociated with flexion/rotation forces. In such cases there may be a temporary reversible loss of cord function. Signs of recovery usually appear within several hours and the persistence of total loss of cord function beyond the first two or three hours is almost always associated with some degree of permanent neurologic deficit. Failure to demonstrate any return of function 24 hours after injury is generally accepted as associated with a poor prognosis for functional recovery.

In the awake, cooperative child, sensory examination enables one reliably to assess the level of cord injury, and in addition provides valuable prognostic information. Preservation of patchy areas of pin sensation and/or the apprecia-tion of deep pain indicate that motor loss may be secondary to spinal shock or cord compression. Spinal shock remains a poorly understood phenomenon that first was brought to clinical attention in 1917 by Head and Riddoch.[13] All deep tendon reflexes are lost, the plantar reflexes cannot be elicited or are downgoing, and there is flaccid paralysis below the level of the lesion. Sphincter tone is generally little affected and there is complete urinary retention. If the injury has not been too severe, reflexes return, voluntary control is reestablished, and motor recovery begins within hours of injury. If cord injury is severe, recovery of reflexes is accompanied by reflex facilitation, which may occur within hours or days unaccompanied by any evidence of improving sensation or voluntary motor activity. In the infant this reflex activity of the isolated cord may be almost indistinguishable from normal motor function.

In assessing the preservation of sensation, two syndromes should be kept in mind. Preservation of sacral sensation is occasionally seen in central cord injuries[30] due to the peripheral location of the sacral portion of the spinothalamic tract. Its predictive value is questionable, but when it is associated with even a flicker of movement in the lower extremities, the patient may go on to complete recovery. In the syndrome of the anterior spinal artery, touch and proprioception are preserved, although there is loss of all other long-tract function.[29] This apparent anomaly is attributable to the fact that the posterior aspect of the cord—that is, dorsal and dorsolateral columns—is supplied by branches of the posterior spinal artery. Preservation of touch and proprioception has no predictive value for motor recovery in this instance, but recognition of the syndrome should alert one to the possibility of disk herniation in the absence of radiologic evidence of anterior cord compression by bone fragments or displaced vertebral body. It should be considered an absolute indication for myelography. Unlike the central cord syndrome in which a high percentage of patients recover useful function, the prognosis for significant neurologic recovery in this group is poor.[3] Assessment of reflexes is helpful in determining the level of the lesion in cervical cord and cauda equina injuries (Table 24-1). Reflex loss is generally appropriate to the degree of motor involvement. In the unconscious or uncooperative child, evaluation of motor function is difficult; however, every effort should be made to obtain a reliable baseline against which progressive neurologic deficit may be measured.

Pain in a radicular distribution may indicate reversible injury to the root at that level, even when associated with sensory-motor reflex loss. The value of functional recovery of even a single nerve root in the brachial plexus cannot be overemphasized.

Table 24-1
Segmental Deficit in Spinal Cord Injury

Spinal Cord Segment	Major Motor Loss	Reflex Loss
Upper limb C4 and C5	Shoulder girdle Deltoid	
C5 and C6	Biceps Brachialis	Biceps
C6 and C7	Triceps	Triceps
C7 and C8	Extensors of hand and wrist	Radial Periosteal
C8 and T1	Intrinsics of hand	
Lower limb T12–L2	Ileopsoas	Cremasteric
L2 and L3	Adductors Quadriceps	Patellar
L4 and L5	Glutei Extensor hallucis longus Peronei	Patellar
L5 and S1	Gastrocnemius Soleus	Ankle
S2	Intrinsics of foot	
S4 and S5		Anal

RADIOGRAPHIC EVALUATION

The stability of the spine is maintained by the posterior ligament complex consisting of the supraspinous and interspinous ligaments along with the ligamentum flavum and capsules of the posterior joints. Disruption of these soft tissue elements rarely occurs without bony injury demonstrable on laminography. An accurate assessment of stability thus usually can be made avoiding undue manipulation, by using either laminography, polytomography, or high resolution computerized axial tomography. Injuries involving the anterior elements (intervertebral disks, periosteum, anterior and posterior longitudinal ligaments) are relatively more stable than those in which both posterior and anterior supporting columns are involved. It is the integrity of the posterior ligament complex that is essential for spine stability. Laminography allows for the delineation of bony injury in those patients in whom conventional spine x-rays are nondiagnostic and in whom special views would require manipulation that might further injure the cord in an unstable spine. In those patients in whom subluxation or fracture is evident on plain x-ray, laminography will help to delineate the full extent of injury. Laminography is also indicated in the patient with persistent radicular back or neck pain with or without neurologic deficit in whom plain x-rays are normal.

If conventional spine films or laminography demonstrate reduction of canal diameter by posterior bony elements or fracture or dislocation of the vertebral body, reduction and/or operative intervention may be carried out without myelography. Computerized axial tomography (CAT) is an additional diagnostic tool that can prove helpful in assessing the degree of disruption of the ring structures of the vertebral column and the presence of bone fragments within the spinal canal.[7,17] Myelography with air or radiopaque contrast material is indicated in patients with neurologic deficit in whom there is no evidence of bone injury and in patients whose neurologic deficit is out of proportion to the bony abnormality demonstrated on laminography. Air or water-soluble contrast myelography allows one to evaluate the upper cord with the patient in the supine position using a C1–2 puncture.[28] Either method requires tomography for good delineation of cord/contrast interface. Cattell and Filtzer[5] have reviewed the problem areas encountered in the interpretation of cervical spine x-rays in young children. Evaluation of the cervical spine in a young child must be done with careful regard for the clinical history and physical examination.

1. In the absence of pain and/or limitation of motion, the normal forward movement of C2 on C3 or C3 on C4 and C5 should not be mistaken for subluxation of clinical significance (Fig. 24-2). Twenty percent of children between 1 and 7 years of age were found to have this type of hypermobility.
2. Atraumatic subluxation of the upper cervical vertebra may present in childhood with the complaint of torticollis. Dislocation most commonly occurs as an anterior unilateral displacement of the atlas upon the axis with turning of the head away from the affected side. It is probable that the pronounced horizontal orientation of the upper cervical facets in the young child contribute to the frequency of this occurrence. Laxity of the transverse ligament must be present to allow the atlas to slide forward on the axis. Atlantoaxial asymmetry produced by such dislocation cannot be counteracted by turning the head as occurs in muscular torticollis. In general a distance of greater than 3.0 mm between the dens and the anterior arch is considered abnormal, although occasional

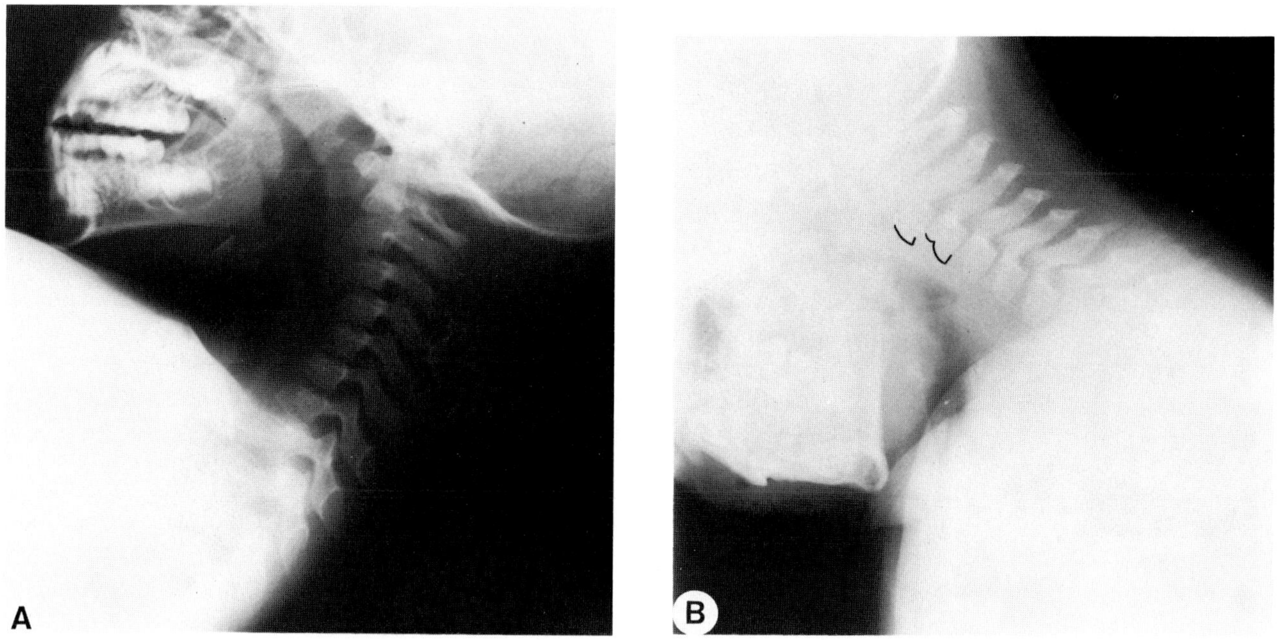

Figure 24-2. A. Forward displacement of C2 on C3 in child with persistent nuchal rigidity following suboccipital craniectomy in C1–3 cervical laminectomy. B. Preoperative film demonstrates similar hypermobility. Symptoms resolved spontaneously over several weeks.

cases have been reported in which a distance of 3.5–4 mm was not associated with symptoms.

3. Variations of the normal cervical spine curve that may resemble spasm were seen in about 15 percent of asymptomatic children.
4. The basilar odontoid cartilaginous plate frequently persists in vestigial form in children under 5 years of age, and occasionally may be seen in the slightly older child. This may be easily mistaken for an undisplaced fracture.

TREATMENT

Treatment of the spinal-cord-injured patient begins at the scene of the accident.[9] Instruction of paramedical personnel in means of transfer and stabilization of the potentially injured spine should reduce the incidence of irreversible spinal cord injury. Autoregulation is lost in the spine-injured patient[31] and so establishment of a good airway and restoration of blood pressure assume added significance. This must be done without movement of possible areas of spinal column instability. Intubation with a cervical spine injury is best accomplished by the nasotracheal route and tracheostomy is indicated if intubation cannot be accomplished without extension and manipulation of the neck. It should also be remembered that "spinal shock" and resulting loss of sympathetic vasomotor tone complicate the general evaluation and may mimic symptoms of shock from internal bleeding. Rapid restoration of normal blood pressure is essential for the preservation of cord function and can be accomplished by vasoconstrictors and/or blood volume expanders. A subsequent drop in blood pressure suggests blood loss rather than a loss of vasomotor tone and the source should be searched for most commonly in the abdominal cavity, thoracic cavity, pelvis, or fractured extremity. It must be remembered that in patients with a high cord lesion, abdominal reflexes may be absent and guarding or complaints of abdominal pain may not occur.

Fractures Involved

Holdsworth's[15] classification for fractures of the vertebral column (Fig. 24-3) divides them into two types—stable and unstable.

Stable

The simple wedge fracture results from flexion forces with impaction of fracture fragments and is rarely associated with neurologic deficit.

A burst fracture results from compression forces with comminution of the body and disruption of the end-plates. The unimpacted fragments, although stable, make this a painful injury that may require rigid external stabilization for comfort. Burst fractures of the cervical spine are frequently associated with severe neurologic deficit.

Extension dislocation fractures are fairly well localized to the cervical spine and the posterior ligaments remain intact so they remain stable in flexion.

Unstable

Dislocation fractures are always accompanied by total rupture of the posterior ligament complex and reduction may be hindered by locking of one or both facet joints.

Rotational fracture dislocations, the most unstable of all vertebral fractures, are a result of a flexion rotation force that disrupts the posterior ligament complex with lateral displacement of the upper vertebral body on the lower. X-rays demonstrate a slice fracture of the upper border of the lower vertebral body with separation of the spinous processes and a lateral shift of the articular processes.

In sheer fracture, which are limited to the thoracic and lumbar regions (e.g., seat-belt injury), there is forward displacement of the body with fracture of the articular processes or pedicles and disruption of all ligamentous support.[10] These are burst fractures associated with fracture of the neural arches.

Regimen

In stable fractures with lesser degrees of cord injury, immobilization in a brace or cast for six to eight weeks is generally all that is required. It should be kept in mind that the young school-age child may not cooperate with this type of

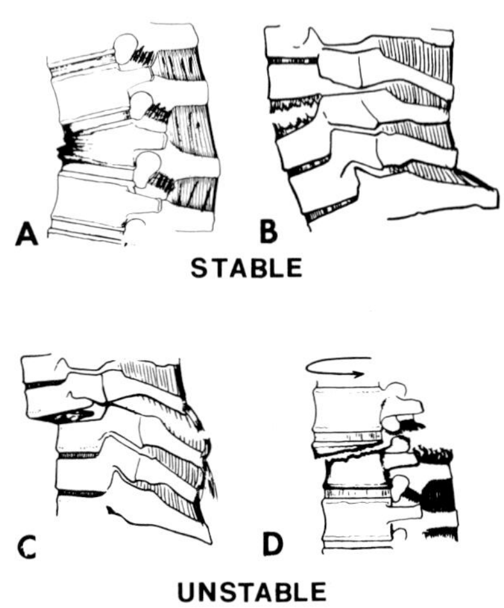

Figure 24-3. A. Wedge compression fracture with preservation of posterior ligament complex. B. Hyperextension dislocation. Because of preservation of posterior ligament complex, this injury is stable in flexion. Often the ruptured anterior longitudinal ligament will avulse a small fragment of bone as it ruptures. This should be evident on plain x-ray. C. Dislocation. Unlike the dislocation in (B), there is often wide separation of the spinous processes secondary to disruption of posterior ligaments. Oblique roentgenograms are advisable to demonstrate displacement and locking of the articular facets. D. Rotation dislocation—rupture of the posterior ligament complex including the posterior articular capsules that allow lateral displacement; slice fracture of the lower vertebral body. Fractures of the posterior elements can usually be well demonstrated by laminography. (Reprinted with permission from Holdsworth F: Fractures, dislocations and fracture–Dislocations of the spine. J Bone Jt Surg 45(B):7–9, 1963.)

program. Not infrequently stability is attested to by the young patient walking home from school, swinging the offending collar that interfered with the day's activities. If continued immobilization is considered imperative, then placement in a lightweight fiberglass cast may be more reasonable than attempts to maintain the child in a removable brace or collar. Stable vertebral fractures in children, in contrast to those in the adult, rarely if ever result in progressive or delayed angulatory deformity. Multiple compression fractures in children have a remarkable tendency toward spontaneous healing and ultimately result in complete restoration of vertebral height. Lateral wedge fractures in children may result in minimal scoliosis but progressive spine deformity is rarely, if ever, observed.[22] Unstable fracture dislocations or stable fractures associated with paraplegia or quadriplegia occurring prior to the adolescent growth spurt, however, will lead to spinal deformity in a large number of patients.[18]

In a patient with an unstable fracture of the cervical spine, traction with increasing weight loads may be required to reduce deformity. In the infant and young child, weight must be added judiciously since the distraction force on the cord may be excessive when ligamentous structures have been disrupted. Braided wire placed between two burr holes on each side of the skull is one means of maintaining traction in the infant whose thin skull will not tolerate the insertion of tongs.[20] In the slightly older child, once adequate reduction of spinal deformity has been attained, rigid external fixation can be obtained by the use of the halo cast. The halo cast offers several advantages over prolonged immobilization in tongs in children with useful cord function. Chief among these is the likelihood that such children will be able to be cared for at home. Secondly, they will be able to participate in active rehabilitation programs at an earlier stage in their recovery. Significant morbidity is infrequent with the use of halo traction in children over 3 years of age.[19] As in the adult, careful attention to the cleanliness of the pin and tong sites is essential and complaints of local pain and headache indicate the possibility of penetration of the inner table or osteomyelitis.

Acute kyphosis and/or disruption of disk material is infrequent in injuries to the thoracic spine and injuries in this region are usually best managed conservatively in the absence of a compound wound. Bracing does not give enough lateral support to maintain the thoracolumbar spine in good condition and casting in patients with anesthetic skin is associated with breakdown and should be undertaken only under close supervision. Treatment for six to eight weeks on a frame followed by bracing allows good repair of supportive structures without the morbidity associated with casting. The need for bracing throughout the adolescent growth spurt in the child with significant neurologic deficit must be emphasized.

Once the diagnosis of spinal cord injury is made, the principle of management and the criteria for operative intervention in the child are not significantly different from the adult. Operation is indicated for the stabilization of an unstable fracture, removal of bone fragments or disk material from the spinal canal, reduction of locked facets, and the debridement of a compound wound. If myelography has demonstrated a widened cord consistent with the diagnosis of either hematomyelia or central cord edema, myelotomy for the evacuation of necrotic material has been suggested. Wagner and Rawe[36] note that myelotomy can be safely accomplished by either the anterior or posterior route. The effectiveness of this procedure in the clinical situation remains largely undocumented. If open reduction or decompression is indicated, consideration of surgical stabilization will depend upon the size and type of bony injury as well as the operative approach used in achieving the decompression.

The posterior approach is indicated in cervical spine injury for reduction of locked facets and the removal of posterior bone fragments or depressed lamina.

Although posterior fusion does not confer the immediate stability gained with anterior fusion, the use of a halo cast will allow early ambulation. Wire fixation, commonly used in atlantoaxial and other fractures of the cervical spine in the adult, may not be tolerated by the young child in whom the lamina and spinous processes are not completely ossified and will be cut through by the wire if additional external fixation is not used. Bony fusion in addition to the wiring is recommended. Posterior dislocation of the vertebral body or myelographic defect suggesting posterior disruption of the disk into the spinal canal are considered indications for the anterior approach in the cervical spine. This approach has found increasing acceptance since its introduction by Bailey and Badgely,[2] Cloward,[6] and Verbiest[34] in the early 1960s. The anterior cervical approach is difficult in the infant because of the small size of the vertebral body and the difficulty in obtaining good tibial cortical bone. Verbiest,[35] however, has reported satisfactory results in four infants using this approach. The management of unstable fracture dislocations of the thoracolumbar or lumbar spine remains controversial, but it appears that the conservative approach favored by Guttman[12] is increasingly being replaced by early surgical intervention, both to decompress the cord and to achieve stability. Stabilization posteriorly followed by anterior decompression and interbody fusion has been reported to be easily accomplished under one anesthetic,[39] although in the young child a two-stage procedure may be necessary to avoid life-threatening blood loss.

It must be remembered that laminectomy converts a stable injury into an unstable injury in those patients in whom the posterior elements are intact. Exploratory laminectomy in this situation to rule out a possible surgically correctable lesion in the paraplegic or quadriplegic child is ill-advised and to be avoided. Long-term management of the paraplegic and quadriplegic child shares many of the problems seen in such adults.

Careful assessment of urinary function is required as soon as the child's condition permits. If urinary tract infection has been avoided and sphincter tone remains intact, that is, the level of injury is above S2, then intermittent catheterization has proved a valuable means of achieving social continence.[11] The use of intermittent catheterization has generally been well accepted by both parents and child, given the proper support and supervision. The older paraplegic child may be interested in self-catheterization. For the quadriplegic and younger paraplegic, instruction of a family member has proved to be relatively easy. Pharmacologic[26] agents and various surgical procedures[16] have wide application. Diversionary procedures that once were used fairly often[27] for the management of older children with bladder dysfunction are used less frequently at present, and generally are reserved for the management of intractable hydronephrosis.

Often diet alone and the establishment of a regular routine are all that is required to keep the child from soiling. The use of a stool softener and/or suppository may be necessary, but laxatives and enemas are to be avoided except under well-defined circumstances.

Decubiti are rarely a significant problem in the bedridden child whose small size makes frequent turning easier than in the adult. The ambulatory child in braces is at risk for the development of decubiti of the heel or other bony prominences, which may significantly interfere with ambulation and rehabilitation. The child must be instructed as to the importance of reporting reddened or ecchymotic areas to the parent. In the younger child, regular inspection of problem areas on a daily or twice-daily basis is mandatory.

Scoliosis is more common in the growing paraplegic child than in the adult with paraplegia. Careful attention to sitting and standing postures is required and exercises to strengthen weakened muscles and decrease asymmetric pull on the spinal column may prevent or retard the development of scoliosis. Bracing is usually required to control progression of the curve. Early recognition and treatment remain the best method of avoiding significant functional deformity. Spinal fusion is indicated in the child in whom kyphosis or scoliosis progresses in spite of bracing.[22]

Regular standing and walking increase the strength of bones in the lower extremities, as well as have a positive psychologic effect on the child's (and family's) outlook. In general rehabilitation is best carried out in a center where a comprehensive program is available. If the child is quadriplegic, special adaptive devices may enable more independent functioning. The occurrence of reactive depression and anxiety about the future is all too often overlooked by staff and family because of the child's inability to verbalize emotions. Failure to deal with the problems of inadequate self-image, sexuality, etc., in the young child and adolescent may lead to life-long dependency.

Recent changes in the law[33] have allowed the paraplegic child to attend regular classes where appropriate. For the young quadriplegic or paraplegic child, involvement with a peer group often requires great determination and creative imagination on the part of the parent. Participation of the handicapped child in the "normal" activities of childhood remains a challenging area for educators, parents, and therapists.

CURRENT RESEARCH

Research efforts in several centers have been directed at elucidation of the pathophysiology of cord trauma and the evaluation of various therapeutic modalities. To date there has been no solid evidence that significant functional recovery can occur if there is immediate complete transverse loss of function that persists for several hours. There is, however, experimental evidence that spinal cord blood flow in the involved area is maintained for one to two hours following an injury[31] that produces paralysis in over 50 percent of animals. This work is quite preliminary but suggests that pharmacologic intervention and consequent preservation of long-tract function may be possible in an indeterminate number of cases now left with permanent neurologic deficit.

Controversy exists concerning the use of corticosteroids and there is no experimental evidence that administration following trauma significantly alters outcome.[8] In other than less severe injuries, clinical reports indicate that "megadose" steroid administration may be of value, but no controlled trials of this regimen have yet been published.

Local hypothermia has been reported to be of value in reducing the degree of neurologic dysfunction but, again, there have been no controlled studies and few centers are presently equipped to carry out this procedure, which requires careful monitoring of cord temperatures.[1,38]

Release of catecholamines in the affected area has been cited as the underlying cause for reduction in spinal cord blood flow[23] but attempts in the laboratory to prevent hemorrhagic necrosis by the use of various blocking agents given shortly after trauma have produced conflicting results.[14,24,25]

It is generally agreed that, in the face of progressive neurologic deficit, surgical decompression and stabilization are indicated and are usually associated with significant functional recovery. Early surgical intervention in patients who have demonstrated no evidence of cord function below the lesion is far less rewarding and controversy exists as to whether or not such intervention is justified in the absence of progression or a compound wound. Epidemiologic research currently underway may provide a definitive answer to this recurring question.[37]

REFERENCES

1. Albin MS, White RJ, Acosta-Rua G, et al: Study of functional recovery produced by delayed localized cooling after spinal cord injury in primates. J Neurosurg 29:113–120, 1968
2. Bailey RW, Badgely CE: Stabilization of the cervical spine by anterior fusion. J Bone Jt Surg 42(A):565–594, 1960
3. Bosch A, Stauffer ES, Nickel VL: Incomplete traumatic quadriplegia—A ten year review. JAMA 216:473–478, 1971
4. Burke DC: Spinal cord trauma in children. Paraplegia 9:1–14, 1971
5. Cattell HS, Filtzer DL: Pseudosubluxation and other normal variations in the cervical spine in children. J Bone Jt Surg 47(A):1295–1305, 1965
6. Cloward RB: Treatment of acute fractures and fracture-dislocations of the cervical spine by vertebral body fusion. J Neurosurg 18:201–219, 1961
7. Colley DP, Dunsker SB: Traumatic narrowing of the dorsolumbar spinal canal demonstrated by computed tomography. Radiology 129:95–98, 1978
8. Ducker TB, Hamit HF: Experimental treatment of spinal cord injury. J Neurosurg 30:693–697, 1969
9. Farrington JD: Death in a ditch. Bull Am Coll Surg May–June, 1967 pp 1–7
10. Fletcher BD, Brogdon BG: Seat belt fractures of the spine and sternum. JAMA 200:177–178, 1967
11. Frankel HL: The development of intermittent catheterization and treatment of the bladder in acute paraplegia, in Proceedings, 18th Veterans Administration Spinal Cord Injury Conference. DC, US Government Printing Office, 1972, pp 132–139
12. Guttman L: Initial treatment of traumatic paraplegia. Proc Roy Soc Med 47:1103–1109, 1954
13. Head H, Riddoch G: The automatic bladder, excessive sweating and some other reflex conditions in gross injuries of the spinal cord. Brain 40:188–263, 1917
14. Hedeman LS, Shellenberger MK, Gordon JH: Studies in experimental spinal cord trauma. Part I. Alternations in catecholamine levels. J Neurosurg 40:37–43, 1974
15. Holdsworth F: Fractures, dislocations and fracture-dislocations of the spine. J Bone Jt Surg 52(A):1534–1551, 1971
16. Kaufman JJ: History of surgical correction of male urinary incontinence. Urol Clin N Am 5:265–278, 1977
17. Kershaw MS, Goodman GA, Perlmutter GS: Computed tomography in diagnosis of atlas fracture. Am J Roent 128:688–689, 1977
18. Kilfoyle RM, Foley JJ, Norton PL: Spine and pelvic deformity in childhood and adolescent paraplegia. J Bone Jt Surg 47(A):659–682, 1965
19. Kopits SE, Steingass MH: Experience with the halo cast in small children. Surg Clin N Am 50:935–942, 1970
20. Matson DD: Spinal cord injury, in Neurosurgery of Infancy and Childhood (ed 2). Springfield, Charles C Thomas, 1969, pp 345–375
21. Melzak J: Paraplegia among children. Lancet 2:45–48, 1969
22. Moe JH, Winter RB, Bradford DS, et al: Spinal injury, in Scoliosis and Other Spinal Deformities. Philadelphia, WB Saunders, 1978, pp 612–624
23. Osterholm JL, Mathews GJ: Altered norepinephrine metabolism following experimental cord injury. Part I. Relationship to hemorrhagic necrosis and post-wounding deficits. J Neurosurg 36:386–394, 1972
24. Osterholm JL, Matthews GJ: Altered norepinephrine metabolism following experimental spinal cord injury. Part II. Protection against traumatic spinal cord hemorrhagic necrosis by norepinephrine synthesis blockade with alpha methyl tyrosine. J Neurosurg 36:395–401, 1972
25. Rawe SE, Roth RH, Collins WF: Norepinephrine levels in experimental spinal cord trauma. Part 2: Histopathological study of hemorrhagic necrosis. J Neurosurg 46:350–357, 1977
26. Raz S: Pharmacological treatment of lower urinary tract dysfunction. Urol Clin N Am 5:323–334, 1978
27. Retik AB, Perlmutter AD, Gross RE: Cutaneous ureteroileostomy in children. N Engl J Med 277:217–222, 1967

28. Rossier AB, Berrey J, Rosenbaum A, et al: Value of gas myelography in early management of acute cervical spinal cord injuries. J Neurosurg 42:330–337, 1975
29. Schneider RC: A syndrome in acute cervical injuries for which early operation is indicated. J Neurosurg 8:360–367, 1951
30. Schneider RC, Cherry G, Pantek H: Syndrome of acute central cervical cord injury with special reference to the mechanisms involved in hyperextension injuries of the spine. J Neurosurg 11:546–577, 1954
31. Senter JH, Venes JL: Loss of autoregulation and post traumatic ischemia following experimental spinal cord trauma. J Neurosurg 50:198–206, 1979
32. Sypert GW, Mozingo GR: A technique for early pantopaque myelography in cervical spinal cord injuries. Surg Neurol 6:221–222, 1976
33. The Education of All Handicapped Children Act of 1975, PL 94–142; 20 USC (40) et seq: Federal Register 42 (163):42474–42518, Aug 23 1977
34. Verbiest H: Anterior operative approach in old irreducible bone displacements and fresh fractures of the cervical spinal cord compression. Excerpta Med Int Cong Ser 36:149, 1961
35. Verbiest H: La chirurgie anterieure et alterale du rachis cervical. Neurochir 16 supp 2:1–212, 1970
36. Wagner FC, Rawe SE: Microsurgical anterior cervical myelotomy. Surg Neurol 5:229–231, 1976
37. Wagner FC: Personal communication
38. White RJ: Current status of spinal cord cooling: Clin Neurosurg 20:400–408, 1974
39. Whitesides TE, Shah SGA: On the management of unstable fractures of the thoracolumbar spine. Spine 1:99–107, 1976

25. Peripheral Nerve Lesions in the Pediatric Age Group

Peter W. Carmel

Trauma to the peripheral nervous system in infants and children is relatively uncommon,[16] and referral centers with great experience with adult nerve injuries have disproportionately small numbers of childhood lesions.[12] The outlook for a child with a properly managed peripheral nerve lesion is better than for similar injury in an adult. Recovery of function following nerve injury in a child is usually faster than in adult years.

The pathologic processes in children are similar to those seen in adults. Division of a peripheral nerve results in retrograde degeneration of the axon toward its neuron of origin, and an antegrade degeneration distal to the site of injury. Following axonal degeneration the myelin sheath condenses into lipid-positive droplets, which undergo phagocytosis. After an initial delay, which may take from several weeks to several months, regenerating axons can be seen bridging the gap of the nerve lesion. As a general rule, nerves regenerate at a rate of 3 to 5 mm per week. Muscles at greater distances from the site of nerve lesions may undergo irreversible atrophy during the period of axonal regeneration.

The reasons for more favorable axonal regrowth in children than adults have not been determined. It has been attributed to rapid axonal regrowth after the suture line or nerve lesion has been bridged.[16] There are little data, however, on the comparative metabolic and growth processes in children and adults.[6] In children the distance between the point of injury and important sensory and motor reinervation sites is usually short, and regenerating axons may be able to reach these sites before irreversible atrophy of the muscle and its end-plate have occurred.

TYPES OF PERIPHERAL NERVE INJURY

In the neonatal period, rare peripheral nerve lesions are seen associated with parturition. These include stretch injuries of either the upper or lower portion of the brachial plexus, and facial nerve palsies due to compression. With improved obstetric technique the incidence of these lesions has fallen rather dramatically.[12]

In later childhood two distinctly different types of injury are seen. The first of these is direct laceration of nerves of the forearm. These injuries can involve the ulnar, radial, or median nerve, or combinations of nerves. The majority of these lesions occur when the arm is thrust through a pane of glass, and the wounds inflicted are usually clean and sharp, and the nerve is smoothly divided. The second important mechanism is damage to nerves by displaced bone fractures. The most common site is the common peroneal nerve due to fracture of the upper fibular. The incidence of this type of nerve lesion seems to have risen with the popularity of skateboarding in the pediatric population. Fractures of the upper extremities may cause damage of the radial nerve by displaced fractures of the humerus, while the ulnar may be injured at the elbow by fractures traversing the medial epicondial.

A third group of nerve injuries in childhood is associated with iatrongenic causes. These include injuries of the sciatic, gluteal, and lateral femoral cutaneous nerves by intramuscular injections.[15] Another iatrogenic group of nerve disorders are those that are caused by compression of the common peroneal nerve at the knee, or of the ulnar nerve at the elbow, secondary to application of plaster casts. Because of the medical–legal implications of these injuries, they are often subjected to unusual delays before proper treatment to restore neural function is instituted.

Finally a disturbing group of injuries is seen with increasing frequency at urban hospital centers. These are nerve lesions seen in early teenage years that are caused by violence, either due to stabbing injuries or to gunshot wounds (see Case 1).

DIAGNOSIS

Diagnosis of peripheral nerve lesions in children is subjected to unusual problems in examination and subjective evaluation because of the patient's age. Perhaps the most important diagnostic test is careful observation of the child at play by an alert observer. Posture of an affected extremity, and use of it in manipulation and handling of objects, as well as any indication of pain on movement should be carefully noted. In lower extremity lesions, the child's gait, both running and walking, may be diagnostic. Peroneal palsies result in a characteristic slapping, drop-foot gait, while a wide swing of the foot may indicate inability to tense the quadriceps muscle secondary to femoral palsy. Abnormal posturing of the extremity because of muscular atrophy or orthopedic deformity also may be characteristic of a given nerve lesion.

Sensory examination can be carried out in most children without unduly alarming the child. The principle of bilateral symmetry of touch is most useful. Finger-touch sensation is reliable in those zones where there is autonomous function of a well-demarcated nerve. Loss of sensation or loss of sweating in an autonomous zone usually indicates injury to the nerve serving that zone. Pin-prick sensation testing is often deferred in the pediatric age group because fear on the child's part may interfere with the rest of the examination.

Motor function may be rapidly assessed by testing the distal-most muscles innervated by the nerve in question. The child is given a simple task that requires use of the muscles involved.

Palpation of the wound or elicitation of Tinel's sign should be left until the end of the examination as it may be painful.

SPECIAL DIAGNOSTIC TESTS

Electrodiagnostic Procedures

Electromyography and recording of nerve conduction speeds and nerve action potentials can be extremely helpful in localizing the level of the lesion and in confirmation of deinnervational changes. These tests, however, are much more difficult to perform in the pediatric population than in adults. Great patience and tact are needed in the electrodiagnostic investigation of most children. The electromyographers' experience in dealing with children may be the limiting factor in employing these tests.[12]

Electrodiagnostic studies may be of little value in the period when the nerve is undergoing Wallerian degeneration. Electromyographic and conduction studies should be deferred for several weeks after injury in order for them to be assessed properly.

Radiologic Tests

Plain films of the injured extremity may easily demarcate the level of nerve interruption by noting the point of fracture. Myelography may be helpful when root involvement is suspected, either following stretch injuries, or in the neonatal type of brachial plexus lesion. Evulsion of nerve roots due to stretch can often be identified by the presence of meningocele or extravasation of contrast. On rare occasions the division of the nerve roots itself may be identified. A normal myelogram, however, does not rule out nerve division secondary to stretch, nor does the presence of a meningocele prove that the nerve root is divided.

MANAGEMENT

Once the diagnosis of nerve injury has been reached and the site of the lesion identified, a choice of management alternatives must be made. Therapy of peripheral nerve lesions is strongly influenced by the type of injury incurred. Special management considerations will come into play in each of four broad categories of injury, which include (1) stretch injuries, including birth palsies; (2) penetrating lacerations and stab wounds; (3) lesions in continuity; and (4) lesions of nerves due to tumors and other masses.

STRETCH INJURIES AND BIRTH PALSIES

"Obstetric paralysis" has been diagnosed since the Middle Ages, but it was not until the studies of Duchenne[5] in 1872 that a precise account of the muscles involved was given. Duchenne felt that injured nerves might regenerate but the prognosis appeared grave in this type of injury. Erb[7] in 1876 gave a detailed analysis of the Duchenne type of brachial plexus injury and his name is now associated with this lesion. This is the most common of the birth palsies, and involves the upper trunk of the brachial plexus, but may include the middle trunk as well. The injury is due to stretching of the upper portion of the brachial plexus secondary to forcible depression of the shoulder. In most cases of common upper arm paralysis, the maximum injury occurs at the point where the fifth and sixth cervical nerve roots join to form the upper trunk of the plexus.[16] This point is distal to the canal and lies approximately at the level of the transverse process of the sixth cervical vertebra. Immediately following the trauma, ecchymosis or hemorrhage may be noted and swelling over this point may be palpable. As time goes by, a noticeable thickening may occur over the scalene tubercle. The muscles of the rotator cuff, the elbow flexors, and even the elbow extensors may be involved. The arm hangs limply by the side in the position of pronation, and the wrist is flexed. This posture has been called the "waiter's tip" position.

This muscle paralysis will lead to early contracture at the shoulder. The arm should be placed in an airplane splint that keeps it in an abducted and laterally rotated position, with the forearm supinated. Range-of-motion exercises must be carried out daily.

Brachial plexus palsy subsequent to the injury of the lower portion of the brachial plexus was described by several authors through the early part of the 19th century. The anatomic basis and pathogenesis of this second type of obstetric palsy, however, was defined and investigated experimentally by Klumpke[14] in 1885. The usual mechanism of this injury is extension and abduction of the forearm within the birth canal while traction is exerted on the infant's body during delivery. The damage here is to the C8 and T1 nerve roots, and results in loss of intrinsic hand function and paralysis of the flexor muscles of the hand. Horner's syndrome may or may not be present.

Although generally regarded as having a poor prognosis, these types of obstetric injuries are not uniformally unfavorable. As Sunderland[20] has described, many of them do show at least partial recovery, particularly upper-trunk injuries. If the root is evulsed or distracted proximally, however, as demonstrated on myelography, the prognosis is much poorer.

Because surgical treatment of birth injuries of the brachial plexus has been generally discouraging, most authors have recommended a period of observation prior to any surgical intervention. During this period it is important to minimize the deformity due to overaction of muscles whose antagonists have been paralyzed. With infants who have been fitted with an airplane splint, it is important to remove them from the splint several times daily for physical therapy. Surgical exploration of these lesions should be delayed as long as there is any evidence of progressive improvement. If no improvement is seen after three to six months, surgical exploration may be of some benefit. In children where ecchymosis or thickening in the supraclavicular fossa has been noted, either in the immediate posttraumatic period or in the subsequent history, neurolysis may help.

The operative procedure in most of the birth paralysis cases that have been explored has been limited to neurolysis. This procedure in upper plexus birth injuries is difficult to assess, but some improvement is seen occasionally. The results of operation in lower trunk injuries are almost universally poor.[16]

Stretch injuries in older children carry a more favorable prognosis. Kline and Bratton[12] recorded that of 15 stretch injuries, significant improvement occurred in 12 children and very satisfactory results were obtained in eight. Several authors have noted fair improvement with several types of procedures, including the use of multiple intrafasicular grafts from an autologous sural nerve.[12,18,21]

Total or partial paralysis of the facial nerve is occasionally seen following difficult obstetric deliveries. This paralysis is a lower motor neuron type of lesion and usually results from undue pressure of an obstetric forceps blade over the nerve, somewhere between its emergence from the skull at the stylomastoid foramen and its sites of innervation of the facial musculature. Forceps marks below and somewhat distal to the ear and extending over the mandible, failure of one eye to close, Bell's phenomenon, drooling from the mouth, or exposure of one alveolar ridge on grimacing should alert one to this possibility. These nerve palsies usually reverse spontaneously in periods of three to six months. Evidence of return of function is often seen within two to three weeks, but even in those cases in which return of function is delayed for many months, the prognosis for eventual return of good function is excellent. On rare occasions peripheral degeneration is complete and permanent.

PENETRATING LACERATIONS AND STAB WOUNDS

The majority of these lesions in the pediatric age group are due to glass penetrating the out-thrust forearm. These are most likely to affect the palmer surface of the forearm and therefore to damage the median and ulnar nerves. Nerve transection is usually noted at the time of the initial emergency visit, and the wound is often clean and neat. In those cases where a "surgically" divided nerve is found, primary repair is certainly indicated. Care must be used, however, in the selection of cases for primary repair. If the wound is contaminated, nerve repair is delayed for a period of two to six weeks or until all signs of infection and inflammation have disappeared. Delayed exploration is also indicated for the blunt and less neat lacerations, as well as for those injuries that leave the nerve in continuity.[16]

Delay of repair carries with it the risk of allowing the scarred nerve stumps to pull further apart and to make reanastosmosis of the severed ends more difficult. In blunt injuries, however, or in those in which the degree of damage to the nerve cannot be adequately assessed at initial observation, a period of delay will allow neuroma formation at the damaged end of the nerve to become well demarcated. This will permit the surgeon to estimate how much nerve to resect to regain healthy neural structure.

LESIONS IN CONTINUITY

Damage to nerve that results in loss of nerve function but without anatomic disruption of the nerve is usually the result of blunt or abrasive types of injuries. It may occur as a result of the "blast effect" from penetrating gunshot wounds. In each of these types of injury, primary repair is not indicated. Sufficient time must be allowed to pass for potential spontaneous recovery of the lesion. Closed injuries of the peripheral nerves, such as those resulting from fracture of fibula or humerus, are also not explored primarily. In these instances the nerve is far more likely to be contused than lacerated. The extremity is put into a cast and braced, and physiotherapy is used to maintain joint movement and prevent orthopedic deformity. In closed injury, and open injuries with the nerve in continuity, frequent examination is necessary. If the most proximately denervated musculature has not regained function over an appropriate period of observation, nerve exploration may be indicated. The length of the observation period will depend upon the distance between the lesion and the proximal musculature. Timing of exploration of these types of injuries has been described by Kline and Hackett.[13] The decision to operate is usually made within three to four months and may be supported by indication of total nerve conduction block, failure on electromyography (EMG) to show reinnervation potential, and lack of Tinel's sign.

Significant improvement will take place without operation in a gratifyingly high number of these patients. Kline and Bratton[12] recently reported on 20 children with nerve lesions in continuity. Ten of these injuries required no surgical intervention and all showed improvement. Of the 10 children who had surgical treatment, eight showed improvement. In the majority of cases, the

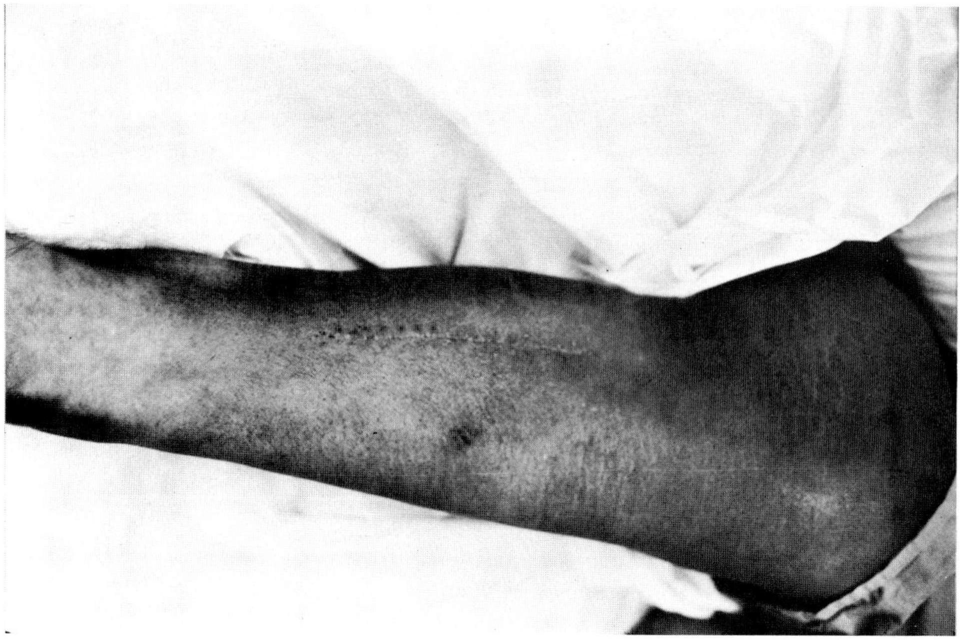

Figure 25-1. Picture of 16-year-old boy showing gunshot wound to the thigh, taken at time of initial neurosurgical evaluation. The bullet had entered the lateral thigh (dark spot) and had lodged in the muscles immediately under the surgical scar.

nerves involved required division and resuture. In several cases neurolysis was carried out without resuturing of the nerve. In this remarkable series, only two of the operated nerves, both of which were sutured, failed to show improvement. The follow-up in these two cases (three months and five months), however was quite short, and it is entirely possible that even these children will show improvement in the future.

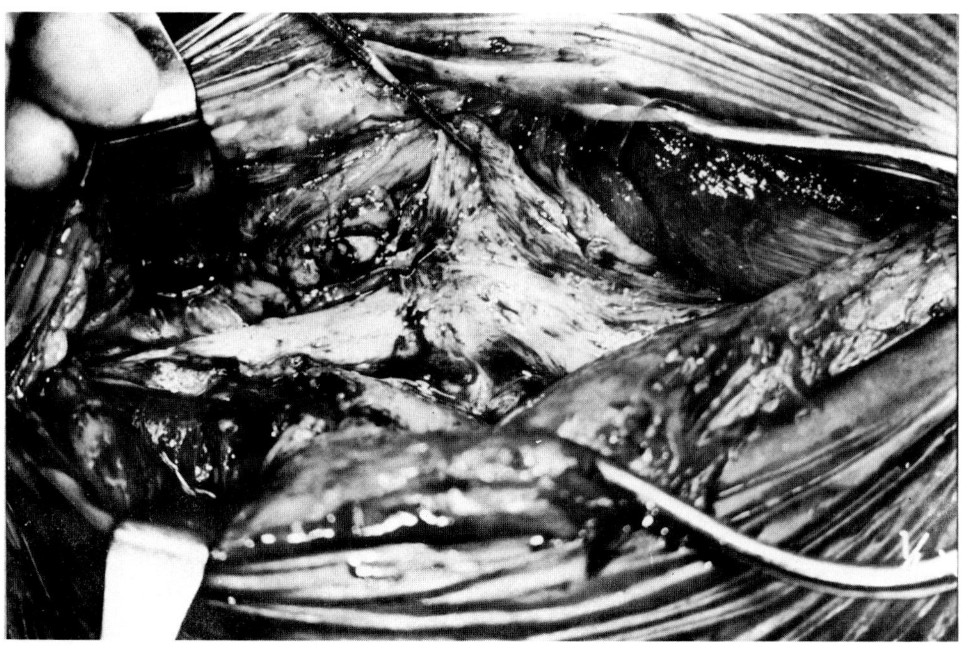

Figure 25-2. Operative photograph showing kinking and scarring of the sciatic nerve. The bullet had not passed through the nerve.

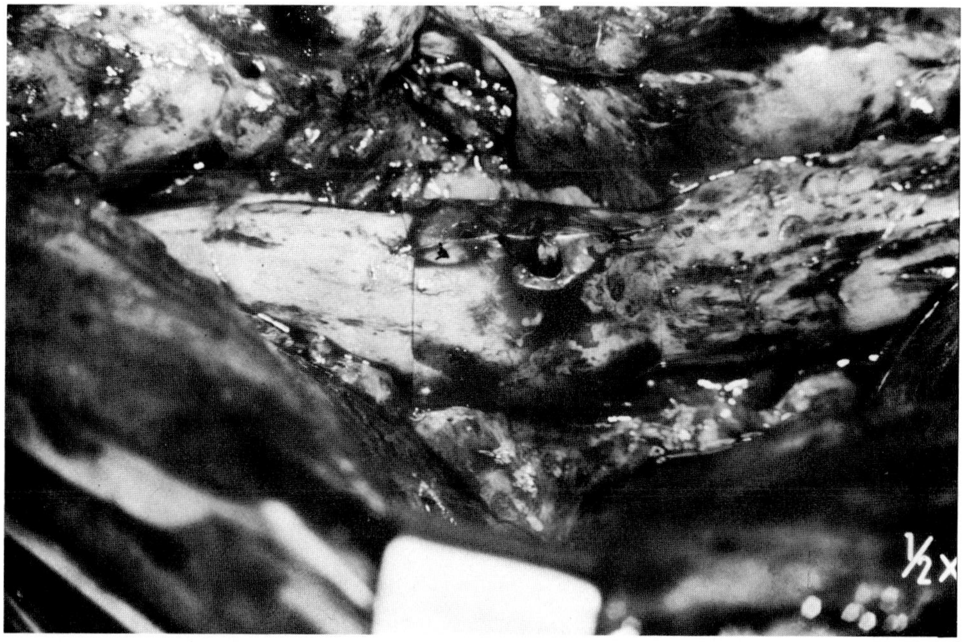

Figure 25-3. Completion of neurolysis. The nerve has been freed of the scar tissue and has resumed a more normal course. A cuff of Silastic has been placed around the area of scarring in an attempt to reduce further scar formation.

CASE 1: E. J.

This 16-year-old boy was involved in a gang fight and sustained a gunshot wound to the thigh. The bullet entered on the lateral aspect of the thigh and traveled in a slightly posterior direction to lodge in the muscles at the posterior thigh. When seen by neurosurgeons, he had already been operated upon by general surgeons and the bullet had been removed (Fig. 25-1). In the four months following operation, there was no evidence of recovery and electrical testing showed a complete block at the level of the bullet wound; operation was elected.

At operation the sciatic nerve was found to be badly kinked and entrapped in dense scar tissue (Fig. 25-2). It did not appear, however, that the nerve was transected and no resection of the nerve was carried out. Instead an extensive neurolysis was done and a Silastic cuff was used to encase the nerve itself (Fig. 25-3).

Three months following operation, conduction across the operative site was found on electrical testing. Recovery progressed slowly, and at six years following operation, there is good posterior tibial nerve function but little common peroneal nerve function. The patient wears a foot brace. Residual numbness to pin prick is present at the lateral border of the foot.

TUMORS AND OTHER MASS LESIONS

The great majority of tumors involving the cranial and peripheral nerves in childhood years are related to von Recklinghausen's disease (also known as Recklinghausen's disease). These tumors are so much more common than others in childhood years as to make any other diagnostic possibility unusual. Other unusual tumors include hemangiomas, glomus tumors, desmoid tumors, and venous malformations. Systemic malignant processes such as lymphomas or carcinomatosis also may infiltrate peripheral nerves. Peripheral nerves may also be damaged by tumors affecting the bony skeleton. These include osteomas, osteoblastomas, osteoid osteoma, and diaphysical aclasis. An unusual case in which a Baker's cyst of the popliteal space compressed the peroneal nerve is reported in Case 2.

Manifestations leading to the diagnosis of von Recklinghausen's disease include multiple café-au-lait spots, subcutaneous and cutaneous neurofibromas, and cystic lesions of the skeleton. Fienman and Yakovac[8] reported that almost half of these children manifest cutaneous stigmata of the disease process at birth. The great majority of these children have shown evidence of the disease before or at the pubertal years. Single neurinomas (neurolemoma, schwannoma), seen in adult years, which are isolated, encapsulated, or partially cystic, are rare in the pediatric age group.

Von Recklinghausen's disease is associated with myriad neurologic defects. The neurinomas may affect the acoustic nerve, segmental nerve roots at all levels intraspinally, nerves to extraocular muscles within the orbit, radial or median nerves in the forearm and upper arm, cervical and brachial plexuses, and sensory nerves within the skin of the scalp, eyelid, cheek, abdomen, neck, and extremities. In addition schwannomas may be located in the gastrointestinal tract, the genitourinary tract, and the respiratory tract, which can cause organ compression symptoms and require excision.

The characteristic lesion is the plexiform neuroma. These lesions extend along many of the fine branches of sensory nerves out into the epithelium itself. Under the skin they are often palpable as a mass of irregular, tubular, structures. Because these tumors tend to stretch along nerves beyond the palpable mass, their true extent may be difficult to assess. Resection frequently leads to further recurrence. Treatment of these tumors is greatly simplified, however, by the absence of axons running through the tumor and is similar in principle to the treatment of solitary benign schwannomas. These children most often are operated upon for cosmetic purposes or because of obstruction in the urinary, alimentary, or respiratory tract.

Intracranial and intraspinal neurinomas should be excised completely as soon as possible as their continued growth may compromise brain or cord function irreversibly.[14] A similar approach should be taken with neurinomas of the orbit, in order to prevent progressive exophthalmus, compression of the optic nerve, or distortion of the extraocular muscles. Lesions of the peripheral nerves in the extremities usually can be removed with sparing of important nerve fibers. Excision of these lesions, using magnification and extreme care, can result in worthwhile relief of nerve compression. The excision may have to be repeated if there is subsequent significant regrowth of the tumor.

Solitary malignant schwannomas, although fortunately rare, do affect those in the pediatric age group. In a large series reported by Brasfield and Das Gupta,[1] 29 of 232 solitary malignant schwannomas occurred before the age of 16. These tumors are generally treated by radical local excision. In addition both radiation therapy and chemotherapy have been reported to be of some value. Das Gupta feels that radical excision is the primary and preferred mode of treatment, to which radiation therapy may be a useful adjunct.[3]

Malignant degeneration in the multiple schwannomas associated with von Recklinghausen's disease in a known common occurrence. Estimates of the rate of malignant degeneration in von Recklinghausen's patients followed for long periods of time run as high as 29 percent.[1] It is generally recognized, however, that most of this malignant transformation takes place in older patients, and it is rare to find a malignant schwannoma in childhood years. Despite the potential for malignant degeneration of each of the plexiform neuromas that a child harbors, radical excision in childhood is not justified on this basis alone.

Neuroma formation following section of a nerve or amputation of a limb may occur in children. A comprehensive clinical review of this entity has been reported by Cieslak and Stout.[2] They found an annoying tendency of these traumatic neuromas to recur after resection. Efforts at stopping this potential for reformation have included caustic and degenerative solutions applied to nerve ends, and wrapping in gold foil, Silastic, etc. The general concensus today is that sharp dissection of the nerve trunk and directing it away from the site of scar formation probably provide as good protection against neuromas as any of the earlier methods.[3,20] When traumatic neuroma follows resection of a nerve tumor, either benign or malignant, it may well be impossible to determine whether mass is a traumatic process or a recurrence of the original tumor.

CASE 2: C. W.

This 12-year-old boy of Chinese extraction first noted a painless swelling behind his knee one year prior to admission. This swelling was located immediately posterior to the head of the fibula, was soft and fluctuant, was not mobile or tender, and had progressively increased in size (Fig. 25-4). During the six months prior to initial evaluation, there had been a gradual but progressive loss of both sensory and motor function of the common peroneal nerve. At initial evaluation there was a complete foot drop and a sensory anesthesia in the peroneal distribution. Electrodiagnostic studies showed denervation in the affected musculature, and there was complete peroneal nerve block at the level of the upper end of the fibula.

At operation a large cystic mass protruding from the posterior surface of the peroneal nerve was found (Fig. 25-5). The cyst was aspirated and approximately 8 cm^3 of light tan, slightly cloudy fluid was removed. Following aspiration greater manipulation of the cyst was possible, and after careful dissection under the microscope it was possible to free the cyst from the surface of the peroneal nerve. The cyst was then found to enter the joint interspace. The diagnosis on pathology examination confirmed the operative impression of Baker's cyst. Recovery in the

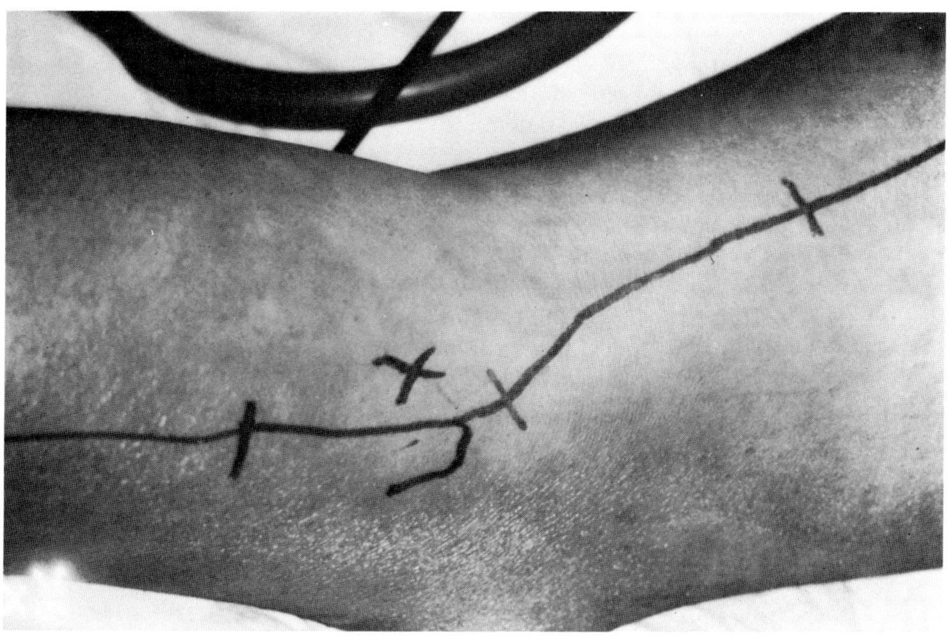

Figure 25-4. Photograph of 12-year-old boy taken at operation, where the "X" represents the top of the fluctuant mass. It is seen to be immediately posterior to the head of the fibula, which is outlined. The linear marking represents the incision that was used to explore this nerve.

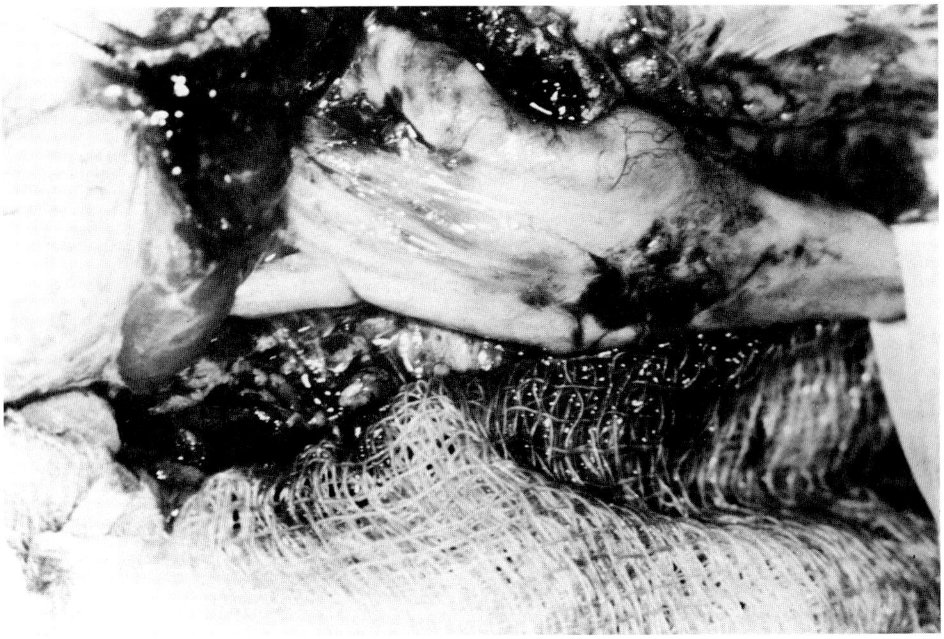

Figure 25-5. Cystic lesion found upon exploration of the peroneal nerve. A tape has been placed around the proximal portion of the nerve (to the right). The cyst was thin-walled and translucent. Nerve kinking distally is noted (to left). With careful dissection the nerve was freed of the cyst, and partial recovery occurred.

peroneal nerve progressed slowly and at three years after operation it was functionally useful but not complete.

IATROGENIC NERVE LESIONS

Iatrogenic nerve lesions may pose difficult diagnostic problems and serious dilemmas for management, as well as embarrassment to the physician. They also provide almost certain medical–legal implication. Inadvertent damage to nerves may occur following application of a cast to an extremity, subsequent to operations for other lesions in the extremities or around the brachial plexus, and as a result of intramuscular injections.

The compressive neuropathy that follows a poorly applied plaster cast usually is seen in the ulnar or peroneal nerves. These lesions are always in continuity and good recovery can be expected if the compression is promptly relieved and the patient carefully followed. In rare cases reinnervation will not take place and these lesions may occasionally need surgical exploration.

Nerve palsy following operation in the extremity or around the brachial plexus may not necessarily indicate that the nerve has been transected. At operation the peripheral nerve may have become involved in abnormal kinking or transposition, or be surrounded by a suture. Late appearance of peripheral nerve lesions may represent involvement of the nerve in a scar formation. When such a lesion is noted immediately following surgery, prompt reexploration is indicated. If the nerve is divided, it is usually a clean and sharp division and immediate resuture is appropriate. Relief of kinking or release of a surrounding ligature will also quickly restore nerve function. When late nerve palsy occurs due to scarring, exploration and resection of the scar and attempt at repositioning the nerve at a distance from the area of scar formation are often helpful.

Nerve lesions following injections are problems that occur almost entirely in childhood years.[15] They occur most frequently in uncooperative squirming infants who move at the last minute as the injection is being administered. The most common nerve involved is the sciatic, usually just distal to the sciatic notch. This lesion generally produces a painful response of tremendous intensity. When this occurs immediate examination will reveal loss of sensory and motor function in the affected nerve distribution. Very often the nerve lesion is discovered only at some time distant to the injection, usually because the child was unable to describe the pain and neural loss. The vast majority of injection injuries are partial and recovery occurs spontaneously.[16] If there is evidence of sensory or motor function through the site of injury immediately following traumatic injection, the prognosis for satisfactory recovery is good. This recovery may take place very slowly and may progress for as long as two years before reaching a maximum. If there is no function at the time of injection, and if this condition persists for three months after the injury, prognosis for subsequent recovery is poor. When this occurs operative exploration should be carried out. While it is always tempting to wait a little longer to see if recovery will occur, little is lost, and possibly substantial gain made, by early careful exploration of the injured nerve.[15]

Matson[15,16] felt that early lysis of perineural scarring was often followed by functional return that was both accelerated in recovery rate and increased in final recovery extent. When total nerve destruction is found at operation, attempt at resuturing and nerve reconstruction should be carried out.

The difficulties in mangement of an iatrogenic lesion are well seen in the following case.

CASE 3: E. W.

This 10½-year-old girl first came to medical attention at the age of 9. At that time she complained of "clicking" in her knee on walking and difficulty with running. She was seen in orthopedic consultation and a diagnosis of lateral meniscus tear was

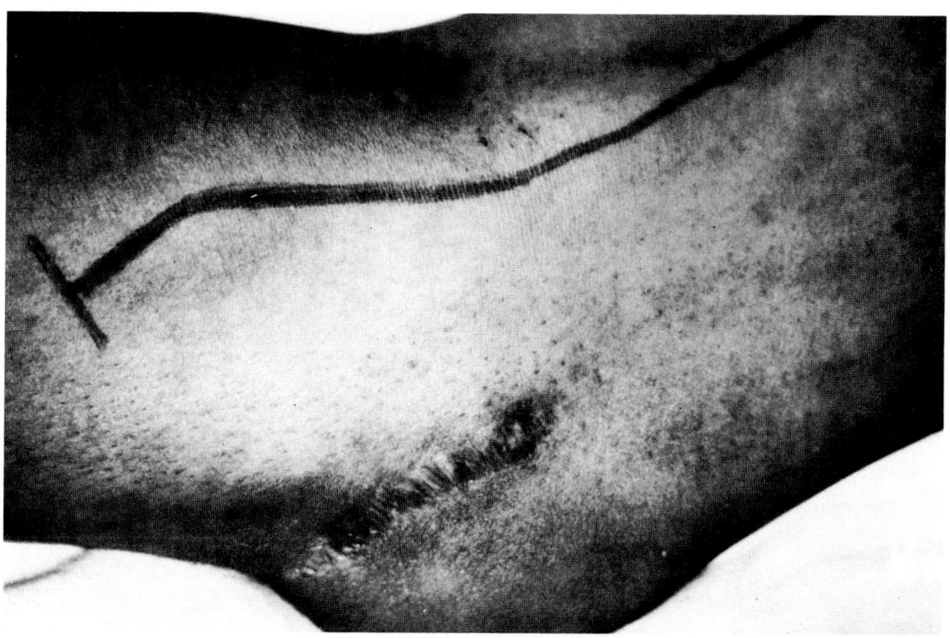

Figure 25-6. Lateral view of knee taken at operation. The surgical scar is the menisectomy incision. Linear mark is the incision to explore the peroneal nerve.

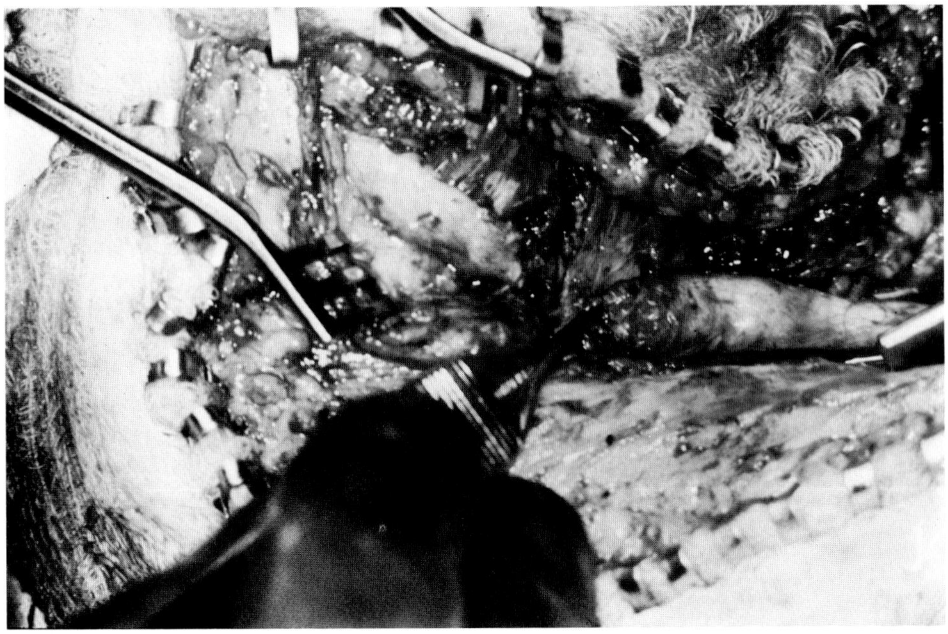

Figure 25-7. Total division of peroneal nerve seen at operation. The nerve is scarred distally (left), and there is a neuroma on the proximal portion (right). The knee has been somewhat flexed to gain length. Greater flexion and dissection into parent nerve were required to bridge the gap. Almost all of the proximal nerve seen in this picture had to be resected to reach healthy neural tissue.

made following diagnostic procedures, including arthroscopy. The child was operated upon and a lateral menisectomy was performed. Following this procedure the leg was placed in a full leg cast. On the morning after operation, it was noted that the child had a complete foot drop and sensory deficits consistent with a common peroneal nerve section. It was felt that this was due to improper casting; the cast was immediately removed, additional padding placed around the leg, and a

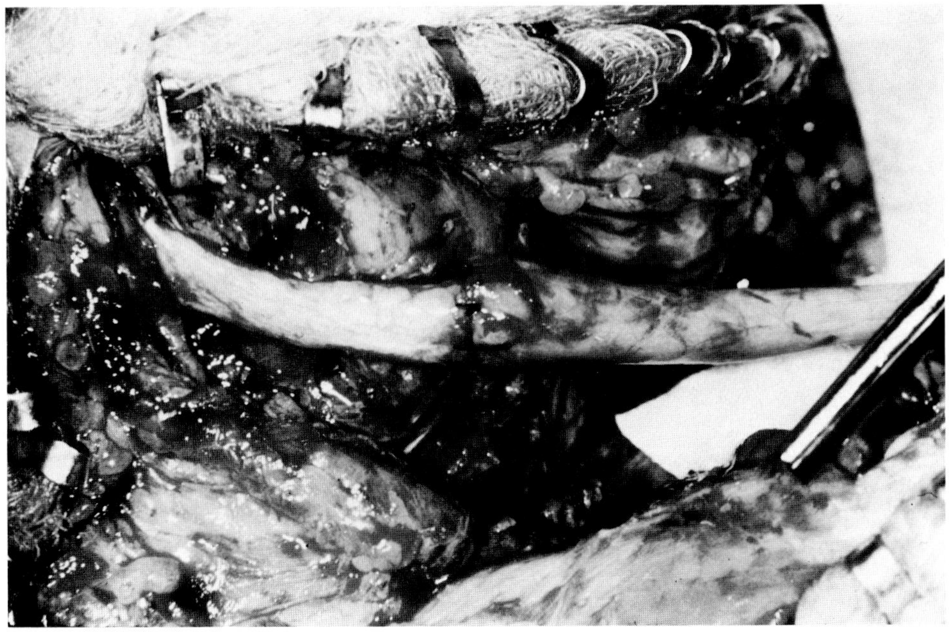

Figure 25-8. Picture taken during epineural repair of peroneal nerve. Several sutures have been placed around nerve, and further sutures are then taken in between these.

new cast applied. There was no recovery in the year following this operation. The postoperative management was complicated by the institution of a lawsuit and the death in a car accident of the orthopedic surgeon involved.

The child was first seen in neurosurgical consultation 19 months following her operation. Total peroneal nerve palsy and sensory loss were found. There was no evidence of reinnervation of EMG of the affected muscles, and there was no nerve conduction across the upper end of the common peroneal nerve. Because of these findings, operation was elected.

At operation (Fig. 25-6) the nerve was found to be completely divided. The distal portion of the nerve was embedded in scar tissue and the proximal portion had retracted well up into the lower thigh and had a large neuroma (Fig. 25-7). The extent of resection necessary to arrive at healthy nerve tissue left a gap of approximately 8 cm. The nerve was dissected well up into the parent sciatic nerve and the knee was flexed at an angle of slightly more than 90 degrees. Epineurial resuturing of the nerve was carried out (Fig. 25-8). The child was placed in a turnbuckle cast, which was gradually lengthened at weekly periods in the ensuing months.

Despite the long length of time after the nerve lesion, clear atrophy of the distal musculature, long nerve gap to be bridged, and unquestionable tension on the nerve following suture, almost complete recovery took place. The child is functionally intact three years after operation, with little or no sensory or motor deficit. This degree of recovery would be surprising in an adult.

TECHNIQUES OF NERVE REPAIR

Recent developments in both microscopic techniques and use of intrafasicular nerve surgery and grafting have radically changed operative approaches (but perhaps not results) following peripheral nerve lesions. The surgical techniques involved in children are identical with those involved in adult years. The techniques of nerve repair recently were excellently reviewed by Kline.[11] He points out that most of the nerve is connective tissue, which constitutes up to 60% of the volume of the nerve. Management of this connective tissue is the key to successful nerve repair. Understanding of the connective tissue structures within the nerve facilitates operative intervention.

Epineurium, a tough sheath of collogen, elastin, and fibroblasts, surrounds the entire nerve. The perineurium surrounds each of the nerve fasicles and may enclose bundles of one to 20 fasicles. Fasicular arrangement is variable at different longitudinal levels within the same nerve. Rearrangement of these fasicles occurs from centimeter to centimeter along the course of the nerve. Sensory and motor fibers are more intermingled proximally than distally.

The endoneurium within the fasicles surrounds each myelinated fiber as well as groups of unmyelinated fibers. The importance of this portion of the connective tissue of the nerve is often overlooked. In Kline's view intrafasicular scar, more than perineural or epineural scar, is responsible for disorganization and poor regeneration seen with most serious nerve injuries.[10,11]

Epineural suture remains the most commonly used operative technique for reconstitution of divided nerves. Despite current enthusiasm for use of the microscope, magnification with 2.5× power loops is usually more than adequate for epineural repair.

Dissection of nerve lesions should always proceed from the normal portion of the nerve toward the abnormal. Intraoperative nerve conduction testing can be extremely helpful in deciding whether or not the nerve is totally divided. Both neurinomas in continuity and stump neuromas or gliomas should be resected carefully until the fasicular structure is healthy. The intrafasicular structures should "pout" from the line of the nerve resection and the epineurium should slip back and forth over the fasicular bundles. Hemostasis must be meticulous and absolute. The fasicular pattern of the divided nerve must be carefully noted and must be matched as closely as possible to the pattern seen in the distal portion of the nerve. The alignment of subepineural blood vessels may be used as a guide in the placement of sutures. Kinking, overriding, and poor alignment of the divided nerves will complicate regeneration of fibers and must be avoided.

Several methods may be employed to gain length of nerve repair. The nerve may be freed longitudinally, and this may be aided by dissection up into parent nerves when necessary. Unimportant nerve branches, such as those to joints, may be sacrificed to gain length. Transposition of nerves may be useful. The extremity may be flexed to a limited extent, usually not to exceed 90 degrees, to gain additional length. Distraction of the sutured nerve is a leading cause of regeneration failure, second only to failure to exclude all of the scarred tissue at the time of nerve resection.

Fasicular repair and interfasicular grafting have an increasing number of proponents.[11,17–19] The introduction of the operating microscope, and familiarity of an increasing number of surgeons with this technique, have aided in the growth of these two methods. Interfasicular nerve grafts are generally reserved for gaps in resected nerves that cannot be made up more easily by classical maneuvers to regain length.[11] Interfasicular grafting usually uses the sural nerve as the grafted element. The technique and results with interfasicular nerve grafting of median and ulnar nerves are well described by Millesi, Meissl, and Berger.[17]

Neurolysis is carried out when nerve resection is not practical or possible. Sharp dissection of epineurial and subepineurial scar can be carried out under loop magnification. Following removal of scar tissue from the perineurial and epineurial spaces, it is important to place the nerve in a healthy bed of muscle or fat in an effort to reduce further scar formation around the nerve.[20] Perhaps the most important factor in reducing scar formation is meticulous hemostasis, as residual blood clot surrounding the nerve will certainly lead to reformation of scar.

REFERENCES

1. Brasfield RD, Das Gupta TK: Von Recklinghausen's disease: A clinicopathological study. Ann Surg 175:86–104, 1972
2. Cieslak AK, Stout AP: Traumatic and amputation neuromas. Arch Surg 53:646–651, 1946
3. Das Gupta TK: Tumors of the peripheral nerves. Clin Neurosurg 25:574–590, 1978
4. Das Gupta TK, Brasfield RD: Amputation neuromas in cancer patients. NY State J Med 69:2129–2132, 1969
5. Duchenne GBA: De l'Electrisation Localisee et Son Application à la Pathologie et a la Therapeutique (ed 3). Paris, JB Bailliere & Fils, 1872
6. Ducker TB: Metabolic factors in surgery of peripheral nerves. Surg Clin N Am 52:1109–1122, 1972
7. Erb WH: Diseases of the peripheral cerebrospinal nerves, in Von Ziemssen H (ed): Cyclopaedia of the Practice of Medicine. New York, William Wood & Co, 1876
8. Fienman NL, Yakovac WC: Neurofibromatosis in childhood. J Pediatr 76:339–346, 1970
9. Kline DG: Operative management of major nerve lesions of the lower extremity. Surg Clin N Am 52:1247–1265, 1972
10. Kline DG: Logical and clinical factors contributing to the timing of nerve repair. Clin Neurosurg 24:425–455, 1977
11. Kline DG: Macroscopic and microscopic concomitants of nerve repair. Clin Neurosurg 26:582–606, 1979

12. Kline DG, Bratton BR: Management of peripheral nerve lesions in infants and children, in O'Brien MS (ed): Pediatric Neurological Surgery. New York, Raven Press, 1978, pp 173–192
13. Kline DG, Hackett ER: Reappraisal of timing for exploration of civilian peripheral nerve injuries. Surgery 78:54–65, 1975
14. Klumpke A: Contribution a l'etude des paralysies radiculaires due plexus brachial. Rev Med 5:591–616, 739–790, 1885
15. Matson DD: Early neurolysis in the treatment of injury of the peripheral nerves due to faulty injection of antibiotics. N Engl J Med 242:973–975, 1950
16. Matson DD: Peripheral nerve injury, in Matson CC (ed): Neurosurgery of Infancy in Childhood. Springfield, Charles C Thomas, 1969, pp 381–400
17. Millesi H, Meissl G, Berger A: The interfasicular nerve grafting of the median and ulnar nerves. J Bone Jt Surg (Br) 54:727–750, 1972
18. Samii M: Modern aspects of peripheral and cranial nerve surgery, in Krayenbuhl H (ed): Advances and Technical Standards in Neurosurgery. New York, Springer-Verlag, 1975, pp 33–80
19. Sunderland S: Fasicular suture and fasicular exclusion in the repair of severed nerves. Br J Surg 40:580–587, 1953
20. Sunderland S: Nerves and Nerve Injuries, London, E & S Livingstone, 1968, chaps 47–51
21. Wickstrom J, Haslam E, Hutchison R: The surgical management of residual deformities of the shoulder following birth injuries of the brachial plexus. J Bone Jt Surg 37A:27–36, 1955

IV NEOPLASMS

26. Survey of Pediatric Brain Tumors

Leonard Bruno
Luis Schut

Pediatric brain tumors constitute a significant portion of neoplasia, or 40 to 50 percent of all solid tumors, in the population under 15 years of age. Incidence figures from population studies in the United States surveyed under auspices of the National Cancer Institute[1] or from tumor registries of states or counties,[2] as well as from population studies in Denmark,[3] Finland,[4] Australia,[5] and other countries,[6] show the incidence to be remarkably consistent from one population group to another, averaging two to five cases per 100,000 per year. This incidence figure compares favorably with that of 2.17 per 100,000 per year reported from the Connecticut Tumor Registry consisting of a large population, whereas a much smaller population in Rochester, Minnesota, yielded an incidence of 5.01 per 100,000 per year.[7] The true incidence is probably between these two figures, emphasizing the influence of sample size. From these incidence figures, approximately 1400 new cases of central nervous system (CNS) malignancy in children can be predicted each year in the United States.

Gliomas are the most common pediatric brain tumors, accounting for greater that 70 percent,[3–6,8–15] or about 1000 cases each year.

Pediatric brain tumors are predominantly infratentorial and differ from those seen in adults. Data from studies with 87 cases,[16] 427 cases,[17] and 750 cases[18,19] all show posterior fossa tumors accounting for 54–70 percent of the pediatric brain tumors with the average at 60 percent.[8–10,16–18,20–24] More recent studies from well-defined population groups in Denmark and Finland indicate the incidence of posterior fossa tumors to be 59 percent and 54 percent respectively.[3,4] Data from the Children's Hospital of Philadelphia for 1968–1977 were compared with data from the Children's Memorial Hospital in Chicago and the Hospital for Sick Children in Toronto.[13–15] Analysis of these data from the total 1350 patients yielded a weighted average for posterior fossa tumors of 54.7 percent of all pediatric brain tumors. Our data from these three major children's hospitals in North America reveal that cerebellar astrocytoma, medulloblastoma, and brain-stem glioma have similar incidences (see Table 26-1). These

Table 26-1
Incidence of Types of Pediatric Brain Tumors

	Children's Hospital of Philadelphia	Children's Memorial Hospital, Chicago	Hospital for Sick Children, Toronto	Walker[9] (from Matson[19])
Dates of survey	10 years, 1968–1977	12 years, 1967–1978	25 years, 1950–1975	
Total number of tumors (1350)	(250)	(305)	(795)	
Average incidence per year	25/year	25.4/year	31.8/year	
Infratentorial—total %	55	46	57	66
Cerebellar astrocytoma	17	12	15	20
Medulloblastoma	13	17	14	18
Brain-stem glioma	17	11	16	10
Ependymoma	3	3	7	8
Other	5	3	5	10
Supratentorial—total %	45	53	43	33
Benign astrocytoma	14	17	12	8
Malignant astrocytoma	11	12	11	6
Ependymoma	5	3	2	6
Craniopharyngioma	6	9	6	5
Dysgerminoma	1	2	2	4
Other	8	10	10	4

figures differ from those review data presented by other authors in the past.[9,18–20] The apparent discrepancy in incidence figures for brain-stem glioma and supratentorial astrocytoma in our data compared with data of Matson[18,19] or Walker[9] may be due in large part to the advent of computerized axial tomographic (CAT) scanning since 1975, which allows more definitive early diagnosis of brain-stem lesions not necessitating autopsy confirmation. The availability of CAT scanning has also caused a change in referral pattern, in that patients with CNS lesions are now more easily diagnosed than with pneumoencephalography and arteriography. They are therefore frequently referred to children's hospitals for definitive neurosurgical treatment after having been correctly diagnosed elsewhere at an earlier stage in their illness than previously. The number and types of pediatric brain tumors found are certainly more accurate than at any time prior to the widespread availability of computerized tomography.

Two further points should be clarified with respect to race and sex as they relate to incidence. Comparison of incidence figures from North America, Europe, Africa, and Asia indicates that while the number of pediatric brain tumors developing in each population group is remarkably similar, that is, 2.1 to 2.5 per 100,000 per year,[1,3–7,11,25,26] the type of tumor diagnosed differs widely from one racial group to another.[6,21,22] In general cerebellar astrocytomas and medulloblastomas are more common in North America and Europe, whereas craniopharyngiomas and pinealoma have a higher incidence in Africa and Japan, with ependymoma more common in India than elsewhere; see Table 26-2.[6] Comparison of North American, European, and African data indicates a significantly smaller incidence of medulloblastoma in blacks (4.5–11 percent) versus whites (14–25 percent), including data gathered in mixed racial populations both in the United States and Africa.[1–7,11,25,26] One study done in the city of Baltimore, Maryland, from 1960 to 1975 showed an incidence of medulloblastoma in black children of 14 percent of all CNS lesions, but again this must be considered in light of possible errors due to sample size and the bias of de facto regionalization of health care in the Baltimore area prior to CT scanning.[27]

Table 26-2
Incidence of Major Tumor Types

Tumor Type	Incidence from Walker[9]	Incidence from Table 26-1	Incidence Worldwide from Survey[6]	Unusual Incidence by Location[6]
Cerebellar astrocytoma	20%	12–17%	All astrocytomas 26–38%	All astrocytomas 15% Japan
Medulloblastoma	18%	13–17%	14–25%	11% Africa
Ependymoma	8%	3–7%	9–11%	19% India
Craniopharyngioma	5%	6–9%	6–9%	18% Africa 16% Japan

Finally overall incidence may be the same for boys and girls if ages 0 to 15 years are included. Males versus females have a 1.2 to 1.0 incidence of brain tumors from age 0 to 10 years, and females predominate 1.1 to 1.0 over males from age 10 to 15.[2,4,18,20] Analysis of population data indicate, however, that tumor incidence is equal for males and females, with sexual predominance merely a reflection of the normal population sex ratio at any point in time.[2,4,7]

Diagnosis of intracranial neoplasms in children has changed dramatically since Harvey Cushing's early report in 1927[20] on the diagnosis and treatment of 18 patients with brain tumors. The diagnosis at that time was predicated on enlargement of the head, positive Macewen's sign on percussion, and the occurrence of malaise and vomiting, failing vision, and gait unsteadiness. His diagnostic armamentarium, which was limited to skull x-rays, along with neurologic examination and examination of the eye grounds for papilledema, was the basis for exploratory surgery. Because of late diagnosis and surgery under local anesthesia, patients frequently had serious neurologic deficit resulting from the surgery even if the disease entity, such as cerebellar astrocytoma, was consistent with long-term survival. Cushing was willing to say that his results were unequivocally excellent, and moreover that his results improved year by year, depending on the sharpening of diagnostic skill and the increased knowledge of the natural history of these lesions.[20] Diagnosis of brain tumors in children improved dramatically with the advent of ventriculography and pneumoencephalography in the 1930s,[24] was refined by the addition of angiography in the 1940s,[21] and was complemented by the widespread use of radionuclide scanning in the 1950s and 1960s.[19] The introduction of CAT scanning in the mid-1970s however, has truly revolutionized the diagnosis of these lesions.[9,28,29] Walker suggested in 1976[9] that CAT scanning has come to be the first, most important, and most useful diagnostic procedure in evaluating children with suspected brain tumors. It is highly accurate in delineating and characterizing new or recurrent tumors.[29] Findings by CAT scan of solid or cystic tumors frequently correlate with histologic categorization and, in such cases, prognostic information can be derived from the CAT scan appearance.[30] Computerized tomography (CT, CAT) is completely replacing pneumoencephalography, myelography, and angiography for the initial evaluation of patients with possible tumors of the posterior fossa.[28] The accuracy of diagnosis and detection of posterior fossa lesions with CT scan is extremely high, between 91 and 98 percent.[28] Although with contrast enhancement characteristics of posterior fossa lesions do *not* correlate with degree of malignancy,[31] overall CT characteristics of posterior fossa lesions, including location, presence of cyst, and enhancement characteristics, allow accurate diagnosis as to histologic type as well as tumor location in greater than 90 percent of all patients examined.[29] If the two most likely histologic diagnoses are considered, the accuracy increases to greater than 96 percent.

The diagnosis and treatment of pediatric brain tumors, and especially infratentorial lesions, previously have been limited because of the difficulty with morbidity of neurodiagnostic procedures and surgical outcome. In the early days of pediatric neurosurgery, there was a reluctance of the medical community to treat children vigorously because of the poor surgical outcome, real or imagined, for what was considered a rapidly progressive malignant process.[9,19–21,24] Since the 1950s our understanding of the natural history of pediatric brain tumors, and marked improvement in surgical technique, anesthesia, and postoperative intensive care of pediatric neurosurgical patients have dramatically changed the outlook and prognosis for this group of patients.[9,19,33–35] Bucy and Thieman[33] in their review of cerebellar astrocytoma patients operated on prior to 1938 revealed a 23 percent operative mortality, which is similar to that reported by Cushing of approximately 30 percent.[21,36] Geissinger and Bucy[32] then reported that their patients operated on after 1938 had a 3.8 percent operative mortality, which is almost twice that of our experience at the Children's Hospital of Philadelphia where operative mortality for posterior fossa surgery since 1968 has been less than 2 percent. Variations of treatment with respect both to surgical technique and to postoperative care are discussed in detail for individual tumor types as defined by histologic criteria in Chapter 27–30.

In summary, pediatric brain tumors constitute a major portion of neoplasia in childhood. Current incidence figures indicate that about 45 percent of all pediatric brain tumors are supratentorial, and 55 percent infratentorial, with gliomas still comprising about 70 percent of all lesions. Computerized tomographic scanning has significantly increased our diagnostic accuracy while lowering both diagnostic and surgical morbidity, and therefore mortality. Advances in anesthetic technique coupled with surgical technical improvements such as bipolar cautery and microsurgical technique, and intensive preoperative and postoperative care, have brought operative morbidity and mortality into a clearly acceptable range of less than 2 percent. Our challenge for the future is in better understanding of the biologic nature of, and therefore in obtaining better control or cure of, the neoplastic process itself, which all too often hampers the lives of our little patients.

REFERENCES

1. Young JL, Miller RW: Incidence of malignant tumors in U.S. children. J Pediatr 86:254–258, 1975
2. Farwell JR, Dohrmann GJ, Flannery JT: Central nervous system tumors in children. Cancer 40:3123–3132, 1977
3. Gjerris F, Harmsen A, Klinken L, et al: Incidence and long-term survival of children with intracranial tumors treated in Denmark, 1935–1959. Br J Cancer 38:442–451, 1978
4. Heiskanen O: Intracranial tumors of children. Child's Brain 3:69–78, 1977
5. Hooper R: Intracranial tumors in childhood. Child's Brain 1:136–140, 1975
6. Dohnmann GJ, Farwell JR: Intracranial neoplasms in children: A comparison of North America, Europe, Africa and Asia. Dis Nerv Syst 37:696–698, 1976
7. Schoenberg BS, Schoenberg DG, Christine BW, et al: The epidemiology of primary intracranial neoplasms of childhood. Mayo Clin Proc 51:51–56, 1976
8. Allen JC: Chemotherapy for primary brain tumors. Ped Annal 7(12):81–85, 1978
9. Walker MD: Diagnosis and treatment of brain tumors. Pediatr Clin N Am 23:131–146, 1976
10. Schiffer D: Morbid anatomy of the tumors of the posterior fossa in childhood. Mod Probl Pediatr 18:3–9, 1977

11. Pasteur DK, Lalitha VS: Pathological analysis of intracranial space-occupying lesions in 100 cases including children. Part 2. Incidence, types and unusual cases of glioma. J Neurol Sci 8:143–170, 1968
12. Cushing H: Experiences with the cerebellar astrocytomas. Surg Gynec Obstet 52:129–201, 1931
13. Raimondi A: Personal communication, 1979
14. Humphreys RP: Posterior cranial fossa tumors in children, in Youmans JR (ed): Neurological Surgery. Philadelphia, WB Saunders, in press
15. Hoffman HJ: Personal communication, 1979
16. Gold JA, Smith KR: Childhood brain tumors: A 15-year survey of treatment in a university pediatric hospital. S Med J 68:1337–1344, 1975
17. Keith HW, Mck Craig W, Kernohan JW: Brain tumors in children. Pediatrics 3:839–844, 1949
18. Matson DD: Neurosurgery of Infancy and Childhood. Springfield, Charles C Thomas, 1969
19. Matson DD: Surgery of posterior fossa tumors in childhood. Clin Neurosurg 15:247–264, 1968
20. Cushing H: The intracranial tumors of preadolescence. Am J Dis Child 33(4):551–584, 1927
21. Walker AE, Hopple TL: Brain tumors in children. J Pediatr 35(6):671–687, 1949
22. Rubinstein LJ: Tumors of the central nervous system, fasc 6, in: Atlas of Tumor Pathology. Washington, Armed Forces Institute of Pathology, 1972
23. Smith WA, Fincher EF: Intracranial tumors in children. S Med J 35(6):547–554, 1942
24. Bailey P, Buchanan DN, Bucy PC: Intracranial Tumors of Infancy and Childhood. Chicago, University of Chicago Press, 1939
25. Levy LF, Auchterlouie MB: Primary cerebral neoplasia in Rhodesia. Int Surg 60:286–292, 1975
26. Templeton AC: Tumours of the brain. Rec Prog Cancer Res 41:200–202, 1973
27. Gold EB, Gordis L: Patterns of incidence of brain tumors in children. Ann Neurol 5:565–568, 1979
28. Nardich TP, Lin JP, Leeds NE, et al: Primary tumors and other masses of the cerebellum and fourth ventricle: Differential diagnosis by computed tomography. Neuroradiology, 14:153–174, 1977
29. Zimmerman RA, Bilaniuk CT, Bruno LA, et al: Computed tomography of cerebellar astrocytoma. Am J Roentgenol 130:929–933, 1978
30. Winston K, Gilles FH, Leviton A, et al: Cerebellar gliomas in children. J Nat Cancer Inst 58:833–838, 1977
31. Butler AR, Horii SC, Kricheff II, et al: Computed tomography in astrocytomas. Radiology 129:433–439, 1978
32. Geissinger JD, Bucy PC: Astrocytomas of the cerebellum in children. Int J Neurol 7(2):103–107, 1970
33. Bucy PC, Thieman PW: Astrocytomas of the cerebellum. Arch Neurol 18:14–19, 1968
34. Elridge AR: Long-term survival in the astrocytoma series. J Neurosurg 25:399–404, 1968
35. Gjerris F: Clinical aspects and long-term prognosis of infratentorial intracranial tumors in infancy and childhood. Acta Neurol Scand 57:31–52, 1978
36. Cushing H: Experiences with the cerebellar astrocytomas. Surg Gynec Obstet 52:129–204, 1931

27. Cerebellar Astrocytoma

Leonard Bruno
Luis Schut
Derek A. Bruce

Cerebellar astrocytoma is one of the more common neoplasms of childhood. Older incidence figures based largely on series of cases from single clinics or hospital populations indicated that posterior fossa tumors in general accounted for two thirds (67 percent) of all pediatric brain tumors, and that cerebellar astrocytoma was the largest single group of tumors in this location, thereby making them the most common brain tumor found in children (Table 27-1).[1–10] Recently gathered more accurate tumor data based on population studies[11–14] and our own collation of 1350 cases of brain tumors in children in North America[15–17] indicate that posterior fossa tumors account for only 54 percent of all intracranial neoplasms in children under 15 years of age throughout the world. In addition cerebellar astrocytoma accounts for less than one third of these posterior fossa lesions in most series, or 12 to 17 percent of all intracranial neoplasia, and is about equal in incidence to medulloblastoma, brain-stem glioma, and benign supratentorial astrocytoma according to our data (Table 27-2).

The clinical presentation of children with cerebellar astrocytoma is the same as that for children harboring any posterior fossa mass lesion, in that symptoms are produced as a result of increased intracranial pressure.[18] Relatively minor focal neurologic deficits tend to be ignored by children and parents alike, and because of the tremendous compensation afforded by the developing brain and cranial structures, tumors often remain asymptomatic until obstruction of cerebrospinal fluid pathways occurs.[5] Prior to diagnosis, cerebellar astrocytomas may produce symptoms over a period of several weeks to three years.[1,3,5,19]

Headache, while perhaps the most common symptom in children with cerebellar tumors, is overlooked because it is a non-specific complaint that in many instances cannot be adequately described by the patient. Sinister features of childhood headache include pain that awakens the patient from sleep, begins

Table 27-1
Incidence of Pediatric Brain Tumors

	Walker[1] (from Matson[2,3])
Total number of tumors	661
Infratentorial—total % 66	
Cerebellar astrocytoma	20
Medulloblastoma	18
Brain-stem glioma	10
Ependymoma	8
Other	10
Supratentorial—total % 33	
Benign astrocytoma	8
Malignant astrocytoma	6
Ependymoma	6
Craniopharyngioma	5
Dysgerminoma	4
Other	4

on awakening, or is confined to early morning and subsides with activity. Examination will reveal papilledema in most children over 2 years of age with these complaints. Cephalgia that presents in this manner warrants further investigation.[1–5,10,18]

Vomiting is common as a presenting complaint of children with cerebellar astrocytoma. Most often such vomiting tends to be confined to early morning and is not associated with nausea.[3,4,10,19] If accompanied by headache, vomiting many times reduces associated head pain that may be a result of hyperventilation during emesis, which in turn reduces intracranial pressure.[18] Vomiting may be due to direct tumor involvement of the fourth ventricle and can be associated with intense and persistent nausea.[5] With present-day diagnostic capability and the relative ease of obtaining computerized tomography (CT), all children with persistent vomiting should be evaluated for the possibility of a brain tumor as part of a thorough workup before a presumptive diagnosis of gastrointestinal or psychiatric disorder can be made.

Gait disturbances, including staggering, frequent falls, or a broad-based stance, are the third most common presenting symptom of children with cerebellar astrocytoma.[1–3,5,10,19] Examination of these children frequently reveals nystagmus, dysmetria, or dysdiadokinesis, some head tilt or neck stiffness, or

Table 27-2
Incidence of Pediatric Brain Tumors

	Children's Hospital of Philadelphia 1968–1977	Children's Memorial Hospital, Chicago 1967–1978	Hospital for Sick Children, Toronto 1950–1975
Total number of tumors (1350)	250	305	795
Infratentorial location (percent of total)	55	46	57
Cerebellar astrocytoma (percent of total)	17	12	15
Medulloblastoma (percent of total)	13	17	14
Brain-stem glioma (percent of total)	17	11	16
Supratentorial benign astrocytoma (percent of total)	14	17	12

truncal ataxia. These signs are obviously of great significance and require that the patient be further evaluated at the earliest convenience.

Presentation of posterior fossa tumors in children under 2 years of age mimics obstructive hydrocephalus.[5,10,18] Head enlargement and a bulging fontanel can be the first signs of a brain tumor, but a careful medical history often reveals that the child is unusually irritable, vomits frequently, and fails to attain normal milestones, especially with respect to motor coordination, standing, and walking. Cerebellar astrocytomas are much less common in children under 2 years of age than other types of tumor,[3,10] but in all instances, despite our present diagnostic capability from CT, definitive diagnoses can be made only at surgery.

Diagnostic procedures for evaluation of patients with suspected cerebellar astrocytoma have been completely revolutionized since the general use of computerized axial tomography (CAT, CT) scanning began in 1975. Procedures used prior to that time included skull x-rays, ventriculography, angiography, and isotope brain scanning.[1,3,18] The majority of our patients are now evaluated by obtaining a history and neurologic examination followed by a CAT scan as the only diagnostic test prior to surgery. Review of our own data[20] and that of other centers[21] indicates a diagnostic accuracy using this format of 96 to 98 percent.

Cerebellar astrocytoma has a characteristic spectrum of CT findings, allowing not only initial correct diagnosis and delineation, but detection of the recurrent tumor long before it produces symptoms.[20] In our series of newly diagnosed patients, we found hydrocephalus present in every case. These tumors appear either cystic or solid by CT and tend to be large at the time of diagnosis, with cystic tumors 4.0 and 5.6 cm in diameter and solid ones 2.0 to 4.8 cm (Figs. 27-1 and 27-2). Half of all cystic cerebellar astrocytomas have a mural nodule of tumor tissue that demonstrates marked contrast enhancement on CT, with the nonenhancing wall of the cyst composed of either a layer of reactive nonneoplas-

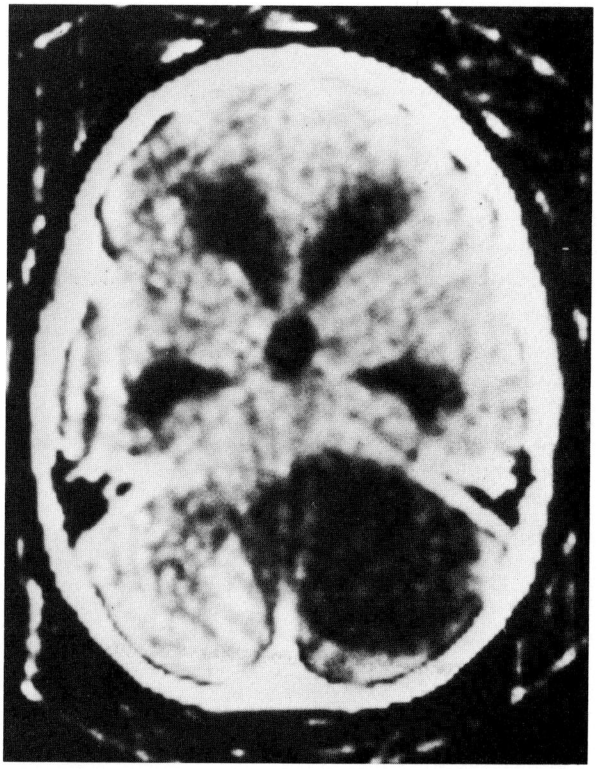

Figure 27-1. A typical cystic cerebellar astrocytoma. Note the presence of a large tumor mass, hydrocephalus, and mural nodule on the lower right side of the cyst wall.

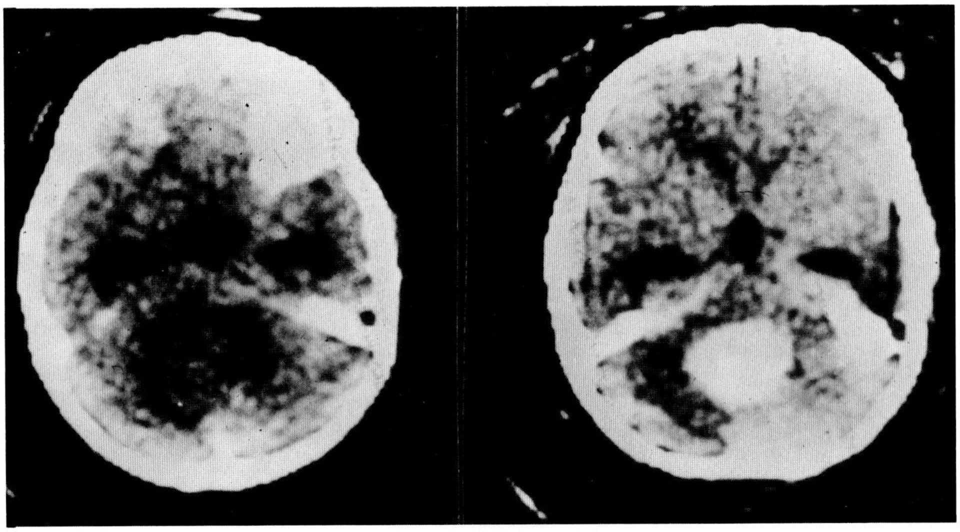

Figure 27-2. Precontrast and postcontrast enhancement appearance of a solid cerebellar astrocytoma. Note the presence of hydrocephalus, decreased tumor density precontrast, uniform enhancement postcontrast, and somewhat smaller tumor size compared with Figure 27-1.

tic cerebellar tissue or ependymal lining. The other half of cystic cerebellar astrocytomas show contrast enhancement in the cyst wall that is composed of poorly cellular tumor lining. Solid cerebellar astrocytoma, which accounts for slightly less than half of this tumor type, has slightly decreased density on initial CT examination and demonstrates uniform enhancement on CT after administration of contrast material (Fig. 27-2).[20]

Recurrent cerebellar astrocytoma is well demonstrated by CT and has the same spectrum of CT findings as the newly diagnosed tumors.[20] Fluid density in CT units within recurrent cystic tumor consistently measures about twice that of cerebrospinal fluid, allowing differentiation of tumor cyst from postoperative surgical defect (Figs. 27-3 and 27-4). In addition compression or distortion of the fourth ventricle and of the cerebellopontine angle or perimesencephalic cisterns is a consistent finding in recurrent cerebellar astrocytoma, despite the occasional absence of hydrocephalus. Computed tomography plays a major role in diagnosis and evaluation of patients with cerebellar astrocytoma preoperatively, immediately postoperatively, and for long-term follow-up.

Cerebellar astrocytoma is the most favorable pediatric brain tumor in any location.[1,18] Improvement in survival since the earliest outcome reports[4,19] is dependent on a number of factors. A better understanding of the natural history and biologic nature of this disease,[10] earlier diagnosis,[20] improved anesthetic and surgical technique,[3] and improvements in preoperative and postoperative care have all contributed to reducing overall mortality of pediatric cerebellar astrocytoma to less than 20 percent. Operative mortality, which ranged from 27 to 40 percent early in this century,[19,22] is now virtually 0 percent in major pediatric neurosurgery centers. This dramatic decrease in mortality is due in part to use of preoperative and postoperative corticosteroids, in part to major advances in endotracheal anesthetic management and intraoperative monitoring of patients, in part to specialized postoperative intensive care unit management of patients, and in part to concomitant development of effective means to combat infection and treat hydrocephalus. Long-term survival of patients with cerebellar astrocytoma ranges from 75 to 90 percent with surgery alone, indicating a generally benign biologic nature of the tumors.[23–27] Recent studies by ourselves and others[28] have also shown histologic variables that may be important prognostic indicators of patients who are at high risk for tumor recurrence and therefore would benefit

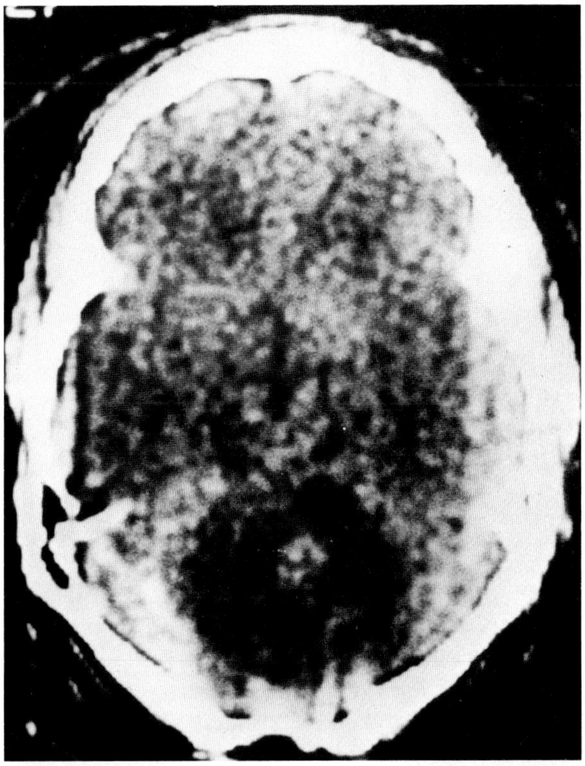

Figure 27-3. Recurrent cystic cerebellar astrocytoma. Note the absence of hydrocephalus. The CT unit density of this cyst is twice that of the cerebrospinal fluid.

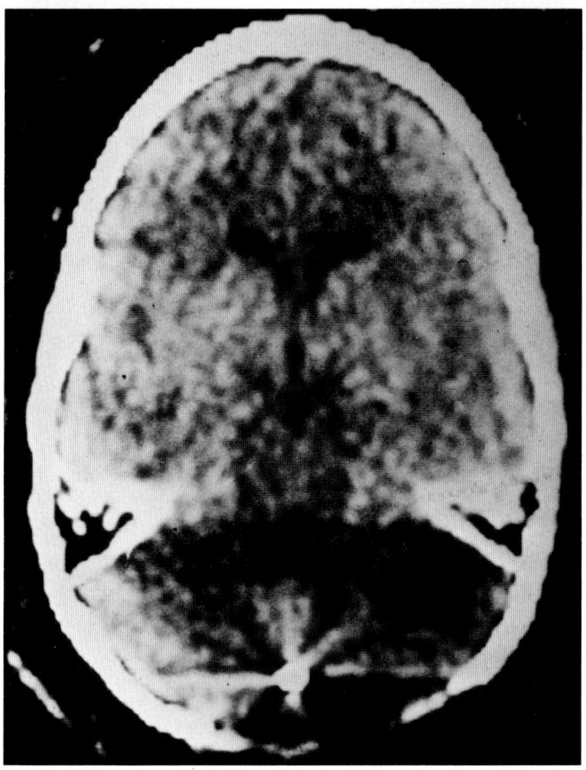

Figure 27.4 Follow-up CT scan for cerebellar astrocytoma with no tumor present. Note the absence of hydrocephalus, normal position of the slightly enlarged fourth ventricle. The CT unit density of the cystic area in the right cerebellar hemisphere is the same as the cerebrospinal fluid, indicating encephalomalacia with no tumor cyst present.

from close follow-up, and possibly repeat surgery, or who might be candidates for prophylactic treatment to prevent tumor regrowth.

We reviewed 41 patients with cerebellar astrocytoma at the Children's Hospital of Philadelphia, who were diagnosed between 1960 and 1976. We sought to determine recurrence rate, long-term morbidity, and mortality, and to establish criteria for early prognostication for individual patients with a confirmed diagnosis of cerebellar astrocytoma. All patients in our review group underwent suboccipital craniectomy and posterior fossa exploration with attempt made for gross total tumor excision in each case, except where tumor was seen to invade the brain-stem or walls of the fourth ventricle. There is a consensus among all pediatric neurosurgeons that tumor excision within these limitations should be carried out for all cases of cerebellar astrocytoma.[1,2,18,19,24–26,29]

Tumor histology from all of our patients was reviewed. The histology of cerebellar astrocytomas classically demonstrates piloid astrocytic cells grouped together in strands or brushes alternating with areas of looser cellular density filled with glial fibrils or ground substance. Prominent features of many cerebellar astrocytomas are areas of microcystic formation with surrounding stellate astrocytes, and areas of Rosenthal fibers, oligodendroglial-appearing cells, and occasionally areas of vascular proliferation and glomeruli formation. Microcysts, Rosenthal fibers, stellate astrocytes, and oligodendroglial change are interpreted by various authors as regressive changes or indications of tumor benignity.[3,4,8,10,28,30] We classified our cerebellar astrocytomas according to a schema introduced by Winston, Gilles, Levitan, et al.[28] Group A tumors should have microcystic formation, Rosenthal fibers, leptomeningeal tumor deposits, or foci of oligodendroglia, whereas Group B tumors must have a high cellular density, mitoses, necrosis, perivascular pseudorosette, or calcification.[28] Tumors that showed features of both Type A and B are classified as Type C.

As discussed by other authors, macrocyst formation seemed to occur in both benign and more aggressive cerebellar astrocytomas.[3,8,24,30] Some 85 percent of our tumors that were seen to have a macrocyst on CT were of Type A histology, whereas 78 percent of tumors purely solid on CT were Type B.[20] Solid tumors with cystic components on CT were all either Type B or C.[20] Rubinstein[30] has said that more invasive cerebellar astrocytomas tend to be midline, and we found that two thirds of the Type B and C tumors in our series were so. We also found that two thirds of our patients with tumor recurrence originally had midline tumors, whereas 85 percent of patients without recurrence began with tumors of the cerebellar hemisphere.[20]

Table 27-3 shows the overall mortality of our review group. Operative deaths, which were responsible for over half of the overall group mortality, all occurred before 1970. There have been *no* operative deaths in the last 35 consecutively operated patients, due to improved operative and anesthetic techniques. The overall recurrence rate in our group of patients was 35 percent and mortality with recurrence was 23 percent. Recurrence presented 5 to 19 months postoperatively with a median time to recurrence of 12 months, and, as mentioned above, occurred more often in patients with solid, midline lesions than

Table 27-3
Cerebellar Astrocytoma Review (CHOP 1960–1975)

Histologic Type	Total	Operative Deaths	Recurrence	Mortality with Recurrence	Overall Mortality
A	28 (68%)	2	8/26 (31%)	2/8 (25%)	4/28 (14%)
B	9 (22%)	1	4/8 (50%)	0/4 (0%)	1/9 (11%)
C	4 (10%)	1	1/3 (33%)	1/1 (100%)	2/4 (50%)
Total	41	4 (10%)	13/37 (35%)	3/13 (23%)	7/41 (17%)

Table 27-4
Cerebellar Astrocytoma Review (CHOP 1960–1975)

	Radiation Therapy		
Histologic Type	Radiated	Recurred Post-Radiation Therapy	Recurred without Radiation Therapy
A	12/26 (46%)	5/12 (42%)	3/14 (21%)
B	4/8 (50%)	2/4 (50%)	2/4 (50%)
C	2/3 (66%)	1/2 (50%)	0/1
Total	18/37 (49%)	8/18 (44%)	5/19 (26%)

in others. We concluded that histologic grouping of these tumors as discussed by Winston et al.[28] along with CT findings, correlates with prognosis. When considered together histologic Type B and C tumors clearly have a worse prognosis than Type A. Long-term survival in our group of patients was 83 percent, or 93 percent excluding operative mortality, with all patients surviving at least four years at the time of review.

Many authors agree that radiation therapy for cerebellar astrocytoma is not indicated.[1,3,18,24,27,29–31] We would agree with this overall statement with slight modification. Of our review group, approximately half of the patients received radiation therapy at the discretion of the responsible surgeon, and half did not. As shown in Table 27-4, the results were not clear. Recurrence of histologic Type A tumors seemed independent of radiation therapy, and there was no clear advantage to radiating Type B or C tumors demonstrated in this small sample. We did not find any retardation of somatic growth, however, in patients who did receive posterior fossa radiation to 4000 rads, and no other correlation between radiation therapy and residual neurologic deficit or functional impairment could be found. While radiation therapy of the posterior fossa therefore seems safe, we reserve treatment now for patients with Type B or C lesions, or documented recurrence and progression of Type A tumors. In two Type B patients radiated postoperatively, we have seen recurrence of tumor as a Type A lesion amenable to resection, which may indicate radiation inhibition of tumor growth.[20]

Mortality from cerebellar astrocytoma is quite low and quality of survival is excellent. Although virtually all patients have hydrocephalus at the time of diagnosis, only 32 percent of our patients required permanent ventriculoperitoneal or lumboperitoneal shunts after tumor resection. Accurate histologic classification of these tumors, along with CT scan information, allows more accurate prognostication than ever before. Any recurrence is usually early and most often seen with solid, midline lesions. We feel that systematic monitoring of postoperative cerebellar astrocytoma patients can further lower mortality and morbidity. We believe it to be desirable that patients with a prior history of cystic or Type A cerebellar astrocytomas have a CT examination one year and three to five years after surgery, even if they are asymptomatic. We prefer closer follow-up for patients with solid or Type B or C cerebellar astrocytomas, obtaining CT examination one month and six months after surgery with reexamination yearly for five years thereafter. With this protocol for follow-up, we can anticipate recurrence or progression of tumor growth and decide to proceed with repeat surgery or radiation therapy before symptomatic worsening occurs.

REFERENCES

1. Walker MD: Diagnosis and treatment of brain tumors. Pediatr Clin N Am 23:131–146, 1976
2. Matson DD: Surgery of posterior fossa tumors in childhood. Clin Neurosurg 15:247–264, 1968

3. Matson DD: Neurosurgery of Infancy and Childhood. Springfield, Charles C Thomas, 1969
4. Cushing H: The intracranial tumors of preadolescence. Am J Dis Child 33(4):551–584, 1927
5. Walker AE, Hopple TL: Brain tumors in children. J Pediatr 35(6):671–687, 1949
6. Smith WA, Fincher EF: Intracranial tumors in children. South Med J 35(6):547–554, 1942
7. Keith HW, McK Craig W, Kernohan JW: Brain tumors in children. Pediatrics 3:839–844, 1949
8. Koos WT, Miller MH: Intracranial Tumors of Infants in Children. St. Louis, CV Mosby, 1971
9. Gold JS, Smith KR: Childhood brain tumors: A 15-year survey of treatment in a university pediatric hospital. So Med J 68:1337–1344, 1975
10. Bailey P, Buchanan DN, Buch PC: Intracranial Tumors of Infancy and Childhood. Chicago, University of Chicago Press, 1939
11. Young J., Miller RW: Incidence of malignant tumors in U.S. children, J Pediatr 86:254–258, 1975
12. Gjerris F, Harmsen A, Klinken L, et al: Incidence and long-term survival of children with intracranial tumors treated in Denmark, 1935–1959. Br J Cancer 38:442–451, 1978
13. Heiskanen O: Intracranial tumors of children. Child's Brain 3:69–78, 1977
14. Hooper R: Intracranial tumours in childhood. Child's Brain 1:136–140, 1975
15. Raimondi A: Personal communication, 1979
16. Humphreys RP: Posterior cranial fossa tumors in children, in Youmans JR (ed): Neurological Surgery. Philadelphia, WB Saunders, in press
17. Hoffman HJ: Personal communication, 1979
18. Carmel PW: Cerebellar tumors in childhood. Dev Med Child Neurol 14:809–811, 1972
19. Cushing H: Experiences with the cerebellar astrocytomas. Surg Cynec Obstet 52:129–204, 1931
20. Zimmerman RA, Bilaniuk CT, Bruno LA, Rosenstock J: Computed tomography of cerebellar astrocytoma. Am J Roentgenol 130:929–933, 1978
21. Nardich TP, Lin JP, Leeds NE, et al: Primary tumors and other masses of the cerebellum and fourth ventricle: Differential diagnosis by computed tomography. Neuroradiology, 14:153–174, 1977
22. Bucy PC, Thieman PW: Astrocytomas of the cerebellum. Arch Neurol 18:14–19, 1968
23. Geissinger JD, Bucy PC: Astrocytomas of the cerebellum in children. Int J Neurol 7(2):103–107, 1970
24. Geissinger JD, Bucy PC: Astrocytomas of the cerebellum in children. Arch Neurol 24:125–135, 1971
25. Gjerris F: Clinical aspects and long-term prognosis of infratentorial intracranial tumors in infancy and childhood. Acta Neurol Scand 57:31–52, 1978
26. Lassman LP: The treatment of posterior fossa tumours in childhood. Mod Probl Paediatr 18:16–22, 1977
27. Elridge AR: Long-term survival in the astrocytoma series. J Neurosurg 25:399–404, 1968
28. Winston K, Gilles FH, Leviton A, et al: Cerebellar gliomas in children. J Nat Cancer Inst 58:833–838, 1977
29. Gjerris R, Klinken L: Long-term prognosis in children with benign cerebellar astrocytoma. J Neurosurg 49:179–184, 1978
30. Rubinstein LJ: Tumors of the central nervous system, Fasc. 6. in: Atlas of Tumor Pathology. Washington, DC, Armed Forces Institute of Pathology, 1972
31. Sheline G: Radiation therapy of tumours of the central nervous system in childhood. Cancer, 5:957–964, 1975

28. Cerebellar Medulloblastoma, Sarcoma, and Hemangioblastoma

Derek A. Bruce
Luis Schut

Medullobastomas account for from 4 to 10 percent[1,2] of all intracranial tumors, and for from 15 to 20 percent of intracranial tumors in children.[3,4] In all reported series, boys have been more frequently affected than girls with a ratio of 4:3[5] to 2:1.[6] These tumors occur from the newborn period to the seventh decade of life with a peak incidence in the first decade—69 percent occurring in children less than 8 years of age. The majority of these tumors occur in the region of the fourth ventricle; the minority occur laterally in the cerebellar hemisphere. These laterally located tumors are more frequent in adults and tend to be desmoplastic in type. They may be well circumscribed and have occasionally been referred to as cerebellar sarcomas.[7] Until recently these tumors appeared to carry a better prognosis than the more medial ones.

The single most frequently encountered symptom is vomiting. This usually occurs in the morning upon rising. Once the vomiting, which is accompanied by hyperventilation, is over, the child feels well, and usually can eat breakfast and go off to school. Because of this pattern, the vomiting is frequently ignored for weeks or months or is assumed to be psychogenic in origin. While the vomiting may occur only once a week in the early stages of the disease, as the tumor and hydrocephalus increase in size, it becomes more frequent. At this stage the complaint of headache is very common. The headache either wakes the child from sleep in the middle of the night or is present upon rising. Like the vomiting this is presumably produced by intracranial hypertension, and like the vomiting is usually relieved after the hyperventilation, which accompanies the vomiting, has reduced intracranial blood volume, thus lowering the intracranial pressure. The symptom that usually triggers the parents or the pediatrician into further investigations is unsteadiness of gait.

Neurologic examination early in the course of the disease may show evidence of papilledema and nothing else. Later ataxia of gait, nystagmus, and less frequently fourth or sixth nerve palsies may be found. If the tumors are eccentrically located, there may be evidence of unilateral cerebellar dysfunction.

In the younger children, a positive crack-pot sound of the skull to percussion may be elicited. The time course from first symptoms to diagnosis varies from six months or more to as short as a few days or hours, with a mean of around two months. Fifteen percent of nontraumatic subarachnoid hemorrhage in children has been found to be due to hemorrhage into tumor,[8] and 40 percent of these hemorrhagic tumors were located in the posterior fossa with a diagnosis of medulloblastoma or primitive neuroectodermal tumors. Occasionally the first symptoms are of spinal cord dysfunction as a result of compression secondary to subarachnoid seeding. Very rarely is an intramedullary spinal cord tumor found to be medulloblastoma, the primary appearing only weeks to months later in the posterior fossa.

NEURORADIOLOGIC STUDIES

Once the clinical diagnosis of a posterior fossa tumor is made, further neuroradiologic investigation is sought. Plain skull x-rays are the first study. These may show clear evidence of splitting of the sutures in the child younger than 7 or 8 years of age. At any age demineralization of the floor of the sella turcica or erosion of the posterior clinoids may be seen, confirming the clinical impression of intracranial hypertension. The next test, if available, is a computerized axial tomographic (CAT) scan with and without contrast enhancement. Medulloblastomas are typically more dense than the surrounding brain on the unenhanced scan and show marked homogeneous enhancement (Fig. 28-1). The accuracy of the CAT scanner is extremely high, 91–98 percent,[9] and not only is the tumor well demonstrated, but the degree of hydrocephalus and any evidence of subarachnoid or supratentorial spread of tumor can readily be seen. It is rare that there is a need to do arteriography or ventriculography after the diagnosis of medulloblastoma is made with CAT scan. We have resorted to further tests only when there has been some unusual appearance on CAT scan or where the clinical

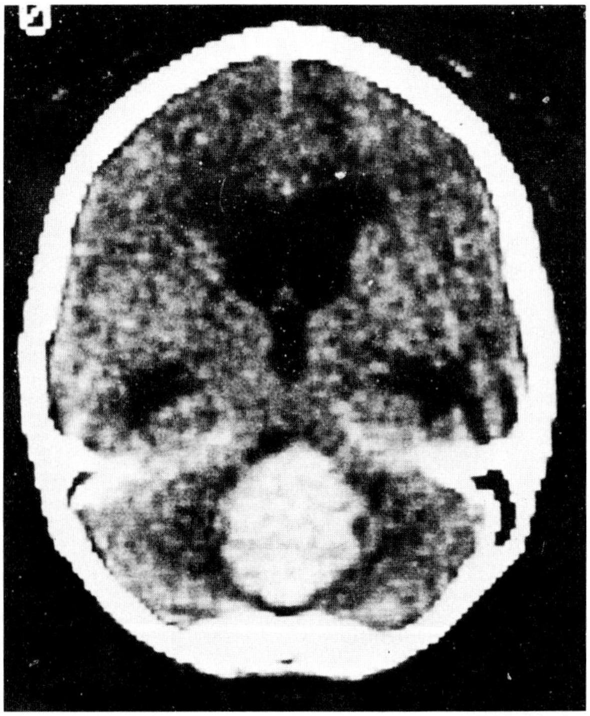

Figure 28-1. Typical medulloblastoma postenhancement.

findings have not correlated with the computerized tomography (CT) picture. We do not perform a lumbar puncture (LP) or myelogram on these patients until after the tumor has been removed.

MANAGEMENT

In children who present in coma or in a severely obtunded and dehydrated state, either a ventriculoperitoneal (VP) shunt with a filter in place or external ventricular drainage is used slowly to reduce the intracranial pressure (ICP). There is a distinct risk of upward herniation at the tentorial notch when large tumors are present, therefore, the ventricles must be drained slowly. In the majority of children, no such emergency intervention is necessary. There are two current ways to handle this latter group of children: One is to shunt all children with hydrocephalus and medulloblastoma. Against this is the fact that only one-third of these children may require a shunt and up to 19 percent may develop shunt-related metastasis.[10] The other regimen is to avoid shunting and to use large doses of dexamethasone, 1 mg/kg/day, for three to four days, to obtain a decrease in ICP[11] and maximum improvement in cerebral compliance.[12] There is frequently complete relief of symptomatology after starting steroids.

The next step in management is posterior fossa craniectomy. The surgery is usually performed with the patient in the prone position. These tumors are usually in the fourth ventricle and the use of the prone position gives the surgeon a good opportunity to visualize the fourth ventricle without the need to split the vermis. The prone position also avoids problems of air embolism, makes control of temperature during surgery in small children easier, and decreases the risk of cells floating down to the lumbar sac. We customarily remove the rim of the foramen magnum and often the arch of Cl as well since the tonsils are frequently herniated. The tumor may be immediately visible between the tonsils or may lie completely within the fourth ventricle. Occasionally diffuse thickening of the arachnoid by tumor spread is seen over the tonsils and cerebellar hemispheres, "sugar coating." Even in those cases, we believe that tumor mass should be removed whenever possible. While the majority of medulloblastomas arise from the region of the posterior medullary velum, they may be intimately attached to the anterior medullary velum, or the region of the aqueduct of Sylvius, or invading the floor of the fourth ventricle. Because of this location, no effort to resect the tumor as a single mass lesion should be made since traction upon these vital structures may produce damage and cause the patient to suffer neurologic signs and symptoms that were not present prior to surgery. There is usually a plane between the tumor and the brain in the midline, but as the dissection is continued laterally and superiorly this plane is usually lost as the tumor begins to infiltrate the cerebellar hemispheres. The major blood vessels can be coagulated on the outside of the pseudocapsule and the mass then decompressed. Bleeding from the tumor bed itself is usually easily controlled. As the tumor mass is debulked, the floor of the fourth ventricle and any invasion of it by tumor can be readily visualized. That portion of tumor can then be removed without traction upon the fourth ventricular floor. The surgical stratagem is grossly to remove all the tumor rather than to just debulk it adequately in order to open the aqueduct of Sylvius. This total gross removal reduces the residual tumor burden and decreases the likelihood of postoperative cerebrospinal fluid (CSF) spread.

Immediately prior to craniotomy in patients with preoperative hydrocephalus, a supratentorial burr hole is always made and a Silastic ventricular catheter inserted into the lateral ventricle. This is tunneled out under the skin in the upper neck and is usually connected to closed drainage and pressure monitoring for two to three days postoperatively. If after two to three days, continued CSF venting is required, the ventriculostomy is readily converted to a VP shunt with millipore filter. If venting is no longer required, the ventriculostomy is removed.

The surgical mortality for this operation should be approaching zero, and certainly should be less than 3 percent. The morbidity from surgery is usually related to excess traction during surgery upon vital structures such as the pons and anterior medullary velum, and usually consists of cranial nerve palsies, particularly sixth, seventh, and fourth; swallowing difficulties; and a nasal-quality slurred speech. Sterile meningitis as a postoperative complication will occasionally occur, though it is much less frequent than with astrocytomas, and is usually treated by increasing the steroid dosage.

PATHOLOGY

This is a highly cellular tumor. The cells are small with dark nuclei and poorly defined cytoplasm. Homer–Wright rosettes are seen in about one-third of tumors but pseudorosettes are more typical. Differentiation to desmoplastic, oligodendroglial, or spongioblastic cell lines may all be seen. Occasionally nonstriated muscle fibers are encountered.

POSTOPERATIVE CARE

Early mobilization is encouraged with sitting out of bed in the second postoperative day. Steroid dosage is slowly decreased over the first 10 days to two weeks, most patients being off steroids within two to three weeks after surgery. A recent study reported a high incidence (43 percent) of unsuspected spinal cord metastasis following the initial surgery and prior to radiation.[13] While this figure seems unusually high, it seems worthwhile to perform routine postoperative myelography prior to radiation therapy. We believe that Pantopaque should be avoided as a myelographic contrast agent because, if any is lost into the head, significant confusion can occur with follow-up scans with the Pantopaque obliterating small amounts of tumor. We thus perform the myelography with Amipaque (metrizamide). Radiation therapy is begun as soon as possible postoperatively and always within the first week. Without radiation therapy these tumors invariably recur and death results within one year.[14] Radiation therapy is designed to include the whole craniospinal axis with a dose of 3500–4000 rads and an additional 1000–1500 rads to the posterior fossa. The axis radiation is usually given first with weekly doses of 800–1000 rads if tolerated. The radiation dosage is modified for the infant. During radiation therapy, throat pain and nonproductive cough are common. About 30 percent of patients will develop a drop in hemoglobin and white cell count and as many as 16 percent will require interruption of radiation because of a low white count.

CHEMOTHERAPY

Vincristine has been the most frequently used chemotherapeutic drug and tumor response has been shown.[15] At present, trials are underway in both Europe and North America to compare the outcome after radiation alone with that after radiation and chemotherapy. The drugs being used are vincristine 1.5 mg/M^2 weekly for three weeks with a three-week rest, CCNU 100 mg/M^2 PO every six weeks, and prednisone 40 mg/M^2 (in the American study) for the first two weeks of each six-week cycle. As yet there is little evidence that the combination therapy is more effective, but the trials are not yet complete. The incidence of moderate to severe complication with the combination of radiation with the chemotherapy, however, is about twice as high.

Most authors[16,17] have stated that after tumor recurrence death occurs within six to nine months. Over the past five years, with an aggressive approach to the recurrent tumor, survivals of four to five years or more have been seen. These patients have also returned to useful independent function. As yet, however, it cannot be stated that cure is possible after the tumor has recurred. The treatment of recurrent disease is dependent upon the site of recurrence and whether recurrence is single or multiple. Recurrences occur most frequently in the posterior fossa. The next most frequent location is spinal, followed by supratentorial space, and finally systemic metastatic disease. The treatment of the recurrence depends upon the site and upon whether recurrence is localized and single or multiple. When there is single posterior fossa recurrence, we believe that the best procedure is repeat surgery with removal of the mass followed by either repeat radiation therapy, if more than a year has expired since the previous therapy, or by chemotherapy. Spinal metastasis may be treated either by repeat local radiation therapy to the metastatic area if they are isolated, or by systemic and intrathecal chemotherapy if widespread. Widespread posterior fossa meningeal recurrence is also treated in this fashion. The mortality for repeat surgery need be no greater than for the initial surgery. Postoperative recovery is usually rapid with immediate resolution of symptoms.

Chemotherapy for recurrent tumors is usually vincristine, CCNU, and procarbazine. If these drugs fail or if the tumor becomes resistant, the use of other chemotherapeutic agents such as cyclophosphamide, VM-26, or dianhydrogalactitol may be tried with the possibility of benefit. Repeat radiation therapy to the whole cranium may be considered, depending on the time from initial radiation to recurrence. While we have not seen evidence of major complications such as stroke, there is no question that intellectual performance will be diminished further by repeat radiation therapy.

Survival rates for this tumor are variously reported from 25 to 70 percent five-year survival.[16–20] There is evidence that total gross tumor removal carries a better prognosis than does simple debulking.[14,19] In the various hospitals specializing in the care of childhood brain tumors, survival rates of 60 percent or more may be expected in children with medulloblastoma following total excision and radiation therapy. While the majority of recurrences occur within the first few years, late recurrences have been reported 8 to 10 years after apparently curative therapy. Children under 2 years of age with medulloblastoma continue to have an almost 100 percent mortality in two or three years.

With longer survival and decreased surgical morbidity, the effects of the tumor, hydrocephalus, surgery, radiation, and chemotherapy plus the social disruption produced in the child and family are taking significant toll. Clinically, growth hormone deficiency can be defined in 80 percent or more of these children, although many of them will apparently continue to grow. The children generally have a poor image of themselves, feel insecure, and frequently show significant change on neuropsychologic testing, particularly in the rate of performance and short-term memory function. These deficits, plus the difficulty of being certain whether or not a cure is obtained, produce significant family and school problems. We believe that it is increasingly necessary to organize a comprehensive clinic with social workers and psychologists to interface between the children, the parents, and the school situation. Other late complications such as thyroid carcinoma have been reported. It is also possible that, with longer survival, second tumors in the areas of radiation may occur.

In conclusion the treatment and outcome for children with medulloblastoma appears to have undergone a significant change in the last five years. At one institution, the Children's Hospital of Philadelphia, there has been only one death in the last 15 medulloblastomas and no evidence of recurrent tumor on CT scan. The CT scan has contributed to the improved results of therapy by (1) early diagnosis, (2) clear definition of the extent of the tumor, (3) better design of the posterior fossa radiation portal, and (4) easy identification of any tumor recurrence. We believe that the concerns of therapy are centered around trying to find the minimum effective dosage for cranial radiation to minimize the neuropsychologic disturbances and to organize a social system that allows the children and their families to cope with the problems and uncertainties of the brain tumor in a more effective fashion. Finally, even when tumor recurrence occurs, as long as the children are in good neurologic condition, an aggressive approach to therapy can prolong useful survival for many years.

SARCOMAS

There is a great deal of disagreement concerning the classification of sarcomas of the brain.[21,22] The tumors that produce least disagreement are the fibrosarcomas of the brain. These account for a very small percentage of tumors and certainly have been seen in children, both in the supratentorial space and the posterior fossa. These tumors have been found, in our experience, in children with neurofibromatosis. Aggressive surgical removal followed by radiation therapy is the treatment of choice of all sarcomas of the brain, sometimes with good tumor control for many years.

Somewhat more controversial is the glial sarcoma. This implies a malignant glioma with significant neoplastic vascular stroma. Since all glioblastomas show some element of vascular proliferation, some pathologists do not recognize the separate entity of glial sarcoma. The behavior of these glial sarcomas is similar to that of other malignant gliomas.

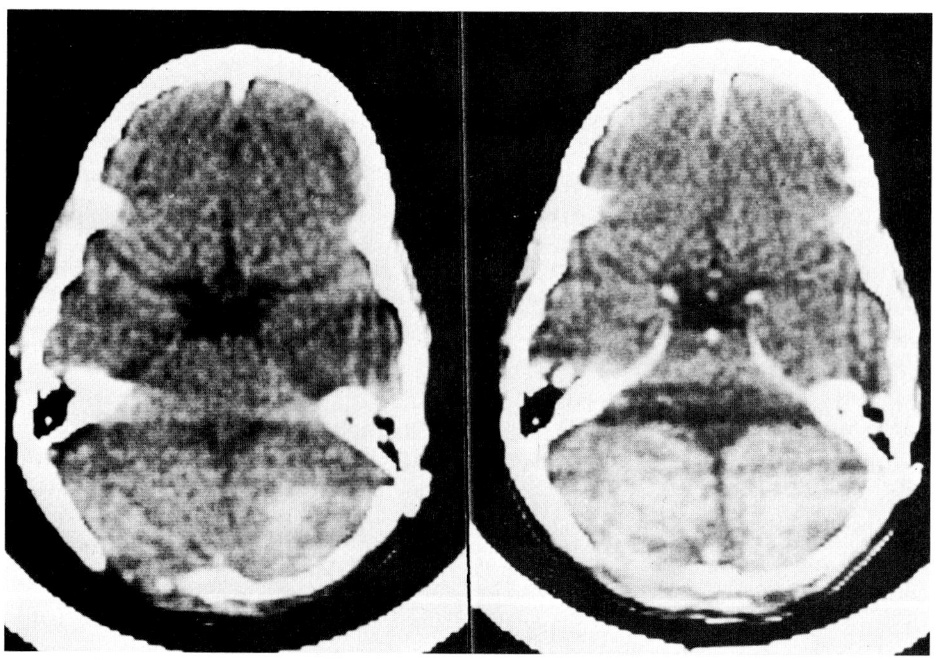

Figure 28-2. Bilateral cerebellar glial sarcoma.

Posterior fossa sarcomas do occur. There is disagreement in the literature as to whether such an entity as a cerebellar exists or whether this tumor is not simply a well-circumscribed lateral medulloblastoma with intense pial reaction. Glial sarcomas occur in the posterior fossa and Figure 28-2 shows such a case. This tumor responded to radiation therapy for several months but then was rapidly fatal.

REFERENCES

1. Tola JS: The histopathological and biological characteristics of primary neoplasms of the cerebellum and the fourth ventricle, with some aspects of their clinical picture, diagnosis and treatment (on the basis of 71 verified cases). Acta Chir Scand, 164(Suppl):1–112, 1951
2. Crue BL, Jr: Medulloblastoma. American Lecture Series. Springfield, Charles C Thomas, 1958
3. Koos WT, Miller MH: Intracranial Tumors of Infants and Children. St. Louis, CV Mosby, 1971
4. Craig WM, Keith HM, Kernohan JW: Tumors of the brain occurring in childhood. Acta Psychiatr Neurol 24:375–390, 1949
5. Bloom HJG, Wallace ENK, Henk JM: The treatment and prognosis of medulloblastoma in children. A study of 82 verified cases. Am J Roentgen 105:43–62, 1969
6. Smith CE, Long DM, Jones TK Jr, et al: Experiences in treating medulloblastoma at the University of Minnesota Hospital. Radiology 109:179–182, 1973
7. Rubinstein LJ, Northfield DWC: The medulloblastoma and the so called "arachnoidal cerebellar sarcoma." A critical re-examination of a nasological problem. Brain 87:379–412, 1964
8. Laurent JP, Bruce DA, Schut L: Hemorrhagic brain tumors in pediatric patients. Child's Brain (submitted)
9. Zimmerman RA, Bilaniuk LT, Pahlajani H: Specifics of meduloblastoma demonstrated by CT. Radiology 126:137–141, 1978
10. Hoffman H: Management of medulloblastoma. Aust Pediatr J 15:55–56, 1979
11. Brock M, Zillig C, Weigand H, et al: The effects of dexamethasone on ICP in cases of posterior fossa tumors, in Beks JWF, Bosch DA, Brock M (eds): Intracranial Pressure III. New York, Springer-Verlag, 1976, pp 236–246
12. Miller JD, Sakalas R, Ward JD, et al: Methylprednisolone treatment in patients with brain tumors. Neurosurgery 1:114–117, 1977
13. Deutsch M, Reigel DH: The value of myelography in the management of childhood and medulloblastoma. Cancer April 15 45(8):2114–2197, 1980
14. Cushing H: Experiences with the cerebellar medulloblastoma. A critical review. Acta Pathol Microbiol Scand 7:150–183, 1930
15. Rosenstock JG, Evans AE, Schut L: Response to vincristine or recurrent brain tumors in children. J Neurosurg 45:135–138, 1976
16. Mealey J Jr, Hall PV: Medulloblastoma in children. Survival and treatment. J Neurosurg 46:56–64, 1977
17. Bloom HJG, Wallace ENK, Henk JM: The treatment and prognosis of medulloblastoma in children. A study of 82 verified cases. Am J Roentgenol Rad Thera Nucl Med 105:43–62, 1969
18. Aron BS: Medulloblastoma in children. Twenty-two years experience with radiation therapy. Am J Dis Child 121:314–317, 1971
19. Raimondi AJ, Tomita T: Medulloblastoma in childhood. Comparative results of partial and total resection. Child's Brain 5:310–328, 1979
20. Hope-Stone, HF: Results of treatment of medulloblastoma. J Neurosurg 42:83–88, 1970
21. Kernahan JW, Uihlein A: Sarcomas of the brain. Springfield, Charles C Thomas, 1961
22. Rubinstein LJ: Sarcomas of the nervous system, in Minckler J (ed): Pathology of the Nervous System, vol. II. New York, McGraw-Hill, 1971, pp 2144–2164

29. Fourth Ventricle Tumors

Tadanori Tomita
Anthony J. Raimondi

ANATOMIC CONSIDERATIONS

The fourth ventricle, located in the center of the posterior fossa, develops from the rhombencephalic cavity. It is bordered by tegmentum of the pons and the upper half of medulla oblongata ventrally, the cerebellar peduncles laterally, and the cerebellum dorsally. The aqueduct of Sylvius opens into it rostrally; it is continuous with the vallecula through the foramen of Magendie posteroinferiorly and the central canal of the spinal cord anteroinferiorly. The lateral extension is into the medullocerebellar cisterns through the lateral recesses, then the foramina of Luschka, on each side. The floor of the fourth ventricle (Fig. 29-1) is rhomboid shaped, and is subdivided by the midline sulcus into two halves, each in turn divided by the sulcus limitans into a median eminence medially and the vestibular area (vestibular nuclei) laterally. Two important landmarks, the facial colliculus (formed by the abducens nucleus and the genu of the facial nerve) and the hypoglossal trigone, lie within the midposition of the floor. The hypoglossal trigone lies at the caudal end of the fourth ventricle and is formed by the underlying hypoglossal nucleus. Lateral to the hypoglossal trigone is the vagal trigone, which overlies the dorsal nucleus of the vagal nerve (ala cinerea). Rostal to the hypoglossal trigone, the striae medullaris (arcuate cerebellar fibers) runs transversely from the median sulcus to the lateral recess. The calamus scriptorius—caudal fourth ventricle—is beneath the obex at the entrance of the fourth ventricle into the central canal. At the lateral wall of the fourth ventricle are the superior cerebellar peduncle (brachium conjunctivum), the brachium pontis, and the inferior cerebellar peduncle (restiform body). The lateral recesses extend, within the fourth ventricle, around the brain stem along the junction of pons and medulla oblongata. Their medial surface is formed by the restiform body, and the lateral surface by the peduncle of the flocculus. It is of importance to note that

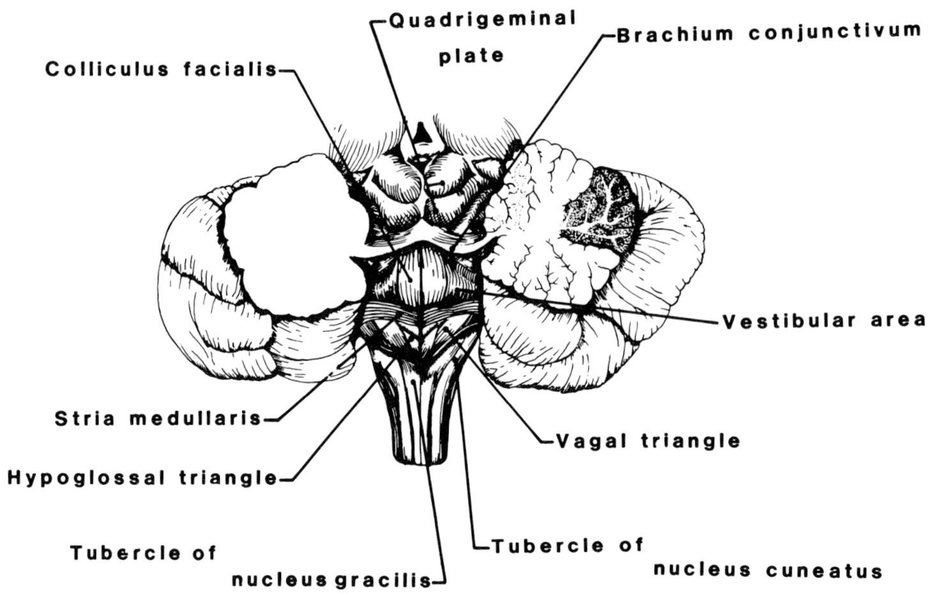

Figure 29-1. Diagrammatic representation of the fourth ventricle and significant neurosurgical structures related to it.

the choroid plexus extends through each lateral recess and appears at the foramen of Luschka.

The fastigium is the dorsal apex of the fourth ventricle, with the roof being the superior medullary velum (medially) and the superior cerebellar peduncles (laterally). The very thin superior medullary velum, located ventral to the lingula, is stretched between the superior cerebellar peduncles. The inferior medullary velum is the tela choroidea of the fourth ventricle.

The choroid plexuses of the fourth ventricle are the paired, T-shaped structures within the caudal half of this chamber, each consisting of vertical and horizontal portions. The posterior layer of the tela choroidea, covering the inferior vermis, is the pia mater. The vertical portions fuse at the cranial margin of the median aperture where they adhere to the vermis. The horizontal portions extend into the lateral recesses and emerge through the lateral apertures, the foramina of Luschka.

The volume of the fourth ventricle is reported to be 0.85 cm^3 in adults,[14] and proportionately smaller in children and infants. From it, cerebrospinal fluid (CSP) flows laterally into the pontocerebellar cisterns through the foramina of Luschka, medially into the cisterna magna, through the foramen of Magendie, and into the central canal of the spinal cord at the calamus scriptorius.

PATHOLOGIC CONSIDERATIONS

Tumors may originate in any part of the above-mentioned structures. Purely intraventricular tumors are choroid plexus papilloma and meningioma.[12,27] Ependymomas or subependymomas originate from the walls of the ventricle, projecting into it, but may grow into the cerebellar parenchyma rather than into the cavity of the fourth ventricle. Cerebellar astrocytomas and medulloblastoma, which have their origin outside of the ventricle, may present as mainly intraventricular masses. It thus is difficult to determine whether a fourth ventricular tumor is intraventricular or paraventricular in origin. By convention, then, one defines a tumor as intraventricular when the majority lies within the fourth ventricle, and as paraventricular when the greater portion lies outside the ventricle.

The choroid plexus papilloma is derived from the epithelium of the choroid plexus. Fifty percent of these tumors occur in the fourth ventricle,[33] though the lateral ventricle papillomas are much more common in children.[23] Very rarely this tumor may occur in the cerebellopontine angle when the tumor arises from tufts of the choroid plexus that project into the lateral recess. They may seed into the spinal subarachnoid spaces. Papillomas are generally well defined, quite separate from the parenchyma, and pedunculated from an arterial–venous pedicle, but they may have a sessile attachment. When they arise within the lateral recess, they compress the adjacent cerebellum, brain stem, and cranial nerves. Intraventricular papilloma originates from the inferior roof, tela choroidea, and stroma of the choroid plexus of the fourth ventricle, in a more inferior location than the medulloblastoma.[28,31]

Dermoid and epidermoid congenital tumors may occur in the fourth ventricle. At approximately the fourth fetal week, the neural tube closes, and the neural ectoderm becomes separated from the cutaneous ectoderm. Retention of fragments of the cutaneous ectoderm within the neural tube may result in midline epidermoid or dermoid tumors later in life. The dermoid is more common intracranially than the epidermoid, and is associated with an occipital dermal sinus.[20] Approximately 10 percent of the intracranial epidermoids occur in the fourth ventricle.[16] Both tumors, by and large, occur more often in adulthood, the epidermoid in more advanced age. Among the congenital tumors, teratoma more often occurs in childhood with benign or malignant teratomas occasionally encountered in the fourth ventricle.[29]

The ependymoma originates from the ventricular wall from which it may occasionally become separated. The most common site of occurrence of the infratentorial ependymoma—as common as the supratentorial location—is in the fourth ventricle, though some have been reported in the pontocerebellar angle. Those in the fourth ventricle almost always attach to the floor at the calamus scriptorius, expanding the cisterna magnum as they surround and compress the dorsolateral aspect of the medulla oblongata and upper cervical cord (plastic ependymoma).[4] It may extend into and plug the aqueduct or lateral recesses. Kahn, Crosby, and DeJonge[13] emphasized that the lateral recesses are invariably involved by ependymoma. When the tumor arises in the region of the apex of the lateral recess, it occupies the cerebellopontine angle and may grow to fill a large part of the ventral half of the posterior fossa without encroaching upon the lumen of the fourth ventricle.[17] According to Goutelle and Fischer,[8] the origin of the ependymoma in the posterior fossa is the floor of the fourth ventricle in 82 percent, roof in 8 percent, lateral recess in 5 percent, and cerebellum without ependymal connection in 5 percent.

Subependymoma, usually an incidental finding at necropsy, occurs in the fourth ventricle of the elderly, rarely causing sysmptoms. Histologically it is a benign tumor.

The posterior fossa hemangioblastoma grows within the cerebellar hemisphere or vermis, and extends into the cavity of the fourth ventricle. Some have been reported to arise also from the medulla oblongata, particularly at the area postrema. It rarely occurs in childhood.

The origin of the medulloblastoma is still controversial. Bailey and Cushing[3] postulated that the medulloblast, a cell of indifferent character derived from the primitive medullary epithelium, remains undifferentiated, particularly in the region of the roof of the fourth ventricle, until it develops into tumor. Stevenson and Echlin[32] suggested that it derives from the remnants of the fetal external granular layer, which normally perists in the infant cerebellum until the end of the first year of life, at which time it begins an inward migration to form the majority of neurons of the internal granular layer. It is presently accepted that this tumor originates from the remnants of cell rests in the posterior medullary velum[22] (and possibly anterior medullary velum[26]) of the roof of the fourth ventricle, that it invades the vermis, and that it fills the fourth ventricle and may spread into the cerebellar hemispheres. The tumor may also, though much less commonly, originate in the cerebellar hemisphere and not extend into vermis. Invasion of the floor of the fourth ventricle or extension into the cerebellar peduncles is not uncommon; 10 percent of our 40 cases. Tumor lobules often plug the aqueduct of Sylvius or protrude through the foramen of Magendie into the cisterna magnum; they rarely occlude the foramina of Luschka.

Cerebellar astrocytoma, located in the cerebellar vermis or hemisphere, may arise from the roof of the fourth ventricle or the calamus scriptorius,[15] invading the fourth ventricle in either event. Though it generally bulges into this cavity, it may grow through the ependymal barrier, fungate within the fourth ventricle, and even become adherent to its floor.[30]

Tumors of the brain stem ventral to the fourth ventricle produce hypertrophy of the pons and medulla oblongata. They deform the shape of the fourth ventricle but rarely present as exophytic growths within its cavity. Instead their exophytic growth extends ventrally or ventrolaterally into the prepontine or cerebellopontine cisterns. "Cystic" collections of necrotic tissue often protrude into the ventricle, presenting as bluish or reddish domes that tempt the surgeon to puncture them with the thought they may be "hematoma."

From the surgical point of view, we follow Möller's[18] classification of fourth ventricle tumors: When the majority of the tumor lies within the fourth ventricle, it is considered to be intraventricular; a tumor is paraventricular when the greatest part of it lies outside the ventricle. This presentation is based on our experiences with 154 posterior fossa tumors at Northwestern University (Children's Memorial Hospital) from 1967 through 1979.

Sixty-two out of 332 brain tumors in infancy and childhood were considered fourth ventricular tumors. These include 40 medulloblastoma, 14 ependymoma (3 were ependymoblastoma), 6 astrocytoma, 1 choroid plexus papilloma, and 1 teratoma. Because of the ill-defined criteria for classifying fourth ventricular tumors, the published literature presented variable results.

The incidence of fourth ventricular tumor in childhood has been reported to range from 8 to 11 percent[15] of all intracranial tumors. Harwood-Nash and Fitz[9] described the ependymoma as a pure intraventricular tumor, the astrocytoma and medulloblastoma as secondary, encroaching neoplasms, growing into the fourth ventricle from the cerebellum. They reported ependymoma, 53 percent; astrocytoma, 20 percent; and medulloblastoma, 14 percent. Craig and Kernohan [5] reported 82 tumors of the fourth ventricle in all age groups: there were 31 medulloblastomas, 21 ependymomas, 19 astrocytomas, 4 oligodendrogliomas, 3 hemiangioepitheliomas, 2 gliomas of granular layers, 1 epidermoid cyst, and 1 choroid plexus papilloma. Mori, Takaku, Mineura, et al.[19] reported 74 intra- and paraventricular tumors including 38 medulloblastomas, 23 astrocytomas, and 13 ependymomas. Medulloblastoma, ependymoma, and astrocytoma thus are the main tumors in this particular location.

Among 56 medulloblastomas of our series, 40 (73 percent) were located in the fourth ventricle. This is in harmony with the 67 to 80 percent reported by various authors. Approximately one half of our series showed some extension into the cerebellar hemisphere; five of our 40 intraventricular medulloblastomas were attached to or invaded the floor of the fourth ventricle, and another six showed extension into the inferior or superior cerebellar peduncles.

Of our 42 cerebellar astrocytomas, six (14.2 percent) were located in the fourth ventricle, two of which were purely intraventricular (one had an attachment to the floor of the fourth ventricle and the other invaded the cerebellar peduncle). Four were benign (two Grade I, two Grade II), and two were malignant (Grade III). All but one showed solid tumor and one was partially cystic at its center. Cushing[6] described the median cerebellar astrocytoma as "so soft and free from cysts as to suggest a medulloblastoma, so vascular as to suggest an angioblastoma, or so disposed as to resemble an ependymoma."

Of our 14 intraventricular ependymomas, 11 were benign and three malignant (ependymoblastoma); 10 were attached to the floor of the fourth ventricle; cerebellar involvement was noted in seven; only one extended into the cerebellopontine angle.

CLINICAL CONSIDERATIONS

Depending upon whether the CSF pathways are obstructed, the cerebellum or its peduncles are infiltrated, the floor of the fourth ventricle is invaded, or the cranial nerves (nuclei) are compressed, the symptoms and signs will vary considerably.

Vomiting, headache, lethargy, papilledema, or a bulging anterior fontanel are more common and rapidly progressive in children with medulloblastoma. Vomiting is unassociated with headache in 50 percent of the cases, suggesting that the lesion causes direct pressure upon the emetic center in the floor of the fourth ventricle. Headaches, intermittent and generalized or localized in frontal or occipital regions, commonly awaken the children from sleep and abate as the day progresses. In young children and infants, the headache is expressed clinically by irritability, head holding, and/or head banging. Fourth ventricular tumors may give rise to Bruns' syndrome:[10] (1) vertigo, vomiting, and nystagmus, sometimes terminating in unconsciousness, or change in position of the head; (2) freedom from symptoms until the head assumes another position; (3) maintenance of the head in lateral or anterior flexion in order to prevent attacks. Unsteadiness of gait, truncal titubation, head tilt, double vision, or squint are commonly present.

The most common and important sign is papilledema, noted in 69 percent of our cases. Since we began shunting routinely—prior to posterior fossa craniotomy—in children with hydrocephalus complicating fourth ventricle tumors, we have never seen a case of postcraniotomy blindness. One patient showed paraparesis and another quadriparesis. The changes of the deep tendon reflexes were of interest: 19 children were hyperreflexic and 15 hyporeflexic. Hyperreflexia results from associated hydrocephalus or brain-stem compression; hyporeflexia, from the disconnection of vestibulocerebellar fibers. Cranial nerve involvement is most commonly of the abducens and facial nerves, most likely due to compression of the colliculus facialis. Only rarely appearing are other cranial nerve signs such as trigeminal, auditory, or vagal-glosso-pharyngeal. In cases with decreased or absent gag reflexes, the ependymoma is attached to the caudal half of the floor of the fourth ventricle. Head tilt and nuchal rigidity indicate tumor extension into the foramen magnum. It is likely that the child with head tilt is compensating for diplopia, headache, vertigo, or vomiting.

The incidence of uptake of radionucleide in fourth ventricular tumors is high. Radioisotope brain scan showed positive findings in three out of four astrocytomas, five out of five ependymomas, and 15 out of 19 medulloblastomas. Air studies, encephalography, or ventriculography, which have been recommended by others, have not been of value to us, except to differentiate brain-stem glioma from fourth ventricular tumor.

Angiography is performed on all children with already (clinical, radionucleide, computerized tomography scan) diagnosed posterior fossa tumors prior to direct surgical attack. The reasons are (1) to evaluate degree of vascularity, (2) to identify origin and location of feeding arteries, and (3) to identify veins and

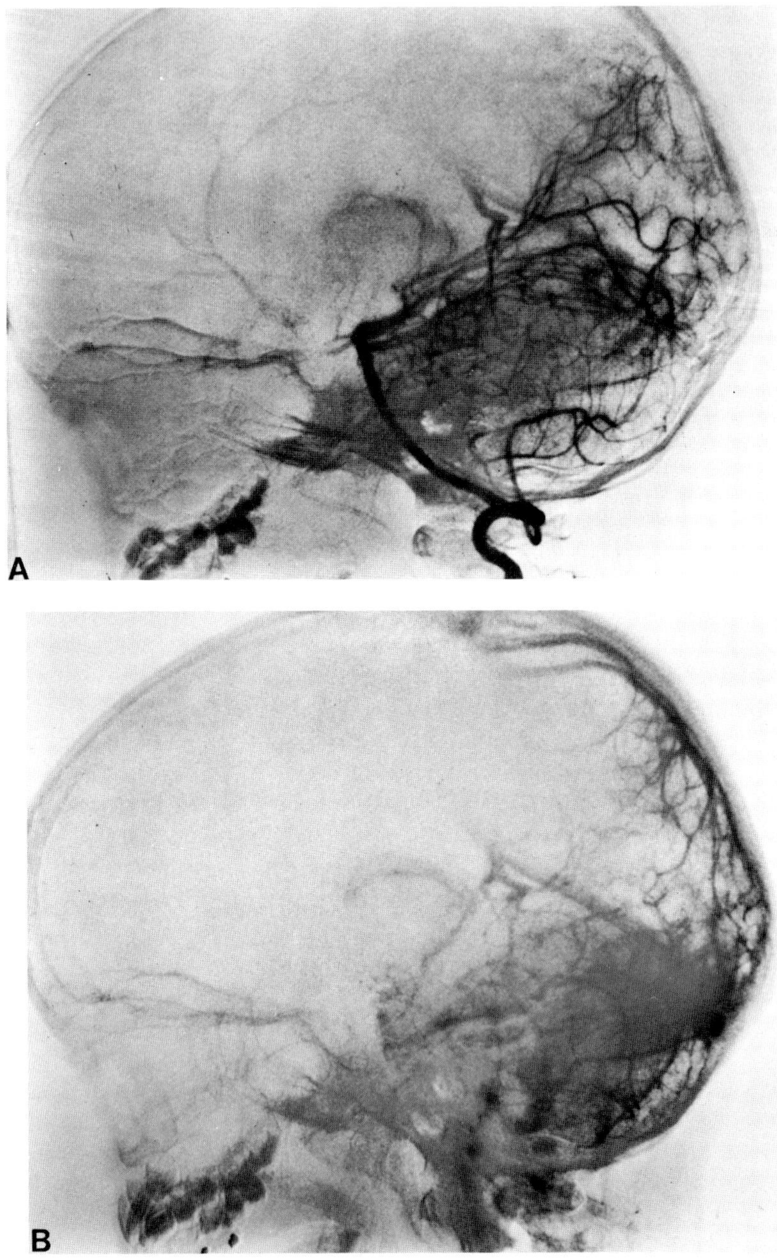

Figure 29-2. Angiographic study of a child with a medulloblastoma who presented clinically with hydrocephalus, and computerized transmission tomographic evidence of a large midline mass in the posterior fossa. A. Arteriography provides specific information concerning arterial supply to the tumor and, in this case, its lack of vascularity. B. The venographic studies identify clearly the venous drainage to be located anterosuperior to the main tumor mass, thus providing the surgeon with essential information to assist in the technical aspects of tumor removal.

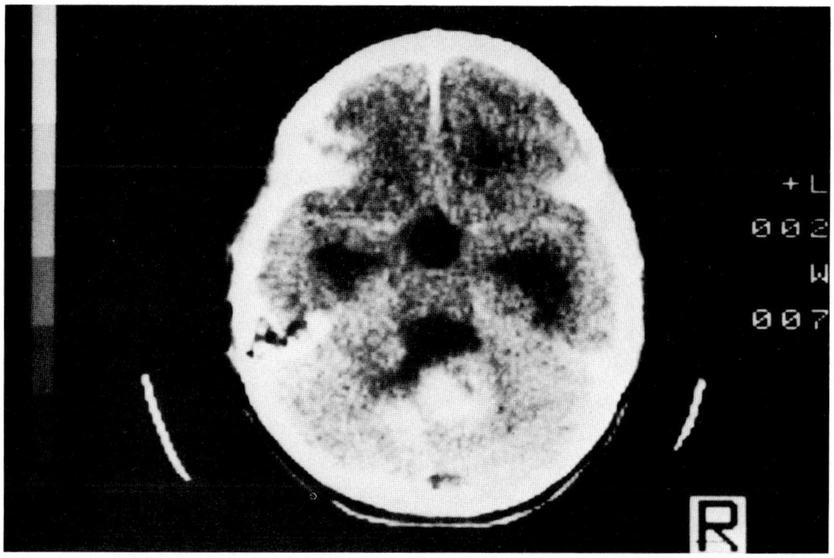

Figure 29-3. Computerized transmission tomogram of a child with medulloblastoma. Note, in this enhancement study, the large mass occupying the region of the fourth ventricle and the halo, cerebellar edema, surrounding it.

sinuses into which the tumor vessels drain (Fig. 29-2 A, B). This facilitates the surgical procedure greatly.

Computerized tomography (CT) scan was obtained in three of our cerebellar astrocytomas, six of our medulloblastomas, and five of our ependymomas of the fourth ventricle. Though CT scans are quite valuable in making the diagnosis of posterior fossa tumor, and of the complicating hydrocephalus, attempts at histologic diagnosis have been less than satisfying. This is not surprising and should, in our opinion, be avoided: histological diagnosis is difficult enough with the light microscope! All tumors were enhanced by the contrast media. The changes of the fourth ventricle are usually central in location and have a lucent halo (Fig. 29-3). There may be evidence of a separate, displaced fourth ventricle. Tumors originating in the cerebellar vermis displace the fourth ventricle anteriorly, and lack a halo in the posterior portion. Occasionally the rostral portion of the fourth ventricle is enlarged by the blockage of the fourth ventricle caused by the caudally located tumor. One may miss the presence of the tumor if a more caudal cut is not obtained.

TREATMENT

The hydrocephalus associated with fourth ventricular tumors is the major cause of the presenting symptoms and signs, and may indeed become the cause of death. It is variable in degree, but invariably symmetric and hypertensive. The treatment of hydrocephalus associated with a posterior fossa tumor is still a matter of debate. Cushing[6] used intraoperative ventricular cannulation in posterior fossa surgery in 1909, "so as to avoid the prolapse of the cerebellar tissue through the dural opening and to control the extracranial venous stasis produced by the increased intracranial pressure." Preoperative external ventricular drainage (EVD) was proposed by Poppen[21] in 1943, "to improve the condition of the patient before posterior fossa surgery." Gol and McKissock[7] stated that "the prognosis is better in preoperative EVD than without it." Subsequently, after improvement of CSF shunting devices, preoperative internal shunts such as ventriculoperitoneal (VP) or ventriculoatrial (VA) have been utilized.[1,2,25]

The majority of symptoms and signs—expressions of increased intracranial pressure—are produced by the complicating and secondary hydrocephalus. For this reason we suggest inserting a VP shunt to compensate the hydrocephalus, and return the intracranial pressure to normal. Subsequent to shunting most of the symptoms and signs secondary to the increased intracranial pressure subside. The definitive posterior fossa surgery is performed when all such signs have subsided. The VP shunt is preferred to EVD because it is a definitive procedure that allows the surgeon the option to perform craniotomy on a purely elective basis, does not require the same close nursing observation to avoid overdrainage, has a much lower (less than 0.5 percent) incidence of infection, and may be kept in situ (since over 30 percent of children with posterior fossa tumors are permanently hydrocephalic). The interval between precraniotomy shunt and definitive surgery for the posterior fossa tumor is usually 7 to 14 days, by which time the papilledema is resolved and the child's physical and neurologic condition becomes stable. This eliminates the risk of postoperative blindness. The internal shunt has theoretic disadvantages: (1) difficulty in regulating the intracranial pressure, with a risk of upward herniation or supratentorial subdural hematoma; (2) risk of systemic dissemination of neoplastic cells through the shunt tube. From our experience upward herniation occurred in 5 percent of the 240 cases shunted and prompt posterior fossa decompression in all instances was followed by full recovery. The risk of upward herniation is the same when EVD is used as when a definitive shunt is inserted. Also, in spite of previous reports regarding shunt-related systemic metastases,[11] we have not observed a single instance in malignant posterior fossa tumors.

The posterior fossa craniotomy is performed in the sitting position for all fourth ventricle tumors, since they invariably occupy the superior cerebellar triangle. Rectal thermocouple, arterial and central venous pressure lines, urinary catheterization, and two intravenous lines are mandatory. Spontaneous respiration is preferred when dissecting the tumor from the floor of the fourth ventricle. In terms of sitting position, several comments may be of value: The head should be fixed rigidly, after maximum distraction, then flexed 30 degrees. Overflexion should be avoided because of resultant impaired venous return, tracheal damage, or pressure sores of the chin from the suprasternal region. The legs should be elevated to the level of the heart, resulting in the patient being in the "horizontal" sitting position (Fig. 29-4). The advantages are a dry field, ease of use of the operating microscope, approachability of the fourth ventricle and the aqueduct of

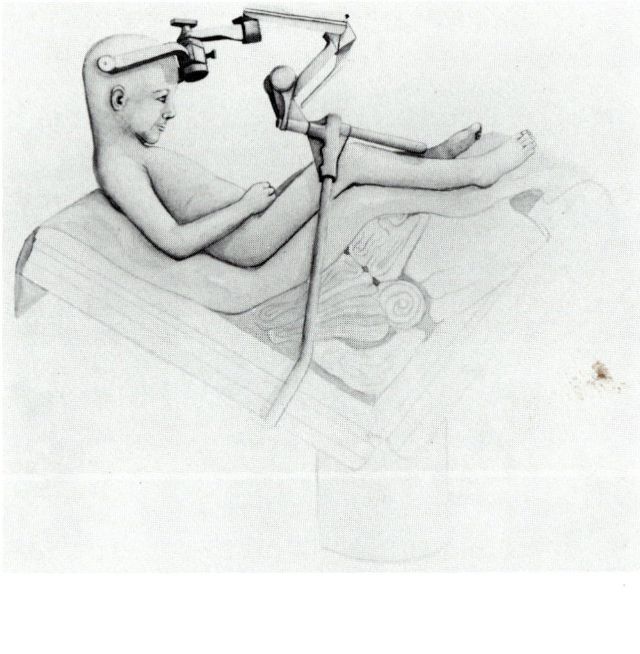

Figure 29-4. The ideal position for posterior fourth ventricular tumor surgery in the child. Particular attention should be given to the position of the head (maximally distracted, flexed 30 degrees, perpendicular to the horizon) since this opens maximally the atlantooccipital space, and puts all cervical vertebra in a verticle plane as it "horizontalizes" the tentorium, giving the surgeon a clear line of vision to the fourth ventricle, cerebellar triangle, and tentorial opening.

Sylvius, and ready access to the culmen monticuli and anterior medullary velum. It also permits the anesthesiologist free access to the nose and mouth of the child.

We routinely use a midline skin incision, extending from 1 cm above the inion to the level of C6 spinal process. The suboccipital muscles are separated subperiosteally from the squamous occipital bone and the arch of the atlas. No muscles are dissected from C2, C3, C4, etc.

The posterior fossa craniotomy is performed by opening bilateral burr holes in the squamous portion of the occipital bone, separating the underlying dura from the inner table of the occipital bone and the foramen magnum with the Gigli saw guide, and making the trapezoid-shaped bone flap connecting the burr holes and foramen magnum. If the tumor extends through the foramen magnum into the upper cervical canal, the arch of C1 should be osteotemized and reflected downward, not removed. This allows the reapproximation of C1 into its normal position and anchoring of this arch by periosteal sutures. If the tumor occupies the superior cerebellar triangle only, the craniotomy is not extended into the foramen magnum. Rather, 2 cm or more of squamous occipital bone are left above the rim. This affords support to the cerebellar hemispheres in the inferior cerebellar triangle.

A posterior fossa craniotomy is preferable to a craniectomy in children since this method permits reconstructing completely the squamous portion of the occipital bone and the suboccipital musculature. In children in general, but in small infants with thin occipital muscle layers in particular, craniotomy prevents postoperative cerebellar protrusion and/or pseudomeningocele through the craniectomy site.

The dural opening is made in a Y-shaped fashion; the occipital sinus clipped and divided. One notices immediately the slack posterior fossa resulting from the precraniotomy shunt. At this point tumor within the cisterna magnum may be identified usually, but tumor entirely within the fourth ventricle is indicated by the downward herniation of the tonsils or bulging of the pyramis of the cerebellar vermis. After opening the arachnoid of the cisterna magnum, the tonsils are separated and the inferior vermis (pyramis) is split in the midline. The inferior vermian veins are coagulated. Subsequently, the fourth ventricle is entered.

The surgical aim is to resect as much of the tumor as possible and to open the CSF pathways. Intraoperative frozen section should be maintained. Every effort should be made to gain access to the angiographically identified vascular supply and drainage of the tumor before undertaking the resection. It is not advisable to work within the tumor mass with the hope of debulking it first, lest the fourth ventricular floor be entered. The first step in the resection is the dissection of the tumor away from the floor of the fourth ventricle, and the placement of a telfa protective covering between it and the tumor. The same is then done for the lateral surfaces of the fourth ventricle. Most of the ependymomas may be attached to the floor of the fourth ventricle. Occasionally, it is possible to tease the fibrous adhesion from the floor. This should be done with meticulous care, under magnification. In most cases, however, complete dissection of the tumor from the floor of the fourth ventricle is dangerous; a thin layer of tumor tissue should be left to avoid the destruction of the cranial nuclei or cerebellar peduncles. Tumors extending to the cerebellopontine angle through the cerebellar hemisphere are resected totally. Tumors such as the ependymoma extending to the cerebellopontine angle through the lateral recess should not be resected, because of attachment to the brain stem and cranial nerves. The aqueduct of Sylvius may be plugged by a peglike extension of the fourth ventricular tumor. These tumors usually do not invade the periaqueductal tissue, however, and the reopening of the aqueduct is possible.

SURGICAL COMPLICATIONS

The most serious complication was postoperative hemorrhage into the fourth ventricle, occurring in 2 patients. Both suffered decreased levels of consciousness, changes of vital signs (particularly hypertension), and seizure activity preceded by headache. Prompt posterior fossa reexploration was life saving in both instances. Transient or permanent palsies of the cranial nerves may occur. The most common complication was external ocular palsy. Horizontal gaze palsy with vertical gaze spared is thought to be due to damage of the pontine paramedian reticular formation. It was experienced in three cerebellar astrocytomas, two ependymomas, and two medulloblastomas. This complication is described by Kahn, Crosby, and DeJonge[13] as "curious staring effect" and may be explained by the bilateral destruction of the medial longitudinal fasciculus. Abducens palsy or skewed eye deviation may also occur. The facial palsy is invariably associated with gaze (abducens) palsy, suggesting damage of the region of the facial colliculi. Decreased or absent gag reflex was noted in three children, who required a tracheotomy and gastrostomy.

Five children died within one month after surgery (four medulloblastoma, 1 malignant teratoma), for a surgical mortality rate of 8 percent. One, three-, and five-year survival rates were 64.7 percent, 40.0 percent, and 23.1 percent in medulloblastoma. The medulloblastoma survival rates are of particular interest, especially in light of ependymoma, which, in spite of its benign histologic nature, shows much poorer survival. One-, three-, and five-year survival rates in this latter tumor were 100 percent, 37.5 percent, and 14.3 percent. All children with astrocytoma and choroid plexus papilloma are still alive over periods ranging from one to 12 years.

In addition to the surgical treatment, "T"-port neuroaxis radiation therapy was given to all medulloblastoma and ependymoblastoma patients. We seriously challenge the widespread use of this form of prophylactic roentgen therapy because of the serious and severe complications.[24]

REFERENCES

1. Abraham J, Chandy J: Ventriculo-atrial shunt in the management of posterior fossa tumor. Preliminary report. J Neurosurg 20:252–253, 1963
2. Albright L, Reigel DH: Management of hydrocephalus secondary to posterior fossa tumor. J Neurosurg 46:52–55, 1977
3. Bailey P, Cushing H: Medulloblastoma cerebelli: A common type of midcerebellar glioma of childhood. Arch Neurol Psychiatr 14:192–224, 1924
4. Courville CB, Broussalian SL: Plastic ependymomas of the lateral recess. Report of eight verified cases. J Neurosurg 18:792–799, 1961
5. Craig W McK, Kernohan JW: Tumors of the fourth ventricle. JAMA 111:2370–2377, 1938
6. Cushing H: Experiences with cerebellar astrocytomas. A critical review of 76 cases. Surg Gynec Obstet 52:129–204, 1931
7. Gol A, McKissock W: The cerebellar astrocytomas. A report in 98 verified cases. J Neurosurg 16:287–296, 1959
8. Goutelle A, Tisher G: Les 'ependymomes intracraniens et intrarachidiens. Neurochirurgie 23(Suppl 7):111–147, 1971
9. Harwood-Nash D, Fitz CR: Neuroradiology in Infants and Children. St. Louis, CV Mosby, 1976
10. Haymaker W, Kuhlenbeck H: Disorders of the brain stem and its cranial nerves, in Baker, Baker LH (eds): Clinical Neurology, vol. 3. New York, Harper & Row, 1971
11. Hoffman HJ, Hendrick EB, Humphreys RP: Metastasis via ventriculoperitoneal shunt in patients with medulloblastoma. J Neurosurg 44:562–566, 1976

12. Hoffman JC Jr, Burkin WJ, Richardson HD: Primary intraventricular meningiomas of the fourth ventricle. Am J Roentgenol Rad Thera Nucl Med 115:100–104, 1972
13. Kahn EA, Crosby EL, DeJonge BR: Tumors of the posterior fossa, in Kahn EA et al (eds): Correlative Neurosurgery. Springfield, Charles C Thomas, 1969
14. Knudsen PA: Ventriklernes Storrelsesforhold: Anatomisk normale njerher fra voksne mennesker Odense, Denmark, Andelsbogtrykkereit, 1958
15. Koos W Th, Miller MH: Intracranial Tumors of Infants and Children. Stuttgart, Georg Thieme Verlag, 1971
16. Mahoney W: Die Epidermoide des Zentral-Nerven Systems. Z Ges Neurol Psychiatr 155:416–471, 1936
17. Matson DD: Neurosurgery of Infancy and Childhood. Springfield, Charles C Thomas, 1969
18. Möller A: Pneumography in paraventricular and intraventricular tumors of the posterior fossa. Acta Radiol 342(suppl):1–145, 1974
19. Mori T, Takaku A, Mineura K, et al: Follow-up study of fourth ventricle tumors in childhood. Neurol Surg 5:965–972, 1977
20. Patriquin H, Melancon D, Bertrand G, et al: Epidermoids of the fourth ventricle. J Canad Assoc Radiol 20:37–42, 1969
21. Poppen JL: Ventricular drainage as a valuable procedure in neurosurgery. Report of a satisfactory method. Arch Neurol Psychiatr 50:587–589, 1943
22. Raaf J, Kernohan JW: Relation of abnormal collections of cells in posterior medullary velum of cerebellum to origin of medulloblastoma. Arch Neurol Psychiatr 52:163–169, 1944
23. Raimondi AJ, Gutierrez FA: Diagnosis and surgical treatment of choroid plexus papillomas. Child's Brain 1:81–115, 1975
24. Raimondi AJ, Tomita T: The Disadvantages of Prophylactic Whole CNS Postoperative Radiation Therapy for Medulloblastoma. Multidisciplinary Aspects of Brain Tumor Therapy. Elsevier/North-Holland, Biomedical Press, 1979
25. Raimondi AJ, Yashon D, Matsumoto S, et al. Increased intracranial pressure, without lateralizing signs: The midline syndrome. Neurochirurgia 10:197–209, 1967
26. Ringertz N, Tola JH: Medulloblastoma. J Neuropath Exp Neurol 9:354–372, 1950
27. Rodriquez-Carbajal J, Palacios E: Intraventricular meningiomas of the fourth ventricle. Am J Roentgenol Rad Ther Nucl Med 120:27–31, 1974
28. Rovit RL, Schechter MM: Choroid plexus papillomas. Observations on radiographic diagnosis. Am J Roentgenol Rad Ther Nucl Med 110:608–617, 1970
29. Rubinstein LJ: Tumors of the Central Nervous System. Washington DC, ATIP, 1972
30. Russell DS, Rubinstein LJ: Pathology of Tumors of the Nervous System. London, Edward Arnold, 1971
31. Stanley P: Papillomas of the choroid plexus. Br J Radiol 41:848–857, 1968
32. Stevenson L, Echlin F: The nature and origin of some tumors of the cerebellum (medulloblastoma). Arch Neurol Psychiat 31:93–109, 1934
33. Van Wagenen WP: Papillomas of the choroid plexus (reports of 2 cases, 1 with removal of the tumor at operation and 1 with "seeding" of tumor in the ventricular system). Arch Surg 20:199–231, 1930

brain tumors. Approximately 12 percent of patients with this lesion, however, may present between the ages of 12 and 20 years.[11] The youngest case reported is that of a 3-year-old child.[13] The younger the age of presentation, the more likely the patient is to have the Von Hipple–Lindau syndrome. This condition either may occur sporadically or be familial; if familial, it is inherited as an autosomal dominant with partial penetrance. The Von Hipple–Lindau syndrome is characterized by at least one hemangioblastoma of the neuraxis combined with one or more of the following: retinal angiomatosis, angiomas of the liver and kidney, renal cell carcinoma, pheochromocytoma, and cysts of the pancreas, kidney, and epididymis.[12]

The majority of hemangioblastomas occur in the posterior fossa. In one series of 76 patients with this tumor, 67 were located in the posterior fossa, five were spinal, and four were supratentorial[13] The tumor may be either cystic or solid, single or multiple, or situated either in the midline or in the hemispheres of the cerebellum. Many of these tumors have meningeal attachment, frequently to the ventral aspect of the tentorium.[28] Erythrocytosis with elevated hemoglobin values is often associated with hemangioblastoma. In one series 18 percent of patients had a hemoglobin level of greater than 18 gm% and in 42 percent the level was greater than 16 gm%. The tumor is believed to secrete erythropoietin, a hormone that has been isolated from the tumor cyst fluid, the tumor tissue, and the plasma of the host patient.[13] In the patient who initially presents with erythrocytosis, postoperative return of hemoglobin values to normal is a good index of total removal of the hemangioblastoma.[14]

Headache is the most common presenting symptom. Papilledema is present in the majority of patients, and ataxia and nystagmus may occur. Skull films rarely show more than changes attributable to increased intracranial pressure. The CT scan may show one or more cysts, but the tumors themselves are rarely visualized on the noncontrast study. Following iodinated contrast administration, the solid tumor and/or mural nodules show distinct enhancement.[10] Cerebral angiography is indicated in all suspected cases of hemangioblastoma. This study usually demonstrates a dense stain of the nodular portion of the lesion, mass effect of the cystic portion, and early filling of draining veins (Fig. 30-1).[1] Angiography also serves to determine whether or not multiple lesions are present.

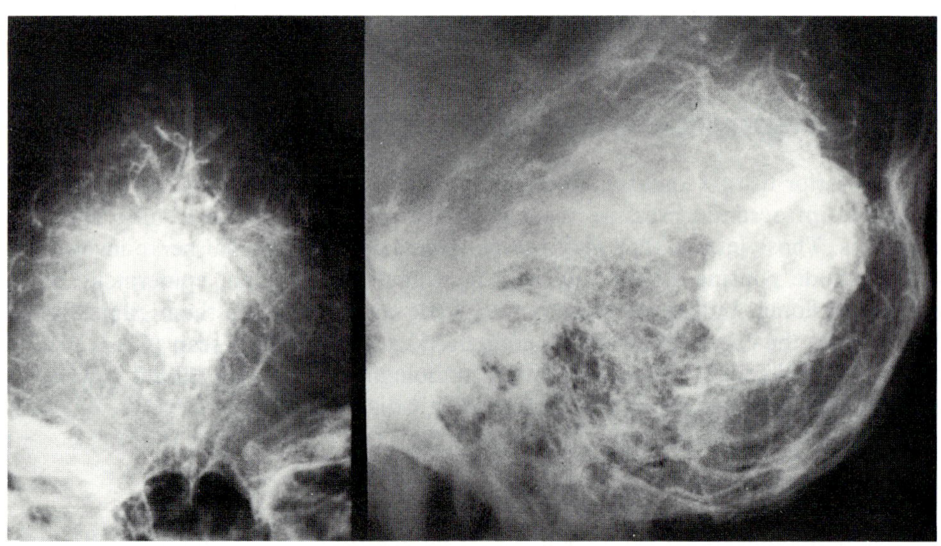

Figure 30-1 Anterior-posterior (left) and lateral (right) vertebral angiogram shows a large, vascular, midline hemangioblastoma in a 13½-year-old male.

The patient with hemangioblastoma should have a thorough evaluation in order to exclude the other stigmata of Von Hipple–Lindau syndrome. In our opinion this should include intravenous pyelography and CT scanning of the abdomen in a search for liver and kidney angiomas, cysts of the pancreas, and kidney and renal carcinoma. Detailed ophthalmologic retinal examination and palpation of the epididymis are an integral part of any such evaluation. Urinary catecholamine levels should be obtained to exclude pheochromocytoma. Some authors propose that spinal angiography and/or myelography should be done on all patients with hemangioblastoma of the cerebellum. We prefer to perform such studies only if the patient shows symptoms of spinal cord involvement.

Total surgical removal is the treatment of choice for hemangioblastoma. The associated cysts should be aspirated. In the event that tumor vascularity or technical problems prevent total removal, radiotherapy can be considered. Radiotherapy probably slows the rate of growth of the tumor and may reduce vascularity, but it will not suppress the erythropoietic activity of the tumor cells.[14]

CHOROID PLEXUS PAPILLOMA

Papillomas of the choroid plexus may occur wherever choroid plexus is located. In adults they are most commonly located in the fourth ventricle. In a series of 141 children with this tumor accumulated from the literature and the experience at the Hospital for Sick Children in Toronto, 97 percent occurred in the lateral ventricle, 7 percent in the third ventricle, and 14 percent in the fourth ventricle.[29] The majority of children presenting with choroid plexus papillomas are less than 5 years of age. The older child is more likely to have a posterior fossa location. In Matson's series of 418 posterior fossa tumors in children, only three were choroid plexus papillomas.[18] Eighty percent of these tumors are pathologically benign but 20 percent demonstrate malignant transformation.[29] Regardless of the pathologic picture, all choroid plexus papillomas have the potential to metastasize via the CSF pathways.[22,29]

The clinical picture of a papilloma of the fourth ventricle is one of increased intracranial pressure without localizing features except for ataxia, nystagmus, and cranial nerve palsies. In infants the symptoms are those of progressive hydrocephalus with enlargement of the head, apathy, irritability, and a failure to thrive.[22] If the lesion is in the fourth ventricle, hydrocephalus is usually of the obstructive variety and overproduction of cerebrospinal fluid (CSF), such as occurs with lesions in the regions of the trigones, is not a contributing factor.[22] Choroid plexus papillomas usually present on noncontrast CT scans as well-circumscribed dense lesions and invariably show contrast enhancement.[4] A tumor stain with well-defined choroidal vessels feeding from the neoplasm is usually demonstrated angiographically. Optimal treatment is total surgical removal of the lesion. Radiotherapy is of questionable benefit and should probably be employed only if there is pathologic malignant transformation, evidence of CSF seeding, or incomplete removal.[22]

DERMOID CYST

Dermoid cysts may occur anywhere within the skull, but their most common single intracranial site is in the posterior fossa at or near the midline. These lesions are the result of incomplete separation of the epithelial ectoderm from the neuroectoderm in the region of the anterior neuropore at the fourth week of gestation. Pathologically the dermoid cyst, and its associated sinus if present, are lined by stratified squamous epithelium and may contain hair follicles, sweat, and sebaceous glands, and other specialized skin structures.[15] The cyst slowly enlarges as a result of the secretion of sebaceous material and the desquamation of epithelium within the lesion. Rupture of the lesion with discharge of the contained material into the surrounding tissue and/or subarachnoid space may occur. Logue and Till[16] divide the cranial dermal lesions into the following four categories: (1) extradural dermoid cysts with complete dermal sinus, (2) intradural dermoid cyst with no dermal sinus, (3) intradural dermoid cyst with an incomplete dermal sinus, and (4) intradural dermoid cyst with a complete dermal sinus. If a congenital dermal sinus accompanies the cranial dermoid lesion, its origin is usually in the midline near the occipital protuberance. The dermal sinus extends inward in a caudal direction penetrating the skull inferior to its site of surface origin.[18] The associated dermoid, if intracranial, may be epidural, in the midline cerebellum, or within the fourth ventricle. Cranial dermoid cysts are rare lesions. The largest personal series is that of Matson who reported 17 cases.[18] Exact incidence figures are not available. Most of the cases in which a cutaneous dermal sinus accompanies the intracranial dermoid present in the early pediatric age groups. If a dermal sinus does not exist, the intracranial dermoid may lie dormant, only to act as an expanding mass lesion in adult life.

Clinically the child harboring this lesion may be noted either at birth or shortly thereafter to have a dimple with associated palpable sinus tract or mass in the midline occipital region. There may or may not be associated telangiectasia or abnormal hair growth. The sinus tract may drain purulent material intermittently and it is not unusual to obtain a history indicating that the cutaneous aspect of this lesion has been surgically "removed," only to result in an open draining wound. Another mode of clinical presentation is repetitive bouts of meningitis. The meningitis may be either aseptic secondary to the inflammatory reaction to cholesterol discharged into the subarachnoid space from the dermoid, or bacterial secondary to organisms entering through the sinus tract.[21] In the latter instance, the organism is usually *Staphylococcus epidermidis*. An abscess may form around or within the substance of the dermoid. Finally the child may present with signs and symptoms of increased intracranial pressure secondary to hydrocephalus. The hydrocephalus may be obstructive due to the effect of the midline posterior fossa mass or communicating secondary to arachnoidal adhesions from repeated bouts of meningeal inflammation.

Investigation of these patients varies and is frequently dictated by the clinical presentation. Repetitive bouts of meningitis or a single bout of meningitis with an unusual organism should arouse suspicion of a dermal sinus. The diagnosis of a dermoid cyst may be made preoperatively by finding cholesterol debris and hair fragments in the CSF. Plain skull films may show an occipital defect with sclerotic borders through which a sinus tract passes (Fig. 30-2).[6] It is not unusual, however, for the skull x-ray to be within normal limits. Currently, few data are available on CT scanning in this condition, but the dermoid should be of lower relative density than brain because of the high lipid and cholesterol content (Fig. 30-3). In addition, hydrocephalus may be present.

The preferred treatment of central nervous system dermoid lesions is total excision of the cyst along with the accompanying sinus tract if present. This procedure may be technically difficult if the child has experienced previous episodes of meningitis, thereby acquiring dense adhesions. For this reason it is our opinion that prophylactic surgical treatment is indicated in infants born with an occipital dermal sinus. It is important to trace any dermal sinus tract to its point of termination and in treating an occipital dermal sinus the neurosurgeon should be prepared to perform a major posterior fossa midline exploration.

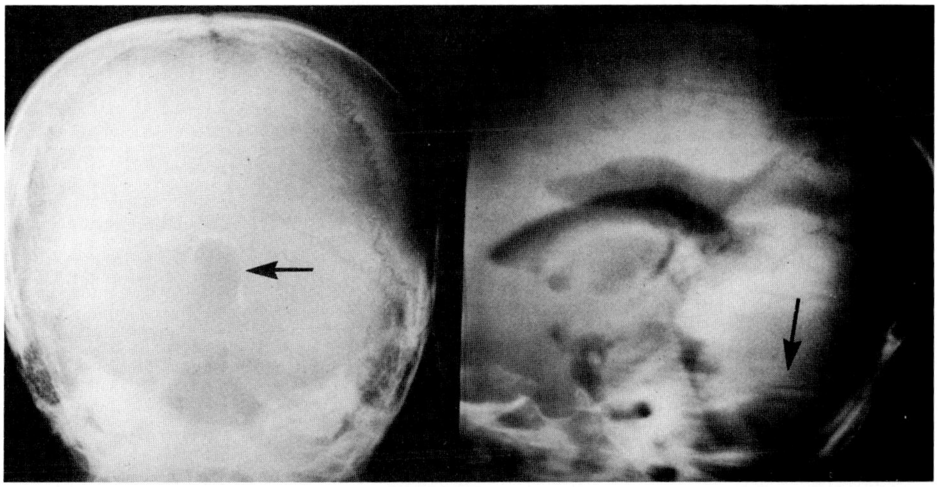

Figure 30-2 Intracranial dermoid cyst in a 4-year-old male. Plain anterior-posterior skull film (left) shows a midline skull defect in the occipital bone with a dense sclerotic margin (arrow). Lateral pneumoencephalogram (right) shows a midline soft tissue mass projecting into the cisterna magna inferiorly (arrow).

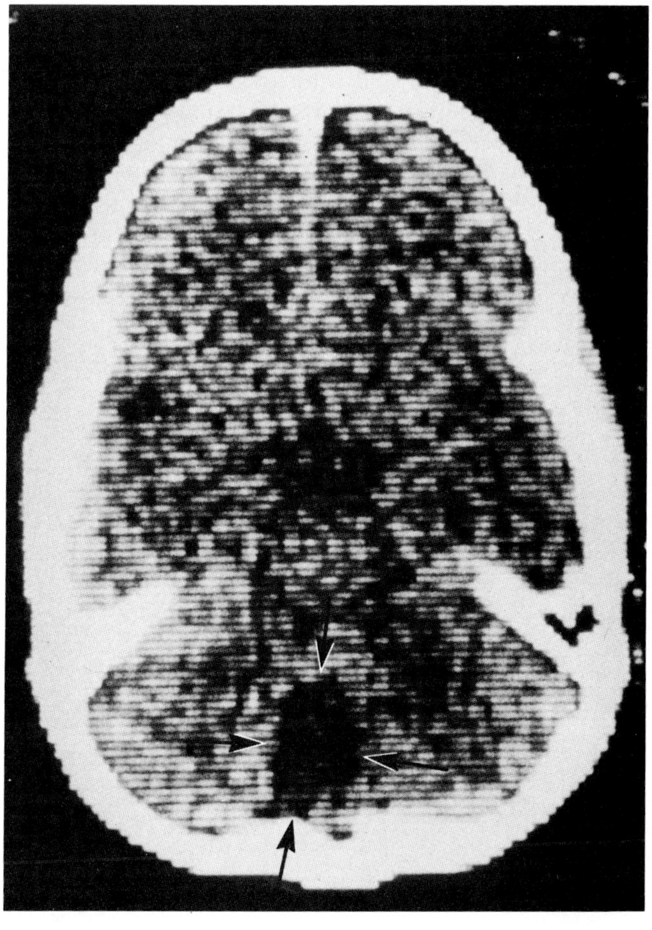

Figure 30-3. A CT scan (noncontrast) in a 4-year-old male with an intracranial dermoid cyst. Original interpretation of the study was "large cisterna magna," but in retrospect the midline rounded area of decreased density was the dermoid cyst (arrows). (Same case as in Fig. 30-2.)

EPIDERMOID CYST

Epidermoid cysts (cholesteatomas) of the posterior fossa are very unusual in the pediatric age group. They are to be distinguished from the previously discussed dermoid lesions in that they contain only the epidermal cell layer in their capsule and are devoid of dermal structures such as hair and sebaceous glands. They arise from epithelial cell rests, usually near the base of the brain, and are considered congenital lesions on this basis, although they may not become clinically apparent until adult life.[30] Epidermoids grow slowly by virtue of collection of desquamating cells of the epithelial wall. Within the posterior fossa, these lesions are usually located either in the cerebellopontine angle or ventral to the brain stem.

Children harboring epidermoid cysts usually present with cranial nerve dysfunction and symptoms and signs suggesting brain-stem compression. The symptom complex associated with these lesions may be easily confused with that caused by pontine glioma. Seizures may occur if the mass grows into the middle fossa. Trigeminal neuralgia in a young person should arouse suspicion of a posterior fossa epidermoid tumor. The clinical history is usually lengthy but occasionally a malignant transformation to an epidermoid carcinoma may result in a fulminating course.[35] Recurrent aseptic meningitis is an unusual manifestation, and occurred in a case of intrinsic pontine epidermoid in a 2-year-old child previously reported from our institution.[27]

Prior to the advent of CT scanning, the diagnosis of epidermoid tumor in the child was difficult and often was not made until operation and/or autopsy. The typical appearance on CT scanning is of a posterior fossa mass lesion usually located in the cerebellopontine angle or adjacent brain-stem region with a low attenuation coefficient of −8 to +32 Hounsfield units (Fig. 30-4). Infrequently these lesions may be relatively dense on the CT scan (i.e., 80–120 Hounsfield

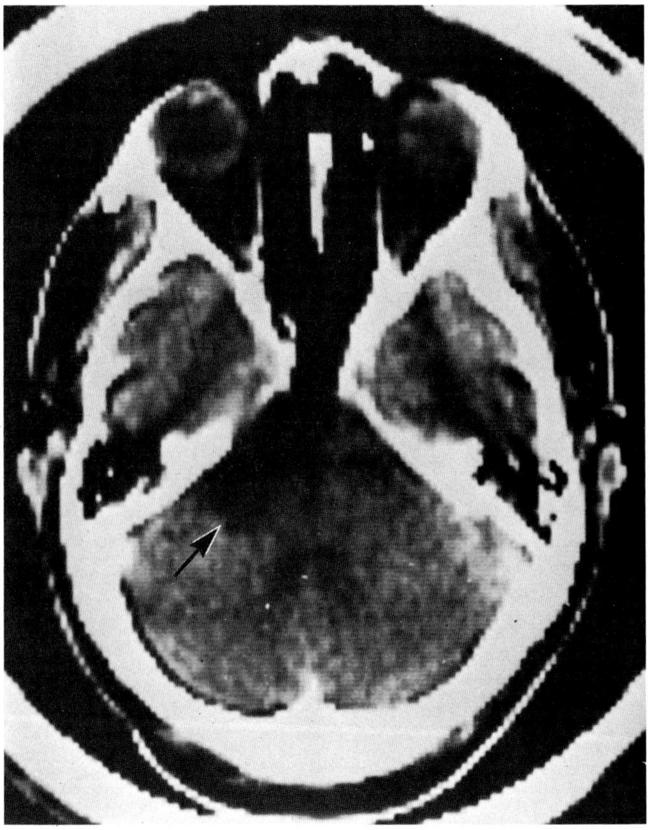

Figure 30-4. A CT scan showing epidermoid tumor of the left cerebellopontine angle. Precontrast scan shows the lesion as an area of decreased attenuation coefficient.

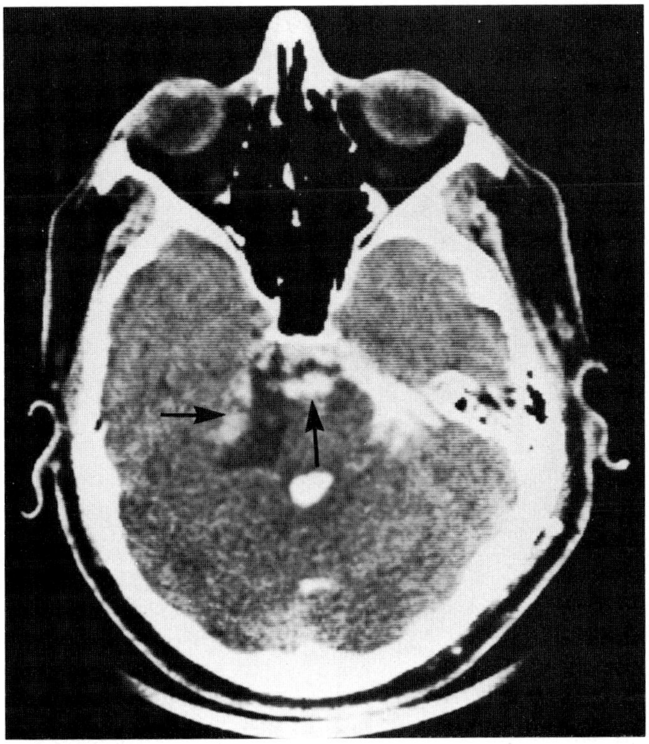

Figure 30-5. Same epidermoid tumor as in Figure 30-4. Metrizamide cisternography shows the contrast agent in the interstices of the lesion (arrows).

units).[4] In either case the lesion does *not* show contrast enhancement. A typical finding of epidermoid on pneumoencephalography is entrapment of air in the tumor interstices, which produces a "foamy" appearance. This appearance was noted in one of our recent adult cases during a metrizamide cisternogram in which the metrizamide became entrapped within the irregular interstices of an epidermoid (Fig. 30-5).

Ideal treatment of this benign lesion is complete surgical removal if possible. Radiotherapy has no role in the treatment of this cyst.

ACOUSTIC NEUROMA

Acoustic neuroma rarely occurs in childhood, and most cases reported in children are in adolescents. Mark and Sweet reported an 8½-year-old boy with a unilateral acoustic tumor whose symptoms started before age 6 years[17] and the Italian literature contains a report of an acoustic neuroma in a 1-year-old girl.[32,36] Although the majority of children presenting with bilateral acoustic neuromas have the stigmata of Ricklinghausen's neurofibromatosis, unilateral tumors are not necessarily associated with this entity. Children usually present with clinical features similar to those of adults harboring this neoplasm, that is, unilateral sensorineural hearing loss, facial weakness, and corneal anesthesia, gait disturbance, and unilateral dystaxia.[7] Signs and symptoms of increased intracranial pressure due to obstructive hydrocephalus may occur later in the course, and are probably a more common presenting symptom complex in children than in adults due to the tendency for unilateral hearing loss to remain unrecognized in the child.

Otologic examination in the majority of patients with acoustic neuroma will show sensorineural hearing loss and vestibular testing usually reveals a reduced caloric response as measured by electronystagmography. Neuroradiologic assessment should include plain skull films, polytomography of the petrous bones, and CT scanning with contrast enhancement. Plain films may show abnormal

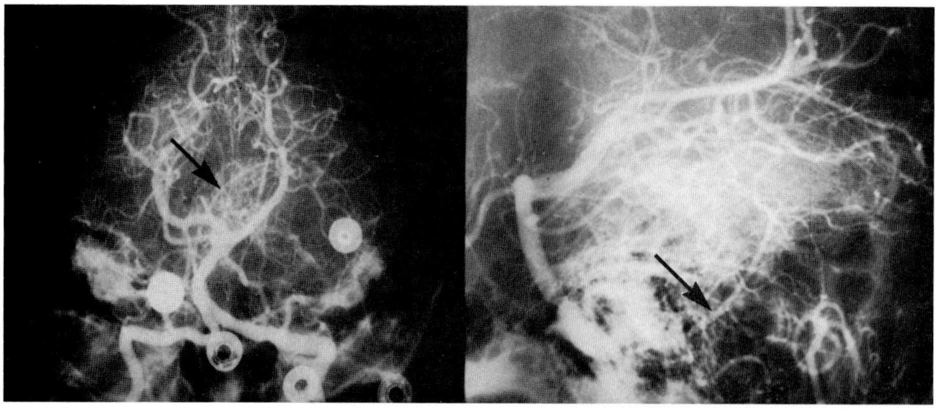

Figure 30-6. Anterior-posterior (left) and lateral (right) vertebral angiogram demonstrating stretching and displacement of the anterior inferior cerebellar artery caused by an acoustic neuroma in a 13-year-old female (arrows).

calcification or changes in the skull base. The internal auditory meatus may be abnormally enlarged on polytomography but not invariably. Precontrast CT scanning usually shows the tumor to be isodense with brain, although its presence may be inferred by shifts of surrounding structures (i.e., mass effect). Following the intravenous injection of iodinated contrast, an acoustic neuroma will usually show dense enhancement, and CT scanning with contrast enhancement will demonstrate greater than 95 percent of acoustic neuromas larger than 1.5 to 2 cm.[9] Vertebral angiography (via transfemoral injection) is indicated only if these studies are either equivocal or atypical; for instance in the case of a positive CT scan and normal internal auditory meati on polytomes, or a CT scan showing increased density before contrast (Fig. 30-6). In both of these latter situations, meningioma is the most likely alternative diagnosis and external carotid selective injection of a contrast medium is valuable in delineating the vascularity of the tumor.

The goal of treatment of acoustic neuroma is total excision with preservation of neurologic function including preservation of facial nerve function and of hearing in some instances. The authors prefer the suboccipital transmeatal approach performed with the patient in the sitting position. The details of this operative approach are well described in other publications.[24]

Bilateral acoustic neuroma is most often seen in adolescents and young adults with Recklinghausen's disease. If the tumors are both large and there is nerve deafness bilaterally, the initial surgical procedure should be directed toward the largest tumor even if cranial nerve deficit is worse on the side of the smaller tumor. The contralateral tumor can then be removed in a second procedure. If one or both of the tumors are small with some preservation of hearing, the decision regarding timing of therapy becomes more difficult. Some authors recommend repetitive internal decompression of the tumor and the internal auditory canal in order to preserve hearing.[23] It is our belief that the postoperative changes from such procedures may preclude eventual total removal of the tumor.

MENINGIOMA

Only approximately 1.5 percent of intracranial tumors of childhood are meningiomas.[19] Reports vary as to the percentage of childhood meningiomas located in the posterior fossa from almost 50 percent in the series of Crouse and

Berg[8] to 19 percent in a series of 75 cases collected from the United States by Merten, Goding, Newton, et al.[20] Meningiomas are seldom found in early childhood, with most of the reported cases occurring in adolescence. Approximately 23 percent of children harboring intracranial meningiomas have the stigmata of Recklinghausen's neurofibromatosis and associated acoustic neuromas are not unusual. Many authors believe that meningiomas in childhood are pathologically more aggressive lesions than in adults, and are prone to sarcomatous change.[5]

Meningiomas of the posterior fossa in children most commonly involve the petrous ridge and cerebellopontine angle. Clinical presentation is usually with nonspecific signs of increased intracranial pressure. Lower cranial nerve deficits, especially hearing loss, may occur and ipsilateral ataxia may be seen. Seizures are an unusual presentation unless the tumor has extended into the middle fossa.

Plain skull films may show calcification within the tumor, hyperostosis of adjacent bone, and/or nonspecific evidence of increased intracranial pressure (i.e., erosion of the dorsum sella and split sutures). Computerized tomographic scanning is the most useful diagnostic test and usually reveals an enhancing mass lesion (Fig. 30-7). Obstructive hydrocephalus may be demonstrated. Currently the necessity for angiography in view of the usually striking CT changes is controversial. If it is performed, it may reveal either a vascular or avascular mass. It may be of benefit in determining predominant blood supply to the tumor. Despite CT scanning and angiography, the differentiation between acoustic neuroma and meningioma may not be possible preoperatively. Cystic areas within the mass favor the diagnosis of acoustic neuroma.

Total resection of a meningioma is the treatment of choice. With the operating microscope, self-retaining retractors, bipolar coagulation, and microtechnique, this should be possible in most instances. Occasionally, because of either excessive size or vascularity, the operative procedure may require staging.

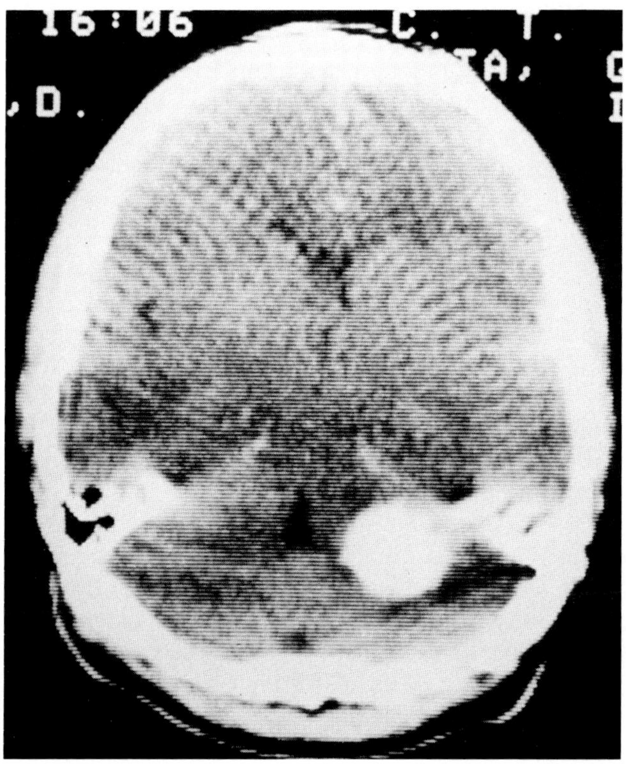

Figure 30-7. CT scan after contrast enhancement in a 16-year-old male showing an enhancing mass (meningioma) in the right cerebellopontine angle.

Meticulous removal of all bone involved by tumor should be carried out. Wara, Sheline, Newton, et al.[34] agree that total resection is the procedure of choice, but point out that if resection is known to be incomplete, radiation therapy may prevent or significantly delay recurrence. In addition they believe that some previously nonirradiated recurrent meningiomas may be decreased in size by preoperative irradiation and that the value of radiation therapy appears unrelated to the histologic type.[34]

CLIVUS CHORDOMA

Clivus chordomas are rare lesions in children, less than a dozen having been reported in the literature prior to 1967.[26] A brief discussion of this lesion is included, however, primarily because of the similarity in clinical presentation to pontine glioma. The youngest case reported was that of a 10-month-old male.[3] Chordomas are twice as common in males as females and originate from notochordal remnants in the clivus. They have the ability to metastasize generally secondary to invasion of dural sinuses, with tumor being carried by venous channels to the lungs.

Clinically the most common early symptoms of a clivus chordoma are headache and diplopia. Cranial nerve involvement is frequent and the sixth cranial nerve is usually affected first. Dysphagia and difficulty with breathing may be attributed both to cranial nerve dificit and/or to growth of the tumor into the nasopharynx. Symptoms of anterior pontine compression such as progressive spastic quadriparesis may occur, and in at least one instance in a child the delay in development of hyperreflexia in spite of a progressive quadriparesis resulted in the erroneous diagnosis of Landry–Guillian–Barre syndrome early in the illness.[2]

Plain skull films may show erosion or expansion of the clivus and arteriography and metrizamide cisternography may demonstrate an extraaxial prepontine mass.

Treatment is difficult primarily because of the relative inaccessability of the clivus surgically. Depending upon the tumor's location within the clivus, a transphenoidal, transoral, or transcervical approach for tumor removal have all been attempted. Craniospinal instability with the necessity for bony fusion is a frequent concomitant problem. In general radiotherapy has not proved to be of any lasting benefit, although sporadic instances of tumor regression with this therapy have been reported.[3]

METASTATIC TUMORS

Metastatic tumors in the posterior fossa may originate either hematogenously or via CSF pathways. The incidence of hematogenous metastases from solid malignant tumors is two to three times greater in adults than children. This is most likely due to the rarity of primary bronchogenic carcinoma in children and the biologic characteristics of the common childhood neoplasms. Vannucci and Baten[31] have found hematogenous cerebral metastasis in children with malignant tumors in 13 (6 percent) of 217 brains examined from the Memorial Sloan-Kettering Cancer Center. Pulmonary involvement by tumor was present before the onset of CNS dysfunction in all cases. Most common tumor types demonstrating brain metastasis were neuroblastoma, embryonal rhabdomyosarcoma, and Wilm's tumor. Only one of their 13 cases had metastases to the posterior fossa—a 10-year-old girl with metastatic ovarian carcinoma to the left cerebellar hemisphere who presented with headaches, clumsiness of the left arm, and gait imbalance.

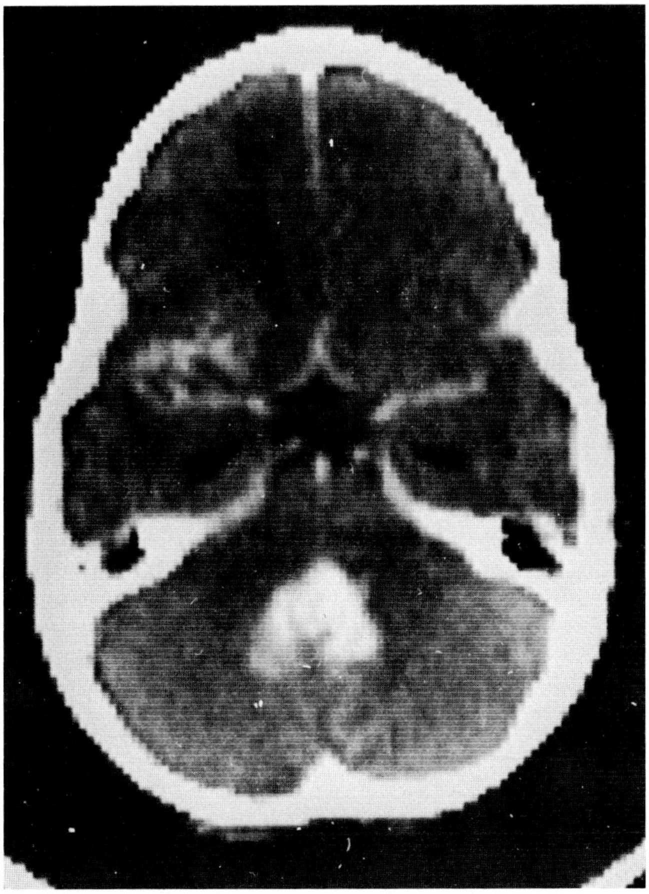

Figure 30-8. CT scan (after contrast enhancement) in a 2-year-old male showing a midline posterior fossa mass and a left temporal mass. The lesion in the posterior fossa midline proved to be an immature teratoma. Presumably both lesions are metastatic from the posterior third ventricular pineal region.

The utilization of CT scanning following the intravenous injection of iodinated contrast agent is currently the appropriate diagnostic procedure for brain metastases, and the use of lumbar puncture as a routine first investigative study should be condemned. Provided the patient is in satisfactory general medical condition, it is the authors' preference surgically to extirpate the solitary metastatic lesion and then employ radiotherapy. In the case of multiple brain metastases, radiotherapy alone is used.

Two of the primary central nervous system neoplasms most commonly associated with metastases via the CSF pathways usually develop in the midline posterior fossa, namely, the medulloblastoma and ependymoma. Other primary central nervous system tumors, however, may show CSF seeding with secondary posterior fossa involvement. Tumors having this capability include choroid plexus papilloma, glioblastoma multiforme, astrocytoma, oligodendroglioma, and primary tumors of the pineal region (Fig. 30-8).[25]

TUBERCULOMA

Intracranial tuberculomas are extremely rare in the United States today, although they made up a sizeable part of all reported brain tumor series during the first half of this century. They still occur with some frequency in India, South America, and some Mediterranean countries. Intracranial tuberculoma is a disease that generally affects young people and more than 50 percent of the lesions in most series occur in the cerebellar hemispheres.[33] Clinical findings are usually related to increased intracranial pressure and/or cerebellar involvement. The chest x-ray shows positive findings for tuberculosis in slightly less than half of the cases and acid-fast bacilli can be isolated from other parts of the body in the majority. Skull films may show signs of increased intracranial pressure, and the CT scan findings are not yet well described. Treatment is surgical extirpation and vigorous triple antibiotic therapy (i.e., isoniazid, rifampin, and streptomycin).

SUMMARY

In children infratentorial tumors other than medulloblastoma, astrocytoma, ependymoma, and pontine glioma are rare, and the alternative diagnostic possibilities are many and varied. A physician who is cognizant of the pathologic possibilities, however, and studies the details of the clinical presentation and radiologic examination, should rarely be deceived regarding the fundamental nature of the lesion.

REFERENCES

1. Archer CR, Roberson GH, Taveras JM: Posterior medullary hemangioblastoma. Radiology 103:323–28, 1972
2. Bartal AD, Heilbronn YD: Transcervical removal of a clivus chordoma in a 2-year-old child. Reversal of quadriplegia and bulbar paralysis. Acta Neurochir 23:127–33, 1970
3. Becker LE, Yates AJ, Hoffman HJ, et al: Intracranial chordoma in infancy. J Neurosurg 42:349–352, 1975
4. Braun IF, Naidich TP, Leeds NE, et al: Dense intracranial epidermoid tumors. Radiology 122:717–719, 1977
5. Cooper M, Dohn DF: Intracranial meningiomas in childhood. Cleveland Clin Q 41:197–204, 1974
6. Corkill G, McCullough GAJ, Tonge RE: Cranial dermal sinus: Valve of plain skull x-ray examination and early diagnosis. Med J Aust 1;885–887, 1974
7. Craig WMcK, Dodge HW, Ross JP: Acoustic neuromas in children. Report of 2 cases. J Neurosurg 11:505–508, 1954
8. Crouse SK, Berg BO: Intracranial meningiomas in childhood and adolescence. Neurology 22(2):135–141, 1972
9. Davis KR, Parker SW, New PF, et al: Computed tomography of acoustic neuroma. Radiology 124:81–86, 1977
10. Gado M, Huete I, Mikhael M: Computerized tomography of infratentorial tumors. Roentgenol XII(2):109–120, 1977
11. Hamer J: Angioblastoma of the posterior fossa in childhood. Mod Probl Paediat 18:27–29, 1977
12. Horton WA, Wong V, Eldridge R: Von Hipple–Lindau disease: Clinical and pathological manifestations in nine families with 50 affected members. Arch Intern Med 136(7):769–777, 1976
13. Jeffreys R: Clinical and surgical aspects of posterior fossa hemangioblastomata. J Neurol Neurosurg Psychiatr 38:105–111, 1975
14. Jeffreys R: Pathological and haematological aspects of posterior fossa hemangioblastomata. J Neurol Neurosurg Psychiatr 38:112–119, 1975
15. Lekias J, Stokes B: Dermoid lesions of the central nervous system in childhood. Aust NZ J Surg 39:335–340, 1970
16. Logue V, Till K: Posterior fossa dermoid cysts with special reference to intracranial infection. J Neurol Neurosurg Psychiatr 15:1–12, 1952
17. Mark VH, Sweet WH: An unusual case of unilateral eighth nerve tumor. J Neurosurg 9:395–397, 1952

18. Matson DD: Neurosurgery of Infancy and Childhood (ed 2). Springfield, Charles C Thomas, 1969
19. Mendiratta SS, Rosenblum JA, Strobos RJ: Congenital meningioma. Neurology 17:914–918, 1967
20. Merten DF, Gooding CA, Newton TA, et al: Meningiomas of childhood and adolescence. J Pediatr 84:696–700, 1974
21. Mount LA: Congenital dermal sinus as a cause of meningitis, intraspinal abscess and intracranial abscess. JAMA 139:1263–1268, 1949
22. Nassar SI, Mount LA: Papillomas of the choroid plexus. J Neurosurg 29:73–77, 1968
23. Ojemann RG: Acoustic neuroma, in Tindall, Long (eds): Contemporary Neurosurgery. Baltimore, Williams & Wilkins, 1979
24. Ojemann RG, Crowell RC: Acoustic neuromas treated by microsurgical suboccipital operations. Prog Neurol Surg 9:337–373, 1978
25. Russell DS, Rubinstein LJ: Pathology of Tumors of the Nervous System (ed 3). Baltimore, Williams & Wilkins, 1971, pp 252–255
26. Sassin JF, Chutorian AM: Intracranial chordoma in children. Arch Neurol 17:89–93, 1967
27. Schwartz JF, Balentine JD: Recurrent meningitis due to an intracranial epidermoid. Neurology 28:124–129, 1978
28. Silver ML, Hennigar G: Cerebellar hemangioma (hemangioblastoma)—A clinicopathological review of 40 cases. J Neurosurg 9:484–494, 1952
29. Thompson JR, Harwood-Nash DC, Fitz CR: The neuroradiology of childhood choroid plexus neoplasms. Am J Roentgenol Radium Ther Nucl Med 118(1):116–133, 1973
30. Toglia JU, Netsky MG, Alexander E.: Epithelial (epidermoid) tumors of the cranium. J Neurosurg 23(4):384–393, 1965
31. Vannucci RC, Baten M: Cerebral metastatic disease in childhood. Neurology 24(10):981–985, 1974
32. Vassilouthis J, Richardson AF: Acoustic neuroma in a child. Surg Neurol 12:37–39, 1979
33. Villarejo F, Soto M, Dabdoub C: Posterior fossa tuberculomas. Mod Probl Paediatr 18:84–89, 1977
34. Wara WM, Sheline GE, Newton H, et al: Radiation therapy of meningiomas. Am J Roentgenol Radium Ther Nucl Med 123:453–458, 1975
35. Wong SW, Ducker TB, Powers JM: Fulminating parapontine epidermoid carcinoma in a four-year-old boy. Cancer 37:1525–1531, 1976
36. Fabiani A, Croveri G, Torta R: Neurinoma della fossa posteriore in un bambino di un anno. Acta Neurol (Napoli) 30:218–222, 1975
37. Koos WT, Miller MH: Intracranial Tumors of Infants and Children. Stuttgart, Germany, Georg Thieme Verlag, 1971

31. Brain-Stem Tumors during Childhood

Donald H. Reigel

Neurorectodermal tumors arising from the brain-stem axis between the thalamus and cervical spinal cord have been called brain-stem gliomas. This group of tumors comprises 10 to 20 percent of all central nervous system tumors during childhood, and they occur most commonly between the ages of 6 and 8 years.[1–5] Congenital forms have been observed and, although less common, the tumor does appear during adulthood.[6] There is no sex or race predilection. Because of the anatomic compactness of the brain stem, intramedullary masses tend to produce a common clinical picture consisting of progressive cranial nerve deficit, alteration in corticospinal tract function, and ataxia.[7] Historically air encephalography was the preferred diagnostic study. Biopsy and incomplete removal of brain-stem masses have been discouraged because of inherent operative risk and failure to alter the generally poor prognosis.[8] Many authors thus have recommended radiation therapy on the basis of clinical and neuroradiologic findings alone. Because of the relative homogeneous clinical and radiographic appearance of these tumors, it has been common to treat all brain-stem gliomas as though they were histologically homogeneous. The results of treatment during the past 30 years have been variable and disappointing.[2,3,9–12] Recently reports have indicated that prognosis may be directly related to tumor type and location.[5,13] Clinical data, biopsy, and treatment results indicate that there may be a more favorable prognosis associated with glioblastoma multiforme of the medulla oblongata.

CLINICAL FEATURES

The most common changes observed are gait disturbance, vomiting, headache, and drowsiness.[3,7,13] As many as 50 percent of the patients will have personality and behavior changes such as irritability, lethargy, and weight loss.[3] Other complaints include facial weakness, diplopia, squint, dysarthria, head tilt, dysphasia, drooling, tinnitus and hearing loss, and change in bladder control. Seizure occurs initially in less than 10 percent of the patients.[4] Approximately one third of the patients will have complaints of focal motor weakness.

The neurologic signs at the time of admission commonly include pyramidal tract signs, cranial nerve deficits, and ataxia. The incidence of papilledema may be as high as 55 percent at the time of initial examination.[14] Other ophthalmologic findings have included horizontal, vertical, and downbeat nystagmus, internuclear ophthalmoplegia, skew deviation, abnormal optokinetic responses, and ptosis.[15–17]

Hemisensory changes and facial hypoesthesia have been reported.[13] Early pyramidal tract signs and cranial nerve deficits may be unilateral but with tumor progression became bilateral. Hydrocephalus has been identified in as many as 65 percent, and skull x-rays show increased intracranial pressure in up to 35 percent of the patients.[7,13,18] The prompt resolution of vomiting, headache, gait disturbance, squint, and papilledema, which often occurs following shunt insertion, suggests that these complaints may often be secondary to hydrocephalus and increased intracranial pressure. With tumor growth, however, many of these observations reappear as a result of tumor growth.

It appears that tumors in the upper brain stem are more likely to be associated with vomiting, drowsiness, cerebellar signs, and hydrocephalus. Children with lower brain-stem tumors are more likely to have multiple lower cranial nerve deficits, dysarthria, head tilt, personality change, and a lower incidence of increased intracranial pressure and hydrocephalus.[13]

The clinical changes occurring in untreated patients are often unrelenting and include progressive cranial nerve deficit, quadriparesis, dysarthria, aphasia, and decreasing level of consciousness to coma, with respiratory and cardiovascular insufficiency terminating life. Although this unrelenting course is characteristic of many brain-stem gliomas, remissions and prolonged survivals have been reported in untreated patients.[19,20]

The differential diagnosis includes brain-stem encephalitis, epidermoid cyst, ependymoma and other posterior fossa tumors, ganglioglioma, basilar meningitis, abscess, tuberculoma, Guillian–Barre syndrome, cerebrovascular disease, hemangioma, arteriovenous malformations and hemorrhage, myasthenia gravis, organic phosphate intoxication, and demyelinating diseases.[21–26]

DIAGNOSTIC STUDIES

Routine laboratory studies have not been particularly helpful in pinpointing a diagnosis of brain-stem glioma. In the future, however, special chemical analyses such as cyclic nucleotides and polyamines may become increasingly useful in the differential diagnosis of tumors of the posterior fossa.[27,28]

Skull x-rays may show signs of increased intracranial pressure in 25 to 35 percent of the patients with brain-stem gliomas.[10,13] Rarely calcification has been observed on skull x-rays or CT scan.[29]

Focal changes in electroencephalography (EEG) such as posterior slowing has been observed, but more often the EEG is normal.

Audiometric testing such as maximum speech intelligibility, performance-intensity functions, synthetic sentence identification, and Bekesy audiometry may help in distinguishing intraaxial brain-stem disorders from extraaxial lesions.[31] Brain-stem auditory evoked potentials, however, appear to hold more promise in the identification of brain-stem lesions. Studies of latencies, amplitude, waveshape, and peeks of responses have enabled identification of brain-stem lesion sites, which subsequently have been varified by radiology and surgery.[32,33] Somatosensory evoked potentials appear to be almost pathognomonic for demyelinating diseases.[34]

Spinal fluid studies have shown normal cell counts, protein, and sugar in a majority of patients. Absence of pleocytosis and elevated protein supports the diagnosis of brain-stem glioma, whereas a lymphocytic pleocytosis with slight protein elevation supports a diagnosis of viral inflammatory disease. Consideration of lumbar puncture should be delayed until after a CT scan has been obtained, thus decreasing the known risks of lumbar puncture (LP) in the presence of a posterior fossa mass. Cytology has generally been negative in the presence of brain-stem glioma.[13]

Radionucleide brain scan has been a useful noninvasive study; however, the success of detection of brain-stem glioma has been variable (5–80 percent).[35,36]

Prior to CT, air or iodine contrast studies (ventriculograms or pneumoencephalograms) were the most accurate methods of making a diagnosis of brain-stem neoplasm. Brain-stem enlargement, posterior–superior displacement of the fourth ventricle and aqueduct, along with narrowing of the pontine cistern, were considered strong evidence for brain-stem neoplasm. Other entities, however, including viral encephalitis, tuberculoma, abscess, meningioma, and arteriovenous malformations are known to produce brain-stem enlargement and cisternal irregularities. Angiography still has an important role in identifying vascular lesions in the posterior fossa or brain stem. The known exophytic and often nodular irregular growth pattern of brain-stem neoplasms may make differentiation between extra- and intraaxial neoplasm difficult. Enlarged, stretched pontine arteries on angiography help eliminate the diagnosis of extraaxial tumor.[37] The location of the basilar artery may not be helpful in this differentiation, but displacement of the anterior pontomesencephalic vein to a position anterior to the basilar artery suggests exophytic brain-stem tumor.[38]

Computerized tomography has replaced air encephalography as the primary study for the diagnosis of brain-stem gliomas. The most common findings are flattening and displacement of the fourth ventricle and changes in the pontine and interpeduncular cisterns.[39] With the newer scanners, density changes and distortion of the basilar and posterior cerebellar arteries can be demonstrated, and as many as 25 percent of the patients may show an area of low density within

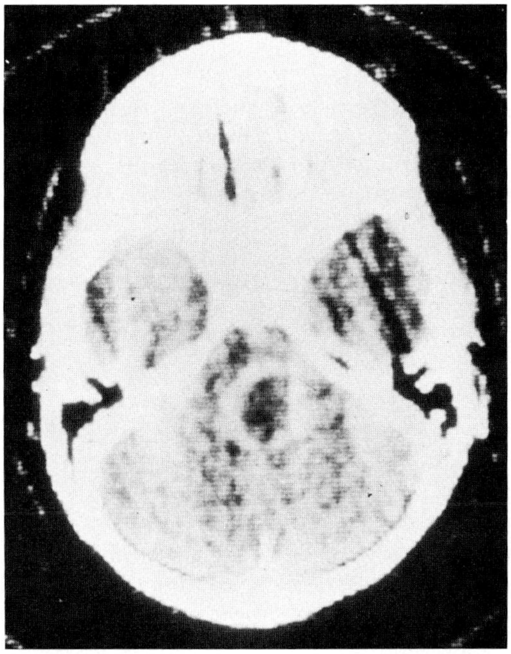

Figure 31-1. CT scan of brain-stem glioma demonstrating enhancing cystic glioblastoma.

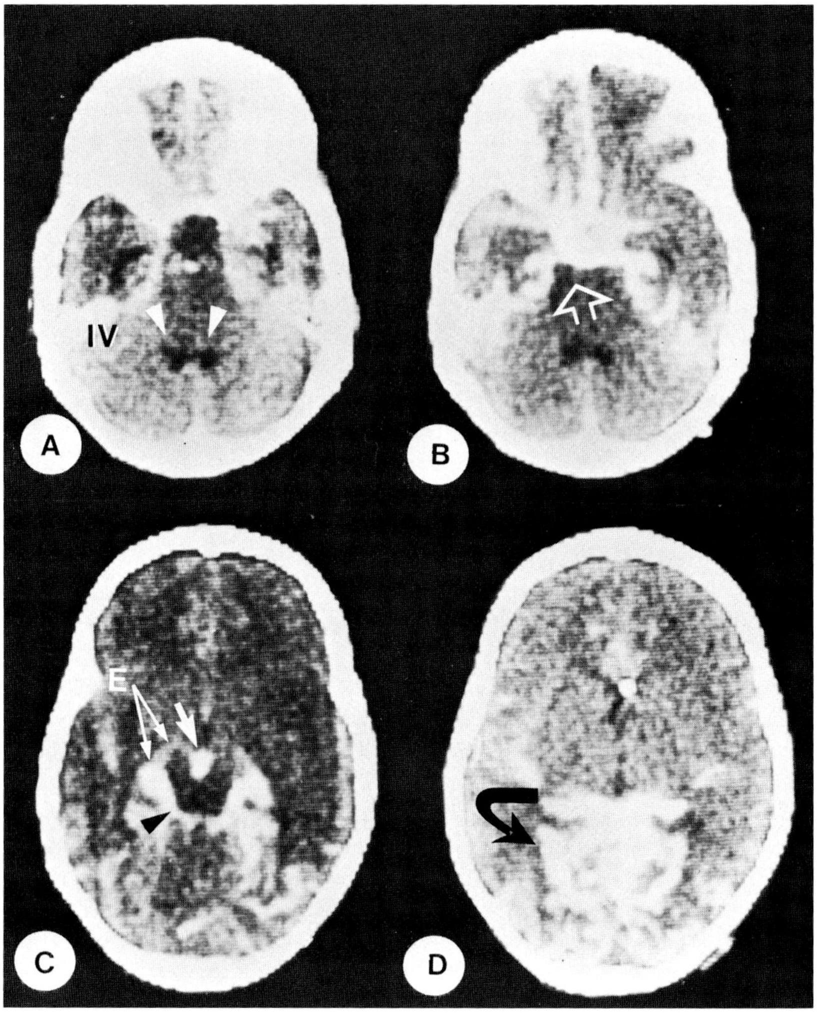

Figure 31–2. Brain-stem glioma. A. Intravenous enhancement: flattening of the fourth ventricle (IV) from an anterior direction. No enhancing mass was noted. B. Intrathecal enhancement: squared appearance of upper pons (arrow). The flattened fourth ventricle did not fill with metrizamide. C. Intrathecal enhancement: characteristic appearance of intraaxial midbrain mass includes "boxy" appearance of tectum (arrowhead) and contiguous tegmentum, displacement of interpeduncular cistern from left to right (arrow), and enlargement of the left cerebral peduncle with exophytic extension (E). This exophytic mass provided the site for surgical biopsy of this glioblastoma. D. Intrathecal enhancement: unusual "chinese letter" pattern (arrow) of accessory posterior subarachnoid spaces is most likely related to midbrain compromise of subarachnoid space. (Courtesy of Dr. Burton P. Drayer.)

a mass in the brain stem (Fig. 31-1).[40] The differentiation of extra- versus intraaxial tumor may be studied with metrizamide CT cisternography (Fig. 31-2).[41]

Finally open biopsy has been demonstrated to be a safe diagnostic procedure for the diagnosis of brain-stem tumors, and the information obtained may contribute to improved understanding and treatment of these tumors.[5,13,42] The CT scan has not provided reliable data on differentiation of low-grade gliomas from more neoplastic tumors such as glioblastoma. Perhaps diagnostic accuracy and histopathologic correlation will be improved with refinement of stereotaxic CT biopsy.[43]

PATHOLOGY

In 1930 Buckley described the pathology of 25 "pontile gliomas" from the Bailey and Cushing series of 1787 intracranial tumors. Ten were classified as glioblastoma multiforme, and their courses were very short. This tumor's gross appearance was that of a large, necrotic hemorrhagic cystic mass involving primarily the base of the pons. Histology demonstrated necrosis, pleomorphism, mitotic activity, and endothelial hyperplasia. Fourteen were classified in the astrocytic series (protoplasmic, fibrillary, or spongioblastic). These tumors were thought to be slower growing and to extend between neurons and nerve fibers (Fig. 31-3).[44] Despite this early description of three or more histologic types of brain-stem glioma, it has been suggested that these tumors have a similar behavior and poor prognosis.[7] Recently authors have called attention to brain-stem glioblastoma with characteristic changes of anaplasia and a rapid, lethal clinical course irrespective of therapy. These tumors seem to have histologic variation from area to area and extend rostrally and caudally along the brain stem.[18,45] Others have pointed to a group of tumors with a varying clinical course specifically associated with prolonged survival and composed predominantly of more uniform-appearing astrocytes without the features of malignant gliomas.[5] Glial tumors of the brain stem have not generally been thought to metastasize; however, intra- and extradural spinal metastases have been described.[46] Spongioblastoma polare is now thought to be a form of astrocytoma and is frequently included in the astrocytoma classification.[18,56] Several rare histologic tumors have been observed in the brain stem, such as astroblastoma, ganglioglioma, and oligodendroglioma.[24]

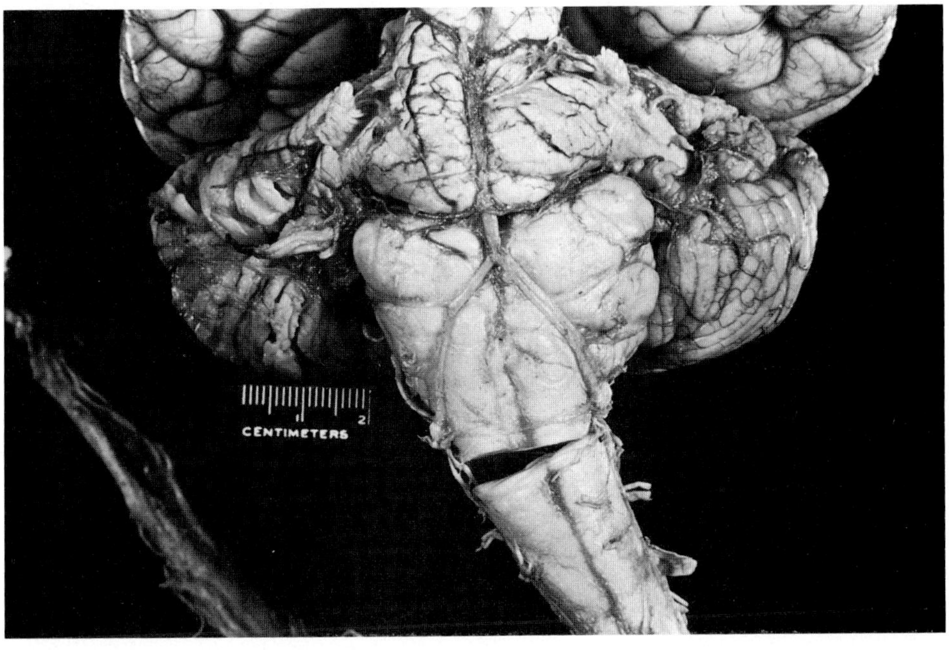

Figure 31-3. External basilar view of a brain-stem astrocytoma demonstrating diffuse, nodular enlargement of the pons, medulla, and spinal cord. The brain stem is deeply grooved by the basilar artery. (Courtesy of the Department of Pathology, the Western Pennsylvania Hospital.)

TREATMENT

Principles of good critical care and pediatric neuroanesthesia are essential for the diagnostic and surgical care of patients with brain-stem tumors. Steroid treatment provides clinically observable benefit.

As many as two thirds of the patients with brain-stem neoplasm may have obstructive hydrocephalus. Cerebral spinal fluid shunt may be associated with prompt, significant reduction of papilledema, ataxia, headache, and vomiting.[13] The risk of metastases is probably small.[47] A more profound, but also probably rare, risk is upward transtentorial herniation of the tumor.[48,57] Although debatable, in our experience the benefits of inserting a cerebral spinal fluid shunt have outweighed the risks associated with other forms of treatment such as external ventricular drainage.

The history of treatment of brain-stem glioma has emphasized the futility of craniotomy and the benefits of radiation therapy. Few people would disagree that most brain-stem neoplasms are not amenable to complete removal and attempts to do so are futile and impractical. Contrary to Menkes,[49] however, surgical approach is possible, and many would agree that operation should be considered in the number of circumstances.

Diagnostic Uncertainty

The decision for surgery as a result of diagnostic uncertainty assumes greater importance when the possibility of benign lesions such as hematoma, abscess, tuberculoma, and dermoid are suggested by CT scan.

Tumor Extending into the Fourth Ventricle

The identification and removal of lesions such as ependymoma, cysts, papillomas, and dermoid may alter the prognosis. Attempts to dissect tumor from within the brain stem at this level are dangerous, however.

Exophytic Tumor

Recently Hoffman, Becker, and Craven[5] identified a group of slow-growing tumors that were astrocytic in origin and tended to fungate out of the brain stem. Excision was associated with survival for 1 to 15 years.[5] In some patients subtotal removal of exophytic mass within the cerebellar pontine angle, third and fourth ventricle, and pineal region may produce significant palliation.

Cyst Aspiration

Lassiter, Alexander, Davis, et al.[42] originally proposed that all patients with brain-stem tumors be explored with "the hope of finding a surgically approachable cyst" that when aspirated would lead to longer, improved survival. These lesions occur in less than 10 to 15 percent of the patients. Unfortunately the benefit of aspiration seems to be limited, but may contribute to less risk with radiation therapy.

Biopsy

Lassman and Arjona[20] reported 4 patients with clinical diagnoses of pontine gliomas and no treatment who were surviving up to 13 years. We reported 3 patients who had no tumor identified at biopsy and no further treatment and are now surviving up to six years.[13] With improved understanding of the risks of radiation therapy during childhood, it may become increasingly important to identify patients without tumor and those with inactive tumors, and therefore either withhold further treatment or modify the dose of radiation treatment.

When the appropriate indications for operation are established and the most accessible apex of growth or exophytic area of tumor is identified by neuroradiologic means, the following operations are commonly chosen.

1. Suboccipital craniotomy for access to the fourth ventricle and cerebellar pontine angles.
2. Supracerebellar subtentorial approach of Krause for the suprapineal and pretectal areas.[50]
3. Frontal parietal craniotomy and transcallossal division for access to the third ventricle region.[51]
4. Stereotaxic biopsy.[13,43]

The mainstay of treatment of brain-stem tumors is radiation therapy. Most therapists recommend 4500 to 5500 rads over four- to six-week periods. We have included the spinal axis of patients with the diagnosis of glioblastoma multiforme. Within four to six weeks, most patients will show arrest of progression and observable improvement. Infrequently deterioration may occur during radiation therapy. Analysis of treatment results indicates improved and prolonged survival following radiation therapy for patients with more cephalad tumors. Three-year survival rates reported in the past 20 years range from 9 to 58 percent and five-year survival rates from 13 to 63 percent.[2,3,9–12] Ten-year survival rates have been reported.[20,52] Clearly treatment results contradict the suggestion that long-term survivals are not possible. Serial CT scan offers the opportunity to follow the results of treatment. Delayed recurrence of tumor may lead to valid considerations of retreatment.

A wide variety of chemotherapeutic drugs have been tried in small studies with limited results and include methotrexate, CCNU, vincristine, procarbazine, 5-fluorouracil, cyclophosphamide, 7-mercaptopurine.[52–54] Finally it may be true that if accurate in-depth stereotaxic access to these tumors is achieved, in-depth radiation therapy or chemotherapy may hold promise.

PROGNOSIS

Contrary to Matson, the prognosis for patients with brain-stem tumors is not hopeless and operation is not necessarily associated with high morbidity, and for many patients survival does extend beyond one year.[8] Pool[55] reported 3 patients who survived 10 to 22 years following radiation therapy. Equally important are the observations that radiation therapy may be associated with significant clinical improvement and the fact that now biopsy and subtotal removal can be safely proposed and in some cases contribute to quality survival.[5,13] Operations prior to radiation therapy do not appear to alter survival. Patients with astrocytomas located more cephalad in the brain stem have more prolonged survival than those with untreated, caudally located anaplastic tumors.[5]

REFERENCES

1. Yates AJ, Becker LE, Sachs LA: Brain tumors in childhood. Child's Brain 5:31–39, 1979
2. Abramson N, Raben M, Cavanaugh PJ: Brain tumors in children: Analysis of 136 cases. Pediatr Radiol 112:669–672, 1974

3. Panitch HS, Berg BO: Brain stem tumors of childhood and adolescence. Am J Dis Child 119:465–472, 1970
4. Walker AE, Hopple TL: Brain tumors in children. J Pediatr 35:671–687, 1949
5. Hoffman HJ, Becker L, Craven MA: A clinically and pathologically distinct group of benign brain stem gliomas. Neurosurgery 7:243–248, 1980
6. Luse SA, Teitelbaum S: Congenital glioma of brain stem. Arch Neurol 18:196–201, 1968
7. Bray PF, Carter S, Taveras JM: Brain stem tumors in children. Neurology (Minneapolis) 8:17, 1958
8. Matson DD: Neurosurgery of Infancy and childhood (ed 2). Springfield, Illinois, Bannerstone House, 1969
9. Greenberger JS, Cassady JR, Levene MB: Radiation therapy of thalamic, midbrain and brain stem gliomas. Ther Radiol 122:463–468, 1977
10. Redmond Jr JS: The roentgen therapy of pontine gliomas. Am J Roentgenol 86:644-688, 1961
11. Lee F: Radiation of infratentorial and supratentorial brain-stem tumors. J Neurosurg 43:65–68, 1975
12. Whyte TR, Colby MY, Layton DD: Radiation therapy of brain-stem tumors. Radiology 93:413–416, 1969
13. Reigel DH, Scarff TB, Woodford JE: Biopsy of pediatric brain stem tumors. Child's Brain 5:329–340, 1979
14. Bucy PC: Ocular Manifestations of brainstem tumors. Arch Ophthamol 62:541; 1959
15. Wolf MS: An unusual case of brain stem glioma with prolonged spontaneous remission and downbeat nystagmus. Bull Los Angeles Neurol Soc 38(4):202–208, 1973
16. Cogan DG, Wray SH: Internuclear ophthalmoplegia as an early sign of brainstem tumors. Neurology 20:629–633, 1970
17. Nair KR, Kutty SJ, Warrier GK: Transient ocular bobbing in a case of brain stem encephalitis. J Assoc Phys Ind 25:573–575, 1977
18. Golden GS, Ghatak NR, Hirano A, et al: Malignant glioma of the brain-stem. J Neurol Neurosurg and Psychiatry 35:743–738, 1972
19. Sarkari NBS, Bickerstaff ER: Relapses and remissions in brain stem tumours. Br Med J 2:21–23, 1969
20. Lassman LP, Arjona VE: Pontile gliomas of childhood. Lancet i:913–915, 1967
21. Dick AR, White HH: Unusual features of brain stem tumors. Postgrad Med 46(4):121–125, 1969
22. Yalaz K, Tinaztepe K: Brain stem encephalitis. Acta Paediatr Scand 63:235–240, 1974
23. Schain RJ, Wilson G: Brainstem encephalitis with radiographic evidence of medullary enlargement. Neurology 21:537–539, 1971
24. Friedman WA, Vries JK, Quisling RG: Ganglioglioma of the medulla oblongata. Surg Neurol 12:105–108, 1979
25. Fisman M: Brain stem encephalitic lesions and schizophrenia. SA Med J 48:1491–1494, 1974
26. Patterson RH, Fraser RAR: Vascular neoplasms of the brainstem: A place for profound hypothermia and circulatory arrest. Am Assoc Neurol Surg 31–36, 1975
27. Gerosa M, Cisotto P, Carteri A: CSF levels of cyclic neucleotides in primary intracranial neoplasms: A preliminary report. Acta Neurochir 50:61–65, 1979
28. Marton LJ: CSF polyamines potential as brain tumor markers. Arch Neurol 38:73–74, 1981
29. Duffner PK, Klein DM, Cohen ME: Calcification in brainstem gliomas. Neurology 28:832–834, 1978
30. Gjerris F: Clinical aspects and long-term prognosis of infratentorial intracranial tumours in infancy and childhood. Acta Neurol Scand 57:31–52, 1978
31. Jerger J, Jerger S: Auditory findings in brain stem disorders. Arch Otolaryngol 99:342–350, 1974
32. Hashimoto I, Ishiyama Y, Totsuka G, et al: Diagnostic significance of brainstem auditory evoked responses in acoustic neurinomas and other posterior fossa lesions. Neurol Med Chir (Tokyo) 19:605–615, 1979

33. Nodar RH, Hahn J, Levine HL: Brain stem auditory evoked potentials in determining site of lesion of brain stem gliomas in children. Lyryngoscope 90:258–266, 1980
34. Baker JB, Larson SJ, Sances Jr A, et al: Evoked potentials as an aid to the diagnosis of multiple sclerosis. Neurology 18:286, 1968
35. Feigin DS, Welch DM, Siegel BA, et al: The efficacy of the brain scan in diagnosis of brainstem gliomas. Radiology 116:117–120, 1975
36. Donahoe CR, Robinson RG, Kishore PRS, et al: Role of the radionuclide brain image in the diagnosis of brainstem gliomas. Radiology 125:735–737, 1977
37. Scotti LN: Pontine arteries in brainstem glioma. Radiology 118:627–632, 1976
38. Sarwar M, Batnitzky S, Schechter MM: Anterior pontomesencephalic vein and basilar artery in exophytic brainstem glioma. Radiology 124:403–407, 1977
39. Bilaniuk LT, Zimmerman RA, Littman P, et al: Computed tomography of brain stem gliomas in children. Radiology 134:89–95, 1980
40. Weisberg LA: Computed tomography in the diagnosis of brain stem gliomas. Comput Tomogr 3:145–153, 1979
41. Drayer BA, Rosenbaum AE, Reigel DH, et al: Metrizamide CT cisternography pediatric applications. Radiology 124:349–357, 1977
42. Lassiter KRL, Alexander Jr E, Davis Jr CH, et al: Surgical treatment of brain stem gliomas. Neurosurgery 34:719–725, 1971
43. Lewander R, Bergstrom M, Boethius J, et al: Stereotactic computer tomography for biopsy of gliomas. Acta Radiol Diag 19:867–888, 1978
44. Buckley RC: Pontile Gliomas: A pathologic study and classification of twenty-five cases. Arch Pathol 9:779–819, 1930
45. Queiroz LS, Neto JNC, Faria JL: Glioblastoma multiforme of the medulla oblangata. Acta Neuropath (Berlin) 29:355–360, 1974
46. Kepes JJ, Striebinger CM, Brackett CE, et al: Gliomas (astrocytomas) of the brain-stem with spinal intra- and extradural metastases: Report of three cases. J Neurol Neurosurg Psychiatr 39:66–76, 1976
47. Hoffman HJ, Hendrick EB, Humphreys RP: Metastasis via ventriculoperitoneal shunt in patients with medulloblastoma. J Neurosurg 44:562–566, 1976
48. Epstein F, Murali, R: Pediatric posterior fossa tumors: Hazards of the "preoperative" shunt. Neurosurgery 3:348–350, 1978
49. Menkes JH: Textbook of Child Neurology. Philadelphia, Lea & Febiger, 1974
50. Krause F: Operative freilegung der vierhugel, nebst Boebachtunger uber hirndruck und de kompression. Zbl Chir 53:2812–2819, 1926
51. Schucart WA, Stein BM: Transcallosal approach to the anterior ventricular system. Neurosurgery 3:339–343, 1978
52. Zaunbauer F, Pichler E, Fodor M: Experiences with radiotherapy and chemotherapy in the treatment of tumors involving the caudal brain stem, in Modern Problems in Paediatrics Pediatric Neurosurgery, vol. 18. Basel, Karger, 1977
53. Rosen G, Ghavimi F, Vanucci R, et al: Pontine glioma high-dose methotrexate and leucovorin rescue. JAMA 230:1149–1152, 1974
54. Rosenstock JG, Evans AE, Schut L: Response to vincristine of recurrent brain tumors in children. J Neurosurg 45:135–140, 1976
55. Pool JL: Gliomas in the region of the brain stem. J Neurosurg 29:164-167, 1968
56. Russell DS, Rubinstein LJ: Pathology of Tumors in the Nervous System (ed 3). Baltimore, Williams & Wilkins, 1971
57. Kessler LA, Dugan P, Concannon JP: Systemic metastasis of medulloblastoma promoted by shunting. Surg Neurol 3:147–152, 1975

32. Ependymoma

Shizuo Oi
Anthony J. Raimondi

DEFINITION

Normal Ependymal Cells

The ependyma is formed by one layer of cuboidal or columnar cells, and has oval or round nuclei that are oriented at right angles to the ventricular surface. The cytoplasm is pale. Along the luminal surface of the intracytoplasmic compartment, one may identify blepharoplasts. The microorganelles are moderate in number. Mitochondria (primarily close to the luminal surface), both smooth and granular endoplasmic reticulum, and a well-developed Golgi complex are the most prominent microorganelles. Along the ventricular surface of the cell, are cilia and irregular patterns of microvilli. There are cytoplasmic glial filaments in normal (and neoplastic) ependymal cells. The subependymal glial layer consists of fibrous astrocytes.[1,2]

Neoplastic Development

Ependymomas are tumors composed of primitive forms of ependyma. This tumor occurs in any part of the ventricular system, in the central canal of the spinal cord, in the cerebral parenchyma remote to the ventricular system (because in the normal development of the cerebrum the subependymal neuroglia continues as streaks, or bands, into adjacent white matter, incorporating nests of polygonal ependymal cells), in the ventral spur of the aqueduct, in the sheet of neuroglial tissue that extends outward about the foramina of Luschka, and in the film terminale. The microscopic diagnostic feature of the ependymoma is the presence of rossettes, cilia, and blepharoplasts. They may show such malignant features as invasive properties, foci of necrosis, anaplasia, increased cellularity, mitotic figures, multinucleation, and giant cell formation.[2] Some pathologists speak of malignant and benign ependymomas, some grade the tumor, some refer to the more primitive appearing form as "ependymoblastoma."[4] Both the benign and malignant ependymomas are invasive tumors, which have a tendency to invade the midline structures, so that the tumor tends to regrow after radical operation. Courville and Brousallian[28] described a characteristic form of ependymoma, the "plastic ependymoma," which may gradually expand within the ventricles or cisterna magna, and protrude into the subarachnoid spaces to form a sizable tongue-like projection. Kim and Fayos[17] reported that 34 percent of patients with posterior fossa ependymoma developed spinal subarachnoid implants, worsening the prognosis significantly. Barone and Elvidge[19] reported 74 ependymomas, in all age groups, with no case of spread within the spinal fluid pathways. Coulon and Till[8] reported five children, of 43 with intracranial ependymoma, who developed positive cytology in the spinal fluid—but none of them showed signs or symptoms of spinal metastases.

Extracranial metastases of intracranial ependymoma have been reported by some to be extremely rare.[29,30] According to Glassauer and Yuan,[31] however, 13 of 89 reported cases of intracranial tumors with extracranial metastases were ependymomas. Among these 13 only one of the tumors was in the posterior fossa. In our series of 30 intracranial and five intraspinal ependymomas in children, we found that 6 patients developed spinal fluid seeding of the tumor documented either at autopsy or by spinal fluid cytology (Table 32-1). Four patients had tumors in the posterior fossa; five of six tumors were malignant, one developed diffuse extracranial metastases from a benign primary site in the lateral ventricle involving cervical and supraclavicular lymph nodes and lung. All 6 patients with postoperative spinal fluid dissemination had prophylactic whole neuroaxis radiation therapy.

NATURAL HISTORY AND INCIDENCE

Incidence

Ependymomas have been reported to comprise from 6.1 to 12.7 percent of pediatric intracranial neoplasms,[6-12] and their relative incidence among gliomas to range from 8 to 20.9 percent. This tumor is more common in children,[14] and it rarely occurs as a congenital tumor,[15] having a peak age incidence under 5 years

Table 32-1
Malignancy and Dissemination/Metastasis

	Malignancy			Metastases		
Location	Malignant Ependymoma	Ependymo-blastoma	Ependymoma (Benign)	CNS	General	Total
Fourth	5			3	0	
ventricle		1		0	0	4
			11	1	0	(4/17 or 23.5%)
Third	1			1	0	
ventricle		2		1	0	2
			1	0	0	(2/4 or 50.0%)
Lateral	4			0	0	
ventricle		0		0	0	1
			5	0	1	(1/9 or 11.1%)
Total	10			4	0	
		3		1	0	7
			17	1	1	(7/30 or 23.3%)

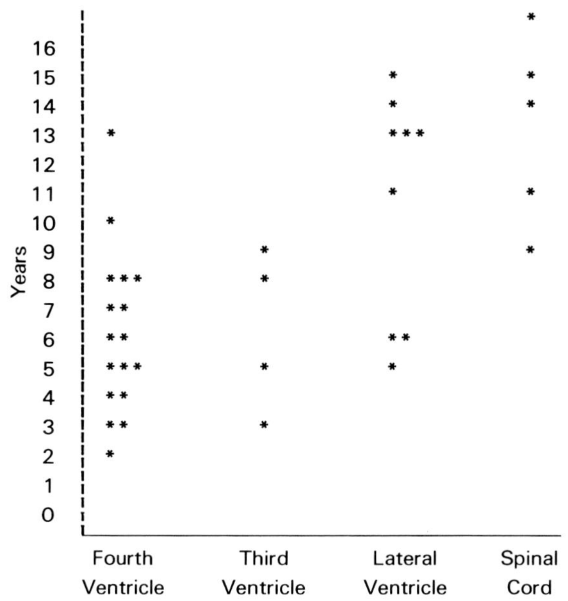

Figure 32-1. Tumor location and age distribution (male; female = 20; 15).

of age.[7,8,9,16] We noted that ependymomas involving the third or fourth ventricles occurred in children under the age of 10, while the older age groups were characterized by lateral (ventricule or hemisphere) and spinal cord tumor growth (Table 32-1). As the medulloblastoma this tumor is more common in male patients and children[8,16] (Fig. 32-1) than in adults.[16–18]

Tumor Location

The majority of authors[2,8,14,16–20] agree that the most common location is in the fourth ventricle, although Koos and Miller[6] reported an equal number of infratentorial and supratentorial ependymomas. Matson[9] and Dohrmann, Farwell, and Flannery[7] report that the ependymoma is the only glioma in childhood

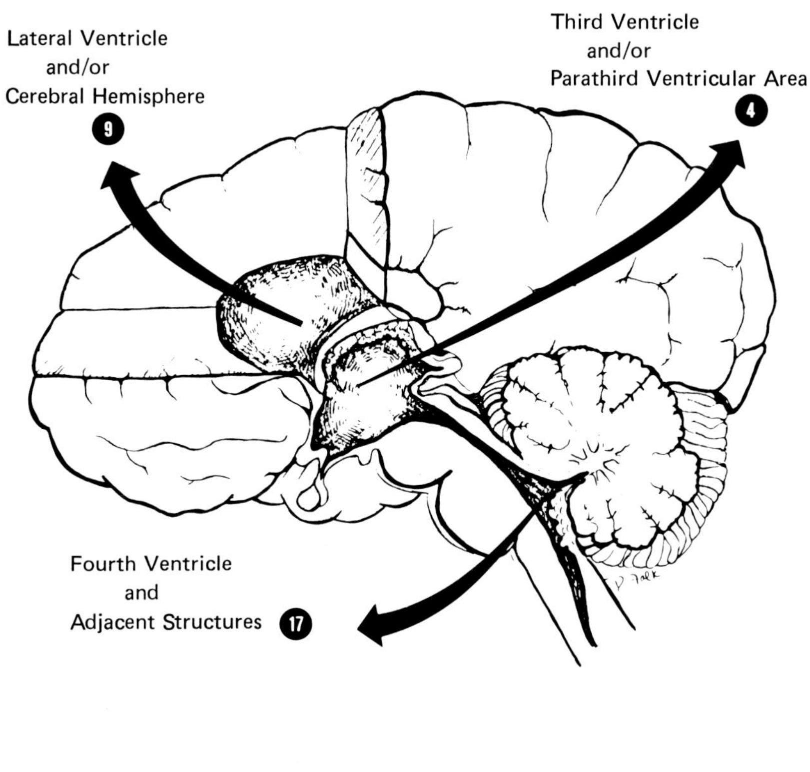

Figure 32-2. Ependymoma—the location of tumor.

that is more common above the tentorium than below it. Eighty-one percent of the ependymoblastomas grow in the supratentorial compartment. Of our 35 ependymomas, either benign or malignant, 13 were located above the tentorium, 17 below it, and 5 in the spinal cord. Among the supratentorial ependymomas, nine were in the lateral ventricle and/or cerebral parenchyma and four in the intra- or parathird ventricular area (Fig. 32-2). Seven of 13 supratentorial ependymomas were malignant, six of 17 in the infratentorial compartment were malignant. It is of value to the neurosurgeon to remember that the ependymoma may grow entirely within the cerebral parenchyma free of any connection to the ventricular system.[8,19]

Signs and Symptoms

The most common symptoms are nausea, vomiting, and headaches,[7,8] occurring with equal frequency in the infra- and supratentorial compartments. In the infratentorial ependymomas, symptoms such as nuchal rigidity and spasm of the head/shoulder muscles, limitation of neck motion, and suboccipital or upper cervical spine tenderness are commonly seen, likely the result of transforaminal tumor extension into the upper cervical canal.[9] Head tilt, gait disturbance, cranial nerve palsies, nystagmus, cerebellar signs (other than truncal ataxia),

Table 32-2
Radiologic Observation of Intracranial Ependymoma

		Location			
		Fourth Ventricle	Third Ventricle	Lateral Ventricle	Total
Angiography	(21 cases)				
Avascular mass		11	1	4	16
Vascular mass		1	1	2	4
Negative		0	1	0	1
Skull x-ray	(16 cases)				
Splitted sutures		4	0	1	5
Calcification		0	0	1	1
J-shaped sella		0	1	0	1
Posterior clinoid erosion		0	0	1	1
Normal		5	0	2	7
Brain scan	(11 cases)				
Positive		6	1	3	10
Negative		0	1	0	1
CT scan	(8 cases)				
Preinfusion density	high	2	0	0	2
	mixed/ISO	3	0	0	3
	low	0	0	2	2
Contrast enhancement	+++	0	0	0	0
	++	3	0	0	1
	+	2	0	2	4
	−	0	0	0	0
Peritumoral edema	+++	0	0	1	1
	++	0	0	2	2
	+	5	0	0	5
	−	0	0	0	0

and papilledema are commonly observed signs. Papilledema is the single most common finding in both infratentorial[8] and supratentorial ependymoma.[7]

Hydrocephalus

The most important complication of ependymoma, supra- or infratentorial, is hydrocephalus: 17 of 19 children with midline tumors, and one of nine with laterally located masses. Though this chapter does not deal with spinal cord neoplasms, we consider it appropriate to comment on the fact that eight of our 61 (13 percent) intraspinal tumors presented with hydrocephalus, three were gliomas, none ependymoma.

Radiologic Observations

Computerized axial tomography, of course, has greatly simplified the diagnosis of all intracranial tumors, and the ependymoma is no exception. We stress the fact, however, that this, as all other radiologic diagnostic studies, does not permit the diagnosis of the histologic nature of the neoplasm, nor does it allow one—with a reliable index of accuracy—to predict vascularity or adherence to the floor of the ventricles. Angiography is essential if one wishes to prepare adequately for the resection of the tumor since it permits the surgeon to identify feeding and draining vessels, degree of vascular stain, and whether the peripheral vascular pattern is well circumscribed or extends diffusely into parenchymal structures (this form is impossible to resect and exceedingly bloody at surgery). We have not been able with pneumoencephalography to learn whether the tumor

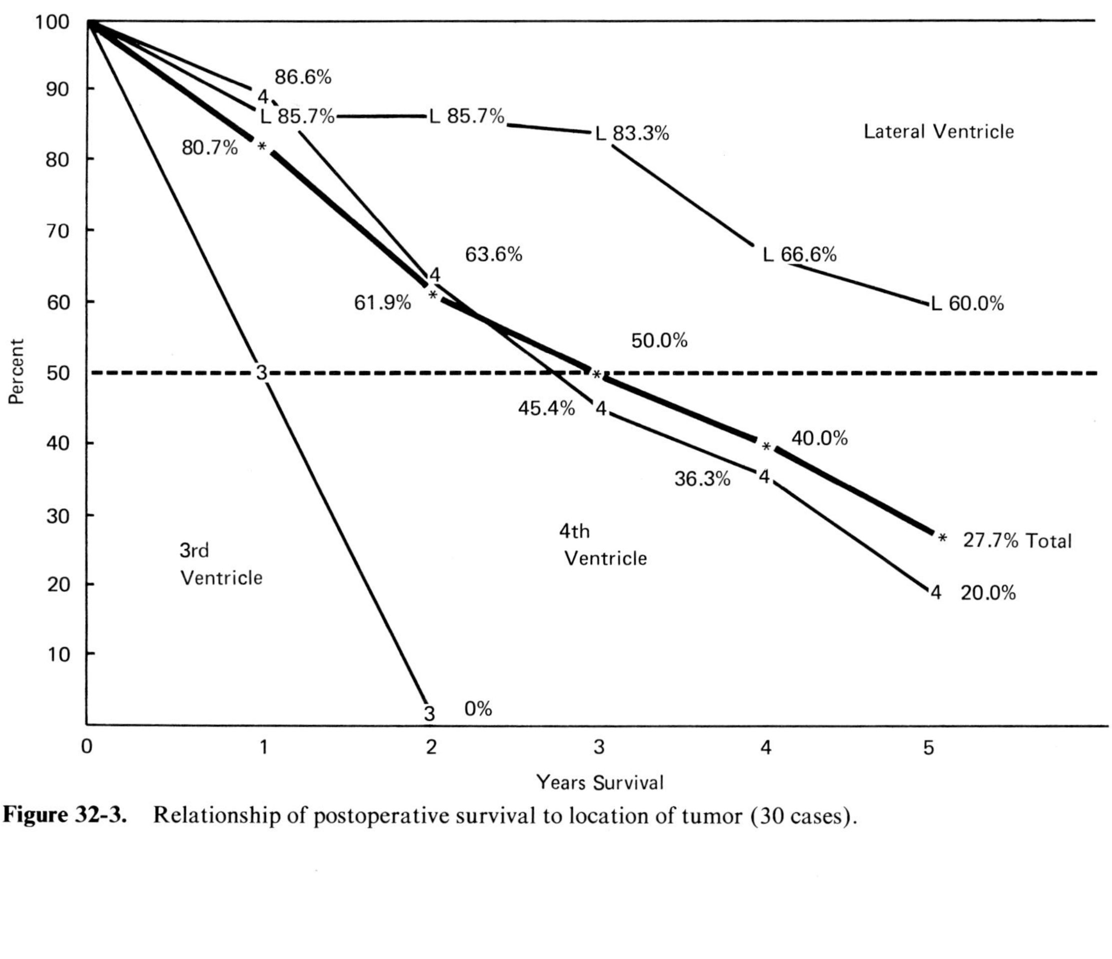

Figure 32-3. Relationship of postoperative survival to location of tumor (30 cases).

is adherent to the ventricular surfaces, and so we do not use this procedure except in the rarest circumstances. We no longer consider nuclear brain scan or plain skull films of value. The observations are compared in Table 32-2.

TREATMENT AND PROGNOSIS

Results of Radical Operation

Mork and Loken[18] reported the prognosis in untreated ependymoma to be extremely poor (no three-year survival in 11 patients).[18] Operative mortality for intracranial ependymoma has been reported to range from 17 to 28 percent in children[7,20,22,23] and 22 to 40 percent in adults[18,19,24] with the overall five-year survival 12.5 to 18 percent[7,8] in children and 41 percent in adults.[25] In our series the operative mortality (four weeks after surgery) was 0 percent, 6.6 percent of the children died of tumor progression before discharge. Our five-year survival is 27.7 percent, three-year survival is 50 percent, and two-year survival is 61.9 percent (Fig. 32-3).

Concerning factors affecting the prognosis, tumor location is extremely important. The five-year survival for third and fourth ventricle lesions is 0 percent and 20 percent respectively, and 60 percent for lateral ventricle and/or cerebral parenchyma lesions (Fig. 32-3). Some authors consider histology important in predicting prognosis.[7,8,17,18] We have observed, however, that the histologic identification of benign or malignant characteristics is not associated with a good or poor prognosis to any degree of consistency (Fig. 32-4). The most important factor is tumor location (Fig. 32-5). The degree of resection affects prognosis directly (Fig. 32-6).

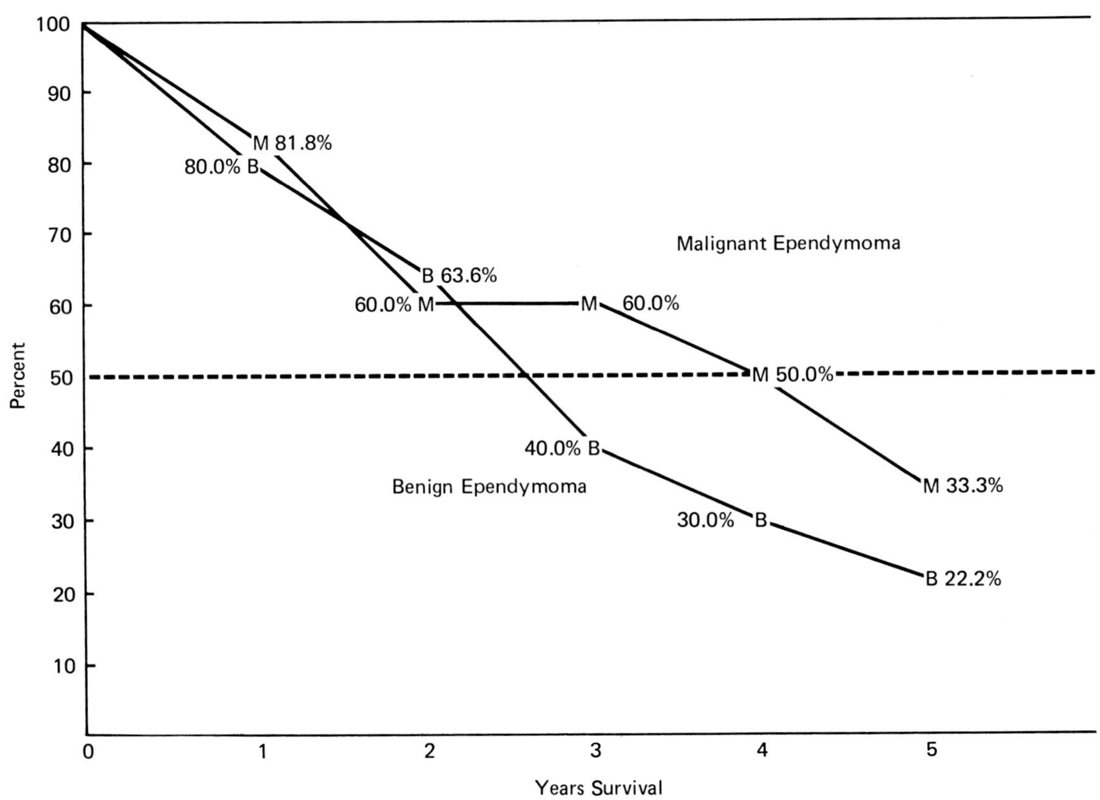

Figure 32-4. Relationship of postoperative survival to histology (30 cases).

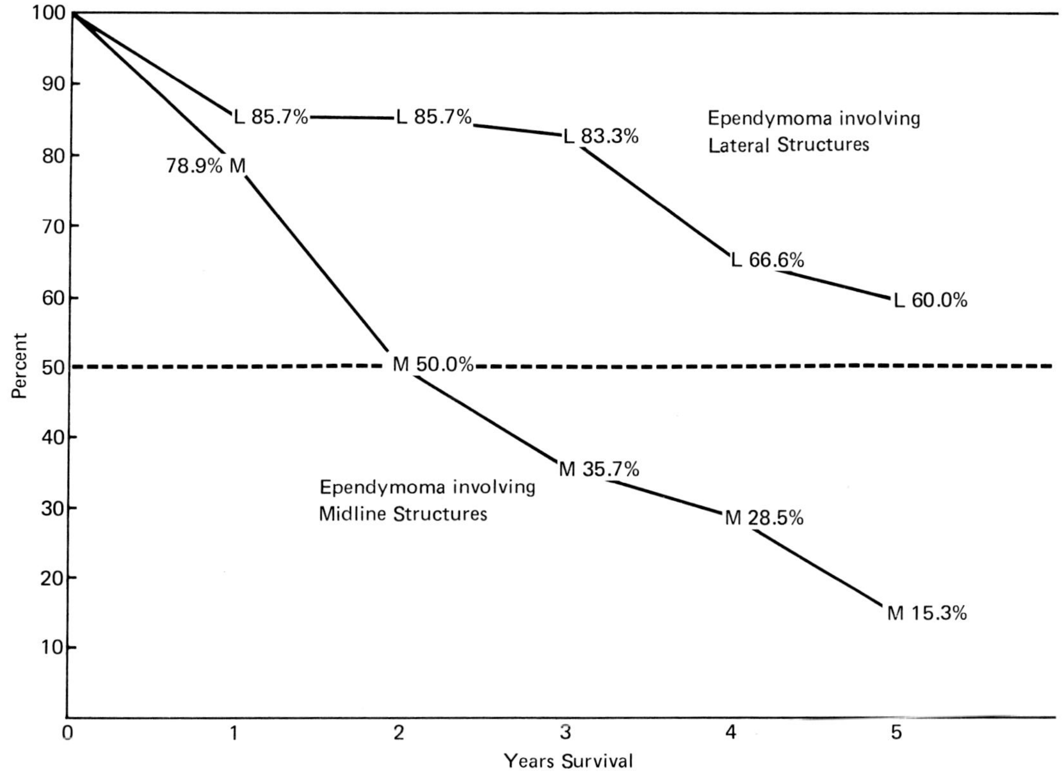

Figure 32-5. Relationship of postoperative survival to location (30 cases).

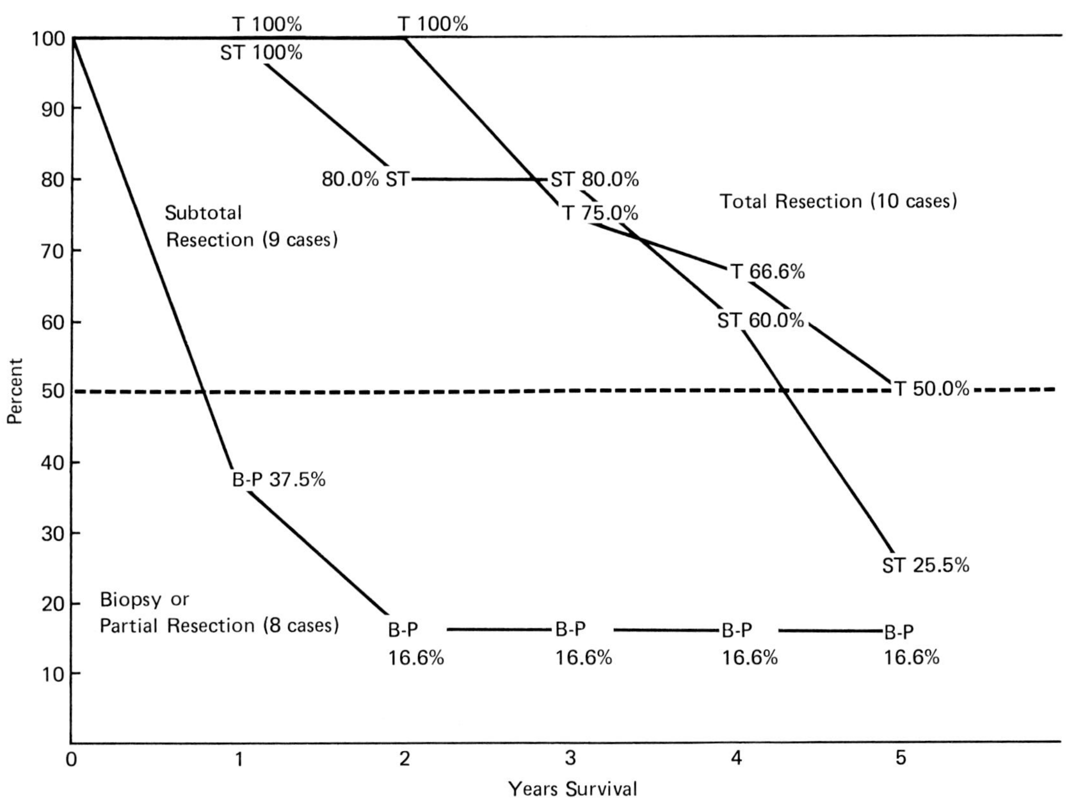

Figure 32-6. Relationship of postoperative survival to degree of surgical resection (27 cases).

Table 32-3
Radiation Therapy and Dissemination/Metastasis

Sites of Radiation	Fourth Ventricle	Third Ventricle	Lateral Ventricle	Total
Whole brain and	**O O O O O**		**O**	**O**; 6
Whole spine	**D* D D D**	**D D**		**D**; 6
Whole brain	**O O O**		**O O O**	**O**: 6 **D**: 0
Area unknown	**O O O**		**O O O O**	**O**: 7 **D**: 0
No radiation therapy	**O**	**O O**	**G**	**O**: 3 **G**: 1

*Dissemination seen before radiation therapy.
D = Tumor cell dissemination. **G** = General metastasis. **O** = No metastasis, no dissemination.

Radiation Therapy

We have given radiation therapy to all but 4 patients. Kam and Fayos[17] concluded that spinal irradiation is required if the tumor is poorly differentiated or located in the infratentorial area. Salazar, Rubon, Bassano, et al.[26] found that elective craniospinal radiation provides longer survival, lower recurrence, good tolerance, no complications, and excellent quality of survival. We have already reported the severe mental retardation, growth stunting, and endocrine deficiencies associated with whole neuroaxis prophylactic radiation therapy for medulloblastoma.[32] One of the radiated patients ("benign" ependymoma, supratentorial) suffered diffuse extracranial metasases. In light of the fact that it is generally agreed that the ependymoma should be treated with radiation after surgical removal,[7] it is of value to note that 6 of 12 patients who received whole neuroaxis radiation therapy developed tumor cell dissemination in the spinal fluid (Table 32-3).

We conclude that histologic characteristics and radiation therapy are of questionable, *if any,* value. Tumor location (lateral rather than midline) and radical resection are associated with most favorable—*less unfavorable,* given the almost invariably fatal outcome—results.

REFERENCES

1. Lewis AJ: Mechanism of Neurological Disease. Boston, Little Brown, 1976
2. Rubinstein LJ: Tumors of the Central Nervous System. Washington, DC, AFIP, 1972
3. Russel DS, Rubinstein LJ: Pathology of Tumours of the Nervous System. Philadelphia, Williams & Wilkins, 1963
4. Rubinstein LJ: The definition of the ependymoblastoma. Arch Pathol 90:35–45, 1970
5. Mabon RA, Svien HJ, Kernohan JW, et al: Symposium on new and simplified concept of gliomas: ependymomas. Proc Staff Meet Mayo Clin. 24:65–71, 1949
6. Koos WT, Miller MH: Intracranial Tumors of Infants and Children. Stuttgart, George Thieme Verlag, 1971
7. Dohrmann G, Farwell JR, Flannery JT: Ependymomas and ependymoblastomas in children. J Neurosurg 45:273–283, 1976
8. Coulon RA, Till K: Intracranial ependymomas in children. Child's Brain 3:154–168, 1977

9. Matson DD: Neurosurgery of Infancy and Childhood. Springfield, Charles C Thomas, 1969
10. Farwell JR, Dohrmann GJ, Flannery JT: Central nervous system tumors in children. Cancer 40:3123–3132, 1977
11. Schoenberg BS, Schoenberg DG, Gomez MR: The epidemiology of primary intracranial neoplasms of childhood. A population study. Mayo Clin Proc 51:51–56, 1976
12. Yates AJ, Becker LE, Sachs LA: Brain tumors in childhood. Child's Brain 5:31–39, 1979
13. Abramson N, Raben M, Cavanaugh PJ: Brain tumors in children: Analysis of 136 cases. Radiology 112:669–672, 1974
14. Jennett B: An Introduction to Neurosurgery. Chicago, Year Book Medical Publishers, 1977
15. Abbott M, Namiki H: Congenital ependymoma case report. J Neurosurg 28:162–165, 1968
16. Harwood-Nash DC, Fitz CR: Neuroradiology in Infants and Children, vol 2. CV Mosby, 1976
17. Kim YH, Fayos JV: Intracranial ependymomas. Radiology 124:805–808, 1977
18. Mork S, Loken AC: Ependymoma. A follow-up study of 101 cases. Cancer 40:907–915, 1977
19. Barone BM, Elvidge AR: Ependymomas. A clinical survey. J Neurosurg 33:428–438, 1970
20. Merritt HH: A Textbook of Neurology, (ed 5). Philadelphia, Lea Fiebiger, 1973
21. Gilday DL, Ash J: Accuracy of brain scanning in pediatric craniocerebral neoplasms. Radiology 117:93–97, 1975
22. Hendrick EB, Hoffman HJ, Humphreys RP: Treatment of intratentorial gliomas in childhood, in Hekmatpanah J (Ed): Current Concepts in Biology, Diagnosis and Therapy. New York, Springer Verlag, 1975
23. Shuman RM, Alvord EC, Leech RW: The biology of childhood ependymomas. Arch Neurol 32:731–739, 1975
24. Ringertz N, Raymond A: Ependymomas and choroid plexus papillomas. J Neuropathol Exp Neurol 8:355–380, 1949
25. Kricheff II, Becker M, Schneck SA, et al: Intracranial ependymomas—Factors influencing prognosis. J Neurosurg 21:7–14, 1964
26. Salazar OM, Rubon P, Bassano D, et al: Improved survival of patients with intracranial ependymomas by irradiation: Dose selection and field extension. Cancer 35:1563–1573, 1975
27. Shalet SM, Beardwell CG, Morris-Jones PH, et al: Pituitary function after treatment of intracranial tumours in children. Lancet 104–107, 1975
28. Courville CB, Broussalian SL: Plastic ependymomas of the lateral recess. Report of eight verified cases. J Neurosurg 18:792–799, 1961
29. Fragoyannis S, Yalcin S: Ependymomas with distant metastasis. Report of 2 cases and review of the literature. Cancer 19:246–256, 1966
30. Wentworth P, Birdsell DC: Intracranial ependymoma with extracranial metastases. J Neurosurg 25:648–651, 1966
31. Glasauer FE, Yuan RHP: Intracranial tumors with extracranial metastases. Case report and review of the literature. J Neurosurg 20:474–493, 1963
32. Raimondi AJ, Tomita T: The Disadvantages of Prophylactic Whole CNS Postoperative Radiation Therapy for Medulloblastoma. Multidisciplinary Aspects of Brain Tumor Therapy. Elsevier/North-Holland, Biomedical Press, 1979, pp 209–218

33. Supratentorial Astrocytoma

Howard M. Eisenberg

Supratentorial astrocytomas arising from the hemispheres or thalamus make up only 10 to 15 percent of all pediatric intracranial tumors. In Matson's[1] series of 750 children with intracranial tumors, there were 118 gliomas that arose from these locations; 40 were benign astrocytomas and a similar number were malignant. The largest portion of the remaining tumors were ependymomas.

The early signs and symptoms of hemispheric tumors found in adults are less commonly found in children. Mild abnormalities of cognition, memory, sensation, and even movement are less obvious in younger children. This may explain the observations in children that many of these tumors reach very large sizes by the time they are diagnosed and that at the time of hospital admission these children frequently have signs of chronically raised intracranial pressure. The first symptom indicating the presence of a tumor, however, is usually focal motor weakness or seizures. Approximately one third of Matson's cases of cerebral gliomas had seizures.

Twenty-three children in this series were identified as having seizures for three or more years prior to the onset of other signs and symptoms of their tumors.[2] Fifteen of these children had astrocytomas, of which 11 were benign. These cases were seen prior to the advent of computed tomography (CT), and since the association of seizures with tumors is uncommon in this age group, they did not have a neuroradiologic workup until they developed other signs. Rarely did the type of seizure at the onset suggest a focal lesion, but in these cases a change in the pattern of the seizures or a change in the electroencephalogram (EEG) was generally one of the first indications of the presence of a focal lesion.

Children with thalamic astrocytomas frequently have a short duration of symptoms and a predominance of motor deficits.[3] Studies of patients of all ages with thalamic tumors indicate that there is a relatively high incidence in childhood.[4,5] Focal motor weakness is a common finding in these children, and in some cases there are also signs of ataxia. Ataxia, nystagmus, and hypoactive reflexes may be found without focal weakness so that some of these children appear initially to have cerebellar mass lesions. Involuntary movements are common, but signs of sensory abnormalities are rare.[3] Anisocoria has been described in children with thalamic tumor, the smaller pupil generally present ipsilateral to the lesion.[4–6]

Skull x-rays in patients with hemispheral or deep astrocytomas are frequently abnormal, generally showing signs of increased intracranial pressure, most often splitting of the sutures. Suture separation occurred in 65 percent of Matson's cases.[1] In addition approximately one quarter had abnormal calcification in the area of the tumor. In some cases skull films showed local erosion of the calvarium adjacent to the mass. Diagnosis of these tumors is now easily made by CT. These tumors generally enhance with contrast, are frequently large (Fig. 33-1), and sometimes contain cysts (Fig. 33-2). Ventricular dilatation is common in patients with deep tumors.[3]

The associated EEG abnormalities include phase reversals, spikes, and focal low-amplitude slow waves (2–3 Hz). Children with thalamic tumors may also have bilateral posterior diffuse slowing, bursts of slow waves, and spindle activity when awake.[3]

Astrocytomas of the cerebrum are generally avascular and frequently infiltrative. They may involve a major portion of the hemisphere or cross the midline. The treatment of those hemispheric tumors that do not cross the midline and are histologically benign is operative resection. In some cases the tumor is surrounded by a pseudocapsule and a plane can be developed between tumor and normal brain. When this is the case, total removal should be attempted, although in actuality it is achieved in only a small number. When the tumor is located near the pole of the frontal, temporal, or occipital lobe, lobectomy is generally the best approach. In some patients with benign tumors, multiple operations may result in total removal.[1,3,7]

The value of resection of deep tumors is more open to question. Those tumors that appear discrete, however, particularly when located in posterior thalamus, should not be considered inaccessible. They can be approached by a posterior cortical incision opening the trigone. The posterior portion of the thalamus is then well visualized and large portions of the tumors can be removed without increasing neurologic deficits. This operation has occasionally resulted in a gross total removal.[3] Biopsy of deep tumors can be made stereotactically or by using an open technique; however, an operation done for biopsy alone when the diagnosis is not seriously in question would seem to have little merit. Many cases of cerebral astrocytoma, particularly those arising from a deep location, are associated with hydrocephalus. In these cases when the hydrocephalus is not

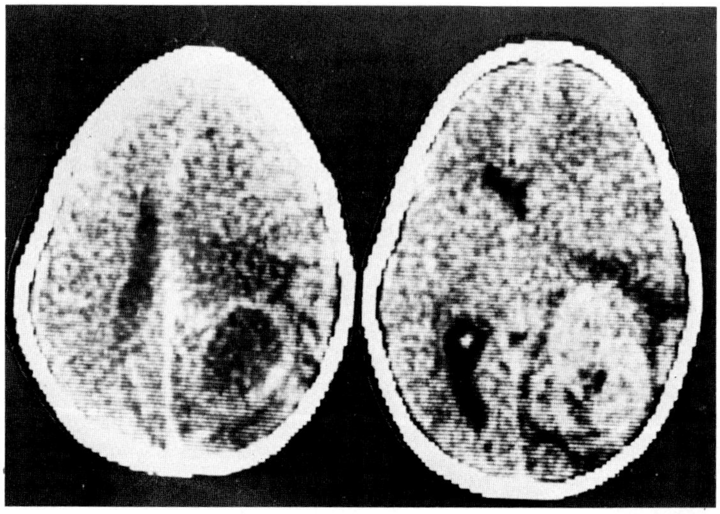

Figure 33-1. Astrocytoma in a 7-year-old girl. A CT scan after contrast enhancement showing the tumor at the level of the body of the lateral ventricles (left) and at a slightly lower level (right). (Courtesy of R. D. Strand, Children's Hospital Medical Center, Boston.)

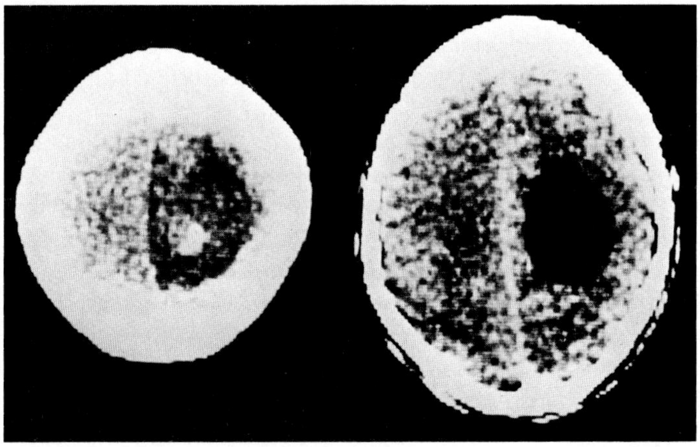

Figure 33-2. Cystic astrocytoma in a 12-year-old girl. A CT scan after contrast enhancement showing a portion of the solid tumor (left) and a large cystic portion (right). The cyst contained xanothochronic fluid. (Courtesy of R. D. Strand, Children's Hospital Medical Center, Boston.)

resolved by resection or resection cannot be done, shunting is generally required.

The value of radiotherapy in the management of benign cerebral astrocytomas has not been established, although the effects of this treatment have been the subject of several studies. These reports imply beneficial effects; however, the number of patients with benign tumors is small in each of the reported series and these studies were done retrospectively without randomization. In one report of 37 children with astrocytomas,[8] it was found that of 15 children with hemispheric astrocytomas given radiation, 11 survived for at least five years. Surprisingly in this series the nine children with deep-seated tumors did as well or even better than those with more superficial lesions. Five of six survived for five years, and of the nine, seven were still living at the time of the report without evidence of disease. A study of 143 patients of all ages with supratentorial astrocytomas showed that those with benign lesions treated with resection and radiation had a five-year survival of 40 percent, whereas of those treated with resection alone, only 20 percent survived for this period.[9] Similar survival figures were determined by Fazekas,[10] but in his study it was found that although five-year survival was more common in radiated patients, at 10 years there was little difference in the percentage of survivors in those radiated and those not radiated. In general it can be assumed that patients with benign supratentorial astrocytomas treated by resection and radiation have a five-year survival of approximately 50 percent.[11]

What then is the best treatment for benign astrocytomas? When should feasible total excision of the tumor be attempted? These tumors may sometimes be safely resected even when they are near important structures such as the motor strip, but even when it appears as though a "gross total removal" has been achieved, the probability of regrowth is high. In those cases, however, in which all visible tumor is thought to be removed, x-ray therapy should be withheld. When a benign tumor thought to be totally removed later regrows, a second operation should be considered. A tumor known to be incompletely removed or malignant should be treated with x-ray therapy. The effects of chemotherapy, particularly for the treatment of benign astrocytomas, are even less certain than are the effects of radiation therapy.

INTRAVENTRICULAR ASTROCYTOMAS IN ASSOCIATION WITH TUBEROUS SCLEROSIS

Although the presence of nodules along the walls of the lateral ventricles of patients with tuberous sclerosis is a common finding, the occurrence of intraventricular tumors is rare. In those patients with tuberous sclerosis and intraventricular tumors, other signs of the syndrome are usually seen. Most frequent are seizures, mental retardation, and adenoma sebaceum. Surprisingly retinal lesions are not common in this group and a clear family history often cannot be obtained.

These intraventricular tumors are histologically different from other astrocytomas and from the tubers found in the cortex. They are usually covered by intact ependyma and are comprised of elongated spindle cells having the appearance of spongioblasts and of plump or large polyhedral cells that resemble giant astrocytes. Those tumors and the subependymal nodules frequently calcify, but while the ventricular nodules have no site of predilection, the intraventricular tumors are almost always located in the region of the foramen of Monro, in the adjacent lateral ventricle or in the anterior third ventricle. They therefore may obstruct the flow of cerebrospinal fluid.[1,12] Although these tumors are almost always benign, one case with malignant features has been reported.[13] Despite the frequency of benign features, many of these tumors cannot be totally removed and the results of treatment even after total removal are often disappointing. In Matson's[1] series of seven cases, one died before operation, and of the six who had operations, four died and two were severely retarded. In Knapp, Paulson, and Odom's[12] series of seven cases, one died before operation, two died after, and three were retarded, two of these requiring institutionalization. When faced with an enlarging intraventricular tumor in a patient with tuberous sclerosis, however, operative resection usually represents the only hope. The indications for operation are symptoms caused by the mass, usually raised intracranial pressure due to the tumor or the associated hydrocephalus. In those patients in whom there are no symptoms attributable to the tumor, particularly when it is small, its growth may be observed using CT. If the rate of growth indicates that symptoms are likely to occur, an operation should be considered.

REFERENCES

1. Matson DD: Neurosurgery of Infancy and Childhood (ed 2). Springfield, Charles C Thomas, 1969
2. Page LK, Lombroso CT, Matson DD: Childhood epilepsy with late detection of cerebral glioma. J Neurosurg 31:253–261, 1969
3. Hirose G, Lombroso CT, Eisenberg HM: Thalamic tumors in childhood. Arch Neurol 32:740–744, 1975
4. Cheek WR, Taveras JM: Thalamic tumors. J Neurosurg 24:505–513, 1966
5. Tovi D, Schisano G, Liljeqvist B: Primary tumors of the region of the thalamus. J Neurosurg 18:730–740, 1961
6. McKissock W, Paine KWE: Primary tumors of the thalamus. Brain 81:41–63, 1958
7. Milhorat TH: Pediatric Neurosurgery. Philadelphia, FA Davis Co, 1978
8. Marsa GW, Probert JC, Rubinstein LJ, et al: Radiation therapy in the treatment of childhood astrocytic gliomas. Cancer 32:646–654, 1973
9. Stage WS, Stein JJ: Treatment of malignant astrocytomas. Am J Roentgenol Radium Ther Nucl Med 120:7–18, 1974
10. Fazekas JT: Treatment of grades I and III brain astrocytomas. The role of radiotherapy. J Radiat Oncol Biol Phys 2:661–666, 1977
11. Bouchard J: Radiation Therapy of Tumors and Diseases of the Nervous System. Philadelphia, Lea & Febiger, 1966
12. Knapp JP, Paulson GW, Odom GL: Brain tumors with tuberous sclerosis. J Neurosurg 26:191–202, 1967
13. Brown JM: Tuberose sclerosis with malignant astrocytoma. Med J Aust 1:811–814, 1975

34. Unusual Tumors of Cerebral Hemisphere

Fred Epstein
Nancy Epstein

There are a constellation of embryonal neoplasms that are uniquely peculiar to children. These include undifferentiated primitive neuroectodermal tumors as well as those neoplasms that manifest varying degrees of cellular differentiation and are classified as neuroblastoma, spongioblastoma, or ependymoblastoma. All of these neoplasms are apparently related to neoplastic proliferation of cells, which, at the inception of gestation, make up the germinal matrix of the evolving neural tube.[1] Rarely these immature embryonal neoplasms undergo progressive maturation and become clinically manifest as mature neuronal tumors (ganglioneuroma, ganglioglioma) or mixed gliomas.

To understand the neuropathologic spectrum of embryonal neoplasms, it is necessary briefly to describe the embryologic events whereby normal primordial neuroectodermal elements evolve to the cellular constituents of the mature brain.

The most immature of the primordial cells is multipotential and referred to as a "matrix cell" or "germinal cell."[2,3] These cells, which are adjacent to the lumen of the neural tube, differentiate to neuroblasts, ependymoblasts, and spongioblasts. It is believed that neuroblasts do not undergo mitoses, nor do they form cells other than neurons. Spongioblasts mature to astrocytes and oligodendrogliocytes while the ependymoblasts remain adjacent to the lumen of the neural tube and become the ependymal lining of the ventricles.[1] The "matrix" cells thus mature to form the three neuroectodermal constituents of the normal brain.

The human brain is immature at birth, and residual matrix cells are normally present until 4 to 9 months of age.[3–6] They are concentrated adjacent to the ventricular system and in the region of the tuber cinereum. Rarely nests of these cells may persist for longer periods of time and become neoplastic, developing into an embryonal neoplasm. The term primitive neuroectodermal tumor is reserved for those embryonal neoplasms that are largely undifferentiated and, therefore, may not be specifically classified according to cell type.[7]

these highly undifferentiated neoplastic precursors undergo maturation that culminates in a normal adrenal gland. In addition there have been rare case reports of cerebral neuroblastoma and many more of peripheral neuroblastoma maturing over a period of many years to ganglioneuromas.[21,22,24–28] Also lending support to this concept is the common presence of immature cells (neuroblasts, spongioblasts) within a highly differentiated neuronal neoplasm.

There thus is a spectrum of neoplasia among cells that are undergoing neuronal differentiation. The neuroblastoma represents the neoplastic transformation among precursor cells while ganglioglioma and ganglioneuroma occur as these more primitive neoplasms undergo progressive differentiation. Interestingly it has been speculated that if maturation continues, the lesion may evolve from a neoplasm to a hamartoma.[4]

As with the immature embryonal tumors, ganglioneuromas occur in relatively deep locations and are commonly adjacent to a ventricular wall.[29] A number have been described in the region of the anterior third ventricle, which is consistent with the observation that it is in the region of the tubor cinereum that immature matrix cells occur in large numbers and may rarely persist for many months after birth. These tumors are usually firm, white or gray in color, and frequently cystic and well demarcated from adjacent brain. Microscopically the ganglioneuroma consists of predominantly mature ganglion cells, whereas the ganglioglioma is associated with glial neoplasia as well. These are slowly growing tumors, and following surgical excision, long-term remission or cure is to be expected.

MIXED GLIAL TUMORS

Although common in children, these neoplasms may occur at any age. They grow slowly, and are grossly identical to a low-grade astrocytoma. Microscopically the combination of astrocytoma and oligodendroglioma is most common, and oligodendroglioma and ependymoma somewhat less so. These neoplasms have been classified as compact or diffuse. The former implies that the tumors are well demarcated from one another, whereas in the latter, the cells are intermingling. It has been well documented that initially slow-growing neoplasms may undergo malignant degeneration to glioblastoma.[30]

The pathogenesis of these tumors is speculative, but it has been suggested that they are a result of differentiation of primitive tumors that originated from the spongioblast cell line. In this regard it is hypothesized that the mixed glioma is the end result of progressive maturation among glial precursors, and in this way is analogous to what has been proposed as the origin of the mature neuronal tumor.

REFERENCES

1. Rubinstein LJ: Presidential address: Cytogenesis and differentiation of primitive central neuroepithelial tumors. J Neuropathol Exp Neurol 31:7–26, 1972
2. Fugita S: The matrix cell and cytogenesis in the developing central nervous system. J Comp Neurol 120:33, 1963
3. Langman J, Guerrant RL, Freeman BG: Behavior of neuroepithelial cells during closure of the neural tube. J Comp Neurol 127:399, 1966
4. Feigin I, Budzilovich GN: Tumors of neurons and their precursors. J Neuropathol Exp Neurol 33:483–506, 1974
5. Jellinger K: Cerebral medulloepithelioma. Acta Neuropathol 22:905–101, 1972
6. Tuthill CR: Medulloblasts of the infant brain. Arch Pathol 26:791–799, 1938

7. Hart MN, Earle KM: Primitive neuroectodermal tumors of the brain in children. Cancer 32:890–897, 1973
8. Hortein BC, Rubinstein LJ: Primary cerebral neuroblastoma, A clinicopathological study of 35 cases. Brain 99:735–756, 1976
9. Kosnik EJ, Boesel CP, Bay J, et al: Primitive neuroectodermal tumors of the central nervous system in children. J Neurosurg 48:741–746, 1978
10. Partier JC, Mortara RH, McCloskey JJ: Biological behavior of the primitive neuroectodermal tumors: Significant supratentorial childhood gliomas. Surg Neurol 4:383–388, 1975
11. Leestma JE, Earle KM: Neoplasms of the central nervous system in infants 2 years of age and under—Analysis of 163 cases. Meeting, American Association Neuropathology, Chicago, June 1972
12. Mabon RT, Svien HJ, Gates EM, et al: Medulloepithelioma. A critical re-evaluation. J Exp Neurol 9:193, 1950
13. March SB, Urich H: Medulloepithelioma: Definition of an entity. J Neuropathol Exp Neurol 31:27–52, 1972
14. Deck JH: Cerebral medulloepithelioma with maturation into ependymal cells and ganglion cells. J Neuropathol Exp Neurol 29:442–454, 1969
15. Jellinger K: Cerebral medulloepithelioma. Acta Neuropathol 22:95–101, 1972
16. Pearson J, Milstoc M, Harris J, et al: Anaplastic neuronal tumors of the brain. Cancer 38:1424–1437, 1976
17. Rubinstein LJ: The definition of the endymoblastoma. Arch Path 90:35, 1970
18. Smith DR, Hardman JM, Earle KM: Metastasizing neuroectodermal tumors of the central nervous system. J Neurosurg 31:50–58, 1969
19. Henriquez AS, Robertson DM, Marshall WJS: Primary neuroblastoma of the central nervous system with spontaneous extracranial metastasis. Case report. J Neurosurg 38:226–231, 1973
20. Beckwith JB, Perrin EV: In situ neuroblastomas: A contribution to the natural history of neural crest tumors. Am J Pathol 43:1098–1104, 1963
21. Liss L: Neuroblastoma. (Malignant gangliocytoma of the parietal lobe.) J Neurosurg 17:529–536, 1960
22. Griffin ME, Bolande RP: Familial neuroblastoma with regression and maturation to ganglioneurofibroma. Pediatrics 43:377–382, 1969
23. Schwartz AD, et al: Spontaneous regression of disseminated neuroblastoma. J Pediatr 85:760–763, 1974
24. Cushing I, Wolbach SB: The transformation of a malignant paravertebral sympathicoblastoma into a benign ganglioneuroma. Am J Pathol 3:203–216, 1927
25. Russell DS, Rubinstein LJ: Ganglioglioma: A case with long history and malignant evolution. J Neuropathol Exp Neurol 21:185–193, 1962
26. Rubinstein LJ, Okazaki H: Gangliogliomatous differentiation in a pineocytoma. J Pathol 102:27–32, 1970
27. Fox F, Davidson J, Thomas LB: Maturation of sympathicoblastoma into ganglioneuroma. Cancer 12:108–116, 1959
28. Chandler FA, Norcress JR: Sympathicoblastoma. JAMA 114:112–117, 1940
29. Courville CB: Ganglioglioma: Tumor of the central nervous system, review of the literature and report of two cases. Arch Neurol Psychiatr 24:439–491, 1930
30. Hart MN, Petito CK, Earle KM: Mixed glioma. Cancer 33:134–140, 1974

35. Chemotherapy of Malignant Glial Tumors of Childhood

Fred Epstein
Abraham Lieberman

Malignant astrocytomas (glioblastomas) represent only 9 percent of all pediatric intracranial tumors, but with each advancing decade, there is a proportional increase in the incidence of malignant gliomas.[5,6]

CLINICAL SYMPTOMS AND SIGNS

Because malignant gliomas are rapidly growing tumors, the antecedent history is commonly four months or less, and is generally characterized by symptoms of increased intracranial pressure and evolving focal neurologic deficits.

While surgery is directed toward achieving a gross total removal of the tumor, it is not curative because microscopic foci of tumor always remain and regrow within a short period of time. Although the combination of surgery and radiation therapy (RT) (5500–6000 rads) has extended postoperative survival, it also is not curative.[1,3,4,11,12,14,17] The explanation for this is, in part, that within the tumor there are necrotic areas in which cells grow in an anaerobic environment where they are more resistant to the effects of ionizing radiation, and a lethal dose of RT cannot be delivered to the tumor without also damaging the surrounding normal brain. Studies currently are underway to evaluate agents such as misonidazale, which sensitize the hypoxic core of the tumor to ionizing radiation,[15] and to evaluate high-energy particle beams (Pi mesons), which may be able to deliver a tumorcidal dose of RT without also damaging the surrounding brain.

While the combination of surgery and RT may eradicate up to 90 percent of tumor (a one-log kill), chemotherapy is required to eliminate the remainder. Chemotherapy thus is not intended to eradicate the bulk of a tumor at present, but only those remnants that survive surgery and RT. Originally it was believed that the ideal chemotherapeutic agent should be of low molecular weight and lipid soluble so as to facilitate its crossing the blood–brain barrier (BBB).[7,13,15] Evidence from experimental animal models, however, as well as from human studies, has documented that in most regions of a malignant brain tumor there is no functional BBB, and that it is only in the brain adjacent to the tumor in which there are clusters of tumor cells that even a partial BBB exists.[16] It is only in these regions of the brain on the periphery of the tumor where a few malignant cells have infiltrated, therefore, that a chemotherapy agent must cross a relatively intact BBB. This is consistent with the clinical observation that most malignant brain tumors are demonstrable by radionucleotide scan and contrast-enhanced computed tomography techniques that require a breakdown in the BBB for tumor visualization. While most currently available chemotherapeutic agents pass directly into the center of a tumor (since there is already a breakdown of the BBB in this region), the oncolytic effect of these agents also depends on their ability to migrate into the tumor cell across the brain–tumor barrier, a property that may be different from the property that facilitated its penetration through the BBB.

It is evident that improvement in patient survival will be a function of increased understanding of the basic pathophysiology of glial neoplasms, and as the biologic behavior of malignant gliomas is probably not age related, it may be valid to draw conclusions regarding the efficacy of chemotherapeutic agents from studies that have been carried out in adults. In order critically to evaluate any drugs, well-designed propsective randomized studies utilizing a sufficiently large number of patients to achieve statistical validity are required. The Brain Tumor Study Group (BTSG) of the National Cancer Institute, a cooperative multi-institutional group, was organized to accomplish this task through a series of carefully designed studies, each involving a minimum of 300 patients, and taking at least three years to complete.

The first study (BTSG 66-01) evaluated Mithramycin.[17] Although there was no significant difference in survival in patients receiving Mithramycin as compared with those not receiving Mithramycin, this study demonstrated the ability of a large multicentered group to accumulate and randomize sufficient numbers of cases to determine statistical signficance, study them according to a uniform protocol, develop accurate recording procedures, and cooperate in the evaluation of treatment.

The second study (BTSG 69-01) evaluated 1-3-*bis*-(2-chloroethyl)-1-nitrosourea (BCNU) and radiotherapy in 303 patients.[17] Patients were randomly assigned to four treatment groups. Group I received radiation therapy (5000–6000 rads to the whole brain) plus BCNU (80 mg per square meter of body surface area per day, on three successive days, every six to eight weeks); Group II received BCNU alone; Group III received radiation therapy alone; and Group IV, surgery alone. The median survival of patients was 14 weeks for surgery alone, 19 weeks for BCNU alone, 35 weeks for RT, and 35 weeks for BCNU plus RT.

The usefulness of RT was unequivocally demonstrated in this study, increasing median survival by 150 percent. Although the addition of BCNU to RT failed to alter median survival, it resulted in an increased number of patients living more than 18 months compared with patients receiving RT alone. The quality of survival among patients receiving RT alone, or RT combined with BCNU, was good; the majority returned to work, or remained independent in activities of daily living for most of their treatment period.

The third BTSG study (BTSG 72-01) evaluated methyl-1-(2-choroethyl)-3-(40, ethyl cyclohexyl)-1 nitrosourea (methyl CCNU) as well as BCNU with and without RT. Patients were randomly assigned into one of four treatment groups: Group I—methyl CCNU alone; Group II—radiation therapy alone; Group III—radiation plus methyl CCNU; and Group IV—radiation plus BCNU. The median survival for each of the four groups was significantly longer than for treatment with surgery alone (using Group IV from BTSG 01 as a historic control). Moreover the median survival for combined therapy with methyl CCNU and RT therapy approached statistical significance when compared with chemotherapy or RT alone. Among patients receiving the full course of RT and two or more courses of chemotherapy (adequately treated group), the figures for BCNU combined with RT reached statistical signficance, and 18-month survival exceeded 30 percent. Quality of survival among patients, as in BTSG 69-01, remained good.

The immediate toxicity of BCNU and methyl CCNU coincident with their administration includes nausea, vomiting, flushing, transient rashes, and diarrhea, none of which are serious. Thrombocytopenia occurs in three weeks, leukopenia in four weeks, and a drop in hematocrit at five weeks. Acute hepatic, renal, and pulmonary toxicity is rare. Serious and often fatal, however, are pulmonary interstitial fibrosis and/or interstitial nephritis that may occur with repeated courses of the drugs. There was a greater improvement in survival among patients receiving BCNU combined with RT (median survival of 52 weeks) compared with the same group in the earlier BTSG (median survival of 35 weeks). This increased survival is attributable to the more aggressive use of BCNU in the later study, which included not modifying individual courses because of relatively minor adverse effects.

The fourth study (BTSG 75-01) evaluated the potential oncolytic effect of corticosteroids compared with BCNU and procarbazine. Corticosteroids ameliorate neurologic signs and symptoms in more than 70 percent of patients with brain tumors, both primary and metastatic. Onset of action is rapid (24 to 48 hours), but is usually short lived (three to six months). Although most investigators postulate that improvement with steroids is secondary to a reduction in cerebral edema, it has been well documented that high doses may inhibit tumor growth both in tissue culture and in some animal models.[9] So suggestive was this evidence for tumor inhibition and/or oncolysis by steriods, that the BTSG undertook a cooperative study to investigate this phenomenon.

Patients after surgery were randomized into four groups: Group I—radiation plus BCNU alone; Group II—radiation plus procarbazine; Group III—radiation plus corticosteroids (methyl prednisolone, 400 mg/M/day, one week out of every three); Group IV—radiation plus corticosteroids plus BCNU.

Unfortunately it does not appear that corticosteroids cause tumor inhibitor and/or oncolysis in humans. Adverse effects with high-dose intermittent methylprednisolone were surprisingly modest, with an incidence of serious infections, gastrointestinal bleeding, myopathy, and endocrine abnormalities of under 5 percent.

The fifth and recently completed study (BTSG 78-01) evaluated a radiation sensitizer, misonidazole, and compared it with the lipid-soluble nitrosourea BCNU, the water-soluble nitrosourea, streptozotocin, and superfractionated RT. Superfractionation utilizes more than one dose of ionizing radiation per day, and has a theretic advantage over single-dose daily RT because it increases the oxygen enhancement ratio of the hypoxic tumor cells and renders them more susceptible to radiation.[2] Patients after surgery were randomized into one of four groups: Group I—radiation plus BCNU; Group II—radiation plus Misonidazole plus BCNU; Group III—superfractionated radiation plus BCNU, and Group IV—radiation plus streptozotocin. Preliminary results of this study indicate no advantage of superfractionated RT, Misonidazole, or streptozotocin over RT plus BCNU.

The sixth, and currently ongoing, study (BTSG 81-01) evaluates combinations of chemotherapeutic agents. Patients after surgery are randomized into three groups: Group I—radiation plus BCNU; Group II—radiation plus BCNU plus procarbazine; and Group III—radiation and cycles of BCNU plus hydroxyurea alternating with cycles of epipodophyllotoxin plus procarbazine. No results of this study are available.

Several studies have been undertaken to evaluate immunologic factors in brain tumors.[10] The underlying assumption of this work is that cancer cells can be distinguished from normal cells by the presence of distinctive antigens. Despite the enormous literature that has centered on the question of tumor-specific antigens, however, the existence of such antigens remains speculative. More sophisticated immunologic studies are now in progress, which are intended to define and exploit suspected antigenic differences.

CONCLUSIONS

Despite the progress in increasing both survival and quality of survival, it is painfully apparent that a malignant glioma is almost always fatal, primarily as a result of our inability to eradicate all of the tumor cells. When a brain tumor develops, it shares its space with the brain, which occupies approximately 1200 ml within the confines of the skull. In this space 100 grams of tumor, equivalent to one hundred billion cells, is usually fatal. Patients who present to a physician because of major symptoms usually have tumors that are 30 grams to 60 grams in size. Assuming an initial tumor burden of 100 grams, or one hundred billion cells, a subtotal surgical resection might at best remove 99 percent of the tumor, leaving behind 1 gram, or one billion cells.[8] It would then be left to chemotherapy and RT further to reduce the population of tumor cells to 0.001 grams, or one hundred thousand cells, a size where the body's own natural immune mechanisms can destroy the tumor. The surgeon is rarely able to do a complete resection, however, and conventional RT and chemotherapy do not suffice to kill the remaining malignant cells, thus permitting the tumor to grow at a rate faster than it can be removed. Improved surgical techniques, RT, perhaps augmented by newer radiation sensitizers, and improved chemotherapy and immunotherapy, including new drugs with optimum combinations and schedules, may in the near future result in more favorable long-term results.

REFERENCES

1. Concannon JP, Kramer S, Berry R: The extent of intracranial gliomata at autopsy and its relationship to techniques used in radiation therapy of brain tumors. Am J Roetgenol 84:99–107, 1960
2. Douglas BG: Preliminary results using superfractionation in the treatment of glioblastoma multiforme. J Canad Assoc Radiolol 28:106–110, 1977
3. Frankel SA, German WJ: Glioblastoma multiforme. J Neurosurg 15:489–503, 1958
4. Jelsma R, Bucy P: The treatment of glioblastoma multiforme of the brain. J Neurosurg 27:388–400, 1967
5. Koos WT, Miller MH: Intracranial Tumors of Infants and Children. St. Louis, CV Mosby 1971
6. Matson DD: Neurosurgery of Infancy and Childhood (ed 2). Springfield, Charles C Thomas, 1969
7. Levin VA, Freeman-Dove M, Landahl HD: Permeability characteristics of brain adjacent to tumors in rats. Arch Neurol 32:785–791, 1975
8. Lieberman A, Ransohoff J: Treatment of primary brain tumors. Med Clin N Am 63:835–848, 1979
9. Lieberman A, LeBrun Y, Glass P: Use of high dose corticosteroids in patients with inoperable brain tumors. J Neurol Neurosurg Psychiatr 40:678–682, 1977

10. Mahaley MD, Brooks WM and Roszman TL: Immunobiology of primary intracranial tumors. J Neurosurg 46:467–476, 1978
11. Ransohoff J, Lieberman A: Surgical therapy of primary malignant brain tumors. Clin Neurosurg 25:403–411, 1978
12. Roth JG, Elvidge AR: Glioblastoma multiforme: A clinical survey. J Neurosurg 17:736–750, 1960
13. Shapiro W: Chemotherapy of nervous system neoplasms, In Scher J, Ford D (eds): Primary Intracranial Neoplasms. New York, Spectrum Press, (in press)
14. Taveras J, Thompson HG, Pool JL: Should we treat glioblastoma multiforme? Am J Roentgenol 87:473–479, 1962
15. Urtasun RR, Band R, Shapman JD: Radiation and high dose metronidazole in supratentorial glioblastoma. N Engl J Med 294:1364–1367, 1964
16. Vick NA, Khandekar JD, Bigner DD: Chemotherapy of brain tumors. The blood–brain barrier is not a factor. Arch Neurol 34:523–526, 1977
17. Walker MD, Alexander E, Hunt WE: Evaluation of mithramycin in the treatment of anaplastic gliomas. J Neurosurg 44:655–667, 1976
18. Wasserman TH, Phillips TL, Johnson RJ: Initial clinical and pharmacologic evaluation of misonidazole (RO-07-0582), a hypoxic cell radiosensitizer. Internat J Radiat Concol Biol Phys (in press)

36. Meningiomas

Kenneth Shapiro
Kenneth Shulman

Meningiomas are relatively common intracranial tumors in adults, but are rare in children, comprising between 0.4 percent and 4.6 percent of all intracranial neoplasms found in children.[4,8] Up to 3 percent of all patients with meningiomas will present in the first decade of life, with an additional 6 percent presenting in the second decade.[4,9] Based on an earlier review of 121 children with meningiomas including our own experience with 9 patients,[8] this chapter describes the clinical characteristics of meningiomas in the pediatric population, including preoperative assessment and intraoperative considerations for the management of these unusual tumors.

It is helpful to separate patients into groups based on age of initial presentation. This distinction is important not only because clinical evaluation is easier in older patients, but, more important, because the clinical presentation and tumor location are often characteristic for specific groups of children.

Even with increased reportage of individual cases, meningiomas presenting in infancy are exceedingly rare with only six case reports found in the literature.[8] Four of these meningiomas had convexity locations; one was intraventricular and another located at the falx-tentorial junction. As is often the case in infants, symptoms and signs of increased intracranial pressure predominated. The majority of these tumors were exceedingly large, suggesting their presence from birth. Calcification occurred in two of these tumors, a feature which, coupled with convexity location on plain skull x-ray films, should suggest a meningioma. Since computed tomography (CT) is now employed routinely for neuroradiologic diagnosis, a mass lesion found in an infant with the CT features associated with meningiomas of adulthood, coupled with appropriate location, should lead to accurate preoperative diagnosis.

A total of 61 children (up to 12 years of age, including three of our own cases) had intracranial meningiomas. The sex distribution was equal, a difference from the strong female predominance found in adults with meningiomas. Onset was insidious with the average duration of symptoms being 1.5 years, compared with only 0.5 year reported in children harboring brain tumors of other types.[2] Clinical signs were usually compatible with the location of the tumor. Twenty-three of the 58 children (40 percent) in whom location was reported had parasagittal or convexity meningiomas. These children had seizures, signs of increased intracranial pressure, and focal paresis, but did not have hemianopsia. By contrast 13 children (22 percent) with lateral ventricle tumors often had seizures, raised intracranial pressure, hemiparesis, and hemianopsia. The presence of hemianopsia helped to distinguish lateral ventricle meningiomas from convexity or parasagittal tumors on clinical grounds. The frequency of these lateral ventricle tumors is striking when contrasted with adult patients, as only 0.2 percent to 4 percent meningiomas are intraventricular.[4–7,9]

When considering lateral ventricle meningiomas overall, 7 to 10 percent occur in patients age 2 to 12 years old.[1,11] Three of 15 third and fourth ventricle meningiomas reviewed occurred in this same age group.[1,4,8] Although sarcomatous degeneration has been associated with meningiomas in children,[13] this occurred in only 14 percent of pediatric meningiomas. Cushing and Eisenhardt[4] described 8 adult patients who had meningiomas with sarcomatous degeneration; 5 lived longer than five years, including one patient who survived 21 years.[4] Since sarcomatous degeneration may not be as ominous as its name implies, it is important to distinguish this tumor from the meningeal sarcoma that carries a less favorable prognosis.[10]

Fifty-four adolescents (aged 13 through 18) were identified with intracranial meningiomas. Forty-one percent were males and 59 percent females. The average duration of symptoms was 2.2 years, compared with 1.5 years in younger children and 2.8 to 3.5 years in adults.[4,7] Clinical signs again correlated with the location of the tumor. When these locations were compared with those commonly found in adults, certain differences were again apparent. Only 8 percent of meningiomas of adolescence had parasagittal and falx attachments compared with 23 percent found in adults.[4] There were two convexity and two sphenoid ridge meningiomas (8 percent), while these locations would be expected in 34 percent of adults.[4] Nine adolescents (17 percent) had tumors in the posterior fossa, compared with about 8 percent in adults.[3,4,7,9] As in children the most striking finding is that 35 percent of meningiomas found in adolescents were located in the lateral ventricles. The clinical signs are similar to children with lateral ventricle meningiomas, with many adolescents also exhibiting extrapyramidal tract signs. Approximately 19 percent of adolescents with meningiomas found in the literature had the central form of Recklinghausen's disease.[8,12] Furthermore almost half of all patients with this phakomatosis became symptomatic in adolescence. Since patients with this disease often have multiple tumors of differing tissue types, they may present with signs referrable to many anatomic sites. This diagnostic confusion may be especially vexing, as we experienced in a patient who had bilateral acoustic nerve tumors, a falx meningioma, a pontine astrocytoma, and a thoracic meningioma, as well as multiple spinal neurofibromata. Cutaneous lesions in these patients may be minimal or absent.

Beginning with adolescence the incidence of meningiomas increases with age.[4,7,9] It is possible, therefore, that meningiomas occurring in adolescent patients in the more common locations are often not reported. Perhaps this partially accounts for the smaller number of meningiomas reported in adolescents compared with the childhood age group and for the predominance of unusual clinical features gleaned from the literature.

The radiographic features of meningiomas in pediatric patients from all three age groups are not different from those found in adults. Plain skull x-ray films in young patients may show calcification (13 percent), hyperostosis (10 percent), or erosion of bone (9 percent). In adolescence sellar erosion due to diffusely elevated intracranial pressure was common (36 percent), while in children suture diastasis was sometimes observed (17 percent). Frequently calcification of an intraventricular meningioma will be seen on plain skull x-ray films of the skull, but calcification of meningiomas in general is unusual in patients less than 5 years of age.[12] Angiography, when performed, often showed a typical sunburst tumor stain and demonstrated the lesion's vascular supply (Fig. 36-1).

Surgical considerations for many meningiomas of childhood must begin at the time of initial diagnosis of the patient's tumor. The ease of diagnosis of an intracranial lesion by CT scan may lull the surgeon into operating without further neuroradiologic investigation. The often immense size of these tumors, however, and the unusual locations of many of them, make angiography extremely important. This is especially so in the relatively common intraventricular tumors. These operations may terminate unfavorably if the vascular pedicle supplying the tumor is beyond the surgeon's control. In one tumor occurring in an adolescent, the preoperative CT was compatible with an intraaxial tumor, although at operation a large frontal convexity meningioma burrowing into the brain but separate from it was found. This intraoperative surprise, which changed the operative approach, could have been avoided with a preoperative angiogram.

Techniques for the removal of the convexity tumors are no different from those employed in adults with meningiomas. Careful dissection within the arachnoid plane under magnification with adequate blood available for replacement should lead to good postoperative results. The tumors of the lateral ventricles may often reach enormous sizes as shown in Figure 36-2. A well-planned approach giving access initially to the vascular pedicle coming from the choroid vessels may turn a potentially difficult operation into one that can be performed in a relatively bloodless field with piecemeal removal of the tumor.

In reviewing the case reports of pediatric meningiomas, operative mortality

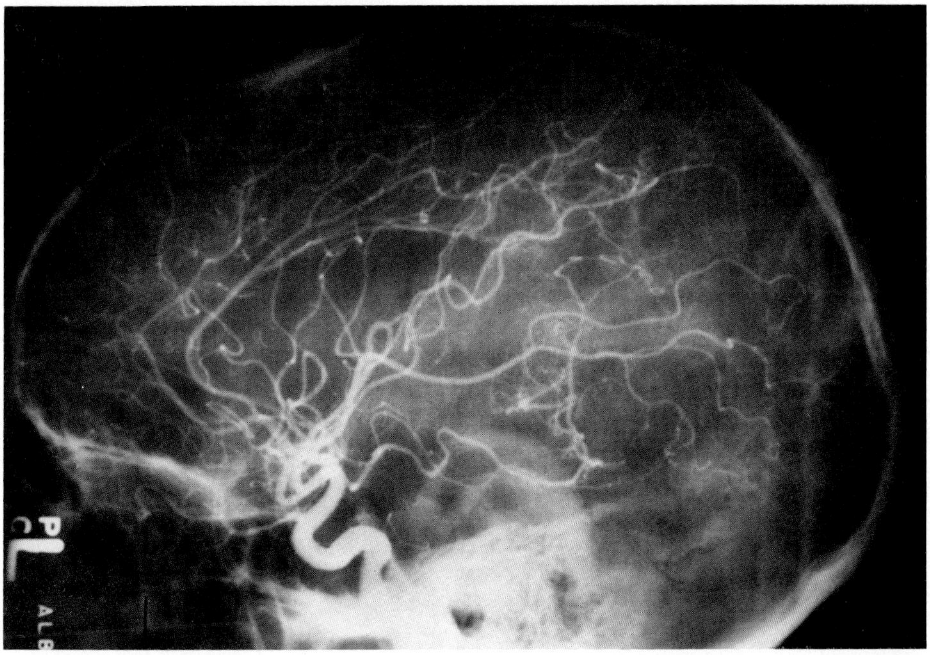

Figure 36-1. Lateral arterial phase of left carotid arteriogram demonstrating a vascular intraventricular mass supplied by a hypertrophied anterior choroidal artery.

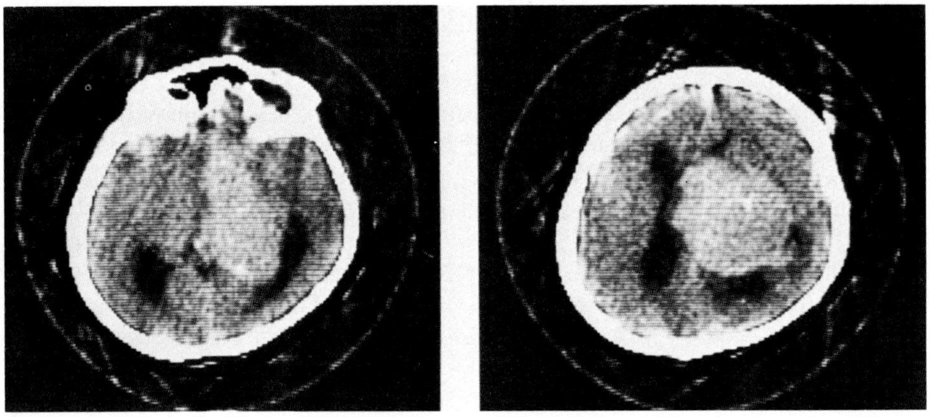

Figure 36-2. CT scan without contrast enhancement demonstrating a mass within the right lateral ventricle. Total removal of this mixed meningioma was accomplished.

approached 40 percent from meningiomas found in infants and children. Since many of these cases were treated before the availability of the present standards of medical and anesthetic support, we believe the mortality figure may overestimate the surgical risks in this age group. Mortality in the adolescent group was also high (33 percent) again a reflection, at least in part, of the large numbers collected before 1960. On the basis of these reports, survival in approximately 90 percent will be useful, with 60 percent of survivors leading reasonably normal lives. We anticipate that this good quality of survival can be maintained, and that operative mortality can be lessened in pediatric patients with meningiomas.

If the goal of improved surgical morbidity and mortality is to be realized for children with meningiomas, one of the major determinants of outcome will be the proper preoperative evaluation of these patients. Since meningiomas are unusual in the pediatric population, we have identified several clinical features that should place meningioma in the differential diagnosis. First, in children presenting with a lateral ventricle syndrome (seizures, hemiparesis, hemianopsia, and papilledema), meningiomas should be considered. Second, children with a central form of Recklinghausen's disease, while clearly at risk of harboring a variety of tumors, often have meningiomas. Third, the finding of an extraaxial tumor in the preoperative evaluation of the child should raise the suspicion of meningioma. Although many of these tumors are quite large, it is clear that cure can be achieved with proper preoperative evaluation and well-planned surgical therapy.

REFERENCES

1. Abbott KH, Courville CB: Intraventricular meningiomas. Review of the literature and report of two cases. Bull LA Neurol Soc 7:12–28, 1942
2. Bodian M, Lawson D. The intracranial neoplastic diseases of childhood: A description of their natural history based on a clinicopathological study of 129 cases. Br J Surg 40:368–392, 1953
3. Castellano F, Ruggiero G: Meningiomas of the posterior fossa. Acta Radiol (Stockholm) suppl 104:70–96, 154–157, 1953
4. Cushing H, Eisenhardt L: Meningiomas: Their Classification, Regional Behavior, Life History, and Surgical End Results. New York, Hafner, 1962
5. Fornari M, Savoiardo M, Morello G, et al: Meningiomas of the lateral ventricles. J Neurosurg 54:64–74, 1981

6. Frazier CH, Alpers BJ: Meningeal fibroblastomas of the cerebrum. A clinicopathologic analysis of 75 cases. Arch Neurol Psychiatr 29:935–989, 1933
7. Grant FC: Intracranial meningiomas, surgical results. Surg Gynec Obstet 85:419–431, 1947
8. Herz DA, Shapiro K, Shulman K: Intracranial meningioma of infancy, childhood and adolescence: Review of the literature and addition of 9 case reports. Child's Brain 7:43–56, 1980
9. Horrax G: Meningiomas of the brain. Arch Neurol Psychiatr 41:140–157, 1939
10. Kernohan JW, Vihlein A: Sarcomas of the Brain. Springfield, Charles C Thomas, 1962, pp 99–107
11. Ladenheim JC: Choroid Plexus Meningiomas of the Lateral Ventricle. Springfield, Charles C Thomas, 1963
12. Merten DF, Gooding CA, Newton TH, et al: Meningiomas of childhood and adolescence. J Pediatr 84:696–700, 1974
13. Turner OA, Craig WM, Kernohan JW: Malignant meningiomas. Surgery 11:81–101, 1942

37. Choroid Plexus Papilloma

Jose Manuel Velasco-Siles

Anthony J. Raimondi

The choroid plexus papilloma, a well-known tumor, was first reported by Guerard[7] in 1833. It has a relatively low incidence: 3 percent in both Matson's series of 408 children under 12 years of age, and Raimondi and Tomita's 332 cases under 16 years.

In general these tumors are noninvasive and slow growing, with only 10 percent of them malignant.[20] Because diagnosis initially was primarily clinical, predicated entirely upon ventriculography or pneumoencephalography, and only recently have angiography and computerized transmission tomography (CTT) become available, this tumor has remained rare and very difficult to diagnose preoperatively.[11,20] In 60 to 70 percent of newborns, infants, and adolescents, the tumor is located in the lateral ventricles,[16,20] though it is more common in the fourth ventricle in adults. Rovit, Schechter, and Chodroff[23] reviewed 234 cases (adding 11 of their own) in all age groups, and noted that 43 percent of the tumors were located in the lateral ventricles, 10 percent in the third ventricle, 39 percent in the fourth ventricle, and 9 percent in the cerebellopontine angle. Though some papers have reported (anecdotally) that the lateral ventricle tumors are more common on the left, and in boys, a careful review of all published cases fails to bear this out.[13,20,21]

Concerning the age of incidence of the choroid plexus papilloma, Herren[9] carefully analyzed cases published prior to 1936, noting that approximately 10 percent of the reported tumors occurred during the first year of life and 30 percent occurred during the first two decades of life. Hydrocephalus is an almost invariable complication of the tumor, often persisting after total resection.[3,4,14–16,21,22]

Seventy percent of the children with choroid plexus papilloma[17,18,19] present either with enlargement of the head or an increase in intracranial pressure (ICP). According to Matson[12] the most common complaint is vomiting. In Raimondi's series[20,21] only 2 patients with papilloma in the lateral ventricles displayed hemiparesis before surgery. The overproduction of cerebrospinal fluid (CSF) in cases of choroid plexus papilloma has been documented[3,4,25] and found to be four times greater than the normal rate. One of our cases, a 9-month-old boy, weighing 7.5 kg, produced 1200 cm^3/day. It seems as though elevation of ICP does not exert a direct influence upon the rate of CSF production if the cerebral perfusion pressure is maintained at a normal level.[26] The question of whether CSF overproduction alone can produce hydrocephalus remains unsettled.[1,3,24] Gudeman, Sullivan, and Royer[6] reported a patient with bilateral choroid plexus papillomas, concluding that elevated CSF production by itself is sufficient to cause hydrocephalus. Kahn and Luros[10] and Matson and Crofton[13] also mentioned that overproduction alone can cause ventricular dilation. If the tumor has recently bled, the fluid may be slightly xanthochronic or display an elevated protein content. Perfectly normal CSF, however, is compatible with the presence of such a tumor (Raimondi,[21] Rovit[23]). Concerning its ultrastructural (Fig. 37-1) and ultracytochemical composition, no obvious distinction has been found between a hypersecreting choroid plexus papilloma and normal choroid plexus tissue.[2,5,15]

Plain skull x-rays usually show evidence of increased ICP. The radioisotope brain scan can be a helpful method for making the diagnosis, especially if blocking agents are used. Negative or positive contrast pneumography or ventriculography is nonspecific, unreliable, and dangerous. Visualization of intraventricular tumors by these studies depends entirely upon adequate coverage of the tumor mass by contrast media.[20]

At the present time, we have two diagnostic procedures of choice. One is CTT scanning, which is able to detect a well-circumscribed mass within a ventricle that appears to have a heterogenous density after infusion, and in most cases discloses asymmetric ventricular dilation (Fig. 37-2). Enhancement is often, but not always, necessary.

The other procedure is cerebral angiography, which, in our experience, is essential in planning the removal of the tumor, since extension is variable and the anatomy of the blood supply is critical to the surgical procedure (Fig. 37-3). Angiographic criteria for diagnosis of this tumor are (1) an asymmetric hydrocephalus with a shift away from the side of the larger ventricle; (2) a vascular deformity suggestive of two tumors, one in the temporal lobe, one in the occipital parietal area; (3) an irregularly outlined granular stain at the trigone, or a dense ventriculothalamic stain fed by newly formed vessels and containing

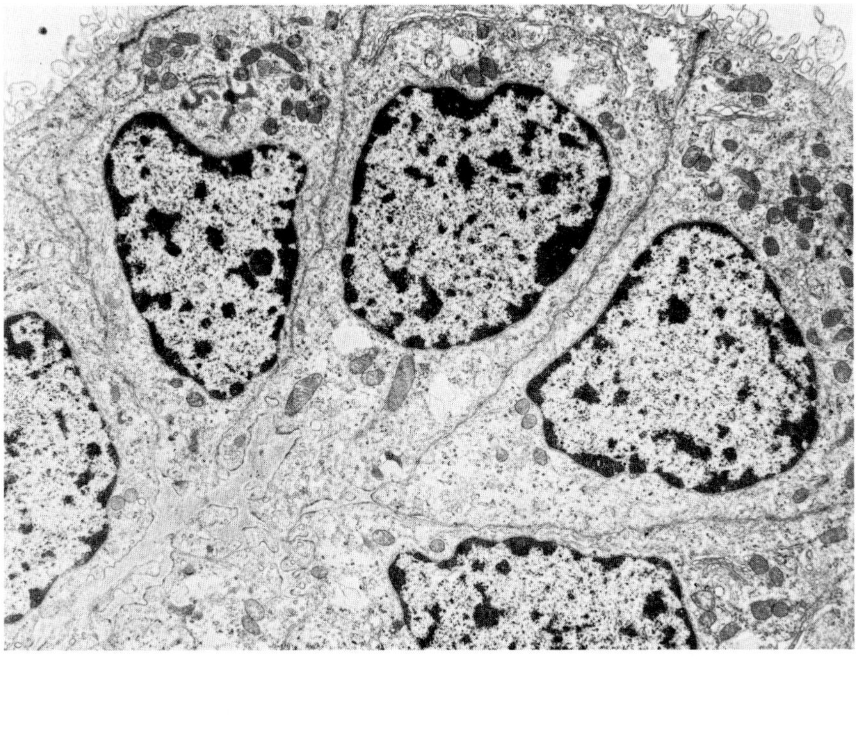

Figure 37-1. Electron micrograph (X6500) shows cuboidal tumor cells that very closely resemble normal choroid plexus.

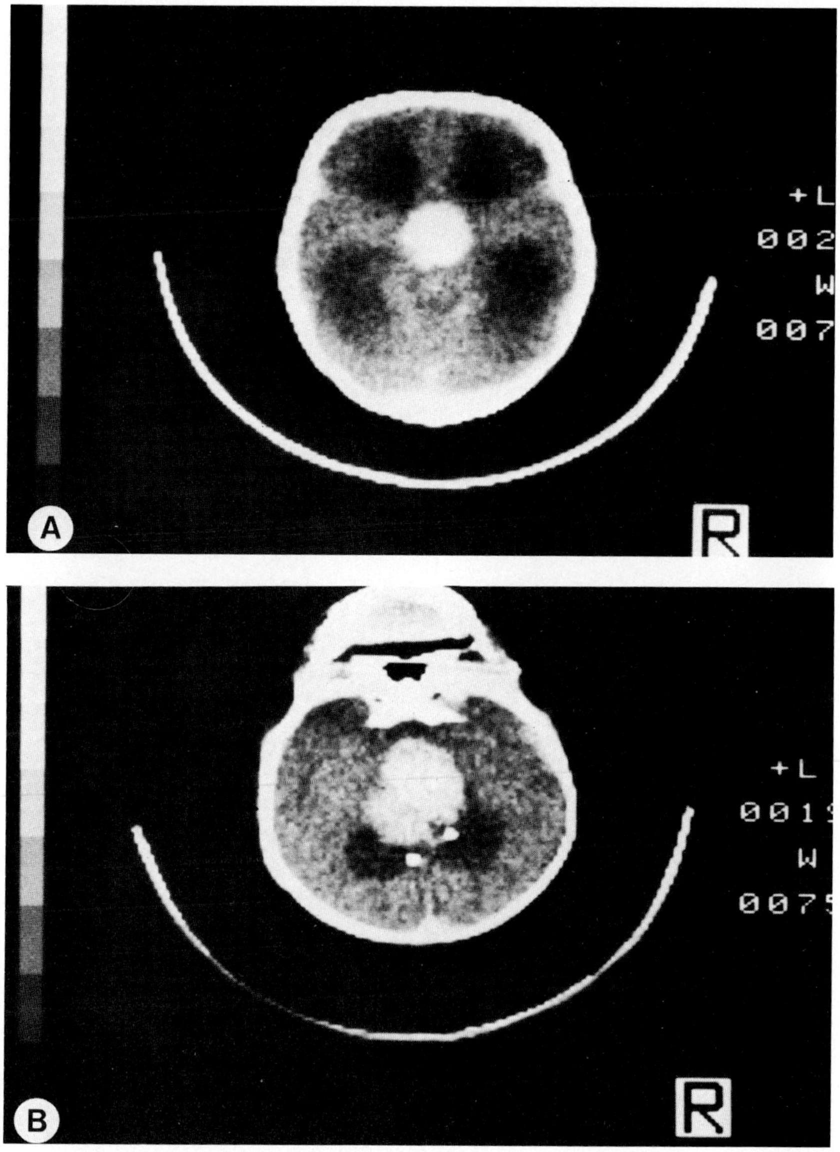

Figure 37-2. Choroid plexus papilloma of the left lateral and third ventricles extending posteriorly to the quadrigeminal cistern. A. Axial cut. B. Coronal cut.

many arteriovenous shunts; (4) hypertrophy of either the anterior choroidal or posterior choroidal arteries; (5) inferior and medial displacement of the internal occipital artery and vein of Rosenthal; (6) anterior and inferior displacement of the thalamic image; and (7) the presence of either an arteriovenous malformation or venous aneurysm on the surface of the tumor.

The angiographic criteria for diagnosing fourth ventricular choroid plexus papillomas[8] are: (1) a symmetric hydrocephalus with dilation of the lateral and third ventricles; (2) the presence of a midline mass occupying the entirety of the fourth ventricle and at times extending into the cisterna magna; (3) the presence of a finely granular stain within the midline of the posterior fossa; and (4) hypertrophy and tortuosity of either the medullary or vermian branches of the posterior inferior cerebellar arteries (Fig. 37-2).

SURGICAL CONSIDERATIONS

Raimondi and Gutierrez[20] personally treated 28 cases of choroid plexus papilloma at the Cook County and Children's Memorial Hospitals from July 1962 through July 1979. The majority were in the lateral ventricles, extending

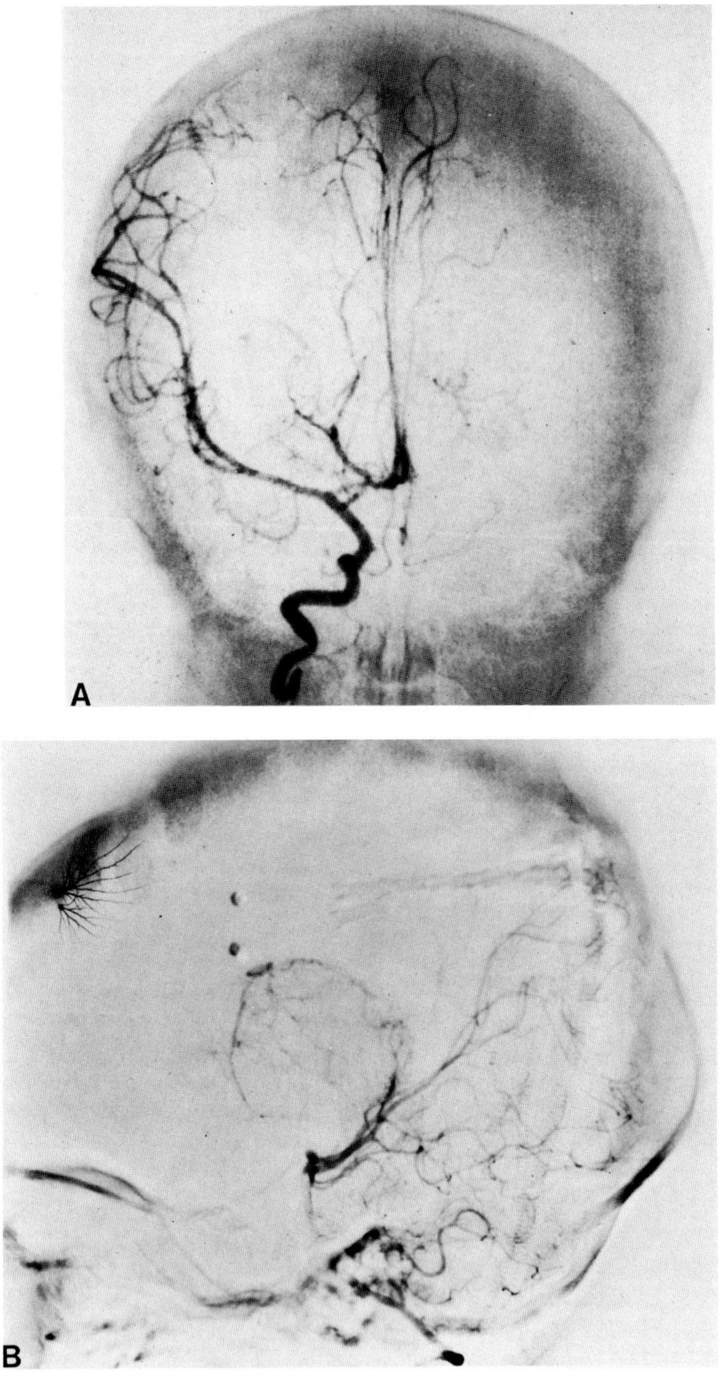

Figure 37-3. A. Lateral displacement of posterior cerebral arteries and left lateral posterior choroidal artery in the quadrigeminal cistern. B. Lateral posterior choroidal artery feeding the tumor. C. Tumor blush with downward displacement of the internal cerebral vein.

along the choroid plexus through the foramen of Monro and down to the tela choroidea of the roof of the third ventricle. Four were primarily within the third ventricle, and three were entirely within the fourth ventricle. None of these latter tumors extended into the pontocerebellar angle through the lateral recesses of the fourth ventricle; two extended into the cisterna magna and upper cervical subarachnoid spaces. One seeded along the CSF pathways into the central canal (thoracic) of the spinal cord. There were three deaths; one followed a third operation for a malignant papilloma of the left lateral ventricle, another (a newborn) died immediately after ventriculography without surgery, and one died of intraoperative bleeding. In 19 cases hydrocephalus persisted following surgery

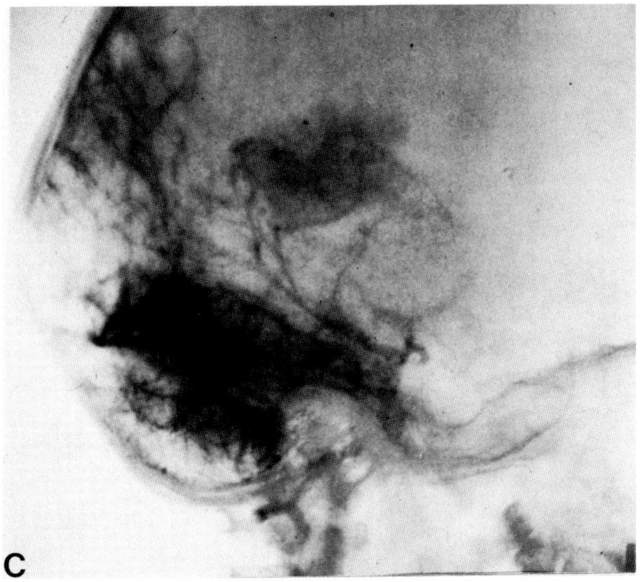

C

and was treated with shunt operations; in 14 patients there was some residual focal neurologic deficit, which had been present preoperatively. In 25 cases the diagnosis was made angiographically and in four cases the diagnosis was made by CTT scan.

The lateral ventricle choroid plexus papilloma blocks the flow of CSF from the temporal lobe, converting this chamber into a cystic cavity holding densely xanthochronic fluid. The mass may extend along the choroid plexus, through the foramen of Monro and into the third ventricle, with resultant obstruction and progressive asymmetric dilatation of both lateral ventricles, one by the tumor and the other by obstruction to the flow of CSF. There is no consistent pattern of ventricular dilatation. One must take care to document carefully which ventricles or ventricular chambers are simply dilated and which hold tumor. Also, these tumors can extend through the choroid fissure into the quadrigeminal cistern, from whence they may enter the opposite lateral ventricle through the choroidal fissure.

Trigone papillomas are best resected through a temporal-parietal flap that is large enough to give access to the temporal pole anteroinferiorly, and the angular gyrus posterosuperiorly (Fig. 37-4). Upon opening the dura, one invariably notes flattening of the gyri. Puncturing the encysted temporal horn before opening the dura, with drainage of its densely xanthochronic ventricular fluid, affords immediate decompression (from 10 to 60 cm^3) (Fig. 37-5). A cerebrotomy within a sulcus located behind the angular gyrus, 3–4 cm in length, provides generous access to the trigone. The dissection through the white matter is best performed with two spatulas, thereby minimizing the area of cerebrotomy, and maximizing the depth of the opening. Once the ependyma over the surface of the tumor is identified, it may be coagulated and sectioned, thereby unsheathing the tumor proper. The collapsed temporal horn and linear cerebrotomy permit ample access to the tumor pedicle. The feeding branches of the anterior choroidal artery enter the tumor at its posteroinferior and medial surfaces. Finger-like pieces of cotton are brought circumferentially over the lobular mass until they surround the pedicle of the tumor at its inferomedial surface, the line of entry of choroidal arteries and exit of draining veins (Fig. 37-6). On occasion the surgeon may remove this tumor piecemeal, coagulating across a lobule of tumor and then cutting it away. En bloc resection, however, after the vascular pedicle has been coagulated and transected, is preferable. This may be done either under direct

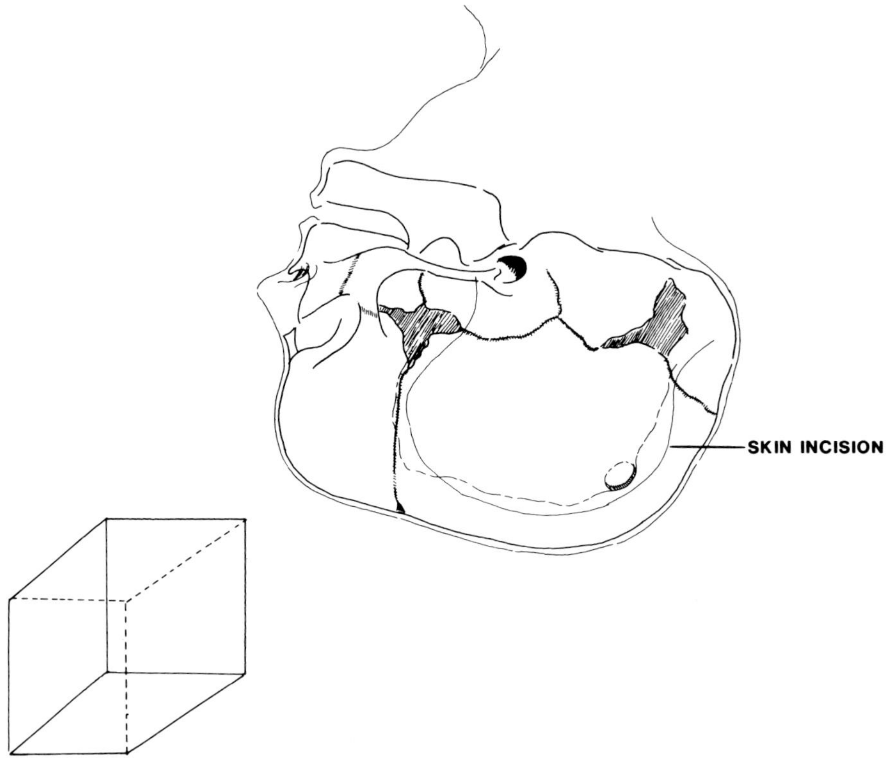

Figure 37–4. Illustration of head position and recommended skin incision.

vision or through digital palpation and "blind" application of hemostatic clips. No surgeon is comfortable with "blind" clip application, but at times it is necessary. The vascular pedicle at the trigone may extend anteroinferiorly along the choroid fissure, toward the hippocampus, or superomedially along the choroid plexus toward the terminal sulcus and foramen of Monro. The draining veins enter the subependymal system, penetrate the choroidal fissure to enter the quadrigeminal and Galenic systems, or may extend downward to enter the supraculminate system. Following en bloc removal of the tumor mass, it is essential to wait for approximately 10 minutes after filling the ventricle with normal saline, to be certain that there is no active bleeding or oozing.

One should inspect the entire lateral ventricle up to the foramen of Monro to assure that tumor is not plugging the outflow of CSF, as this is another extension of the choroid plexus papilloma: along the choroid plexus as far lateral as the terminal sulcus and anteriorly through the foramen of Monro and into the third

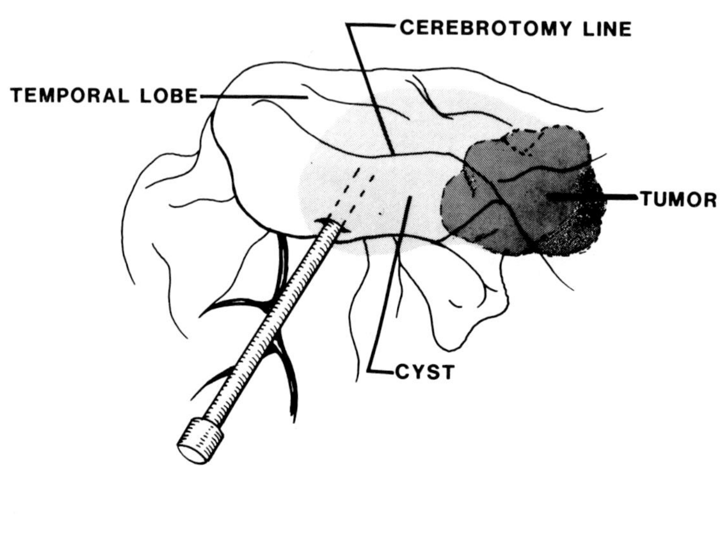

Figure 37-5. Drawing illustrating drainage of encysted temporal horn.

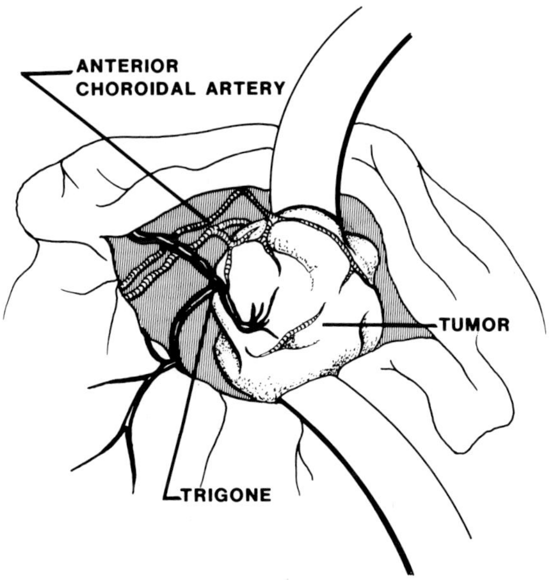

Figure 37-6. Drawing illustrating resection of papilloma at trigone.

ventricle. When this occurs and the foramen of Monro is occluded, one may encounter the encysted temporal, occipital, and frontal horns, as the mass occludes the trigone and enters the third ventricle. A temporal–frontal–parietal flap, allowing access to the angular gyrus posteriorly, the middle frontal convolutions anteriorly, the rostrum and genu of the corpus callosum anteromedially, and the temporal pole anteroinferiorly, is necessary. Before opening the dura, the temporal horn is punctured, followed by the frontal horn, to allow egress of the encysted ventricular fluid. A cerebrotomy 3–4 cm in length is made behind the angular gyrus, and the tumor is isolated prior to sectioning its vascular pedicle. This allows one to clip and section the feeding branches of the anterior choroidal artery at the trigone prior to lifting the tumor from its bed in the terminal sulcus, advancing toward the foramen of Monro and obliterating minute perforating feeders along the bed. This anteromedial dissection is not carried beyond the point at which the body of the fornix bifurcates into the crus fornicis. At this time a cerebrotomy is made in the middle gyrus of the frontal lobe so as to gain access to the encysted frontal horn. The foramen of Monro is identified and the obliteration of the perforating feeders to the tumor is carried out by proceeding posteriorly from the foramen of Monro to approximately the point at which the body of the fornix ends. This frees the tumor from the point of its attachment to the floor of the trigone and the body of the lateral ventricle.

Extension of the tumor from the lateral ventricle into the third ventricle through the foramen of Monro has been in our experience, variable in the amount, vascularity, and adhesions to the foramen of Monro, roof of the third ventricle, and anterior surface of the third ventricle. There has always been a constricted area at the foramen on Monro, however, which has allowed us either to coagulate or clip across it, so as to separate the main tumor mass from its extension into the third ventricle, permitting removal of the tumor in two portions rather than one. After this is done, a large piece of fluffy cotton is placed in the lateral ventricle at the foramen of Monro, and the line of dissection is moved from transventricular to parasagittal by retracting the frontal lobe laterally so as to gain access first to the genu and rostrum of the corpus callosum, and then to the lamina terminalis as far inferiorly as the supraoptic recess. The third ventricle is then entered through its anterior margin by performing a cerebrotomy extending from the rostrum of the corpus callosum, inferomedially along the fornix, and then through the lamina terminalis as far inferiorly as the supraoptic recess. The tumor is removed through this opening by beginning dissection along the roof of the third ventricle, separating it from the choroid plexus located within the tela choroidea. It is recommended that the entire ventricular system be filled with normal saline to minimize stretching of the bridging veins.

Another extension of the lateral ventricle papilloma is through the choroidal fissure into the quadrigeminal cistern and contralateral ventricle. The tumor compresses the quadrigeminal plate, becomes adherent to the commissure of the fornix, and elevates the splenium of the corpus callosum. There is obstruction of the passage of CSF from the ambient cisterns into the quadrigeminal cistern, forward displacement of the pineal gland and suprapineal recess of the third ventricle, and, to some extent, extension of the tumor along the anterior surfaces of the culmen monticuli and lobulus centralis of the vermis. The tumor is fed through the medial and lateral branches of the posterior choroidal arteries on both sides, the quadrigeminal arteries and the inferior retrosplenial arteries (inferiorly and posteriorly). It drains into the internal cerebral veins (lesser galenic system), the veins of Rosenthal, the greater galenic system, the supraculminate system, and anteromedial occipital veins. A biparietal craniotomy through a vertex S-shaped incision is preferred, since it affords excellent exposure, has minimal blood loss, and does not present problems for revascularization and healing. After puncture of the bilateral horns, the dura is opened and the tumor is dissected free from its ventricular adhesions and to its pedicle at the choroidal fissure, from the pes hippocampus anteriorly to the collateral eminence posteriorly. The section of the tumor within the quadrigeminal cistern is performed by the parasagittal approach, coming down bilaterally on either side of the falx cerebri. The anterior and posterior branches of the lateral posterior choroidal artery going to the tumor, as well as the quadrigeminal and inferior retrosplenial arteries, are identified as a group, occluded, and transected. This dissection is carried out from side to side, and forward from behind. It is necessary to identify the anterior choroidal artery coming posterolaterally through and over the tela choroidea of the third ventricle. Venous drainage into the lesser and greater galenic system and its tributaries diminishes considerably once these last feeding vessels are transected.

The fourth ventricle choroid plexus papilloma invariably produces symmetric obstructive hydrocephalus, superimposed upon communicating hydrocephalus, requiring a shunting procedure immediately after the diagnosis is made. We allow the patient to stabilize for 7–14 days prior to posterior fossa surgery, and remove the shunt three to five days after excision of the tumor.

Choroid plexus papillomas in the fourth ventricle grow from the glomus and establish adhesions within the entirety of the anterior and inferior medullary velum and the fastigium. They may extend anterolaterally into the lateral recess of the fourth ventricle, and often do extend posteriorly, elevating the anterior medullary velum and displacing the lingula and lobulus centralis of the vermis. This compresses the colliculus facialis and medial eminence of the floor of the fourth ventricle. In some circumstances this tumor sends digital extensions into the floor of the fourth ventricle or fungates into either cerebellar hemisphere. When there is extension through the foramen of Magendie and into the cisterna magna, the tumor may engulf the posterior inferior cerebellar artery and push downward through the foramen magnum into the upper cervical canal.

We prefer to perform a posterior fossa craniotomy, rather then craniectomy, in children, since this permits us to reconstruct completely the squamous portion of the occipital bone and the suboccipital musculature. The arch of C1, similarly, is not resected; rather it is incised at its junction with the lateral mass. Subsequent to this osteotomy of the arch of C1, at the lateral mass on either side, it is retracted posteroinferiorly, exposing the dura down to C2, but not breaking the continuity of the periosteum around C1. This allows for the reapproximation of C1 into its normal position and anchoring of this arch by periosteal sutures. The dura is then opened, exposing the vermis, cisterna magna, and upper cervical cord. Before dissecting the tumor from the posterior inferior cerebellar or vertebral arteries, it is dissected from the nodulus and uvula of the vermis, displacing the tonsils laterally, allowing access to feeding vessels coming from tonsilar and vermian branches of pica. A cerebellar incision is then made in a limbic fashion extending from the medial surface of one tonsil over the nodulus to the medial surface of the contralateral tonsil, exposing tenia of the fourth ventricle at the calamus scriptorius, and thereby permitting complete isolation of most of the blood supply to the tumor. Fluffy cotton is used to separate the lobular papilloma from adhesions that connect it to the surrounding wall of the fourth ventricle. One is advised to exert particular caution in removing the tumor from the fourth ventricle when it appears to be completely free, lest feeding vessels coming from branches of the precentral system be torn prior to occlusion and transection. If one has been able to identify these vessels angiographically prior to surgery, this danger will be minimized.

REFERENCES

1. Cutler RWP, Page L, Galicich J, et al: Formation and absorption of cerebrospinal fluid in man. Brain 91:707–720, 1968
2. Davis LE, Cushing H: Papillomas of the choroid plexus with the report of 6 cases. Arch Neurol Psychiatr 13:681–710, 1925
3. Eisenberg HM, McComb JG, Lorenzo AV: Cerebrospinal fluid overproduction and hydrocephalus associated with choroid plexus papilloma. J Neurosurg 40:381–385, 1974
4. Fairburn B: Choroid plexus papilloma and its relation to hydrocephalus. J Neurosurg 17:166–171, 1960
5. Ghatak NR, McWhorter JM: Ultrastructural evidence for CSF production by a choroid plexus papilloma. J Neurosurg 45:409–415, 1976
6. Gudeman S, Sullivan HG, Rosner NJ: Surgical removal of bilateral papillomas of the choroid plexus of the lateral ventricles with resolution of hydrocephalus. J Neurosurg 50:677–681, 1979
7. Guerard: Tumeur fongueuse dans de ventricule droit du cervau chez une petite fille de trois ans. Bull Soc Anat Paris 8:211 (1832–1833; cited by Dairs and Cushing)
8. Hammon WK, Kempe LG, Hayes GJ: Angiographic appearance of a papilloma of the choroid plexus of the lateral ventricle. J Neurosurg 20:711–714, 1963
9. Herren RY: Papilloma of the choroid plexus. Arch Surg Chicago 42:758–774, 1941
10. Kahn EA, Luros JT: Hydrocephalus from overproduction of cerebrospinal fluid (and experiences with other papillomas of the choroid plexus). J Neurosurg 9:59–67, 1952
11. Laurence KM, Hoare RD, Till K: The diagnosis of choroid plexus papilloma of the lateral ventricle. Brain 84:628–641, 1961
12. Matson D: Case reports and technical notes. Hydrocephalus in a premature infant caused by papilloma of the choroid plexus with report of surgical treatment. J Neurosurg 10:416–420, 1953
13. Matson D, Crofton FDL: Papilloma of the choroid plexus in childhood. J Neurosurg 17:1002–1027, 1960
14. Milhorat TH: Hydrocephalus and the cerebrospinal fluid production. Science 166:1514–1516, 1969
15. Milhorat TH, Davis DA, Hammock MK: Choroid plexus papilloma II. Ultrastructural and ultracytochemical localization of Na-K-ATPase. Child's Brain 2:290–303, 1976
16. Milhorat TH, Hammock MK, Davis DA, et al: Choroid plexus papillomas. I: Proof of cerebrospinal fluid overproduction. Child's Brain 2:273–289, 1976

17. Nassar S, Mount LA: Papillomas of the choroid plexus. J Neurosurg 29:73–77, 1968
18. Norlen G: Papillomas of the choroid plexus. With a report of a successfully removed tumour of the left lateral ventricle in a 7 month old child. Acta Chir Scand 98:273–279, 1949
19. Portnoy HD, Croissant PD: A practical method for measuring the hydrodynamics of cerebrospinal fluid. Surg Neurol 5:273–277, 1976
20. Raimondi AJ, Gutierrez FA: Diagnosis and surgical treatment of choroid plexus papilloma. Child's Brain 1:81–115, 1975
21. Raimondi AJ, Tomita T: Personal communication
22. Ray BS, Peck FC Jr: Papilloma of the choroid plexus of the lateral ventricles causing hydrocephalus in an infant. J Neurosurg 13:405–410, 1956
23. Rovit RL, Schechter MM, Chodroff P: Observations on radiographic diagnosis. Am J Roentgenol 110:608–661, 1970
24. Russell DS: Observations on the pathology of hydrocephalus. Special reports, series no. 265, Medical Research Council. London; His Majesty's Stationary Office, 1949
25. Vigoroux A: Ecoulement de liquide cephalorachidien. Hydrocéphalie papillome des plexus choroides du IV ventricle. Rev Neurol 16:281–285, 1908
26. Weiss MH, Wertman N: Modulation of CSF production by alterations in cerebral perfusion pressure. Arch Neurol 35:527–529, 1978

38. Third Ventricle Tumors

William A. Shucart

Tumors of the third ventricle in childhood are stated to be rare, but in some series the reported incidence has been as high as 15 to 20 percent of supratentorial brain tumors.[4,9] Confusion stems from the fact that many neoplasms arise in surrounding structures and extend into the ventricle whereas few actually arise within it.[2,6,8] If craniopharyngiomas are excluded, as they are rarely solely in the ventricle, the most common tumors in the anterior third ventricle are astrocytomas. Tumors that occur less commonly include epidermoids, dermoids, teratomas, germinomas, and choroid plexus papillomas.[3] Colloid cysts are much more common in adults than in children and are discussed elsewhere in this text. Other mass lesions that may rarely involve the third ventricle are abscesses, arteriovenous malformations, and harmartomas.

Historically attempted removal of third ventricular lesions has been associated with significant morbidity and mortality. A philosophy of nonoperative treatment utilizing either stereotactic needle biopsy or radiation therapy gained wide acceptance. In recent years a more aggressive surgical philosophy has evolved because newer surgical techniques allow operative treatment with much lower morbidity and mortality rates.[1,2,5,7,10]

PREOPERATIVE EVALUATION

The clinical presentation of lesions involving the anterior third ventricle is variable. Neoplasms involving the thalamus may cause motor and, less commonly, sensory impairment; lesions of the diencephalon often do not cause any endocrinologic abnormalities until they are well advanced, but may cause a syndrome in young children of cachexia associated with hyperactivity and an unusually alert facial expression (diencephalic syndrome). Many times the lesions are clinically silent until they cause compromise of the foramina of Monro, leading to hydrocephalus. Some hypothalamic gliomas merge into the optic chiasm and visual field defects may be part of the clinical picture, but generally visual field defects suggest a mass outside the third ventricle.

Plain skull radiographs have few findings diagnostic of anterior third ventricular tumors. In those occasional tumors that are exophytic and extend to the area of the optic chiasm, there may be local erosive changes of the skull in the region of the sella turcica. If hydrocephalus is present, there may be changes of generalized increased intracranial pressure including suture separation, head enlargement, and enlarged emissary venous channels. Computerized tomography (CT), especially if coronal and sagittal views are available, yields the most information in regard to tumor location and ventricular size. It should be kept in mind that some craniopharyngiomas and epidermoids may have a density close to that of cerebrospinal fluid and astrocytomas of lower grade may resemble normal brain tissue.

In cases where there are questions as to the actual presence of a lesion, the nature of the lesion, or its exact location, angiography may be helpful. Masses originating below the third ventricle but growing up into it may cause elevation of the horizontal portion of the anterior cerebral arteries and lateral displacement of the distal portion of the internal carotid arteries. Lesions within the third ventricle generally tend to displace the anterior choroidal and posterior communicating arteries in such a way that their normal curvature is reversed. Changes in the septal vein are not helpful in differentiating extraventricular from intraventricular masses. It is not uncommon for lesions in the anterior third to show no significant arteriographic findings.

Air constrast studies are helpful in demonstrating the presence of a mass, but less informative in showing its origin.

SURGICAL OBJECTIVES

The primary objectives of surgery in this area are to (1) make a diagnosis, (2) remove resectable lesions, and (3) provide symptomatic relief. If hydrocephalus with increased pressure is a prominent part of the patient's symptomatology, a ventriculoperitoneal shunt should probably be the initial treatment with definitive surgery being done one to two weeks later. If the transcallosal approach is used, the decrease in ventricular size subsequent to shunting does not make the surgery more difficult.

There is some debate as to the appropriate treatment for astrocytomas. Most surgeons agree that in Grade III and Grade IV astrocytomas little more than a biopsy is worthwhile. It is doubtful that any astrocytoma can be totally removed but there are some surgeons who advocate "gross total removal" of Grades I and II astrocytomas. In our experience total removal of low-grade astrocytomas has not been feasible technically because the differentiation between neoplasm and surrounding normal tissue is so difficult. The prognosis following attempted total removal or biopsy followed by radiation therapy is much the same; several-year survivals are seen in both groups.

With extraaxial masses such as epidermoids, a complete removal of the lesion should be possible. For those few craniopharyngiomas that arise solely within the third ventricle, total removal may be possible; in our experience with three cases, complete removal was possible in only one. Ependymomas, because of their radioresistance, should be diligently pursued in an attempt to effect a surgical cure.

OPERATIVE TECHNIQUES

There are alternative operative approaches to the anterior third ventricle. If visual field defects are present, we prefer a subfrontal approach. If visual fields are normal, a transventricular approach is used. Occasionally a combined approach is necessary.

Transcallosal Approach

The transcallosal approach is best for dealing with lesions in the depths of the anterior third ventricle. This approach has several advantages over the frontal transcortical method: the risk of seizures is markedly reduced, the ventricles can be easily dealt with regardless of size, and, most important, the depths of the third ventricle can be well visualized with greater operative mobility.

The patient is placed in the supine position with the head straight and elevated 15 to 20 degrees. Although the lateral position has been advocated, orientation to the anatomic structures is most easily maintained with the head straight. No advantage is gained in regard to hemispheral retraction or field of vision by using the lateral position. A coronal skin incision is made 2–3 cm behind the coronal suture extending toward the zygoma and to the level of the top of the ear bilaterally (Fig. 38-1). The skin flap is reflected anteriorly to expose 6–7 cm in front of the coronal suture. Two burr holes are made, one just behind the coronal suture and one approximately 6 cm anterior to the coronal suture. Both are placed so that their medial margin is on the edge, or slightly on top of, the sagittal sinus. A third burr hole is placed equidistant to the other two, 6–7 cm lateral to the midline (Fig. 38-2). The triangular free bone flap is then removed. The dura is opened along the anterior and posterior bone margins and carefully lifted from the underlying cortex toward the sagittal sinus (Fig. 38-3). A cortical vein draining into the sinus may have to be divided to allow reflection of the dura to the midline. The operating microscope is then introduced.

An imaginary line drawn from the coronal suture at the midline to the external auditory meatus will roughly bisect the corpus callosum. Keeping this line in mind, the frontal lobe is retracted from the falx until the corpus callosum is identified by its white color. Division of the corpus callosum should be confined to the area in front of the "line." If the exposure is too anterior, abundant adhesions will be encountered between the frontal lobes.

The inexperienced surgeon may mistake the cingulate gyrus for the corpus callosum, particularly if the pericallosal artery and callosal marginal artery are mistaken for the two pericallosal arteries. With experience the marked difference in color makes the distinction straightforward. If wider exposure is desired, a retractor may be placed along the falx, but care must be taken not to occlude the

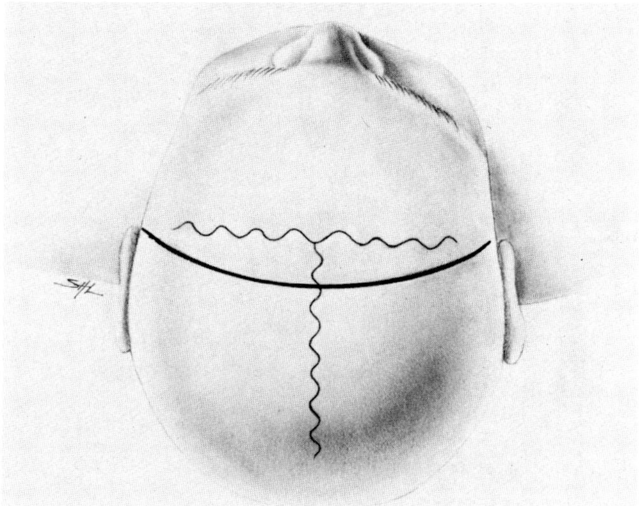

Figure 38-1. Extent of scalp incision.

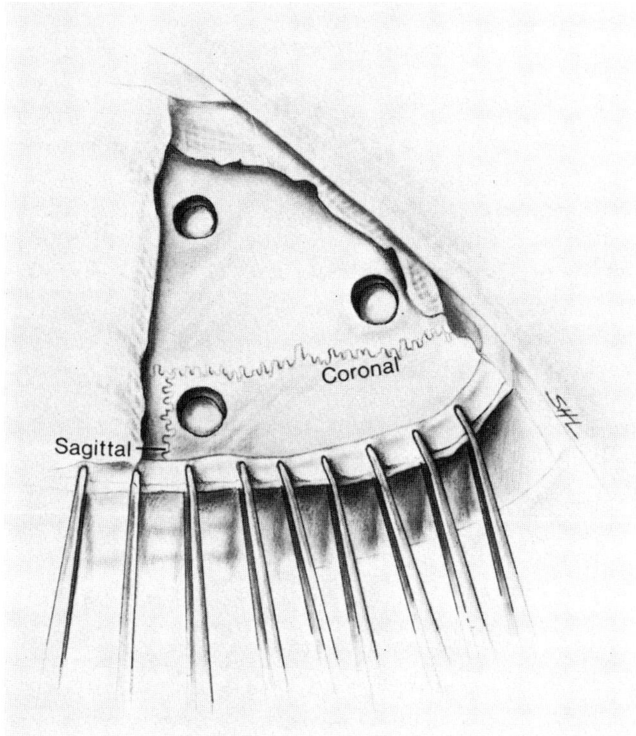

Figure 38-2. Position of burr holes for transcallosal exposure.

sagittal sinus. Both pericallosal arteries are generally seen and it is usually easiest to go between them to divide the corpus callosum; if both arteries are retracted to one side, penetrating branches going to the medial aspect of a hemisphere may have to be divided. The corpus callosum is divided for 2–3 cm using blunt dissection, suction, and bipolar cautery. As soon as the corpus callosum has been divided, cerebrospinal fluid escapes from the ventricle. If there is hydrocephalus, the corpus callosum may be very thin.

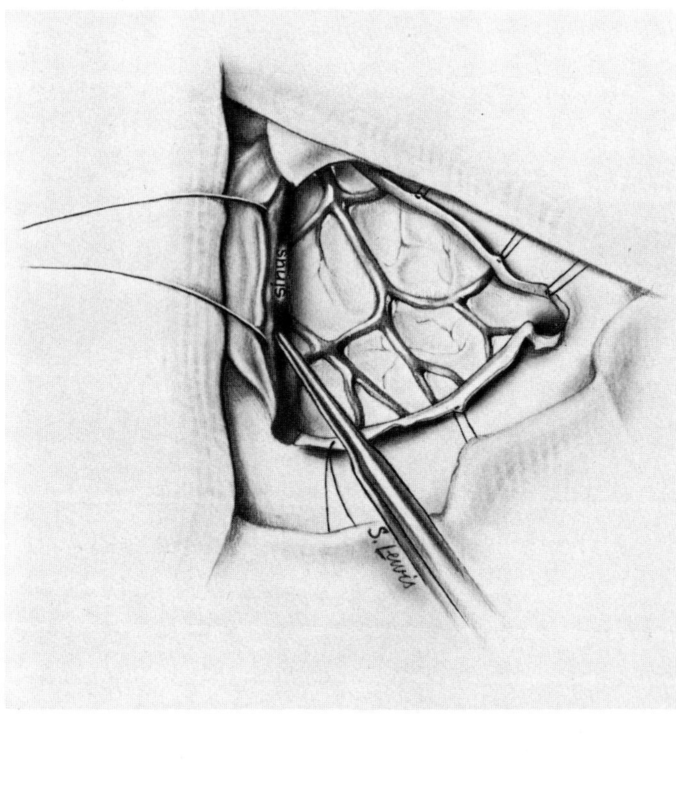

Figure 38-3. Bone flap removed, showing location of sagittal sinus.

The retractor along the right frontal lobe is then placed over the cut edge of the corpus callosum. Orientation is achieved by identifying the structures within the ventricle: the choroid plexus, the thalamostriate vein, and the septal vein. The foramen of Monro is found by following the choroid plexus and thalamostriate vein anteriorly. It is not uncommon to enter the left rather than right lateral ventricle, which will be apparent from the anatomy. A cavum septum pellucidum may be entered and cause confusion until it is realized that no intraventricular structures are present.

Third ventricular lesions are usually easily seen through a dilated foramen of Monro (Fig. 38-4). The column of the fornix is the anterior boundary of the foramen and the anterior commissure is located anteriomedially. Although these structures are not easily visualized, they must be kept in mid. Enlargement of the foramen may be necessary, in which case gentle pressure with a small blunt dissector in all directions except medially is helpful. Further enlargement is rarely necessary, but it can be done by removing a small portion of the posterior rim formed by the thalamus or incising in an anterior and slightly lateral direction through one column of the fornix. Recently it has been shown that an interfornicial approach gives excellent visualization of the third ventricle with no significant physiologic consequences. It is also possible to gain entry to the third ventricle by going through the avascular plane between the thalamus and the fornix. The advantages of these latter two approaches are that they are not limited by the size of the foramen of Monro, and there is no destruction of normal neural tissue. The septum pellucidum should be fenestrated if there is obstruction at a foramen of Monro.

Extraaxial tumors such as epidermoids and craniopharyngiomas are easy to distinguish visually from the surrounding third ventricle. Careful piecemeal

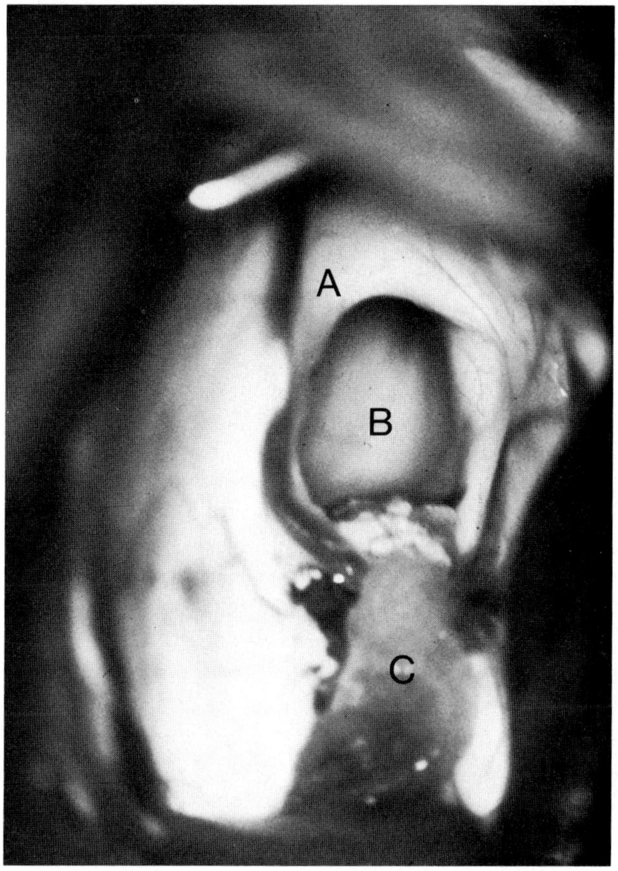

Figure 38-4. Third ventricular astrocytoma seen through dilated foramen of Monro. A. Septal vein. B. Tumor. C. Choroid plexus.

removal of these tumors can be very rewarding. Low-grade astrocytomas are recognizable primarily because of their bulk and distortion of normal anatomy; the lack of clear differentiation from normal tissue may make only a biopsy possible. More malignant astrocytomas usually have abnormal features, making recognition easier. In all cases frozen section studies of the biopsies are helpful to make certain that appropriate tissue is obtained.

When the intraventricular surgery is complete, the ventricles are filled with irrigating solution. In cases where the ventricles are normal in size, the use of dehydrating agents intraoperatively is helpful in lessening the amount of hemispheral retraction required. In patients with hydrocephalus or previously placed shunts, dehydrating agents are not necessary. Prophylactic antibiotics are not necessary and anticonvulsants are not used unless the patient has a previous history of seizures. Patients seem to benefit from treatment with corticosteroids beginning one day preoperatively and continuing through at least the fourth postoperative day.

Subfrontal Approach

If visual field defects are present, the subfrontal approach should be used first and may be the only approach necessary. The exposure must be carried back to the optic chiasm. If nothing is seen in the vicinity of the chiasm, the lamina terminalis should be opened. This opening provides a limited look into the third ventricle and exploration of this area is essential before one can conclude that a subfrontal exploration is negative.

Transcallosal and Subfrontal Approach

If the origin of the tumor is questionable, or if it appears large enough that there might be both significant subfrontal and intraventricular components, a larger bone flap should be made to allow both transcallosal and subfrontal exposure. In this case the more anterior midline burr hole is placed just above the right frontal sinus and a fourth burr hole is placed in the most anterior portion of the temporal line. A quadrangular free bone flap is then removed and exploration of the third ventricle can be carried out by either or both routes.

COMPLICATIONS

The complications of surgery are primarily related to the nature and extent of infiltration of the primary disease process. The complications directly related to the transcallosal approach to the third ventricle generally result from compromise of the sagittal sinus and should be avoidable. There are no significant complications secondary to dividing the anterior third of the body of the corpus callosum. The most common complication of the subfrontal approach is damage to the optic chiasm. An aseptic meningitis may occur with any intraventricular surgery and is usually responsive to cortiscosteroid therapy. Diabetes insipidus, at least transiently, will almost always be present following a subfrontal approach, and is frequently present following a trancallosal approach if significant manipulation is performed in the area of the floor of the third ventricle. Gastrointestinal hemorrhage has been reported as a complication by some. Akinetic mutism may also be a complication of extensive surgery in the anterior third ventricle.

SUMMARY

By utilizing the transcallosal approach to the anterior third ventricle and the operating microscope, excellent exposure of the depths of the anterior ventricle with low operative morbidity and mortality can be obtained. Despite the fact that the majority of tumors in this area are infiltrating and not completely removable, there are enough lesions that are resectable to merit obtaining a tissue diagnosis in all patients.

REFERENCES

1. Apuzzo MLJ, Chikovani OK, Gott PS, et al: Transcallosal interfornicial approaches for lesions affecting the third ventricle. Neurosurgery 10:547–554, 1982
2. Greenwood J Jr: Radical surgery of tumors of the thalamus, hypothalamus, and third ventricle area. Surg Neurol 1:29–33, 1973
3. Izquierdo JM, Rougerie J, Lapras C, et al: The so-called ectopic pinealomas. Child's Brain 5:505–512, 1979
4. Jeeves MA, Simpson DA, and Geffen G: Functional consequences of the transcallosal removal of intraventricular tumors. J Neurol Neurosurg Psychiatr 42:134–142, 1979
5. Long DM, Chou SN: Transcallosal removal of craniopharyngiomas within the third ventricle. J Neurosurg 39:563–567, 1973
6. Menezes AH, Bell WE, Perret GE: Hypothalamic tumors in children. Child's Brain 3:265–280, 1977
7. Shucart WA, Stein BM: Transcallosal approach to the anterior ventricular system. Neurosurgery 3:339–343, 1978
8. Snyder RD: Diencephalic neoplasms. Am J Dis Child 110:109–119, 1965
9. Stein B, Fraser R, Tenner M: Tumors of the midventricle in children. J Neurol Neurosurg Psychiatr 35:776–788, 1972
10. Winston KR, Cavazzuti V, Arkins T: Absence of neurological and behavioral abnormalities after anterior transcallosal operation for third ventricular lesions. Neurosurgery 4:386–393, 1979

39. Colloid Cysts of the Third Ventricle in Infancy and Childhood

Kenneth Shulman
Kenneth Shapiro

Since colloid cysts comprise less than 1 percent of series of intracranial tumors, the number of cases available for review that affect the pediatric age group is limited. The present review is based upon 13 infants and children with colloid cysts reported in the literature, three from the Albert Einstein College of Medicine, in New York.

SYMPTOMS

Three symptom complexes have been described that should make one suspect the diagnosis of colloid cyst. The first one is that of sudden headache due to acute obstruction of cerebrospinal fluid (CSF). Such a symptom causes the patient to seek medical attention as an emergency and this type of headache may be confused with that of subarachnoid hemorrhage. Within hours there are vomiting and lethargy. Finally there are collapse and unconsciousness. In the majority of patients, the obstruction is less complete and the increasingly intensive headache is relieved by assuming the supine position.

There is yet a second headache complex, one of truly episodic nature with a longer headache-free interval. The time course of this headache suggests that the colloid cyst moves in and then out of the foramen on its pedicle, blocking, and then being forced out of, the foramen, leaving the passage clear for some time. Since children rarely complain of headache, the pediatrician may discount this symptom. The resulting delay in diagnosis can be considerable. In Table 39-1 it can be seen that the length of time of headache before diagnosis is nearly six months; this is a longer interval than in the adult cases.

The third symptom complex described first by Riddoch[10] is that of an organic dementia due to a more gradual development of hydrocephalus. Bizarre

Table 39-1
Colloid Cyst of Third Ventricle in Children

Case No.	Author and Year of Report	Age of Child at Time of Diagnosis	Sex	Clinical Observations	Treatment and Results
1	Dandy, W. E. 1933	11	F	Eight months history of repeated headaches and diplopia, episodic, lasting two to three days. One seizure during most recent attack of headache, tonic, and with eyes staring. Increased head size (55.5 cm) with bilateral papilledema.	Right frontal craniotomy with tumor removal. Well.
2	McLean, A. J. 1936	16	F	Four months' headache. Intermittent blindness with changes in head position.	Operated. Well, after stormy course.
3	Greenwood, J., Jr. 1949	14	M	Severe headache and vomiting 18 days p.t.a. cleared with lumbar puncture. Encephalogram showed poor ventricular filling. Six weeks later symptoms recurred and with papilledema. Diagnosis made by ventriculogram.	Cortical resection and cyst removal. Living and well.
4	Greenwood, J., Jr. 1949	8	M	One day of convulsions and loss of consciousness.	Died within 24 hours.
5	Cairns, H., and Mosberg, W. H., Jr. 1951	18	F	At age of 8 years attack of vomiting and unconsciousness. For six weeks prior to diagnosis, headache, vomiting, blurred vision, bilateral papilledema, and sixth nerve paralysis. (Total length of history, 10 years.)	Removal of cyst with recovery; 11-year follow-up. Married with one child.
6	Gemperlein, J. 1960	2/12 mos.	F	Progressive hydrocephalus. Ventriculography showed a mass at foramen of Monro.	Craniotomy and cyst removal. Well.
7	Gemperlein, J. 1960	6/12 mos.	F	Progressive hydrocephalus. Ventriculography showed "obstructive hydrocephalus."	Torkildsen shunt. Died at 16 mos. Cyst, lined by ciliated columnar epithelia, arising in third ventricle.
8	Matson, D. D. 1967	11	N.R.*	Acute headache with decerebration and apnea responding to ventricular drainage.	Tumor removal. Stormy course. Well.
9	Buchsbaum, H. W., and Colton, R. P. 1967	2/12	N.R.	Progressive hydrocephalus. Tense fontanel. Head circumference 51 cm. PEG showed extensive hydrocephalus with tumor in anterior third ventricle.	VJ Shunt. Craniotomy three weeks later with colloid cyst removal. Well.
10	Batnitzky, S., et al. 1974	13	F	Six months of intense intermittent headache associated with dizziness and vomiting. Poor coordination of right upper extremity for one month. Bilateral papilledema.	Right frontal craniotomy and cyst removal. Well.

Case No.	Author and Year of Report	Age of Child at Time of Diagnosis	Sex	Clinical Observations	Treatment and Results
11	Batnitzky, S., et al. 1974	9	F	Three-year history of intermittent attacks of frontal headache with vomiting relieved by assuming supine position. Diplopia 10 days. Bilateral papilledema. Left 7, Right Left 6th N. palsy.	Right frontal craniotomy and cyst removal. Well.
12	Batnitzky, S., et al. 1974	9	M	Six weeks' severe frontal headache with nausea and vomiting. Bilateral papilledema. Left hemiparesis with bilateral upgoing toes.	Right frontal craniotomy and cyst removal. Well.
13	Sackett, J. F., et al. 1975	13	F	Two months of intermittent headache leading to unconsiousness after a possible seizure. Midline density on CTT scan.	Right frontal craniotomy and cyst removal. Well.

*N.R. = No record.

behavior may ensue with the child becoming a behavior problem with the suggestion that a psychiatrist be consulted. Gait apraxia may develop so that the differential diagnosis of a posterior fossa tumor pertains.

SIGNS

The colloid cyst produces no disturbance of neurologic function because there is no direct effect on nerve fiber tracts or nuclei. Experience indicates, however, that patients harboring brain tumors, with head enlargement and suture separation, will have papilledema, as opposed to infants with nontumor hydrocephalus. Papilledema and sixth nerve palsy will develop. Neuroendocrine signs have not been reported.

DIAGNOSTIC PROCEDURES

Plain skull x-rays will show signs of generalized intracranial pressure, with suture separation and demineralization of the sella turcica and amputation of the posterior clinoid process. Colloid cysts do not calcify and the presence of calcium in a tumor presenting in the region of the foramen of Monro should lead one away from the diagnosis of colloid cyst and toward other tumors of the anterior third ventricle—ependymoma, tuberous sclerosis, craniopharyngioma.

It is presently clear that computed transaxial tomography (CTT) scanning is extremely useful and will be diagnostic in most, if not all, cases of colloid cyst of the third ventricle.[11] The lesion will enhance after injection of a contrast agent (Fig. 39-1). The ventriculographic diagnosis of colloid cyst has been well described.[7]

Many papers have been written by neuroradiologists to emphasize the importance of angiography in the diagnosis of tumors around the foramen of

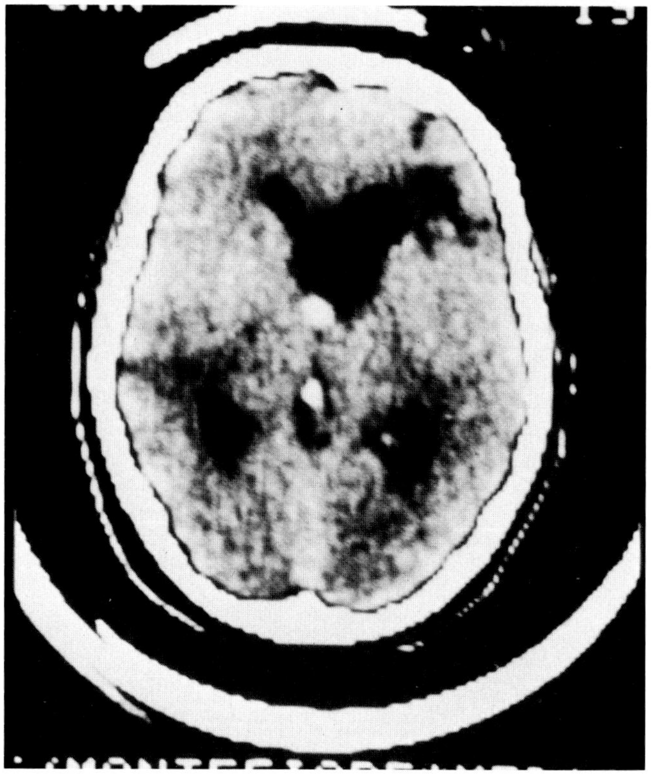

Figure 39-1. Unenhanced CT scan showing colloid cyst at the foramen of Monro.

Monro.[2] Angiography will demonstrate hydrocephalus as evidenced by an increased sweep of the pericallosal artery in the lateral arterial phase and outward bowing of the thalamostriate vein of the frontal venous phase. In nearly all cases studied angiographically, the internal cerebral vein as seen in the lateral venous phase was flattened and depressed in its posterior two thirds with elevation of its anterior third describing a curve concave downward (humping) around the cyst. Sackett, Messina, and Petito[11] have reported a case of colloid cyst causing acute angulation of the basilar artery.

DIFFERENTIAL DIAGNOSIS

Other tumors in childhood occurring at this location include craniopharyngioma and subependymal gliomas, either as a single lesion or as the first lesion of the tuberous sclerosis complex. Craniopharyngioma nearly always will show calcification on the plain films with or without primary changes in the sella turcica. The child with craniopharyngioma or pituitary adenoma will usually have neuroendocrine symptoms or signs on clinical or laboratory data. We have encountered subependymal glioma of the fibrillary astrocytic variety obstructing the foramen of Monro. Ependymoma of the anterior third ventricle is also a consideration. All such lesions, specifically located at the foramen of Monro and not involving the intrinsic walls of the third ventricle, warrant exploration.

SURGICAL MANAGEMENT OF COLLOID CYST, COMPLICATIONS, PATHOLOGY, RESULTS

The treatment of colloid cyst of the third ventricle is in each instance surgical. In reviewing cases of children, it seems that prior shunting would be useful in the infants presenting with colloid cyst and that this shunting procedure should involve ventricular catheters in each of the lateral ventricles with a low-pressure valve and drainage into the peritoneal cavity. Subsequent to shunting the child should have a CTT scan performed and definitive surgery planned when the cortical mantle has reached a width of 3 to 4 cm.

Ventricular drainage of one lateral ventricle as a temporizing procedure in order to delay surgery has led to catastrophe with brain shifts and further brain-stem compression. It is best, therefore, with the presumptive diagnosis of colloid cyst on CTT scanning to confirm this with angiography and avoid air study.

Historically the approach developed by Dandy[5] between 1922 and 1932 through the right frontal lobe and the anterior horn of the right lateral ventricle has proved to be simple and satisfactory. The alternative is that of midline approach through the anterior copus callosum first suggested and performed by Greenwood,[7] and subsequently by Shucart and Stein.[12] In most instances the cyst presenting in the foramen of Monro can be opened and its contents aspirated, permitting delivery of the cyst wall and bipolar coagulation of the cyst wall attachment to the roof of the third ventricle and vellum interpositum. If the foramen of Monro has to be enlarged, it should be done in the anterior direction with separation or manipulation of the columns of the fornix rather than posteriorly since the posterior limit of the foramen is defined by the confluence of veins which form the internal cerebral vein. A colloid cyst generally has a greenish-gray appearance and will be seen within the foramen of Monro. With minimal coagulation of the dorsal surface of the cyst, a small window can be made within the cyst and the contents of the cyst aspirated. To avoid bleeding from veins in the roof of the third ventricle, the anterior and lateral portions of the cyst should be delivered first after aspiration of its contents.

Review of the 13 cases in the pediatric population (Table 30-1) in the literature reveals that one infant died without definitive cyst surgery after a prior Torkildsen shunt,[6] and a second death was that of a 4-year-old operated upon in coma. The children arriving at surgery in poor condition had a stormy postoperative course but eventually recovered. Neurologic deficit or mental abnormality precluding normal schooling and occupation in later life does not seem to be a major problem in children with colloid cyst. The major complication with the transventricular approach has been the development of seizures. It is estimated that perhaps as many as 20 percent of patients operated upon for colloid cysts will have an early or late seizure. We have adopted the policy of one-year prophylaxis anticonvulsants in all patients having transcortical approach to the ventricle, with seizures occurring in less than 10 percent. This is a major reason to adopt the transcallosal approach.

Although there is nearly universal acceptance of the idea that colloid cysts are congenital lesions, they ordinarily do not present until early adult life. The size of the foramen of Monro approaches 1 cm in diameter and colloid cysts do not become symptomatic until they become large enough to obstruct a lumen of this size. Two types of cells, a ligher ciliated cell and a denser, nonciliated cell, form the single-layered epithelial lining. The surface of the nonciliated cell is coated with an electron-dense material. The fine structure of the cyst epithelium has suggested that cysts were derived from a nonneural epithelial structure.[4,8,9] In the opinion of Hirano and Ghatak,[8] the structure of the cyst epithelium differs from that of the ependyma in at least two very important ways. The secretory-like cells of the epithelium are covered by an electron-dense surface coat. Such deposits are not found associated with ependyma or any neuroepithelium at any stage of development. Second, the cyst epithelium is provided with prominent basement lamina that is not found in ependyma that directly abuts on brain parenchyma. The third possible source of colloid cysts is the paraphysis as suggested by Ariens Kappers.[1]

Results of treatment of colloid cysts are rewarding. Although they are rare tumors, they are benign in histology and benign in location, and if diagnosed before coma or other irreversible neurologic deficit occurs, produce long-term useful survival. The major long-term residua are seizures in a few patients, related to cortical excision for approach to the tumor. Recognition of the presence of such tumors at the extremes of childhood, that is, in infancy and young adult life, plus the newer modes of early diagnosis, namely, CTT scanning, should permit earlier diagnosis and a wider experience in the treatment of colloid cysts by pediatric neurosurgeons.

REFERENCES

1. Ariens Kappers J: The development of the paraphysis cerebri in man with comments on its relationship to the intercolumnar tubercle and its significance for the origin of cystic tumors in the third ventricle. J Comp Neurol 102:425–509, 1955
2. Batnitzky S, et al: Colloid cyst of the third ventricle. Radiology 112:327–341, 1974
3. Bull JWD, Sutton D: The diagnosis of paraphyial cysts. Brain 72:487–516, 1949
4. Coxe WS, Luse SA: Colloid cyst of the third ventricle. An electroc microscopic study. J Neuropathol Exp Neurol 23:431–445, 1964
5. Dandy WA: Benign Tumors in the Third Ventricle of the Brain: Diagnosis and Treatment. Springfield, Charles C Thomas, 1933
6. Gemperlein J: Paraphysical cysts of the third ventricle. Report of cases in infants. J Neuropathol Exp Neurol 19:133–134, 1960
7. Greenwood J Jr: Paraphysical cysts of the third ventricle with report of 8 cases. J Neurosurg 6:153–159, 1949
8. Hirano A, Ghatak NB: The fine structure of colloid cysts of the third ventricle. J Neuropathol Exp Neurol 33:333–341, 1974
9. Landhold-Weber UM: Ultrastructur einer kolloidcysts des driten ventrikels. Acta Neuropathol 26:59–70, 1973
10. Riddoch G: Progressive dementia, without headache or changes in the optic discs, from tumors of the third ventricle. Brain 59:225–233, 1936
11. Sacket JF, Messina AJ, Petito CK: Computed tomography and magnification vertebral angiography in the diagnosis of colloid cysts of the third ventricle. Radiology 116:95–100, 1975
12. Shucart WA, Stein BM: Transcallosal approach to the anterior ventricular system. Neurosurgery 3:339–343, 1978

40. Pineal Region Tumors

Bennett M. Stein

Neoplasms arising in the pineal region are rare, except where the statistics are somewhat skewed in those institutions that have demonstrated a special interest in these tumors. In most active neurosurgical practices, these tumors comprise approximately 1 percent of all brain tumors.[1,2] In Japan, for unexplained reasons, there is a much higher incidence of pineal tumors, especially those of the germinoma variety.[3,4] Ueki and Tanaka[5] report an incidence of 4.2 percent of all intracranial tumors in that country. Some clinics in Japan, however, have an incidence of pineal region tumors as high as 10 percent. Similarly they report the germinoma-type pineal tumor as being more common in males with a ratio of 20:1 to females. Pineal region tumors are not exclusive to childhood.[6] In our experience of 26 tumors, 15 patients were 16 years old or under. In other series the peak incidence is about 12 to 15 years, with the pineal germinoma occurring in the older child or adult and teratomas occurring in younger children.[5,6]

The pineal problem has stirred the interest of many medical disciplines for decades. Although the occurrence of such tumors is rare, their endocrinologic implications and a continuing dilemma regarding the best form of therapy have created an extensive literature on the subject. Early endocrinologic interest was centered around the association of pubertas praecox and diabetes insipidus with pineal tumors.[7,8] It was assumed that either the pineal gland or tumors derived from it had a stimulatory effect on gonadal development, however, experimental data were inconclusive. Kitay[9] hypothesized a direct relationship between the type of tumor and the presence of precocious puberty. He found that those tumors that destroyed the pineal gland were most frequently associated with this syndrome and suggested that the normal gland was inhibitory to sexual maturation. Recently because of more sophisticated endocrinologic assays a renewed interest in pineal physiology in the human, and especially in neoplasms of this region, has developed.[2,7,10–12] The general theory of pineal function now dictates that pinealocytes synthesize and release melatonin in response to norepinephrine released from postganglionic sympathetic nerves with an inverse response to light. In addition there is evidence that melatonin has antigonadal properties, and hence the term *Keuschleitsdrüse,* or "chastity gland."

Early surgical endeavors to remove or decompress pineal region tumors resulted in disasters, with high morbidity and mortality.[1,13–15] Subsequently a strong plea for a more conservative approach consisting of procedures to relieve hydrocephalus followed by radiotherapy was made and substantiated with clinical cases.[15–18] The pendulum has swung again, however, and with the use of the operating microscope and improved surgical techniques, a number of recent reports have proposed that all tumors of this region be operated on directly.[19–22] While surgeons[1,2,19,22–25] espousing this more radical management debate the efficacy of their surgical approaches, others advocate a preoperative trial of radiotherapy or stereotaxic biopsy of the region.[16–18,26]

A factor that has tantalized surgeons is the deep location of these tumors. From appropriate surgical entries into the cranium, the pineal tumor is situated equidistant. These tumors are usually overlaid by the important deep venous system consisting of the internal cerebral veins and vein of Galen. It has been suggested that injury or destruction of this venous plexus results in diencephalic and midbrain edema and coma. In addition ventral to the tumor is situated the important quadrigeminal or tectal region of the midbrain. The control of eye movements and pathways activating consciousness are intrinsic to this region. Although, as a group, tumors of this region are not highly vascular, their deep location and adherence to surrounding structures make their removal treacherous.

Terminology of pineal tumors is confusing and complicated by a plethora of terms. Some authors refer to many tumors in this region as pinealomas.[27] The common tumor that comes to mind is a rapidly growing malignant invasive lesion that has a tendency to seed throughout the central nervous system. This tumor has a characteristic appearance, being composed of small lymphocyte-like cells and larger cells with clear cytoplasm and dense nuclei. This tumor has been identified under the broad term of "pinealoma,"[27] but more specifically as an atypical teratoma,[28] and more recently as a germinoma because of its similarity to the seminoma of the testes and the dysgerminoma of the ovaries.[2] It appears that this last term will become the common parlance. Besides this tumor and other malignant tumors arising from glial cells, however, there is a 25 percent incidence of tumors comprising a heterogeneous benign histologic group.[1,19,20,29,30] These tumors are generally radioresistant and have features of encapsulation that permit surgical resection. Teratomas, dermoids, epidermoids, cysts, meningiomas, and pinealcytomas make up this group.

With improved surgical techniques that permit the safe exposure of this region and the removal of certain benign tumors, it has become imperative that operation be carried out and a histologic diagnosis obtained.[1,19,21,25] Futhermore, chemotherapeutic techniques are being developed that offer additional hope in dealing with malignant germinomas of this region.[31]

CLINICAL PRESENTATION

Tumors of this region produce symptomatology by two basic mechanisms: (1) the indirect effects of hydrocephalus created by occlusion or compromise of the aqueduct of Sylvius, and (2) the direct effect of the tumor on the cerebellar outflow pathways and the tectum of the midbrain. In the former instance, the presentation is usually with signs of raised intracranial pressure, including papilledema, headaches, and vomiting. The routine workup, including plain skull x-rays, shows the characteristic features of unlocalized raised intracranial pressure. In this instance the classic Parinaud's syndrome may be seen. Components of this syndrome are often fragmentary and the fully developed syndrome

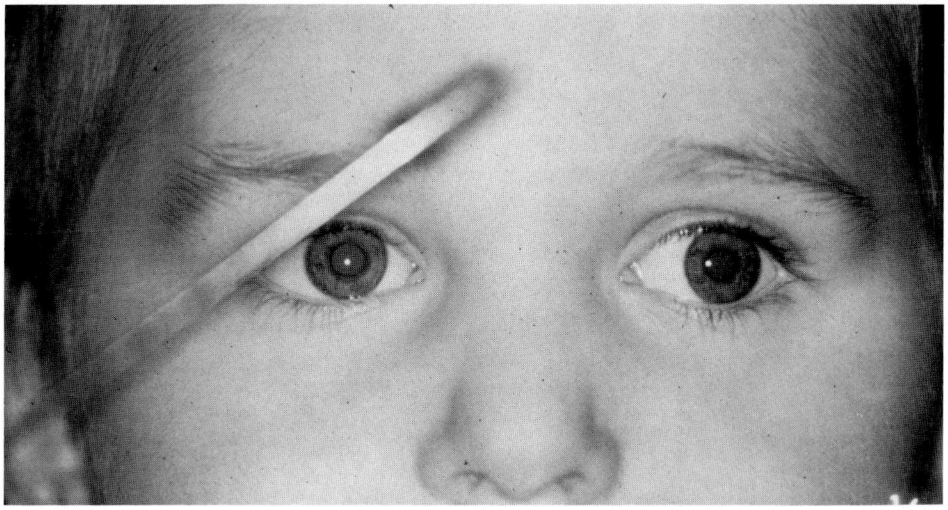

Figure 40-1. Photograph of a patient with a large pineal tumor showing failure of attempted upward gaze.

as described by Parinaud is uncommon (Fig. 40-1). The examiner thus may witness all or some of the components: failure of upward gaze, convergence, the near pupillary reflex, and pupils that react sluggishly to light and are irregular. In cases with extensive involvement, downward gaze may also be affected. Ataxia is a common component of the clinical syndrome and may be due to involvement of the anterior lobe of the cerebellum or to the main outflow pathway through the superior cerebellar peduncle via the midbrain. The disturbances in endocrine function previously mentioned may be due to direct or indirect involvement of the hypothalamus and/or the pineal gland. It should be noted that both diabetes insipidus and precocious puberty have been described in hydrocephalus alone, without the presence of a pineal tumor.

DIAGNOSIS

Plain skull x-rays, in addition to showing the generalized signs of raised intracranial pressure, may give a clue to the diagnosis through the presence of calcification in the pineal region. An area of calcification greater than 5 mm in diameter or dense calcification occurring before the age of 10 is considered abnormal.

Until recently the definitive diagnosis of these tumors rested with contrast ventriculography, either with air or with positive contrast. This technique discloses the involvement of the posterior third ventricle and the displacement or obliteration of the aqueduct of Sylvius. By decompressing the ventricular system and placing air through the lumbar route, an appraisal of the cisterns in the quadrigeminal region may be accomplished if the tumor has not already obliterated them.

Angiography has limited value in definitive diagnosis of these tumors or in demonstrating their exact size and location unless they are extremely vascular. In a young child with hydrocephalus and a mass lesion in this region, with or without intracranial bruit, a vein of Galen aneurysm must be considered in the differential diagnosis and therefore angiography in this instance would be mandatory. Since most of the tumors are not highly vascular, however, the angiographic findings are primarily those of displacement of the deep venous system and posterior choroidal arteries.

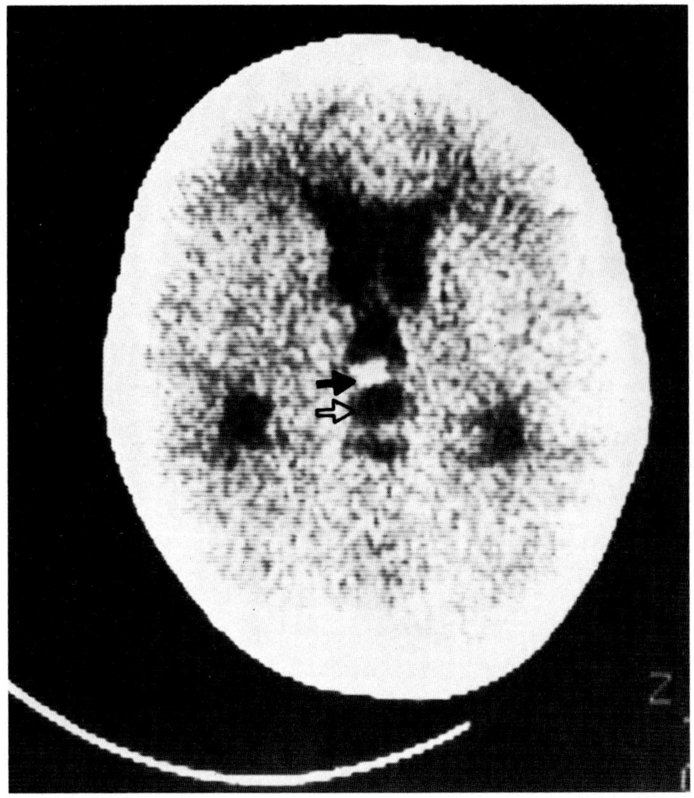

Figure 40-2. Contrast-enhanced CT scan of a pineal tumor subsequently identified as a teratoma. This tumor was both solid (closed arrow) and cystic (open arrow).

With the advent of computerized tomography (CT) scanning, a more accurate diagnosis of the tumor location and extent may be obtained (Fig. 40-2). Of paramount consideration, however, is the ability to make a consistently accurate histologic diagnosis on the basis of the preoperative radiographic studies. Ueki and Tanaka[5] reported a high degree of accuracy in the CT diagnosis of germinomas. They find that these lesions deform the posterior third ventricle and adjacent cisterns on the non-contrast-enhanced scan and on the enhanced scan are homogenous, fairly well-defined masses that moderately enhance. In one of their cases, there appeared to be a small cyst. It has been pointed out by Camins and Schlesinger[16] that CT scanning is valuable in determining the presence of a dermoid tumor with characteristic low-density values, often in the minus range, and that other fluid-filled cysts will have small positive tissue absorption coefficients. The presence of calcification on the CT scan that may not have been recognized on the plain skull x-rays is not of significance since many of these tumors have contained a degree of calcification that may not be picked up on the CT scan alone. In our experience we have not been able to make accurate histologic diagnoses on the basis of combined ventriculographic studies, arteriograms, and CT scans with and without contrast. We have observed large cysts occurring in the germinoma type of tumor, which presumably would lead to the diagnosis of cystic astrocytoma or some cystic type of tumor other than germinoma, which do not commonly have gross cysts (Fig. 40-3). In other instances we have mistaken benign posterior third ventricular meningiomas for malignant tumors because of their high vascularity and contrast enhancing on CT scan as well as discrete borders,[32] fitting all of the criteria reported by Ueki and Tanaka[5] for the germinoma. We thus feel that given the current state of technology, it is impossible consistently to make an accurate histologic diagnosis without biopsy.

The role of cerebrospinal fluid (CSF) cytologic evaluation remains obscure.

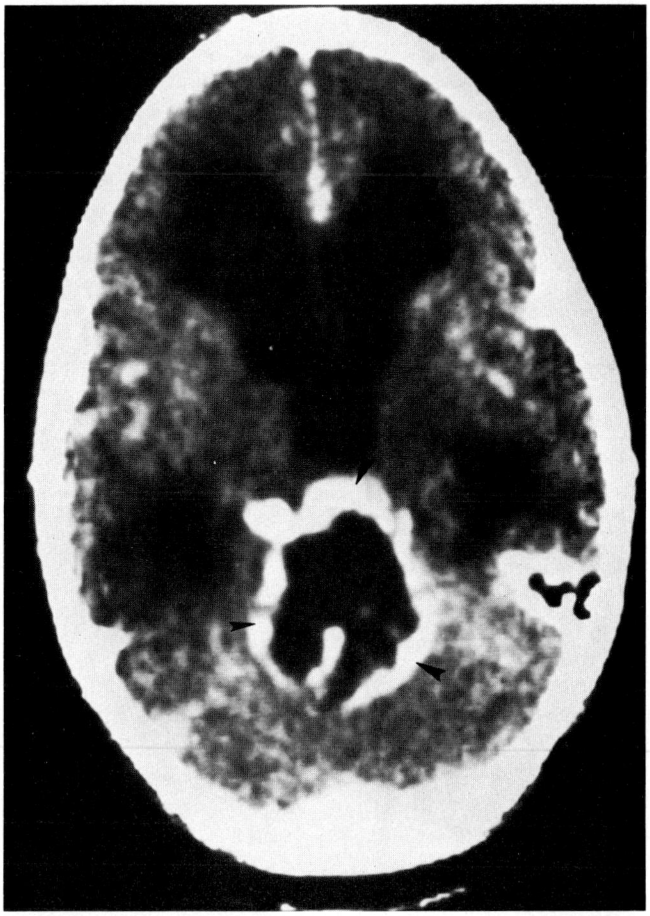

Figure 40-3. CT scan of a patient who had a large cystic pinealoblastoma. The contrast-enhancing portion of the tumor is outlined by arrows.

Ueki and Tanaka[5] report a high incidence of epithelioid-like cells in the lumbar CSF of patients with germinomas. But, even with this high retrieval, they have not correlated the presence of these cells with current or subsequent seeding of the tumor. They do rely upon the presence of these cells, however, to make the histologic diagnosis of germinomas of the pineal with credible accuracy. Sano[6] reported 60 percent accuracy in diagnosing "pinealomas" by CSF cytologic culture.

Abnormally high serum levels of human chorionic gonadotropin have been observed in patients with germinomas and terablastomas of the pineal,[5,31] while Wurtman and Kammer[11] report melatonin synthesis by pineal germinomas. If these evaluations prove to be consistently accurate, biologic tagging may be the only way to make a histologic diagnosis short of biopsy.

TREATMENT

Given the fact that the current mortality rate for exposure of tumors in this region is under 5 percent,[33] and the fact that approximately 25 percent of neoplasms in this region are radioresistant and potentially resectable, the two basic therapeutic regimes offered in the treatment of these tumors must be reexamined.

The first treatment program, a conservative approach,[15,16,18] was an alternative to heretofore prohibitive surgical mortalities (well over 40 percent). In the time of Cushing[13] and Dandy,[14] most patients undergoing pineal tumor surgery were postoperative mortalities. Conservative management consists of an extracranial shunting procedure followed by radiotherapy.

Unfortunately, as this therapy became the norm, there was little control over histology diagnosis, and therefore many of the results could not be correlated with specific tumor types. Recently Camins and Schlesinger[16] reviewed a large series of cases consisting of posterior third ventricular and pineal tumors, with histologic verification in many. They have shown long-term survival in the germinoma type of tumor treated by radiotherapy and shunting.

As an alternative to direct approach to the tumor, stereotaxic biopsy has been utilized in a limited number of cases.[34] Experimental technology to combine this technique with CT scan control carries potential for the future.

The second treatment program is based on an initial exposure of the tumor, with histologic identification of all tumors, and removal of benign encapsulated tumors. Support for this program is a marked reduction in surgical mortality and the need to tailor therapy to a specific tumor type.[19,31,33]

Malignant tumors can now be treated specifically by multidisciplinary approaches using not only radiotherapy but chemotherapy in some instances.[31,35–37] Although controversy still exists, there is strong support for the management of the germinoma-type tumor by local radiation plus entire neural radiation combined with chemotherapy. Embarking on such a program of therapy cannot be done without histologic verification of the tumor type.

On the basis of our experience with 26 patients who have had pineal region tumors, we feel that an aggressive surgical approach to this problem is the logical

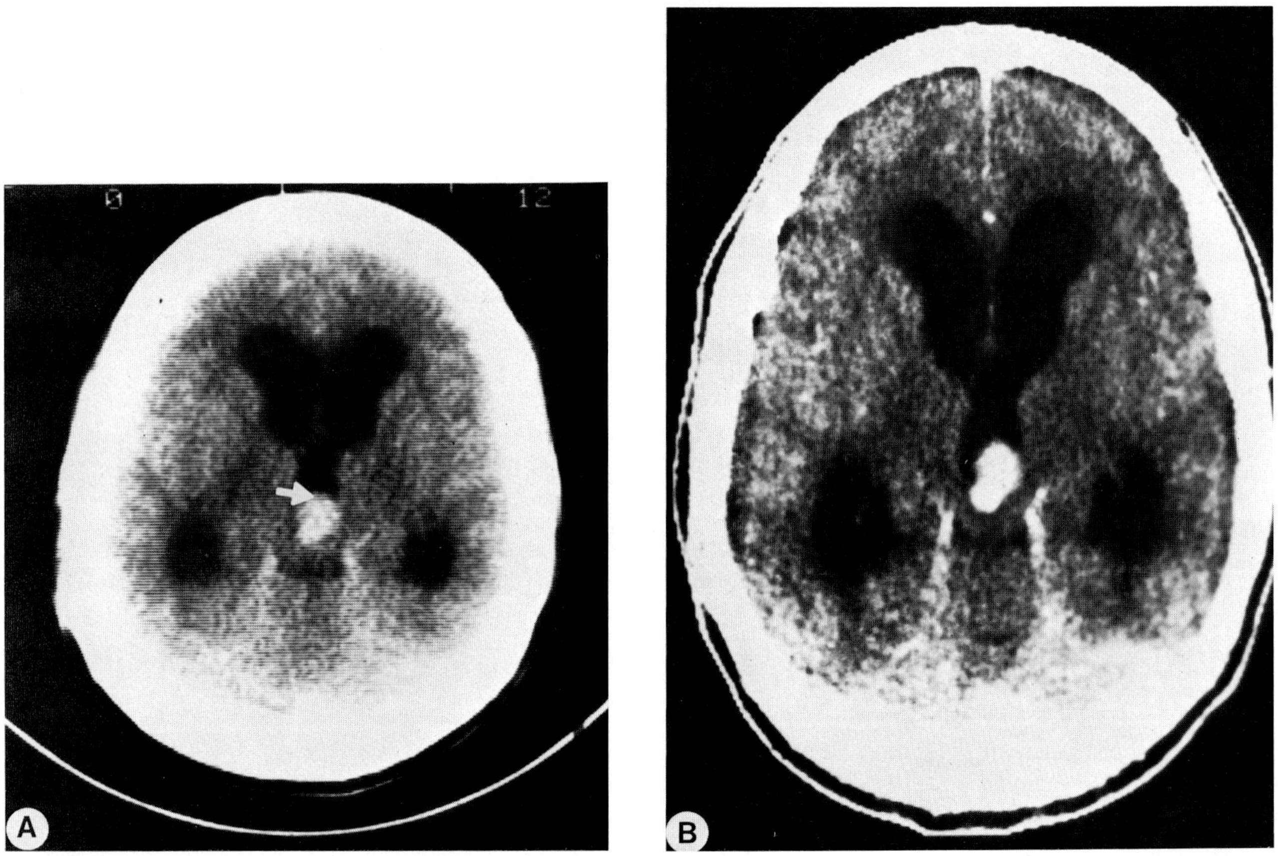

Figure 40-4. A. CT scan of a patient with a solid pineal cytoma indenting the posterior portion of third ventricle (arrow). B. CT scan on the same patient seven months later and two months following a radiation dose of 5500 rads to the tumor. There is no apparent change in this contrast-enhancing tumor.

conclusion to a review of current factual information. Unfortunately a number of our tumors have received prior radiotherapy. A CT follow-up in many instances has shown no change in tumor size or continued growth in spite of radiation therapy, and therefore surgical exploration has been requested (Fig. 40-4). It would seem that the radiation therapy makes the primary approach to these tumors more difficult because of its effect on the normal brain and the creation of vascular and cicatrix changes.

In those cases that have not been previously treated, it has been our policy to relieve the hydrocephalus by a CSF diversionary procedure prior to the direct exposure of the tumor.

Operation on the pineal region has been carried out by a multitude of surgical exposures (Fig. 40-5).[1,2,14,22,25,33,38–41] The basic ones are supra- or infratentorial. In the former group, Dandy's[14] operation was interhemispheric with section of the posterior corpus callosum. Poppen[40] modified this to approach the tumor under the occipital lobe and in many instances sectioned the anterior portion of the tentorium. We have preferred the posterior fossa or infratentorial approach to these tumors since it allows the surgeon to approach the tumor under the important deep venous system, is the same distance from the cranial entry, and permits a wide exposure of the pineal region.[33] The anterior aspect of the third ventricle is well visualized, enabling the removal of tumors that have extended anteriorly into the third ventricle (Fig. 40-6).

An operating microscope is used and the patient is placed in a sitting position with the head well flexed so that the tentorium is relatively horizontal. A long midline incision is made and a craniectomy performed to include the occipital bone over the torcula and lateral sinuses. It is not necessary to extend the craniectomy to the region of the foramen magnum. If the patient has had a CSF diversionary procedure, the cerebellum is usually slack; however, in some

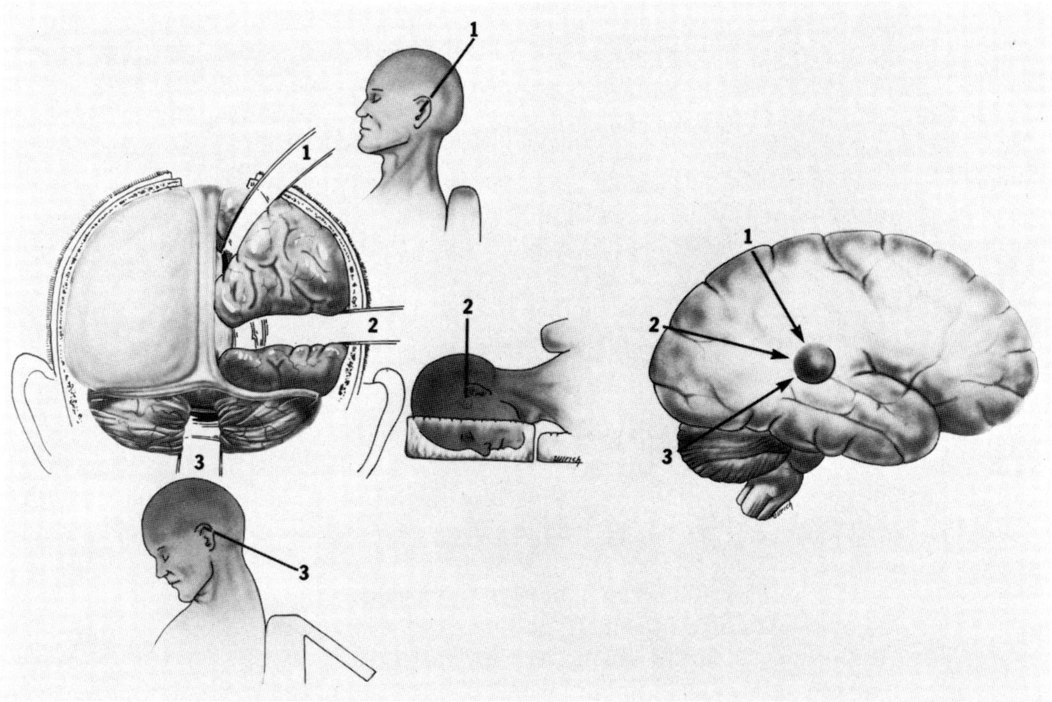

Figure 40-5. Drawing of the basic operative exposures for pineal region tumors: (1) Dandy approach, (2) the occipital approach of Poppen and Horrax, and (3) the suboccipital approach of Krause and Stein. (Reprinted with permission from Stein B: Supracerebellar infratentional approach to pineal tumors. Surg Neurol 11:331–337, 1979.)

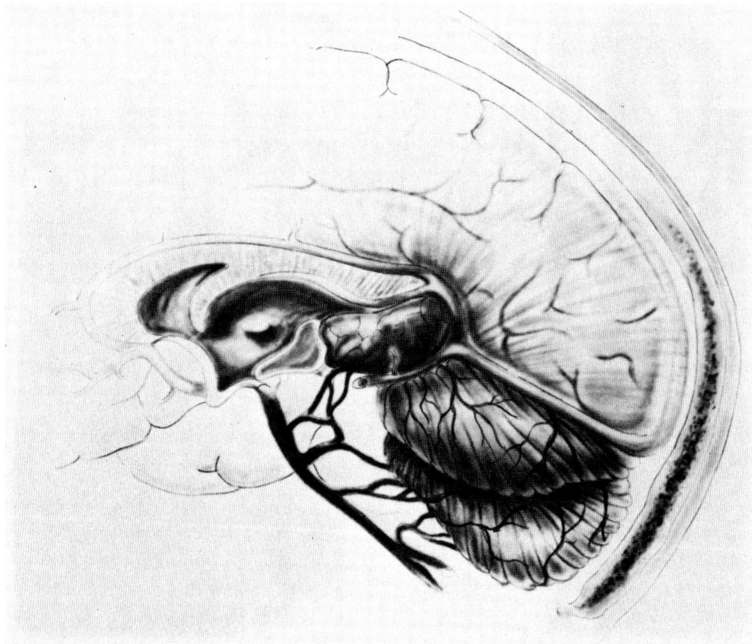

Figure 40-6. Drawing showing the situation of the usual pineal tumor ventral to the deep venous system, which is approached through the posterior fossa.

instances the addition of a dehydrating agent may be beneficial. All veins over the superior surface of the cerebellum and the precentral cerebellar vein are cauterized and divided to gain maximum exposure. Tumors in the pineal region create arachnoidal thickening in the quadrigeminal region, which must be opened by a sharp dissection to reach the capsule or surface of the tumor. At this point a biopsy is taken. If the tumor is of a malignant variety, little more than a modest decompression may be carried out; in some instances an opening through the center of the tumor into the posterior third ventricle is created to provide space for the positioning of a ventricular catheter, which may then be brought distally into the cisterna magna.[19] In the presence of benign and encapsulated tumors, the entire tumor may be removed successfully. Even in some cases of germinoma, the majority of the tumor is encapsulated, and can be removed, and in rare instances large cysts within the tumor may be evacuated. No attempt is made to remove infiltrating tumors from the midbrain or walls of the third ventricle. Care must be taken to preserve the deep venous system and in no instance of benign tumor have we found the tumor to encircle these veins, but rather to attach to their undersurface where the tumor can be resected.

RESULTS OF TREATMENT

We have had under a 5 percent operative mortality and no significant morbidity utilizing this technique. The types of tumors and their outcome are summarized in Table 40-1.

Long-term follow-up indicates a moderate degree of success following radiation of the germinoma-type tumor. In some cases,[1,5,16,17,26,35–37] which have been confirmed histologically, survivals exceeding 10 and 20 years have been reported following radiation therapy alone, and Sano[6] reports a 50 percent five-year survival. Our experience, however, had been less optimistic, with frequent recurrence of these tumors, especially in the form of seeding. Apparently this experience is shared by others, since additional therapy for these tumors has been proposed. This includes radiation of the entire central nervous system and insitution of chemotherapy comprising bleomycin, vinblastine, and

Table 40-1
Pineal Tumors

No.	Age (Yrs)	Diagnosis	Follow-up
1	8	Teratoma	Normal
2	24	Cystic astrocytoma	D.D.*
3	⅔	Arachnoid cyst	Normal
4	12	Epidermoid	Normal
5	9	Teratoma	Unchanged
6	4	Teratoma	Improved
7	5	Germinoma	D.D.
8	25	Astrocytoma	D.D.
9	10	Astrocytoma	Unchanged
10	8	Glioblastoma	O.D.‡
11	12	Germinoma	D.D.
12	37	Germinoma	D.D.
13	35	Astrocytoma	D.D.
14	16	Germinoma	Improved
15†	43	Germinoma	Improved
16	18	Germinoma	Improved
17	22	Colloid cyst	Unchanged
18	15	Germinoma	D.D.
19	15	Pinealcytoma	Improved
20	28	Meningioma	Improved
21	29	Meningioma	Improved
22†	44	Germinoma	Deteriorating
23	5	Teratoma	Normal
24	16	Gernimona	Deteriorating
25	28	Pinealcytoma	Improved
26	11	Pinealblastoma	Improved
27	32	Astrocytoma	Improved
28	19	Germinoma	Deteriorating
29	12	Cystic astrocytoma	Unchanged
30	17	Germinoma	Unchanged
31	16	Astrocytoma	Deteriorating
32	33	Germinoma	Unchanged
33	¾	Astrocytoma	D.D.
34	12	Cystic astrocytoma	Improved
35	38	Pinealcytoma	Improved
36	7	Pinealblastoma	Unchanged
37	49	Astrocytoma	O.D.

*D.D. = Dead from disease.
†Case #15 and 22 the same.
‡O.D. = Operative death.

cis-platinum currently being utilized in the treatment of seminomas.[31] Encouraging reports of the effect of such combined therapy on tumors that have already spread have been reported. In our estimation the most fortunate course of events has been the institution of unnecessary radiation to tumors recognized to be benign, radioresistant, and possibly resectable by surgery. There is therefore a strong case to be made for histologic verification of virtually all pineal tumors. It should be emphasized that we are not comparing pineal region tumors with those of the third ventricle, either anterior or mid, most of which arise from the thalamus and are glial in origin. These tumors have been included with reports of pineal tumors and are of a more homogeneous nature, follow different growth patterns, and thereby may respond to treatment in an entirely different fashion. Similarly their surgical exposure carries a higher risk and is generally performed through other routes.

REFERENCES

1. Obrador S, Soto M, Gutierrez-Diaz JA: Surgical management of tumours of the pineal region. Acta Neurochir 34:159–171, 1976
2. Schmidek HH: Pineal Tumors. New York, Masson, 1977
3. Araki C, Matsumoto S: Surgical reevaluation of pinealoma and related tumors in Japan. J Neurosurg 30:146–149, 1969
4. Katsura S, Suzuki J, Wada T: A statistical study of brain tumors in the neurosurgical clinics in Japan. J Neurosurg 16:570–580, 1959
5. Ueki K, Tanaka R: Study on treatment and prognosis of pineal neoplasms. Seara Med Neurocir 8:279–315, 1978
6. Sano K: Pinealoma in children. Child's Brain 2:67–72, 1976
7. Kappers JA: The mammalian pineal gland, a survey. Acta Neurochir 34:109–149, 1976
8. Krabbe KH: The pineal gland, especially in relation to the problem of its supposed significance in sexual development. Endocrinology 7:379–414, 1923
9. Kitay JI: Pineal lesions and precocious puberty: A review. J Clin Endocrinol Meta 14:622–625, 1954
10. Nir I, Reiter RJ, Wurtman RJ: The pineal gland, in Proceedings of the International Symposium, Jerusalem, November 14–17, 1977. Vienna-New York, Springer-Verlag, 1978
11. Wurtman RJ, Kammer H: Melatonin synthesis by an ectopic pinealoma. N Engl J Med 274:1233–1237, 1966
12. Wurtman RJ, Moskowitz MA: The pineal organ. N Engl J Med 296:1329–1333, 1383–1386, 1977
13. Cushing H: Intracranial Tumors: Notes Upon a Series of Two Thousand Verified Cases with Surgical Mortality Pertaining Thereto. Springfield, Charles C Thomas, 1933
14. Dandy WE: Operative experience in cases of pineal tumor. Arch Surg (Chicago) 33:19–46, 1936
15. Horrax G, Daniels JT: The conservative treatment of pineal tumors. Surg Clin N Am 22:649–659, 1942
16. Camins MB, Schlesinger EB: Treatment of tumours of the posterior part of the third ventricle and the pineal region: A long term follow-up. Acta Neurochir 40:131–143, 1978
17. Cummins FM, Taveras JM, Schlesinger EB: Treatment of gliomas of the third ventricle and pinealomas With special reference to the value of radiotherapy. Neurology (Minneapolis) 10:1031–1036, 1960
18. Poppen JL, Marino R Jr: Pinealomas and tumors of the posterior portion of the third ventricle. J Neurosurg 28:357–364, 1968
19. Page, LK: The infratentorial supracerebellar exposure of tumors in the pineal area. Neurosurgery 1:36–40, 1977
20. Stein BM: The infratentorital supracerebellar approach to pineal lesions. J Neurosurg 35:197–202, 1971
21. Stein BM: Supracerebellar approach for pineal region neoplasms, in Current Techniques in Operative Neurosurgery. Schmidek HH, Sweet WH (eds): New York, Grune & Stratton, 1977
22. Suzuki J, Iwabuchi T: Surgical removal of pineal tumors (pinealomas and teratomas). Experience in a series of 19 cases. J Neurosurg 23:565–571, 1965
23. Jamieson KG: Excision of pineal tumors. J Neurosurg 35:550–553, 1971
24. Lazar ML, Clark K: Direct surgical management of masses in the region of the vein of Galen. Surg Neurol 2:17–21, 1974
25. Reid WS, Clark K: Comparison of the infratentorial and transtentorial approaches to the pineal region. Neurosurgery 3:1–8, 1978
26. DeGirolami U, Schmidek H: Clinicopathological study of 53 tumors of the pineal region. J Neurosurg 39:455–462, 1973
27. Globus JH: Pinealoma. Arch Pathol 31:533–568, 1941
28. Russell D: The pinealoma: Its relationship to teratoma. J Pathol Bacteriol 56:145–150, 1944

29. Haldeman KO: Tumors of the pineal gland. Arch Neurol Psychiatr (Chicago) 18:724–754, 1927
30. Ringertz N, Nordenstam H, Flyger G: Tumors of the pineal region. J Neuropathol Exp Neurol 13:540–561, 1954
31. Neuwelt EA, Smith G: Presence of lymphocyte membrane markers on small cells on a pineal germinoma. Ann Neurol (in press)
32. Rozario R, Adelman L, Prager RJ, et al: Meningiomas of the pineal region and third ventricle. Neurosurgery (in press)
33. Stein BM: Supracerebellar-infratentorial approach to pineal tumors. Surg Neurol 11:331–337, 1979
34. Backlund E-O, Rahn T, Sarby B: Treatment of pinealomas by stereotaxic radiation surgery. Acta Radiol 13:369–376, 1974
35. Sund DI, Harisiadis L, Chang CH: Midline pineal tumors and suprasellar germinomas: Highly curable by irradiation. Ther Radiol 128:745–751, 1978
36. Wara WM, Fellows CF, Sheline GE, et al: Radiation therapy for pineal tumors and suprasellar germinomas. Ther Radiol 124:221–223, 1977
37. Waga S, Handa H, Yamashita J: Intracranial germinomas: Treatment and results. Surg Neurol 11:167–172, 1979
38. Glasauer FE: An operative approach to pineal tumors. Acta Neurochir (Vienna) 22:177–180, 1970
39. Krause F: Operative frielegung der vierhugen, nebst beobachtungen uber hirndruck und dekompression. Zentbl Chir 53:2812–2819, 1926
40. Poppen JL: The right occipital approach to a pinealoma. J Neurosurg 25:706–710, 1966
41. Van Wagenen WP: A surgical approach for the removal of certain pineal tumors. Report of a case. Surg Gynec Obstet 53:216–220, 1931

41. Suprasellar Germinomas

Harold J. Hoffman

Suprasellar germinomas are a rare group of tumors that occur predominantly in childhood. In Schmidek's[1] review of suprasellar germinomas, 74 percent were under the age of 16. Whereas pineal germinomas tend to occur predominantly in boys, suprasellar germinomas occur more frequently in girls (Table 41-1).

PATHOLOGY

The germinomas are poorly defined infiltrating lesions that have a soft, grayish-pink appearance. They are highly malignant, and not only infiltrate widely at their site of origin, but can also spread by cerebrospinal fluid (CSF) pathways to other parts of the brain and spinal cord. They may also spread systemically by means of CSF bypass shunts (Fig. 41-1).[6] In a review of suprasellar germinomas treated at Columbia University, Chang[7] reported a 32 percent incidence of CSF metastases as compared with a 6 percent incidence with pineal germinomas.

Microscopically these tumors are composed of large polygonal cells, as well as smaller cells that resemble lymphocytes. Mitotic figures are common in the large cells. Occasionally a germinoma may contain areas of differentiation into a typical teratoma.

In the past suprasellar germinomas were termed "ectopic pinealomas" because they had the same histologic appearance as pineal germinomas, which were then called "pinealomas." We now know that a pinealoma is a germ cell tumor that can arise primarily in the suprasellar area or can spread to the suprasellar area from the pineal region. (Fig. 41-2). The pineal and suprasellar germinomas are histologically identical to the seminoma of the testicle and the dysgerminoma of the ovary.

Because of their location in the suprasellar area, germinomas can infiltrate the optic chiasm (Fig. 41-3) and optic nerves, thickening these structures and giving them the appearance of an optic nerve glioma at the time of surgical exploration (Fig. 41-4).[8]

Table 41-1
Sex Incidence of Suprasellar Germinomas

Author	Males	Females	Total
Schmidek[1]	12	11	23
Takeuchi et al.[2]	9	9	18
Jenkin et al.[3]	3	3	6
Izquierdo et al.[4]	10	5	15
Hoffman[5]	0	4	4
Total	34	32	66

CLINICAL FEATURES

By virtue of their location, suprasellar germinomas have a characteristic presentation. In children involvement of the floor of the third ventricle produces diabetes insipidus as a very early sign. Infiltration of the optic nerves and chiasm leads to visual field defects and eventually blindness. Extension into the parasellar area can produce oculomotor palsies, and obstruction of the third ventricle can produce hydrocephalus, with characteristic signs of raised intracranial pressure. The history is usually short and the patient is frequently a young girl.

INVESTIGATION

Plain skull x-rays may show nothing more than signs of raised intracranial pressure. A computerized tomography (CT) scan, however, will typically show a solid, contrast-enhancing suprasellar mass that is difficult to differentiate from a solid craniopharyngioma or an optic nerve glioma (Fig. 41-5). Cerebral angiography will frequently show pathologic vessels within the tumor parenchyma.

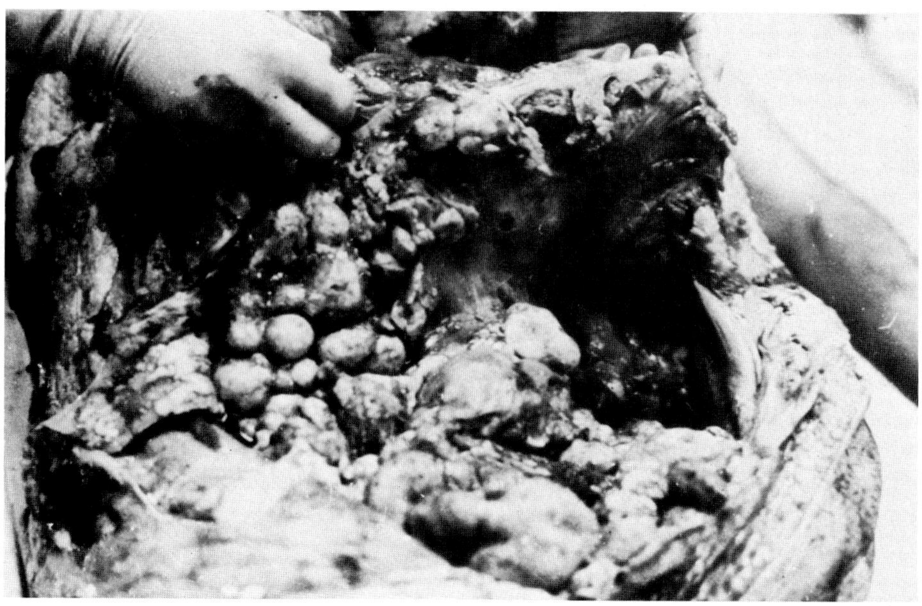

Figure 41-1. Metastatic deposits from germinoma in peritoneal cavity in patient with VP shunt.

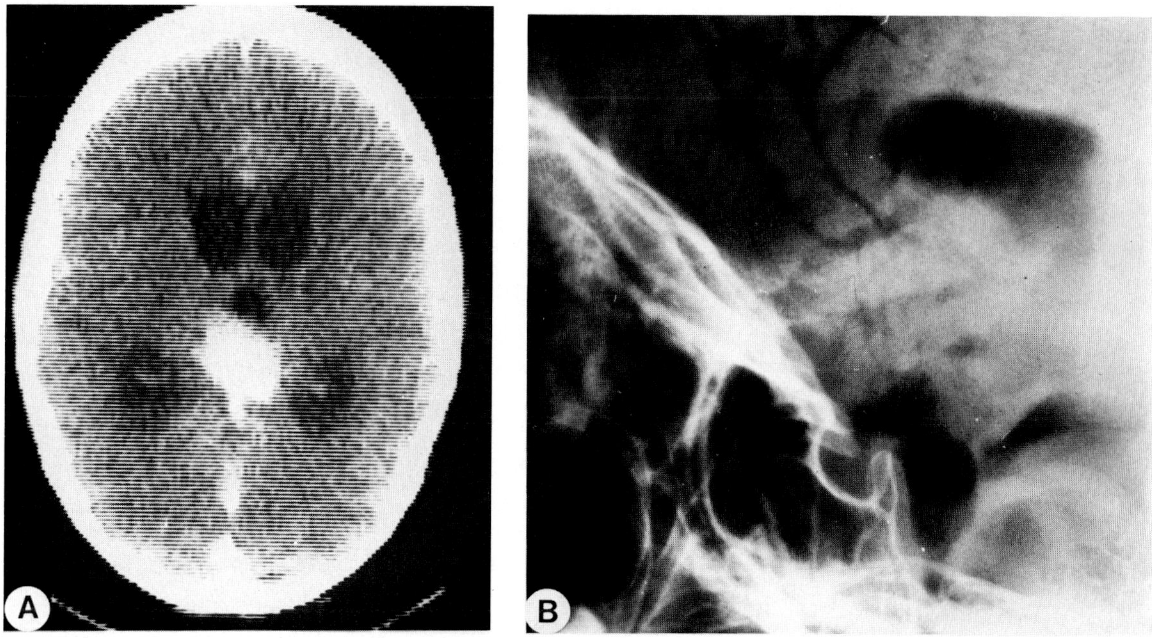

Figure 41-2. A. CT scan (contrast-enhanced) showing pineal germinoma. B. Pneumoencephalogram in same patient showing irregular anterior third ventricle due to spread of germinoma to suprasellar region.

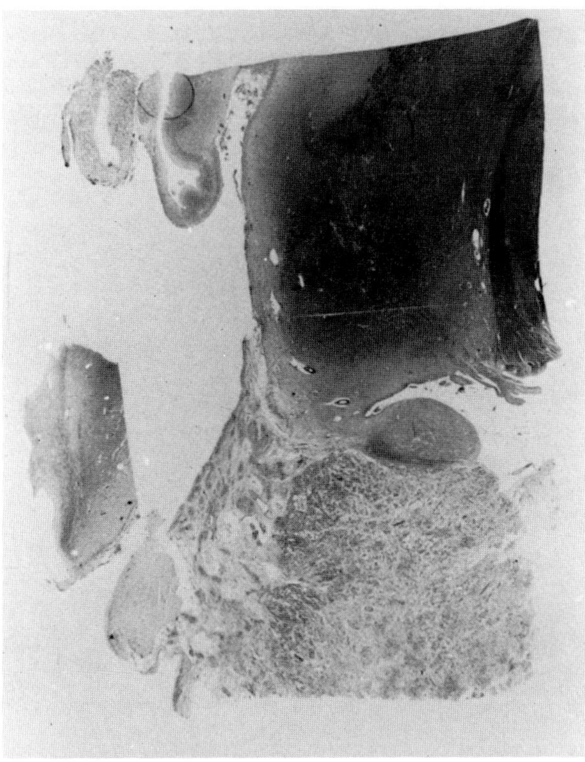

Figure 41-3. Histologic slice through suprasellar germinoma showing infiltration of hypothalamus and optic tract (H&E × 1).

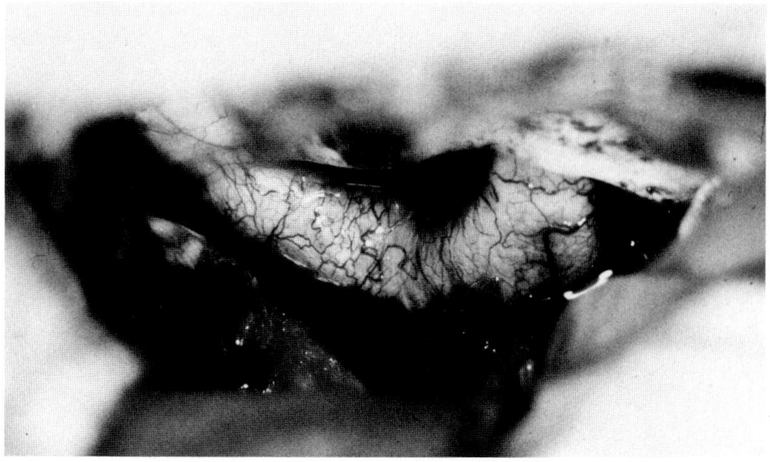

Figure 41-4. Optic chiasm thickened by infiltration with germinoma.

TREATMENT

Because it is difficult preoperatively to distinguish between suprasellar germinomas and craniopharyngiomas or optic nerve gliomas, a subfrontal approach should be used. In 50 percent of the suprasellar germinomas surgically treated in our institution, the optic nerves and chiasm had the thickened appearance of an optic nerve glioma. Once the tumor is exposed, therefore, biopsy must be taken to confirm the diagnosis.

If the tumor is proved to be a suprasellar germinoma, then radiotherapy must be directed to both the primary tumor site and the entire craniospinal axis.

If the tumor has caused obstruction of the third ventricle, then a preopera-

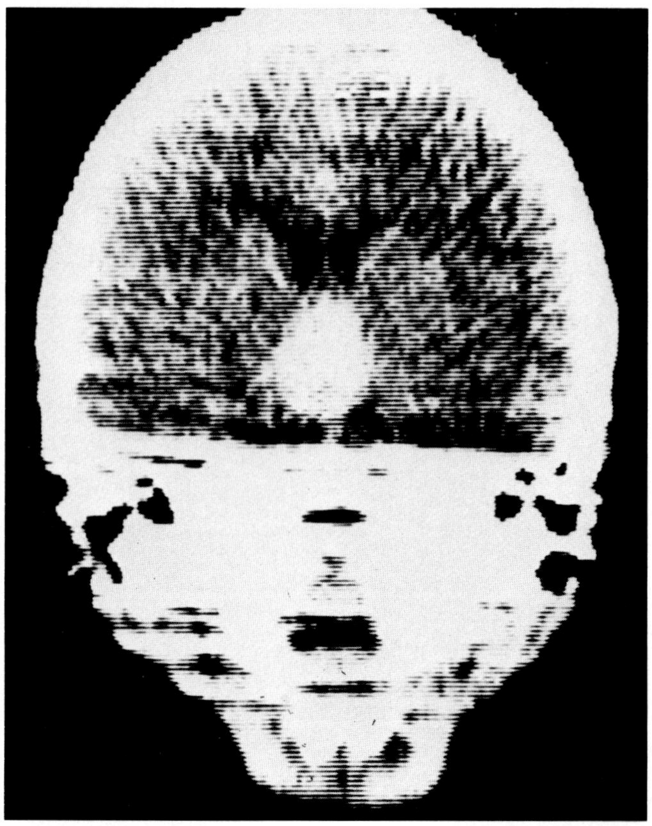

Figure 41-5. CT scan (contrast-enhanced) showing suprasellar germinoma.

tive bypass shunt is useful in improving the patient's clinical status prior to surgical exploration. Because these tumors can spread by CSF bypass shunts, a millipore filter should be incorporated in the shunt to prevent metastases.[9]

PROGNOSIS

Despite the fact that these tumors are histologically identical to pineal germinomas, suprasellar germinomas have a much worse prognosis. The vast majority of pineal germinomas can be cured by radiotherapy; this has not been true in the case of suprasellar germinomas, where the majority of patients eventually die. In our institution five suprasellar germinomas were treated by surgical biopsy and postoperative radiation; only one patient has survived. This low survival rate is reflected in Chang's report[7] of a 20 percent survival rate in suprasellar germinomas as compared with a 60 percent survival rate in pineal germinomas.

CONCLUSIONS

Suprasellar germinomas are a rare but lethal group of tumors that respond poorly to therapy. Although they share common histologic features with pineal germinomas, suprasellar germinomas have a different sex preference and a much less favorable prognosis. This disparity indicates that the histologic features of this tumor do not necessarily coincide with its biologic characteristics.

REFERENCES

1. Schmidek H: Suprasellar germinomas in pineal tumors, in Schmidek, H (ed): USA Masson, 1977, pp 115–126
2. Takeuchi J, Handa H, and Nagata I: Suprasellar germinoma. J Neurosurg 49:41–48, 1978
3. Jenkin RDT, Simpson JK, Keen CW: Pineal and suprasellar germinomas. J Neurosurg 48:99–107, 1978
4. Izquierdo JM, Rougerie J, Lapras C, et al: The so-called ectopic pinealomas. Child's Brain 5:505–512, 1979
5. Hoffman HJ: Supratentorial Tumors in Childhood, in Youmans, J (ed): Neurological Surgery (ed 2). Philadelphia, WB Saunders, 1982 pp 2702–2732
6. Wilson ER, Takei Y, Bikoff WT, et al: Abdominal metastases of primary intracranial yolk sac tumors through ventriculoperitoneal shunts: Report of 3 cases. Neurosurgery 5:356–364, 1979
7. Chang CH: Findings presented at seminar, American Association of Neurological Surgeons, New York, April 22, 1980
8. Cohen DH, Steinberg M, Buchwald R: Suprasellar germinomas. Diagnostic confusion with optic gliomas. Case report. J Neurosurg 41:490–493, 1974
9. Hoffman HJ, Hendrick EB, Humphreys RP: Metastasis via ventriculoperitoneal shunt in patients with medulloblastoma. J Neurosurg 44:562–566, 1976

42. Pituitary Adenomas

Harold J. Hoffman

Pituitary adenomas are an extremely rare tumor of childhood. Ingraham and Matson[1] reported only two pituitary adenomas out of a total of 313 intracranial tumors in children, and Koos and Miller[2] had 10 pituitary adenomas in their series of 700 tumors in children. In a series of 344 supratentorial tumors treated at the Hospital for Sick Children during the years 1950 to 1975, there were four pituitary adenomas.[3]

PATHOPHYSIOLOGY

The anterior pituitary gland is conventionally regarded as being composed of three types of cells: chromophobe (50 percent); acidophil (35 percent); and basophil (15 percent). In recent years this rough classification has been subjected to close scrutiny using immunochemical and electron microscopic examination, resulting in the discovery of at least five cell types that actively produce trophic hormones, as well as two types of endocrine inactive cells.

The anterior pituitary gland secretes the following trophic hormones: prolactin (PRL), somatotropin (human growth hormone, HGH), adrenocorticotrophic hormone (ACTH), melanocyte-stimulating hormone (MSH), thyrotropin (thyroid-stimulating hormone, TSH), follicle-stimulating hormone (FSH), and luteinizing hormone (LH). There are individual cell types that produce PRL, HGH, and TSH; one cell type that produces both ACTH and MSH; and a second cell type that produces FSH and LH. There thus can be PRL, HGH, TSH, ACTH-MSH, and FSH-LH adenomas.

In the past the endocrine inactive chromophobe adenoma was the most common type of pituitary adenoma. Since the more recent discovery of the microadenoma, however, the most common pituitary adenoma has become the HGH adenoma, a tumor that comprises 33 percent of Wilson and Dempsey's series.[4] In this same series, endocrine-inactive adenomas accounted for 28.8

percent, PRL adenomas for 23.6 percent, and ACTH adenomas for 14.4 percent of the cases. The TSH and the FSH-LH secreting adenomas are rare in all series and have not been reported in children.

Cushing[5] initially described the syndrome that bears his name in 1932, and felt it was due to a basophil tumor of the pituitary gland. Although it has been long known that Cushing syndrome is the result of ACTH overproduction, this was felt to be hypothalamic in origin and the treatment for Cushing's disease until recent years was pituitary irradiation or adrenalectomy. In 1958, however, Nelson, Meakin, Dealey, et al.[6] described the development of a pituitary gland tumor in a patient who had undergone previous bilateral adrenalectomy for Cushing's syndrome. This particular patient presented with hyperpigmentation, headaches, visual impairment, and enlarging sella, with the hyperpigmentation attributable to overproduction of MSH. Recently the first case of Nelson's syndrome was described in a child.[7] Now patients with Cushing's syndrome are being explored transsphenoidally even when the sella is perfectly normal, and ACTH adenomas are being found.[8] In one such case in our institution, the syndrome completely reversed with removal of the adenoma.

Large pituitary adenomas expand the sella tursica and can rise above the diaphragm to encroach on brain. The tumors can be dumbbell in shape, with the constriction being due to the diaphragma sellae and the circle of Willis. The main direction of suprasellar expansion is in the midline, with impingement and/or extension into the third ventricle, resulting in hydrocephalus. Adenomas can also push in a lateral direction into the middle fossa, and their intrasellar portion can cause erosion of neighboring bone as far as the cavernous sinus, where the dural capsule of the gland is frequently breeched by the tumor. Secondary changes due to degeneration or spontaneous hemorrhage are often found in the tumor, and as a result it may be largely cystic. Ortiz-Suarez and Erickson[9] demonstrated that pituitary adenomas in children are aggressive and have a high incidence of extrasellar extension.

Pituitary carcinomas are extremely rare. In all cases metastases or direct evidence of blood-borne spread of the tumor must be present, but the tumor can be endocrinologically active or inactive. A pituitary carcinoma with distant metastases has been reported in a 7½-year-old child.[10]

CLINICAL SYMPTOMATOLOGY

Headache is a frequent symptom in a patient with a pituitary tumor. It can be due to raised intracranial pressure, but is more frequently due to traction on pain-sensitive dura of the diaphragma sellae or cavernous sinus. Visual field defects and visual loss may be present in 25 percent of patients with pituitary adenomas.

Endocrinopathy as a result of a functionally active tumor or impairment of pituitary function by an endocrinologically inactive tumor can be present. The endocrinologically active tumors commonly seen in children include the ACTH-producing tumor, which results in Cushing's syndrome, and the rarer HGH-producing tumor, which causes giantism. The PRL-secreting tumors produce galactorrhea and amenorrhea; these have been recognized only in recent years and we have had one such example at our institution. The endocrinologically inactive tumors will give rise to amenorrhea, delayed puberty, and evidence of hypothyroidism.

RADIOLOGIC INVESTIGATION

Routine skull x-rays will show the sella tursica on anteroposterior (AP) and lateral planes. The upper limit of normal for the sella tursica is an AP diameter of 17 mm, a depth of 14 mm, and a width of 10–15 mm (Fig. 42-1). In cases where the sella is perfectly normal, AP and lateral polytomograms will show small areas of erosion and/or asymmetry of the sella tursica, and alterations in the clinoid processes, together with other important changes that may not be seen on routine skull x-rays.

Air encephalography will determine the extent of suprasellar extension and will exclude the possibility of an empty sella syndrome as part of the etiology of the enlarged sella.

Cerebral angiography is valuable in establishing the extent of suprasellar extension. This test will also exclude the possibility of intracranial aneurysm with

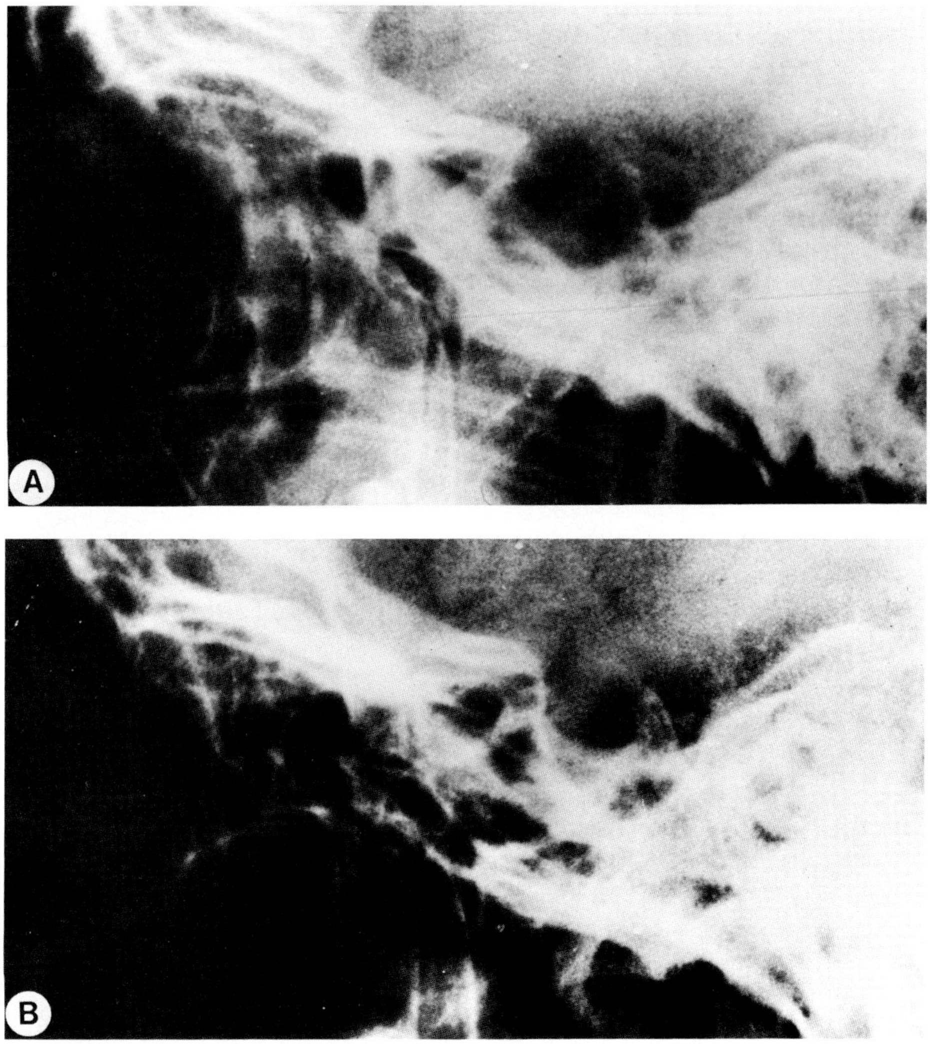

Figure 42-1. A. View of enlarged sella with thinned-out dorsum in child with pituitary adenoma. B. Sella of same child two years after removal of adenoma showing reconstitution of sella. (Reprinted with permission from Hoffman HJ: Youmans J (ed): Neurological Surgery (ed 2). Philadelphia, WB Saunders, 1982, p 2727.)

intrasellar extention and may show a blush in a small adenoma in the pituitary gland.

Pituitary adenomas of significant size will appear on computerized tomography (CT) scan as contrast-enhancing masses within and above the sella. A CT scan with small slices through the sella will identify the possibility of an empty sella.

ENDOCRINOLOGIC TESTING

Endocrinologic testing should be performed before and after surgery in all patients with pituitary tumors. Endocrine investigation includes studies of all of the trophic hormones of the pituitary gland as well as the hormones produced by their target organs.

EMPTY SELLA SYNDROME

The term "empty sella syndrome" was first used in 1962 when Colby and Kearns[11] described the following situation: "A rather rare complication of irradiation is the empty sella syndrome in which a patient treated a number of years previously with improvement in vision, later experiences visual impairment and when operated on with the presumption that this tumor is growing again at operation no tumor is found."

They felt that with the enlarged sella empty of tumor, the optic nerves and chiasm fell into the sella and were subsequently strangulated. In a series of 89 autopsies reported by Kaufman and Chamberlain[12] in 1972, 72 percent of diaphragms had allowed cisternal herniation and sellar remodeling, resulting in 37 percent with a partially empty sella and 6.7 percent with a completely empty sella. Pituitary adenomas may be found in conjunction with a partially empty sella, a situation that can create difficulties when these tumors are approached transsphenoidally and the optic chiasm and nerves are encountered within the sella.[13]

SURGICAL MANAGEMENT

Transsphenoidal surgery for pituitary tumors was used early in the development of neurosurgery by Hirsch[14] and Cushing.[15] Poor illumination and lack of magnification, however, together with imprecise intraoperative localization within the sella tursica, led to a high incidence of recurrence. As a result a subfrontal approach became the approach of choice for pituitary tumors. Guiot,[16] and later Hardy and Wigser,[17] rekindled interest in the transsphenoidal operative technique by adopting two major innovations for this purpose:—the operating microscope and televised fluoroscopy. The problem of infection that plagued the earlier pioneer surgeons was overcome by modern-day antibiotics, and the era of transsphenoidal surgery finally emerged in the late 1960s.

Because transsphenoidal surgery for pituitary tumors is safer and less troublesome than craniotomy, even patients with small tumors causing only minimal symptoms are now operated upon with relative safety and effectiveness. In many cases complete tumor removal can be accomplished without compromise of the normal pituitary gland, and the patient will not require replacement hormone therapy.

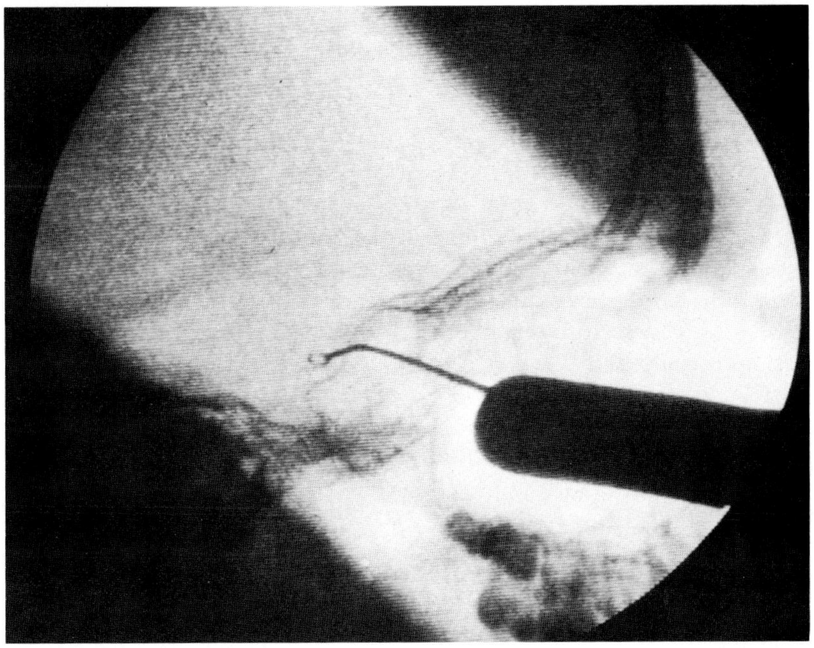

Figure 42-2. View on image intensifier showing curette in sella during removal of pituitary adenoma.

The operative procedure is performed under general anesthesia. The head is extended and the upper lip is retracted. An incision is made in the gingival mucosa, and the soft tissues are separated from the maxilla. With the mucosa of the nasal passages exposed, a submucosal dissection plane is developed along each side of the nasal septum. The lower portion of the septum is excised and the anterior wall of the sphenoid sinus (vomer) is removed. Televised fluoroscopy is used to identify the limits of the floor of the sella tursica (Fig. 42-2). With the aid of the operating microscope and the image intensifier, the operation is continued within the sphenoid sinus. The floor of the sella is then removed and the dura mater is opened (Fig. 42-3). The tumor may extrude into the operative wound. If a large tumor is removed, it is wise to place muscle or fat taken from the abdominal wall or thigh into the sella to prevent prolapse of the optic chiasm into the sella tursica. Freeze-dried dura is packed into the sella and held in place by a

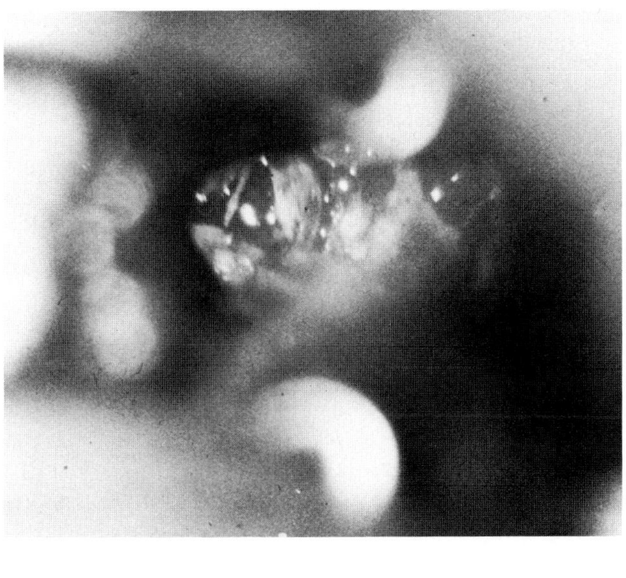

Figure 42-3. View of pituitary adenoma after opening of dura—transsphenoidal route.

plaque of nasal septum to help prevent a cerebrospinal fluid leak. Soft airway tubes are inserted into each nostril to reapproximate the nasal mucosa, and the wound is closed with absorbable sutures. Antibiotics are continued postoperatively for five days.

The sphenoid sinus is well developed by adolescence, and as most pituitary adenomas occur in children older than 10 years, transsphenoidal resection can be performed with ease. Since 1975 all pituitary adenomas seen at the Hospital for Sick Children have been successfully treated by transsphenoidal resection using the technique described by Hardy and Wigser.[17]

In the case of intrasellar adenomas having a diameter of 5 mm or less, Wilson and Dempsey[4] described a technique of making one horizontal and three vertical incisions through the pituitary gland in order to search for the microadenoma. They felt that multiple incision of the anterior pituitary did not produce impairment of function. They also found that selective transsphenoidal removal of microadenomas had a high probability of accomplishing endocrine cure with preservation of normal pituitary function.

RADIATION THERAPY

Several forms of irradiation, including proton beam therapy, have been used for pituitary tumors. In the case of secreting tumors with irradiation of any type, there is a significant delay from the time radiation is begun until a beneficial lowering of trophic hormones is achieved. Further, the normal pituitary gland may be damaged by irradiation, particularly when the high-energy proton beam is used.

In cases in which the tumor is grossly totally removed, radiotherapy should not be instituted. In those cases, however, in which obvious gross tumor is left behind or there is evidence of rapid tumor recurrence, radiotherapy is useful.

In recent years, attention has been drawn to the oncogenic effects of pituitary region irradiation.[18,19]

CONCLUSIONS

Refinement of transsphenoidal technique has revolutionized the surgical approach to pituitary adenomas, and has encouraged the vigorous investigation and treatment of these tumors, which now have such gratifying results.

REFERENCES

1. Ingraham FD, Matson DD: Neurosurgery of Infancy and Childhood. Springfield, Charles C Thomas, 1954, p 223
2. Koos WT, Miller MH: Intracranial Tumors of Infants and Children. Thieme G (ed): Classification of Tumors. Stuttgart, Verlag 1971, p 11
3. Hoffman HJ: Supratentorial Tumors in Childhood, in Youmans J (ed): Neurological Surgery (ed 2). Philadelphia, WB Saunders, 1982, pp 2702–2732
4. Wilson CB, Dempsey LC: Transsphenoidal microsurgical removal of 250 pituitary adenomas. J Neurosurg 48:13–22, 1978
5. Cushing H: The basophil adenomas of the pituitary body and their clinical manifestations (pituitary basophilism). Bull Johns Hopkins Hosp 50:137–195, 1932
6. Nelson DH, Meakin JW, Dealy JB, et al: ACTH-producing tumor of the pituitary gland. New Engl J Med 259:161–164, 1968

7. Formi C, Giovanelli MA: Nelson's syndrome in the paediatric age. Child's Brain 3:309–314, 1977
8. Tyrrell JB, Brooks RM, Fitzgerald PA, et al: Selective transsphenoidal resection of pituitary microadenomas. New Engl J Med 298:753–758, 1978
9. Ortiz-Suarez H, Erickson DL: Pituitary adenomas of adolescents. J Neurosurg 43:437–439, 1975
10. Graf C, Blinderman EE, Terplan KL: Pituitary carcinoma in a child with distant metastases. J Neurosurg 19:254–259, 1962
11. Colby MY Jr, Kearns TP: Radiation therapy of pituitary adenomas with associated visual impairment. Proc Staff Meet Mayo Clin 37:15–24, 1962
12. Kaufman B, Chamberlain, WB, Jr: The ubiquitous "sella" tursica. Acta Radiol (Diagn) 13:413–425, 1972
13. Dominque JN, Wing SD, Wilson CW: Coexisting pituitary adenomas and partially empty sellas. J Neurosurg 48:23–28, 1978
14. Hirsch D: Endonasal method of removal of hypophyseal tumors. With report of two successful cases. JAMA 55:772–774, 1910
15. Cushing H: Intracranial Tumors. Notes Upon a Series of Two Thousand Verified Cases with Surgical-Mortality Percentages Pertaining Thereto, vol 12. Springfield, Ill., Charles C. Thomas, v 1932, p 75
16. Guiot G: Adenomes Hypophysaires. Paris, Masson, 1958, pp 165–178
17. Hardy J, Wigser SM: Radiofluoroscopic control in trans-sphenoidal surgery. J Neurosurg 23:612–619, 1965
18. Waltz T, Brownell B: Sarcoma: A possible late result of effective radiation therapy for pituitary adenoma. J Neurosurg 24:901–907, 1966
19. Amine ARC, Sugar O: Suprasellar osteogenic sarcoma following radiation for pituitary adenoma. J Neurosurg 44:88–91, 1976

43. Craniopharyngiomas

Harold J. Hoffman

Craniopharyngiomas are the most common suprasellar neoplasm in children. They comprise 9 percent of all intracranial tumors in Matson's pediatric series,[1] and in our own institution, they account for 6 percent of brain tumors and 14 percent of supratentorial tumors.[2] Despite their benign histologic appearance, many of these tumors follow a malignant course and result in significant disability and a high mortality rate. Controversy continues to surround the issue of their management, whether it be radical removal, radiotherapy, or a combination of these modalities.

PATHOLOGY

Most authorities agree with Erdheim's[3] statement that craniopharyngiomas arise from embryonic squamous cell rests of an incompletely involuted hypophyseal-pharyngeal duct. These rests are found within the pituitary stalk extending from the infundibulum down to the pituitary gland itself. As a result the tumor is closely adherent to the area of the tuber cinereum, from which point it can insinuate itself into brain parenchyma. Elsewhere the tumor is covered with meninges and hence is distinct from brain tissue. It is in the tuber cinereum that tumor nests surrounded by glial tissue are found (Fig. 43-1). Concern has been expressed that surgical removal always leaves nests of tumor cells behind in this region.[4] It would seem, however, that these so-called "nests" are always continuous with the main tumor capsule, which sends fingers of tumor into the adjacent tuber cinereum. When sectioning the hypothalamus, the pathologist cuts these fingers transversely, and the resultant specimens appear to contain isolated tumor cells. Further, Sweet[5] has pointed out that these nests of tumor cells cause an intense glial reaction, which itself helps to effect a total removal of the tumor: as the surgeon pulls on tumor capsule, the glial tissue containing the tumor nests come with the capsule. In some patients, however, nests of cells may be left behind; these are no doubt the source of tumor recurrence in cases where

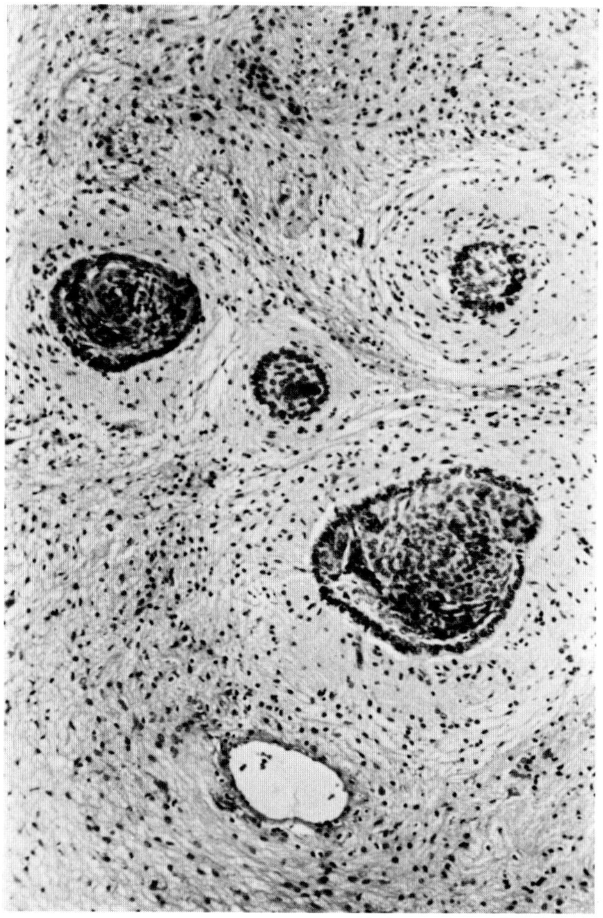

Figure 43-1. Finger-like processes of craniopharyngioma in substance of tuber cinereum, which on section look like nests of tumor cells (H&E × 100). (Reprinted with permission from Hoffman HJ. Craniopharyngioma. The continuing controversy on management, in American Society of Pediatric Neurosurgeons (eds): Concepts of Pediatric Neurosurgery II. New York, S. Karger Publishers, Inc. 1982.)

the surgeon feels a total removal has been accomplished and where the postoperative computerized tomography (CT) scan shows no evidence of residual tumor.

Most craniopharyngiomas are partly cystic, with large solid components. By virtue of their location, they compress the optic chiasm anteriorly, the diaphragma sellae and pituitary gland inferiorly, and the third ventricle superiorly. They can protrude posteriorly and lie ventral to the pons. The free surfaces are smooth, often irregularly lobulated, and vary from thin translucent membrane over the cystic portions to a grayish-white opaque surface over the firm and often calcified solid parts. Where there is no meningeal plane of cleavage, the tumor is ill defined and firmly adherent to adjacent brain by gliosis. The cysts contain yellow opalescent fluid in which glittering cholesterol crystals are present. The solid sections are granular and pale, with minute cysts, cholesterolamatous deposits, and craggy foci of calcium.

Craniopharyngiomas are entirely suprasellar tumors arising in the pituitary stalk. They can enlarge the sella, however, and push the diaphragma sellae and pituitary gland inferiorly. At our institution we have not encountered a craniopharyngioma below an intact diaphragma sellae, but dumbbell-shaped tumors in which the suprasellar portion is typical craniopharyngioma and the intrasellar portion is lined by simple cuboidal or ciliated epithelium have been described.[6] Such infradiaphragmatic intrasellar cysts are found only in adults.

The lining of the cystic portion of a craniopharyngioma is composed of simple stratified squamous epithelium supported by a collagenous basement membrane that separates it from the adjacent gliosis or meninges. The more solid portions of the tumor are sometimes called adamantinomas; here the trabeculae are supported by a loose and scanty cellular vascularized stroma of connective tissue.

CLINICAL FEATURES

More than 50 percent of craniopharyngiomas are diagnosed in children and adolescents. They are rarely seen in young children, however, a fact that attests to their slow growth. Our youngest patient was 2 years of age, and only four cases have been reported in the neonatal period.[7] Craniopharyngiomas demonstrate no sex preference.

Evidence of visual disturbance is present in nearly all patients with craniopharyngioma. The most common visual finding is a bitemporal hemianopia, but signs of intracranial pressure, including papilledema, can occur in as many as 25 percent of patients. Seesaw nystagmus in which one eye moves upward and the other downward—and conversely—in continuously repetitive fashion is characteristic of a parasellar tumor and can be found in 5 to 10 percent of patients with craniopharyngiomas.[8]

Endocrine symptomatology is common; more than 50 percent of patients have diabetes insipidus, excessive shortness due to inadequate growth hormone, obesity, hypothyroidism, or sex hormone deficiency at the time of presentation.

RADIOLOGY

Plain skull radiographs will reveal calcification of the tumor in more than 50 percent of patients, but the CT scan will both delineate the mass and indicate its cystic areas. With the advent of CT scanning, we are now beginning to see craniopharyngiomas that are small in size and where symptoms are minimal (Fig. 43-2). Several of our recent patients have had no visual findings, and little, if any, in the way of endocrine findings, and presented with headaches that led to a CT scan, which showed the suprasellar tumor.

Angiography still remains essential in the preoperative evaluation of a patient with a craniopharyngioma. The position of the two internal carotid arteries, and anterior cerebral and anterior communicating arteries, and the posterior communicating arteries and basilar artery are essential to a proper plan for operative attack on the tumor. In children angiography requires general anesthesia and premedication with steroids.

NEUROENDOCRINOLOGY

A preoperative endocrine workup should include tests for diabetes insipidus, for impairment of adrenocorticortrophic hormone (ACTH) release, and for hypothyroidism. Urine specific gravities, urine osmolarity, and 24-hour urine volume check should be performed to determine the presence of diabetes insipidus.

Serum cortisol levels should be measured preoperatively. The normal serum cortisol level is usually 15–30 mg at 8 A.M. and 5–15 mg at 8 P.M. Impairment of ACTH release may effect not only an absolute reduction of cortisol levels, but also a change in the diurnal variation. Since so many of these patients are hypoadrenal preoperatively, it is essential that they be premedicated with steroids (dexamethasone 0.2 mg/kg to a maximum of 10 mg as a loading dose,

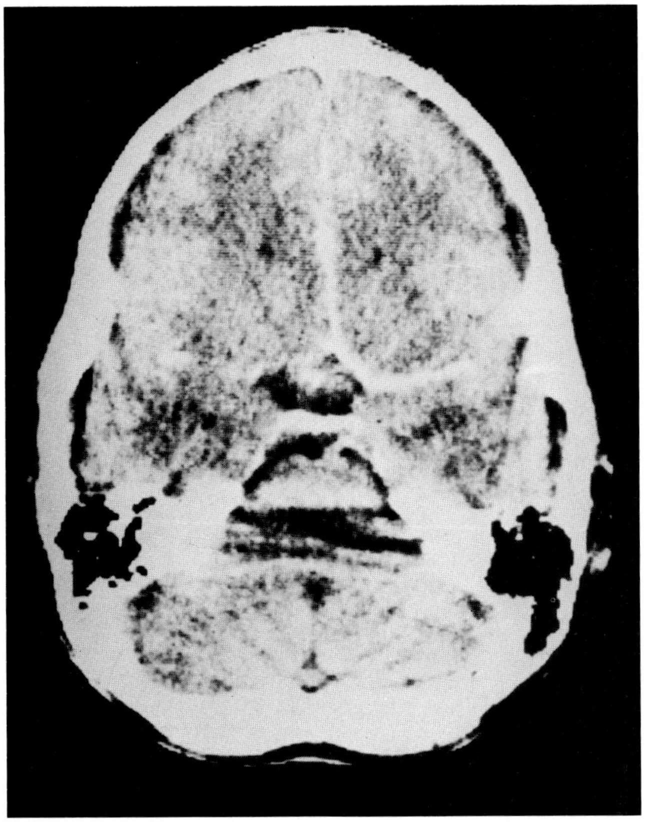

Figure 43-2. CT scan (contrast-enhanced) showing small suprasellar craniopharyngioma in child who presented with headache.

and then 0.1 mg/kg q.6.h. to a maximum of 4 mg as a maintenance dose) prior to any stressful procedures, such as angiography and finally surgery.

Serum electrolytes should be measured and corrected preoperatively if gross imbalances are found.

Hypothyroidism is common in patients with craniopharyngiomas; serum thyroxin levels, together with serum thyroid stimulating hormones (TSH) should be determined. Should hypothyroidism be present, therapy with L-thyroxine should be started.

SURGICAL MANAGEMENT

With the advent of steroid therapy in 1950, Matson began to attempt complete removal of every craniopharyngioma.[9] In recent years better endocrinologic management, together with the accuracy afforded by the operating microscope and the earlier diagnosis made possible by CT scan, should have greatly reduced the operative mortality and permitted a much higher incidence of complete excision. A commonly accepted view of craniopharyngiomas, however, is that there is no line of cleavage between tumor and adjacent brain and that forcible removal of the tumor is accompanied by severe damage to the hypothalamus and the optic apparatus.[10] This belief still restrains many surgeons and encourages such palliative procedures as partial removal and radiotherapy as popular methods of management.[11]

Because the suprasellar region lies quite literally in the center of the head, exposure is difficult, and a wide variety of approaches have been devised to deal with mass lesions in this area: subfrontal, subtemporal, transpterional, transventricular, transcallosal, transphenoidal, and transpalatal.

Primary pituitary adenomas should be approached by a transsphenoidal route even when they extend above the level of the sella. Craniopharyngiomas, however, require meticulous dissection from the adjacent optic nerves, optic chiasm, and internal carotid arteries, as well as the overlying hypothalamus, and must be approached subfrontally so that all of these structures are well exposed and can be safely separated from the tumor. Any other approach, in the case of a craniopharyngioma, may result in an incomplete removal and a high risk of symptomatic regrowth. Completely intrasellar craniopharyngiomas amenable to a transsphenoidal approach have been described, but they are rare and occur only in adults.

For the subfrontal approach, the patient should be positioned supine with the head in a pin fixation head rest, neck extended, and the nose pointing directly upward. This position avoids distortion of anatomic relationships and facilitates the surgeon's orientation to the optic nerves, the internal carotid arteries, and the hypothalamus. Rotating the head toward one side may improve visualization of one optic nerve and internal carotid artery but makes the contralateral nerve and artery less accessible. A right-sided approach to the tumor is initially preferable, in that the right hemisphere is usually nondominant and consistency of approach facilitates anatomic orientation. If a significant portion of the tumor extends along the clivus into the posterior fossa, the scalp incision and bone flap are in a frontotemporal position and the pterion is removed. This exposure allows one to approach the tumor not only subfrontally, but along the pterion, with retraction of the temporal pole for exposure of any tumor that lies behind the chiasm and the internal carotid artery, and thus allows for extraction of any posterior fossa extension of the tumor.

The dura is opened along the supraorbital ridge from the pterion medially to the sagittal sinus. The frontal lobe is then elevated and any veins draining from the frontal pole into the sagittal sinus are coagulated and divided.

The olfactory nerve is coagulated and divided just behind the olfactory bulb. The frontal lobe is then elevated to expose the chiasmatic cistern. At this point the operating microscope is brought in and the more delicate maneuvers begin. The arachnoid overlying the optic nerve and chiasm is cut and split. The frontal lobe can then be retracted away from the optic nerve and chiasm to allow full visualization of both of these structures together with the contralateral optic nerve. Typically, the craniopharyngioma capsule can now be seen between the two optic nerves, protruding below the right optic nerve and impinging bilaterally on the internal carotid arteries. In cases where the optic chiasm is prefixed or pushed forward (Fig. 43-3) by a posteriorly placed tumor, the frontal lobe must be lifted off the lamina terminalis and the lamina terminalis incised. This will allow tumor to be removed between the optic tracts as well as between the optic nerves. With more posteriorly placed tumors, it is advantageous to go between the frontal and temporal lobes along the pterion to expose the internal carotid artery and the structures directly behind it. This allows one to deal with tumors extending back over the dorsum sellae into the posterior fossa. Patterson and Danylench[12] advocate an approach through the tuberculum sellae into the sphenoid sinus in addition to the route through the lamina terminalis to deal with those craniopharyngiomas in which the chiasm is prefixed.

Once the craniopharyngiomas is visualized, the capsule is incised, fluid contents are aspirated with suction tip, and solid elements are removed by curettage. When the tumor contains large amounts of solid material, the Cavitron® (Medical Systems Group, 43-30 38th St., Long Island City, N.Y. 11101) is useful for delicate removal of intracapsular solid contents.

Once the craniopharyngioma has been collapsed by removal of both cystic and solid contents, traction can be applied to the capsule and the filmy adhesions between tumor and adjacent structures can be released.

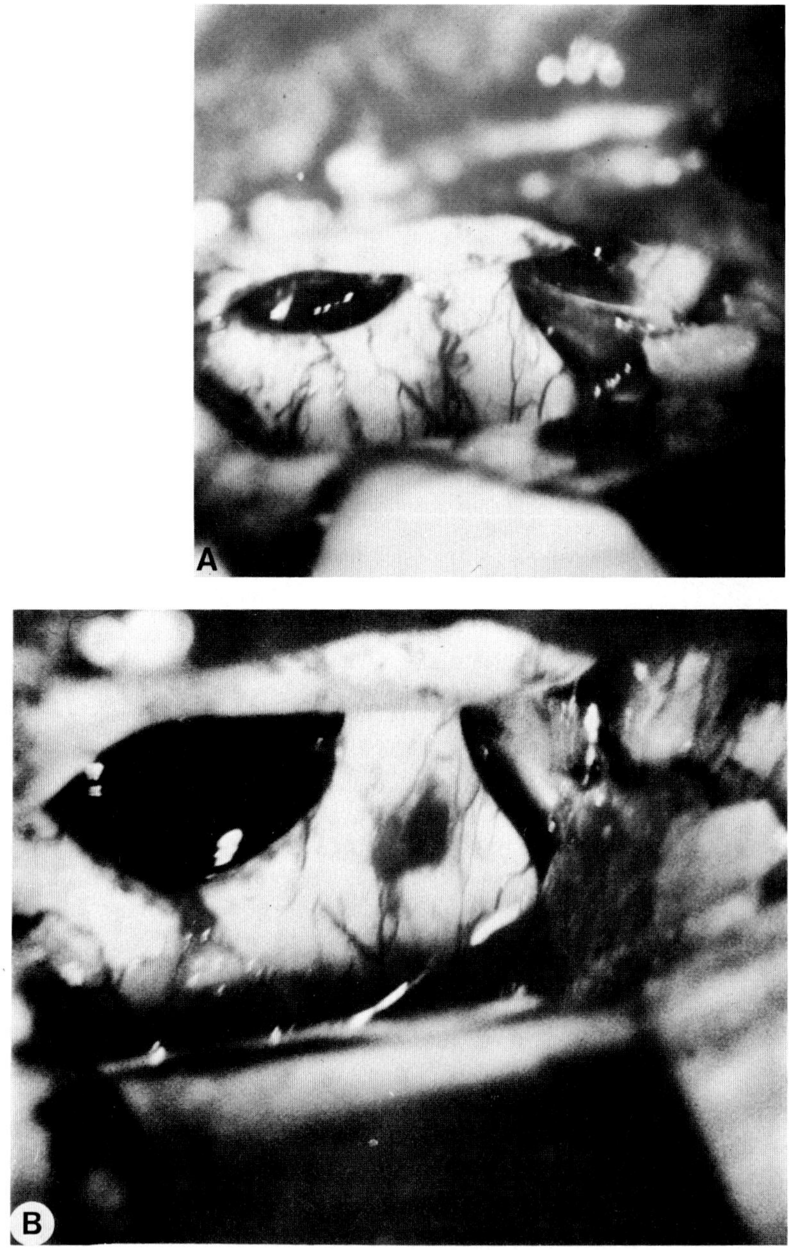

Figure 43-3. A. Chiasm pushed forward by craniopharyngioma. B. With removal of craniopharyngioma, chiasm assumes normal position.

The tumor will usually separate easily from optic nerves and chiasm, but may occasionally adhere with particular tenacity to the internal carotid arteries. In some cases small fragments of capsule have to be left behind to avoid massive hemorrhage from these important vessels, thus accounting for cases of subtotal removal. In most cases, however, it can be freed from these vessels and from the posterior communicating artery with ease. Once the tumor has been dissected off the carotid vessels and the optic apparatus, the tumor capsule can be forcibly pulled off the hypothalamus (Fig. 43-4). The glial reaction of the hypothalamus to the invaginating tumor prevents damage, except in the region of the tuber cinereum. The very nature of the tumor necessitates sacrifice of the pituitary stalk. Inferiorly the tumor may be adherent to the diaphragma sellae, from which it must be excised, and any remaining tumor elements on the diaphragma can be cauterized to prevent recurrence at this site.

In cases where the craniopharyngioma has been large enough to produce

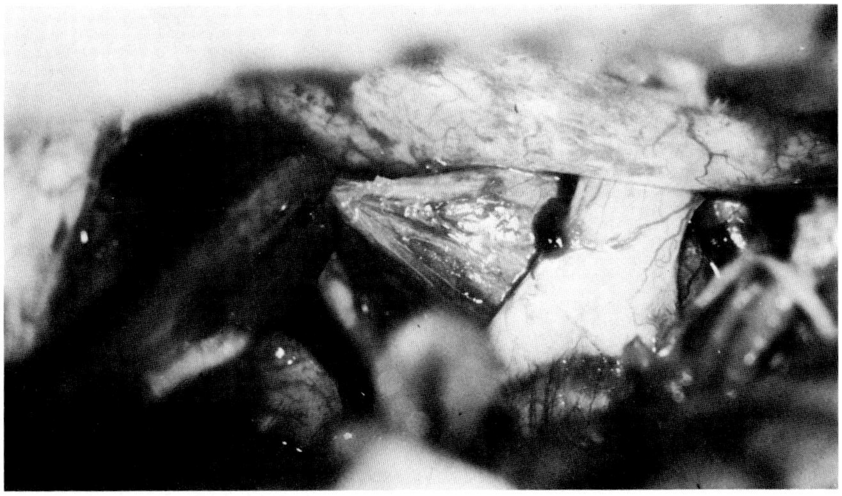

Figure 43-4. Traction being applied to capsule of craniopharyngioma. (Reprinted with permission from Hoffman HJ. Craniopharyngioma. The continuing controversy on management, in American Society of Pediatric Neurosurgeons (eds): Concepts of Pediatric Neurosurgery II. New York, S. Karger Publishers, Inc. 1982).

obstruction of the third ventricle and hydrocephalus, we have found that insertion of a shunt as a preliminary step has improved both the patient's functional status and tolerance of the surgical removal of the tumor.

Postoperatively the patient must be monitored closely. Surgical retraction of the frontal lobe may result in seizure activity and prophylactic doses of dilantin should accordingly be administered for a period of 7–10 days (5–7 mg/kg/24 hr). Preoperative doses of dexamethasone are continued for 48–72 hours postoperatively, at which point maintenance doses of cortisone (25 mg/m^2) are substituted. Eventually the cortisone should be reduced to the lowest effective level with a warning to the patient that an increase in dosage may be necessary to avoid possible Addisonian crises during periods of stress or infection.

If the sphenoid sinus has been entered during a surgical approach through the tuberculum sellae, then prophylactic antibiotics should be administered to prevent a postoperative meningitis.

Total removal of a craniopharyngioma almost invariably leads to diabetes insipidus. This condition normally becomes manifest during the first 24–48 hours postoperatively. Treatment is now very simple and effective. DDAVP (desmopressin) is administered by nasal instillation in doses of 5–20 mg (contained in 0.05–0.2 cc) every 12–24 hours. This material is extremely effective for postoperative as well as long-term management.

Thyroid studies should be repeated after surgery; if there is evidence of hypothyroidism, thryoid treatment should be instituted. Similarly gonadotrophic hormones should be assessed in pubertal children and appropriate replacement therapy begun if sex hormone levels are found to be depressed.

Finally, clinical monitoring of the patient's growth, together with growth hormone studies, should begin six months postoperatively. If growth slows or halts entirely, and if growth hormone levels are significantly depressed, replacement therapy is begun. In some cases, however, normal growth continues despite the absence of growth hormones.[13] Therapeutic intervention in such cases is obviously unnecessary.

DISCUSSION

Despite the best of surgical management, craniopharyngiomas can recur. Amacher's review[4] indicates that even after excision, there is still an 18.5 percent risk of recurrence. These figures should be considered, however, in light of the fact that most of the patients he describes had their surgery performed during the years when the microscope was not routinely used and when postoperative CT scanning was not available to ascertain whether total removal had indeed been achieved. With the use of the operating microscope and the availability of the postoperative CT scan, confirmation of total removal is easier and more accurate, and the risk of recurrence is far lower. At the Hospital for Sick Children, the risk of recurrence after confirmed total excision is less than 10 percent.

When the surgeon believes a total removal has been achieved, and yet CT scan shows residual tumor, the risk of recurrence is of course higher. If the surgeon finds it impossible to remove all visible tumor, the incidence of recurrence may reach 60 percent.[14] It is for this group that radiotherapy on a prophylactic basis is advocated by many surgeons.[4] At our institution we do not use prophylactic radiotherapy for the following reasons: (1) there is a significant chance that the tumor will not recur despite the fact that tumor has been left behind, (2) radiotherapy in itself carries risk, and (3) there is no guarantee that radiotherapy will prevent recurrence.[4]

In those recurrent craniopharyngiomas where the initial surgeon has really made no attempt at total resection, a concerted effort should be made to remove the tumor using a different operative approach. If there has been no significant postoperative bleeding of adhesions, 50 percent of such cases will result in a successful secondary procedure. In the small group of patients where the surgeon feels a total removal has been achieved and where the postoperative CT scan has indeed shown no evidence of tumor, if there is recurrence, reexploration is worthwhile; as Amacher[4] points out, the source of recurrence may be residual islets of cells in the hypothalamus. These "recurrences" should be considered primary lesions, since they can be removed with the same degree of ease as a fresh case.

RADIOTHERAPY FOR CRANIOPHARYNGIOMAS

Radiotherapy appears to have some destructive influence on craniopharyngioma epithelium in spite of the fact that craniopharyngioma epithelium consists of stratified squamous epithelial cells that should be resistant to a dose that will be harmless to surrounding brain parenchyma. Unlike conventionally radiosensitive tumors, however, craniopharyngiomas never completely resorb after radiation, and Amacher[4] has demonstrated that the residual mass left after radiotherapy can be largely necrotic with some viable tumor cells that can lead to tumor recurrence (Fig. 43-5).

Radiotherapy, however, is not completely benign. The toxic effects of radiation on the brain are well known.[15-20] They are usually dose related, but one must also consider the fractionation of the dose and the elapsed time over which the course of radiotherapy is given.

In order to avoid damage to the brain, the nominal standard dose (NSD) must be less than 1760 rets. To ascertain the NSD, the following formula is used:

$$D = NSD \times n^{0.24} \times t^{0.11}$$

where D = the total dose in rads, NSD = nominal standard dose, n = number of fractions, t = elapsed time in days over which the radiation is given.[13] Thus for a dose of 5500 rads given over six weeks, with treatment being given five of seven days of the week (30 fractions over 42 days), the NSD would be 1610 rets.[15]

Although neural tissue is relatively radioresistant, glial tissue and cerebral

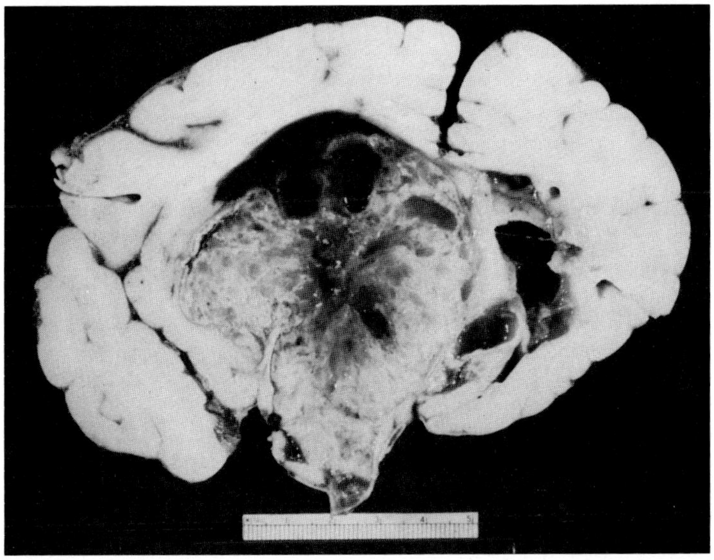

Figure 43-5. Large recurrent craniopharyngioma in child treated by partial removal and radiotherapy.

vasculature are much more susceptible. Long-term effects of radiation therapy on major blood vessels include hypoplasia, stenosis, and premature arteriosclerosis. Even in patients who have received doses well within the therapeutic range, occlusion of the large vessels may eventually produce cerebral infarction.[15]

Delayed radiation necrosis of the brain is also a well-recognized entity that may result from too large a dose of radiation or too short an interval between exposure. This type of delayed cerebral necrosis has been reported in all parts of the brain, including the optic nerves (Fig. 43-6).[16,17]

Finally there is risk of radiation-induced tumor. The most common radiation-induced tumor is a sarcoma. Waltz and Brownell[18] presented a series of

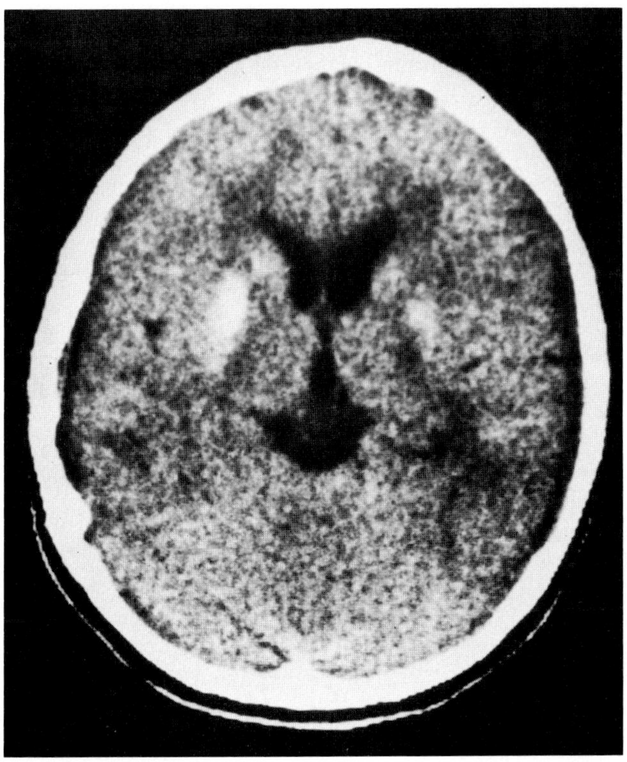

Figure 43-6. Calcification in basal ganglia in patient, two years after radiotherapy for craniopharyngioma. (Reprinted with permission from Hoffman HJ. Craniopharyngioma. The continuing controversy on management, in American Society of Pediatric Neurosurgeons (eds): Concepts of Pediatric Neurosurgery II. New York, S. Karger Publishers, Inc. 1982.)

radiation-induced sarcomas that developed anywhere from 2½ to 20 years after radiation with dosages that always exceeded 3000 rads. Recently Spallone, Gagliarde, and Vagnozzi[19] reported the development of multiple meningiomas following low-dose radiation for tinea capitis of the scalp. Allen[15] reports that children who receive low-dose scalp irradiation for fungal infections have a sevenfold greater likelihood of acquiring malignant brain tumors up to 16 years following therapy, and Waga and Handa[20] report a tentorial meningioma occurring 12 years after radiotherapy for a craniopharyngioma. Considering the seriousness of these potential complications, radiotherapy should be approached cautiously and reluctantly.

CONCLUSIONS

Total excision can be achieved in over 80 percent of children with craniopharyngioma. Modern technical aids eliminate any significant surgical morbidity or mortality and reduce the risk of recurrence after total excision to less than 10 percent. In those few cases where tumor adherence to surrounding vessels prevents total excision, radiotherapy should not be instituted prophylactically. Postoperatively these patients can be followed with CT scan, and only if there is clinical and/or radiologic evidence of a recurrent suprasellar mass lesion should irradiation be undertaken.

REFERENCES

1. Matson DD: Neurosurgery of Infancy and Childhood, vol 2. Springfield, Charles C Thomas, 1969, p 545
2. Hoffman HJ: Supratentorial tumors in childhood, in Youmans J (ed): Neurological Surgery (ed 2). Philadelphia, WB Saunders, 1982, pp 2702–2732
3. Erdheim J: Über hypophysengangsyesehwülste und Hirncholesteatome. Sitzungsb Akad Wissensch 113:537–726, 1904
4. Amacher AL: Craniopharyngioma: The controversy regarding radiotherapy. Child's Brain 6:57–64, 1980
5. Sweet WH: Craniopharyngioma: Radical surgery. Clin Neurosurg 23:52–79, 1975
6. Russell DS, Rubinstein LJ: Pathology of Tumours of the Nervous System (ed 4). Baltimore, Williams & Wilkins, 1977, p 35
7. Azar-Kia B, Kreshnan UR, Schecter MM: Neonatal craniopharyngioma: Case report. J Neurosurg 42:91–93, 1975
8. Drachman DA: See-saw nystagmus. J Neurol Neurosurg Psychiatr 29:356–361, 1966
9. Matson DD, Crigler JF Jr: Management of craniopharyngioma in childhood. J Neurosurg 30:377–390, 1969
10. Rougerie J: What can be expected from the surgical treatment of craniopharyngiomas in children? Child's Brain 5:433–449, 1979
11. Kramer S, Southard M, Mansfield CM: Radiotherapy in the management of craniopharyngiomas. Further experiences and late results. Am J Roentgenol Radium Ther Nucl Med 103:44–52, 1968
12. Patterson R, Danylevich A: Surgical removal of craniopharyngiomas by a transcranial approach through the lamina terminalis and sphenoid sinus. Neurosurg 7:111–117, 1980
13. Holmes LB, Frantz AG, Rabkin MT, et al: Normal growth with subnormal growth hormone levels. N Engl J Med 279:559, 1968
14. Hoffman HJ, Hendrick EB, Humphreys RP, et al: Management of craniopharyngioma in children. J Neurosurg 47:218–227, 1977
15. Allen J: The effects of cancer therapy on the nervous system. J Pediatr 93:903–909, 1978

16. Di Lorenzo N, Nolletti A, Palma L: Late cerebral radionecrosis. Surg Neurol 10:281–290, 1978
17. Ross HS, Rosenberg S, Friedman AH: Delayed radiation necrosis of the optic nerve. Am J Ophthalmol 76:683–686, 1973
18. Waltz TA, Brownell B: Sarcoma: A possible late result of effective radiation therapy for pituitary adenoma. Report of two cases. J Neurosurg 24:901–907, 1966
19. Spallone A, Gagliarde FM, Vagnozzi R: Intracranial meningiomas related to external cranial irradiation. Surg Neurol 12:153–159, 1979
20. Waga S, Handa H: Radiation-induced meningioma: With review of literature. Surg Neurol 5:215–219, 1976

44. Optic Nerve Gliomas

Martin Peter Sayers

INCIDENCE

Optic nerve gliomas represented 1 percent of Harvey Cushing's tumor experience,[38] and were 4 percent on a typical pediatric neurosurgery service in central Ohio. They were 10 percent of the astrocytomas at the Columbus Children's Hospital from 1950 to 1981 (Table 44-1).

DEFINITION

These tumors encompass gliomas in (1) the prechiasmatic and retroorbital optic nerves, (2) the optic chiasm, and (3) some that involve nerve, chiasm, and hypothalamus. Despite controversy we look upon these tumors as variations of pilocytic astrocytoma.[1,2,11,14,15,32,35,37,45,51,54,59,60,65] In the author's experience with 36 of these tumors, 36 percent were diagnosed in patients with recognizable neurofibromatosis (Table 44-2).

PATHOLOGY

There is evidence confirmed by tissue culture that midline and paramedian pilocytic astrocytomas represent the same entity whether located anteriorly in the visual apparatus or posteriorly in the brain stem and cerebellum.[27,28,33,45,65] The contention that these tumors may be hamartomas[1,24,30,42,54,55,64] tends to be refuted by morphologic and tissue culture data and well-documented multidecade follow-up.

Optic gliomas characteristically show spindle cells variable to multipolar with Rosenthal fibers (cytoid bodies) (Fig. 44-1).[59,60] The background is microcystic to honeycombed with some degree of vascular proliferation. The consis-

Table 44-1
Astrocytomas—Columbus Children's Hospital (1950–1981)

Brain stem	98
Cerebellum	77
Optic nerve gliomas	36
Thalamus	23
Frontal	22
Third ventricle	21
Hypothalamus	17
Parietal	13
Temporal	13
Tuber sclerosis	12
Lateral ventricle	7
Occipital	5
Pineal	2
Total	346

tency may be solid, gelatinous, or grossly cystic. The cells invade the pia mater and have extended into both subarachnoid space and the ventricle. Local invasion and spread are described.[50,51] Verhoeff felt there was contiguous activation by tumor of surrounding glial elements into neoplastic cells, rather than replication.[59,60] Others have presented evidence that the process is potentially multicentric with or without neurofibromatosis.[12,15,44,55] Malignant degeneration has been documented but is not common.[6,63]

With or without macrocysts, the tumor has frequently enlarged enough to block the foramen of Monro.

Eight of 36 patients in our series developed hydrocephalus. Five had

Table 44-2
Optic Nerve Gliomas—The Columbus Children's Hospital (1950–1981)

Patients	
Total	36
Survivors	31
Surgically verified	34
Surgical mortality	0
Subsequent mortality	5
Neurofibromatosis	14 (36%)
Location	
Prechiasmatic	11
Chiasmatic	20
Chiasmatic/hypothalamic	5
Age at Diagnosis	
Average age	6 yr, 2 mo
Oldest	16 yr
Youngest	16 mo
Sex incidence	
Male	18
Female	18
Hydrocephalus	
Shunted	10
Aqueduct stenosis	3

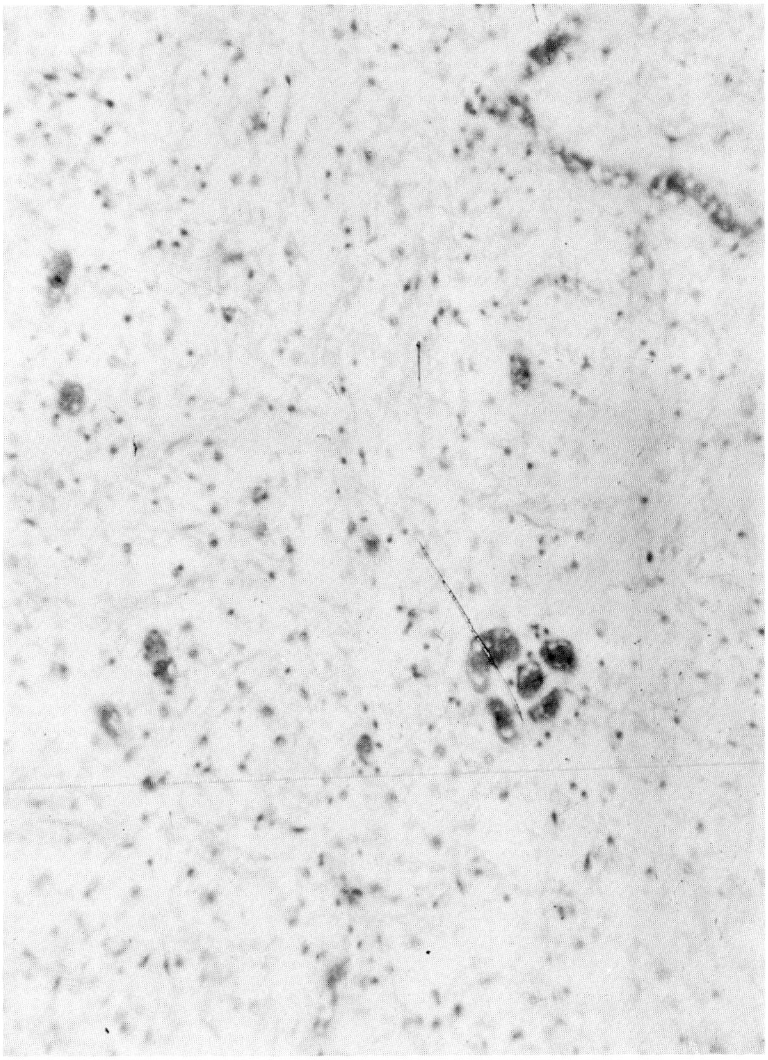

Figure 44-1. Pilocytic astrocytoma in optic chiasmatic glioma.

obstruction in the third ventricle and 3 patients (all with neurofibromatosis) had aqueduct stenosis.

NATURAL HISTORY

This is predominantly a childhood disease. All of our patients had become symptomatic by the age of 16 years; the youngest was 16 months old. As in most published series, 75 percent of our patients were diagnosed prior to 10 years of age.[11,17,21,22,30,32,41] It is probable that 40 to 50 percent have minimal diagnostic features for neurofibromatosis, although these are not always sought out and documented accurately.

Visual loss is the most common presenting symptom. Optic atrophy is always visible but is too easy to miss in the early stages. In fact 38 percent of our patients were not seen until they manifested increased intracranial pressure. Forty percent had complained of headache. Thirteen of 36 patients showed proptosis or lid tumor (Figs. 44-2 and 44-3). Twenty percent had clinical evidence of impaired hypothalamic function, all with small stature and retarded

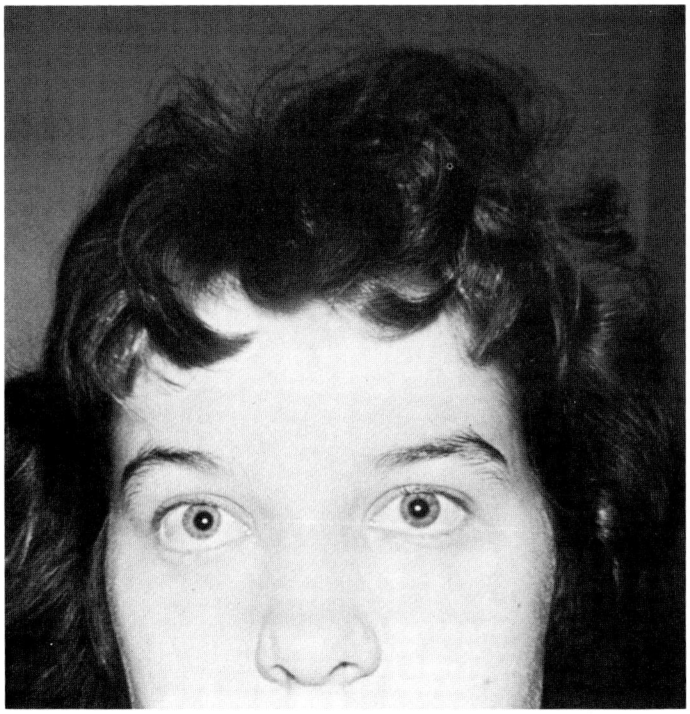

Figure 44-2. Early proptosis of right eye caused by optic nerve glioma.

development of secondary sexual characteristics. Four presented with diabetes insipidus.

In our series of 36 patients, it appears that 11 tumors had not involved the optic chiasm at the age of diagnosis. Of the remaining 25 chiasmatic lesions, five had invaded into the hypothalamus. We have seen an additional 17 hypothalamic astrocytomas with no apparent involvement of the optic nerves or chiasm.

The most frequent presenting symptoms are loss of vision, headache, and proptosis. Strabismus and nystagmus develop in the children under 10 years of age, with significant visual loss.

We have experienced no operative mortality, but 5 patients died subse-

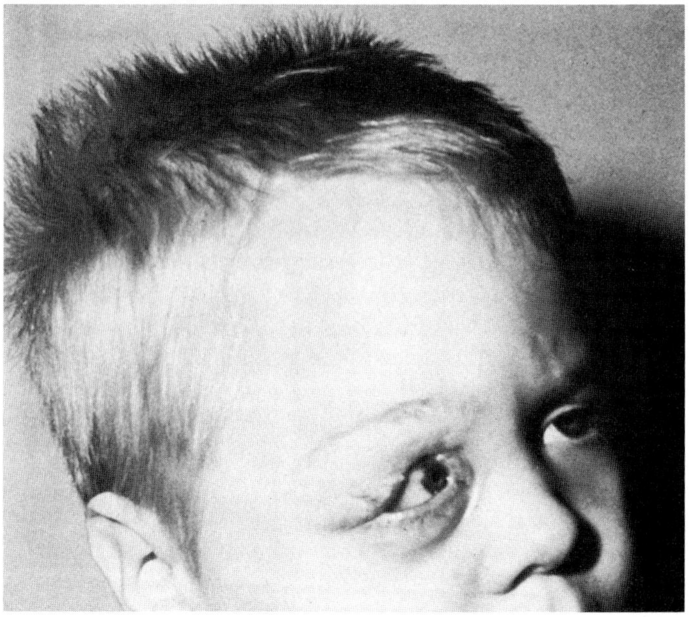

Figure 44-3. Neurofibromatosis in eyelids associated with optic nerve glioma.

quently (four months, two years, five years, five and a half years, and nine years after craniotomy). Three deaths occurred in patients who had at first appeared to have tumor limited to the nerves and chiasm, two more were from the chiasmal/hypothalamic group. Two of the fatalities had neurofibromatosis.

Another of the patients with neurofibromatosis experienced documented further loss of vision.

The foregoing data further refute the hamartoma–static lesion arguments. We have documented progression of the lesion with loss of function in 9 patients. On the other hand, none of the cases has expired after age 13 years (deaths at 2½ years, 11 years, 12 years, 12 years, and 13 years). Our experience and review of literature[11,16,17,21,22,30,32,41,45] suggest gradually slowed tumor growth after the first 15 years of life.

DIAGNOSIS

The diagnosis is presently established in an orderly progression of testing:

1. Fundoscopic examination has always shown some degree of optic nerve pallor (atrophy). The atrophy may be somewhat masked by papilledema.
2. Visual fields are always incongruous because of the tendency to greater involvement of one or the other of the optic nerves. In advanced lesions all crossing fibers may be destroyed, resulting in total loss of the temporal fields. Complete blindness may be present. Involvement of only one field suggests that the lesion may be prechiasmatic and requires intensive investigation regarding the threat of spread to the chiasm.
3. Plain skull x-rays may show enlarged J-shaped sella turcica and flecks of calcium in the suprasellar tumor. The "J" is backward and titled anteriorly and results from depression of the posterior margin of the planum sphenoidale (Fig. 44-4). The sella and dorsum sella may be further eroded and the cranial sutures separated with a very large tumor and in the event of hydrocephalus.
4. X-rays of the optic foramena are suspect if any dimension of the forman exceeds 7 mm or if there is a difference of 2 mm or more in any dimension between the right and the left foramen.

   Lateral and anteroposterior tomography of the optic nerve canals is invaluable in demonstrating a lesion impinging on either end of the canal and in placing the bulk of the lesion in either the orbit or the intracranial cavity.
5. Computerized tomographic (CT) brain scanning may demonstrate the tumor clearly in the orbit, the optic canal, the chiasm, and hypothalamus, or following the optic tracts posteriorly.

   Coronal and sagittal cuts are often more diagnostic than the conventional angulation of the beams.
6. If doubt remains concerning hypothalamus involvement, positive contrasting of the third ventricle with fluoroscopy, x-ray, and CT scanning for visualization of the chiasmatic and infundibular recesses of the ventricle and of the aqueduct of Sylvius can be valuable.
7. Angiography is not always necessary but may be helpful in the differential diagnosis and in planning surgery.
8. Evaluation of endocrine function should be routinely utilized, initially and in follow-up.

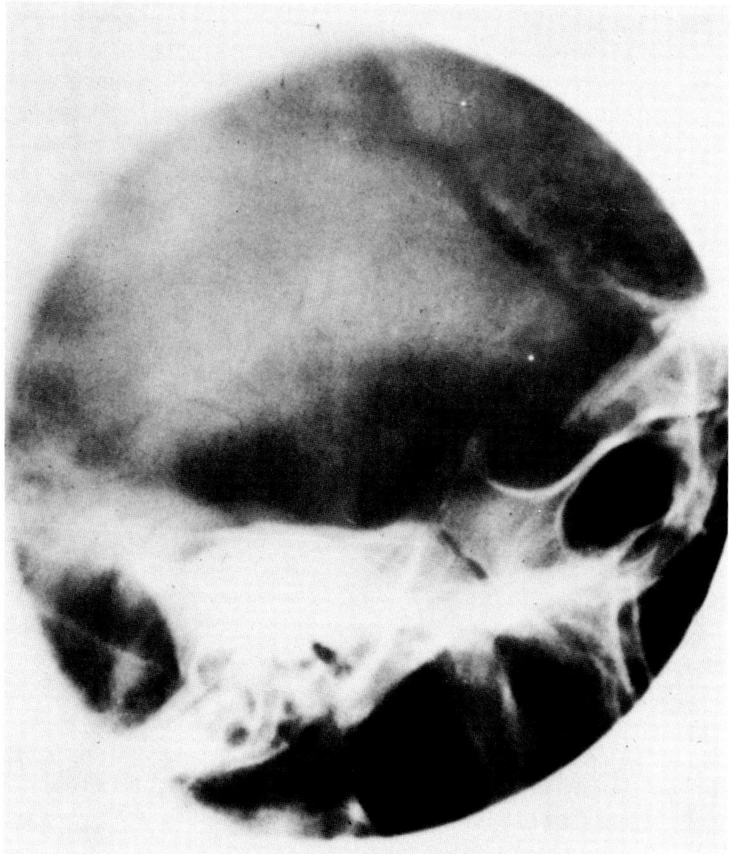

Figure 44-4. J-shaped sella turcica.

TREATMENT

A number of resectable and radiation-sensitive lesions has simulated optic nerve glioma, even with neurofibromatosis. A very definitive diagnosis is needed if one elects to withhold treatment and observe optic nerve lesions.

A prechiasmatic (unilateral) optic nerve glioma should be explored if it exists in any part intracranially. In a patient under 15 years of age, we resect the tumor if it is within 1 cm of the chiasm. If the eye is blind or amblyopic, it is safer to resect at any age. If the tumor is in the optic canal, the progression of optic atrophy may be slowed by uncapping the foramen and linear decompression of the sheath. If the tumor is in the foramen, it may be necessary to view it to rule out cuff meningioma.

It is feasible to remove an intracranial-orbital or solely orbital optic nerve glioma transcranially through the roof of the orbit. If CT scan or tomograms show the tumor to be intracranial, it is mandatory to remove the intracranial portion, despite the fact that there are recorded cases of subtotal removal without chiasmatic spread or recurrence. There are recorded instances of spread from the nerve to the chiasm[47] and into the opposite nerve.[66] There have been well-documented reports of orbital recurrences.[10,34,55,57]

The orbital roof bone should be saved and replaced as a mosaic. The bulb and extraocular muscles are carefully preserved. The annulus of Zinn should be incised between the medial rectus muscle and the superior rectus and retracted laterally. It is later resutured to preserve nerve supply and ocular motility. The nerve to the medial rectus muscle passes under the optic nerve.

If the orbital roof bone is replaced, there rarely will be postoperative pulsating exopthalmos.

It is not necessary to remove an orbital glioma with preserved vision, but marked proptosis and prolonged disagreeable diplopia are acceptable indications for resection. An orbital tumor with extension into the foramen should not be resected extracranially.

Three times in our experience it has been possible to accomplish total resection of an optic nerve tumor that had extended to within 0.5 cm of the optic chiasm. When the optic nerve tumor is invading the chiasm, we do not resect if there is preserved vision in that eye. We unroof that optic foramen. If the eye is blind, the tumor is resected.

The approach to chiasmal involvement is for diagnosis and may be therapeutic. If any question exists regarding the character of a chiasmatic or anterior hypothalamic tumor, exploration should be undertaken to rule out meningioma, germinoma, craniopharyngioma, dermoid cyst, teratoma, and epithelioma. If there is preserved vision, extension into an optic foramen should be unroofed and decompressed. Occasionally a cyst can be drained and fenestrated.

In one instance a soft gelatinous extension of the chiasmatic tumor was encountered in the subarachnoid space. This tumor was removed, and there has been no further loss of vision in a 15-year follow-up period. Obstruction at the foramen of Monro requires fenestration of the septum pellucidum, as well as lateral ventricle shunt. Only 2 of our 8 shunted patients have died—both with very extensive hypothalamic tumor.

Improvement of visual acuity and regression of mass have been frequently demonstrated following radiation therapy for optic nerve gliomas.[11,19,36,56,62] Further impairment of hypothalamic function due to radiation should be avoided in a growing child, if at all possible. It is advisable to wait for repeated evidence of undeniable progressive loss of visual acuity, peripheral vision, or hypothalamic function before radiating.

Chemotherapy has been used for optic gliomas, but as yet has shown little benefit.

Careful multidiscipline long-term follow-up is an absolute necessity for these patients. Individualization of patient care is especially important when confronted with this tumor of indeterminate natural history and potential for multidecade survival. Both the patient and physicians need encouragement for many tedious visual tests, x-rays, and laboratory procedures.

PROGNOSIS

The average age at diagnosis of our 36 children with optic nerve gliomas was 6 years and 2 months. Thirty-four were operated upon one or more times, with no surgical mortality. Five subsequently died four months to nine years later. The average age of the patients now is 16 years and those over 30 years of age show no evidence of progressive disease.

Patients with chiasmatic and hypothalamic tumor are smaller than average in stature and somewhat underdeveloped, but have normal intelligence.

Very few new optic nerve gliomas are seen after age 20 years and reviews of available long-term series show rare mortality between 30 and 50 years of age.

REFERENCES

1. Anderson DR, Spencer WH: Ultrastructural and histochemical observations of optic nerve gliomas. Arch Ophthalmol 83:324–335, 1970
2. Arkhangelsky VN: Neoplasms of the optic nerve, Ophthalmologica 151:260–271, 1966

3. Bailey P, Buchanan DN, Bucy PC: Intracranial Tumors of Infancy and Childhood, Chicago, The University of Chicago Press, 1939, pp 114–188, 242–298
4. Bernell WR, Kepes JJ, Seitz EP: Late malignant recurrence of childhood cerebellar astrocytoma, Report of two cases, J Neurosurg 37:470–474, 1972
5. Block MA, Goree JA, Jimenez JP: Craniopharyngioma with optic canal enlargement stimulating glioma of the optic chiasm. J Neurosurg 39:523–527, 1973
6. Brooks WH, Parker JC Jr, Young AB, et al: Malignant gliomas of the optic chiasm in adolescents. Clin Pediatr 15:557–561, 1976
7. Bucy PC, Thieman PW: Astrocytomas of the cerebellum, Arch Neurol 18:14–19, 1968
8. Bucy PC, Gustafson WA: Structure, nature, and classification of the cerebellar astrocytomas, Am J Cancer 35:327–353, 1939
9. Byers WGM: Primary intradural tumors of the optic nerve: Fibromatomis nervi optici. Stud Roy Victoria Hosp Montreal 1:3–82, 1901
10. Christensen E, Andersen SRy: Primary tumours of the optic nerve and chiasm. Acta Psychiatr Neurol Scand 27:5–16, 1952
11. Chutorian AM, Schwartz JF, Evans RA, et al: Optic gliomas in children. Neurology (Minneapolis) 14:83–95, 1964
12. Condon JR, Rose FC: Optic nerve glioma. Br J Ophthalmol 51:703–706, 1967
13. Cushing H: Experiences with the cerebellar astrocytomas, A critical review of seventy-six cases. Surg Gynec Obstet 52:129–204, 1931
14. Dandy WE: Prechiasmal tumors of the optic nerve. Am J Ophthalmol 5:169–188, 1922
15. Davis FA: Primary tumors of the optic nerve. Arch Ophthalmol 23:735–821, 957–1022, 1940
16. DeSousa AL, Muller JL, Kolsbeck JE, et al: Histology and prognosis of opticochiasmatic gliomas. Am Ophthalmol 3:376–381, 1979
17. Dodge HW, Love JG, Craig WM, et al: Gliomas of the optic nerves. Arch Neurol Psychiat 79:607–621, 1958
18. Dyke CG, Davidoff LM: Roentgen Treatment of Diseases of the Nervous System. Philadelphia, Lea & Febiger, 1942, pp 100–103
19. Eggers H, Jakobiec FA, Jones IS: Tumors of the optic nerve. Doc Opthalmol 41:43–128, 1976
20. Elvidge AR: Long-term survival in the astrocytoma series, J Neurosurg 28:399–404, 1968
21. Fog J, Seedorff HH, Vaernet K: Optic glioma, clinical features and treatment. Acta Opthalmol 48:644–653, 1970
22. Fowler FD, Matson DD: Gliomas of the optic pathways in childhood. J Neurosurg 14:515–528, 1957
23. Geissinger JD, Bucy PC: Astrocytomas of the cerebellum in children. Arch Neurol 24:125–135, 1971
24. Glaser JS, Hoyt WF, Corbett J: Visual morbidity with chiasmal glioma. Arch Opthalmol 85:3–12, 1971
25. Gol A: Cerebellar astrocytomas in children. Am J Dis Child 106:21–24, 1963
26. Grinker RR: Tumors of the optic nerve. Arch Opthalmol 4:497–508, 1930
27. Gullotta F, Kreutzberg G: Das Gliom des Opticus, Morphologische and Histochemische Untersuchungen am Schnittpraparat und der Gewebekultur. Acta Neuropathol (Berlin) 2:413–424, 1963
28. Cullotta F, Fliedner E: Spongioblastomas, astrocytomas, and rosenthal fibers. Ultrastructure, tissue culture, and enzyme histochemical investigations. Acta Neuropathol (Berlin) 22:68–78, 1972
29. Housepain EM: Surgical treatment of unilateral optic nerve gliomas. J Neurosurg 31:604–607, 1969
30. Hoyt WF, Baghadassarian SA: Optic glioma of childhood. Br J Opthalmol 53:793–798, 1969
31. Hoyt WF, Meshel LG, Lessell S, et al: Malignant optic glioma of adulthood. Brain 96:121–132, 1973
32. Hudson AD: Primary tumors of the optic nerve. Roy London Opthalmol Hosp Rep 18:317–439, 1912

33. Kersting G: Tissue culture of human gliomas. Progr Neurol Surg 2:165–202, 1968
34. Lloyd LA: Gliomas of the optic nerve and chiasm in childhood. Trans Am Ophthamol Soc 71:488–535, 1973
35. Lundberg A: Ueber di primaren Tumoren des Sehnerven und der Sehnerven Kreuzung. Inaug Dissert, Karolinisches Institut, Stockhold, Nordiska Bokhandeln, 1935
36. MacCarty CS, Boyd AS Jr, Childs DS: Tumors of the optic nerve and optic chiasm. J Neurosurg 33:439–444, 1970
37. Marshall D: Glioma of the optic nerve, as a manifestation of von Recklinghausen's disease. Am J Opthalmol 37:15–36, 1954
38. Martin P, Cushing H: Primary gliomas of the chiasm and optic nerves in their intracranial portion. Arch Opthalmol 52:209–241, 1923
39. Matson DD: Neurosurgery of Infancy and Childhood, Springfield, Charles C Thomas, 1969, pp 436–448
40. Matson DD: Cerebellar astrocytoma in childhood. Pediatrics 18:150–158, 1956
41. Miller NR, Iliff WJ, Green WR: Evaluation and management of gliomas of the anterior visual pathways. Brain 97:743–754, 1974
42. Miller NR: Optic nerve glioma and cerebellar astrocytomas in a patient with von Recklinghausen's neurofibromatosis. Am J Opthalmol 79:582–588, 1975
43. Mohan J, Sen DK: Astrocytoma of the optic nerve. Br J Opthalmol 54:284–286, 1970
44. Myles ST, Murphy SB: Gliomas of the optic nerve and chiasm, Canad J Opthalmol 8:508–514, 1973
45. Oxenhandler DC, Sayers MP: The dilemma of childhood optic gliomas. J Neurosurg 48(1):340–341, 1978
46. Pfaffenbach DD, Kearns TP, Hollenhorst RW: An unusual case of optic nerve-chiasmal glioma. Am J Opthalmol 74:523–525, 1972
47. Rand CW, Irvine R, Reeves DL: Primary glioma of the optic nerve. Arch Opthalmol 21:799–816, 1939
48. Reese AB: Tumors of the Eye. New York, Harper & Row, 1963, pp 162–179
49. Ringertz N, Nordenstam H: Cerebellar astrocytoma. J Neuropathol Exp Neurol 10:343–367, 1951
50. Rubinstein LJ: Tumors of the Central Nervous System. Washington, DC, Armed Forces Institute of Pathology, 1972, pp 9–15, 19–39
51. Russell DS, Rubinstein LJ: Pathology of Tumors of the Nervous System. Baltimore, Williams & Wilkins, 1972, pp 115–123, 137–142, 230, 233, 246–252
52. Scott RM, Ballantine HT Jr: Cerebellar astrocytoma: Malignant recurrence after prolonged postoperative survival. J Neurosurg 39:777–779, 1973
53. Sen DK, Mohan H: Glioma of optic nerve (record of an unusual case). EENT Monthly 51:273–275, 1972
54. Spencer WH, Borit A: Diffuse hyperplasia of the optic nerve in von Recklinghausen's disease. Am J Opthalmol 64:638–642, 1967
55. Spender WH: Primary neoplasms of the optic nerve and its sheaths: Clinical features and current concepts of pathogenetic mechanisms. Trans Am Opthalmol Soc 70:490–528, 1972
56. Taveras JJ, Mount LA, Wood EH: The value of radiation therapy in the management of glioma of the optic nerves and chiasm. Radiation 66:518–528, 1956
57. Tym R: Piloid gliomas of the anterior optic pathways. Br J Surg 49:322–331, 1961
58. Udvarhelyi GB, Kodadoust AA, Walsh FB: Gliomas of the optic nerve and chiasm in children: An unusual series of cases. Clin Neurosurg 15:204–237, 1966
59. Verhoeff FH: Primary intraneural tumors (gliomas) of the optic nerve, a histological study of eleven cases, including a case showing cystic involvement of the optic disk, with demonstration of the origin of cytoid bodies of the retina and cavernous atrophy of the optic nerve. Arch Opthalmol 51:120–140, 239–254, 1922
60. Verhoeff FH: Tumors of the optic nerve, in Penfield W (ed): Cytology and Cellular Pathology of the Nervous System, vol 3. New York, Paul B Hoeber, 1932, pp 1029–1039
61. Wagener HP: Gliomas of the optic nerve. Am J Med Sci 237:238–261, 1961

62. Walsh FB: The ocular signs of tumors involving the anterior visual pathways. Am J Opthalmol 42:347–377, 1956
63. Wilson WB, Feinsod M, Hoyt WF, et al: Malignant evolution of childhood chiasmal pilocytic astrocytoma. Neurology (Minneapolis) 26:322–325, 1976
64. Wong IG, Lubow M: Management of optic glioma of childhood: A review of 42 cases. Neuro-opthalmology, Symposium of the University of Miami and the Bascom Palmer Eye Institute, 1972, pp 51–60
65. Zulch KH: Brain Tumors. New York, Springer, 1965, pp 147–152
66. Jain I: Optic gliomas. Br J Opthalmol 45–54, 1961

45. Pseudotumor, Fibrous Dysplasia, and Leukemia

David M. Klein

PSEUDOTUMOR CEREBRI

Pseudotumor cerebri (benign intracranial hypertension) is a clinical syndrome of elevated intracranial pressure without focal neurologic findings, cerebrospinal fluid (CSF) abnormality, ventricular enlargement, or other evidence of a localized intracranial mass lesion. The diagnosis ultimately is made by excluding other possibilities. The condition tends to remit spontaneously after several weeks to months.

The syndrome is attributed to a wide variety of etiologic factors that are not easily explained by a common pathophysiology. In fact cerebral edema, CSF malabsorption, and increased intracranial vascular volume have all been suggested as mechanisms, variably documented,[1–5] and can be related to known precipitating factors. Precipitants include otitis media, mastoiditis, and superior vena cava syndrome; adrenal cortical insufficiency or withdrawal of steroid therapy that has suppressed endogenous secretion; and pregnancy, menstrual irregularity, oral contraception, and female obesity, perhaps related to adrenal insufficiency through estrogenic abnormality.[6,7] Pathophysiology is even less clear in cases associated with excessive or inadequate vitamin A intake, hypoparathyroidism, or iron deficiency anemia.[8] In children otitis and mastoiditis have been the most common precipitants identified, but recently there has been an increase in the syndrome associated with the treatment of other diseases. Although chronic use of topical steroids can provide sufficient absorption, particularly in children, to suppress endogenous secretion, the absorbed steroid itself is inadequate for metabolic maintenance and so intracranial hypertension can result while steroid treatment is in progress.[9–11] Pseudomotor cerebri has been reported with the use of hyperalimentation catheters in infants.[12] The mechanism may be one of obstructed venous drainage, but could also be the result of "catch-up cerebral growth," with the rapid correction of malnutrition.[13]

Sydenham's chorea, pertussis immunization, and antibiotic therapy (tetracyclines and naladixic acid) also have been implicated.[8] No precipitating factor can be identified in approximately 50 percent of cases.

The symptoms and signs are those only of increased intracranial pressure. While infants may become irritable or somnolent, most patients remain bright despite some headache or vomiting. Papilledema and abducens palsy can develop insidiously. Computed tomography (CT) is the most useful current procedure for excluding other diagnoses. Angiography may be required if a diagnosis of venous sinus obstruction is to be established. Lumbar puncture should be performed only after the possibility of a mass is excluded. Under these circumstances, drainage of fluid for both diagnostic and therapeutic purposes does not carry the usual risks of herniation, despite a high opening pressure.

The condition tends to be self-limited in children and frequently no other treatment is required if causative factors are eliminated.[14–16] Occasionally more active treatment is necessary to prevent optic atrophy and permanent visual loss. Periodic lumbar puncture may be sufficient to keep pressure under control. Corticosteroid therapy can be effective, and steroids should be reinstituted and their use tapered very gradually in cases where their withdrawal initiated the problem. If symptoms persist despite these treatments, lumboperitoneal shunt can be considered.[17] Although intracranial hypertension recurs only rarely, close neurologic and ophthalmologic supervision should be maintained for many months after initial symptoms subside.

FIBROUS DYSPLASIA

Fibrous dysplasia is a chronic condition of unknown etiology characterized by the localized development of benign fibro-osseous tissue within one or more bones. Involved areas tend to expand during childhood and then to stabilize after puberty, although this is not invariable.[18] The condition probably represents a nonhereditary developmental defect in bone formation. Changes may be seen in only one bone (monostotic) or in many bones (polystotic) in an individual. As many as 50 percent of those with polystotic disease have craniofacial lesions.[18,19] Of 67 monostotic cases, Schlumberger found 14 (21 percent) to involve the skull.[20] Here the process may extend across suture lines to become regional, but single lesions of this sort are still classified as monostotic. The frontal, sphenoid, and facial bones most often are involved, and basal structures more often than vault.

Involved areas may be grossly enlarged. Fibro-osseous tissue masses usually are grayish, somewhat gritty, and solid, except for small degenerative cysts. Histologically there are fibroblasts, mature collagen, variable new bone formation, occasional islands of cartilage, and scattered giant cells. Vascular supply is usually prominent. The radiographic picture varies accordingly. There may be thickening in contour, with fibrous tissue islands demonstrated as "cystic" areas, and irregular radiolucency, varying with the density of new bone content. Some areas therefore appear sclerotic; this is particularly true of the involved skull base in children. Normal bony landmarks and cavities may become obliterated.

The most common complaints are of craniofacial asymmetry or deformity, headache, and local tenderness.[21–23] Fibro-osseous expansion can produce proptosis. Optic canal encroachment can result in visual loss and optic atrophy.[21,24] Deafness is reported as a result of similar encroachment upon the middle ear or external auditory canal.[21,25,26] A diagnosis of tumor may be suggested by these developments or by seizures, which are observed with higher than usual incidence in fibrous dysplasia.[21,27] The reason for this is unclear. Hemorrhage or cyst formation, with sudden enlargement, tenderness, or fluctuance over the skull, can suggest sinusitis, osteomyelitis, or malignancy.[25] Malignant degeneration is observed in both monostotic and polystotic fibrous dysplasia, and craniofacial sites are common. Prior irradiation or surgery probably is not contributory.[29]

The radiographic picture must be differentiated from that of tumor or osteomylelitis. Hyperostotic basal meningioma may present particular difficulty, unless there are other stigmata of fibrous dysplasia. In the vault, this distinction is easier; the bony reaction of meningioma is usually enostotic whereas that of fibrous dysplasia more often is cystic and tends to expand outwards.[22]

Cranial nerve compression may develop insidiously in children. Those with basicranial disease should have interval examinations and x-rays, particularly where there is potential for spheno-orbital expansion. Prompt decompression may reverse proptosis and arrest optic nerve damage, but lost vision is seldom recovered. Successful otologic decompression has been described. Radical craniofacial excision and reconstruction can be considered in cases of gross deformity, but there may be recurrence unless the affected area is totally removed. Diagnostic questions may require bone biopsy. Treatment is otherwise expectant. Radiotherapy is not effective.

Lesions of the vertebral column are uncommon, but cases of spinal cord compression can result from either fibro-osseous encroachment of pathologic fracture.[30,31]

LEUKEMIA

Childhood leukemias are usually acute, with about 80 percent of cases identified as lymphoblastic, 15 percent as myeloblastic, and the remainder as undifferentiated or chronic. Central nervous system (CNS) symptoms develop in 20 to 50 percent of patients and may appear at any time in the leukemic course. The involvement can be asymptomatic.[32,33]

The primary CNS infiltration is usually subarachnoid. Proliferating blast cells extend along perivascular spaces and may perforate the pial barrier to invade underlying brain. Cranial nerves are often involved, most commonly the sixth, seventh, and eighth. Obliteration of CSF pathways can lead to hydrocephalus and signs of increased intracranial pressure.[34,35] Hypothalamic infiltration can result in hyperphagia and obesity.[33,35] Subarachnoid bleeding occurs, particularly during episodes of thrombocytopenia. Massive intracerebral hemorrhage is usually associated with *blastic crisis,* a situation of uncontrolled peripheral leukocytosis, with the formation of cerebrovascular leukemic nodules and ultimately vascular erosion.[34,36]

Present-day systemic chemotherapy can usually produce bone marrow remission, but diffusion of drugs across the blood–CSF barrier is inadequate to eliminate all residual blast cells in the meninges. Central nervous system relapse can be followed by blast-cell recirculation, and generalized recurrence may follow from this. Blast cells packed in deep Virchow–Robin spaces can also remain insulated from agents delivered into the CSF. The most successful treatment programs to date therefore include prophylactic CNS radiation as well as chemotherapy.[37,38]

A CNS relapse must be differentiated from the complications of treatment, which can be significant. Leukoencephalopathy following systemic chemotherapy, particularly methotrexate, can present as generalized ventricular dilatation and focal periventricular encephalomalacia. It is unclear whether this is

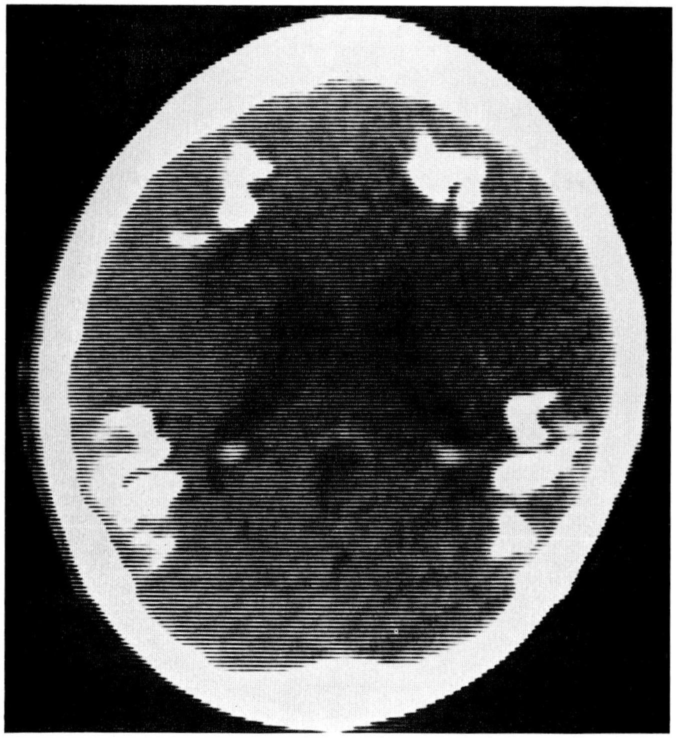

Figure 45-1. Computed tomography in a 5-year-old male treated with both radiation and chemotherapy for acute lymphoblastic leukemia. There are areas of periventricular leukomalacia and laminar calcification as well as mild ventricular dilatation.

produced by chemotherapy alone or by chemotherapy in conjunction with radiation. Radiation itself can result in cerebral angiopathy and laminar calcification in cortex and basal ganglia (Fig. 45-1).[39–42]

The neurosurgeon may be called upon to insert an Ommaya reservoir for intraventricular chemotherapy, but with present-day treatment, hydrocephalus and intracranial hemorrhage seldom reach proportions requiring surgical intervention while the leukemia itself is still responsive to treatment.

REFERENCES

1. Sahs AL, Joynt RJ: Brain swelling of unknown cause. Neurology 6:791–803, 1956
2. Johnston I, Paterson A: Benign intracranial hypertension. II. CSF pressure and circulation. Brain 97:301–312, 1974
3. Martins AN: Resistance to drainage of cerebrospinal fluid: Clinical measurement and significance. J Neurol Neurosurg Psychiatr 36:313–318, 1973
4. Gucer G, Viernstein L: Long-term intracranial pressure recording in the management of pseudotumor cerebri. J Neurosurg 49:256–263, 1978
5. Dandy WE: Intracranial pressure without brain tumor. Diagnosis and treatment. Ann Surg 106:492–513, 1937
6. Greer M: Benign intracranial hypertension. IV. Menarche. Neurology 14:569–573, 1964
7. Greer M: Benign intracranial hypertension. V. Menstrual dysfunction. Neurology 14:668–673, 1964
8. Greer M: Management of benign intracranial hypertension (pseudotumor cerebri). Clinical Neurosurg 15:161–174, 1968
9. Munro DD: The effect of percutaneously absorbed steroids on hypothalamic-pituitary-adrenal function after intensive use in in-patients. Br J Dermatol 94(suppl 12):67–76, 1976
10. Sparkes CG: Measuring adrenal function in out-patients using topical steroids. Br J Dermatol 94(suppl 12):77–82, 1976

11. Hosking GP, Elliston H: Benign intracranial hypertension in a child with eczema treated with topical steroids. Br Med J 1:550–551, 1978
12. O'Tuama LA, Kirkman HN, James PM: Raised intracranial pressure after hyperalimentation. Lancet 2:1101, 1973
13. Bray PF, Herbst JJ: Pseudotumor cerebri as a sign of "catch up" growth in cystic fibrosis. Am J Dis Child 126:78–79, 1973
14. Grant DN: Benign intracranial hypertension. A review of 79 cases in infancy and childhood. Arch Dis Child 46:651–655, 1971
15. Rose A, Matson DD: Benign intracranial hypertension in children. Pediatrics 39:227–237, 1967
16. Weisberg LA, Chutorian AM: Pseudotumor cerebri of childhood. Am J Dis Child 131:1243–1248, 1977
17. Vander Ark GD, Kempe LG, Smith DR: Pseudotumor cerebri treated with lumbar-peritoneal shunt. JAMA 217:1832–1834, 1971
18. Grabias SL, Campbell CJ: Fibrous dysplasia. Orthop Clin N Am 8:771–783, 1977
19. Windholz F: Cranial manifestations of fibrous dysplasia of bone. Am J Roentgenol Radium Ther Nucl Med 58:51–63, 1947
20. Schlumberger HG: Fibrous dysplasia of single bones (monostotic fibrous dysplasia). Milit Surg 99:504–527, 1946
21. Sassin JF, Rosenberg RN: Neurological complications of fibrous dysplasia of the skull. Arch Neurol 18:363–369, 1968
22. Leeds N, Seaman WB: Fibrous dysplasia of the skull and its differential diagnosis. Radiology 78:570–582, 1962
23. Ramsey HE, Strong EW, Frazell EL: Fibrous dysplasia of the craniofacial bones. Am J Surg 116:542–547, 1968
24. Finney HL, Roberts TS: Fibrous dysplasia of the skull with progressive cranial nerve involvement. Surg Neurol 6:341–343, 1976
25. Basek M: Fibrous dysplasia of the middle ear. Arch Otolaryngol 85:4–7, 1967
26. Wong A, Vaughan CW, Strong MS: Fibrous dysplasia of temporal bone. Arch Otolaryngol 81:131–133, 1965
27. Bertoni JM, Kooi KA: Fibrous dysplasia of the skull, with seizures and focal electroencephalographic findings. Dev Med Child Neurol 20:483–493, 1978
28. Pyke R, Cope JR, Doshi R: Fibrous dysplasia mimicking intracranial tumour. J Laryngol Otol 87:1233–1238, 1973
29. Schwartz DT, Alpert M: The malignant transformation of fibrous dysplasia. Am J Med Sci 247:1–20, 1964
30. Montoya G, Evarts CM, Dohn DF: Polyostotic fibrous dysplasia and spinal cord compression. J Neurosurg 29:102–105, 1968
31. Rosencrantz M: A case of fibrous dysplasia (Jaffe–Lichtenstein) with vertebral fracture and compression of the spinal cord. Acta Orthop Scand 36:435–440, 1965
32. Sullivan MP: Intracranial complications of leukemia in children. Pediatrics 20:757–781, 1957
33. Hardisty RM, Norman PM: Meningeal leukemia. Arch Dis Child 42:441–447, 1967
34. Moore EW, Thomas LB, Shaw RK, et al: The central nervous system in acute leukemia. Arch Intern Med 105:451–468, 1960
35. Shaw RK, Moore EW, Freireich EJ, et al: Meningeal leukemia. Neurology 10:823–833, 1960
36. Fritz RD, Forkner CE, Freireich EJ, et al: The association of fatal intracranial hemorrhage and "blastic crisis" in patients with acute leukemia. N Engl J Med 261:59–64, 1959
37. Pinkel D: Treatment of acute lymphocytic leukemia. Cancer 43:1128–1137, 1979
38. Jenkin RDT: Radiation in the treatment of meningeal leukemia. Am J Pediatr Hematol/Oncol 1:49–58, 1979
39. Price RA: Histopathology of CNS leukemia and complications of therapy. Am J Pediatr Hematol/Oncol 1:21–30, 1979
40. Griffen TW, Rasey JS, Bleyer WA: The effect of photon irradiation on blood–brain barrier permeability to methotrexate in mice. Cancer 40:1109–1111, 1977
41. Peylan-Ramu N, Poplak DG, Pizzo PA, et al: Abnormal CT scans of the brain in

asymptomatic children with acute lymphocytic leukemia after prophylactic treatment of the central nervous system with radiation and intrathecal chemotherapy. N Engl J Med 298:815–818, 1978

42. Ochs JJ, Berger P, Brecher ML, et al: Computed tomography brain scans in children with acute lymphocytic leukemia receiving methotrexate alone as central nervous system prophylaxis. Cancer (in press)

46. Intramedullary Tumors of the Spinal Cord

Fred Epstein
Nancy Epstein

INCIDENCE

Intramedullary spinal cord tumors constitute approximately 6 percent of all neoplasms of the central nervous system, and 31.4 percent of all primary intraspinal tumors of childhood. They occur most frequently between the ages of 10 and 16, and are equally divided between the sexes.[1,3]

PATHOLOGY

Unlike the adult population in which ependymomas account for 50 percent of intramedullary tumors, approximately 58.7 percent of pediatric intramedullary tumors are astrocytomas. Furthermore, in pediatric patients "pure" intramedullary ependymomas represent only 28.1 percent of all intramedullary lesions (excluding conus of filum terminale tumors that extend into the lumbar sacral subarachnoid space).

When evaluating intramedullary lesions in children, further diagnostic considerations include "cystic lesions" (hydromyelia, syringomyelia), which have a reported incidence of 4.7 percent, and congenital dermoid or epidermoid tumors at 5.8 percent. Additional lesions may include metastatic medulloblastomas among others (Table 46-1).[1,2,8,10,16,17,20,22,28,32–34]

There is a definite predisposition for pediatric tumors to be rostrally located compared with the adult population. Forty-six percent of pediatric intramedullary tumors are cervical and cervicothoracic, whereas in adults only 28 percent of these tumors occur in the cervical or cervicothoracic cord (Table 46-2).[1,3,8,10,21,22,28,29] Intramedullary tumors generally occupy many cord segments (average six), and rarely, the entire length of spinal cord from the cervicomedullary junction to the conus may be involved.[1,2,5,8,17,21,29]

Table 46-1
Pathology of Pediatric Intramedullary Tumors: Compilation of 13 Reported Series[1,2,8,10,16,17,20,22,28,32–34]

Total	Astrocytoma	Ependymoma	"Cyst"	Dermoid Ependymal Teratoma	Others
128	74 (58.7%)	36 (28.5%)	6 (4.7%)	5 (5.5%)	3 (2.6%)

CLINICAL MANIFESTATIONS

Clinical symptoms are commonly present for months, or even years, prior to neurosurgical consultation.[1,2,8,13,23,26,29,32] In some situations the course may be punctuated by exacerbations and remissions that are possibly related to alterations in edema surrounding the neoplasm.[1,2] On occasion the onset of symptomatology may be associated with a trivial spinal injury. It has been suggested that in rare cases "injury" may precipitate peritumoral edema and result in the relatively rapid progression of symptoms.[2,17,29]

Pain is the initial symptom in more than one half of children with intramedullary spinal cord tumors. The type of pain may be classified as (1) root, (2) spinal, and (3) tract.

Root pain occurs in 20 percent of children with an intramedullary tumor. It is commonly referred over a single cervical dermatoma, and is indistinguishable from root pain that occurs in association with the more typical extramedullary disease processes. It is unclear as to whether the pain is caused by swelling of the spinal cord with distortion of the root, or if the root entry zone is actually infiltrated by tumor.

Spinal pain, localized to bony segments adjacent to tumor, occurs in 70 percent of these patients.[29] The pain is dull and aching in quality, and may be secondary to dural tube distention produced by a swollen spinal cord.

Tract pain, vague and burning in quality, as well as parasthesias may reflect peritumoral edema or frank infiltration of the lateral spinal thalamic tracts. Although these symptoms typically occur caudal to the tumor, their "locale" bares no anatomic relationship to the spinal segments that are infiltrated by tumor.[1,17,20]

Children in different age groups with intramedullary tumors may present with very different clusters of symptoms. In the absence of obvious neurologic dysfunction,[1–3,8,28] infants and younger children may manifest severe pain, rigidity, and paraspinal spasm. Conversely the primary presenting symptom complex in older children may be the presence of a progressive scoliosis or gait impairment.[1–3,8,17,29,32]

In cervical tumors the neurologic examination commonly discloses mild weakness of the upper extremities with or without associated weakness of the lower extremities. Muscle atrophy may be present in the upper extremities. Sensory examination may disclose a "waistcoat" type of sensory impairment, a finding most suggestive of an intramedullary spinal cord tumor.[23,29] A well-defined sensory level is slightly less common with intramedullary than extramed-

Table 46-2
Location of Pediatric Intramedullary Tumors: Compilation of Eight Reported Series[1,3,8,10,21,22,28,29]

Total	Cervical	Cervical Thoracic	Thoracic	Thoracolumbar	Lumbar	Lumbar Sacral
102	39 (38.2%)	7 (6.8%)	21 (20.5%)	23 (23.0%)	4 (3.9%)	8 (7.8%)

ullary tumors. In addition sphincter dysfunction may be present, but these problems more typically occur later in the course of the illness with intramedullary than extramedullary lesions[1,2,8,17,29,32]

Increased intracranial pressure may complicate the clinical manifestation of intramedullary tumors in as many as 12.5 percent of patients. The computerized axial tomography (CAT) scan may disclose a normal or markedly dilated ventricular system. Although the etiology of the increased pressure has not been established, some authors have noted a dense arachnoiditis at the outlets of the fourth ventricle, while others have maintained that the greatly elevated cerebrospinal fluid (CSF) protein interferes with normal circulatory dynamics.[2,8,23]

Even more rarely, severely increased intracranial pressure in the absence of other neurologic signs may be the presenting symptoms of an intramedullary tumor. It must be suspected if the CSF protein is markedly evaluated in the absence of demonstrable introcranial pathology.

NEURODIAGNOSTIC STUDIES

Abnormal plain x-ray examinations have been reported in up to 50 percent of patients with intramedullary and extramedullary spinal lesions. Those most frequently associated with intramedullary tumors include an abnormal widened spinal canal with medial erosion of the pedicles, and posterior scalloping of the vertebral bodies (Fig. 46-1).[1,2,8,17,29]

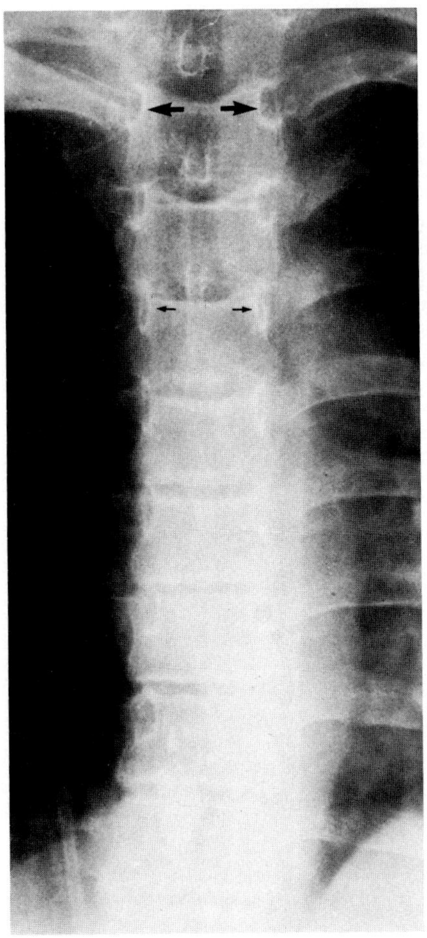

Figure 46-1. Widened spinal canal associated with flattened pedicles (small arrows) is suggestive of intramedullary tumor. Note normal pedicles for comparison (large arrows).

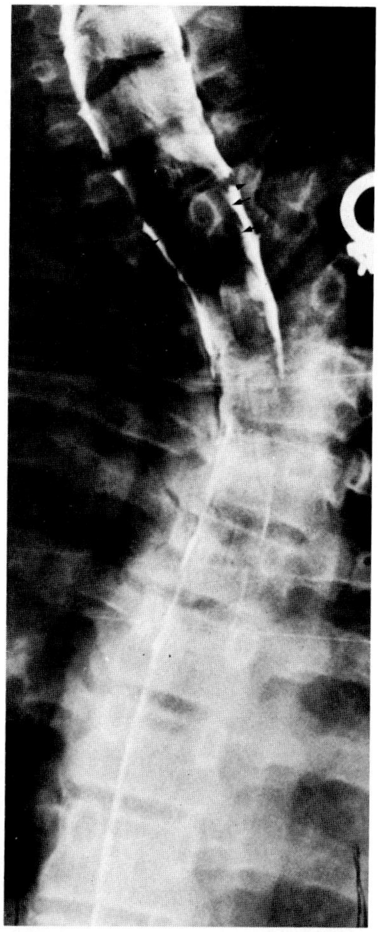

Figure 46–2. Widened cervical spinal cord with associated scoliosis, which is diagnostic of long-standing intramedullary mass.

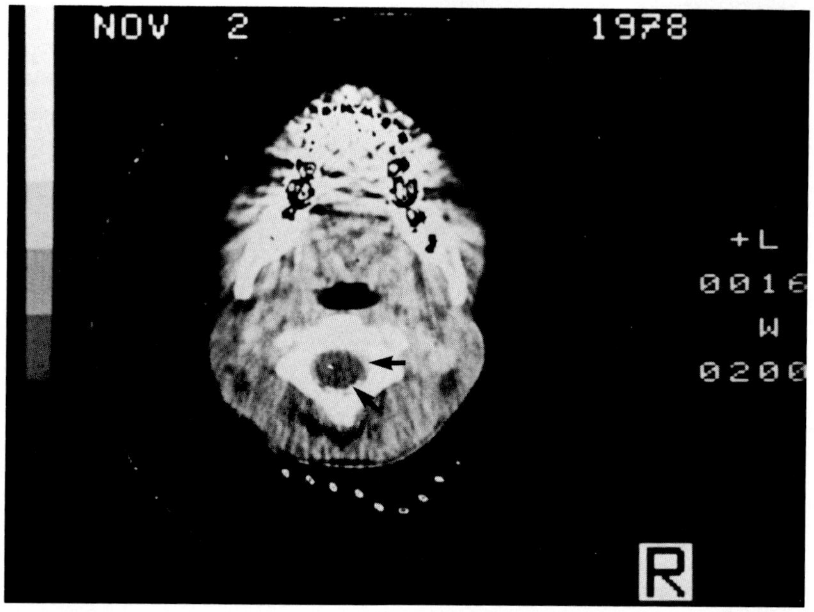

Figure 46-3. Cervical CAT scan disclosing widened spinal cord. Note metrizamide in adjacent subarachnoid space, which is essential to visualization of cord (arrow).

Myelography typically reveals a widened spinal cord in both anterior and lateral projections, with a high incidence of partial or complete block (Fig. 46-2). In the event that total block is demonstrated from below, a C1–C2, or cisternal injection of positive contrast, is absolutely mandatory to define the most rostral extent of the tumor and avoid a poorly planned and incomplete operation.

The spinal CAT scan has also been utilized as a diagnostic adjunct for these neoplasms. It is necessary to utilize intrathecal positive contrast material inasmuch as the cord is not visualized without opacification of the adjacent subarachnoid space. Because the CAT scan only demonstrates a widened spinal cord, it is not yet superior to myelography for intrinsic spinal cord tumors (Fig. 46-3).

DIFFERENTIAL DIAGNOSIS

Although an intramedullary neoplasm is the most common cause of a widened spinal cord, it must be differentiated from hydromyelia, which may occasionally cause identical signs and symptoms but mandate a different surgical approach. Almost invariably hydromyelia is associated with bony anomalies at the cranial–vertebral junction, or within the vertebral bodies (Klippel–Feil syndrome) (Fig. 46-4).[3] Air myelography, in the sitting position, may disclose "collapse" of the spinal cord in the sagittal plane as compared with positive contrast studies that document a markedly swollen cord in the same region.[12] In addition one may occasionally document reflux of contrast material into the hydromyelic cavity via the fourth ventricle.[12] Also, hydrocephalus, which is often present with hydromelia, suggests the diagnosis. When one of these abnormalities is present in association with a progressive neurologic deficit and a widened spinal cord, hydromyelia is a more likely diagnosis than intramedullary spinal cord neoplasm. Unfortunately the resolution of the spinal CAT scan is not consistently sufficient to identify the intramedullary cystic lesion, and for this reason the neurodiagnostic studies are identical irrespective of the primary intramedullary pathology.

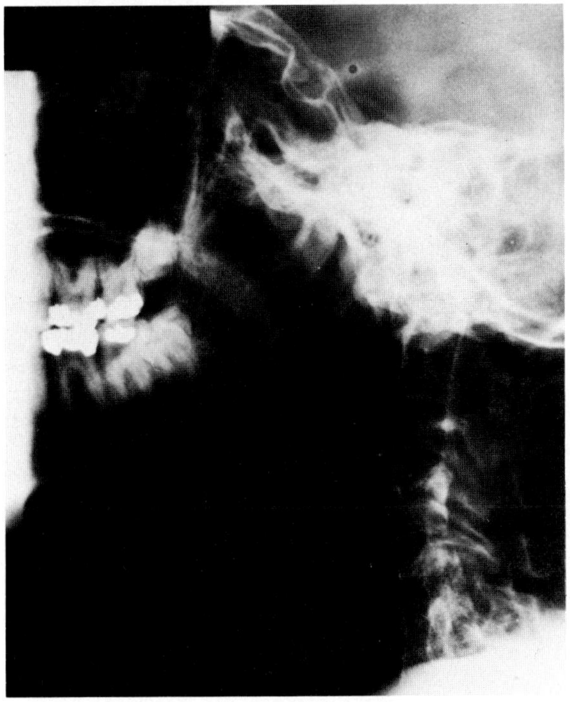

Figure 46-4. Increased sagittal diameter of spinal canal is associated with fusion of posterior elements of C1 and C2, and vertebral bodies of C4–5. When associated with an intramedullary mass, the most common diagnosis is hydromyelia.

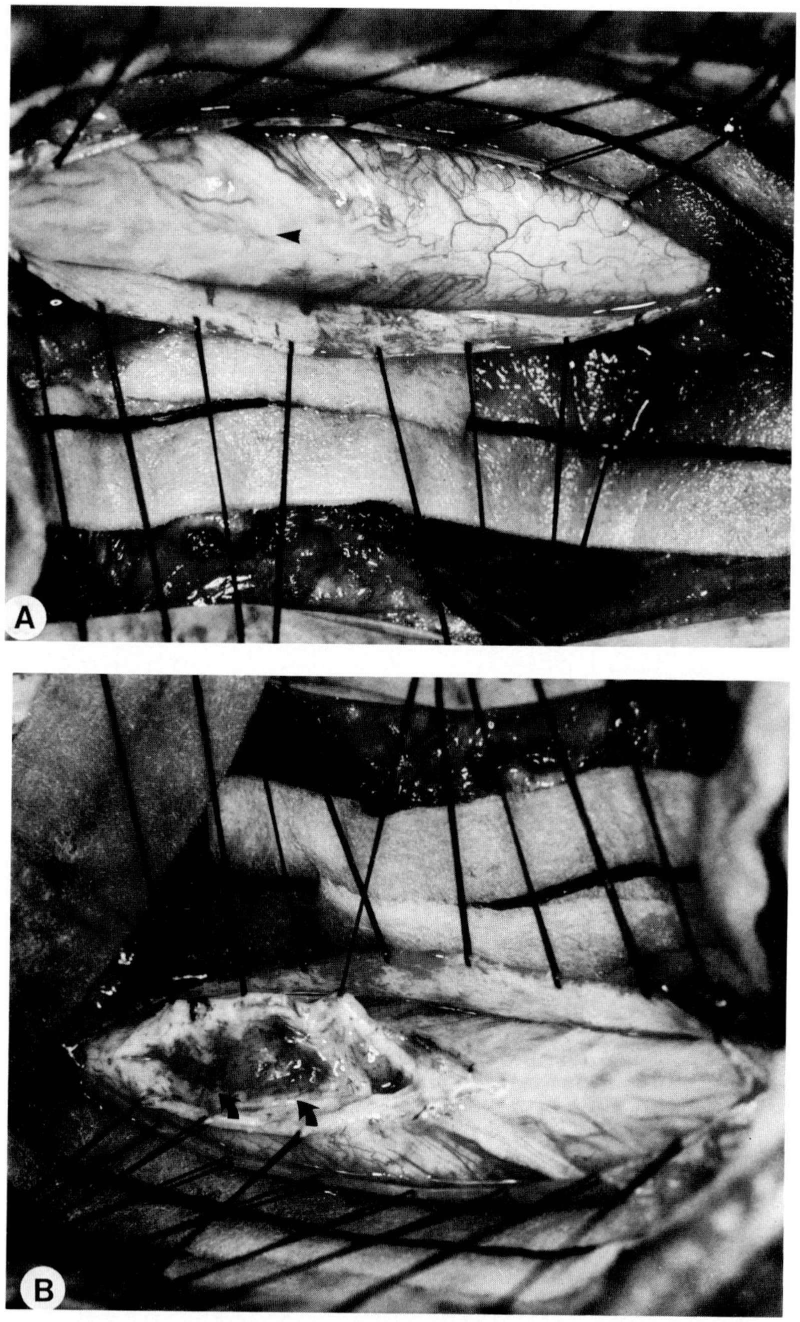

Figure 46-5. A. Swollen spinal cord is shown with abundant abnormal surface vasculature and thickened opalescent arachnoid (arrow). B. Following midline posterior myelotomy, tumor is clearly demarcated from adjacent spinal cord (arrow). C. Radical removal terminates at anterior pial surface (small arrow). Note that traction sutures through pia maintain exposure of tumor cavity (large arrows). D. Pia traction sutures have been removed, permitting reapproximation of posterior spinal cord elements. Patient had no postoperative neurologic deficit other than preoperatively present monoparesis of the right upper extremity, which returned to normal over the ensuing few weeks.

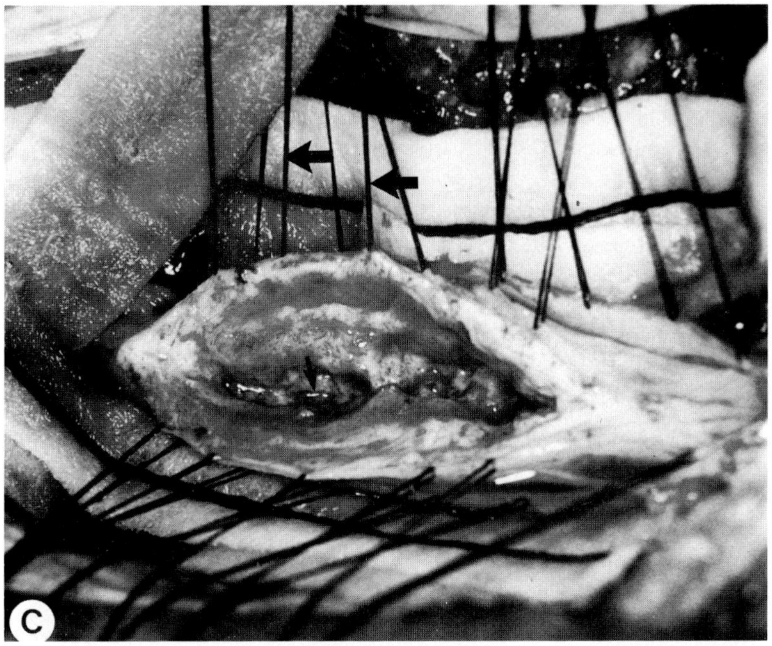

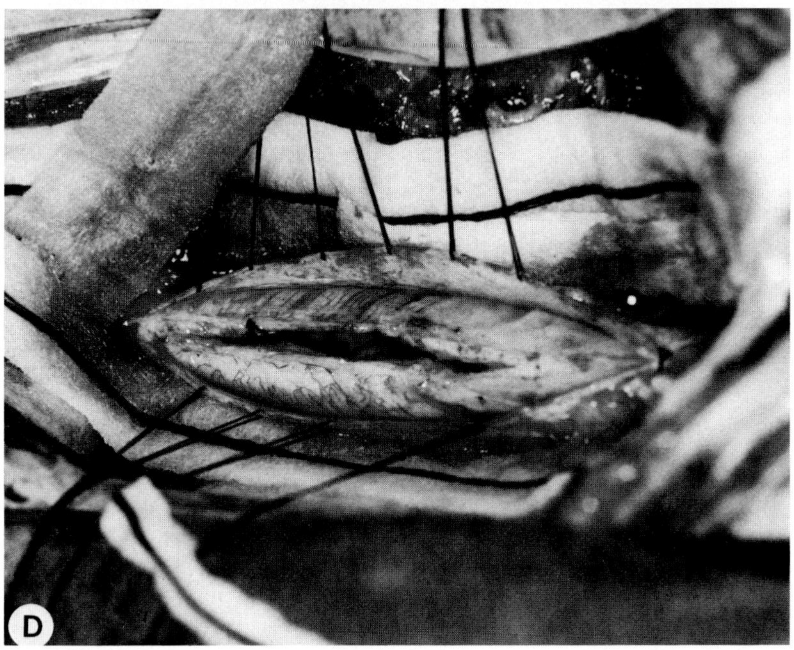

TREATMENT

Elsberg[13] and Elsberg and Beer[14] first advocated radical removal of intramedullary tumors in classical reports in which a two-stage procedure was described. At the first surgery, a long midline posterior myelotomy overlying the tumor was performed, following which the dura was not closed. One week later the wound was reopened and a large volume of tumor was extruded through the myelotomy, facilitating the establishment of a clear plane of cleavage and total tumor excision. Since that time, Elsberg's underlying thesis concerning the feasibility of total tumor removal has been established by many neurosurgeons, although utilization of the operating microscope has obviated the need for a two-stage procedure.[1,5,8,16,18,19,25,26,32,36]

Surgical exploration is mandatory for any child with a progressively symptomatic intramedullary mass. There is no justification for giving radiation therapy without obtaining a definitive tissue diagnosis. Furthermore, in most situations surgery should be directed toward total or radical removal of the tumor; there is no acceptable rationale for intending only to obtain a biopsy specimen and then automatically administering a full course of "postoperative" radiation therapy.

The contemporary neurosurgeon must have a clear understanding of the necessity for pursuing radical or even total tumor excision when technically possible. Ependymomas are clearly demarcated from adjacent normal cord, and therefore in most circumstances may be totally extirpated. Even with an astrocytoma, there is often an interface between the pseudocapsule and normal spinal cord, which serves as a cleavage plane facilitating radical, or occasionally "total," removal.[16]

When dealing with an intramedullary congenital tumor (dermoid, teratoma), it is safest to evacuate its contents while leaving the anterior cyst wall, which is often inseparable from normal neural tissue, intact.

Inasmuch as these tumors commonly grow over multiple spinal segments, it is essential that the laminectomy be of sufficient length to expose the mass completely. The facets must be undisturbed inasmuch as injury potentiates the likelihood of postoperative spine deformity.[34]

The operating microscope and the bipolar cautery are indispensable adjuncts to spinal cord surgery.

After the dura is opened, the surgeon will observe a swollen cord with abnormal surface vasculature. Rarely, when hydromyelia is present, the cord is collapsed secondary to the escape of CSF on opening the subarachnoid space. In some situations it is possible to identify the anatomic midline of the spinal cord by the median vein that traverses it. Occasionally careful inspection of the surface of the cord will disclose an area in which tumor is close to the surface. The surface vasculature is coagulated over the midline, or just adjacent to the median vein, and the pia is incised and retracted with 7–0 sutures, exposing the interior of the cord. It is essential that the myelotomy, which will not result in permanent neurologic deficit, extend over the entire length of the tumor, as a limited exposure will only permit biopsy or inadequte tumor removal.

Occasionally the myelotomy will open into a large cystic cavity, which must be differentiated from hydromyelia. In the latter situation, the fluid is crystal clear whereas a cyst adjacent to a tumor, which occurs in approximately 20 percent of intramedullary neoplasms, contain deeply xanthochromic fluid.[29]

Utilizing microdissectors and very fine suction, the thin layer and white matter overlying the tumor is removed. When the tumor is exposed, an attempt is made to define a cleavage plan between it and the surrounding cord. During the tumor excision, the small vessels that pass from the spinal cord into the tumor are coagulated with the bipolar coagulator under constant saline irrigation, which prevents the current from passing into adjacent spinal cord. Occasionally the pursuit of the tumor will terminate at the anterior pial surface along the entire length of the myelotomy. Although a huge cavity appears with little functional residual cord tissue, most of the dorsal lateral spinal cord is intact but compressed, and in most cases no permanent injury results from a radical exturpation (Fig. 46–5).

Following total or radical removal of the tumor, the dura is tightly closed. If total removal was not technically feasible and the cord remains swollen, the dura is left open and sutured to the adjacent muscles. A dural substitute is utilized to prevent the evolution of a large postoperative pseudomeningocele.

For cases in which hydromyelia is encountered, there are a spectrum of

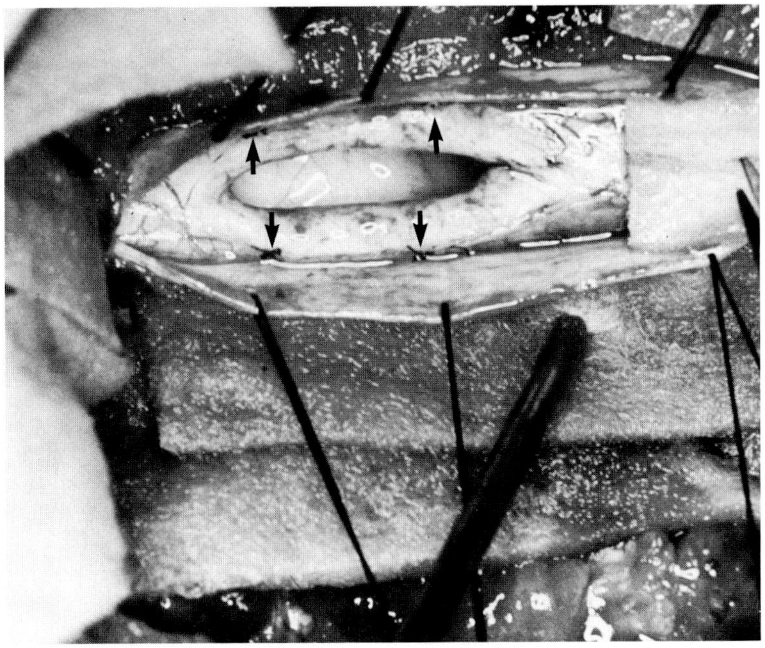

Figure 46-6. Classical, massively dilated, cystic central canal, which is pathognomonic of hydromyelia. Note sutures that pass from pia to anterior lateral dura (arrows), marsupializing cyst to spinal fluid circulation.

procedures that have been advocated by various authors[4,7,15,24,31,35,37] It would seem that, as the first endeavor, the simplest and least hazardous technique should be employed. If the diagnosis is made preoperatively, the hydrocephalus is present, a shunting procedure is indicated. If the hydromyelia is operated on directly, the cavity must be opened over an extensive length and the pia sutured to the anterior lateral margin of the dura along the entire myelotomy (Fig. 46-6). In this way a large segment of the hydromyelic cavity is marsupialized to the spinal fluid circulation. The dura may then be closed, or left open, at the discretion of the surgeon.

Another equally rational technique in dealing with large hydromyelic cysts is continuous drainage via a shunt within the cyst cavity, with the distal tubing terminating in the pleural cavity.

One may conclude with some certainty, however, that given the large number of techniques that have been advocated for this condition, the ideal one has yet to be discovered.

POSTOPERATIVE COURSE

Although commonly there is a transient increase in motor dysfunction, this usually improves rapidly and, often within a few days, the patient is as strong as, or stronger than preoperatively. Steroids (solumedral, medral, prednisone 2 mg/kg/24 hr, or the equivalent), which are a mandatory adjunct to surgery, may be discontinued over 10 days to two weeks. It is essential that patients be followed closely from an orthopedic perspective, as kyphosis as well as scoliosis may be a late complication of the combination of laminectomy and intrinsic spinal cord pathology.

In the cervical region, kyphosis develops in approximately 26 percent of patients.[34] Elsewhere in the spine, scoliosis and lordosis may occur, and frequent x-ray examination in combination with orthopedic evaluation and utilization of postoperative support to the spine is essential in children who have yet to pass through rapid growth.[6,30,34] Rarely, cervical kyphosis may become so advanced

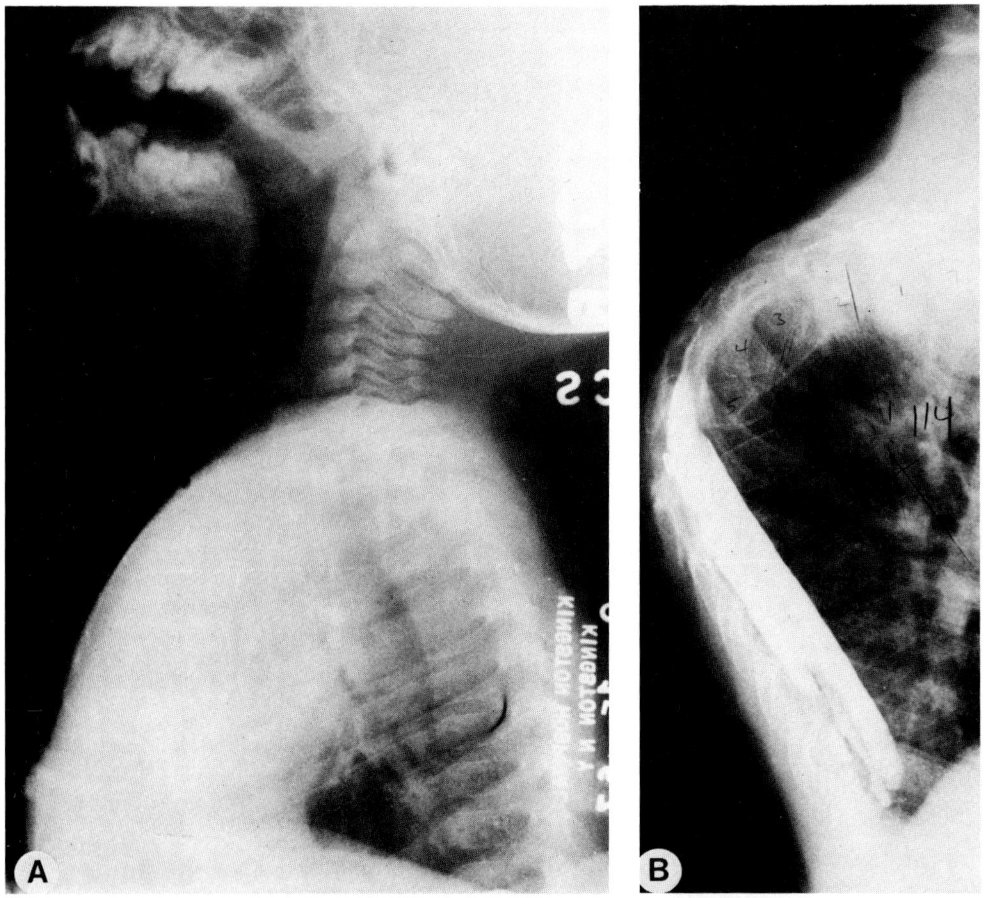

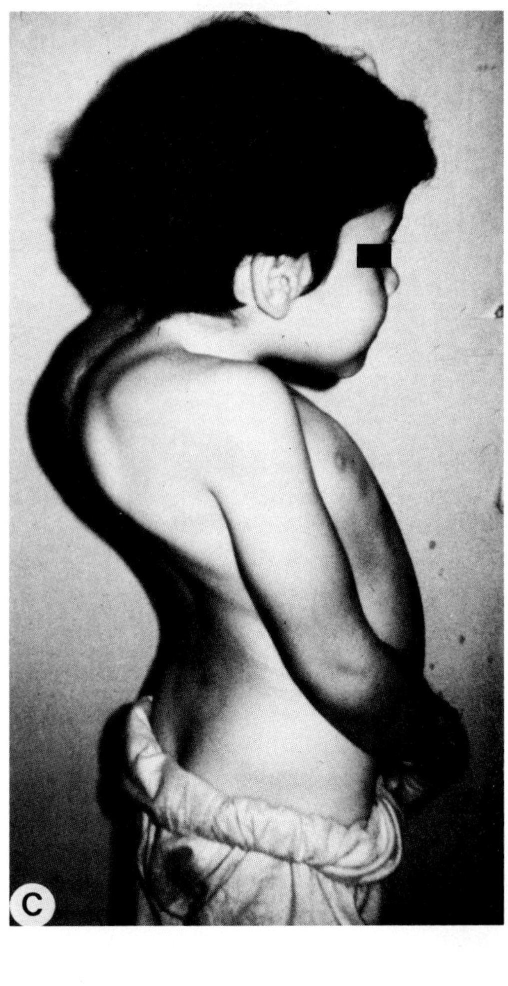

Figure 46-7. A. Preoperative plane x-ray of 5-year-old child with cervicothoracic intramedullary astrocytoma. B. Same child four years following cervicothoracic laminectomy. Note marked kyphosis with complete myelographic block. C. Same patient showing classical postlaminectomy "swan neck" deformity.

that it causes cord compression, and many years later may masquerade as recurrent tumor for which inappropriate surgery is undertaken (Fig. 46-7).

The place of radiation therapy as a postoperative adjunct is controversial.[1,8,16,18,19] Low-grade astrocytomas elsewhere in the nervous system are relatively insensitive to radiation therapy, and although more often than not it has been utilized in this patient population, there is no well-documented evidence that it is effective. The biologic behavior of intraspinal low-grade astrocytomas, with or without radiotherapy, is quite unpredictable; in many cases the tumor recurs and results in complete disability, but in a few it remains static or does not recur.[22] There have been long-term survivals with myelotomy and biopsy as well as with biopsy plus radiation.[1,2,18,19,36] One must conclude that although many of these patients have been radiated, there is no clear evidence that this is entirely responsible for the occasional favorable long-term results that may follow subtotal surgical excision of intramedullary astrocytomas. At the present time, it would seem that a radical or "total" excision of a spinal cord tumor makes postoperative radiation a controversial adjunct, while following a subtotal removal or biopsy, it would seem a reasonable undertaking.

REFERENCES

1. Anderson FM, Carson JJ: Spinal cord tumors in children: A review of the subject and presentation of 21 cases. J Pediatric 43:190–207, 1953
2. Arseni C, Horvath L, Iliescu D: Intraspinal tumors in children. Psychiatr Neurol Neurol Neurochir 70:123–133, 1976
3. Banna M, Gryspaerat GL: Review article: Intraspinal tumors in children (excluding dysraphism). Radiology 22:17–32, 1971
4. Bertrand B: Dynamic factors in the evolution of syringomyelia and syringobulbia. Clin Neurosurg 20:322–333, 1973
5. Cairns H, Riddoch G: Observation in the treatment of ependymal gliomas of the spinal cord. Brain 14: 117, 1931
6. Catell HS, Clark GL Jr: Cervical kyphosis and instability following multiple laminectomies in children. J Bone Jt Surg 49-a:713–720, 1967
7. Conway LW: Hydrodynamic studies in syringomyelia. J Neurosurg 27:501–514, 1967
8. Coxe WS: Tumors of the spinal canal in children. Am Surg 27:62–73, 1961
9. Craig J, Mitchell A: Spinal tumors in childhood. Arch Dis Child 6:11-16, 1931
10. DeSousa AL, Kalseech JE, Mealey J Jr, et al: Intraspinal tumors in children: A review of 31 cases. J Neurosurg 51:437-445, 1979
11. Eden K: Dissemination after gliomas of the spinal cord in the leptomeninges. Brain 61:298, 1938
12. Ellertson AB, et al: Myelocystographic and fluorescein studies to demonstrate communication between intramedullary cysts and the cerebrospinal fluid space. Acta Neurol Scand 45:418–430, 1969
13. Elsberg CA: Diagnosis and Treatment of Surgical Diseases of the spinal cord and Its Membranes. Philadelphia and London, WB Saunders, 1916, pp 288–289
14. Elsberg CA, Beer R: The operability of intramedullary tumors of the spinal cord. A report of two operations with remarks upon the extrusion of intraspinal tumors. Am J Med Sci 142:636–647, 1911
15. Gardner WJ, Angel J: The mechanism of syringomyelia and its surgical correction. Clin Neurosurg 6:131–140, 1959
16. Garrido, E., Stein, B.M.: Microsurgical Removal of Intramedullary Spinal Cord Tumors. Surg. Neurol. 7:214–219, 1977
17. Grant FC, Austin GM: The diagnosis, treatment and prognosis of tumors affecting the spinal cord in children. J Neurosurg 13:535–545, 1956
18. Greenwood J: Surgical removal of intramedullary tumors. J Neurosurg 26:276–283, 1967

19. Guidetti B: Intramedullary tumors of the spinal cord. Acta neurochir 17:7–23, 1967
20. Haft H, Ransohoff J, Carter S: Spinal cord tumors in children. Pediatrist 23:1152–1159, 1959
21. Hamby WB: Tumors in the spinal canal in childhood. J Neuropathol Exp Neurol 3:347–412, 1944
22. Ingraham FD: Intraspinal tumors in infancy and childhood. Am J Surg 39:342–376, 1938
23. Kernohan JW, Woltman HW, Adson AW: A review of 51 cases with an attempt at histological classification. Arch Neurol Psychiatr 25:679–710, 1931
24. Love JG: Syringomyelia: A look at surgical therapy. J Neurosurg 24:714–718, 1966
25. Mork SJ, Liken AC: Ependymoma: A followup study of 101 cases. Cancer 40:907–915, 1977
26. Pool JL: The surgery of spinal cord tumors. Clin Neurosurg 17:310–330, 1970
27. Rasmussen TB, Kernohan JW, Adson AW: Pathologic classification with surgical consideration of intraspinal tumors. Ann Surg 3:513–530, 1940
28. Richardson FL: A report of 16 tumors of the spinal cord in children: The importance of spinal rigidity as an early sign of disease. J Pediatr 57:42–54, 1960.
29. Shenkin HA, Alpers BJ: Clinical and pathologic features of gliomas of the spinal cord Arch Neurol Psychiatr 52:87-105, 1944
30. Sim FH, Svien HJ, Bickel WH, et al: Swan-neck deformity following extensive cervical laminectomy. J Bone Jt Surg 49-A:564–579, 1967
31. Singouras EG, et al: Terminal ventriculostomy in syringomyelia. Acta Neurochir (Vienna) 46:293–295, 1979
32. Stookey B: Tumors of the spinal cord in childhood. Am J Dis Child 36:1184–1203, 1928
33. Svien HJ, Thelen EP, Keith HM: Intraspinal tumors in children. JAMA 155:959, 1954
34. Tachdjian MO, Matson DD: Orthopedic aspects of intraspinal tumors in infants and children. J Bone Jt Surg 47-A:223-248, 1965
35. Wetzel N, Davis L: Surgical treatment of syringomyelia. Arch Surg 68:570–573, 1954
36. Woltman HW, Kernohan JW, Adson AW, et al: Intramedullary tumors of the spinal cord and gliomas of the intradural portion of the filum terminale. Arch Neurol Psychiatr 65:378–395, 1951
37. Worster-Drough C, Wakeley LPG, Shafar J: The surgical treatment of syringomyelia. Br J Surg 29:56–73, 1941

47. Extramedullary Spinal Tumors

Robert L. McLaurin

Extramedullary tumors constitute approximately two thirds of all intraspinal tumors occurring in childhood. There are several methods of classifying such lesions but we shall classify them as discussed in the following section. It must be noted that because of the relative rarity of intraspinal tumors in this age group, no single author has had wide experience and the material presented has been obtained from a review of several authors.[1–5]

Clinically extramedullary spinal tumors present with signs of progressive loss of cord junction. Although frequently difficult to recognize in younger age groups, motor weakness is probably the most common symptom. Pain is another frequent symptom, and is more likely to be present than with intramedullary tumors of the cord. Other symptoms that are recorded in all major series include torticollis, scoliosis, weakness of upper extremities, and urinary incontinence. The type of tumor is generally not predictable on the basis of its clinical presentation.

TUMORS ASSOCIATED WITH CONGENITAL SPINAL DYSRAPHISM

These tumors, histologically benign, include dermoids, epidermoids, teratomas, and neurenteric cysts, usually accompanied by dysraphism, and lipomas, which may occur with or without associated structural defect.

Dermoids and epidermoid tumors are frequently, but not always, associated with a dermal sinus opening on the skin surface and occur most commonly in the lumbosacral region.[6] As with cranial dermal sinuses, the surface opening is quite small, and frequently difficult to detect, but may be accompanied by discoloration or thickening of the adjacent skin. Occasionally the tumor may occur without a dermal sinus, although it is generally assumed that the sinus and tumor arise from incomplete separation of the cutaneous and neuroectodermal cells.

The principal complication of the sinus tract is that it acts as a source of meningeal infection. The dermoid or epidermoid tumor, however, acts as an

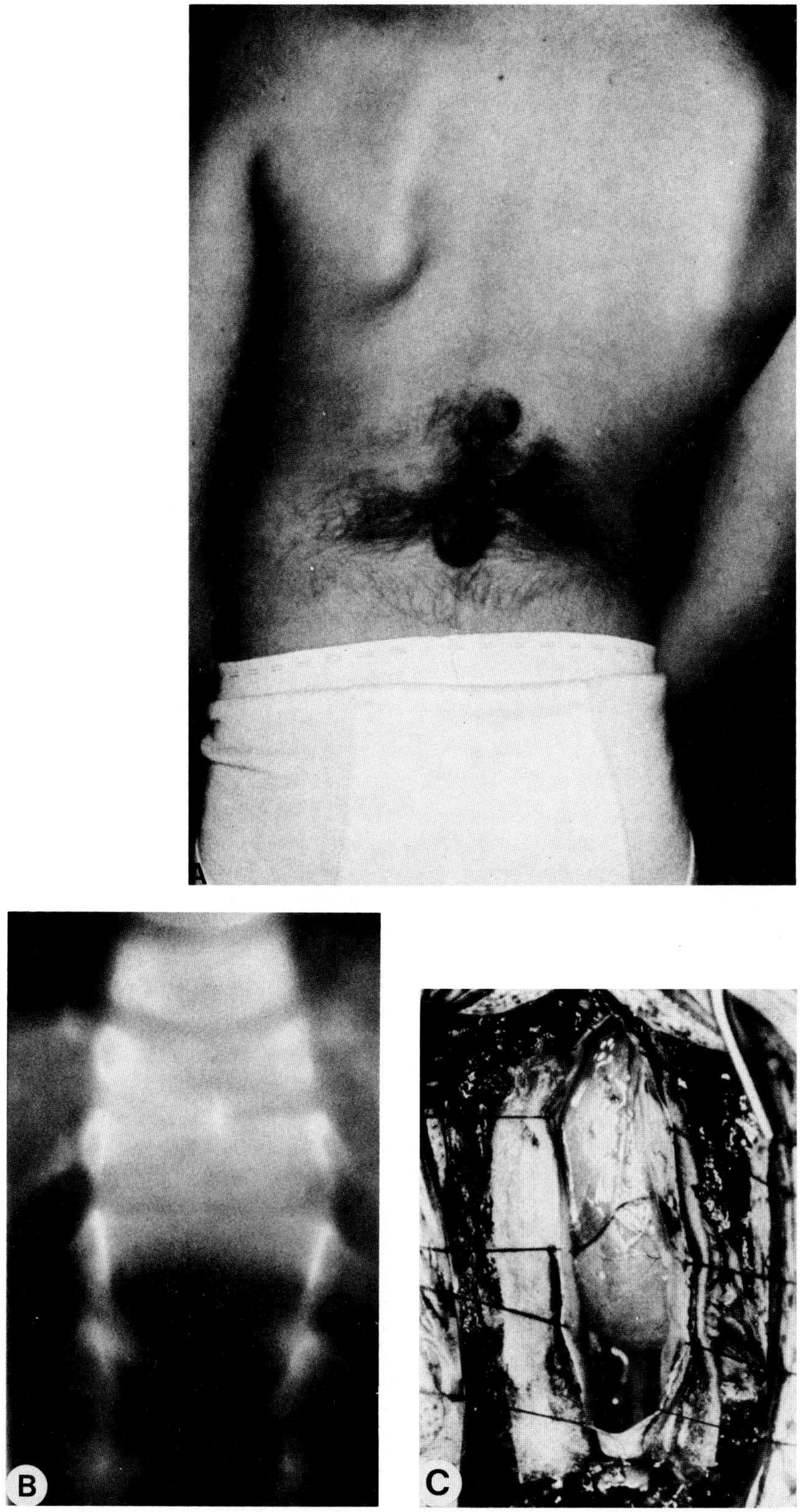

Figure 47-1. Teratoma in 8-year-old male. A. Hirsute area in lumbodorsal region associated with scoliosis. B. Laminogram showing widening of spinal canal, flattening of pedicles, and midline bony spicule. C. Teratoma below level of diastematomyelia.

expanding intraspinal mass. The tumor may be extradural, intradural, or intramedullary. Dermoids, however, are rarely intramedullary. The tumors may present, therefore, with evidence of neurologic deficit superimposed on a past history of episodic meningitis. Pain and stiffness of the spine are common symptoms with these lesions. Rarely the tumor may present as clinical meningitis, presumably due to the irritant effect of the cyst contents in the subarachnoid space.[7]

The diagnosis is usually evident from the surface manifestation and confirmed by dysraphism on x-ray examination. Evidence of raised intraspinal pressure, as indicated by scalloping of the posterior margins of the vertebral bodies and widening of the interpedicular distance, is usually present. Treatment is designed to remove the sinus tract as well as the intraspinal tumor cyst. Unless the cyst is intramedullary, this usually can be accomplished without neurologic trauma. There is no role of radiation therapy in the management of these lesions.

Teratoid tumors, including derivatives of two or three primitive cell layers, are less commonly accompanied by a dermal sinus (Fig. 47-1). The sacrococcygeal region is the most frequent site of teratomas related to the spine but is not truly an intraspinal lesion. As with other congenital lesions, the lumbosacral level is the most common intraspinal site. The tumors are intradural and can usually be completely excised.

The neurenteric cyst represents a special type of congenital tumor (Fig. 47-2). Although the precise embryologic basis is not well understood, it is presumed to arise from entodermal remnants that have failed to separate from notochord. The notochordal plate is initially in close contact with the entoderm and normally separates from the entoderm and becomes surrounded by mesodermal cells. If separation fails to occur, entodermal cells are drawn into the spinal

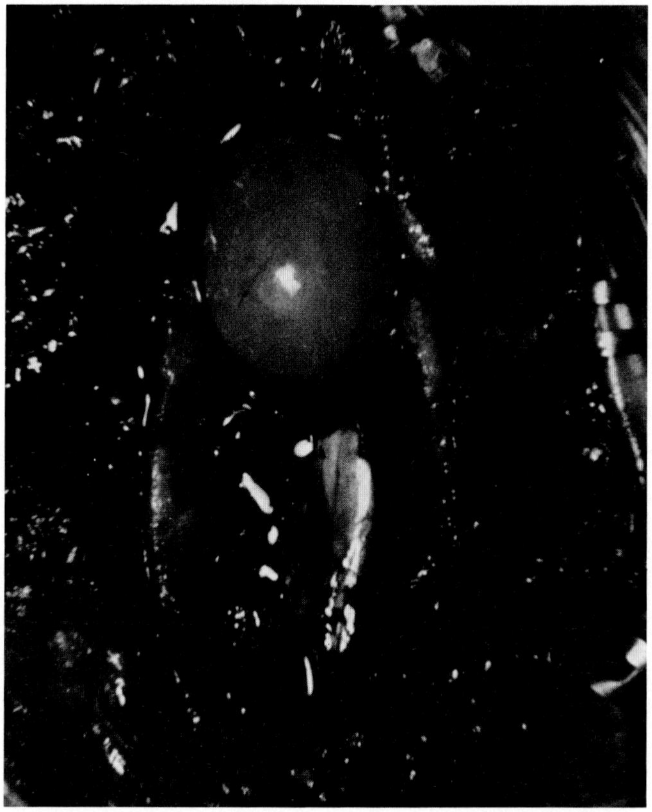

Figure 47-2. Neurenteric cyst in 5-year-old male presenting with pain and spasm of spine.

canal anteriorly, similar to the development of a dermal sinus and dermoid posteriorly.[8] The most common site is the dorsal region and the intraspinal component may be extradural or intradural. The signs depend on the level of cord compression. Histologically the cyst is lined by cuboidal cells or mucus-secreting epithelium. The most characteristic diagnostic feature is the presence of a defect in the vertebral body anterior to the canal; such a defect, however, is not necessarily present. Excision usually can be accomplished, although an extraspinal component may require a separate surgical procedure.

Lipomas most often occur in association with developmental defects of the spine but occasionally occur as discrete lesions.[9,10] In the latter form, they constitute approximately 5 percent of intraspinal tumors in childhood. When part of a dysraphic state, they are accompanied by neurologic signs that usually do not progress. Lipomas are most commonly found in the lumbar spine entwined among the roots of the cauda equina. The tumor may be attached to the conus, the filum terminale, or the cauda equina. The neurologic signs are not correlated with the site of tumor attachment. Even with the assistance of magnification, complete removal is usually not possible, and may be unnecessary as clinical experience has demonstrated a frequent lack of neurologic progression after partial excision. There is no evidence that radiation treatment has any beneficial effect.

TUMORS SEEDING VIA CEREBROSPINAL FLUID

Metastatic tumors within the subarachnoid space are more frequently seen in the pediatric age group than in adults. Although the reasons for the tendency to "seed" within the nervous system demonstrated by some tumors are not understood, there are, nevertheless, certain histologic types that are noteworthy in this regard.

The most frequent metastatic tumor of the nervous system is the medulloblastoma. McFarland, Horwitz, Saenger, et al.[11] reviewed a series of 430 medulloblastomas in the literature and found an incidence of 33 percent with metastasis. The metastases were distinguishable from recurrences within the posterior fossa. Ninety-four percent of the metastases were spinal. The development of spinal metastases after an interval of apparent freedom from disease worsens the overall prognosis. The frequency of spinal metastases occurring with this tumor is the basis for the current practice of radiating the entire spine after confirming the type of tumor in the posterior fossa. Occasionally the initial presentation of medulloblastoma will be the effect of a metastatic spinal lesion.

Ependymomas also may spread throughout the subarachnoid space. This tendency is shared with choroid plexus papillomas, which are closely related to the ependymomas. Since many spinal metastases may not be recognized prior to the patient's death from the intracranial tumor, the true incidence of spinal metastases can only be determined by routine examination of the spinal cord at necropsy. Using this method, Svien and Gates[12] found an incidence of 31.6 percent in a series of 19 cases. Further, spinal implantation occurs only from ependymomas that arise below the tentorium within the fourth ventricle. As with medulloblastomas the spinal metastases may be clinically silent or may be responsible for the initial presentation of the tumor. Choroid plexus papillomas have shown spinal seeding in approximately 20 percent of cases.[13]

Russell and Rubenstein[14] reported 21 cases of pineocytoma with widespread metastases in 10 (seven were pineoblastomas and three malignant pineocytomas). They concluded that the more primitive forms of pineal parenchymal tumors are probably related to medulloblastoma. Germinomas, occurring in the pineal region, also may metastasize to the spinal cord.

There are basically two types of spinal subarachnoid metastases. The more common type consists of discrete nodular implants on the cord and spinal nerve roots. The implants may be few or may be profusely seeded throughout. It is reported that more lesions are seen on the dorsal surface of the cord, reflecting the pattern of cerebrospinal fluid flow from the fourth ventricle. The discrete metastases are seen as filling defects on myelography while large coalescent aggregates may cause complete obstruction. The second type of metastasis consists of diffuse meningeal involvement, which may give a myelographic picture similar to adhesive arachnoiditis.

TUMORS OF THE MENINGES

Meningeal tumors presenting in childhood are more rare than in adulthood. In this respect they are similar to nerve root tumors. Matson[4] reported three such tumors in his series of 134 intraspinal tumors. The histologic, clinical, and therapeutic features are similar to the lesions presenting in later life; they are generally single, benign, and surgically correctible.

Arachnoidal cysts, not a true neoplasm, may occur in childhood and act as an expanding lesion with gradual cord compression. Nugent, Odom, and Woodhall[15] found that 19 of 45 patients with this lesion were between 11 and 20 years of age. The cysts may be intradural or extradural and most often occur dorsal to the cord in the thoracic region. The extradural cyst is thought to represent a herniation through a congenital dural defect. The origin of intradural cysts is not clear. In children a high incidence of kyphoscoliosis is present. The principal complaint is intermittent pain and weakness, which may be accentuated in the upright posture and which is thought to be related to gravitational filling of the cyst and cord compression. The diagnosis can usually be substantiated preoperatively by filling of the cyst on myelography when the patient is supine and emptying when prone. Treatment is by excision of the cyst and repair of the dural defect if present.

TUMORS OF NERVE ROOTS

Pathologists are not agreed on the terminology of tumor of the spinal nerve roots. Russell and Rubenstein[14] (1977) separate the solitary encapsulated lesions, which they call schwannomas, from the tumors that are associated with Recklinhausen's disease. Other authors do not make this distinction.

Unlike its incidence in adults, in whom it is probably the most common intraspinal tumor, neurofibroma is quite rare in childhood. In Matson's series[4] it constituted about 5 percent of intraspinal tumors. Clinically the presence of progressive scoliosis in a young child suggests this type of tumor whereas the x-ray characteristic is erosion of an intervertebral foramen as the tumor extends along the spinal nerve to become a "dumbbell" lesion. Total excision of the tumor is necessary to prevent recurrence and separate operative approaches may be needed for the intraspinal and extraspinal components. Radiation has no role in the management of this lesion unless elements of neurofibrosarcoma are present.

In the largest series thus far reported, Gautier-Smith[16] found, in a series of 115 spinal neurofibromas, that 11 were in patients under 20 years of age and one occurred in the first decade. Those in childhood were equally distributed through the cervical, thoracic, and lumbar spine. The majority of tumors were intradural, with occasional extensions to the extradural space or through the intervertebral foramen.

TUMORS OF BONE

Primary tumors of the vertebrae are rare in infancy and childhood. Any tumor, whether primary or metastatic, however, may compromise the spinal canal and lead to compression myelopathy or radiculopathy.

The aneurysmal bone cyst occurs most commonly in children and young adults and the vertebral column is one of the common sites.[17] The neural arch is the most frequently involved portion of the vertebra, although the body occasionally may be affected. The cyst is characterized by localized distention and destruction of bone and is limited by a thin shell. Radiographically the lesion appears as an expansile lytic process surrounded by a thin cortical shell (Figure 47-3). Clinically the patient usually has pain and stiffness of the affected portion of the spine associated with evidence of cord compression in more advanced cases.

The aneurysmal bone cyst is a benign lesion that is not a true neoplasm but rather a vascular malformation. Treatment should be instituted promptly since the lesion may enlarge rather rapidly. The preferred treatment is curettage of the bone cyst; even incomplete curettage may result in progressive obliteration of the cyst and healing. Radiotherapy has also been used effectively in patients resistant to surgical cure.

Osteogenic sarcoma, while rare, may cause extensive destruction of the bodies and neural arches. Fragmentation and collapse of a body may result. In addition to the bony changes seen by x-ray, there is likely to be seen a paraspinal

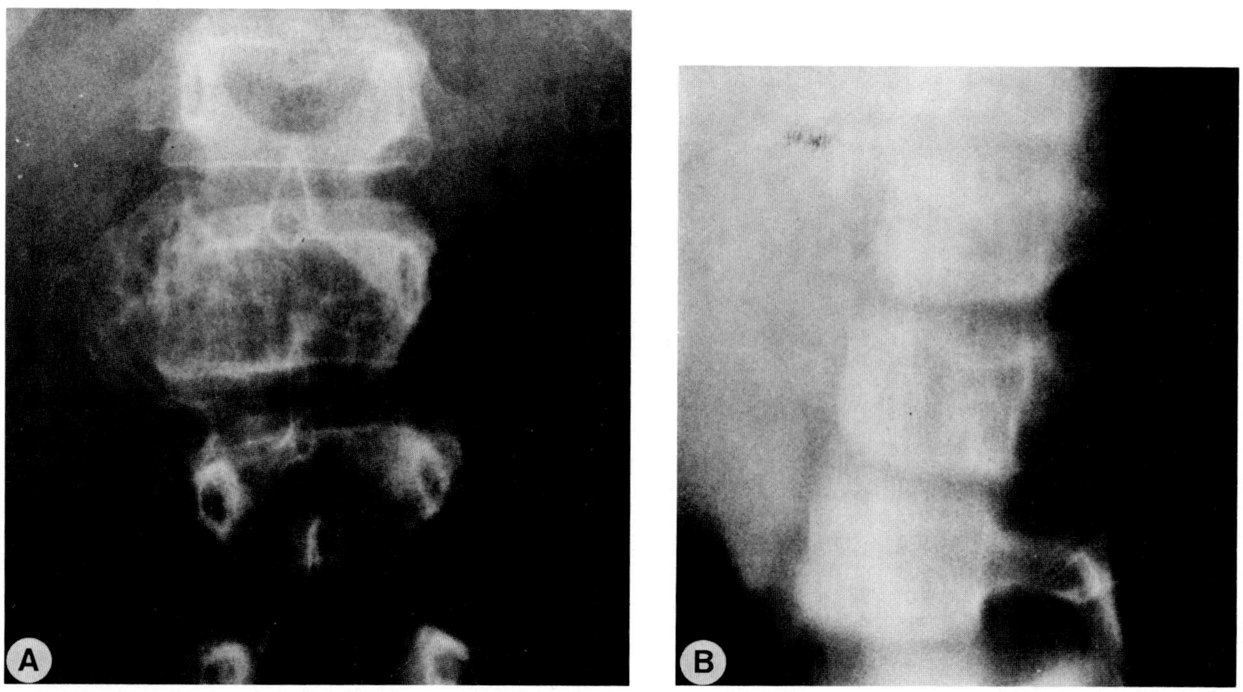

Figure 47-3. Aneurysmal bone cyst. A. Characteristic radiologic appearance in anteroposterior projection. B. Expanded lytic lesion of pedicle as seen in lateral laminogram.

neoplastic mass. Giant cell tumors may also cause destruction and vertebral collapse with consequent compromise of the spinal cord. Hemangioma, probably the most common tumor of the spine, usually produces no symptoms. Radiologically it is characterized by a spongy or honeycomb osteoporosis.

Chordomas are extremely rare in the spinal canal of children, although approximately half of chordomas seen in all ages occur in the sacrococcygeal region. The tumor is considered to arise from notocordal remnants and grows by erosion and compression of adjacent structures rather than by invasion. Such tumors do not metastasize. The signs are those of slowly progressive compression of the cauda equina associated with destructive changes in the sacrum. Treatment is mainly surgical, although radiation therapy has been used with some prolongation of the disease course.

TUMORS INVADING THE EPIDURAL SPACE

Tumors of the autonomic nervous system may enter the spinal canal through an intervertebral foramen and result in a "dumbbell" tumor. These tumors are of the neuroblastoma–ganglioneuroblastoma–ganglioneuroma spectrum.[18] There is a 2:1 ratio of male to female incidence in all series published.

It is important to note that a 10 percent spontaneous cure rate has been seen with neuroblastomas of childhood. Some authors feel that the sympathetic tumors all arise originally as neuroblastomas. Maturation of some of these lesions would be consistent with a spontaneous cure.

The prognosis of the sympathetic tumor spectrum is obviously quite variable. The ganglioneuroma is a benign tumor and is generally surgically curable. The neuroblastoma, on the other hand, is highly malignant but may run a benign course with surgical and radiation treatment. The prognosis for neuroblastomas occurring in the first year of life is significantly better than for those occurring later. If there is evidence of distant metastases, particularly in bone or bone marrow, the prognosis is extremely poor. If there is no evidence of distant metastases, every effort should be made to remove the tumor totally.

The roentgenographic appearance of a dumbbell autonomic tumor is basically that of a paraspinal mass with associated changes in adjacent ribs and spinal canal. The mass may or may not contain calcium and, if located in the supra- or pararenal region, may result in displacement of the kidney. The skeletal changes include separation and erosion of the posterior aspects of adjacent ribs, localized scoliosis of the spine, erosion or flattening of the pedicles, widening of the spinal canal, and scalloping of the posterior aspect of the vertebral bodies. Sclerosis and enlargement of the intervertebral foramen may be noted. Myelography shows a partial or complete block (Figure 47-4).

Surgical treatment should consist of staged intraspinal and extraspinal approaches. The sequence of these procedures depends primarily on the neurologic state and the rate of deterioration at the time the diagnosis is made. The lesion, which is extradural, can generally be completely excised to its point of entrance into the spinal canal. The remaining extraspinal portion is then excised as a separate operation. If the tumor is a neuroblastoma or ganglioneuroblastoma, the surgical excision is followed by radiation and chemotherapy.

Chemical markers of autonomic tumors include several catecholamines. The urinary excretions of these substances are important in the initial diagnosis and also in the postoperative period as indicators of recurrence or metastases.

Although leukemia only rarely causes mass lesions in the spinal canal, Hodgkin's granuloma is not so uncommon.[19] It invades the extradural space and results in cord compression. Although the tumor is responsive to radiation

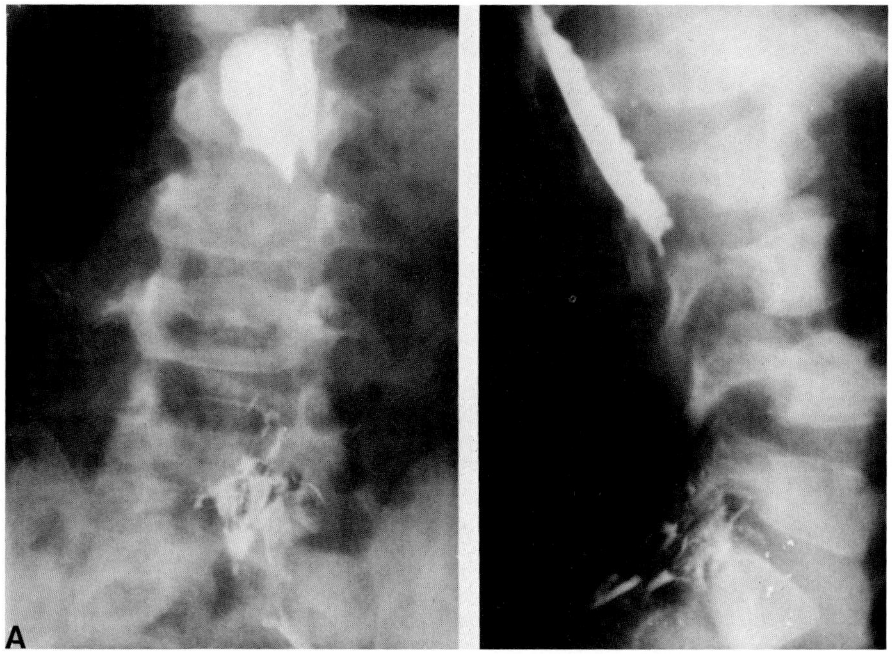

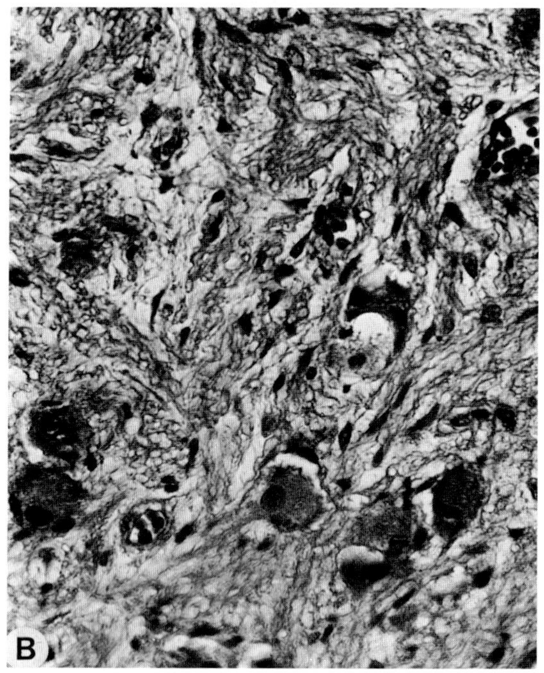

Figure 47-4. A. Anteroposterior and lateral views of myelogram of patient with dumbbell ganglioneuroma. The intraspinal portion of tumor is characterized by interpedicular widening, scalloping of vertebral bodies, and myelographic blockage at L2–3. B. Histologic appearance of benign ganglioneuroma showing mature neuronal cell bodies in fibrous stroma.

therapy, the presence of rapidly progressive paralysis may make surgical decompression necessary. Steroids are usually effective in reversing and slowing the neurologic deterioration temporarily.

Wilhyde, Jane, and Mullan[20] reviewed 42 cases of spinal epidural leukemia and reported that two thirds of these were in patients less than 20 years of age. The tumors were found at all levels of the epidural space and varied from discrete localized deposits to sheets of tumor extending over many spinal segments. The most common location seems to be in the posterior epidural space. It has been noted that if epidural tumor formation does occur in the course of leukemia, it is the initial manifestation in two thirds of the cases. Otherwise, it appears early in the course of leukemia.

REFERENCES

1. Hamby W: Tumors in the spinal canal in childhood. J Neuropath Exp Neurol 3:397–412, 1944
2. Haft H, Ransohoff J, Carter S: Spinal cord tumors in children. Pediatrics 23:1152–1159, 1959
3. Coxe W: Tumors of the spinal canal in children. Am Surg 27:62–73, 1966
4. Matson DD: Neurosurgery of Infancy and Childhood (ed 2). Springfield, C Thomas, 1969, p 934
5. Banna M, Gryspeerdt G: Intraspinal tumours in children (excluding dyspaphism). Clin Radiol 22:17–32, 1971
6. Bailey I: Dermoid tumors of the spinal cord. J Neurosurg 33:676–681, 1970
7. Decker R, Gross S: Intraspinal dermoid tumor presenting as chemical meningitis. J Neurosurg 27:60–62, 1967
8. Dorsey J, Tabrisky J: Intraspinal and mediastinal foregut cyst compressing the spinal cord. J Neurosurg 24:562–567, 1966
9. Rogers HM, Long DM, Chou SN, et al: Lipomas of the spinal cord and cauda equina. J Neurosurg 34:349–354, 1971
10. Thomas J, Miller R: Lipomatous tumors of the spinal canal: A study of their clinical range. Mayo Clin Proc 48:393–400, 1973
11. McFarland DR, Horwitz H, Saenger EL, et al: Medulloblastoma—A review of prognosis and survival. Br J Radiol 42:198–214, 1969
12. Svien H, Gates E: Spinal subarachnoid implantation associated with ependymoma. Arch Neurol Psychiatr 62:847–856, 1949
13. Herren R: Papilloma of the choroid plexus. Arch Surg 42:758–774, 1941
14. Russell D, Rubinstein L: Pathology of Tumours of the Nervous System (ed 4). Baltimore, Williams & Wilkins, 1977, p 448 (see p 293)
15. Nugent G, Odom G, Woodhall B: Spinal extradural cysts. Neurology 9:397–406, 1959
16. Gautier-Smith P: Clinical aspects of spinal neurofibromas. Brain 90:359–394, 1967
17. McArthur R, Fisher R: Aneurysmal bone cyst involving the vertebral column. J Neurosurg 24:772–776, 1966
18. Balakrishnan V, Rice M, Simpson D: Spinal neuroblastomas. Diagnosis, treatment and prognosis. J Neurosurg 40:631–638, 1974
19. Hunt W, Bouroncle B, Meagher J: Neurologic complication of leukemias and lymphomas. J Neurosurg 16:135–151, 1959
20. Wilhyde D, Jane J, Mullan S: Spinal epidural leukemia. Am J Med 34:281–287, 1963

48. Neurofibromatosis

David M. Klein

Neurofibromatosis (Recklinghausen's disease) is the most common of the neurocutaneous syndromes (phakomatoses), a group of conditions characterized by cutaneous and neural manifestations typical for each, familial predisposition, and dysplastic involvement of other organ systems. Although there may be some overlap of manifestations, the pattern of affectation is almost always diagnostic for each condition.

Neurofibromatosis is distinguished by cutaneous café-au-lait spots and central and peripheral neurofibromas, with the latter frequently emerging as subcutaneous nodules. Crowe, Schull, and Neel[1] found an incidence in Michigan of one case in every 2500 to 3300 births. There is simple autosomal dominant inheritance with variable penetrance. As many as 50 percent of cases arise without familial history, thus suggesting a high rate of new genetic mutation. Increased serum levels of nerve growth factor are detectable but the significance of this remains unclear.[2,3] Miller and Hall[4] find greater morbidity in cases born to affected mothers than in those involving affected fathers or with new mutation, which suggests humoral meditation. Central neurofibromas are also reported to develop earlier where transmission is maternal.[5] A high incidence of associated tumor and malformation, not only of the central nervous system (CNS) but also of connective tissue throughout the body, is offered as evidence of disordered development originating independently in more than one germinal layer.

The severity and distribution of manifestations vary within the individual, with no consistency seen among affected relatives. New lesions can present at any time in life, but it is probable that a majority of those with severe impairment will show evidence of this by 10 years of age.[6] Café-au-lait spots are oval, flat, light-brown skin blemishes, which usually increase in size and number from the time of birth to maturity, and then recede slightly. Subcutaneous neurofibromas appear relatively later. They are shotty, nodular, ropy, or plexiform, and usually painless. Pedunculated lesions are uncommon in childhood. The skin may be thickened and fixed where infiltrated by a plexiform lesion. Patients with multiple superficial stigmata tend to have fewer CNS manifestations; those with "central neurofibromatosis" may show little or no superficial disease.

Neurofibroma or schwannoma can involve any part of the peripheral nervous system, including sensorimotor and visceral plexuses and spinal nerve roots, with the development of intraspinal or dumbbell tumors. Plexiform involvement of neck, scalp, or eyelids is common. Similar intraorbital infiltration can produce proptosis. Among cranial nerves, eighth nerve involvement predominates, and although acoustic neurinomas are mainly an adult development, they are occasionally noted in children, both with and without other stigmata and neurofibromatosis.[7–12]

A wide range of CNS abnormalities is found. Primary tumors can be single or multiple. Gliomas are most common in children but any type or combination of tumors may occur. Optic glioma is highly characteristic. Approximately 25 percent of children bearing this tumor are found to have neurofibromatosis; however, the true incidence may be considerably higher, since optic glioma can be the initial manifestation.[7,8,13,14] Stern, DiGiacinto, and Housepian[13] find a higher incidence of neurofibromatosis where the glioma involves one optic nerve (70 percent) or is multicentric (100 percent) than where the chiasm is involved (7 percent). Nontumoral CNS abnormalities include vascular malformations, syringomyelia, aqueduct stenosis, hydrocephalus, choroid plexus calcifications, and chorioretinal malformations.[15,16] Seizures and psychomotor retardation may relate to developmental abnormalities in cerebral cytoarchitecture, rather than to neoplasm.[17] Occlusive cerebrovascular disease is reported.[18,19]

Skeletal abnormalities are frequent. Scoliosis is reported by Fienman and Yakovac[20] in 20 percent of children under 12 years of age with neurofibromatosis, and in Holt's series[7] in 36 percent of those under 15 years of age. Three percent of all scoliosis patients have neurofibromatosis, according to Rezaian.[21] Sharp thoracic angulation is common, but spinal cord compression as a consequence of this condition alone is rare.[7,22–24] Congenital bowing of tibia and fibula, craniomegaly, localized gigantism, and circumscribed radiolucent defects are noted.[7,20]

Isolated mesodermal defects typical for neurofibromatosis may produce x-ray changes similar to those found with tumors that are also typical for neurofibromatosis, giving rise to a unique series of self-contained differential diagnoses. Calvarial defects, frequently lambdoid in location, need not be associated with local tumor; an enlarged optic foramen or chiasmatic sulcus (*J-shaped sella*) may be present without optic glioma; and a defect in the greater sphenoid wing, with or without pulsating exophthalmos, could suggest tumor to the unwary. Dysplastic scalloping of vertebral bodies and enlargements of intravertebral foramina can be indistinguishable from secondary changes seen with intraspinal tumor. The condition may or may not be associated with a thinned, greatly dilated dural sac and root sleeves (dural ectasia) (Fig. 48-1).[7,25] In turn the protrusion and dilatation of such a root sleeve, usually at the apex of a scoliotic curve (*intrathoracic meningocele*), can mimic mediastinal or dumbbell tumor.[26–28] Enlarged internal acoustic canals associated with similar ectatic root sleeves can suggest bilateral acoustic tumors on plain x-rays.[29,30]

Disturbances in sexual maturation may or may not be associated with pituitary-hypothalamic tumor.[20] Pheochromocytoma, a well-known development during adult years, is generally not the cause of hypertension seen in these children. Here the problem is usually related to renal artery stenosis. There is an increased incidence of nonneurologic tumors and leukemia.[31–34]

Sarcomas, arising either from malignant degeneration in existing neurofibromas or from primary new growth, are variously estimated to occur in from 3 to 29 percent of patients.[1,33–35] Brasfield and Das Gupta[34] suggest that for those surviving Recklinghausen's disease for 50 years or more, the chance of developing a malignant nerve tumor may be as great as 50 percent, but malignancy is

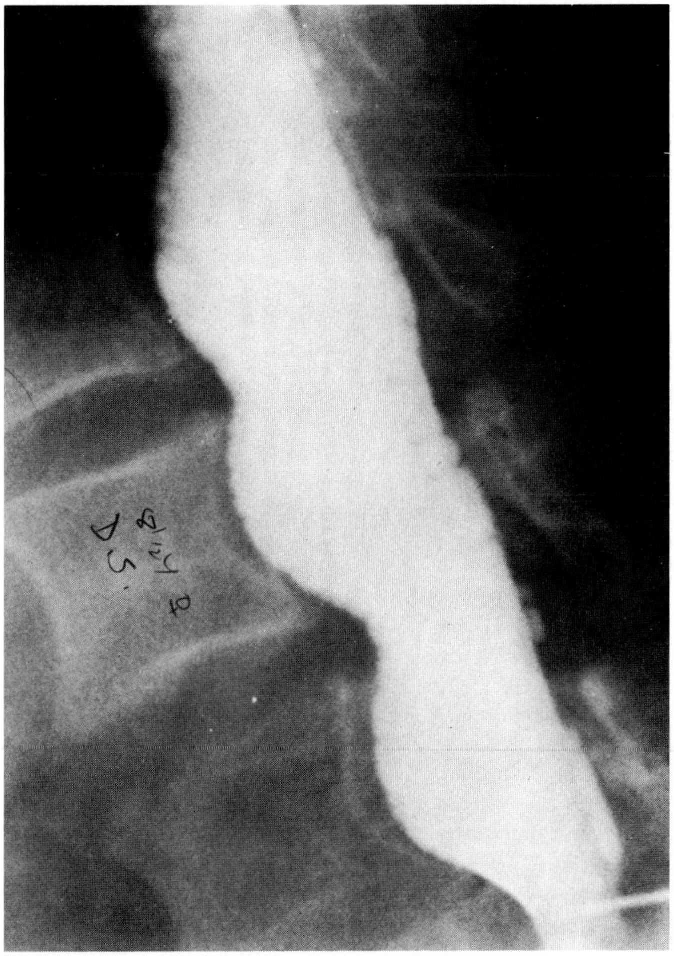

Figure 48-1. Lateral view of lumbar myelogram in an 8-year-old girl with neurofibromatosis. Note ectatic dural sac whose anterior border follows the scalloped posterior margins of corresponding vertebral bodies. No tumor was found.

uncommon in children. Childhood neurofibromas therefore can be considered benign until proved otherwise.

For diagnosis in children under 5 years of age, Whitehouse[36] found five or more cafe-au-lait spots, each at least 0.5 cm in greatest diameter, to be statistically significant. Over this age, six or more spots, each 1.5 cm or greater in diameter, were found diagnostic by Crowe and associates.[1] True neoplasms of peripheral nerves are rare in children, except where associated with generalized neurofibromatosis. Recklinghausen's disease therefore should be suspected whenever solitary neurofibroma is found in childhood, particularly if it is plexiform. Multiple subcutaneous nodules with biopsy confirmation, or the finding of multiple separate manifestations as noted, should be sufficient diagnostically. A positive family history is confirmatory. Computed tomography (CT) with or without intravenous or subarachnoid contrast enhancement is particularly helpful in distinguishing tumor from nontumor dysplasia. Radionuclide scanning has been reported to be useful in detecting malignant degeneration in neurofibromas.[37]

The outlook for a child with neurofibromatosis is difficult to estimate, but the prognosis is clearly poorer for those showing widespread, serious manifestations earlier in childhood.[6,34] The early emergence of central tumors, even if initially benign, suggests a potential for accelerated neoplasia that is frequently realized by late adolescence.

Treatment is that of individual manifestations, considered in the context of the overall disease state. Radical surgery may be justified when solitary lesions are progressive and potentially curable; a more conservative approach may be indicated for the same patient when lesions are static, profuse, or recurrent. Superficial tumors should be excised if mechanically symptomatic and well localized, or if rapid progression suggests malignancy.

Neurofibromatosis is a dynamic process. Every patient should have routine neurologic evaluations at scheduled intervals, including CT of appropriate body areas.

REFERENCES

1. Crowe FW, Schull WJ, Neel JV: Multiple Neurofibromatosis. Springfield, Charles C Thomas, 1956, p 181
2. Schenkein I, Bueker ED, Helson L, et al: Increased nerve-growth-stimulating activity in disseminated neurofibromatosis. N Engl J Med 290:613–614, 1974
3. Fabricant RN, Todaro GJ: Increased levels of a nerve-growth-factor cross-reacting protein in "central" neurofibromatosis. Lancet 1:4–7, 1979
4. Miller M, Hall JG: Possible maternal effect on severity of neurofibromatosis. Lancet 2:1071–1073, 1978
5. Kanter WR, Eldridge R: Maternal effect in central neurofibromatosis. Lancet 2:903, 1978
6. Riccardi VM, Kleiner B: Neurofibromatosis: A neoplastic birth defect with two age peaks of severe problems. Birth Defects 13:131–138, 1977
7. Holt JF: Neurofibromatosis in children. Am J Roentgenol Radium Ther Nucl Med 130:615–639, 1978
8. Harwood-Nash DC, Fitz CR: Neuroradiology in Infants and Children. St. Louis, C.V. Mosby, 1976, p 1227
9. Craig WM, Dodge HW, Ross PJ: Acoustic neuromas in children. Report of 2 cases. J Neurosurg 11:505–508, 1954
10. Mark VH, Sweet WH: An unusual case of eighth nerve tumor. J Neurosurg 9:395–397, 1952
11. Bjorkesten G: Unilateral acoustic tumours in children. Acta Psychiatr Neurol Scand 32:1–5, 1957
12. Moyes PD: Familial bilateral acoustic neuroma affecting 14 members from four generations. J Neurosurg 29:78–82, 1968
13. Stern J, Di Giacinto GV, Housepian EM: Neurofibromatosis and optic glioma: Clinical and morphological correlations. Neurosurgery 4:524–528, 1979
14. Chutorian AM, Schwartz JF, Evans RA, et al: Optic gliomas in children. Neurology 14:83–95, 1964
15. Walsh FB, Hoyt WF: Clinical Neuroophthalmology (ed 3). Baltimore, Williams & Wilkins, 1969, p 2754
16. Cotlier E: Café-au-lait spots of the fundus in neurofibromatosis. Arch Ophthalmol 95:1990–1992, 1977
17. Rosman NP, Pearce J: The brain in multiple neurofibromatosis (von Recklinghausen's disease): A suggested neuropathological basis for the associated mental defect. Brain 90:829–837, 1967
18. Tomsick TA, Lukin RR, Chambers AA, et al: Neurofibromatosis and intracranial arterial occlusive disease. Neuroradiology 11:229–234, 1976
19. Levisohn PM, Mikhael MA, Rothman SM: Cerebrovascular changes in neurofibromatosis. Dev Med Child Neurol 20:789–793, 1978
20. Fienman NL, Yakovac WC: Neurofibromatosis in childhood. J Pediatr 76:339–346, 1970
21. Rezaian SM: The incidence of scoliosis due to neurofibromatosis. Acta Orthop Scand 47:534–539, 1976
22. Chaglassian JH, Riseborough EJ, Hall JE: Neurofibromatous scoliosis. J Bone J Surg 58-A:695–702, 1976
23. Curtis BH, Fisher RL, Butterfield WL, et al: Neurofibromatosis with paraplegia. J Bone J Surg 51-A:843–861, 1969

24. Scott JC: Scoliosis and neurofibromatosis. J Bone J Surg 47-B:240–246, 1965
25. Heard G, Payne EE: Scalloping of the vertebral bodies in von Recklinghausen's disease of the nervous system (neurofibromatosis). J Neurol Neurosurg Psychiatr 25:345–351, 1962
26. Leech RW, Olafson RA, Gilbertson RL, et al: Intrathoracic meningocele and vertebral anomalies in a case of neurofibromatosis. Surg Neurol 9:55–57, 1978
27. del Buono MS, Osacar EM: Intrathoracic meningocele associated with cutaneous neurofibromatosis. Acta Neurochir 9:561–580, 1961
28. Shealy CN, LeMay M: Intrathoracic meningocele. J Neurosurg 21:880–883, 1964
29. Hill MC, Oh KS, Hodges FJ: Internal auditory canal enlargement in neurofibromatosis without acoustic neuroma. Radiology 122(suppl 2):730, 1977
30. Sarwar M, Swischuk LE: Bilateral internal auditory canal enlargement due to dural ectasia in neurofibromatosis. Am J Roentgenol Radium Ther Nucl Med 129:935–936, 1977
31. Bader JL, Miller RW: Neurofibromatosis and childhood leukemia. J Pediatr 92:925–929, 1978
32. Reich SD, Wiernik PH: Von Recklinghausen neurofibromatosis and acute leukemia. Am J Dis Child 130:888–889, 1976
33. Knight WA, Murphy WK, Gottlieb JA: Neurofibromatosis is associated with malignant neurofibromas. Arch Dermatol 107:747–750, 1973
34. Brasfield RD, Das Gupta TK: Von Recklinghausen's disease: A clinicopathological study. Ann Surg 175:86–104, 1972
35. D'Agostino AN, Soule EH, Miller RH: Sarcomas of the peripheral nerves and somatic soft tissues associated with multiple neurofibromatosis (von Recklinghausen's disease). Cancer 16:1015–1027, 1963
36. Whitehouse D: Diagnostic value of the café-au-lait spot in children. Arch Dis Child 41:316–319, 1966
37. Hammond JA, Driedger AA: Detection of malignant change in neurofibromatosis (von Recklinghausen's disease) by gallium-67 scanning. J Can Med Assoc 119:352–353, 1978

V Infections

49. Central Nervous System Infections in the Newborn

Mark S. O'Brien
James F. Schwartz

Central nervous system infections in the newborn may present as acute fulminating illness with bulging fontanel, seizures, fever, coma, and focal neurologic deficits, particularly with bacterial meningitis. Many infants, however, particularly premature or small-for-gestational-age infants, do not show evidence of their neurologic disorder with classic signs of meningeal or cerebral disease, even with bacterial infection. With central nervous system (CNS) infections attributable to viruses, protozoa, etc., the classic neurologic signs may be much less prominent, particularly in the first days or weeks of life. Initially these infants may appear to have primarily systemic disease, with rash, jaundice, hepatomegaly, and anemia, without obvious neurologic impairment. Neurologic manifestations, if present neonatally, may include seizures and inactivity, or structural changes such as microcephaly or hydrocephalus, indistinguishable from those seen with noninfectious causes. Many of these perinatal CNS infections are silent or subclinical in the neonate, despite serologic or cerebrospinal fluid (CSF) evidence of infection. Clinical evidence of the infection may not be apparent until the child is of preschool or school age and is found to have intellectual impairment or a specific sensory deficit. Timing of the infection, route of acquisition, and virulence of the infecting organism can vary widely with the various perinatal infections involving the central nervous system. Neurologists and neurosurgeons should be aware of these problems, as well as of the advances in laboratory diagnosis and treatment; with the improvement in neonatal and perinatal care, more such infants may be expected to be seen.

PATHOGENESIS AND EPIDEMIOLOGY

Maternal infection is the major source of infection of the infant with nonbacterial and some of the bacterial agents. Maternal host defenses may be protective, but the mother may be the host, frequently without being clinically ill, for a number of agents, particularly the so-called TORCH complex (T—toxoplasmosis, O—other, including syphilis and *Listeria,* R—rubella, C—cytomegalovirus, and H—herpes simplex viruses). These may infect the fetus transplacentally, by ascending infection from the genital area, or at the time of delivery, or postpartum. Toxoplasmosis, rubella, and cytomegalovirus are probably transplacentally transmitted. Genital herpes virus infection provides a particularly good example of infant exposure and contagion during the birth process, with subsequent development of disease postpartum. Similarly, some *Listeria* and Group B streptococcal infections may be acquired in transit through the birth canal. Disseminated neonatal Coxsackie virus infection and other bacterial infections of the CNS may be acquired in the nursery. Other avenues for introduction of infection in the newborn's CNS have resulted from recent advances in perinatal care, including intrauterine transfusion or amniocentesis, fetal scalp electrocardiographic monitoring, and scalp puncture for fetal blood sampling, all of which may be sources of entry of organisms for the fetus.

Data regarding incidence of maternal and chronic perinatal infections for some organisms are given in Table 49–1.[2] Maternal infection rates markedly exceed fetal infection rates, and both vary widely, depending on geographic locale and social class.

Cytomegalovirus (CMV) infection occurs as a primary cervical infection in about 1 percent of pregnant women in early gestation and increases during pregnancy so that approximately 10 percent of pregnant women are infected at term. The newborn acquires CMV in the presence of maternal cervical infection in an estimated 50 percent of cases. Neonatal CMV infection, which can be acquired at birth—that is, during descent through birth canal—is never a cause of symptomatic CNS or systemic disease in the newborn. More significant CMV infection that may affect the newborn's brain is probably acquired early in pregnancy, reaching the fetus either via placental infection or through infection of endometrial vessels, during the viremic phase of primary maternal infection.[8] Timing of maternal primary infection appears to be important in determining severity and prognosis of neonatal CMV infection. Early infection, as documented by maternal seroconversion, is more commonly responsible for symptomatic neonatal infection, whereas infection in late pregnancy is more likely to result in silent subclinical newborn infection.

The timing of maternal rubella infection with respect to fetal and neonatal disease is also of paramount importance. Rubella virus is transmitted transplacentally to the fetus during maternal viremia, whether the mother has clinical or subclinical infection. As was shown originally by Gregg in 1941, and confirmed

Table 49-1
Incidence of Certain Maternal and Chronic Perinatal Infections

	Mother per 1,000 Pregnancies	Fetus—Intrauterine per 1,000 Live Births	Newborn—Acquired at or Just Prior to Delivery per 1,000 Live Births
Cytomegalovirus	30–150	5–15	50–100
Rubella			
Epidemic	20–40	4–30	0
Interepidemic	0.1–1.0	1.5	0
Toxoplasmosis	1.5–6.4	0.75–1.3	0
Herpes	10–15	Rare	0.03–0.33
Syphilis	0.2	0.1	0

in the rubella epidemic of 1964–1965, when approximately 20,000 babies were born with congenital rubella, the frequency of congenital rubella syndrome with CNS involvement is highest with maternal infection in the first eight weeks. But some danger to the fetus occurs with maternal infection as late as the 16th week.[3] Hearing loss, now well documented as the most frequent sequela of maternally transmitted rubella, may be the only overt manifestation, especially if maternal infection occurs after the first eight weeks.

Herpes simplex virus genital infection of the pregnant woman, usually with herpes simplex virus type 2, is most commonly, although not exclusively, the source of neonatal herpes infection, resulting in systemic disease with or without CNS involvement. The maternal source may be a subclinical infection, with either herpes simplex virus type 1 or 2. In over one third of the total reported cases of neonatal herpes, there is good presumptive evidence for maternal genital infection being the source of virus infection in the newborn, with infection being acquired at the time of birth.[13] In two large hospital surveys, one documented clinical case of herpes infection in the newborn was noted per 7500 deliveries. Maternal herpes genital infection is about three times more common during pregnancy, and approximately 1 percent of women in the lowest socioeconomic group have evidence of such infection. Unlike the other TORCH agent infections, neonatal herpes infection is almost never subclinical or asymptomatic.

Neonatal toxoplasmosis is the result of maternal primary infection during pregnancy, which is usually clinically inapparent. In the United States, six to seven per 1000 mothers have acquired toxoplasmosis, as documented by serological surveys during pregnancy. Infection is transmitted to the fetus in over one half of the cases, although the transmitted infection is usually subclinical in the newborn. Again, as with the other agents, timing of maternal infection in relation to the severity of congenital infection is extremely important. Although the last months of pregnancy are the period of most frequent transmission to the fetus, newborn infection acquired at that time is usually subclinical. Maternal infection and transmission to the fetus by the third month of pregnancy, although less common, much more frequently results in severe neonatal disease. Desmonts and Couvreurs documented a 17 percent transmission rate to fetus with first trimester infection; 25 percent transmission rate with second trimester infection; and third trimester transmission and fetal infection rate of 65 percent with these last cases being almost all subclinical, at least in the neonatal period.

NEONATAL ILLNESS AND DELAYED SEQUELAE

Cytomegalovirus

Neonatal CMV illness probably occurs in no more than one out of 10 infected infants, that is, infants with viruria. Virus recovery or cytopathologic changes in urinary sediment and clinical disease thus are not equivalent. The classic neonatal manifestations of symptomatic CMV disease share many of the clinical features of severe illness manifested in congenital rubella and toxoplasmosis, for which cytomegalic inclusion disease was frequently mistaken initially. The systemic manifestations include hepatomegaly, jaundice, hepatitis, thrombocytopenia with petechiae and purpura, microcephaly, chorioretinitis, and optic atrophy. Seizures, lethargy, and hypotonia may occur in the acute neonatal CNS infection. If fetal infection has occurred early in pregnancy, during the period of organogenesis, allowing the virus to interfere with the process of differentiation and development, microcephaly, optic atrophy, microophthalmia and aplasia of various parts of the brain microgyria, cerebellar hypoplasia, micropolygyria), and subependymal calcification are more likely to occur. Most congenitally infected infants do not subsequently develop CNS disease severe enough to become microcephalic, but when microcephaly occurs, it is usually associated with mental retardation. The chorioretinitis of CMV infection cannot be differentiated from toxoplasma chorioretinitis on the basis of location or appearance. Cerebral calcifications, although usually subependymal in location and therefore periventricular, may be diffuse at times, simulating the radiographic pattern seen usually with congential toxoplasmosis. The intracranial calcifications occur in less than 1 percent of all CMV infected infants, so their absence does not exclude the diagnosis. Deafness, which is a result of viral infection of the inner ear, is most commonly bilateral and may not be suspected until the second year of life.

Hanshaw,[8] reporting on a serologic survey of 8644 consecutive infants, using a sensitive CMV-IGM specific antibody test, found 53 patients with positive sera, or one in 163. Forty-four of these patients were evaluated at school age for school progress and intellectual abilities. Increased CMV antibody levels were found in the lower socioeconomic class, and there was an association of CMV antibody with variable intellectual impairment that was not documented in matched controls. Although none of the patients had documented neonatal clinical disease, hearing impairment was documented bilaterally in 5 of 40 or 12.5 percent and questionable hearing loss in 6 of 40 (15 percent).[8]

Similarly, Stagno, Reynolds, Amos, et al.[18] found significant sensorineural hearing loss in 10 of 59 (17 percent) patients with congenital CMV infection; 3 of 8 had been symptomatic as newborns, and 7 of 51 had subclinical infection. The hearing deficits were associated with severe impairment of verbal communication in 3 patients with profound, severe bilateral loss, with mental retardation of 2 patients, and with a gross behavior disorder in one patient. Of further interest was the finding that the auditory impairment progressed many months after delivery in one patient born with subclinical infection for whom other causes of progressive deafness could be excluded. Ocular complications, including chorioretinits, optic atrophy, and strabismus, were usually present at or shortly after birth as part of symptomatic neonatal CMV disease. Chorioretinitis does not usually develop later if absent in the neonatal period, but it has been documented as a "new" clinical finding at 9 to 10 months of age.

Rubella

The congenital rubella syndrome includes systemic manifestations almost identical to CMV infection, with additional findings of heart defects, cataracts, glaucoma, a rather characteristic salt and pepper retinopathy, and radiolucent lesions in the long bones. The neurologic findings are also similar to those of CMV infection, with deafness and microcephaly that may be apparent in the neonatal period. Additionally some infants have evidence of an active encephalitis. Desmond, Wilson, Melnick, et al.[4] documented neurologic manifestations occuring between birth and 18 months in 81 of 100 patients with congenital rubella infection. They describe three groups of patients with abnormal neurologic findings and their progression. The largest group of infants initially were lethargic and hypotonic, and had large anterior fontanels at birth or in the first few weeks; this was followed by increasingly irritability, restlessness, and constant crying. They gradually developed increasing hypertonicity and transient opisthotonus in response to stimulation; some developed persistent opisthotonus. About one half of these infants later improved, whereas the others showed persistent delayed motor development. A second, smaller group of infants was, in contrast, unusually quiet, inactive, and hypotonic; "good babies," but with hyperactive reflexes. These infants also had intermittent opisthotonic posturing, but this group showed improvement at about 9 to 12 months. The third group of patients had an acute onset of seizures in the first week and a "meningitis-like" picture at 2½ months. Altogether seizures were observed in about a quarter of the 100 infants, beginning either shortly after birth to as late as 16 months. The most prominent neurologic manifestation described in the 100, however, was abnormal posture, with head retraction, with or without opisthotonus in 49 percent of the total. Increased CSF protein and moderate pleocytosis were also frequently noted, with CSF protein diminishing to normal levels by the age of 3 months. Rubella virus was present in the CSF in 28 patients and persisted there throughout the first year in 9 patients.

Hearing deficits may not be apparent on neonatal examination, and clinical assessment of infants born of mothers with gestational rubella exposure, if performed only in the neonatal period, has been shown to underestimate to a significant degree the possible consequences of this infection. Psychomotor retardation and deafness may later be apparent despite absence of characteristic congenital rubella at birth. With time, in addition to these chronic neurologic sequelae, behavior disorders and learning disabilities have been documented in many children with congenital rubella.

An even later consequence of congenital rubella infection has now become apparent with the reports of Townsend, Baringer, Wolinsky, et al.[20] and Weil[21] in 1975. These investigators reported four children, with varied but mild signs of congenital rubella, with sensorineural hearing loss but intellectual function within normal limits, and then, after a stable period of 8 to 14 years, progressive deterioration with progressive dementia, motor involvement with both spasticity and ataxia, myoclonus in one patient, and elevated CSF gamma globulin with high titers of rubella antibody. The pathologic changes were those of an inflammatory panencephalitis.

Toxoplasmosis

Congenital toxoplasmosis may present in the early neonatal period as a generalized systemic disease with predominant manifestations being fever, jaundice, anemia, hepatosplenomegaly, and lymphadenopathy. If the predominant involvement is of CNS or eye, the onset may be delayed for several months after birth. Most children with congenital toxoplasmosis involving the CNS are described as being normal at birth. This may reflect not delayed onset of disease, but delayed recognition. Delayed onset at several months of life clearly does occur, however, and may be severe, particularly with premature infants in whom the severe neurologic manifestations of convulsions, abnormal CSF, and intracranial calcifications may not be evident until three months after birth. The full-term infant is said to have an earlier but also delayed onset, with perhaps milder manifestations. The largest series of patients with congenital toxoplasmosis, 152 patients described by Eichenwald,[6] could be divided into two groups: the dominant neurologic disease that affected 69 percent, and the generalized systemic form that occurred in 28 percent. Abnormal CSF was noted in 69 percent, convulsions in 34 percent intracranial calcifications in 27 percent, and hydrocephalus is only 14 percent of the entire series.

The most common manifestation was chorioretinitis, noted in 80 percent of the entire group of 152 patients. Chorieretinitis can occur months after birth in babies whose fundi have been checked repeatedly, and on occasion it may first be noted at school age. Similarly late aqueductal stenosis leading to hydrocephalus may not become evident until early childhood. The important point is that infants totally asymptomatic at birth may develop chorioretinitis, strabismus, blindness, hydrocephalus, microcephaly, mental retardation, seizures, or deafness months or years later.[1] As with CMV infection, however, most asymptomatic infants suffer no sequelae. At present there is no way to predict outcome of infection in an asymptomatic newborn, but *if* severe disease is present in the early months, prognosis is poor. A four-year follow-up study of children with symptomatic congenital toxoplasmosis in infancy revealed that 89 percent of those who had neurologic manifestations in infancy were mentally retarded, as compared with 81 percent who had only systemic disease. Seizures later occurred in 83 percent of those with early neurologic involvement and in 77 percent of those with systemic manifestations. Spasticity occurred in 76 percent of the former and 48 percent of the latter, and decreased vision of severe degree was noted in 69 percent of those with neonatal neurologic disease and 42 percent of those with generalized systemic infection in infancy. Hydrocephalus or microcephaly was a sequela in 44 percent of those with neonatal CNS disease, but in only 6 percent of those with systemic disease. Only 9 percent of the survivors who had neurologic findings in the first few months of life were ultimately normal.[16]

Chorioretinitis appears to increase with age during the early years. It usually begins as a focal necrotizing retinitis, which is commonly bilateral. The earliest overt sign may be searching nystagmus or strabismus. Other ocular features can include optic atrophy, microophthalmia, papilledema, and even cataracts. Mental retardation can also occur as a sequel to subclinical congenital infection. Cerebrospinal fluid protein is commonly increased, and there is a pleocytosis.

Herpes Simplex

Congenital herpes infection has received increasing attention in recent years as its epidemiology and mode of clinical presentation have become better understood. As noted in the foregoing, neonatal infection is usually acquired from silent or asymptomatic maternal genital infection, most frequently with herpes simplex virus type 2. A few cases of transplacental infection with either type 1 or 2 have been documented. Unlike toxoplasmosis or CMW newborn infection, herpes infection in the newborn is almost always symptomatic, with either disseminated infection involving primarily liver and adrenals, and also other organs, including the brain, or as localized infection affecting only the skin and/or the eye, or infection involving primarily the brain, usually associated with cutaneous and/or ocular disease. The ocular involvement can be a conjunctivities, keratitis, cataract, or chorioretinitis. Cutaneous disease may consist only of a few discrete vesicles or bullae, but crops and clusters of skin lesions are not infrequent, and may be a recurring problem if the infant survives, with recurrence being at either the same or different sites.[13]

Neurologic manifestations occur with disseminated disease in about one half of the cases, with focal or generalized seizures, irritability, bulging fontanel, opisthotonus, spasticity or marked flaccidity, and coma. Of those infants whose CNS infection is not associated with disseminated systemic involvement, onset of clinical symptoms is at about 10 days of age, which is slightly later than the disseminated disease. With the primary CNS infection, seizures, lethargy, irritability, and tremors occur in 50 percent as initial symptoms. Microcephaly has been noted at birth in a few, and intracranial calcifications have been noted as early as two months of age. The course of the untreated illness is rapid, with death from the disseminated disease within a few hours to a few weeks after onset, with the median duration from onset to death being about seven days, and median age at death 14 days. Mortality rate of the disseminated disease is 82 percent. In the primary CNS infection, without dissemination, there is a progressive neurologic deterioration, with a mortality rate of about 40 percent. Sequelae can include severe psychomotor retardation, microcephaly, hydrocephalus, porencephalic cysts, cataracts, and corneal scars. Cerebrospinal fluid changes are variable, with pleocytosis of 50 to 200 cells, with a peak cell count of $2500/mm^3$ in one; CSF protein can be markedly elevated to levels as high as 1000 mg/100 ml. The diagnosis thus must be made early, and the clinical similarities with the other members of the TORCH complex should be noted, as well as features common to some bacterial infections, including *Escherichia coli* and Group B streptococcal meningitis of the newborn, although those are more readily diagnosed by routine bacteriologic tests.

OTHER VIRAL INFECTIONS

Infection of the central nervous system with other nonbacterial agents in the newborn period is extremely uncommon. Neonatal polimyelitis, once an extremely serious illness, with high mortality, is now nonexistent. Coxsackie virus infections, acquired transplacentally, have been reported on rare occasion. Perhaps more common, although still very infrequent, are postnatally acquired infections with Coxsackie B viruses (B_2, B_3, B_4, B_5), which may produce an aseptic meningitis or meningoencephalitis, usually with a moderate degree of lethargy, fever, diminished or absent Moro reflex irritability, and occasionally twitching, with elevated CSF protein and mononuclear pleocytosis. When associated with myocarditis, as has been reported in a few epidemics, this may be a very serious illness, but the myocardial disease is the most prominent aspect. Echoviruses 3, 9, 11, and 17 have been reported as causes of aseptic meningitis of a mild nature in newborn infants in epidemic situations.

LABORATORY DIAGNOSIS

Diagnosis of a TORCH agent infection depends in large measure on the selection of appropriate laboratory tests and their interpretation. The many common clinical manifestations of the TORCH infections make it difficult, if not impossible, to arrive at a specific etiologic diagnosis without laboratory testing. Furthermore, in view of the potential of treating some of these infections, particularly at an early stage and thereby improving outcome, specific etiologic determination becomes more than an academic exercise.

One widely advocated screening test is the total serum IgM determination in all instances of suspected newborn infection. IgM is always of fetal and not maternal origin, and elevated levels, greater than 20 mg/100 ml, were thought to be indicative of intrauterine or early postnatal infection. This test has its limitations, however, because not all infected infants have elevated serum IgM, and some infants with elevated IgM levels do not have infection. There thus are false negatives as well as false positives. More useful as a screening test is the rheumatoid factor test. About one third of babies tested before a week of age, when infected with intrauterine-acquired TORCH agents, have been found to have positive rheumatoid factor tests, whereas none of 600 controls had a positive reaction.[19] Even when IgM specific assays to an infective agent are performed, false negative tests may occur, as with toxoplasmosis or cytomegalovirus, and false positive reactions also may occur.

RUBELLA

Most normal babies will have levels of maternally derived antibody (IgG) to rubella comparable to those of rubella-infected infants because of transfer of maternal antibody to rubella to the fetus. This transplacentally acquired maternal antibody generally disappears from the infant's serum by the age of 4 to 6 months. At the present time, the Center for Disease Control recommends serial testing by the hemagglutination inhibition (HI) serologic method of a suspected rubella infant's sera in the newborn period and again at 4–6 months of age. Persistence of HI antibody beyond the age of 6 months is significant.

In older infants and children who have not received rubella vaccine, a positive HI test only indicates that there has been infection with rubella at some undetermined time in the past. It is often impossible to establish the diagnosis of congenital rubella when a child is first seen at 15 months of age or older.

Specific IgM antibody to rubella virus can be detected in the serum in approximately 60 percent of infected infants in the first four months of life, and in about 40 percent by 8–12 months, but is entirely gone by 2 years of age. This test may be useful in some instances.

CYTOMEGALOVIRUS

In the newborn infant, congenital CMV infection may be diagnosed most readily by identification of the virus in fresh urine specimens. This may be accomplished most rapidly, within about 30 minutes, by identifying the viral particles by electron microscopy using the pseudoreplica method.[9] Cytologic examination using Papanicolaou staining may be performed on fresh urine sediment, and characteristic "owl's eye" intranuclear inclusions can be seen in the renal epithelial cells in about one third of those infants whose kidneys are infected with the virus. Clinical specimens, such as urine and throat secretions, may be cultured for cytomegalovirus. Culture is the definitive method for the diagnosis of CMV in the newborn, but it may take four to six weeks for the virus to grow in tissue culture. In infants beyond 6–8 weeks of age and in young children, although isolation or identification of CMV from fresh urine specimens or throat secretions may establish that CMV infection has occurred, this is not diagnostic of intrauterine-acquired infection. Furthermore, as noted above, infection with virus may not be associated with disease.

Serologic tests are of little help in diagnosing CMV in the newborn. Complement fixation (CF) and passive hemagglutinating antibody (PHA) titers, which may be present in infected as well as in noninfected newborns, may represent maternally transmitted antibody. Maternally transmitted antibody titers, however, will show significant declines by 6 months of age. Fluorescent antibody tests (FA) using specific CMV-IgM antibody conjugates are difficult to perform and are less sensitive than viral cultures.

TOXOPLASMOSIS

Serologic studies for toxoplasmosis are also confusing because of maternal IgG antibody transfer to the fetus, in the absence of infant infection. The time-honored Sabin–Feldman dye test, which measures IgG antibody, is used infrequently today. Now more commonly employed are the indirect hemagglutination (IHA) test and indirect fluorescent antibody (IFA) techniques for IgG and IgM antibodies. Serum obtained from both mother and infant should be tested for both IFA-IgG and IFA-IgM antibodies. It is usually necessary to test sequential serum specimens from both mother and infant every 7 to 10 days, until a significant rise in the infant's IFA-IgG titer is documented or IFA-IgM is detected. It is recommended that consultation be obtained from experts in the field in interpreting toxoplasma antibody titers, since early diagnosis is mandatory if therapy is to be of value in these infants.

HERPES SIMPLEX VIRUS

Neonatal herpes simplex virus infection can be readily suspected when characteristic herpetic lesions (skin vesicles, mouth ulcers, or keratoconjunctivitis) are present. Aspirated vesicle fluid may be examined for viral particles by electron microscopy as well as cultured in a variety of tissue culture cells. The virus readily grows in tissue culture in one to five days. Other sites in the newborn that often yield herpes simplex virus in culture include the conjunctivae, throat, nasopharynx, urine, and occasionally CSF and buffy coat lymphocytes. Such sites should be cultured even in the absence of clinical findings of keratonconjunctivitis or mouth ulcers.

Cytologic examination is the most readily available rapid diagnostic tool for the identification of herpes virus in scrapings of skin, eye, or mouth lesions, particularly when Pap staining is used. An experienced cytopathologist can readily identify the characteristic multinucleated giant cells with intranuclear inclusions diagnostic of herpes simplex virus. Fluorescent antibody can also be applied to scrapings of skin, oral, or ocular lesions, using type-specific herpes antiserum. Serologic testing as a means of diagnosing herpes infection is indicated only as an adjunct to culture, cytologic examination, electron microscopy, and fluorescent antibody techniques in suspected neonatal infection. Attempting to diagnose neonatal herpes infection by serologic methods alone is inadvisable, as it may take approximately three to four weeks for the infant to develop serum IgM antibody to herpes virus, and precious time will be lost as this is currently a potentially treatable infection.

In highly suspect neonates with a meningoencephalitic illness, if there are no ocular cutaneous, or mouth lesions characteristic of herpetic infection, and if bacterial infection as well as other TORCH agent infections have been ruled out, a brain biopsy is recommended if a computerized tomography scan or radioisotopic brain scan shows a focal temporal lesion.[14] Such illness does occur and is particularly difficult to diagnose in the absence of skin, oral, or ocular lesions. A history of genital herpes in the mother or her sexual contact is important to ascertain, but the absence of such a history does not exclude the diagnosis of neonatal herpes.

TREATMENT OF VIRAL INFECTIONS

Although there is at present no specific antiviral therapy for congenital CMV or rubella infection, it is important to diagnose these infections for prognostic reasons. Long-term follow-up is necessary in both infections, since hearing defects and neurologic or retinal damage may not become apparent until several years of age. Moreover these infants will continue to shed virus for many months or even years, and contact with pregnant women should be avoided.

Toxoplasmosis, if diagnosed early, is treatable. Treatment should be initiated promptly with a combination of pyrimethamine and sulfadiazine. Since pyrimethamine is a folic acid antagonist that produces reversible and gradual bone marrow suppression, all patients should have white blood cell and platelet counts twice a week. It is advisable to give folinic acid twice weekly during pyrimethamine therapy to reverse the toxic effects of the latter drug. Herpes virus infection in the newborn should be diagnosed promptly and treatment initiated without delay. Vidarabine (adenine arabinoside) has been found in controlled studies to decrease significantly the mortality of neonatal herpetic infections. The drug is given at a dosage of 15 mg/kg/day intravenously over a 12-hour period each day for 10 days.[14]

BACTERIAL MENINGITIS

Bacterial meningitis in the newborn is a disease with high morbidity and mortality, due in great part to the fact that it occurs much more frequently in low-birth-weight infants who are simultaneously subject to adverse effects from hypoxia and acidosis, and whose immune mechanisms are either incompletely developed or functional. Other factors operative in the pathogenesis of bacterial sepsis and meningitis in the low-birth-weight infant are related to maternal infection, especially with prolonged rupture of membranes; respiratory depression at birth, necessitating resuscitation and intubation that may introduce infection; and the use of inhalation and humidification therapy equipment and various monitoring devices including arterial catheters, which may also provide ready access for bacterial invasion and colonization. The incidence of bacterial meningitis in infants below 2500 grams is greater than three times that observed in those over 2500 grams. Finally the large numbers of medical and nursing personnel involved in the neonatal intensive care unit increase in the likelihood of exposure to infection for the very small newborn.

Another reason for the high morbidity and mortality of neonatal meningitis may relate to the difficulty of establishing the diagnosis clinically, in the absence of classic signs of meningeal infection. Nuchal rigidity is rare, and a bulging fontanel is present in no more than 25 percent of cases. Although the newborn or small-for-dates infant with meningitis may have fever, frequently the baby is afebrile, or even hypothermic. Lethargy is perhaps the most common clinical sign, and also common are nonspecific manifestations such as failure to feed, hypotonia, irritability of modest degree, or respiratory distress. Convulsions, tremors, or simply agitation and constant movements have been noted in approximately 40 percent of such infants. Apnea does occur, but is a late manifestation. Meningitis must therefore be suspected in the premature or full-term infant on the basis of minimal criteria or these nonspecific manifestations. The rapid course of bacterial meningitis in the small infant and the sudden deterioration make early diagnosis mandatory. In addition to obtaining blood cultures, a readiness to perform lumbar puncture on any infant who deviates in almost any fashion from the child's usual state is the only way to diagnose meningitis at this age.[7]

To evaluate CSF in the premature or full-term infant, the physician must be aware of normal values for cells, glucose, and protein. In the premature infant, the mean cell count, reported by Sarff, Platt, and McCracken,[17] was 9/mm^3, with a range of 0–30, and CSF protein values from 65 to 150 mg/dl, with a mean of 115. Others have quoted peak CSF protein in the preterm infants as high as 180 mg/dl. Full-term infants have a mean of 8.2 cells/mm^3, with a range of 0–32, and reaching levels of approximately 15–20 mg/dl by age 6 months. Cerebrospinal fluid glucose values are low in infants, related to the lower blood glucose levels, which may be 30 mg/dl or above in the full term, and as low as 20 mg/dl in the preterm or small-for-dates infant.

Laboratory diagnosis of bacterial meningitis in the newborn in most hospitals must rely on classic methods of analysis, using Gram and methylene blue stained smears of cerebrospinal fluid, chemical determinations of glucose and protein, and appropriate culture techniques. New techniques that have been advocated and are under trial by some investigators include counterimmunoelectrophoresis (CIE), and the limulus lysate test. A CIE evaluation of cerebrospinal fluid that depends on the migration of the capsular antigens of the CSF bacteria in the presence of specific antisera appears to be accurate in providing rapid etiologic diagnosis within one hour after spinal tap. Specific antisera available for use in CIE include *Hemophilus influenzae* type B, pneumococcus, meningococcus, and some serotypes of Group B streptococcus; and Group B meningococcal antisera have been used to detect K1 strains of *E. coli.* At present CIE does not appear to yield results better than those obtained with conventional Gram stain smear. The limulus lysate test, which detects the presence of endotoxin in CSF in cases of gram negative organisms, including *E. coli, Serratia, Salmonella, Proteus mirabilis,* and *Pseudomonas.* This test was found by McCracken and Sarff[10] to be positive in 72 percent of patients with gram negative meningitis. They also established a definite relationship, using this test, between presence and persistence of endotoxin with prognosis, with longer persistence of endotoxin indicative of poorer clinical outcome. In addition to these or conventional examinations of CSF, blood cultures should be obtained when meningitis is suspected, since they are positive in approximately 60 percent of cases of neonatal meningitis.

The etiology of neonatal meningitis is of importance in selecting antibiotics and method of therapy, and also in determining the length of treatment. For many years coliform organisms were implicated as the principal etiologic agents. In most nurseries they are still important, but not the leading cause. Within the past few years, specific serotypes of *E. coli* have been found to be of particular significance. *E. coli* with K1 capsular polysaccharide antigen is associated with a higher incidence of neonatal meningitis than *E. coli* within K1 antigen. It has also been shown that *E. coli* with K1 antigen produces meningitis with a greater morbidity and mortality, and prognosis has been related to both amount and persistence of K1 antigen in serum and cerebrospinal fluid.

Group B beta-hemolytic *Streptococcus* accounts for a significant proportion of cases of neonatal meningitis, and is not only the most common gram positive organism causing meningitis in the first month of life, but in many geographic areas is the cause of more cases than the coliforms. There appear to be two clinically distinct patterns of illness with Group B *Streptococcus:* "early" disease, occurring under 10 days of age, and "late" disease, with onset after 10 days of age. The former is associated with more systemic manifestations, with respiratory distress simulating hyaline membrane disease, unexpected apneic episodes that occur in approximately 80 percent, seizures in about 50 percent, and fever in only 33 percent. Lethargy is the most common manifestation in the "late" disease; apneic spells and respiratory symptoms are uncommon, but fever is common, and bulging fontanel occurs in almost two thirds of the patients. Early-onset streptococcal disease has a considerably higher mortality than late-onset meningitis.

Listeria monocytogenes meningitis is the second most common gram positive organism causing meningitis in infancy, occurring not only in the immediate neonatal period, but also in the first few months of life, and, in our experience, is the third most common agent associated with bacterial meningitis in infancy. Onset is usually in the second week of life, and the disease is more common in full-term infants. In general the disease has a more favorable outcome than other types of neonatal meningitis. The diagnosis of *Listeria* meningitis can be suspected in some infants who have monocytosis, with increased monocyte levels (greater than 6 percent) in peripheral blood, although CSF cell count usually shows predominance of polymorphonuclears in over 70 percent of patients, along with depressed glucose concentration and elevated protein. Gram stain smears have been particularly helpful in our institution in diagnosing *Listeria,* and blood cultures have been positive in less than one third of cases.

TREATMENT OF BACTERIAL MENINGITIS

Although most attention is focused on identification of organism and sepcific antimicrobial therapy, other problems requiring attention during therapy include seizures, shock (for which either plasmanate or other volume expanders must be utilized), and careful attention to fluid and electrolyte balance, since inappropriate antidiuretic hormone secretion has been a common problem in our nursery. Other forms of neonatal support—that is, temperature, respiration, cardiovascular—are obviously continued, as with other sick newborns.

Choice of antibiotics and route of administration are clearly based on identity of the organism, sensitivity of the organism in the particular geographic locale or institution, and the method necessary to provide adequate antibiotic concentration in the subarachnoid space and ventricular system.[12]

The initial choice of antibiotics, prior to identification of the organism, consists of the following: ampicillin 100 mg/kg/day in two divided doses (i.e., every 12 hours) intravenously; gentamicin 5 mg/kg/day in two divided doses (i.e., every 12 hours) intramuscularly. After 1 week of age, these dosages are increased to ampicillin 200 mg/kg/day in three divided doses (i.e., every 8 hours) intravenously; gentamicin 7.5 mg/kg/day, in three divided doses, intramuscularly.

If *E. coli* in a community or hospital is sensitive to kanamycin, that antibiotic can be used instead of gentamicin. The combination of ampicillin and gentamicin or kanamycin is advocated for *E. coli.* Because of unacceptably high rates of treatment failure, with high morbidity and mortality rates, there has been considerable question regarding alternative methods or routes of administration of the aminoglycosides. In an 18-institution collaborative study of the efficacy of combined therapy, comparing intravenous and intrathecal gentamicin in gram negative bacterial neonatal meningitis, there was no significant difference in morbidity, mortality, or days of CSF culture remaining positive between the two treated groups, with a case fatality rate of 32 percent.[11] A subsequent similar multi-institutional collaborative study of the effects of intraventricular administration of aminoglycosides, either by direct needle ventricular puncture, or by instillation of the antibiotic into ventricular reservoirs, compared with systemic (intravenous) administration of the same antibiotics showed no significant advantages accruing from intraventricular antibiotic therapy, and a higher rate of complications. As a result current recommendations for the treatment of gram negative organism meningitis in the newborn do not include either intrathecal or intraventricular routes of administration.

Recommended antibiotic therapy for Group B streptococcal meningitis consists of aqueous penicillin 150,000 units/kg/day in two divided doses for the first week of life, and 250,000 units/kg/day in three or four divided doses for one additional week.

Ampicillin is the recommended drug of choice for *Listeria* and also for *P. mirabilis.* For pseudomonas meningitis the recommended treatment is carbenicillin. Dosage for infants under 2000 grams of weight is 200 mg/kg/day in three divided doses during the first week of life, and 300 mg/kg/day in four divided doses (every six hours) for infants over 2000 grams in the first week of life. The carbenicillin is combined with gentamicin 5 mg/kg/day in three divided doses. After the first week of life, and carbenicillin dosage is increased to 400 mg/kg/day in four divided doses (every six hours), and gentamicin is increased to 7.5 mg/kg/day.

For staphylococcal meningitis in the newborn, methicillin, nafcillin, or oxycillin should be administered at a dosage of 50 to 75 mg/kg/day in two divided doses (every 12 hours) for the first week of life, and the dosage is increased to 75 to 100 mg/kg/day in three divided doses after the first week of life.

Current recommendations for duration of therapy are for two weeks for the gram positive organisms, and a minimum of three weeks, or until the cerebrospinal fluid has been sterile for at least two weeks (whichever is longer), with gram negative organism meningitis.[15]

REFERENCES

1. Alford CP, et al: Congenital toxoplasmosis: Clinical laboratory therapeutic considerations with special reference to subclinical diseases. Bull NY Acad Med 50:160, 1974
2. Alford CP, Reynolds DW, Stagno S: Current concepts of chronic perinatal infections, in Gluck L (ed): Modern Perinatal Medicine. Chicago, Year Book Medical Publications, 1975, pp 285–306
3. Cooper, LZ: Congenital rubella in the United States, in Kraugman S, Gershon AS (eds): Infections of the Fetus and the Newborn Infant. New York, Alan R Liss, 1975, pp 1–22
4. Desmond NM, Wilson GS, Melnick JL, et al: Congenital rubella encephalitis. J Pediatr 71:311–331, 1967
5. Desmonts G, Couvreur J: Toxoplasmosis in pregnancy and its transmission to the fetus. Bull NY Acad Med 50:146–159, 1974
6. Eichenwald HF: A study of congenital toxoplasmosis with particular emphasis on clinical manifestation, sequelae and therapy, in Siim JC (ed): Human Toxoplasmosis. Copenhagen, Munksgaard, 1959
7. Feigin RD: Bacterial meningitis in the newborn infant. Clin Perinatolog 4:103–166, 1977
8. Hanshaw JB: Cytomegalovirus, in Remington JS, Klein JO (eds): Infectious Diseases of the Fetus and the Newborn Infant. Philadelphia, WB Saunders, 1976, pp 107–155
9. Lee FK, Nahmias AJ, Stagno S: Rapid diagnosis of cytomegalovirus infection in infants by electron microscopy. N Engl J Med 299:1266–1270, 1978
10. McCracken GH Jr, Sarff, LD: Neonatal *E. Coli* meningitis. Hosp Pract 9:57, 1974
11. McCracken GH Jr, Mize SG: A controlled study of intrathecal antibiotic therapy in gram negative enteric meningitis of infancy. J Pediatr 89:66, 1976
12. McCracken GH Jr: Clinical pharmacology of antibacterial agents in Remington JS, Klein JO (eds): Infectious Diseases of the Fetus and Newborn Infant. Philadelphia, WB Saunders, 1976, pp 1020–1067
13. Nahmias AJ, Visintine AM: Herpes simplex in Remington JS, Klein JO (eds): Infectious Diseases of the Fetus and Newborn Infant. Philadelphia, WB Saunders, 1976, pp 156–190
14. Nahmias AJ, Whitely RJ: Herpes simplex virus encephalitis in pediatrics. Pediatrics (in press)
15. Nelson JD: Pediatric Antimicrobial Therapy (ed 3). Dallas, Jodone Pub Co, 1979
16. Remington JS, Desmonts G: Toxoplasmosis, in Remington JS, Klein JO (eds):

Infectious Diseases of the Fetus and Newborn Infant. Philadelphia, WB Saunders, 1976, pp 191–332

17. Sarff LD, Platt LH, McCracken GH Jr: Cerebrospinal fluid evaluation in neonates: A comparison of high risk infants with and without meningitis. J Pediatr 88:473, 1976
18. Stagno S, Reynolds DW, Amos CS, et al: Auditory and visual defects resulting from symptomatic and subclinical congenital cytomegaloviral and toxoplasma infections. Pediatrics 59:669–687, 1977
19. Stagno S, et al: Comparative study of diagnostic procedures for congenital cytomegalovirus infection. Pediatrics (in press)
20. Townsend JJ, Baringer JR, Wolinsky JS, et al: Progressive rubella panencephalitis. Late onset after congenital rubella. N Engl J Med 292:990, 1975
21. Weil ML: Chronic progressive panencephalitis due to rubella virus simulating subacute sclerosing panencephalitis. N Engl J Med 292:994, 1975

50. Suppurative Cranial and Intracranial Infections

William R. Cheek

The treatment of suppurative cranial and intracranial infections continues to be a challenge, although the overall incidence of this disorder in the United States undoubtedly has decreased since the advent of antibiotics. Improved diagnostic methods and more sophisticated techniques of culturing purulent material have influenced certain aspects of management. The importance of early recognition of these infections cannot be overemphasized. The basic therapeutic principles of removing the inoculum from the host and administering antibiotics in sufficient amount and type to achieve systemic sterilization must be observed.

BRAIN ABSCESS

Brain abscess fortunately is not common in children. In the pediatric age group, 1 to 3 patients are all that one would expect to see in a year on a busy neurosurgical service.[1–6] This disorder occurs approximately twice as often in males as in females. The development of antibiotics seems to have decreased the incidence of brain abscess,[7,8] but there is not universal agreement on this point.[1,2] This reduction in incidence logically is attributed to a decrease in the number of patients with sinusitis, mastoiditis, and otitis[7] (all of which are frequently associated with the development of brain abscess) due to the general use of antibiotics. Significant reduction in intracranial complications secondary to otitic infection following the development of antibiotics has been well documented by Proctor.[9] The incidence of brain abscess relative to the total incidence of complications in his series increased, however. Brain abscesses are caused by a variety of sources: (1) contiguous infection such as sinusitis or mastoiditis by direct extension or by propagation through venous channels; (2) direct introduction via penetrating wounds; (3) hematogenous spread from a distant focus of infection or hematogenous origin without known infection elsewhere, as is frequently the case with congenital heart disease; or (4) intracranial abscess formation as a result of an infected dermoid in the frontal lobe or the cerebellum.

The pathologic characteristics of the mature lesion in children do not differ significantly from those in adults. Initially the organism produces an inflammatory reaction consisting of congestion and outpouring of polymorphonuclear leukocytes, toxic changes in the neurons, and perivascular infiltration of the polymorphonuclear leukocytes. Next the involved tissues become necrotic, accompanied by liquefaction and pus formation. The brain attempts to wall off the necrotic purulent material. Since fibroblasts in the brain arise from the vessels, this occurs best in the gray matter where they are most common. The wall is composed of fibroblasts, capillaries, and collagen similar to granulation tissue elsewhere in the body. As the collagen deposition increases, the wall becomes thicker and more fibrous. Edema of varying degree and swollen glial elements appear in the brain tissue surrounding the capsule. As the lesion matures, astrocytes proliferate and produce a gliotic zone externally to the fibrous capsule (Fig. 50-1). This process usually takes a few weeks. Grant,[10] in a clinical study during the preantibiotic era of patients with brain abscess, showed that a capsule was present in all of them after a period of six weeks. Clinical differences in brain abscesses in children from those in adults have been observed. The lesions are larger, have thinner walls, and more edema is present in the surrounding brain tissue than is the case in adults.[2] Pathologic differences have not been documented.[11]

Brain abscess is a rare occurrence in infants and prior to the development of antibiotics was always fatal.[12] In more recent reports, Munslow, Stovall, Price, et al.[13] and Hoffman, Hendrick, and Hiscox[14] showed gram negative organisms to be the cause of these large lesions, but their source was not known. One of the reasons why infants are believed to be subject to gram negative brain abscess is that the M fraction of immunoglobulins does not pass across the placenta. The development of paranasal sinuses and mastoid air cells after 1 year of age eliminates infection in these areas as a source of brain abscess in young infants.

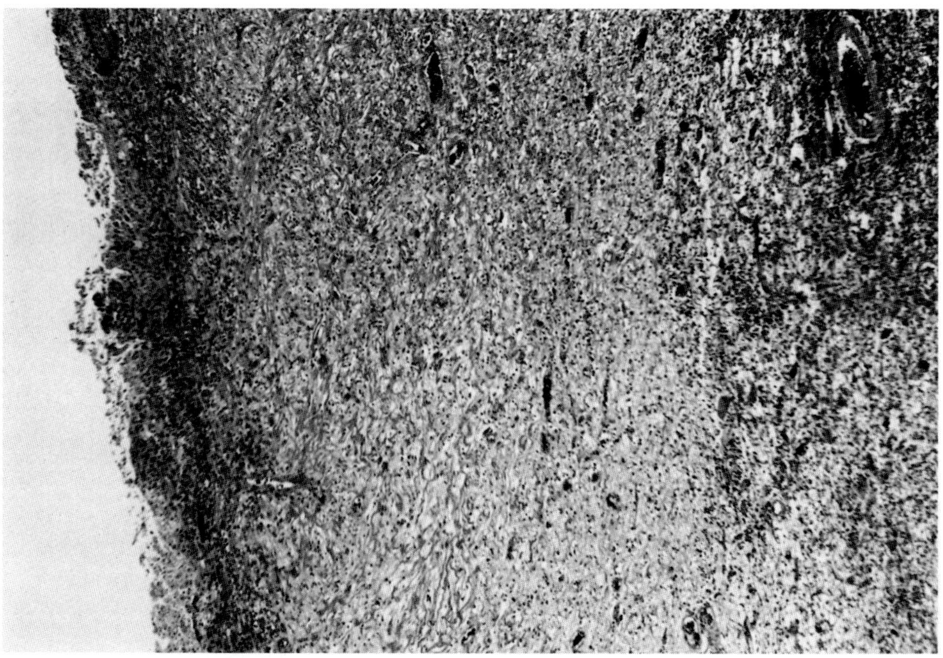

Figure 50-1. Photomicrograph of section of wall of brain abscess showing the different layers. To the left is that portion of the lining next to the cavity (50×).

Idriss, Gutman, and Kronfol[3] reported meningitis to be frequently associated with these abscesses. The failure of the infection to become well encapsulated, together with few clinical signs, accounts for the large size of the lesion by the time a diagnosis is made.[13,14] The rare disorder of pyocephalus in newborns is secondary to cerebral abscess 50 percent of the time.[15]

The incidence of brain abscess is 4 to 7 percent in patients with congenital heart disease.[16–18] Lesions from this source almost never occur in infants under 2 years of age. Tetralogy of Fallot that has not been totally corrected surgically is the most common underlying cardiac anomaly.[18–20] A right-to-left shunt is always present, causing the pulmonary bed to be bypassed and allowing circulating bacteria direct access to the cerebral circulation. The majority of these children are cyanotic, but the first reported cure was that of a girl with noncyanotic disease.[21] Decreased oxygen saturation to the brain and focal encephalomalacia may set the stage for focal infection,[19] but since these conditions occur with other diseases such as sickle cell disease, which has no particular propensity to brain abscess,[22] the right-to-left shunt is the primary etiologic factor. Studies of acute bacteremia support this reasoning.[23] Brain abscess also can occur in a child with a right-to-left shunt caused by pulmonary arteriovenous aneurysm.[24] Subacute bacterial endocarditis is rarely a factor in brain abscess.

Any area of the brain may become involved, but rarely the brain stem.[25,26] Hematogenous lesions usually are located in the distribution of the middle cerebral artery,[2,27,28] whereas those secondary to otitic or sinus infections are invariably in the adjacent areas of the brain, that is, the temporal lobe or frontal lobe respectively.[2,5,29] Direct penetration of the dura can be caused by many types of wounds during childhood, and the abscess may not form for such a prolonged period that the initial injury will be unknown or forgotten.[30] Minor wounds about the eye, in particular, must be examined carefully since puncture of the orbital roof requires little force in children.[31,32]

Clinical Features

Awareness that a brain abscess may be present is extremely important since early diagnosis is the best way to achieve low morbidity and mortality. The clinical picture in infants consists of an enlarging head and full fontanel without localizing neurologic signs. Fever is seldom present, but should such a lesion exist, the peripheral white blood cell count will be $18{,}000/mm^3$ or greater.[14] Infants usually do not have a history of infection.

In children the presence of cyanotic heart disease or a history of one of the following conditions should alert the physician to the possibility of brain abscess: (1) purulent infection such as sinusitis, mastoiditis, or chronic otitis media; (2) penetrating head wound, even in the remote past;[30,31] (3) nasal or occipital dermal sinus tract; or (4) esophageal stricture and subsequent dilatations.[33] The primary infection may have been treated with antibiotics and no longer be present. Fever is usually a symptom at some phase of the illness[3,28,34] and should suggest the possibility of brain abscess. The interval between the primary infection and abscess formation may be many months but usually is one to four weeks.[5,19] The early symptoms are those common to many infectious processes, such as malaise, fever, irritability, lethargy, and anorexia. Although usually present at some phase of the illness,[6,27] the absence of these symptoms does not rule out brain abscess. By the time the child is admitted, the peripheral white blood count usually is greater than 10,000 per cubic millimeter[3,27,28] and the sedimentation rate is almost always elevated.[22] Blood cultures are invariably negative.[3,27]

Neurologic signs and symptoms are those related to increased intracranial pressure and those secondary to focal effects of the mass. Headache, vomiting,

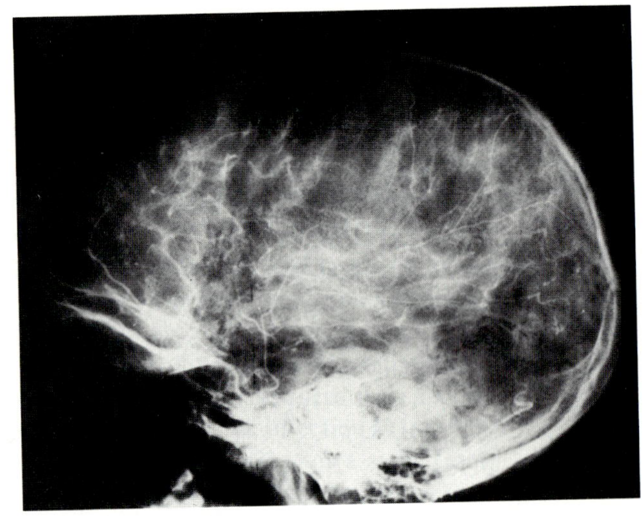

Figure 50-5. Right lateral angiogram showing avascular mass effect of right parietal abscess in a 12-year-old boy with tetralogy of Fallot.

enhancement, and 80 to 90 percent will show a ring with enhancement on the initial study.[42,46] Correlation of this ring with capsule formation is not yet completely known.[47] Increased uptake of contrast material by the ependyma may indicate the presence of ventriculitis and signal the need for appropriate therapy.[42] Computerized tomographic scanning should be done immediately on any child in whom brain abscess is a possibility or any infant with an enlarging head and full fontanel.

Treatment

Treatment of brain abscess consists of surgery for evacuation of the purulent material and systemic antibiotic therapy appropriate to the organisms cultured. If diagnosed during the cerebritic stage, the disease may be cured by antibiotic therapy.[48] Cure of abscess has been reported without surgery,[49] but this mode of therapy must be used with great caution because without surgery mortality is generally 100 percent.[28] Clinical and experimental evidence has shown the relative ineffectiveness of antibiotics in killing bacteria in suppurative lesions even though apparently adequate levels of drug are present.[50,51]

The availability of CT scanning has made it possible to diagnose brain abscesses earlier and more accurately than was heretofore possible, which should help to decrease morbidity and mortality. Instillation of radiopaque substances is now unnecessary in following the progress of the lesion during treatment.

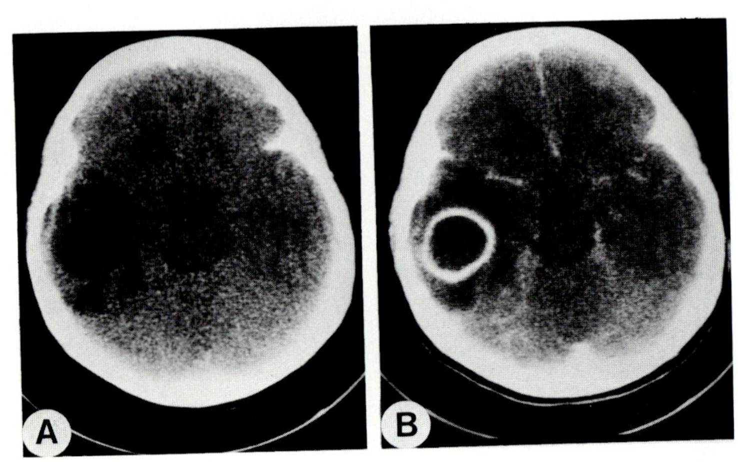

Figure 50-6. CT scan in 10-year-old boy. A. Before contrast injection. B. After contrast injection. Note edema surrounding the abscess and typical ring enhancement after contrast injection.

Surgical treatment is of three types: (1) catheter drainage; (2) tapping, single or multiple; and (3) excision. Catheter drainage is the oldest successful method[52] and continues to be used with good results.[10,53,54] This method consists of making a burr hole over the most insensitive portion of the cortex where the abscess is superficial, opening the dura, and making a small cortical incision. The abscess is palpated with a brain cannula and then punctured with a small soft catheter (no. 10 French) over a stylet. The catheter is anchored loosely into place with a suture through the scalp. Pus usually flows spontaneously from the tube. Gentle aspiration with a syringe can be performed at the operating table and saline irrigation used to help empty the cavity. Instillation of local antibiotics probably is unnecessary if the organism is sensitive to an antibiotic that perfuses well into the brain from the blood. The catheter is usually left in place for about seven days until drainage ceases and then is removed. This method is best suited for supratentorial lesions relatively near the surface.

Tapping usually is done through a burr hole also, and has been a useful method since first described in 1926 by Dandy.[55] It is the preferred method for evacuating deep collections or those in sensitive areas,[56,57] as well as those in children with congenital heart disease.[22] With the sophisticated methods of localization and follow-up currently available (CT scanning) and antibiotic therapy, tapping may be the treatment of choice for any brain abscess. The procedure can be performed using local anesthesia, and a single aspiration is frequently all that is required.[27,55] Follow-up by CT scanning must be done in every child. Repeated tapping may be done should material reaccumulate.

Excision of the entire abscess is best accomplished after the formation is encapsulated, but removal of deep lesions or those in critical areas of the cortex is not advisable. Whether excision offers any advantages over the other methods is open to serious question.[37,58–60] Damage to surrounding brain from the dissection may increase morbidity.[56] Certainly if excision is carried out, dissection must be done carefully to produce only minimal trauma to surrounding brain. Surrounding white matter should not be resected as was advised in the past.[61] Excision is performed in the usual manner for removing a mass lesion. The bone opening is centered over the most superficial part of the abscess, and a cortical incision is made through the closest silent area after palpation of the capsule with a blunt cannula. The lesion is resected intact if possible. If the lesion is large, deflating it by aspiration may be advisable prior to removal so as to decrease trauma to the surrounding brain. When resection is completed, the area is irrigated copiously with saline and the wound closed as is done following removal of any other intracranial mass. No drain is left in the brain. Good results can be achieved by resection.[1,2]

Any focus of infection elsewhere must be eradicated as soon as possible by appropriate therapy. Regardless of the mode of surgical treatment contemplated, as soon as the possibility of a brain abscess arises the patient should be started on dexamethasone to reduce cerebral edema and be given antibiotics. Because of appropriate antibiotic coverage, dexamethasone can be given in the usual doses without increasing the risk of spreading the infection. If the organism is unknown prior to surgery because a focus of infection such as mastoiditis or sinusitis is not present to culture, then antistaphalococcal penicillin, penicillin, and chloramphenicol should all be started in doses appropriate for treating meningitis. Pretreatment with antibiotics[5] probably accounts for some of the 15 to 40 percent sterile cultures of the abscess contents[27,56,60] but is still mandatory. When laboratory information is available regarding organism sensitivities, the antibiotic regimen can be altered appropriately. If one expects a high rate of positive findings, material from the abscess must be cultured meticulously for aerobes, anaerobes, and fungi as soon as possible. System antibiotics should be continued for three to six weeks, depending on clinical response. With intensive antibiotic therapy, rupture of the abscess into the ventricular system need not be fatal; but, of course, this can be avoided if drainage is done early. The reasons for failure of treatment are late recognition and inadequate antibiotic therapy.[59] Anticonvulsant medication should be given to all patients.

Results

The long-term results in infants cannot be expected to be as good as those in older children. The enormous size of the abscess and relatively poor host resistance makes for greater brain damage; in addition, almost all these infants have hydrocephalus.[13,14,62] Early recognition and referral for neurosurgical treatment will improve their prognosis. Early diagnosis and surgical drainage or excision combined with intensive antibiotic therapy should reduce mortality in older children to nearly zero. The neurosurgeon must be prepared to perform emergency surgery if the level of consciousness is poor or deteriorating since the death rate in comatose patients is high.[2] This approach also will decrease morbidity, which may tend to be greater in children than in adults.[64] One must remember that every brain abscess causes some degree of destruction to brain tissue. An increasing number of survivors experience seizures as time passes (up to 72 percent). These are not related to age, type of surgical treatment, site of abscess (except for the cerebellum), or residual neurologic deficit. Presence or absence of preoperative seizures does not necessarily predict that a patient will develop seizures postoperatively.[65] The interval between treatment and seizure development is longest in children who are less than 10 years of age. The seizures usually occur infrequently and can be controlled by anticonvulsant medication, which should be given prophylactically to all patients.[18,64] A follow-up electroencephalogram in patients with seizures almost invariably shows a localized sharp and slow wave complex.

SUBDURAL EMPYEMA

Subdural empyema of the intracranial space is an uncommon disorder that occurs principally in children and adolescents. The incidence is approximately one fifth that of brain abscess.[66] This disorder is usually secondary to paranasal sinus or middle ear infections, but also may be a complication of purulent scalp infection, osteomyelitis of the skull, or secondary to a hematogenous infection in a subdural hematoma. The pathway from contiguous infection can be through infected venous channels or a bone defect. The collections are located most often over the frontoparietal convexities and may involve the interhemispheric space. Bilateral or posterior fossa spread is rare. These lesions may become very large before they are diagnosed. In patients with subdural empyema who also have meningitis, brain abscess, or extradural abscess, the prognosis is worsened. Signs and symptoms consist of headache, vomiting, signs of infection, and nuchal rigidity.[67] The history may be as long as six months. Sedimentation rate and peripheral white blood count are elevated. Infants will have increasing head size and bulging fontanel, and seizures are common.[68] Focal signs may develop late in the disease process, often accompanied by a deteriorating level of consciousness, indicating the need for rapid institution of treatment. If symptoms are suggestive of subdural empyema, spinal puncture should not be done because of the danger of precipitating brain herniation. The fluid will show only elevated protein and pleocytosis, usually of lymphocytes, and hence is not of diagnostic value. The diagnosis of subdural collection can be made by CT scanning or angiography

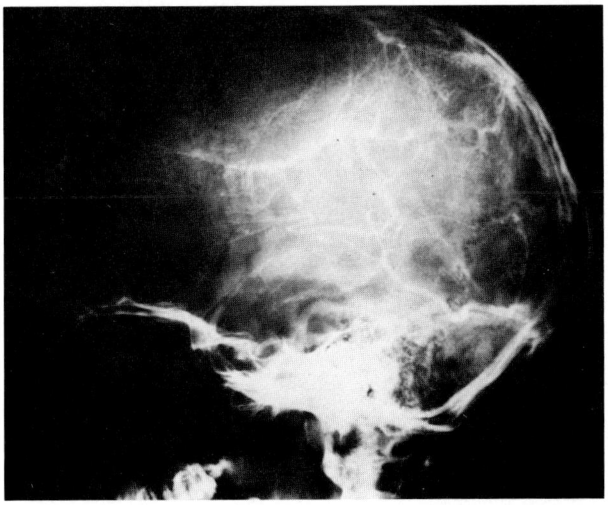

Figure 50-7. Left lateral angiogram of a 12-year-old boy with subdural empyema. Note hypervascular rim.

(Fig. 50-7). An interhemispheric spread should be noted, as well as the presence of a brain abscess. The empyema can be seen easily on CT scan as an extracerebral mass and any interhemispheric spread can be readily observed. The injection of contrast medium enhances the cortical membrane (Fig. 50-8). Lateral displacement of the pericallosal and callosomarginal branches present on the anteroposterior angiogram indicates the existence of an interhemispheric collection. Plain skull roentgenograms may reveal sinusitis, mastoiditis, or skull osteomyelitis.

Treatment consists of an antibiotic regimen similar to that for brain abscess, and local antibiotics usually are not necessary.[66] Steroids are administered to control increased intracranial pressure, and anticonvulsants should be given to prevent seizures. A focus of infection identified elsewhere should be eradicated as soon as possible. After surgery a follow-up CT scan should be obtained to rule out the presence of an intracerebral abscess not seen on the initial examination.

Surgical drainage must be done in all cases of subdural empyema.[68] Evacuation and irrigation through multiple burr holes are adequate if the pus is thin and there is no interhemispheric collection. If the pus is thick or an interhemispheric collection is present, a craniotomy should be performed and the infected material removed as completely as possible. Drains usually are not necessary, but catheters may be left in the subdural space for a few days for irrigation. At the time of surgery, pus should be taken in an airtight container directly to the bacteriology laboratory for Gram stain and culture. Particular

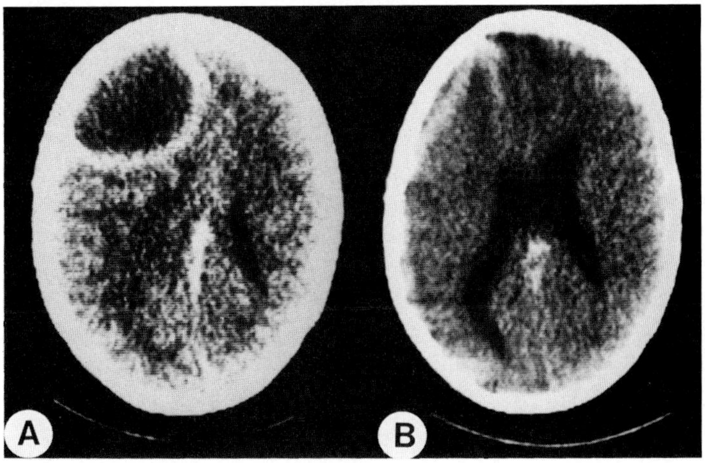

Figure 50-8. CT scan of the patient in Figure 50-7. A. Preoperative scan with enhancement. B. Ten days postoperative with enhancement.

attention to isolation of anaerobic organisms is important since these bacteria frequently are present in paranasal sinus infection.[70] Mortality remains about 40 percent[69] even with treatment. Complications such as cortical thrombophlebitis, brain abscess, and meningitis decrease the success rate. Early diagnosis and therapy together with meticulous attention to bacteriologic studies should improve the prognosis. Seizure incidence in long-term survivors is about 26 percent,[71] and consequently anticonvulsants should be continued for at least two years after surgery. If after this time no seizures have occurred and the electroencephalogram shows no epileptogenic focus, the patient can be taken off anticonvulsant medication on a trial basis.

EPIDURAL ABSCESS

Epidural intracranial abscess is virtually always secondary to or associated with another infection such as mastoiditis, sinusitis, postoperative flap infection, or osteomyelitis of the skull (Fig. 50-9). This abscess also may result from infection of compound wounds of the head. A purulent extradural collection without osteomyelitis of the skull is rare.[72] Increased intracranial pressure from this lesion alone is uncommon as the mass effect is usually not great, but it can be associated with subdural empyema or brain abscess. Hence these conditions must be ruled out in all patients by CT scanning or some other means. Epidural abscess serves as a focus of infection and may cause septicemia, which cannot be successfully treated until the epidural infection is eradicated. Plain skull roentgenograms often will show osteomyelitis or air in the subdural space.[72]

The patient frequently manifests few specific clinical signs, except those due to infection, such as fever or malaise. Peripheral white blood cells are increased. Local findings of scalp redness, swelling, and tenderness, together with focal headache secondary to sinus infection, mastoiditis, or skull osteomyelitis, are usually present. If neurologic signs and symptoms do occur, they usually appear late in the course of the disease and when a large lesion is present.

Therapy consists of evacuation of the epidural collection through burr holes or by craniectomy if osteomyelitis is present. All epidural granulations should be removed as thoroughly as possible.[72] A catheter drain may be left in the epidural space for the first few days, and is desirable if the cavity is large. The bone should be treated as described in the following section. Any associated problem such as sinusitis or brain abscess must be treated promptly. Antibiotics should be started

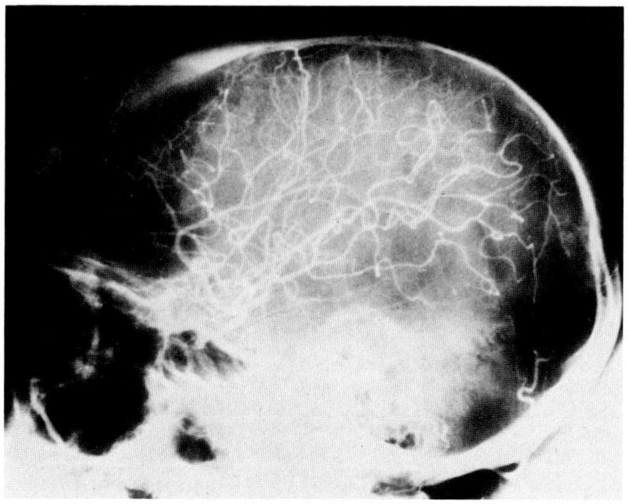

Figure 50-9. Left lateral angiogram of 15-year-old boy with frontal osteomyelitis and epidural abscess.

when the condition is first believed to be present, and, of course, cultures should be done carefully for aerobes, anaerobes, and fungi so that appropriate drugs can be selected. Before the culture results are available, the antibiotics used in the initial treatment of a brain abscess are given. Follow-up CT scans should be done until the patient recovers in order to follow the progress of the lesion or to detect the presence of the more serious brain abscess or subdural empyema.

OSTEOMYELITIS OF THE SKULL

Osteomyelitis of the skull is most commonly a complication of a compound skull wound, either postoperatively or posttraumatic. It can occur in the frontal bone secondary to sinus infection or in the parietal and temporal bones from ear infection.[73] Osteomyelitis may develop in the skull of a newborn as a complication of an infected scalp wound from forceps or secondary to intrauterine monitoring.[74]

Clinical signs consist of local heat, swelling, tenderness, and redness. In the postoperative period, poor healing of the suture line or a draining sinus of the wound may alert one to the problem. The patient may not have fever.[75] If the infection is severe, the patient will have high fever, will suffer prostration, and peripheral white blood cells will be elevated. In this last situation, blood cultures are indicated. *Staphalococcus aureus* is the most commonly associated organism in postoperative and posttraumatic wounds. The disease may progress rapidly if an epidural abscess is also present.[73] Meningitis almost never occurs unless the dura is open from previous surgery or has been lacerated from a compound wound.

X-ray examination of the skull may show no change for the first 10 to 14 days. The classic picture is a "moth-eaten" appearance (Fig. 50-10). Radionuclide scan with technetium-labeled organic phosphate can show changes as soon as the infection is present, and scalp artifact is not a problem with current scintillation cameras.

Treatment consists of debridement of the area and antibiotic therapy. In a postoperative wound, the bone flap must be removed but the pericranium should be preserved. Poorly vascularized and infected bone surrounding the craniotomy must be rongeured back to well-vascularized bone. If surgical therapy is done promptly and antibiotic treatment is adequate, it is rarely necessary to remove bone other than that already devitalized, that is, the flap or a sequestrum. All

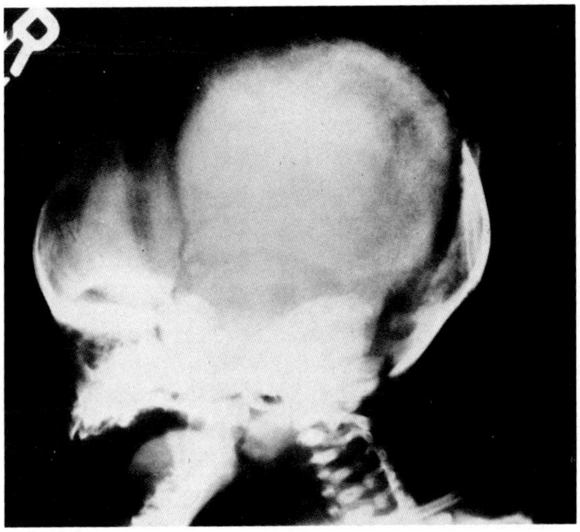

Figure 50-10. Typical "moth-eaten" appearance of osteomyelitis of the skull.

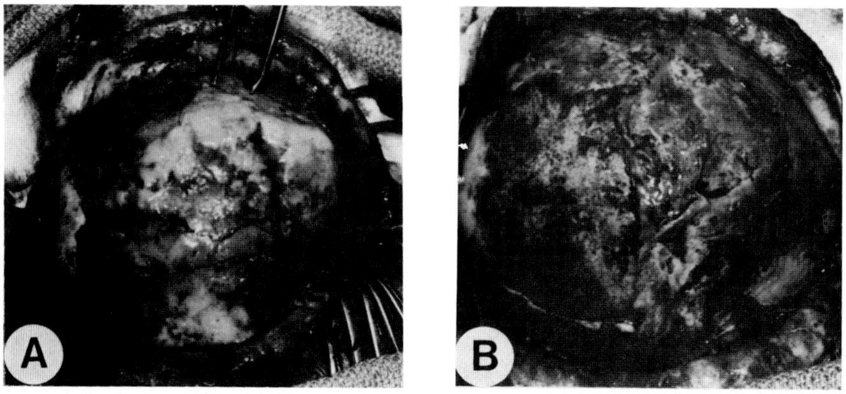

Figure 50-11. Ten-day-old girl with extensive staphylococcal osteomyelitis of the skull. A. Before debridement. Note forceps pointing to infected granulations. B. After debridement. Well-vascularized bone was preserved. Wound subsequently healed without incident.

infected granulation tissue should be curretted away and any epidural abscess treated as described. Care should be taken not to penetrate the dura. By removing any infected granulation tissue attached to the skull that is producing bone destruction, the process can be stopped and make removal of the underlying bone unnecessary (Fig. 50-11). Copious irrigation with saline solution is done throughout the procedure, and the wound is closed in one layer with nylon or stainless steel sutures. A drain may be left in place for 24 hours. Local antibiotics usually are not indicated. These same principles are used in treating skull osteomyelitis from other causes. If debridement is done early, rapid resolution of the process can be expected. Cranioplasty should not be done for at least six months.

REFERENCES

1. Wright RL, Ballantine HT: Management of brain abscess in children and adolescents. Am J Dis Child 114:113–122, 1967
2. Arseni C, Horvath L, Dumitrescu L: Cerebral abscesses in children. Acta Neurochir (Vienna) 14:197–224, 1966
3. Idriss ZH, Gutman LT, Kronfol NM: Brain abscesses in infants and children. Clin Pediatr (Philadelphia) 17:738–746, 1978
4. Loeser E, Scheinberg L: Brain abscesses: A review of 99 cases. Neurology (Minneapolis) 7:601–609, 1957
5. Samson DS, Clark K: A current review of brain abscess. Am J Med 54:201–210, 1973
6. Beller AJ, Sahar A, Praiss I: Brain abscess. J Neurol Neurosurg Psychiatr 36:757–768, 1973
7. Matson DD: Brain abscess, in Matson DD: Neurosurgery of Infancy and Childhood. Springfield, Charles C Thomas, 1969, pp 708–715
8. McClelland CJ, Craig BF, Crockard HA: Brain abscesses in Northern Ireland. J Neurol Neurosurg Psychiatr 41:1043–1047, 1978
9. Proctor CA: Intracranial complications of otitic origin. Laryngoscope 76:288–308, 1966
10. Grant FC: The mortality from abscess of the brain. JAMA 99:550–556, 1932
11. Friede RL: Developmental Neuropathology. New York/Vienna, Springer-Verlag, 1975, pp 175–176
12. Sanford HM: Abscess of the brain in infants under 12 months of age. Am J Dis Child 35:256–261, 1928

13. Munslow RA, Stovall VS, Price RD, et al: Brain abscess in infants. J Pediatr 51:74–79, 1957
14. Hoffman HJ, Hendrick EB, Hiscox JL: Cerebral abscess in early infancy. J Neurosurg 33:172–177, 1970
15. Izquierdo JM, Sanz F, Coca JM, et al: Pyocephalus of the new-born child. Child's Brain 4:129–136, 1978
16. Maronde RF: Brain abscess and congenital heart disease. Ann Intern Med 33:602–606, 1950
17. Newton EJ: Hematogenous brain abscess in cyanotic congenital heart disease. Q J Med 25:201, 1956
18. Taussig HB, Crocetti A, Eshaghpour E, et al: Long-time observations on the Blalock–Taussig Operation. III: Common complications. Johns Hopkins Med J 129:274–289, 1971
19. Matson DD, Salam M: Brain abscess in congenital heart disease. Pediatrics 27:772–789, 1961
20. Tyler HR, Clark DB: Incidents of neurological complication in congenital heart disease. Arch Neurol Psychiatr 77:17–22, 1957
21. Smolik EA, Blattner RJ, & Heys FM: Brain abscess associated with congenital heart disease. JAMA 130:145–147, 1946
22. Raimondi AJ, Matsumoto S, Miller RA: Brain abscess in children with congenital heart disease. J Neurosurg 23:588–595, 1965
23. Wood WB, Smith MR, Perry WD, et al: Studies on the cellular immunology of acute bacteremia. J Exp Med 94:521–534, 1951
24. Meacham WF, Scott HW: Congenital pulmonary arteriovenous aneurysm complicated by bacteriodes abscess of brain. Ann Surg 147:404–408, 1958
25. Danziger J, Allen KL, & Block S: Brain stem abscess in children. J Neurosurg 40:391–393, 1974
26. Robert CM Jr, Stern WE, Brown WJ, et al: Brain stem abscess treated surgically. Surg Neurol 3:153–160, 1975
27. McGreal DA: Brain abscesses in children. Can Med Assoc J 86:261–268, 1962
28. Eberhard SJ: Diagnosis of brain abscess in infants and children: A retrospective study of 26 cases. NC Med J 30:363–369, 1969
29. Shaw MD, Russell JA: Cerebellar abscess: A review of 47 cases. J Neurol Neurosurg Psychiatr 38:429–435, 1975
30. Mikhael MA, Mattar AG: Case report: Chronic graphite granulomatous abscess stimulating a brain tumor. J Comput Assist Tomogr 1:513–516, 1977
31. Miller CF, Brodkey JS, Colombi BJ: The danger of intracranial wood. Surg Neurol 7:95–103, 1977
32. Fanning WL, Willett LR, Phillips CF, et al: Puncture wound of the eyelid causing brain abscess. J Trauma 16:919–920, 1976
33. Kolter R, Schild JA, Holinger PH: Delayed CNS complications. Largyngoscope 85:1379–1386, 1975
34. Torales A, Franco FR, Calderon E: Intracranial abscesses in children. Bol Med Hosp Infant Mex 35:33–43, 1978
35. Snyder BD, Farmer TW: Brain abscess in children. South Med J 64:687–690, 1971
36. DeVio DC: Cerebral abscess in children. Dev Med Child Neurol 13:800–804, 1971
37. Morgan H, Wood MW, Murphey F: Experience with 88 consecutive cases of brain abscess. J Neurosurg 38:698–704, 1973
38. Norrell H, Howieson J: Gas-containing brain abscesses. Am J. Roentgenol 109:273–276, 1970
39. Russell JA, Taylor JC: Circumscribed gas-gangrene abscess of the brain. Br J Surg 50:434–437, 1963
40. Morte PD, Brannon WL, Furlow TW Jr: Case report: Evolution of cerebral abscess. Disparity between radionuclide and CT scans. Postgrad Med 63:226,229–230, 1978
41. Waxman AD, Siemsen JK: Gallium scanning in cerebral and cranial infections. Am J Roentgenol 127:309–314, 1976
42. Nielson H, Gyldensted C: Computed tomography in the diagnosis of cerebral abscess. Neuroradiology 12:207–217, 1977

43. New PFJ, Davis KR, Ballantine HT: Computed tomography in cerebral abscess. Radiology 121:641–646, 1976
44. Zimmerman RA, Patel S, Bilaniuk LT: Demonstration of purulent bacterial intracranial infections by computed tomography. Am J Roentgenol 127:155–165, 1976
45. Stephanov S: Experience with multiloculated brain abscesses. J Neurosurg 49:199–203, 1978
46. Price H, Danziger A: The role of computerized tomography in the diagnosis and management of intracranial abscess. Clin Radiol 29:571–577, 1978
47. Enzmann DR, Britt RH, Yeager AS: Experimental brain abscess evolution; computed tomographic and neuropathologic correlation. Radiology 133:113–122, 1979
48. Heineman HS, Braude AJ, Osterholm JL: Intracranial suppurative disease. JAMA 218:1542–1547, 1971
49. Berg B, Franklin G, Cuneo R, et al: Neurosurgical cure of brain abscess: Early diagnosis and follow-up with computerized tomography. Ann Neurol 3:474–478, 1978
50. Black P, Graybill RJ, Charache P: Penetration of brain abscess by systemically administered antibiotics. J Neurosurg 38:705–709, 1973
51. Smith MR, Wood WB: AN experimental analysis of the curative action of penicillin in acute bacterial infections. J Exp Med 103:509–521, 1956
52. Macewen W: Pyogenic Infective Diseases of the Brain and Spinal Cord. Glasgow, James Maclehose & Sons, 1893
53. Mount L: Conservative surgical therapy of brain abscesses. J Neurosurg 7:385–389, 1960
54. Selker RG: Intracranial abscess: Treatment by continuous catheter drainage. Child's Brain 1:368–375, 1975
55. Dandy WE: Treatment of chronic abscess of the brain by tapping. JAMA 87:1477–1478, 1926
56. Jooma OV, Pennybacker JB, Tutton GK: Brain abscess: Aspiration, drainage, or excision? J Neurol Neurosurg Psychiatr 14:308–313, 1951
57. Ballantine HT Jr, White JC: Brain abscess. N Engl J Med 248:14–19, 1953
58. Liske E, Weikers NJ: Changing aspects of brain abscesses. Neurology (Minneapolis) 14:294–300, 1964
59. Garfield J: Management of supratentorial intracranial abscess. Br Med J 2:7–11, 1969
60. Alphen, HAM von, Dreissen JJR: Brain abscess and subdural empyema. J Neurol Neurosurg Psychiatr 39:481–490, 1976
61. Le Beau J: Radical surgery and penicillin in brain abscess. J Neurosurg 3:359–374, 1946
62. Butler NR, Barrie H, Paine KWE: Cerebral abscess as a complication of neonatal sepsis. Arch Dis Child 32:461–465, 1951
63. Carey ME, Chou SM, French LA: Long term neurological residua in patients surviving brain abscess with surgery. J Neurosurg 34:652–656, 1971
64. Legg NJ, Gupta PC, Scott DF: Epilepsy following cerebral abscess. Brain 96:259–268, 1973
65. Kerr FWL, King RB, Meagher JN: Brain abscess: A study of 47 consecutive cases. JAMA 168:868–872, 1958
66. Bhandari YS, Sarkari NBS: Subdural empyema: A review of 37 cases. J Neurosurg 32:35–39, 1970
67. McLaurin RL: Subdural infection, in Gurdjian ES (ed): Cranial and Intracranial Suppuration. Springfield, Charles C Thomas, 1969, pp 73–88
68. Rao S, Dinakar I: Subdural empyema in infants. Indian J Pediatr 38:358–361, 1971
69. Glasauer FE, Coots D, Levy LF, et al: Subdural empyema in Africans in Rhodesia. Neurosurgery 3:385–391, 1978
70. Yoshikawa TT, Chow AW, Guze LB: Role of anaerobic bacteria in subdural empyema: Report of 4 cases and review of 327 cases from the English literature. Am J Med 58:99–104, 1975
71. Hitchcock E, Andreadis A: Subdural empyema: A review of 29 cases. J Neurol Neurosurg Psychiatr 27:422–434, 1964

72. Woodhall B: Osteomyelitis and epi-, extra- and subdural abscesses, in Clinical Neurosurgery, Vol 16. Baltimore, Williams & Wilkins, 1967, pp 239–255
73. Gurdjian ES: Cranial and Intracranial Suppuration. Springfield, Charles C Thomas, 1969, pp 59–72
74. Overturf GD, Balfour G: Osteomyelitis and sepsis: Severe complications of fetal monitoring. Pediatrics 55:244–247, 1975
75. Matson DD: Osteomyelitis, in Matson DD: Neurosurgery of Infancy and Childhood. Springfield, Charles C Thomas, 1969, pp 701–704

51. Intraspinal Infections

James H. Salmon

Neurosurgical infections of the spine are rare in children. The symptoms are nonspecific. Prompt diagnosis and treatment can provide an excellent result. A successful program must include a high index of suspicion; myelography to confirm the diagnosis and localize the abscess; surgical drainage; culture of the abscess for aerobic, anaerobic, fungal, and acid-fast organisms; and appropriate antibiotics.

EPIDURAL ABSCESS

Diagnosis

An epidural abscess is most likely to cause neurologic dysfunction. This is rare and in a 1971 review[1] only eight reported primary cases could be found. The presenting symptoms are fever and back pain. The infant is particularly irritable when handled. The older child may localize the back pain and will limp or refuse to bear weight at all. The patient seen in a later stage has root pain, weakness, or paraplegia. Heusner[2] described the four developmental phases in the adult as spinal ache, root pain, weakness, and paralysis. The rate of progression is very variable and paraplegia may occur within hours of the onset of root pain.

On examination the child usually is febrile, but may not be. There is tenderness over the involved portion of the spine, and sometimes rigidity. Focal neurologic signs help to localize the lesion. In the afebrile child, the symptoms mimic those of an epidural spinal cord tumor.

Typically there is an increased white blood cell count with an increased percentage of polymorphonuclear leukocytes. The sedimentation rate is markedly elevated. Blood cultures are frequently normal.

Radiologic examination of the spine can be diagnostic for certain spinal infections. Disk space inflammations in children are the best example. A paraspinal mass may suggest the likely location for a secondary epidural abscess.

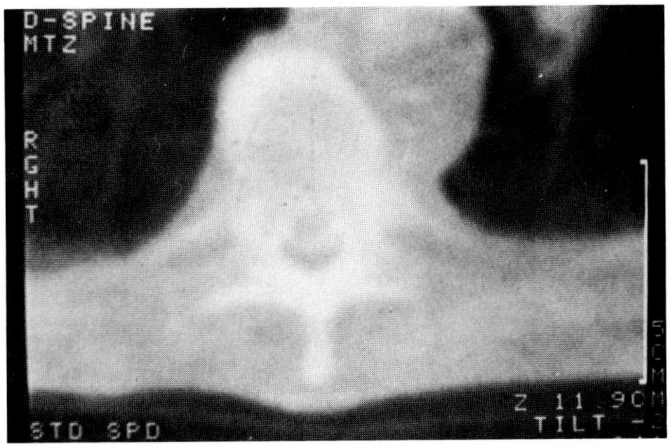

Figure 51-1. CT scan of dorsal epidural abscess. Metrizimide outlines the cord shadow that has been displaced ventrally by the crescent-shaped epidural abscess. (Courtesy of Dr. D. J. Millet.)

Primary epidural abscess and intramedullary abscess typically have x-rays that appear normal.

A child with a fever and these findings is usually diagnosed as having meningitis and lumbar puncture is done. If an epidural abscess is suspected, the puncture should be done at the time of myelography. A collection of pus may be encountered in the epidural space if the stylet is removed periodically during introduction of the needle. Many abscesses, however, are remote from the usual puncture site. There may be pleocytosis of the cerebrospinal fluid, and the culture ordinarily grows *Staphylococcus aureus*. In nearly half of the cases, however, the cerebrospinal fluid (CSF) will be entirely normal. Manometric study is frequently unreliable for detecting a spinal block, and this is particularly true in a struggling infant. Myelography, preferably with a water-soluble agent, is the definitive diagnostic tool The myelogram will demonstrate the epidural mass and localize the spinal level, which is usually in the lumbar area but may occur anywhere in the spine. To aid in the laminectomy, the skin should be marked. A transverse needle scratch away from the line of incision is preferred. Some authors have stated that myelography is not indicated and the diagnosis should be made by laminectomy. The myelogram, however, permits the surgeon to restrict the laminectomy to the involved area, and this may decrease the possibility of future scoliosis. Transventricular spinal myelography[3] may be used to localize the upper level of the lesion or when lumbar puncture is unsuccessful. Pantopaque is placed in the lateral ventricle and manipulated into the spinal canal with fluoroscopic control.

Computer-assisted tomography (CAT) of the spine shows great promise (Fig. 51-1). Current-generation scanners require the injection of contrast material in the subarachnoid space to define the abscess. The CAT scan can show the state of the canal between two levels of myelographic blockage. The myelogram only demonstrates the poles of the lesion.

Treatment

Laminectomy should be performed as soon as the diagnosis is made. Recovery from paraplegia is possible. Most of the pus will be in the dorsal half of the spinal canal because of the configuration of the epidural space. The purulent material should be promptly cultured for aerobic, anaerobic, fungal, and acid-fast organisms. A stained smear, done while surgery is in progress, may aid antibiotic selection. Multiple abscesses may be encountered. All purulent material should be removed and thorough irrigation is done prior to closure. Diluted (1.5 percent) hydrogen peroxide may be used.

In chronic cases granulation tissue may be encountered. This is gently dissected from the dura. Thrombosed vessels may be seen. Involvement of the segmental vessels by vasculitis or compression can cause spinal cord infarction and a permanent deficit.

The wound is drained and closed in layers. Stainless steel is the preferred suture material.

A penicillinase-resistant penicillin and a broad spectrum antibiotic are given intravenously during the operation. The culture report will dictate further antibiotic treatment. Antibiotic therapy is continued for an arbitrary time, usually three weeks. Determination of the minimal inhibitory concentration is a useful guide to antibiotic dosage. Although *Staph. aureus* is the most common organism, the incidence of other organisms is increasing.[4] This is particularly true if the child is immuno-suppressed or a narcotics abuser.

Secondary epidural abscess from a puncture wound, following surgery, or osteomyelitis of an adjacent vertebra can occur.

In summary a child or infant may present with fever, irritability when handled, or a limp. Myelography is the definitive diagnostic tool. Normal CSF and blood cultures should be anticipated. Laminectomy with drainage of the abscess is the definitive treatment and should be carried out promptly. The occasional occurrence of an unusual organism mandates careful and thorough culturing of the abscess.

SPINAL CORD ABSCESS

Fifty-five cases of spinal cord abscess were reported between 1830 and 1977.[5] The peak age incidences were between a few days and 10 years and between 20 and 30 years.

The symptoms of spinal cord abscess are very similar to those of epidural abscess—fever, spinal ache, root pain, and paraparesis. The progression may be rapid. A source of infection was found in 80 percent of cases. *Staphylococcus* is the most frequent organism. Multiple abscesses are sometimes encountered.

Cerebrospinal fluid studies may be completely normal and myelography is the definitive diagnostic procedure.

The treatment is exposure by laminectomy and aspiration of the swollen spinal cord to localize the abscess. A longitudinal dorsal myelotomy is needed for adequate drainage. Relapse is common without proper treatment. The dura is closed about a small, soft drainage catheter. Four weeks of intravenous antibiotic therapy are recommended.

CONGENITAL DERMAL SINUS

This entity is of particular interest to pediatric neurosurgeons as they are frequently asked for an opinion regarding the management of an asymptomatic dermal sinus. The sinus results from a failure of separation of the cutaneous epithelial ectoderm from the neuroepithelial ectoderm during the first month of intrauterine life. Meningitis is the most common infection from the source, but subdural abscesses and a rare intramedullary abscess have been reported.[6] The sinus is usually in the sacral area but may occur in the cervical spine.[7] The presentation is the same as described for epidural abscess. The treatment is laminectomy and drainage. As the sinus may connect with the central spinal canal, a very extensive abscess may be found. The best treatment is prophylactic. Every congenital dermal sinus tract should be totally excised as soon as the condition is recognized.[8] "Dimples" may harbor a tract and probably should be excised.

DISK SPACE INFECTIONS

Infection of the disk space in children is a benign disease of unknown etiology. Disk space inflammation[9] may be the appropriate term. It has characteristic clinical and roentgenographic findings. This disorder may be considered the childhood equivalent of vertebral osteomyelitis in adults. The latter is extremely rare in children since the widespread use of antibiotics and the control of tuberculosis; not a single case was encountered in a series of 93 children with acute osteomyelitis.[10]

Diagnosis

The symptoms resemble those of epidural abscess. The child, usually between 1 and 4 years of age, may refuse to walk, stand, or even sit. Older children complain of back or hip pain. Fever and malaise occur. Back pain or rigidity is present. There are no signs of spinal cord or nerve root involvement and the spinal fluid examination is always negative. Blood cultures are almost always normal. The sedimentation rate is elevated.

The radiologic picture is typical. There is disk space narrowing and sometimes irregularity of the vertebral end-plate. The lumbar spine is the most common site and it does not occur above the mid-dorsal area.

Immobilization for 10 to 20 weeks is the definitive treatment. Antibiotics may be given if the patient has a recurrence of symptoms or is not improving as rapidly as expected. Needle biopsies occasionally are done.

Patients with disk space inflammations are cared for by an orthopedic surgeon after the diagnosis has been established.

REFERENCES

1. Baker CJ: Primary spinal epidural abscess. Am J Dis Child 121:337–339, 1971
2. Heusner AP: Nontuberculous spinal epidural infections. N Engl J Med 239:845–854, 1948
3. Salmon JH: Transventricular spinal myelography in the infant. Radiology 91:1041, 1968
4. Guerrero IC, Slap GB, MacGregor RR, et al: Anaerobic spinal epidural abscess: Case report. J Neurosurg 48:465–469, 1978
5. Menezes AH, Graf CJ, Perret GE: Spinal cord abscess: A review. Surg Neurol 8:461–467, 1977
6. Gind SE, Fairburn B: Intramedullary spinal abscess as a complication of congenital dermal sinus. J Neurosurg 30:494–497, 1969
7. Bean JR, Walsh JW, Blacker HM: Cervical dermal sinus and intramedullary spinal cord abscess: Case report. Neurosurgery 5:60–62, 1979
8. Matson DD, Jerva MJ: Recurrent meningitis associated with congenital dermal sinus tract. J Neurosurg 25:288–297, 1966
9. Spiegel PG, Kengla KW, Isaacson AS, et al: Intervertebral disc-space inflammation in children. J Bone J Surg 54-A:284–296, 1972
10. Mollan RAB, Piggot J: Acute osteomyelitis in children. J Bone J Surg 59-B:2–7, 1977

52. Antibiotic Therapy in Central Nervous System Infections

Peter T. Frame
Robert L. McLaurin

Antibiotics have made a significant impact on the therapy of infections in the central nervous system. The mortality rate for meningitis, for example, has dropped from virtually 100 percent to as low as 5 percent for *Neisseria meningitidis* infection. Concomitant with the development of effective therapy for bacterial meningitis, however, more sophisticated neurosurgical techniques have developed that have broadened the spectrum of infections in the central nervous system. Also, antibiotic therapy of brain abscess has not provided such a dramatic reduction in mortality rate, which remains approximately 40 percent during the antibiotic era.

Antibiotic therapy for infections in the central nervous system (CNS) is complicated by the fact that penetration of most antibiotics into the compartments of the CNS is considerably reduced by the blood–cerebrospinal fluid (CSF) and blood–brain barriers. In general terms the blood–CSF barrier is composed of the cells of the choroid plexus, which act as a selective barrier to the diffusion of molecules into the subarachnoid space. Most antibiotics are excluded from the spinal fluid by an active transport mechanism, and achieve significant concentrations in the CSF only when the choroid plexus is impaired by inflammation. The blood–brain barrier is composed of the interface between the capillaries and the glial stroma of the brain. The capillary network in the brain differs from that in other tissues, with a very tight union between endothelial cells preventing ready egress of substances into the brain tissue. Movement of antibiotics through these two barriers is also affected by a number of physicochemical and physiologic parameters. Among these are the lipid solubility of the antibiotic, the state of ionization of the molecules at physiologic pH, the acid-base status of the individual, serum protein binding of the antibiotic, and most important, the extent of inflammation present at the barrier site.

Since the anatomic and physiologic structures of the two barriers are different, it is easy to understand the empiric observations that penetration of various antibiotics into normal spinal fluid, inflamed spinal fluid, normal brain tissue, brain abscesses, and brain tumors is variable. Antibiotic penetration of CSF has been fairly well studied for many antibiotics, both in the presence and absence of signs of inflammation in the spinal fluid. Antibiotic penetration into brain tissue, however, has been studied infrequently, although recently there have been a number of attempts to investigate this problem. Measurement of antibiotic concentrations in CSF are fairly simple, being done mainly by applying the same techniques used for measurement of antibiotic concentrations in serum. Measurement of antibiotic concentrations in brain tissue has been done by a number of different methods, which are not always comparable. This lack of uniformity of technique and the scarcity of brain tissue specimens make these data difficult to find.

It is common practice when measuring antibiotic concentrations in spinal fluid or in brain tissue to express the antibiotic concentration in the CNS as a percentage of the serum concentration of antibiotic. This practice has led to considerable confusion and the generation of relatively useless data for the purpose of ascertaining whether the antibiotic concentration in the CNS is in a therapeutic range or not. The difficulty with this approach is that the denominator (the serum concentration of antibiotic) is quite variable and changes rapidly with time as the antibiotic is administered, distributed, metabolized, and excreted. Since very few studies relate the timing of specimen collections, it is impossible to derive any meaningful data from a ratio of a randomly obtained serum and spinal fluid or brain tissue specimen. For example, a CSF containing 1 μg/ml of an antibiotic contains 1 percent of the serum concentration if the serum contains 100 μg/ml, and 100 percent of the serum concentration if the serum contains 1 μg/ml, yet the CSF concentration is no different. During a single dose of an antibiotic, each of these serum concentrations may well be present early and late in the course of the dose. Data reporting penetration of antibiotics into brain compartments, therefore, must be critically evaluated in terms of the antibiotic concentration actually detected in the brain tissue or spinal fluid, and how that concentration relates to the antibiotic's effectiveness against specific organisms.

Several recent reviews have thoroughly summarized data regarding penetration of antibiotics into brain tissue and CSF.[1–4] Comments on specific antibiotics will be made where appropriate in the recommendations that follow.

RECOMMENDATIONS FOR ANTIBIOTIC USE IN NEUROSURGERY

Infections of the central nervous system can be roughly divided into three clinical syndromes: meningitis, meningitis with foreign bodies such as CSF shunts, and brain abscess. Table 52-1 outlines the antibiotic therapy for these three syndromes and Table 52-2 gives recommended dosage of the various antibiotics in infants, children, and adults.

Meningitis

The therapy of meningitis of unknown origin is designed to cover the most common pathogens at the various age groups. In newborns the most common pathogens are *Escherichia coli,* Group B streptococcus, *Listeria monocytogenes,* and *Streptococcus pneumoniae.* Although aminoglycosides do not easily penetrate the CSF in adults, apparently the blood–CSF barrier in newborns is not fully developed, and adequate antibiotic is delivered by the parenteral route. In fact the Cooperative Neonatal Meningitis Study Group has shown that intralumbar and intraventricular therapy in infants with gram negative meningitis did not improve survival.[5]

Between the ages of 2 months and 10 years, the most common organism is

Table 52-1
Selection of Antibiotics in Neurosurgery*

Meningitis without *foreign body*

Empiric therapy of meningitis of unknown origin

- Newborns up to 60 days: ampicillin, IV, plus kanamycin, gentamicin, or tobramycin, IV
- Children, age 2 months–10 years: ampicillin, IV, plus chloramphenicol, IV
- Patients over 10 years: ampicillin, IV
- Penicillin allergic patients: chloramphenicol, IV

Therapy for specific organisms

- *Strep. pneumoniae:* penicillin G, IV (second choice: chloramphenicol, IV)
- *N. meningitidis:* penicillin G, IV (second choice: chloramphenicol, IV)
- *H. influenzae*
    - Non-penicillinase-producing: ampicillin, IV
    - Penicillinase-producing: chloramphenicol, IV
- Group B streptococcus: ampicillin, IV
- *L. monocytogenes:* ampicillin, IV
- *Staph. aureus*
    - Infants less than 7 days: methicillin, IV
    - All others: nafcillin, IV
    - Penicillin allergy: vancomycin, IV; or cefazolin, IV *plus* cephalothin, IT
    - Methicillin resistant: vancomycin, IV *plus* rifampin, PO, *plus* trimethoprim PO
    - Aerobic gram negative rods
    - Moxalactam IV, or cefotaxime IV. Adjust drugs according to susceptibility testing.
    - If aminoglycoside therapy is required, intraventricular therapy is indicated beyond the newborn period.

CSF shunt infections

Staph. aureus and *Staph. epidermidis*

- If sensitive (MIC 1.0 μg/ml or less): nafcillin, cefazolin, cephalothin, or cephapirin IV, IT, plus gentamicin, IT.
- If resistant to nafcillin, cephalothin, or cephapirin: rifampin, PO, plus trimethoprim, PO, plus vancomycin, IV and IT.

Enterococcus: ampicillin IV, IT, plus gentamicin IT. If distal shunt is intravascular, gentamicin IV also.

Other streptococci: either a staphylococcal or enterococcal regimen.

Aerobic gram negative rods: according to susceptibilities; both a beta-lactam and aminoglycoside IV and IT should be used.

Corynebacterium sp. and *Propionobacterium sp.* (diphtheroids)

- Penicillin sensitive: use enterococcal regimen.
- Penicillin resistant: vancomycin IV, plus IT.

Brain abscess

Unknown organisms: penicillin G, IV, *plus* chloramphenicol, IV, add nafcillin, IV, if staphylococcus is suspected.

Staphylococcal: nafcillin IV.

Antibiotic prophylaxis for complicated procedures and microsurgery

Cefazolin, 2 g IV, 60 minutes before surgery begins. Repeat six hours after the first dose, then no further antibiotics.

Also acceptable: nafcillin, 2 g IV, 60 minutes before surgery begins. Repeat at four and eight hours after the first dose. No further antibiotics.

Shunt placement: either above regimen, *plus* gentamicin, IT, one dose.

*See text for additional discussion of recommendations.

Table 52-2
Starting Doses of Antibiotics in Neurosurgery*

Antibiotic	Adult	Children	Newborn (0–7 Days)	Intrathecal
		Intravenous		
Penicillin G	5 M units/6h	50,000 units/kg/6h	50,000 units/kg/8h	
Ampicillin	3 g/6h	50 mg/kg/6h	50 mg/kg/12h	50 mg/24h
Carbenicillin	5 g/4h	100 mg/kg/6h	100 mg/kg/12h	50 mg/24h
Cefotaxime	2 g/4h			
Ticarcillin	3 g/4h	75 mg/kg/6h	50 mg/kg/8h	
Methicillin			25 mg/kg/8h	50 mg/24h
Moxalactam	2 g/6h			
Nafcillin	2 g/6h	25 mg/kg/6h		50 mg/24h
Chloramphenicol	1 g/6h	15 mg/kg/6h		
Gentamicin	1.7 mg/kg/8h	2.5 mg/kg/8h	2.5 mg/kg/12h	8 mg/24h
Tobramycin	1.7 mg/kg/8h	2.5 mg/kg/8h	2.5 mg/kg/12h	8 mg/24h
Kanamycin	7.5 mg/kg/12h	7.5 mg/kg/8h	7.5 mg/kg/12h	12 mg/24h
Amikacin	7.5 mg/kg/12h	7.5 mg/kg/8h	7.5 mg/kg/12h	12 mg/24h
Vancomycin	1 g/12h	15 mg/kg/8h	15 mg/kg/12h	20 mg/24h
Cefazolin	2 g/8h	30 mg/kg/8h	20 mg/kg/12h	
Cephalothin	2 g/4h	50 mg/kg/6h	20 mg/kg/12h	50 mg/24h
Cephapirin	2 g/4h	50 mg/kg/6h	20 mg/kg/12h	50 mg/24h
		Oral		
Rifampin	10 mg/kg/12h	10 mg/kg/12h		
Trimethoprim	5 mg/kg/6h	5 mg/kg/6h		

*These are very high doses and should be monitored with measured serum concentrations for toxicity. Blood counts, renal function, and hepatic function should also be monitored. All but chloramphenicol and rifampin must have dosage adjusted in renal failure. See reference 18 for an excellent review of antibiotic therapy in renal failure.

Hemophilus influenzae, with other common pathogens being *Strep. pneumoniae* and *Neisseria meningitidis*. Because approximately 5 percent of *H. influenzae* are resistant to ampicillin, most experts are now recommending that chloramphenicol be started empirically until susceptibilities are known.

For *Staphylococcus aureus* CNS infections, nafcillin is recommended because it is somewhat more active than methicillin against the staphylococci. Kane, Parker, Jordan, et al.[6] have shown that nafcillin achieves adequate antistaphylococcal concentration in the CSF. Frame, Watanakunakorn, McLaurin, et al.[7] also have shown that the two drugs achieve similar concentrations in brain tissue, but since nafcillin is more active, it is preferred for brain abscesses. Methicillin is recommended for younger infants because nafcillin displaces bilirubin from serum albumin more readily than methicillin, and thus is theoretically more likely to predispose the infant to kernicterus.

Methicillin-resistant staphylococci (MRSA) are becoming an increasingly important problem in the United States. Clinical laboratories sometimes erroneously report these organisms as being susceptible to cephalosporins, which they are not. Rifampin and trimethoprim in conjunction with vancomycin for MRSA infections have been used with some success in our patients. Neither trimethoprim nor rifampin should be given alone because staphylococci develop resistance to these drugs rapidly through single-step mutation.

For patients with gram-negative rod meningitis, two new cephalosporins, cefotaxime and moxalactam, quickly have become the drugs of choice. These cephalosporins achieve therapeutic concentrations in CSF, and they have excellent activity against most Enterobacteriaceae, as well as *H. influenzae.* Since these antibiotics are not as active against *Pseudomonas aeruginosa,* additional therapy with systemic gentamicin or tobramycin should be given to patients with suspected gram-negative sepsis as well as meningitis, or to those with a documented *Ps. aeruginosa* infection. If susceptibility tests indicate that only the aminoglycosides are effective against the organism, intrathecal therapy may be indicated. Unlike gram negative meningitis in the newborn period, adult gram negative meningitis has never been subjected to a clinical trial to ascertain whether intrathecal therapy is advantageous. Intrathecal therapy by the lumbar or intraventricular route is usually advocated for these infections. If there is evidence of ventriculitis, then an intraventricular reservoir for daily injection of aminoglycoside is probably appropriate.[8–10]

Antibiotic Management of CSF Shunt Infections

Infection of CSF shunts is a common problem and there is disagreement about its management. Some groups feel that surgical removal of all CSF shunts, in conjunction with systemic antibiotic therapy, is required.[11] Others feel that some CSF shunt infections can be managed by systemic and intrathecal antibiotics alone, if the shunt itself continues to function. We are in the latter group, having had considerable success in clearing shunt infections with individualized antibiotic regimens that optimized the killing of the offending organisms.[12,13] Only with shunt malfunction has surgical revision of the shunt hardware been found necessary. Then the indicated procedure may be replacement of part of the shunt or of all of the shunt, or sometimes temporary external drainage.

Because penetration of most antibiotics into the ventricular CSF is poor, especially as the inflammation subsides, we feel that direct instillation of antibiotics into the ventricular system via a shunt reservoir is necessary. If there is no reservoir, then revision of the shunt with placement of a reservoir is necessary. If the distal end of the shunt is intravascular, then intravascular or intracardiac vegetations are possible, and antibiotic therapy should be directed toward endocarditis as well as the shunt infection. This usually requires extending the duration of systemic therapy for four to six weeks.

The organisms causing CSF shunt infections are for the most part skin organisms such as *Staph. epidermidis, Staph. aureus,* the viridans streptococci, and diphtheroids. In the newborn period, infections with enteric organisms are common, and these organisms are also seen more often with ventriculoperitoneal shunts. The most common enteric organisms are *E. coli, Klebsiella, Enterobacter,* and the enterococcus. Not infrequently CSF shunts infected with enteric organisms are infected concomitantly with other organisms, and thus require considerable manipulation of the antibiotic regimen to effect a cure.

There are three general principles of antibiotic therapy for CSF shunt infections that are similar to the principles for antibiotic treatment of bacterial endocarditis: (1) In endocarditis, the neutrophils do not migrate to the depths of the vegetation and in CSF shunt infections, the neutrophils do not phagocytize effectively in the presence of a foreign body. Since neutrophils are playing a less important role in eradication of organisms, bactericidal antibiotics or antibiotic combinations become an important factor in sterilizing the infection. (2) High concentrations of antibiotic must be delivered to the infected site. (3) Antibiotic therapy must continue for an extended period of time to achieve sterilization.

To design optimum antibiotic regimens, it is necessary to have accurate antibiotic susceptibility tests, and it is desirable to have laboratory capability for doing quantitative antibiotic susceptibilities, also known as minimal inhibitory concentrations (MICs). The MIC is defined as the minimum concentration of a specific antibiotic necessary to inhibit the growth of the organism in vitro. It is not to be confused with inhibitory titer discussed below. The MIC reflects only the relationship of a population of the cultured organism to the antibiotic being tested in an artificial system, and does not include any serum or CSF from the patient. Qualitative susceptibility testing, as done routinely in all clinical microbiology laboratories, can predict with reasonable accuracy the range within which the MIC of an antibiotic for the cultured organism falls, if quantitative testing is unavailable. For example, if an *E. coli* is determined as being sensitive to ampicillin in qualitative test, the MIC of ampicillin for that specific organism is probably less than 8 μg/ml. The recommendations in Tables 51-1 and 51-2 can be used with either qualitative (sensitive or resistant) or quantitative (MIC) test results.

Antibiotic synergism (bacterial inhibition, or killing, which is greater than the effect of either antibiotic alone) is an important part of the antibiotic therapy of CSF shunt infections. As a general rule, synergism occurs between a beta-lactam antibiotic (a penicillin or a cephalosporin) and an aminoglycoside (gentamicin, tobramycin, kanamycin, amikacin, streptomycin). Antibiotic synergism can be tested in sophisticated clinical microbiology laboratories, but as a general rule synergistic activity is usually present if the organism is sensitive to both the beta-lactam and aminoglycoside being given to the patient. For example, a *Klebsiella* sensitive to both cephalothin and gentamicin most likely would be synergistically inhibited by a combination of the two drugs. Antibiotic synergistically inhibited by a combination of the two drugs. Antibiotic synergism has been studied less well with other combinations of antibiotics, and in fact antibiotic antagonism has been demonstrated with some combinations. Antibiotic antagonism is generally seen when one antibiotic of the combination is a bacterostatic antibiotic such as chloramphenicol or tetracycline. For this reason we try not to use these drugs for therapy of CSF shunt infections because antibiotic killing rather than inhibition is required.

A test of antibiotic effectiveness that can be done in some clinical microbiology laboratories is the CSF (or serum) inhibitory and bactericidal titer. In this test spinal fluid (or serum), containing whatever antibiotics have been given to the patient, is serially diluted in a twofold manner and inoculated with the patient's own infecting organism, along with some nutrient broth. After overnight incubation the dilution of spinal fluid (or serum) that inhibits the growth of the organism is termed the "inhibitory titer" of the specimen. Subcultures of the dilutions that inhibited growth of the organism will reveal whether the bacteria were actually killed, and a second value termed "bactericidal titer" indicates the highest dilution of the specimen that will actually kill organisms. These tests have been in use for the management of endocarditis for many years, and infectious disease consultants usually consider a serum inhibitory titer of 1:8 or greater as being adequate for the therapy of endocarditis. There is some disagreement about whether a bactericidal titer would be more useful, but there are fewer data available about that part of the test. At the University of Cincinnati Medical Center, we have been using the inhibitory and bactericidal titers of the spinal fluid to evaluate the effectiveness of our antibiotic regimens. Because we are injecting antibiotics daily into the shunt reservoir, we have the opportunity to withdraw ventricular fluid 24 hours after each injection. We strive to achieve a "trough" CSF inhibitory titer of greater than 1:8 by manipulating the antibiotic combination and dosages, and prefer to have a bactericidal titer of 1:8 or greater, if possible.

Table 51-1 outlines antibiotic regimens for the most common organisms causing CSF shunt infections.

For both *Staph. aureus* and *Staph. epidermidis,* we have felt that combination therapy has given better results than single-drug therapy. If the regimen containing trimethoprim/sulfamethoxazole, vancomycin, and rifampin is used for resistant staphylococci, serum sulfamethoxazole concentrations must be monitored to maintain concentrations between 80 and 150 $\mu g/ml$. Higher sulfa concentrations may lead to bone marrow suppression and neurologic complications. This becomes of particular importance in the presence of renal failure, such as might be seen with shunt nephritis.

With the Group D enterococcus, antibiotic susceptibility testing is unreliable and does not predict the relative efficacy of antibiotics against this organism. The appropriate therapy for entercoccal infection, regardless of susceptibility results, is ampicillin plus gentamicin. Other streptococci are more susceptible but also require an aminoglycoside for synergistic killing.

Therapy for aerobic gram negative rod shunt infections should include both an aminoglycoside and a beta-lactam antibiotic if possible. Both drugs should be given systemically and intrathecally. In some cases it is possible to improve inhibitory or bactericidal titers in the spinal fluid by using a beta-lactam antibiotic with an aminoglycoside even if the infecting organism is considered resistant to one of the drugs. An empiric trial can be done in which the aminoglycoside is begun, CSF inhibitory and bactericidal titers are obtained, and then a second drug is added to see whether inhibitory or bactericidal titers improve.

Empiric therapy of CSF shunt infections prior to the identification of the infecting organism should include therapy for both staphylococci and gram negative rods. An appropriate regimen thus would include a cephalosporin and aminoglycoside both systemically and intraventricularly.

We have elected to treat patients until there are two weeks of negative CSF cultures. Because we are using CSF cultures as a test of cure, we feel that CSF should be cultured each day when it is withdrawn for antibiotic tests. If shunt malfunction occurs and surgery is required during that period, we generally continue the therapy for two weeks after the surgical procedure.

After antibiotics are discontinued, the patient should be observed for 48 hours and the ventricular fluid aspirated at this time for culture. In addition to culturing the ventricular fluid, antibacterial titers should be performed to assure that culture negativity is due to the absence of organisms rather than to the retained effect of antibiotics.

Most failures to eradicate infection in CSF shunts are related to shunt malfunction. On occasion a particularly resistant organism cannot be eradicated by antibiotics alone. In this situation complete removal of shunt hardware, in conjunction with external drainage of the CSF, may be necessary. After one to two weeks of continued antibiotic therapy and external drainage, a permanent ventricular shunt can be replaced and antibiotics continued for an additional one to two weeks.

Brain Abscess

The most common organisms causing brain abscesses are streptococci, gram negative and gram positive anaerobes, and *Staph. aureus*. Occasionally aerobic gram negative rods may also be involved. Unfortunately specific culture data from most brain abscesses are not available at the time therapy is begun. Appropriate empiric therapy is outlined in Table 51-1. In patients with unknown organisms, when there is suspicion of staphylococcal involvement, nafcillin may be substituted for penicillin G.

Recent case reports have indicated that some brain abscesses can be cured with antibiotic therapy alone. Patients successfully treated in this manner have been neurologically stable and have generally had susceptible organisms. Nonsurgical therapy of brain abscess requires careful and frequent follow-up of clinical condition and repeat computerized tomographic scanning to follow the progress of the lesion. Nonsurgical therapy may be the most appropriate approach for multiple small abscesses such as those due to endocarditis.

Metronidazole has been successfully used in Europe for the treatment of brain abscesses, but experience in the United States is limited.

Antibiotic Prophylaxis for Neurosurgical Procedures

General Principles of Antibiotic Prophylaxis

The administration of antibiotics preoperatively to patients undergoing surgical procedures who are *not otherwise infected* is termed antibiotic prophylaxis. The administration of antibiotics to infected patients who are being operated on is not prophylaxis and is not being considered in this discussion. An example of such a case would be surgical drainage of a brain abscess.

Administration of prophylactic antibiotics to patients undergoing surgery has been advocated for many surgical procedures but has proved to be of benefit in relatively few of them. In general terms antibiotic prophylaxis has been shown to be useful only in procedures that have a high postoperative infection rate. For neurosurgical procedures only one prospective controlled study has been performed,[15] and in that study clindamycin was shown to be associated with a reduced incidence of *Staph. aureus* infection. There was an epidemic of staphylococcal infection in that hospital, however, which was related to a markedly increased surgical load, and during that time almost all patients received placebo. As a result, during the outbreak, the hypothesis that clindamycin given prophylactically would prevent infection was not adequately tested. There thus remain few hard data supporting the efficacy of prophylactic antibiotics in neurosurgical procedures. In a review of 840 CSF shunting procedures, George, Leibruck, and Epstein[16] demonstrated that surgical technique might be the most important determinant of shunt infections.

All studies demonstrating the efficacy of prophylactic antibiotics in reducing the incidence of wound infection also demonstrate two other principles of antibiotic prophylaxis: (1) Tissues must contain adequate concentrations of antibiotics prior to the onset of surgery and that the tissue concentrations of antibiotics should be maintained during surgery. This requirement means that if prophylactic antibiotics are to be used, they must be given prior to the surgical procedure and must be given in doses that achieve adequate tissue concentrations of the drug. In addition the pharmacology of the agents must be such that adequate concentrations are maintained during surgery or doses must be repeated during the surgical procedure to maintain adequate levels. (2) Many studies have demonstrated that, after the procedure, prolonged administration of antibiotics is not required. In fact it is the patients who receive extended courses of antibiotic who are likely to be colonized by antibiotic-resistant hospital-associated organisms. These patients are also at added risk for toxic complications of antibiotics.

In summary, although antibiotic prophylaxis for neurosurgical procedures has not been demonstrated to be efficacious, it is not unreasonable to give antibiotic prophylaxis to uninfected patients who are about to undergo an extended neurosurgical procedure or one in which microscopy is to be used. It is also appropriate to provide antibiotic prophylaxis to patients in whom a prosthesis is to be implanted. If antibiotic prophylaxis is administered, the drugs must be given prior to the surgery, adequate concentrations of antibiotics should be present in the tissue at the time of surgery, and antibiotics should be stopped within 24 hours following the surgery.

Antibiotic Recommendations for Prophylaxis

Postoperative infections from neurosurgical procedures are most often caused by skin organisms, in particular *Staph. aureus, Staph. epidermidis,* streptococci, and *Cornyebacterium* species. Prophylactic antibiotic regimens that would be appropriate are outlined in Table 51-1. Although older cephalosporins have not been successful in the therapy of meningitis because of poor penetration into CSF,[17] we have shown that cefazolin achieves high concentrations in brain tissue of patients undergoing elective craniotomy (Frame, P., McLaurin, R., Khodadad, G., Watanakunakorn, C.; unpublished observations). This is probably related to the very high and sustained serum concentration after 2 grams are given.

REFERENCES

1. Everett ED, Strausbaugh LJ: Antimicrobial agents and the central nervous system. Neurosurgery 6:691–714, 1980
2. Norrby R: Penetration of antimicrobial agents into cerebrospinal fluid: Pharmacokinetic and clinical aspects, in Wood JH (ed.): Neurobiology of Cerebrospinal Fluid, New York, Plenum, 1980
3. deLouvois J: The bacteriology and chemotherapy of brain abscess. J Antimicrob Chemother 4:395–413, 1978
4. Barling RWA, Selkon JB: The penetration of antibiotics into the cerebral spinal fluid and brain tissue. J Antimicrob Chemother 4:203–227, 1978
5. McCracken GH Jr, Mize SG, Threlkeld N: Intraventricular gentamicin therapy in gram-negative basillary meningitis of infancy: Report of the Second Neonatal Meningitis Cooperative Study Group. Lancet 1:787–791, 1980
6. Kane JG, Parker RH, Jordan GW, et al: Nafcillin concentration in cerebrospinal fluid during treatment of staphylococcal infections. Ann Intern Med 87:309–311, 1977
7. Frame PT, Watanakunakorn C, McLaurin RL, et al: Methicillin concentrations in human brain tissues, in Nelson JD, Grassi C (eds): Current Chemotherapy and Infectious Disease. Washington, DC, American Society for Microbiology, 1980, pp 641–643
8. Kaiser AB, McGee ZA: Aminoglycoside therapy of gram-negative bacillary meningitis. N Engl J Med 293:1215–1220, 1975
9. Mangi RJ, Holstein LL, Andriole VT: Treatment of gram-negative bacillary meningitis with intrathecal gentamicin. Yale J Biol Med 50:31–41, 1977
10. Rahal JJ Jr, Hyams PJ, Simberkoff MS, et al: Combined intrathecal and intramuscular gentamicin for gram-negative meningitis. N Engl J Med 290:1394–1398, 1974
11. Schoenbaum SC, Gardner P, Shillito J: Infection of cerebrospinal fluid shunts: Epidemiology, clinical manifestations, and therapy. J Infect Dis 131:543–552, 1975
12. McLaurin RL: Treatment of infected ventricular shunts, in O'Brien MS (ed): Pediatric Neurologic Surgery. New York, Raven Press, 1978
13. Wald SL, McLaurin RL: Cerebrospinal fluid antibiotic levels during treatment of shunt infections. J Neurosurg 52:41–46, 1980
14. Rosenblum ML, Hoff JT, Norman D, et al: Nonoperative treatment of brain abscesses in selected high risk patients. J Neurosurg 52:217–225, 1980
15. Savitz MH, Malis LI: Prophylactic clindamycin for neurosurgical patients. NY State J Med 76:64–67, 1976
16. George R, Leibrock L, Epstein M: Long-term analysis of cerebrospinal fluid shunt infections: A 25 year experience. J Neurosurg 51:804–811, 1979
17. Fisher LS, Chow AW, Yoshikawa TT, et al: Cephalothin and cephaloridine therapy for bacterial meningitis. Ann Intern Med 82:689–693, 1975
18. Bennett WM, Muther RS, Parker RA, et al: Drug therapy in renal failure: Dosing guidelines for adults. Part 1: Antimicrobial agents, analgesics. Ann Intern Med 93:62–89, 1980

53. Reye's Syndrome

Joan L. Venes

In 1963 Reye, Morgan, and Baral,[26] reporting in *Lancet* and Johnson, Scurleitis, and Carroll,[11] reporting in the *North Carolina Medical Journal,* described a distinctive clinical syndrome that they characterized as an acute encephalopathy with fatty degeneration of the viscera. Initially thought to be an uncommon disorder, it is now recognized as one of the most common neurologic disorders of childhood.[3]

CLINICAL PRESENTATION

Reye's syndrome is characteristically preceded by a nonspecific viral illness, most commonly influenza B or varicella.[6] Although reported in all age groups from infancy to late adolescence, there appears to be a peak incidence in the 6–10-year age group. No sexual predilection has been identified.

Typically the child appears to be recovering from the initial illness when he or she is noted to become increasingly lethargic or irritable, followed soon after by the onset of persistent vomiting. Often a hyperexcitable state supervenes with disorientation and restlessness. Drug intoxication may be suggested by the tachypnea, sweating, and pupillary dilatation that accompany this stage.

Rapidity of progression after this stage is variable and may have prognostic significance.[14] A number of staging criteria have been developed. The two most widely used are those of Huttenlocher (Table 53-1)[9] and Lovejoy, Smith, Bresnan, et al. (Table 53-2).[14]

The syndrome in infants usually presents with respiratory distress and coma and often is misdiagnosed as pneumonia.[10] Chest x-ray is usually normal and moderate to severe hypoglycemia is present in all cases. Apneic episodes are not uncommon and seizures usually occur at some time in the course of the disease. Unlike the older child in whom control of intracranial hypertension plays a major role in determining outcome, elevated intracranial pressures are not a feature of the disease in the first months of life. Prognosis for survival and full neurologic recovery is much grimmer in this age group.

Table 53-1
Huttenlocher Classification[9]

Stage I	Stupor (aroused with vigorous stimulus)
Stage II	Decorticate (pain produces flexion arms)
Stage III	Decerebrate (pain produces extension)
Stage IV	Light fixed pupils, flaccidity, apnea

LABORATORY FINDINGS

The triad of hypoglycemia, hyperammonemia, and prolonged prothrombin time has long been considered diagnostic of Reye's syndrome if present with the history of a viral prodrome and the symptoms of vomiting and obtundation. Hypoglycemia is particularly dangerous in the infant and young child where serum levels of less than 10 mg/dl have been reported.[37] Liver dysfunction is also reflected in the elevation of serum transaminases (the only laboratory abnormality required by the National Center for Communicable Disease Control for the diagnosis of Reye's syndrome).[18]

Elevation of serum ammonia concentration is presumptive evidence for Reye's syndrome in the clinical situation. Markedly reduced activities of hepatic carbamyl phosphate synthetase and ornithine transcarbamylase are seen early in the course of the disease and are probably responsible for the inability to detoxify ammonia in these patients.[34] Rose, Schonberger, Gelbach, et al.[27] demonstrated elevation of creatine phosphokinase (isozymes MM and MB) and suggested that the pattern of enzyme elevation might have prognostic significance. Abnormalities of serum lactic dehydrogenase reported by Roe and his group confirmed an earlier report by Thaler, Bruh, Appelbaum, et al.,[36] who suggested that their findings were consistent with significant involvement of skeletal muscle. The profound hypotonia noted in some of these patients may be a clinical reflection of this involvement.

Disturbed amino acid metabolism is characteristic of the disorder, and

Table 53-2
Lovejoy et al. Classification[14]

Stage I	Abnormal liver function, lethargy, and vomiting. EEG—rhythmic slowing, dominant theta.
Stage II	Abnormal liver function, delirium, hyperventilation, and hyperreflexia. EEG—dysrhythmic slowing, dominant delta.
Stage III	Abnormal liver function, decorticate, hyperventilation. EEG—dysrhythmic slowing, dominant delta.
Stage IV	Minimal liver dysfunction (typical), decerebrate, loss of oculocephalic responses, dysconjugate cold coloric responses. EEG—disorganized monorhythm or polyrhythm dominant low-voltage delta with burst supression.
Stage V	Normal liver function (typical), flaccid (no DTRs), apnea. EEG—isoelectric, occasional seizure activity.

aminoaciduria was first noted by Reye. The marked hyperaminoacidemia probably reflects a general insult to cellular integrity rather than specific enzyme disturbance. There appears to be a correlation between high levels of plasma amino acid and poor clinical outcome.[7] Disturbances of this magnitude, however, may be seen in fulminant liver failure of any cause.[16] Excessive lipolysis of unknown cause and associated free fatty acidemia may be responsible for the encephalopathic features of the disease.[2]

Elevations of homovanillic acid have been reported in the ventricular fluid of children with Reye's syndrome and may reflect cerebral ischemia. Results from one laboratory suggest that cerebral dopamine rather than alterations in serotoergic mechanisms are most important since 5-HIAA appears to be unchanged.[32]

PATHOLOGY

Fatty infiltration has been reported in liver, kidney, and myocardium.[21] Electron microscopic examination of liver biopsy material shows the hepatocytes to be diffusely affected by a process that results in swollen pleomorphic mitochondria, as well as small droplet triglyceride accumulation.[23] Acute brain biopsies in three children with Reye's syndrome demonstrated similar changes in neuronal mitochondria associated with myelin bleb formation. Recovery brain biopsies in these three children demonstrated reversibility of the mitochondrial injury with morphologic evidence for repair and regeneration of myelin.[22] Other and more severe changes reported in necropsy studies may occur secondary to ischemia associated with cerebral edema or to prolonged severe hypoglycemia.

DIFFERENTIAL DIAGNOSIS

Rapidly progressive liver failure may be confused with Reye's syndrome and liver biopsy may be the only means by which these two entitites can be separated. The risk of such a procedure in the patient with clotting abnormality must be considered.[5] Elevation of serum transaminases can be seen in the patient with salicylate levels greater than 25 mg/dl.[29] Hyperpnea, a mixed disturbance of acid-base metabolism and a confusional state, makes the differentiation from Reye's syndrome difficult. Again while liver biopsy is the definitive diagnostic procedure, consideration must be given to the risk involved. Other causes of encephalopathy—for example, viral encephalitis, insulin shock or diabetic coma, drug ingestion—may be excluded by the absence of significant liver dysfunction in most instances. Many neonatal disorders associated with hypoglycemia, lactic acidemia, and fatty infiltration of the viscera may present special diagnostic problems.[20,28]

TREATMENT

Attempts to lower serum ammonia and other nondefined toxic substances by means of exchange transfusion or peritoneal dialysis have met with variable success.[9,30] Although diminution in delta activity with associated increase in theta and alpha activity has been reported during and following exchange transfusion,[13] measurement of intracranial pressure during exchange transfusion has failed to demonstrate any consistent relationship between changes in intracranial pressure and falling ammonia levels.[37] Decompressive craniectomy, introduced by Partin,[22] has been advocated as a life-saving measure in those children in whom medical management has failed to control intracranial hypertension. It can be seen that therapy is symptomatic, directed at protecting the brain from the secondary effects of hypoglycemia and hypoperfusion resulting from cerebral edema and/or shock. Although the methods by which this goal is achieved may differ, several principles appear to be generally accepted.

Early diagnosis and prevention of hypoglycemia, particularly in the young infant, are essential to good outcome. For this reason the administration of a bolus of intravenous glucose is advised as soon as appropriate blood studies have been obtained.

Intubation and controlled ventilation enable one more easily to control intracranial pressure and allow for the maintenance of adequate levels of oxygenation. Even at low baseline levels of arterial p-CO_2, manual hyperventilation can effect a prompt, albeit transient, reduction in intracranial pressure.[4] Prolonged or frequent profound hypocarbia, however, may result in significant hypoxemia and a potentially deleterious effect on cerebral metabolism. The use of pancuronium is helpful in maintaining a stable respiratory pattern and avoiding the increase in intracranial pressure that may be seen secondary to a rise in intracranial venous pressure associated with laryngeal irritation and "bucking" on the endotracheal tube. Treatment of cerebral edema by hyperosmolar agents (mannitol), furosemide, and proper fluid restriction is helpful in preventing the herniation syndrome that often heralds death in these children. Serum osmolarity should be maintained between 310 and 320 mOsm, and to avoid hypovolemia, one third of the daily fluid replacement should be in the form of colloid solution. Fresh frozen plasma, in addition to its colloidal properties, may be helpful in correcting coagulation deficits associated with this disorder. The use of dexamethasone is predicated on its ability to shift the ventricular pressure response curve to the right.[12] The cytotoxic nature of the cerebral edema in Reye's syndrome with the apparent preservation of cerebral microvascular integrity suggests that hyperosmolar agents may be more effective in this disorder.

It is generally agreed that in patients with low intracranial compliance, stimulation, even of a non-noxious nature, may produce a significant and sustained pressure elevation (Fig. 53-1). Analgesic agents in general use are morphine and fentanyl. Consideration should be given to the need for appropriate analgesia prior to performance of any traumatic procedure, such as tracheostomy or placement of an arterial line (Fig. 53-2).

The degree of effectiveness of barbiturates in reducing brain injury secondary to ischemia remains highly controversial.[1,33,35] Their value, however, in the prompt reduction of intracranial hypertension in a variety of conditions has been well demonstrated.[8,31] The presumed mechanism by which barbiturates acutely lower intracranial pressures is by an increase in cerebral vascular resistance with reduction in cerebral blood volume by about 50 percent through a combination of direct action on the vascular tree[25] and a reduction of cerebral metabolic rates.[19] Although no controlled studies exist to prove definitively the value of barbiturate coma in Reye's syndrome, there are several reports[17,37] in which mortality and morbidity appear to have been significantly improved by the use of aggressive management including barbiturate coma (defined as a serum level of greater than 3.0 mg/dl). The increased lipid solubility of sodium pentothal and its rapid action make this the preferred agent for the induction of coma although its short half-life contraindicates its use for maintenance in most units. Pentobarbital and phenobarbital are useful long-term agents. It must be emphasized, however, that

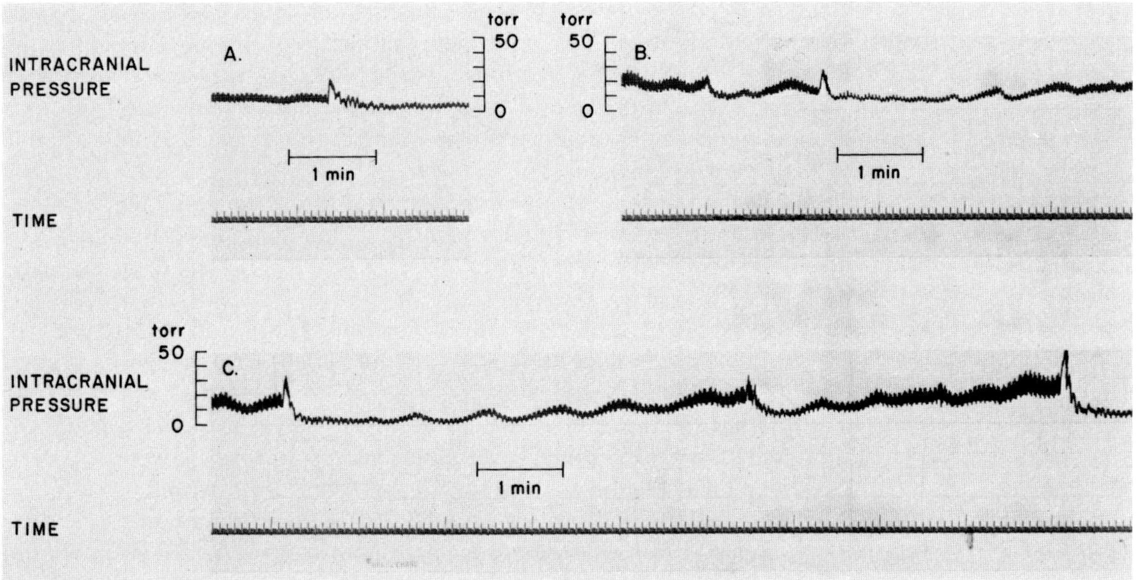

Figure 53-1. A. Brief "spontaneous" rise in intracranial pressure. B. Brief transient in response to pupil checks. C. Gradually increasing intracranial pressure during parents' visit in a curarized, sedated child. Note the reduction in pulse pressure that follows the transients in all these episodes. The physiologic explanation for the transients and the reduction in pulse pressure is unknown. (Reprinted with permission from Venes JL et al: The management of severe cerebral edema and metabolic encephalopathy of Reye-Johnson syndrome. J Neurosurg 48:903–915, 1978.)

the use of barbiturate coma should be limited to those centers in which serum levels are rapidly available.

The loss of neurologic parameters through curarization, narcotization, and/or deep sedation mandates careful continuing assessment of intracranial pressure. It is generally accepted that prevention of intracranial hypertension is more easily managed than the treatment of pressure waves. Monitoring of intracranial pressure should not be considered as a form of therapy, however, but as a guide to treatment in much the same way as the measurement of arterial blood pressure or pulmonary wedge pressure. With this in mind, it can be seen that the institution of intracranial monitoring by whatever means should not significantly alter treatment outcome unless it leads to changes in treatment protocol. Intracranial pressure can be monitored using the extradural, subdural,

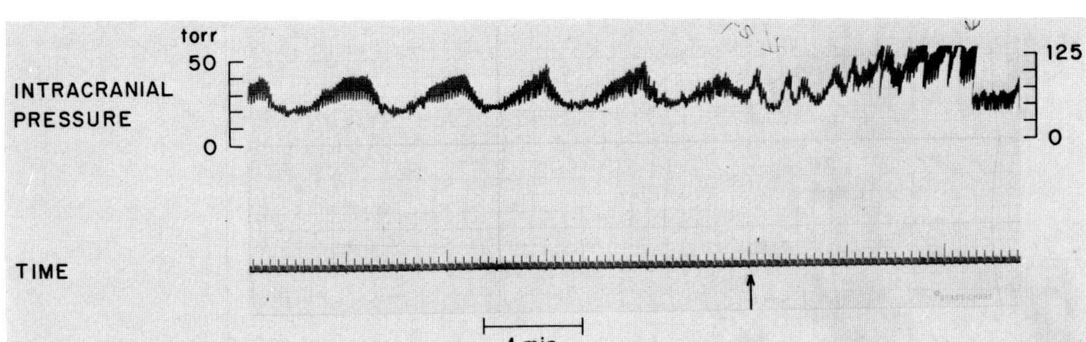

Figure 53-2. Sustained increase in intracranial pressure following noxious stimulation in curarized, sedated patient. (Reprinted with permission from Venes JL et al: The management of severe cerebral edema and metabolic encephalopathy of Reye-Johnson syndrome. J Neurosurg 48:903–915, 1978.)

subarachnoid, or intraventricular compartments, and each method has certain advantages and limitations.[15] Each of these methods requires careful monitoring of the tracing to ensure that readings obtained are an accurate reflection of intracranial events. Failure to recognize that the pressure wave is dampened in a patient in whom other parameters for neurologic assessment are not available may have tragic consequences.

The decision to terminate intracranial monitoring is generally made following an 18–24-hour period in which mannitol or a similar agent has not been required for control of pressure. The following protocol is recommended.

1. Arterial p-CO_2 is brought into normocarbic range, and if well tolerated, curarization is discontinued. No child should be left unsedated and curarized.
2. If intracranial pressure remains between 15 and 20 torr, analgesia and sedation are discontinued. Spontaneous respiration recovers at a variable time depending on the duration of barbiturate coma.
3. Extubation should not take place until adequate spontaneous ventilation is established as determined by assessment of vital capacity, tidal volume, and monitoring of arterial blood gasses. Prior to extubation as the child awakens, it is to be expected that intracranial pressure will increase and that there will be brief elevations to the hypertensive range with straining or stimulation. A sustained rise, however, in the baseline intracranial pressure above 20 torr, accompanied by plateau waves, is an indication for reinstitution of therapy.
4. Intracranial pressure is monitored for several hours following extubation, and if it remains acceptable, the catheter is removed.

Upon using this protocol in 21 consecutive cases of Reye's syndrome, deterioration was not seen in any child following removal of the ventricular catheter.

RESULTS

In a series of 19 severely ill children with serum ammonia of 300 mg/dl or greater and a history of rapid progression to Stage III coma (Lovejoy) reported from the Yale University School of Medicine, 12 (60 percent) recovered without significant neurologic deficit and there was one death reported.[37] Marshall, Shapiro, and Rauscher[17] have reported similar promising results in 7 patients with raised intracranial pressure resistant to steroids and osmotic agents. All survived following the addition of pentobarbital to their therapy and 6 of the 7 survived without significant residua.[17]

The etiology of Reye's syndrome remains unknown and definitive therapy is therefore lacking. Although the role of barbiturate coma as a specific therapy remains to be documented, it is clear that aggressive management of intracranial pressure and attention to those parameters consistent with standard intensive therapy of the critically ill child will produce a good outcome in the majority of these patients.

REFERENCES

1. Arnfred I, Secher O: Anoxia and barbiturates. Arch Intern Pharmacol 139:67–74, 1962

2. Brawn RE: Excessive free fatty acidemia and the encephalopathy in Reye's syndrome. N Engl J Med 292:1297–1298, 1975
3. Corey L: Reye's syndrome—An epidemotogical approach, in Pollack JD (ed): Reye's Syndrome. New York, Grune & Stratton, 1975, pp 179–187
4. Czernicki Z, Jurkiewicz E, Kunicki A: The effect of hypocapnia on normal and elevated intracranial pressure in cats and rabbits, in Lundberg N, Ponten V, Brock M (eds): Intracranial Pressure, vol II. New York, Springer-Verlag, 1975, pp 471–473
5. Devivo DC, Keating JP: Reye's syndrome. Adv Pediatr 22:175–229, 1976
6. Glick TH, Likowsky WH, Levitt LP, et al: Reye's syndrome: An epidemilogical approach. Pediatrics, 46:371–377, 1970
7. Hitty MD, Romshe CA, Delameler PV: Reye's syndrome and hyperammoacidemia. J Pediatr 84:362–365, 1974
8. Horsley JS: The intracranial pressure during barbiturate narcosis. Lancet 141–143, 1937
9. Huttenlocher RR: Reye's syndrome: Relation of outcome to therapy. J Pediatr 80:845–850, 1972
10. Huttenlocher PR, Travner DA: Reye's syndrome in infancy. Petiatrics 62:84–90, 1978
11. Johnson GM, Scurleitis TD, Carroll NB: A study of sixteen fatal cases of encephalitis-like disease in No. Carolina children. NC Med J 24:464–473, 1973
12. Leech PJ, Miller JD: Intracranial volume pressure relationships during experimental brain compression in primates. Neurol, Neurosurg Psychiatry 37:1093–1111, 1974
13. Lewis DJ, Varma RR, Harrington G, et al: Exchange transfusion for Reye's syndrome. J Surg Research 18:327–329, 1975
14. Lovejoy FJ, Smith AJ, Bresnam MJ, et al: Clinical staging in Reye's syndrome. Am J Dis Child 128:36–41, 1974
15. McGraw CP: Continuous intracranial pressure monitoring: Review of techniques and presentation of method. Surg Neurol 6:149–155, 1976
16. Marks MI, Mauer SM, Goldman H: Exchange transfusion in the treatment of hepatic coma. J Pediatr 75:418–430, 1969
17. Marshall LF, Shapiro HM, Rauscher A: Pentobarbital therapy in intracranial hypertension in metabolic coma, Reye's syndrome. J Crit Care Mont 6:1–5, 1978
18. National Center for Disease Control: Reye's syndrome and viral infections. Morbidity Mortality Weekly Rep 23:58–60, 1974
19. Nordstrom CH, Rhencrona S: Reduction of cerebral blood flow and oxygen consumption with barbiturate anaesthesia and hypothermia in the rat. Acta Anes Scand 22:7–12, 1978
20. Parr J, Teree TM, Larner J: Symptomatic hypoglycemia, visceral fatty metamorphosis and aglycogenosis in an infant lacking glycogen synthetase and phosphorylase. Pediatrics 35:770–777, 1965
21. Partin JC: Reye's syndrome (encephalopathy and fatty liver). Gastroenterology 69:511–518, 1975
22. Partin JS, McAdams AJ, Partim JC, et al: Brain ultrastructure in Reye's disease II. J Neuropath Exp Neurol 37:796–819, 1978
23. Partin JC, Schubert WK, Partin JS: Mitochondrial ultrastructure in Reye's Syndrome (encephalopathy and fatty degeneration of the viscera). N Engl J Med 285:1339–1343, 1971
24. Pierce EC: Cerebral circulation and metabolism during theopental anesthesia and hyperventilation in man. J Clin Invest 41:1664–1771, 1962
25. Price ML, Price HL: Effects of general anesthetics on contractile responses of rabbit aortic strips. Anesthesiology 23:16–19, 1962
26. Reye RDK, Morgan G, Baral J: Encephalopathy and fatty degeneration of the viscera: A disease entity in childhood. Lancet 2:749–752, 1963
27. Roe CR, Schonberger LB, Gelbach SH, et al: Enzymatic alterations in Reye's syndrome: Prognostic implications. Pediatrics 55:119–126, 1975
28. Ruebner BH, Bhagavan BS, Greenfield AJ, et al: Neonatal hepatic necrosis. Pediatrics 43:963–970, 1969
29. Russell AS, Sturge RA, Smith MA: Serum transaminases during salicylate therapy. Br Med J 2:428–429, 1974

30. Samaha FJ, Blau E, Berardinelli: Reye's syndrome: Clinical diagnosis and treatment with peritoneal dialysis. Pediatrics 53:336–340, 1974
31. Shapiro HM, Galindo A, Wyte SR, et al: Rapid intraoperative reduction of intracranial pressure with thiopentone. Br J Anes 45:1057–1062, 1973
32. Shaywitz BA, Venes JL, Cohen DJ, et al: Monoamine metabolite concentrations in ventricular spinal fluid in children with Reye's syndrome. Neurology 29:467–472, 1979
33. Simeone FA, Frazer G, Lawner P: Ischemic brain edema: Comparative effects of barbiturates and hypothermia and stroke. 10:8–12, 1979
34. Snodgrass PJ, DeLong GR: Urea-cycle enzyme deficiencies and an increased nitrogen load producing hyperammonemia in Reye's syndrome. N Engl J Med 294:855–867, 1976
35. Steen PA, Milde JH, Michenfelder JO: Cerebral metabolic and vascular effects of barbiturate therapy following complete global ischemia. J Neurochem 31:1317–1324, 1978
36. Thaler MM, Bruh FW, Appelbaum MN, et al: Reye's syndrome in twins. J Pediatr 77:638–646, 1970
37. Venes JL, Shaywitz BA, Spencer DD: The management of severe cerebral edema in the metabolic encephalopathy of Reye-Johnson syndrome. J Neurosurg 48:903–915, 1978

VI VASCULAR DISEASE

54. Strokes in Children

A. Loren Amacher

To juxtapose the words "stroke" and "children" seems almost a contradiction in terms. After all, strokes are events that occur within the human nervous system during its long years of decline. Yet strokes in children, defined as apoplectic events occurring within central nervous system parenchyma in response to vascular occlusion, rupture, or anomalies, are a significant cause of disability and loss of human potential.

The incidence of stroke in children is unknown, in part because of uncertainty relating to the relationship of intrauterine and perinatal vascular events to cerebral palsy and intellectual/cognitive disabilities.[4] Even such an exhaustive survey as that carried out by the Joint Committee for Stroke could find no reliable figures for any of the causes of stroke in children.[10] Death from stroke occurs in about 15 per million children less than 5 years of age per year, and in seven per million in the 5 to 14 age group. Overall the incidence is *probably* less than 1 per 100,000 per year,[10] although a more recent survey from community cases in Rochester, Minnesota, ages 0 to 14 years, from the decade 1965 through 1974, suggests an incidence of 2.52 per 100,000 per year with 95 percent confidence limits, 0.69–6.45 per 100,000 per year. In this survey 55 percent were occlusive, and 45 percent hemorrhagic, although birth incidents, infection, and trauma as etiologies were excluded.[12]

Prevalence of stroke in the pediatric age group is equally uncertain. One cerebral palsy survey suggested that 4 percent of cases reflected a postnatal vascular catastrophe, while another community survey suggested a figure of just over 12 per 100,000 for hemiplegia due to stroke, ages 0 to 15.[5,20]

To be useful a classification of such a nebulous and diffuse problem as stroke in childhood must be simple and easily remembered. We shall not concern ourselves—in any detail, at least—with stroke syndromes arising from parenchymal sequelae of direct trauma, brain loss due to necessary access to mass or vascular lesions, the very rare apoplectic presentation of tumors because of hemorrhage, the rupture of angiomas or aneurysms, or the ingravescent "stroke" syndromes associated with neurocutaneous disorders or slowly progressive degeneration of brain parenchyma.

AN ETIOLOGIC CLASSIFICATION OF STROKE IN CHILDREN

An old obstetric classification lends itself admirably to our purposes.[16]

Abnormalities of the Pump (Heart)

Neurologic sequelae of congenital heart disease (CHD) are less common now than formerly, thanks to earlier surgical correction of heart defects associated with severe cyanosis and to precise surgical techniques. The principal villains associated with cyanotic CHD were (and are) prolonged episodes of hypoxemia, embolism (spontaneous, or induced at surgery), and hypercoaguable states due to hyperviscosity. The old teaching still holds, that stroke associated with cyanotic CHD in children less than 2 years old is usually due to thrombosis, whereas that occurring beyond 2 years of age is the result of brain abscess until proven otherwise.[7,11]

The noncyanotic cases of CHD that are most likely to produce stroke syndromes are those associated with conductive defects in the ventricular/atrial cushion where paroxysmal cardiac arrhythmias and standstill are prone to occur, cases of tight aortic stenosis or severe aortic/mitral regurgitation, and tight coarctations of the aorta.[11]

Because bacterial endocarditis is an eternal hazard in the child with CHD, embolic stroke and cerebral hemorrhage due to ruptured mycotic aneurysm and infected embolus must be kept in mind constantly in such children.

The prolapsing mitral valve has been shown to be a source of cerebral emboli, even in children.[1] Cardiac myxoma must be considered in this context as well.

Abnormalities of the Passages (Arteries)

Congenital

There may be some true examples of congenital stroke. A 3-month-old full-term girl died of uncontrolled seizures. The left cranial vault transilluminated. At autopsy only a short stump of the left middle cerebral artery was found, and the parenchyma nourished by this artery was absent.

Porencephaly replacing part or all of an arterial territory may represent the end result of congenital stroke. Why a specific artery should fail to develop is unknown. Perhaps hydrancephaly is an extreme example of widespread cerebral vascular occlusion at an early embryonic age; some cases of moya-moya may represent intrauterine occlusion or maldevelopment of cerebral vasculature, although progression of the lesion during childhood has been demonstrated.[18]

In addition to the evidence cited, the fact that children with cerebral palsy have a higher incidence of neonatal asphyxia and difficult labor and delivery suggests vascular involvement in the etiology of at least some of these states.[9]

The advent of neonatal intensive care and of expert neonatologists have made premature, tiny survivors of ventricular hemorrhage common problems in management of hydrocephalus and childhood stroke syndromes or movement disorders. This subject is dealt with in Chapter 65.

Traumatic

Injury to vessels supplying the brain may occur directly or indirectly, in the neck or in the head. Stroke may be the result of arterial or venous thrombosis, artery-to-artery embolism, or dissecting aneurysm. Rupture of posttraumatic aneurysms may occur days to months after even relatively minor head injury.

Figure 54-1 is a posterior fossa angiogram from a 10-year-old healthy boy

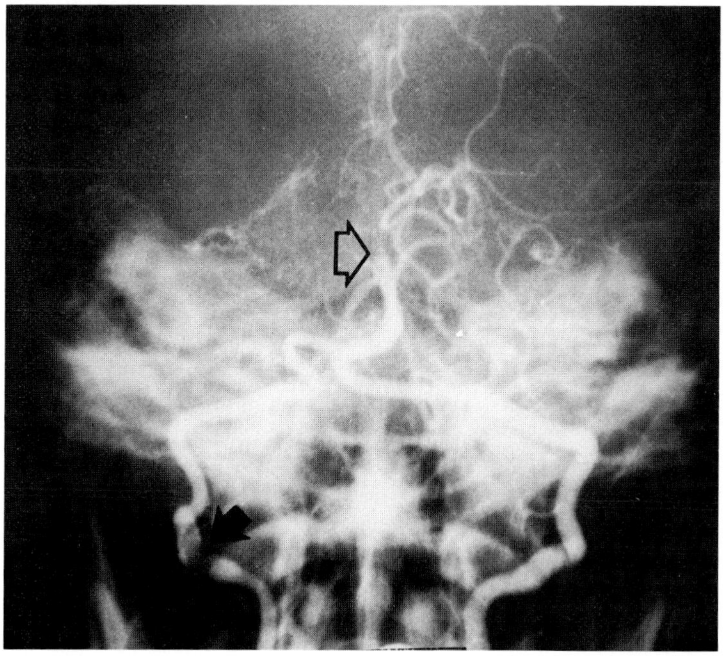

Figure 54-1. Towne's view posterior fossa angiogram. Closed arrow indicates source of artery—artery emboli in the extracranial vertebral artery at C1, constant filling defect on all views; open arrow indicates partially plugged basilar tip.

who began to throw emboli to his basilar bifurcation (open arrow) following a twisting injury to his neck. The site of embolus formation is in the right vertebral artery (dark arrow) just below the arch of the atlas, presumably on the basis of intimal injury.

Cortical vein thrombosis and major sinus occlusions occasionally occur following concussive or penetrating head injury, or in association with nearby sepsis. The latter are frequently devastating in their consequences, whereas residua from the former are often quite mild. It has been suggested that venous strokes are more common in children than in adults.[6]

Infective/Inflammatory

Severe attacks of purulent meningitis may induce occlusion of smaller distributing or perforating arteries because of inflammatory arteritis. Similarly, a nearby focus of pus—as in the tonsillar fossa—may be responsible for stroke if the cervical carotid becomes occluded.[15]

Infective masses—abscesses or parasitic cysts—may induce stroke by mass effect. Neglected or improperly treated facial infections may result in a spreading septic thrombophlebitis, which may, in turn, stimulate thrombosis of the cavernous sinus, usually with devastating consequences.

In generalized sepsis stroke may occur secondarily to hypercoaguability, thrombocytopenia, or disseminated intravascular coagulation (DIC).

Among drug abusers arterial thrombosis may result from progressive vasospasm or vascular hypersensitivity when alkaloids or heroin are involved, from vasculitis when methamphetamine alone or with LSD or heroin is taken intravenously, from emboli—often infected—from subacute bacterial endocarditis (SBE) or contaminated diluents. Cerebral hemorrhage may occur with repeated intravenous amphetamine usage, probably because of hypertensive crises.

Radiation vasculitis is seldom demonstrated. Figure 54-2 is a Towne's view angiogram from a boy 6 years of age who began having transient ischemic attacks related to anterior and middle cerebral artery territories some six months following completion of radiotherapy for recurrent cystic craniopharyngioma. The diagnosis of radiation vasculitis of the anterior cerebral arteries was feared,

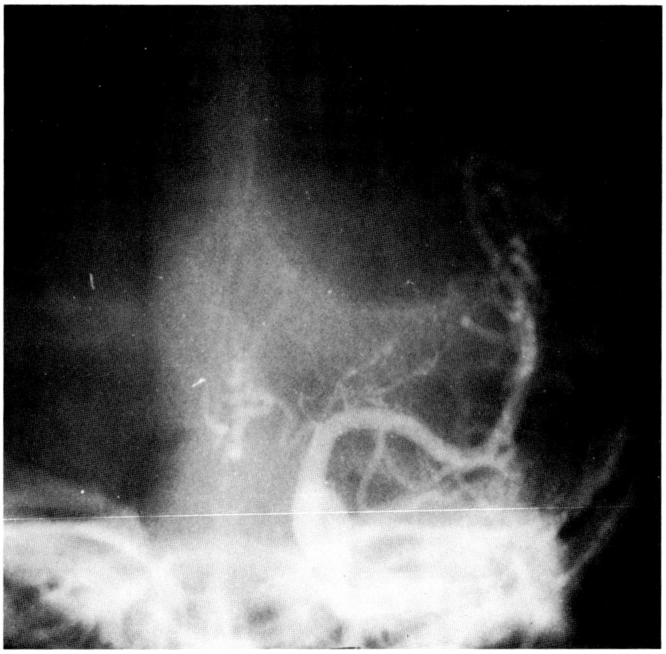

Figure 54-2. Towne's view left carotid angiogram. Note the narrowed, tatty appearance of the A1 segment.

until comparison with the pretreatment angiograms revealed no change in the vessel appearance. A cardiac origin of emboli was later proved to be the cause of his transient cerebral ischemias.

The catastrophic, diffuse cerebral involvement that may occur following some types of viral infections, termed acute hemorrhagic leukoencephalopathy, certainly represents an apoplectic event within the brain on the basis of diffuse, poorly understood, vascular disease.

Fibromuscular hyperplasia (FMH) has been demonstrated in children.[14] Changes similar to those of FMH have been seen in vascular occlusive disease associated with sickle cell disease.[13] The collateral vessel appearance in the deep ganglia following internal carotid occlusion has been noted to resemble moyamoya, suggesting perhaps that the latter process may be related to progressive vascular occlusion.[8]

External Pressure

In certain well-defined situations, pressure from a nearby static or expanding mass may induce vascular symptoms or stroke.

Figure 54-3 shows an exostosis arising from the medial aspect of the right occipital condyle of a healthy 6-year-old boy. He would suffer sudden respiratory arrest, tetraparesis, and loss of consciousness during extreme flexion of his neck. At operation the dominant vertebral artery was found to be thinned as it passed around the mass. Excision of the exostosis cured him.

The pattern of medial occipital lobe infarction induced by posterior cerebral artery occlusion at the incisura, caused by mass lesions or severe edema, is well known.

Systemic Arterial Disease

Among the diffuse collagen inflammatory diseases that may be associated with stroke in children are systemic lupus erythematosis, polyarteritis nodosa, granulomatous angiitis, and dermatomyositis. Some drugs are thought to be capable of inducing SLE, among them dilantin, a common childhood anticonvulsant.

Although there are no good data to indicate that hypertension on the basis of

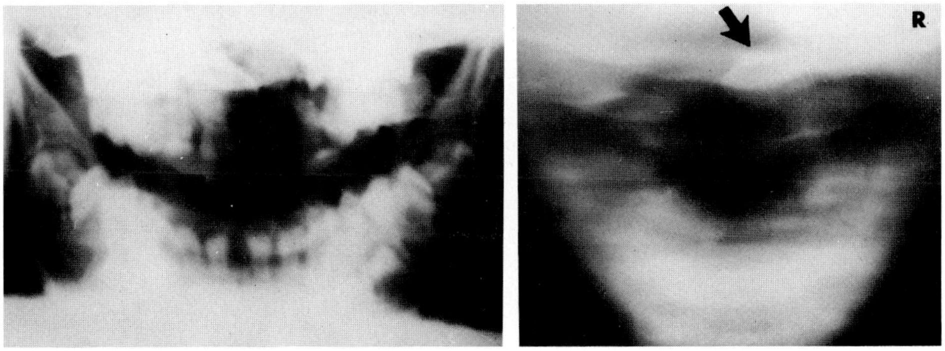

Figure 54-3. Anteroposterior plain film and PA tomogram, foramen magnum. Arrow indicates large bony exostosis contiguous with foramen magnum rim.

atherosclerosis and arteriosclerosis is a problem in children, there are three situations in which hypertensive cerebral vascular events may arise in the young. Coarctation of the aorta and systemic polycystic disease have an unusual association with cerebral hemorrhage from aneurysm, or spontaneously. Catechol-secreting tumors such as pheochromocytoma and neuroblastoma may present as stroke.

Developmental and Miscellaneous

Stroke associated with *angioma* and *aneurysm* is dealt with in Chapters 55 and 56. Sufficient here to say that stroke from such lesions is usually the result of one or more of rupture, vasospasm, "steal" phenomena, or mass effects.

The hemiplegia, hemiconvulsion, and epilepsy (HHE) syndrome of Gastaut is associated with arterial, venous, or sinus occlusions intracranially. Prolonged febrile seizures may be associated with postictal hemiplegia, the deficit probably always only transient.[19] Davidson and Falconer[3] suggest, however, that prolonged febrile seizures may produce permanent cerebral damage, particularly within the medial temporal lobes.

The vasospastic episodes associated with migraine aura may rarely leave permanent residua in terms of motor control and intellect. The classical migrainous aura may be regarded as a transient ischemic episode.

Abnormalities of the Passengers (Blood and Blood Elements)

Red Cells

Strokes associated with red blood cell failure arise because of hypoxemia, secondary to one or more of sudden reduction in red cell mass (shock and hemolytic crises), abnormal adhesiveness and fragility of red cells (sickle cell disease), or hemoglobinopathies (such as thalassemia or red cell poisoning as in methemoglobinemia). In such situations watershed cortical and nuclear areas and certain specially vulnerable neurones such as Purkinje and Ammon's horn cells may be most severely affected. Small vessel occlusions and periarteriolar hemorrhages may also occur.[17]

White Cells

In general terms stroke syndromes are less common now than formerly in leukemic children. Cerebral hemorrhage and small, low-pressure vessel occlusions may occur because of abnormalities of other blood elements and sludging.[2]

Platelets

Stroke syndromes related specifically to platelets may occur from intimal injury (emboli), sludging (thrombosis), abnormalities of platelet number such as ideopathic thrombocytopenic or thrombotic thrombocytopenic purpuras and consumption coagulopathies (thrombosis and hemorrhage) or thrombocytosis (thrombosis), and abnormalities of platelet adhesiveness.

Clotting Factors

Especially notable are deficiencies of Factors VIII and IX, though recent advances in management of hemophiliacs have made cerebral hemorrhage rather unusual.

Hypercoaguable States

Arterial thrombosis related to hypercoaguable states may occur whenever blood viscosity, and hence internal vascular friction and sludging, is increased. Such include severe dehydration, polycythemia vera or secundus, postsplenectomy syndrome, certain cases of sepsis, and some of the states mentioned previously.

Substrate Failure

Neurones are capable of switching to anaerobic metabolic pathways, but they cannot produce sufficient high-energy phosphate to maintain their membrane systems, hence their function. In addition gluconeogenesis within neurones destroys the very machinery that supports the life of the cell. In fact neurones may be able to survive total circulatory arrest for a longer period than they can survive severe hypoxemia and hypoglycemia. Substrate failure tends to strike most savagely at the cortical and nuclear watersheds, and at the susceptible neuronal populations in the medial temporal lobes and cerebellum as indicated previously.

Miscellaneous Conditions

Worth mentioning are the hemolytic–uremia syndrome, where stroke is most likely to be related to thrombotic thrombocytopenic purpura, and stroke associated with increased platelet adhesiveness associated with estrogen ingestion for birth control. One of the more common aminoacidurias, homocystinuria, may carry a 10 percent risk of stroke in affected children, probably on the basis of platelet abnormalities, although intimal hyperplasia and fibrosis may be operant as well.

SPECIAL CONSIDERATIONS

The effects of stroke upon the maturing brain vary with the age of the child (or fetus) at the time of the event. Certainly below the age of 2 years, cerebral dominance can be transferred from a damaged to an intact cerebral hemisphere and speech development remain relatively unaffected.

Strokes that involve the parietal parenchyma seem to have a more noticeable effect upon growth of bone and muscle. Aside from problems associated with hypotonia or spasticity, the loss of trophic neuronal influence upon the contralateral limbs may give rise to special orthopedic difficulties related to limb length and stability. This effect is greater the younger the child at the time of the event.

Strokes due to cortical infarction at a very early age may not be recognized for some months, and often it is the grandmother or aunt who first notices that something is amiss. So it is that infantile hemiplegia frequently becomes apparent between 6 and 12 months of age, when cortical control of movement fails to develop.

Seizures that are triggered from a damaged cerebral hemisphere may be very difficult to control in children. Where high doses of anticonvulsants are required, the effect of sedation may be piled upon preexistent cognitive and perceptual handicaps. In some cases temporal lobectomy, hemispherectomy, or commissurotomy may be the most effective means of seizure control.

Where stroke leaves the residual of profound alterations in tone, cognitive-perceptual handicap, or movement disorder, rehabilitation becomes the most urgent and difficult aspect of the ongoing care of the child. Undoubtedly the young and adaptable brain can overcome major insults, but only with optimum assistance.

PRINCIPLES OF DIAGNOSIS AND TREATMENT

In long-standing cases the hallmark radiologic features include small hemicranial volume and bone thickening, elevation of the sphenoidal and petrous ridges, and foreshortening of the middle fossa on plain films, and unilateral ventriculomegaly or porencephaly, small hemisphere size, reduced cortical mantle or deep nuclear bulk, and unexpected metal depositions in deep cortex or basal grey structures on computerized tomographic (CT) scanning. Typical patterns of metal deposition or radiolucent cerebral lesions may be seen with a variety of conditions such as the craniofacial angiomatoses, toxoplasmosis, cytomegaloviral infestation, parasitic cysts, indolent tumors, Hallervorden–Spatz disease, postkernicterus states, post-hypoxic states, and so on.

In the acute situation, CT scanning and angiography may localize the areas of infarction, hemorrhage, vessel cut-off or narrowing, source of emboli, vasculitides, mass lesions, or vascular anomalies or aneurysms.

Strokes in children are seldom preventable, if only because they are usually unanticipated. Minimization of risk is feasible when predisposing causes are recognized, as with congenital heart disease and transmitted disorders of blood elements. Recurrence or progression of stroke occasionally is possible by removal of angiomas, embolic sources, or mass lesions. Minimization of residua, which are found in over 90 percent of children with occlusive stroke,[12] remains the major consideration of stroke therapy in children. Whether or not revascularization procedures are applicable in any stroke states in children—as for moyamoya—is an open question.

We have discussed some of the aspects of stroke in children. Awareness is the first step toward understanding.

REFERENCES

1. Barnett HJM, Jones MW, Boughner DR, et al: Cerebral ischemic events associated with prolapsing mitral valve. Arch Neurol 33:777–782, 1976
2. Crosley CJ, Rorke LB, Evans A, et al: Central nervous system lesions in childhood leukemia. Neurology (Minneapolis) 28:678–685, 1978
3. Davidson S, Falconer MA: Outcome of surgery in 40 children with temporal-lobe epilepsy. Lancet 1:1260–1263, 1975
4. Dykes J: Ten Thousand Severely Handicapped Children in New South Wales and the Australian Capital Territory. Canberra, Australian Government Publishing Service, 1978, p 120

5. Health Statistics from the U.S. National Health Survey. Origin and Program of the U.S. National Health Survey. PHS Publication 584, Series A-1.
6. Humphreys RP, Hendrick EB, Hoffman HJ: Cerebrovascular disease in children. Canad Med Assoc J 107:774–781, 1972
7. Matson DD: Neurosurgery of Infancy and Childhood. Springfield, Charles C Thomas, 1969, p 934
8. Merkel KH, Ginsberg PL, Parker JC, et al: Cerebrovascular disease in sickle cell anemia: A clinical, pathological and radiological correlation. Stroke 9:45–52, 1978
9. O'Brien MJ, Ash JM, and Gilday DL: Radionuclide brain scanning in perinatal hypoxia/ischaemia. Dev Med Child Neurol 21:161–173, 1979
10. Report of Joint Committee for Stroke Facilities, Gold AP (chairman): IX. Strokes in children (Part 1). Stroke 4:835–858, 1973
11. Rudolf AM: Congenital Diseases of the Heart. Chicago, Year Book Medical Publishers, 1974 p 646
12. Schoenberg BS, Mellinger JF, Schoenberg DG: Cerebrovascular disease in infants and children: a study of incidence, clinical features, and survival. Neurology (Minneapolis) 28:678–685, 1978
13. Seeler RA, Royal JE, Powe L, et al: Moyamoya in children with sickle cell anemia and cerebrovascular occlusion. J Pediatr 93:808–810, 1978
14. Shields WD, Ziter FA, Osborn AG, et al: Fibromuscular dysplasia as a cause of stroke in infancy and childhood. Pediatrics 59:899–901, 1977
15. Shillito J: Carotid arteritis: A cause of hemiplegia in childhood. J Neurosurg 21:540–551, 1964
16. Spence JD: Personal communication, 1979
17. Stockman JA, Nigro MA, Mishkin MM et al: Occlusion of large cerebral vessels in sickle-cell anemia. N Engl J Med 287:846–849, 1972
18. Suzuki J, Takaku A: Cerebrovascular "moya-moya" disease: Disease showing abnormal net-like vessels in base of brain. Arch Neurol 20:288–299, 1969
19. Tibbles JAR, Brown BStJ: Acute hemiplegia of childhood. Canad Med Assoc J 113:309–314, 1975
20. Weinstein BJ, Epstein FH: Comparability of criteria and methods in the epidemiology of cardiovascular disease. Circulation 30:643–653, 1964

55. Aneurysms in Children and Adolescents

Kenneth Shulman

It is difficult to answer the question, "Are aneurysms congenital lesions?" Intracranial aneurysms are seen infrequently in children despite their reputed congenital origin from defects of the media of the cerebral arteries. Autopsy studies have shown no or very few aneurysms in the brains of children.[5,12,25,33] There are a number of clinical series and isolated case reports permitting a review of some 300 patients with aneurysms presenting as diagnostic and therapeutic problems during the first two decades of life.[1-3,7,11,14-19,21,22,27,28,30,31,32,36] Childhood intracranial aneurysms have been reported to account for 1.3 percent of aneurysms for all ages.[14] Fifteen percent of aneurysms occurring in the pediatric population have been seen in the first decade of life; 30 percent from age 11 through 14, and 55 percent in adolescence and young adulthood, from 15 to 20 years of age. In the series of cases reported in which data on age and sex are available, there is a prevalence of cases in males, approaching a ratio of 2:1. This fact is surprising since aneurysms for all ages have a predominant incidence in females.

CLINICAL PRESENTATION

Patients with intracranial aneurysms rarely have symptoms or signs referable to the aneurysm prior to the initial rupture. In three personal cases and a number of children and adolescents reported by others,[2,3,35,36] however, the aneurysm did, in fact, act as a mass lesion causing cranial nerve or brain-stem compression. The third cranial nerve is most often affected. Causes of third nerve palsy in children include congenital palsy, trauma, meningitis, and parasellar tumors, as well as aneurysms. Posterior communicating artery aneurysms with sudden expansion result in pain about the eye and a third nerve palsy, which usually begins with diplopia followed by ptosis. The rare instance of an aneurysm of the superior cerebellar artery in a 7-year-old recently was cited.[36] Amacher and Drake[3] have noted cranial nerve or brain stem compression in 9 of their 32 aneurysm patients. In 6 of 8 such patients, the aneurysm was giant, and in a further two giant aneurysms, compression and subarachnoid hemorrhage occurred so that a total of 34.5 percent of their unique series had features of neural compression. In the child presenting to the pediatrician with subarachnoid hemorrhage, one encounters an irritable, somnolent child with nuchal rigidity and photophobia. There is excruciating headache. The spinal fluid will be bloody, ordinarily containing a large number of red blood corpuscles, in contradistinction to blood-tinged fluid seen after a head injury. The clinical issue is to recognize that the child or adolescent complaining of sudden severe headache has indeed suffered a subarachnoid hemorrhage, and to confirm the clinical impression by lumbar puncture. Too often such headaches and findings are not properly appreciated, leading to a second and more severe or fatal bleed. In general terms a child with initial subarachnoid hemorrhage is more apt to have an early second hemorrhage than the adult, making recognition and diagnosis after the first bleed of the utmost importance.

Aneurysmal subarachnoid hemorrhage in children results from an aneurysm of the circle of Willis in the majority of cases. The anatomic distribution of juvenile aneurysms of the circle of Willis is unique in that over 20 percent of cases occur at the carotid bifurcation.[22,28,32] The more unusual sites away from the circle, and of unusual etiology, are of considerable interest. Mycotic aneurysms occur in association with bacterial endocarditis and result from small infarctions of the arterial wall with infected emboli. Such lesions may rupture, but the vessel wall injury has a tendency to repair with appropriate antibiotic therapy. Indeed the incidence of mycotic aneurysms has been markedly reduced since antibiotics have been available, with McDonald and Korb[19] reporting 34 percent in their 1939 series, and McNeel, Evans, and Ory[20] reporting 9 percent of mycotic aneurysms in 1969. Traumatic aneurysms are the result of a penetrating head injury with the indriven object causing an incomplete tear of the vessel wall. This injury causes dissection of the blood into the vessel wall with aneurysmal dilatation. There is little tendency for healing of such an injury and enlargement of the aneurysm leads to rupture. Traumatic aneurysms tend to occur along the course of the anterior cerebral artery and its distal branches where there is vascular contiguity to dural edges. Aneurysms may occur also in peripheral cortical vessels involved in skull fracture[26] and a number are associated with orbitofrontal vessels.[9] It is good clinical practice to perform an angiogram prior to discharge of a child who has had a major penetrating injury; if an aneurysm is found, it should be surgically corrected, often simply by excision of the small distal vessel or reinforcement of the wall with a muscle stump or plastic adhesive.

There are a number of cases in the older literature describing children with aneurysms associated with unrepaired coarctation of the aorta. These aneurysms are about equally distributed to the major sites of aneurysmal formation. Of 13 patients described with coarctation, there were 10 males. Correction of the aneurysm followed by attention to the coarctation is the recommended treatment.

MANAGEMENT

Based upon clinical experience, the child or adolescent presenting to the pediatrician with spontaneous subarachnoid hemorrhage will have either an arteriovenous malformation or aneurysm. Immediate computerized tomographic (CT) scanning should be done followed by a CT scan with contrast enhancement. On the unenhanced scan, the presence and site of subarachnoid or intraparenchymal bleeding can be determined (Fig. 55-1); on the enhanced scan, a giant

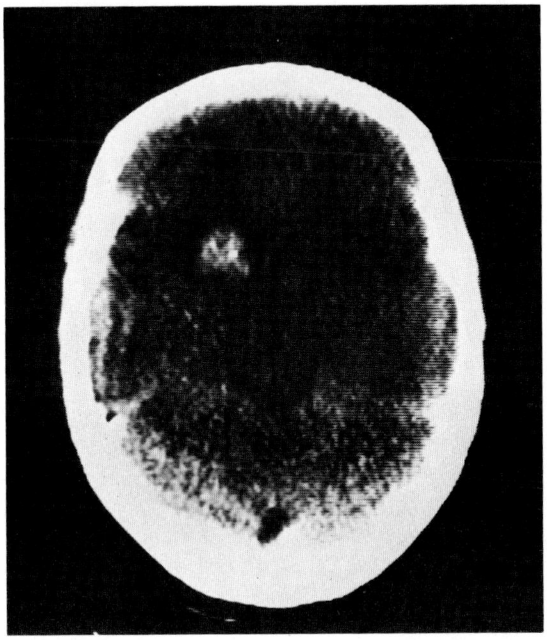

Figure 55-1. CT scan obtained eight hours after rupture of a bifurcation aneurysm in a 16-year-old. Hemorrhagic density is noticed in the left parasellar region.

aneurysm may be seen. The child's clinical condition should then be graded using the schema of Hunt and Hess.[13] Patients in Grades 0 to 2 should be considered for early angiography and surgery prior to day 3 after the hemorrhage. Those children in Grades 3 and 4 with large hematomas should have immediate angiography and surgery. The exact timing of the angiogram will depend a good deal upon the neurosurgeon's practice in the timing of surgery. Timing of surgery is presently an area of intense discussion, between advocates of early surgery and equally strong voices recommending delayed surgery in the second week.[34] It would seem that early surgery is ideal for a child or adolescent who presents with neurologic findings without aneurysmal rupture and those patients with subarachnoid hemorrhage in Grades 0 and 1 who do not demonstrate vasospasm on the first angiogram. If there is clear neurologic deficit or altered states of consciousness, a degree of cerebral ischemia is implied and delayed surgery, so as not to enhance this ischemia, seems best. If surgery is delayed, epsilon aminocaproic acid (EACA, Amicar®—Lederle Laboratories, Pearl River, New York 10965) should be administered intravenously in a dosage of 24–36 g/day until the child is taken to the operating room. In addition absolute bed rest, a quiet environment, and limited visiting should be enforced in the setting of an intensive care unit to prevent rebleeding. Four-vessel angiography is mandatory to visualize the offending aneurysm and to rule out the possibility of multiple aneurysms or the presence of an aneurysm and a concurrent arteriovenous malformation. Since polycystic kidney disease may occur with congenital aneurysms,[4,10] an intravenous pyelogram can be obtained following the contrast injection at the appropriate time.

Surgical technique for all aneurysms is a direct microsurgical approach and has been described by specific site. In general terms the fronto-temporo-sphenoidal (pterional) approach as advocated by Yasargil and Fox[38] is used for all aneurysms of the anterior circle of Willis and for selected aneurysms of the basilar tip. Drake's subtemporal approach is applicable also to aneurysms of the upper basilar artery.[8] For either approach this writer prefers to use spinal drainage, to confine coagulation to the bipolar unit, and to depend upon sodium nitroprusside for induced hypothermia to facilitate dissection of the aneurysmal neck while at the same time preventing or minimizing bleeding from ruptures of

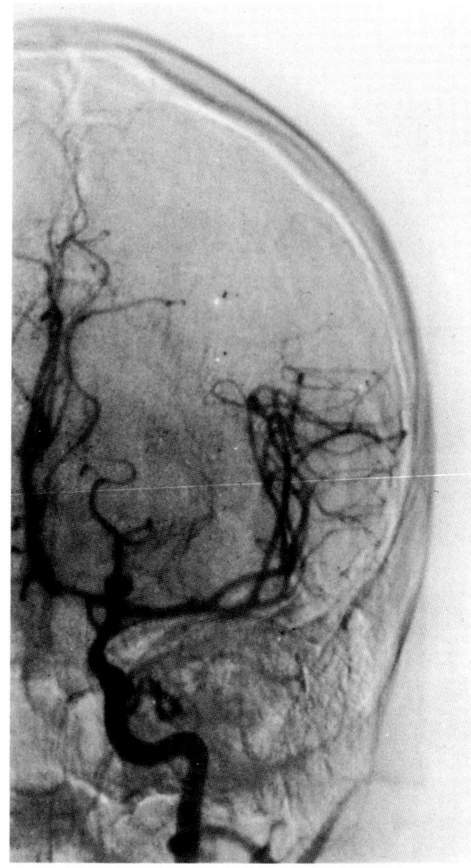

Figure 55-2. Angiogram showing left carotid bifurcation aneurysm that appears to arise on the anterior cerebral side of the bifurcation.

the aneurysm during surgery. Since aneurysms of the internal carotid bifurcation represent only 4 to 8 percent of all aneurysms for all ages, whereas such aneurysms represent over 20 percent in childhood, the surgical treatment of this peculiar aneurysm seems appropriate. There have been discussions by a few authors.[6,23,24,29] The angiographic study and the finding at surgery permit grouping into two varieties (Figs. 55-2, 55-3, and 55-4). In the first the aneurysm

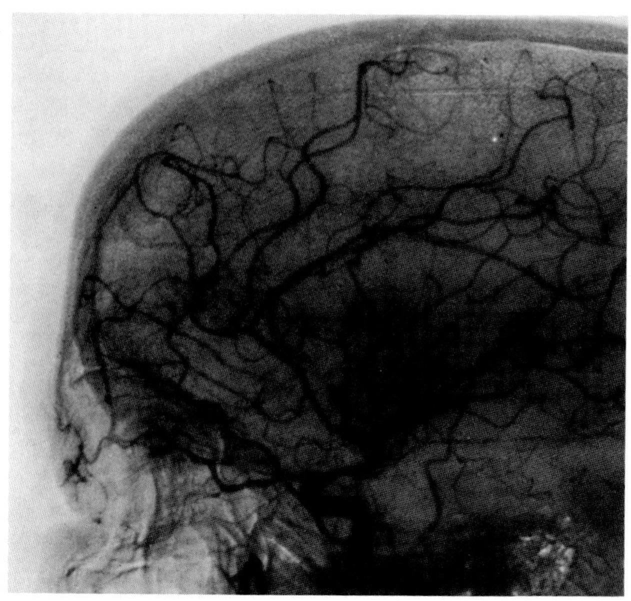

Figure 55-3. Lateral angiogram of same patient demonstrating aneurysm in up and forward position.

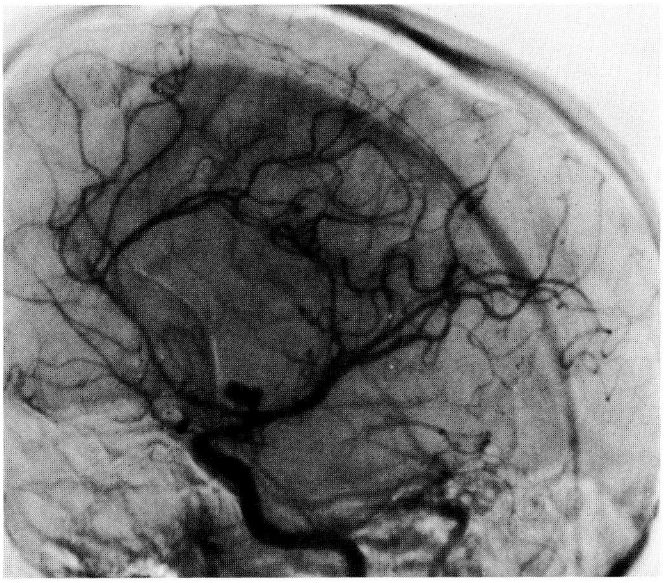

Figure 55-4. Oblique view of small neck of aneurysm with perforating vessels passing behind neck and fundus.

forms a direct continuation of the main internal carotid trunk, projecting upward and backward. Rarely are the neck and fundus symmetric, but rather usually the fundus points toward the anterior cerebral artery. In the second variety, the neck is located at the underside of the bifurcation, but clearly distal to the anterior choroidal artery. This aneurysm is directed backward and again it is most usual to have its fundus on the anterior cerebral side of the bifurcation. DaPian has described a rarer aneurysm with the sac being large and projecting anteriorly. With bifurcation aneurysms special attention must be paid to the relationship of the aneurysm neck to the perforating vessels coming off as does the aneurysm from either the anterior or middle cerebral artery. The essential steps in the dissection include splitting of the sylvian fissure so that the bifurcation can be exposed with the frontal lobe, since the largest number of fundi point upward into the frontal lobe. After identification of the middle and anterior cerebrals, the neck of the aneurysm is dissected with adequate visualization of the medial side of the middle and posterior surface of the anterior cerebral for identification of perforating vessels. Such vessels, no matter how small, should be moved off the neck prior to clipping.

RESULTS

The results of modern microsurgical treatment of juvenile aneurysms is good. As with all aneurysms, the grade of the patient and the location of the aneurysm affect results. For good-risk aneurysms (Hunt grade 0, 1, 2), the surgical death rate has been less than 10 percent.[3,32] Since the spontaneous hemorrhage, a sudden enlargement of a juvenile aneurysm causing neurologic deficit, occurs in the child during a comparatively stress-free and nonhypertensive period of life, it is reasonable to assume that the risk of recurrent hemorrhage and death far exceeds this surgical mortality.

REFERENCES

1. Almeida GM, Pindaro J, Plese P, et al: Intracranial arterial aneurysms in infancy and childhood. Child's Brain 3:193–199, 1977

2. Amacher AL, Drake CG: Cerebral artery aneurysms in infancy, childhood and adolescence. Child's Brain 1:72–80, 1975
3. Amacher AL, Drake CG: The results of operating upon cerebral aneurysms and angiomas in children and adolescents.1. Cerebral aneurysms. Child's Brain 5:151–165, 1979
4. Brown AP: Polycystic diseases of the kidneys and intracranial aneurysms; the etiology and interrelation of these conditions: Review of recent literature and report of seven cases in which both conditions coexisted. Glasgow Med J 32:333–348, 1951
5. Chason JL, Hindman WM: Berry aneurysm of the circle of Willis. Neurology 8:41, 1958
6. DaPian R, Pasqualin A, Scienza R: Direct microsurgical approach to aneurysms of the internal carotid bifurcation. Surg Neurol 13:27–37, 1980
7. Davadiga KV, Mathai KV, Chandy J: Spontaneous cure of intracavernous aneurysms of the internal carotid artery in a 14-month old child. J Neurosurg 30:165–168, 1969
8. Drake CG: The treatment of aneurysms of the posterior cranial fossa, in Progress in Neurological Surgery, vol 9. Basel, Karger, 1978
9. Ferry DJ, Kempe LG: False aneurysm secondary to penetration of brain through orbitofacial wounds, report of two cases. J Neurosurg 36:503, 1972
10. Forster FM, Alpers BJ: Aneurysm of circle of Willis associated with congenital polycystic disease of the kidneys. Arch Neurol Psychiat 50:669–676, 1943
11. Garcia-Chavez C, Mossy J: Cerebral artery aneurysm in infancy: Association with agenesis of the corpus callosum. J Neuropath Exp Neurol 24:492–501, 1965
12. Housepian EM, Pool JL: A systematic analysis of intracranial aneurysms from the autopsy file of the Presbyterian Hospital, 1914–1956. J Neuropath Exp Neurol 17:409, 1958
13. Hunt WE, Hess RM: Surgical risk as related to time of intervention in the repair of intracranial aneurysms. J Neurosurg 28:14–20, 1968
14. Leitinen L: Subarachnoid hemorrhage from arterial aneurysms in children. Nord Med 71:329–333, 1964
15. Lemmen LJ, Schneider RC: Aneurysm in the third ventricle. Neurology 3:474–476, 1953
16. Locksley HB: Aneurysm study, Sec V, part 1. Natural history of subarachnoid hemorrhage, intracranial aneurysms and arteriovenous malformations. J Neurosurg 25:219–239, 1966
17. Matson DD: Intracranial aneurysms in childhood. J Neurosurg 23:578–580, 1965
18. Matson DD: Neurosurgery in Infancy and Childhood (ed 2). Springfield, Charles C Thomas, 1969, p 754
19. McDonald CA, Korb M: Intracranial aneurysms. Arch Neurol Psychiatr 12:298–328, 1939
20. McNeel D, Evans RA, Ory EM: Angiography of cerebral mycotic aneurysms. Acta Radiol (Diag.) 9:407–416, 1969
21. Nibbelink DW: Intracranial hemorrhage, in Cerebrovascular Survey Report NINCDS (revised). Jan 1976, p 172
22. Patel AN, Richardson AE: Ruptured intracranial aneurysms in the first two decades of life. J Neurosurg 35:571–576, 1971
23. Perria L, Rivano C, Rossi GF, et al: Aneurysms of the bifurcation of the internal carotid artery. Acta Neurochir 19:51–68, 1968
24. Pool JL, Potts DG: Aneurysms and Arteriovenous Anomalies of the Brain: Diagnosis and Treatment. New York, Harper & Row, 1965, p 57
25. Riggs HE, Rupp C: Miliary aneurysms: relation of anomalies of the circle of Willis to formation of aneurysms. J Neuropath 1:442, 1942
26. Rumbaugh CI, Bergeren RT, Talalla A, et al: Traumatic aneurysms of cortical cerebral arteries. Radiology 96:49–54, 1970
27. Saha AL, et al: Intracranial Aneurysms and Subarachnoid Hemorrhage: A Cooperative Study. Philadelphia, Lippincott, 1969
28. Sedzimir CB, Robinson J: Intracranial hemorrhage in children and adolescents. J Neurosurg 38:269–287, 1973
29. Sengupta RP, Lassman LP, DeMoraes AA, et al: Treatment of internal carotid bifurcation aneurysms by direct surgery. J Neurosurg 43:343–351, 1975

30. Shucart WA, Wolpert SM: An aneurysm in infancy presenting with diabetes insipidus. J Neurosurg 37:368–371, 1972
31. Shucart WA, Wolpert SM: Intracranial arterial aneurysms in childhood. Am J Dis Child 127:288, 1974
32. Shulman K, Tabaddor K: Intracranial vascular disease in childhood, in O'Brien M (ed): Pediatric Neurological Surgery. New York, Raven Press, 1978, p 45
33. Stehbens WE: Pathology of the Cerebral Blood Vessels. St. Louis, CV Mosby, 1972
34. Sundt TM Jr, Whisnant JP: Subarachnoid hemorrhage from intracranial aneurysms. N Engl J Med 299:116, 1978
35. Thompson RA, Pribam HFW: Infantile cerebral aneurysm associated with ophthalmoplegia and quadriparesis. Neurology 19:785–789, 1969
36. Vincent FM, Zimmerman JE: Superior cerebellar artery aneurysm presenting as an oculomotor nerve palsy in a child. Neurosurgery 6:661, 1980
37. Yasargil MG, Beohm WB, Ho REM: Microsurgical treatment of cerebral aneurysms at the bifurcation of the internal carotid artery. Acta Neurochir 41:61–72, 1978
38. Yasargil MG, Fox JL: The microsurgical approach to intracranial aneurysms. Surg Neurol 3:7–14, 1975

56. Arteriovenous Malformations of the Brain and Spinal Cord

Robin P. Humphreys

What can I know?
What ought I to do?
What may I hope?

I. Kant

CEREBRAL ARTERIOVENOUS MALFORMATION

Children do suffer strokes.[7,10] A child's exclamation about the sudden onset of headache, which is followed by lapse into coma, heralds spontaneous intracranial hemorrhage. Notwithstanding published opinion to the contrary, that hemorrhagic event in children is more likely to be due to rupture of a cerebral arteriovenous malformation (AVM) than aneurysm.[8,22] The material reported here surveys 70 children with arteriovenous malformations of the brain admitted to the Hospital for Sick Children (HSC), Toronto, from 1954 to 1979.[12] As this hospital serves widespread regional needs, it is concluded that subarachnoid hemorrhage from ruptured AVM is at least twice as common as ruptured aneurysm. During the period of review, only 26 patients under 17 years of age were admitted and treated for intracranial aneurysm.

Pathogenesis and Pathology

The imperfect formation of the primitive arteriolar-capillary network normally interposed between brain arteries and veins results in a tangle of arteriovenous communications, which, because of their low resistance, attract exaggerated blood flow. Given enough time the malformations do have the capacity to expand their bulk by enlarging and increasing the tortuosity of the feeding and draining channels. The number of fistulous connections likely does not change, however, and some lesions (such as those of the brain stem) may always remain small.[4,16]

As a rule 90 percent of the malformations are found supratentorial, most frequently within the distribution of the middle cerebral artery.[18,19] But any intracranial artery can be associated with the malformation (hence the advisability of total cerebral arteriography to study all components of the identified malformation), and in the HSC study, 16 patients (23 percent) had malformations located below the tentorium.

The conglomeration of turgid, tortuous vessels covered by opacified and thickened arachnoid on the brain's surface is easily recognizable as the classic AVM. Sometimes the malformation is hidden in a sulcus or the subcortical tissues, and served by a straightened, dilated anomalous artery that acts as its only surface hallmark. The nearby cerebral convolutions show variable degrees of atrophy and there may be local rusty staining from previous hemorrhage. The tough texture of the adjacent gray and white matter is due to gliosis, which permits dissection of the lesion through this relatively inert tissue. Although some malformations are globular in shape, most describe a course to the subjacent ventricle in a wedge-shaped fashion.[6] The component vessels show variation in their numbers, caliber, and thickness of their walls. Normal lamination of elastic and muscle fibers in the arteries is altered; the media varies in thickness and substantial thinning of some vessels can result in marked aneurysmal dilatation of the structure.[16,19]

The AVM, although of congenital origin, does not necessarily declare itself at birth or in the early childhood years. The fact that most lesions become symptomatic between the ages of 20 and 40 years suggests a latency in the malformation's usual evolution. While there is a certain age bias in the reporting of series from predominantly adult units, we have made a striking observation at the Hospital for Sick Children. Approximately 10,000 cerebral arteriograms have been performed in our hospital and not one incidental aneurysm or AVM has been uncovered.[9] The 70 patients reported thus are comprised of 67 studied for specific neurologic symptoms. An additional three children died of other causes and their malformations were discovered incidentally at autopsy.

Natural History

Matched trials of nonoperative and operative management programs for patients with cerebral arteriovenous malformations have understandably not been reported. Papers by Forster, Steiner, and Hakanson,[5] by Schatz and Botterell,[21] by Svien and McRae,[24] and by Troupp, Marttila, and Halonen[25] have analyzed nonoperative treatment methods. It is worth remembering that these experiences were gathered at a time when operative and anesthetic techniques were not as precise as those available currently, and that the patients relegated to a nonoperative program were often those whose lesions were considered inoperable.

There are no figures available that document the natural history of cerebral AVMs in children. The present study, however, which agrees with that of Mori, Murata, Hashimoto, et al.[15] indicates that children are more liable to hemorrhage (79 percent risk) from their malformation than adults (68 percent risk), and that there is a threat of repeat hemorrhage. Eight children with confirmed brain-stem AVMs (four in the midbrain and four in the pons), for example, have suffered a total of 14 bleeding episodes.

If it is agreed that the operative treatment of cerebral AVMs, if undertaken, should, as Drake states, "carry a very low mortality and morbidity, certainly lower than that of the natural history," then operative care for children's arteriovenous malformations is recommended.[4,13,23,27] Not only is there a greater risk of hemorrhage as the first symptom in children, but also the mortality from the *first* hemorrhage in the HSC series is 27 percent, substantially greater than the 6 to 10 percent rate quoted for adults.[16,18] The HSC operative mortality is 8 percent and represents patients who were Grade IV or V category at the time of emergency measures to evacuate clot or place an external ventricular drain. Operative treatment of children's AVMs thus adheres to Drake's principle. It also supports Matson's stance on operative care, recommended because "there is expectation of many years in which these lesions may enlarge and cause increasing disability and the resiliency of the cerebral circulation is better."[14]

Initial Clinical Assessment

Symptoms

The symptoms of a cerebral AVM, whenever they appear, are representative of the structural defects in the vessels of the malformation, and the sump effect of the direct arteriovenous shunting. Perhaps the progressive biologic activity of the malformation accounts for a greater percentage of children (than adults) suffering intracranial bleeding from the lesion, whereas relatively larger numbers of adults display the presumed ischemic symptoms of headache, dementia, and slowly progressive neurologic dysfunction.

Spontaneous subarachnoid, or more frequently intracerebral, bleeding is the most common cause of symptoms experienced by children.[14,15,23] In our review 55 patients (79 percent) experienced spontaneous intracranial hemorrhage as determined by the syndrome of headache, with bloody spinal fluid and/or blood clot recovered at operation or autopsy. The ictus is often explosive, when the previously well child screams out about sudden headache, then clasps the side of the head and collapses. Not surprisingly, therefore, the subarachnoid grading reflects the critical nature of the children at the time of first assessment (Table 56-1). Altered consciousness, meningism, and appropriate lateralized motor and sensory signs are present. Rapidly deepening stupor usually occurs when blood bursts into the ventricular system.

Children seem liable to hemorrhage repeatedly.[15,23] This may be manifest by the "warning leak" that historically has preceded the present ictus by weeks or months, or by a second hemorrhage that appears 48 to 72 hours after the initial flamboyant event. The headache of AVM hemorrhage is characteristic only of intracranial bleeding. Occasionally a severe migraine headache, particularly if it is the first such attack, will mimic subarachnoid hemorrhage, and can be differentiated from the latter only by specialized neuroradiologic evaluation.

Epilepsy, which presumably results from gliosis of brain because of chronic ischemia adjacent to the arteriovenous shunt, occurs as a presenting symptom in 20 to 25 percent of adult patients with AVM.[14,18] While "acute" seizures occurred at the time of, or shortly after, the hemorrhage in nine of our children, "chronic" seizures were the presenting problem in only seven (10 percent). Of the remaining eight children who had neither hemorrhage nor epilepsy in their

Table 56-1
Botterell* Grading of 55 Children with Intracranial Hemorrhage from AVM

Grade I	7 Patients
Grade II	13 Patients
Grade III	16 Patients
Grade IV	9 Patients
Grade V	10 Patients

*Botterell, Lougheed, Scott, et al.[2]

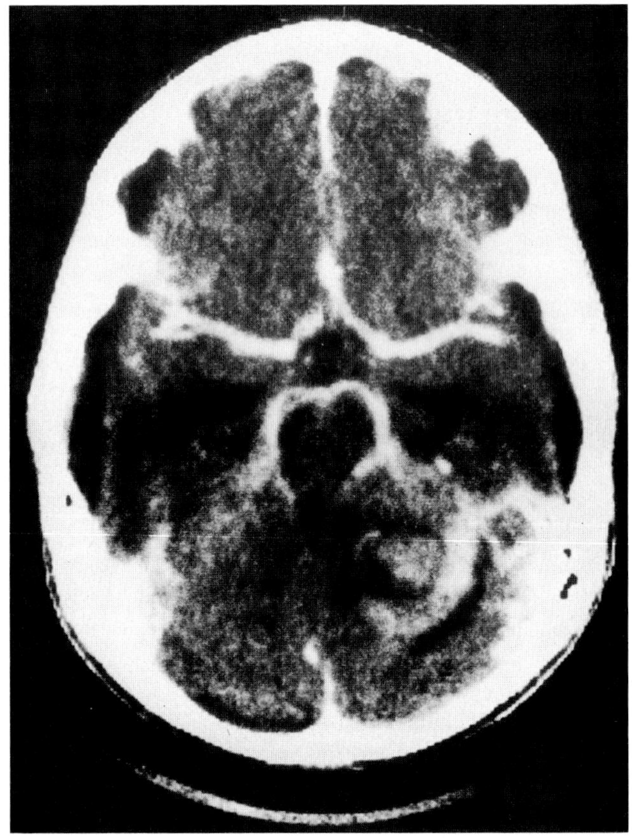

Figure 56-1. CT scan showing left cerebellar hematoma extending into region of dentate nucleus and middle cerebellar peduncle. With peripheral enhancement and vessel-like structures noted after contrast injection, a ruptured AVM is suggested.

profile, four presented with delayed development, one with congestive heart failure, and three with incidental AVM, discovered at necropsy.

Investigations

When the child presents with the typical headache–hemorrhagic ictus, the surgeon should directly proceed with computed tomography (CT) and cerebral arteriography. Lumbar puncture serves no useful purpose and may be dangerous.[11]

The CT head scan will outline blood clot and calcification if present, and on enhanced study detail the dilated vascular channels and large blood-containing varices. (Fig. 56-1) It will thus provide a clue to the site and side of the brain to be studied first with cerebral arteriography.

By means of selective internal carotid and vertebral artery injections, the numbers and location of the arterial feeders can be examined by cerebral arteriography (Fig. 56-2). The numbers of arterial contributors can be determined by properly timed sequential films processed with subtraction techniques. Seldom is a malformation served by only one arterial channel. There may be only one *major* artery contributing to the lesion, but the surgeon should anticipate any number of minor vessels coming from dural, pial, or deep perforating sources. On the other hand, the venous drainage is frequently through a solitary channel via either a large cortical vein or the deep venous system, and is usually precisely defined on arteriography. The geography of the lesion is carefully studied on the arteriogram and its operability thus determined. If the operation proceeds, then the surgeon must be able to match the vascular findings at craniotomy with those on the arteriogram.

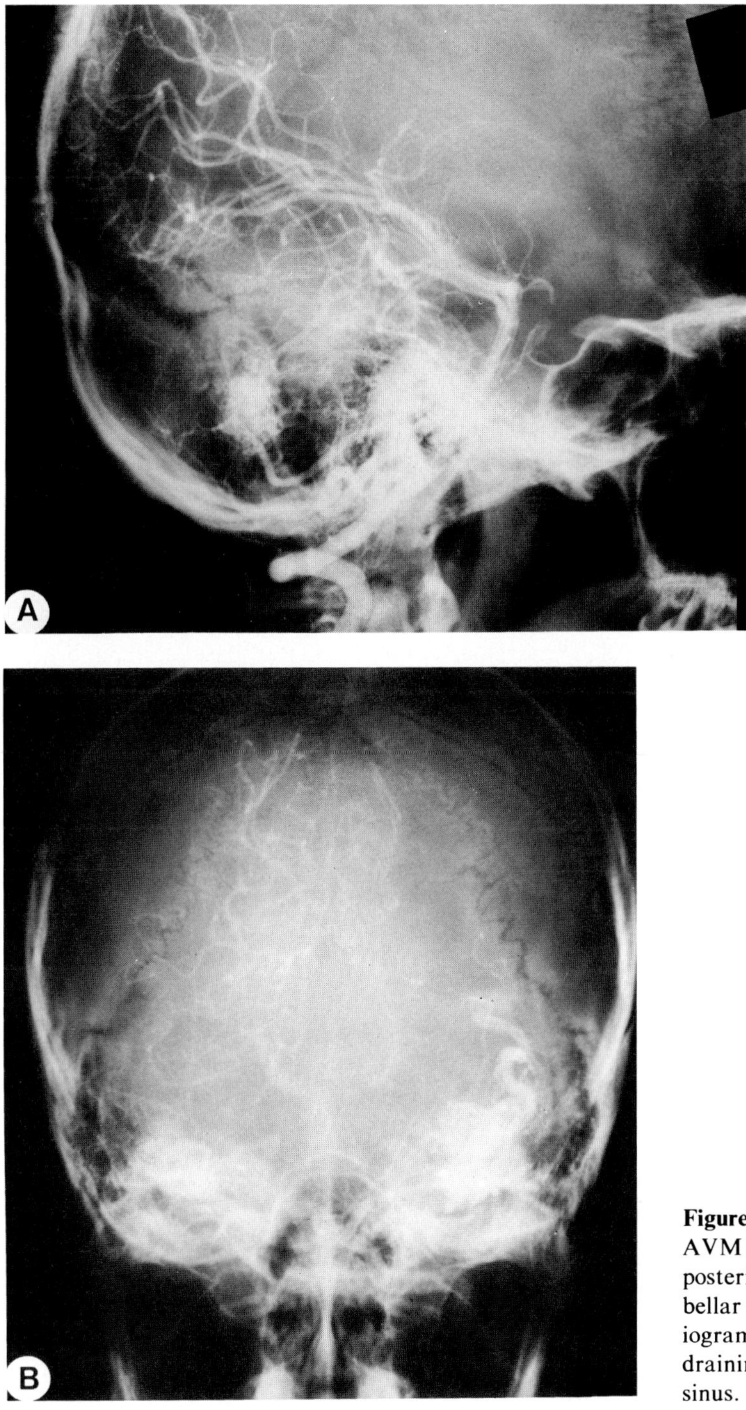

Figure 56-2. A. Lateral left vertebral arteriogram. AVM in left cerebellar hemisphere fed by vessels from posterior inferior cerebellar artery and superior cerebellar artery. B. Anteroposterior left vertebral arteriogram for same patient. There is only one large draining vein emptying directly into the transverse sinus.

Preoperative Management

The luxury of a planned, elective operation for a child with a ruptured AVM may be seldom realized. When 80 percent of the lesions first present with spontaneous intracranial hemorrhage, then urgent neurodiagnostic assessments and operative care are usually undertaken to identify and release the associated clot. The AVM surgery can be tedious and protracted, and is therefore not ideally begun as an emergent procedure late at night. If only subarachnoid hemorrhage has occurred, or if the intracerebral hematoma is small and the patient's condition stable, interval surgery may be staged after a few days' wait. During that time the child is monitored carefully by a "subarachnoid routine" in an intensive care unit. Cerebral vasospasm is seldom a problem in children with AVMs, but rebleeding during the interval frequently is. Antispasm, antihypertensive pharmacologic measures thus are not required, but drug and nursing care for the restless or bored child will be an equal challenge. If the operation can possibly be delayed for three to seven days after the hemorrhage, then the surgeon will be rewarded with a properly prepared patient whose relaxed brain contains a liquefying hematoma.

There is not the same urgency for the 20 percent of patients who present with symptoms other than spontaneous hemorrhage. This group has been investigated in a traditional fashion for headaches, seizures, developmental delay, etc., and the malformation discovered during that testing or even at an elective operation. The clinical challenge will be to determine in advance whether operative obliteration of the malformation will influence the headache, seizure, or developmental problem, and thus whether it should even be undertaken.[26,29]

Surgery

The ideal treatment for a brain AVM is its total excision.[4,6] This has now been achieved in almost all eloquent regions of brain (motor, basal ganglia, brain stem), as well as in less critical areas. With the exception of those lesions that penetrate the brain stem or basal ganglia, it is thus not so much the anatomic location of the lesion in the child that restrains the surgeon, as its size. As the large, lush, and thirsty AVMs are not common in children, and as it is usually the small malformations that produce hemorrhage, then paradoxically it may be the small, awkwardly positioned AVM that will present the greatest operative challenge.[28] Those lesions about 1.0 cm across and located adjacent to or within a ventricle, or positioned deeply along the medial face of the hemisphere, can be difficult to isolate, particularly if the hemorrhage has been in a direction away from the malformation. Moreover the lateral hemispheral AVM may not always be found classically curled on the cortex. Instead it may be hidden subcortically and bear as its only surface landmark an unusually straightened feeding artery running a nonanatomic course, or a red draining vein striking out toward an adjacent venous sinus.

The operative management of a child with an AVM requires all of the major anesthetic and pharmacologic techniques currently available. Curiously AVMs are less prone to bleed during surgery from their original site or hemorrhage than are aneurysms, and thus the various vascular coils and varices can be gently manipulated aside. When bleeding does occur, it tends to be less torrential than with aneurysm rupture, and the bleeding usually represents transgression into the malformation itself. This can be controlled with gentle packing while dissection proceeds at a more remote site.

The operating microscope is almost always an ally, although it may be disadvantageous when working upon large convexity or cerebellar lesions. In these circumstances the surgeon may lose sight of the perimeter of the AVM even when working with the lowest magnifications. Magnifying loupes and a fiberoptic headlight can thus provide more mobility, permitting the surgeon to stay just at the margin of the malformation in its glial plane. A parenchymal clot, if present, can create much autodissection of the AVM. Following clot removal the surgeon will recognize the AVM hanging like a chandelier from the wall or roof of the clot cavity. On other occasions the clot can be located "downstream" from the AVM, which often is isolated before the hematoma is reached.

The dissection proceeds with microinstruments in an organized circumferential fashion about the malformation, preserving until the end one or two major draining veins. As a rule the feeding and draining vessels run a straight course to and from the malformation but become coiled within it. These vessels can be freed by dissecting along their long axis and isolating them with a blunt hook before applying the bipolar coagulation forceps. It is not unusual for an accompanying artery or vein to be hidden immediately deep to the vessel about to be severed, and manipulation with the blunt hook will bring this surreptitious neighbor into view for its coagulation too. Most AVMs describe a wedge or torpedo profile toward the adjacent ventricle, and the surgeon should not be content that a total excision has been achieved until the ventricular wall has been visualized. Once the malformation dissection has been completed, then bleeding has ceased in its bed and the brain is considerably relaxed. If operation has been decided upon, then the surgeon should be satisfied with nothing less than total excision, even if this is achieved in two stages. Proximal vessel ligation can be dangerous and is an inadequate solution; subtotal excision is not only messy, but the shunt remains served by newly recruited contributors.

The embolization of particulate material into the feeding channels of AVMs has been advocated during the past 20 years. While these techniques have been used in patients with dural and extracranial vascular malformations in our hospital, they have not been tried in the cerebral lesions.

Postoperative Care and Results

The child's biologic plasticity is such that the degree of postoperative recovery can be as complete and gratifying as the preoperative deterioration was rapid and dramatic. The experienced surgeon who attempts total excision of the malformation will usually know whether that goal has been achieved at the conclusion of the first craniotomy. If there is some doubt about the completeness of excision, especially after prolonged surgery, and if the operative region is neither bleeding nor swelling, then it may be advisable to close the wound, allow the child to recover, and study the situation further with repeat arteriography. One or two strategically placed metallic hemostatic clips will permit identifica-

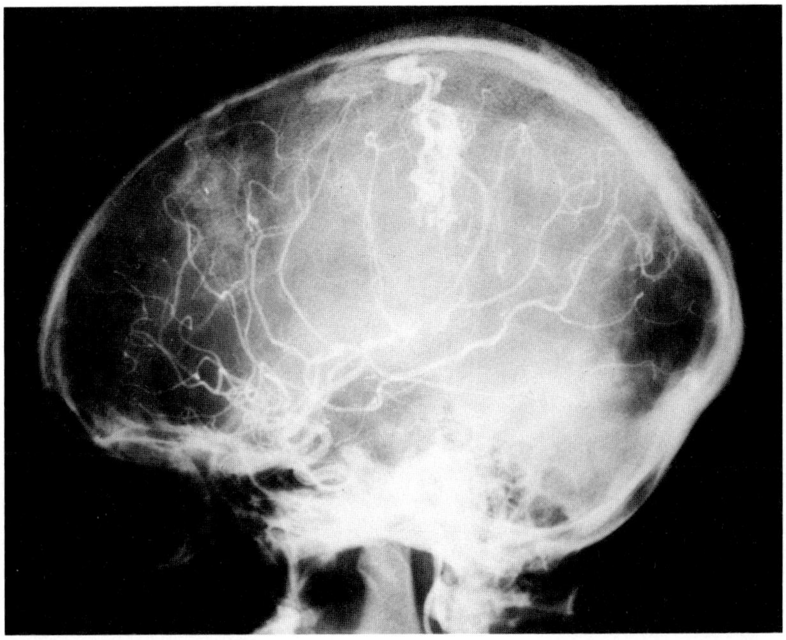

Figure 56-3. Lateral right carotid arteriogram. AVM in right postcentral gyrus, fed by parietal branch of middle cerebral artery and two small branches of anterior cerebral artery.

tion of the area of surgery and serve as coordinates for the further radiologic and operative examination of the malformation that remains.

Whether one or two procedures are required to obliterate the lesion, the surgeon cannot be satisfied that total excision has been achieved until postoperative arteriography confirms this (Figs. 56-3, 56-4). It also happens to show a diminished size of the proximal contributing arteries.[1] Thereafter convalescence depends only on the child's rehabilitation needs, if any. Prophylactic anticonvulsant medication will usually be required for 6–24 months following AVM excision.

In the HSC series, 67 patients received definitive care (three children with incidental malformations discovered at necropsy have thus been excluded). Eighteen children received nonoperative treatment, and 13 died (66 percent mortality). A majority of this group were Grade V category at the time of admission. There were 49 patients who were operated upon and any one or a combination of complete or incomplete AVM removal, obliteration of feeders, evacuation of hematoma, or shunting procedures were achieved. Four patients in this group died, all of whom were Grade IV or V at the time of first assessment.

A chronic seizure disorder was the reason for neurologic evaluation in 7 patients. All of these children were operated upon and none had a lingering convulsive problem during the follow-up period. Paradoxically 6 patients who had been operated upon, and who did not have any preoperative seizure disturbance, were subject to this malady during the follow-up period. All 6 patients had intracerebral clots.

Excluding the patients with incidental malformations and those who have died or are lost to follow-up, there are 46 patients available for follow-up examination three months to 10 years after treatment. An arbitrary scaling of their result according to their neurologic deficit is outlined in Table 56-2.

Conclusions

Arteriovenous malformation is more common than ruptured intracranial aneurysm as a cause of subarachnoid hemorrhage in children, and is especially prevalent between 7 and 13 years of age. Almost 80 percent of children with arteriovenous malformation present with intracranial hemorrhage. Repeat hem-

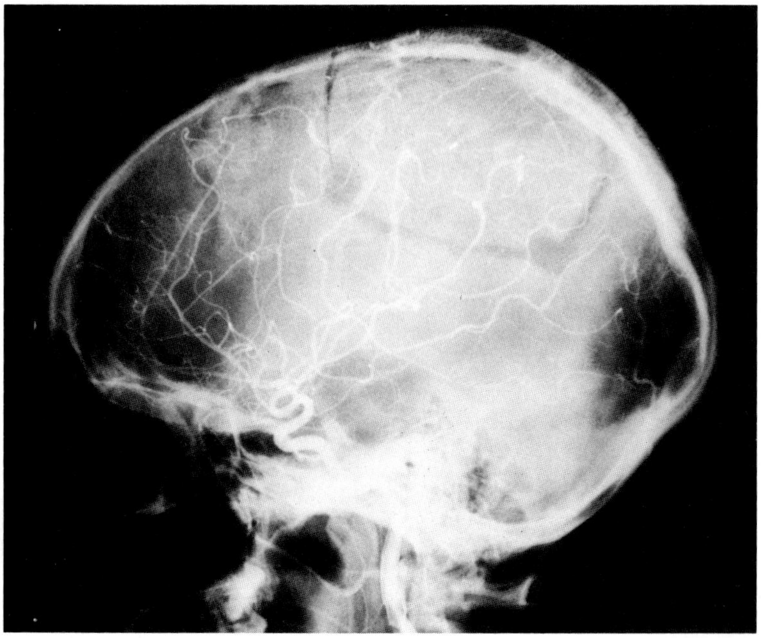

Figure 56-4. Same patient as in Figure 56-3. Postoperative arteriogram ensures complete excision of AVM.

Table 56-2
Results of Treatment—46 Children Treated for Cerebral AVM[12]

Grading	Nonoperative Treatment	Operative Treatment
I Neurologically intact	1	28
II Focal neurologic deficit without limitation of activity and/or epilepsy	1	8
III—Partial disability with focal deficit or mild retardation	1	7
IV Totally disabled	0	0

orrhage from the untreated malformation is a threat. The mortality for the *first* hemorrhage is 27 percent, more than double the 10 percent mortality reported in adults. Chronic epilepsy occurs about half as frequently in children as in adults prior to the diagnosis of the malformation, and responds quite favourably to the excision of the lesion.

As with intracranial aneurysms, AVMs in children can be scattered throughout the brain, often in awkward locations. By contrast with adult experience, there is an unusual preponderance (23 percent) below the tentorium. Wherever possible total excision of the malformation must be attempted, with the expectation that the child's brain vasculature may be more resilient to operative intrusion. The operative mortality is 8 percent, occurring primarily in subarachnoid Grade IV or V patients. Sixty-five percent of patients receiving operative care can be expected to be neurologically intact following surgery.

SPINAL ARTERIOVENOUS MALFORMATION

There has not been enough reported or personal experience with arteriovenous malformations of the spinal cord in children clearly to enunciate proper treatment plans and anticipated results. Scarff and Reigel,[20] however, have surveyed 64 cases reported in patients under 18 years of age, and their observations as well as those obtained in eight children treated at the Hospital for Sick Children (HSC) are examined in the following.

The arteriographic designation of the Type III "juvenile" vascular anomaly is appropriate when examining the experience with children.[17] While AVMs of the cord may be focal (usually at the thoracolumbar junction), they are often more extensive, and penetrate cord substance, so that significant components of the lesion are intramedullary and fed by many arteries that display a rapid flow of contrast. Flamboyant vascular abnormalities with intramedullary aneurysmal dilatations have been described, and were encountered in four children in the HSC series.[20]

Children's spinal AVMs tend to be as theatric in their presentation as those within the brain. Their most outstanding feature is pain, which is sudden in onset, radicular in distribution, intense, and frequently burning in quality. The pain syndrome is usually a manifestation of hemorrhage, which itself may be repetitive. The accompanying sensory dysesthesiae and progressive motor impairment in the hours after the hemorrhagic ictus incriminate involvement of nervous tissue.

Two other syndromes have been described.[20] One is characterized by a subacute or chronic course of progressive motor and sphincter impairment, and the other by episodic exacerabations and remissions of symptoms. The quality of the pain notwithstanding, there is not much that will distinguish the spinal AVM from the far more common problem of an intraspinal tumor. Myelography is frequently the first and only neurodiagnostic procedure performed. The presence of bloody or xanthochromic cerebrospinal fluid recovered during myelography may be the first suggestion that the intraspinal lesion is vascular, and the subsequent myelogram will outline the external vessels on the cord surface. Regrettably it does not show feeding arteries or abnormalities within the cord.[9]

Spinal arteriography is always recommended, and can be scheduled electively for those patients with a chronic history. Ideally every patient should be studied in this fashion, but the surgeon may have to decide whether a child with rapidly deteriorating function should be subjected to several more hours of detailed arteriographic study (probably under anesthesia) before operation commences. Myelography confirms the nature of the lesion but not its true extent, whereas arteriography provides the artistic details of the malformation, sometimes to the point of intimidation. Moreover, as Ommaya states, a patient with an appropriate clinical presentation, equivocal myelogram, and negative arteriogram must still be subjected to exploratory laminectomy for "absolute confirmation."[17]

As with cerebral AVMs, an ambitious operative approach to a child's spinal AVM is recommended, as the recovery may be far more gratifying than anticipated. Some lesions lie in part within the cauda equina and can be vigorously removed from there. Others are associated with dilated intramedullary vascular conglomerates, the excision of which confirms Doppman's thesis[3] that the majority of spinal cord arteriovenous malformations possess a "nidus" that is the crucial zone of arteriovenous transition, and that alone needs to be removed. Decompressive laminectomy by itself is of little benefit, and, for lesions with multiple arterial feeders, partial or subtotal obliteration of the malformation may be all that can be achieved. But the child's recovery from AVM microsurgery can be astonishing, even with interruption of the arterial supply.[20] An ambitious rehabilitation program is essential.

REFERENCES

1. Amacher AL, Allcock JM, Drake CG: Cerebral angiomas: The sequelae of surgical treatment. J Neurosurg 37:571–575, 1972
2. Botterell EH, Lougheed WM, Scott JW, et al: Hypothermia, and interruption of carotid, or carotid and vertebral circulation, in the surgical management of intracranial aneurysms. J Neurosurg 13:1–42, 1956
3. Doppman JL: The nidus concept of spinal cord arteriovenous malformations: A surgical recommendation based upon angiographic observations. Br J Radiol 44:758–763, 1971
4. Drake CG: Cerebral arteriovenous malformations: Considerations for an experience with surgical treatment in 166 cases. Clin Neurosurg 26:145–208, 1979
5. Forster DMC, Steiner L, Hakanson S: Arteriovenous malformation of the brain. A long-term clinical study. J Neurosurg 37:562–570, 1972
6. French L, Seljeskog EL: Arteriovenous malformations of the brain, in Youmans JR (ed): Neurological Surgery, vol 2. Philadelphia, WB Saunders, 1973, pp 827–836
7. Gold AP, Challenor YB, Gilles FH, et al: Report of the Joint Committee for Stroke Facilities. IX. Strokes in children (part 1). Stroke 4:835–858, 1973
8. Gold AP, Hammill JF, Carter S: Cerebrovascular disease, in Carter S, Gold AP (eds): Neurology of Infancy and Childhood. New York, Appleton-Century-Crofts, 1974, p 115
9. Harwood-Nash DC, Fitz CR: Neuroradiology in Infants and Children, vol 3. St. Louis, CV Mosby, 1976, pp 907, 913–929, 1164

10. Humphreys RP, Hendrick EB, Hoffman HJ: Review article: Cerebrovascular disease in children. Canad Med Assoc J 107:774–781, 1972
11. Humphreys RP: Computed tomography and the early diagnostic lumbar puncture. Canad Med Assoc J 121:150–151, 1979
12. Humphreys RP, Garrido E, Hendrick EB, et al: Cerebral arteriovenous malformations in childhood. Annual Meeting, American Association of Neurological Surgeons, New York, 1980
13. Luessenhop AJ: Operative treatment of arteriovenous malformation of the brain, in Morley TP (ed): Current Controversies in Neurosurgery. Philadelphia, WB Saunders, 1967, pp 203–209
14. Matson DD: Neurosurgery of Infancy and Childhood (ed 2). Springfield, Charles C Thomas, 1969, pp 749–766
15. Mori K, Murata T, Hashimoto N, et al: Clinical analysis of arteriovenous malformations in children. Child's Brain 6:13–25, 1980
16. Northfield DWC: The Surgery of the Central Nervous System. A Textbook for Postgraduate Students. Oxford, Blackwell, 1973, pp 402–420
17. Ommaya AK: Arteriovenous malformations of the spinal cord, in Youmans JR (ed): Neurological Surgery, vol 2. Philadelphia, WB Saunders, 1973, pp 852–862
18. Perrett G, Nishioka H: Report on the cooperative study of intracranial aneurysms and subarachnoid hemorrhage. Section VI Arteriovenous malformations. J Neurosurg 25:467–490, 1966
19. Russell DS, Rubinstein LJ: Pathology of Tumors of the Nervous System (ed 4). London, Edward Arnold P, 1977, pp 136–138
20. Scarff TB, Reigel DH: Arteriovenous malformations of the spinal cord in children. Child's Brain 5:341–351, 1979
21. Schatz SW, Botterell EH: The natural history of arteriovenous malformations, in Milliken C (ed): Cerebrovascular Disease, Proceedings of the Association for Research in Nervous and Mental Diseases, vol XLI, Baltimore, Williams & Wilkins, 1974, pp 180–187
22. Sedzimir CB, Robinsin J: Intracranial hemorrhage in children and adolescents. J Neurosurg 38:269–281, 1973
23. So S Cho: Cerebral arteriovenous malformations in children. Child's Brain 4:242–250, 1978
24. Svien HJ, McRae JA: Arteriovenous anomalies of the brain. Fate of patients not having definitive surgery. J Neurosurg 23:23–28, 1965
25. Troupp H, Marttila I, Halonen V: Arteriovenous malformations of the brain: Prognosis without operation. Acta Neurochir 22:125–128, 1970
26. Troupp H: Arteriovenous malformations of the brain: What are the indications for operation?, in Morley TP (ed): Current Controversies in Neurosurgery. Philadelphia, WB Saunders, 1967, pp 210–216
27. Trumpy JH, Eldevik P: Intracranial arteriovenous malformations: Conservative or surgical treatment. Surg Neurol 8:171–176, 1977
28. Waltimo O: The relationship of size, density and localization of intracranial arteriovenous malformations to the type of initial symptom. J Neurol Sci 19:13–19, 1973
29. Wilson CB, Sang UH, Dominque J: Microsurgical treatment of intracranial vascular malformations. J Neurosurg 51:446–454, 1979

57. Vein of Galen Malformations: Combined Neurosurgical and Neuroradiologic Intervention

Alex Berenstein

Fred Epstein

Over the past decades, surgical techniques have evolved to the point that it is within the expertise of contemporary neurosurgeons to extirpate most of the common cortical vascular malformations. Unfortunately vein of Galen malformations are anatomically adjacent to vital brain parenchyma, and in this specific condition, the surgeon must balance the morbidity and mortality of surgery against the natural history of this particular disease.[1,2]

It is the purpose of this chapter to illustrate some of the therapeutic options that interventional neuroradiology contributes to the management of vein of Galen malformations.

Rapidly evolving interventional neuroradiologic techniques utilizing flow-guided catheters and detachable balloons may be directed toward occlusion of the major arterial supply of a wide variety of vascular malformations.[3,4] Flexible flow-guided catheters that utilize balloons of different designs can reach small distal vessels for the deposition of fluid embolic agents of low viscosity such as isobutyl-2-cyanoacrylate (IBCA), a tissue adhesive that can be made radiopaque.[5,6] Detachable balloons,[7,8] which are flow-guided to distal and tortuous arteries, may be used to occlude arteriovenous fistulas, or to occlude a vessel, or trap a segment of a vessel. In addition flow-directed emboli can be utilized to reduce the flow to some lesions.

Depending on the vascular anatomy and the hemodynamic characteristics, embolization with flow-guided catheters or flow-directed emboli may be utilized in one of three ways: (1) preoperatively, with the intention of obstructing the less accessible feeding vessels, thereby making dissection less extensive, and reducing surgical morbidity; (2) Postoperatively, as following surgical ligation of major feeding vessels the blood flow through the remaining arteries to the malformation is increased, thereby rendering them more accessible to distal catheterization for embolic obliteration; and (3) as the only therapeutic endeavor. In this situation the optimal goal is obliteration of all of the feeding arteries. Falling short of this, it may serve as a palliative procedure, stabilizing the cardiovascular status pending future definitive therapy.

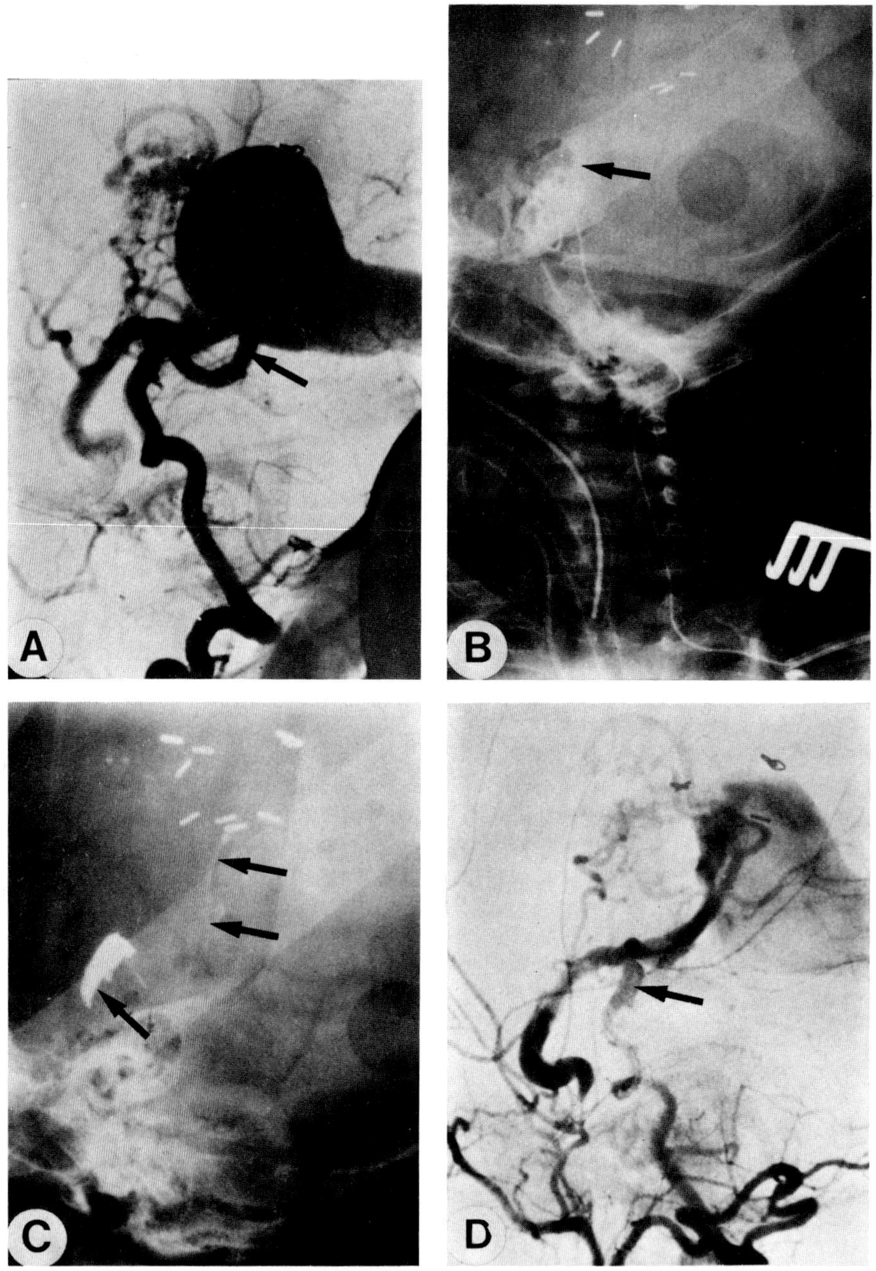

Figure 57-1. A. Lateral subtraction angiogram of the selective left vertebral injection in a 3-month-old infant following surgical ligation of feeding vessels entering the lesion from above. Note the multiple surgical clips and reflux into the carotid circulation. There is a prominent choroidal artery (arrow) that represents a direct arteriovenous fistula. B. Superselective microballoon catheterization of the abnormal choroidal artery. The arrow points to the tip of the microcatheter. C. Radiopaque cast of IBCA (arrows). D. Control postembolization angiogram. The arrow points to the subtracted IBCA case. Note that there is no filling of the choroidal artery to the vein of Galen fistula. The angiogmatous complex from the carotid (MCA) circulation is still seen (compare with A). (Reprinted with permission from Berenstein A, Kricheff II; Catheter and material selection for transarterial embolization: Technical considerations: II. Materials. Radiology 132:631–641, 1979.)

CASE 1

A 3-month-old infant was admitted with progressive macrocephaly, cardiac failure, and a cranial bruit. Angiography disclosed a vein of Galen malformation with multiple feeding arteries from anterior, middle, and posterior cerebral arteries. At craniotomy multiple vessels entering the superior and more superficial part of the aneurysm were clipped. One week postoperatively subselective catheterization of the posterior choroidal artery that represented a direct arteriovenous fistula was occluded with 0.2 cc of radiopaque IBCA (Fig. 57-1). The bruit decreased significantly, and the cardiac failure remitted. A second-stage craniotomy was performed one month later, and the lesion was completely obliterated (Fig. 57-2).

CASE 2

A 14-month-old child was admitted with a cranial bruit and borderline compensated cardiac failure. The diagnosis of vein of Galen malformation had been made previously, and a shunting procedure performed to relieve the hydrocephalus. A repeat arteriogram discosed multiple arterial feeders from both the anterior and posterior circulations. It was believed that obliterating the anterior cerebral artery component would increase the "sump" effect of the posterior supply and thereby render subsequent embolization more effective. At craniotomy the anterior cerebral arteries, both of which entered the lesion, were clipped superficial to the corpus callosum. One week postoperatively, utilizing a nontapered catheter, silicone balls were flow-directed via the vertebral artery to the feeding posterior cerebral branches, which were obliterated (Fig. 57-3).

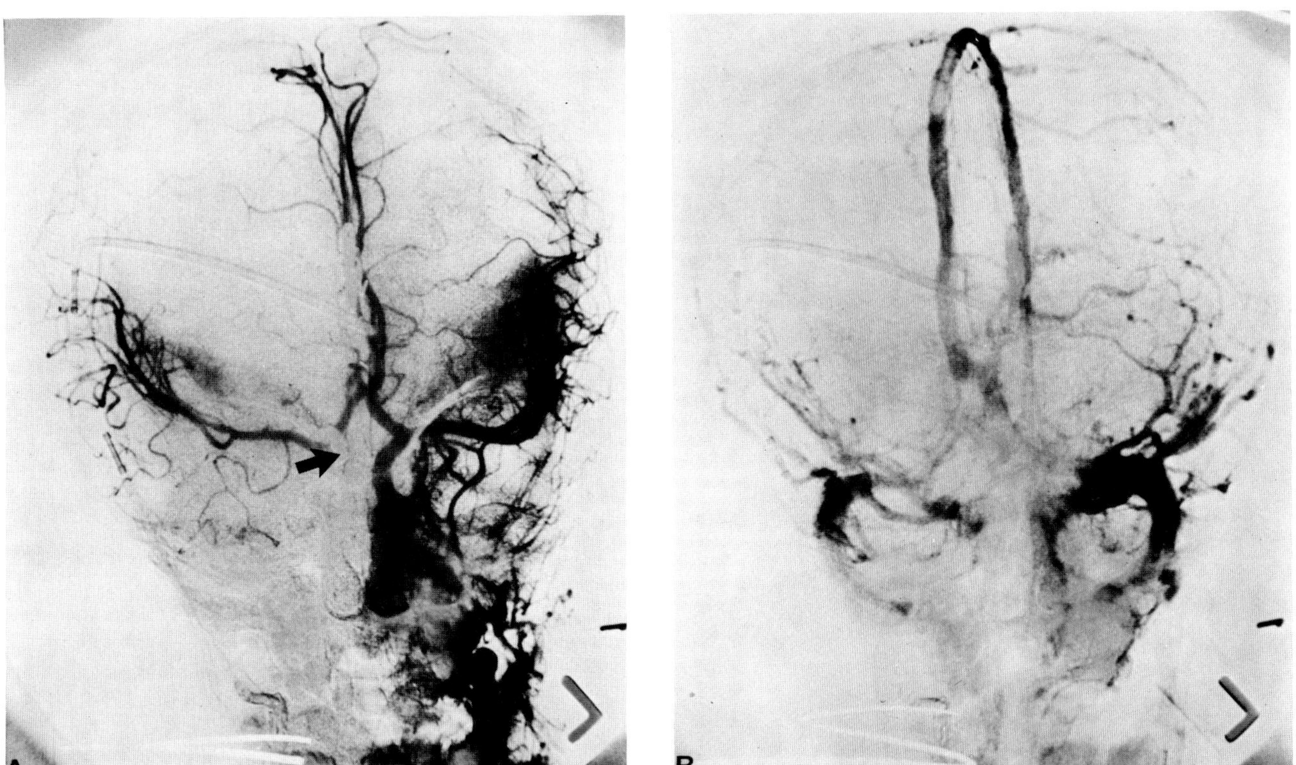

Figure 57-2. Control angiogram after the second craniotomy. There is no remaining lesion. A. Frontal angiograms in the midarterial phase. The arrow points to the subtracted IBCA cast of the abnormal choroidal artery. B. Frontal subtraction angiogram in the venous phase. No filling of the deep venous system, including the vein of Galen.

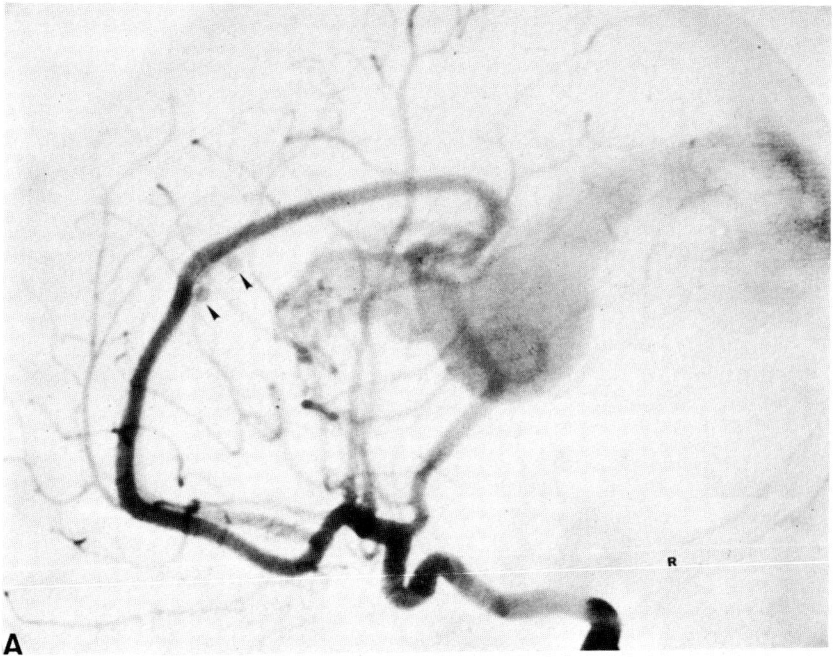

A

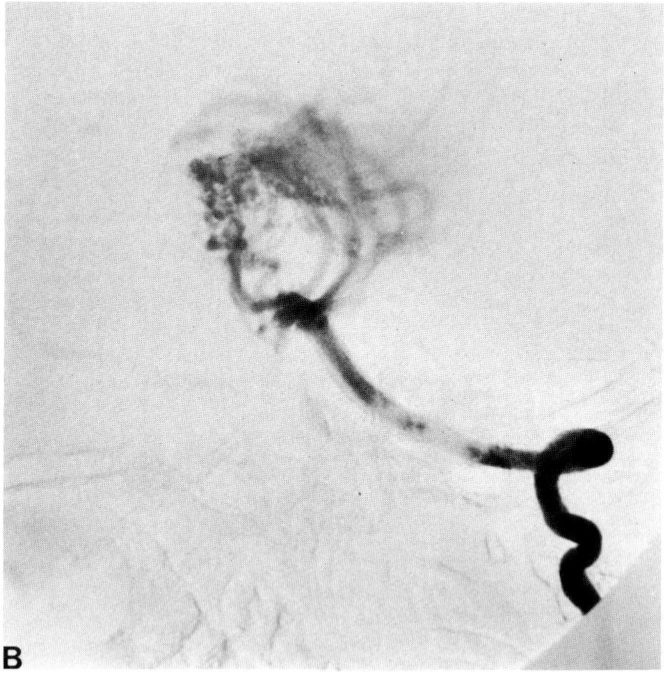

B

Figure 57-3. A. Lateral subtraction angiogram of the right internal carotid artery. The right pericallosal artery is hypertrophied and supplies the malformation. There is filling of the left (contralateral) pericallosal artery (arrowheads) that also supplies the lesion. A prominent choroidal artery is also involved. B. Lateral subtraction angiograms of the selective left vertebral artery early arterial phase shows an angiomatous complex draining into the vein of Galen. Note the poor filling of the normal posterior fossa vessels. C. Lateral subtraction angiogram following surgical clipping of both pericallosal arteries as they reach the vein of Galen. No change in the angiomatous complex filling from the vertebral system. D. Plain film of the skull in the lateral view following silicone sphere embolization via the vertebral basilar system. E. Lateral subtraction angiogram in late arterial phase following embolization. Note the decrease in the angiomatous complex, and the significantly better filling of the normal posterior fossa vessels. (Compare with B and C.)

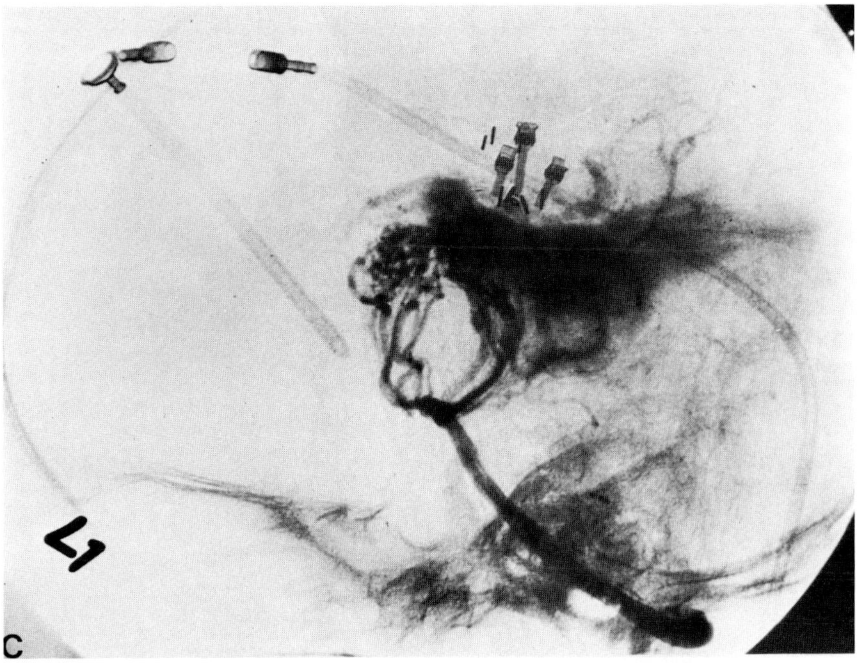

C

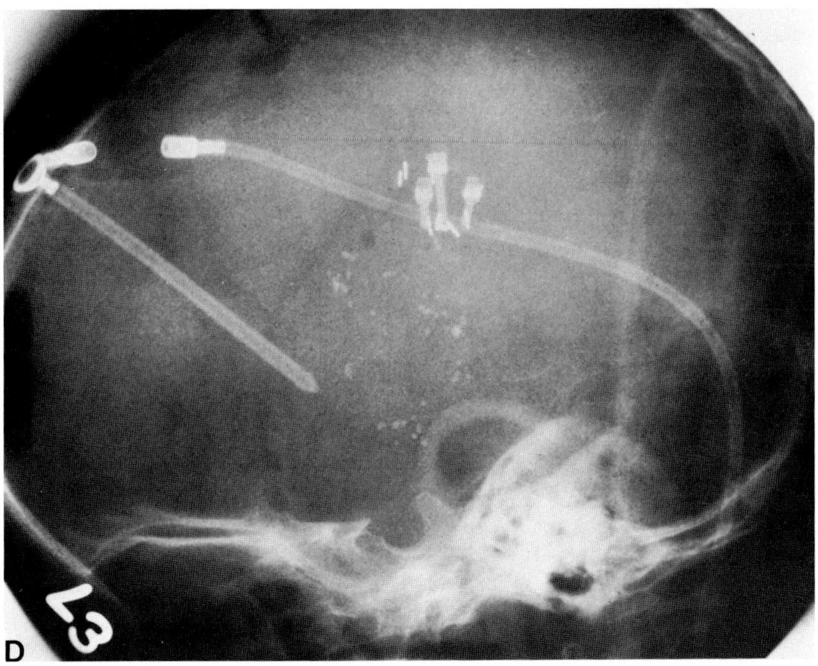

D

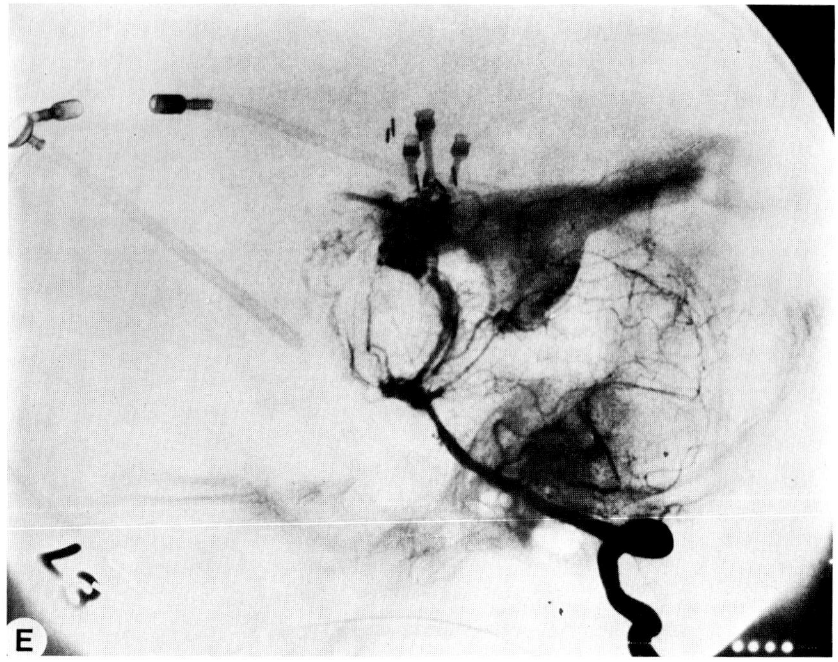

CASE 3

A 6-month-old female was admitted with macrocephaly and papilledema. Angiography disclosed an arteriovenous malformation supplied by hypertrophied posterior choroidal arteries that were opacified from the carotid and vertebral injections, and supplied a small vessel angiomatous network that entered the vein of Galen on its right inferior lateral aspect (Fig. 57-4). The lesion was occluded in two separate embolization procedures using flow-guided microballoon catheterization and IBCA deposition (Fig. 57-5).

Embolization of vascular anomalies has become an established therapeutic modality as newer techniques of transvascular occlusion have evolved. When utilized as a preoperative surgical adjunct, embolization is directed toward relatively less accessible feeding arteries. This may be done with silicone spheres alone, or detachable balloons. In addition, to facilitate surgery, the partial obstruction of the arterial supply may prevent a postoperative hyperemic edema syndrome by more gradual staged vascular occlusions.[9,10]

Perhaps application of embolization techniques of vein of Galen malformations will radically alter the significant morbidity and mortality that are attendant with surgery alone. It is clear that the best long-term results are in that select group that present in later infancy with macrocephaly and a bruit, but stable cardiovascular status.[1] Conversely the poorest results are in that large group of neonates that present with intractable heart failure. This is almost certainly more related to the unstable cardiovascular status than the brain surgery per se. It would seem reasonable, therefore, that converting the former group to the latter may reduce subsequent surgical morbidity and mortality. Embolization of some major feeding arteries accomplishes this goal by greatly reducing the arteriovenous shunt, thereby facilitating medical management and contributing to the relative safety of delayed elective rather than emergent intracranial surgery.

Although there is a large body of literature describing the various surgical techniques that may be utilized to obliterate vein of Galen aneurysms,[1,2] it is

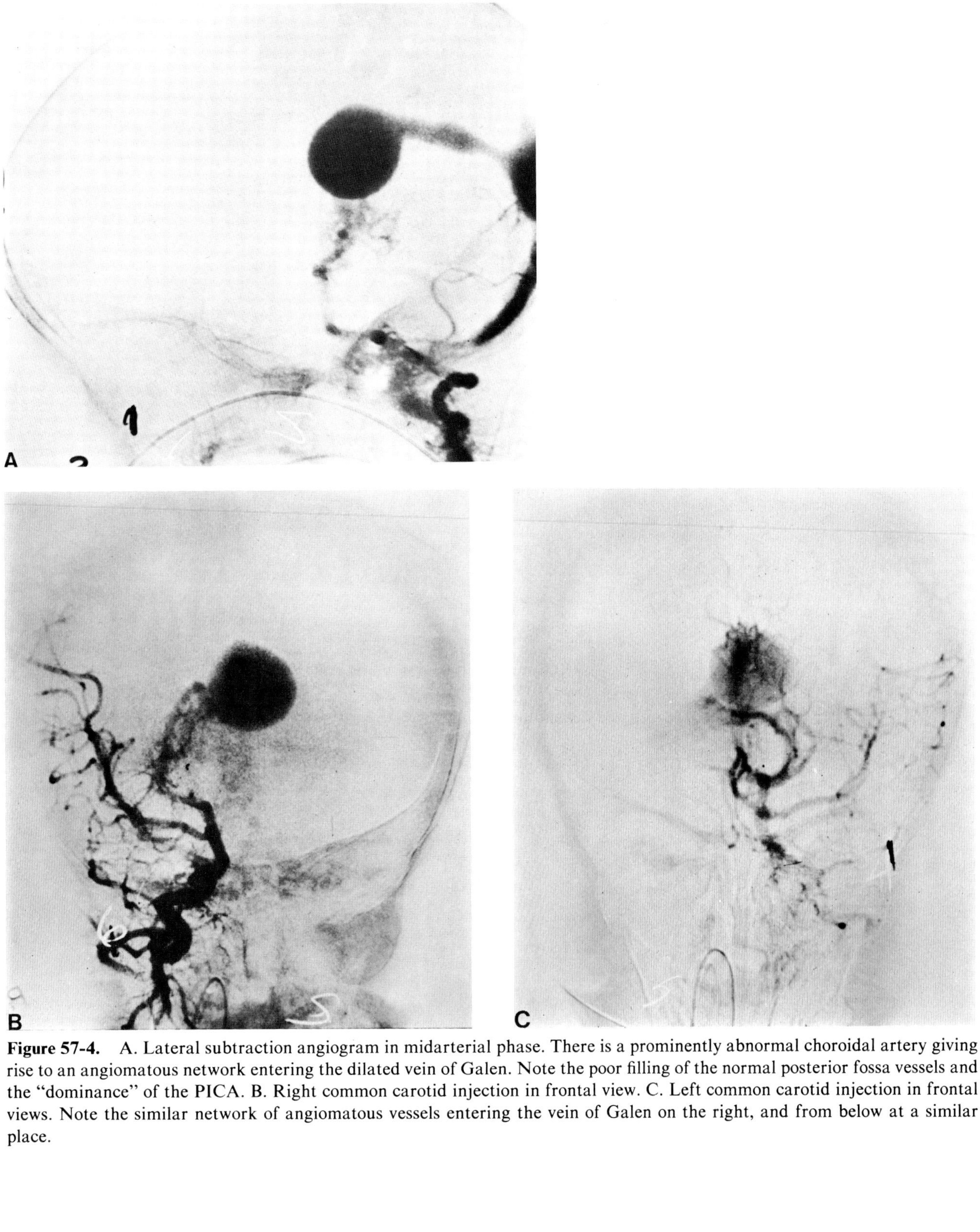

Figure 57-4. A. Lateral subtraction angiogram in midarterial phase. There is a prominently abnormal choroidal artery giving rise to an angiomatous network entering the dilated vein of Galen. Note the poor filling of the normal posterior fossa vessels and the "dominance" of the PICA. B. Right common carotid injection in frontal view. C. Left common carotid injection in frontal views. Note the similar network of angiomatous vessels entering the vein of Galen on the right, and from below at a similar place.

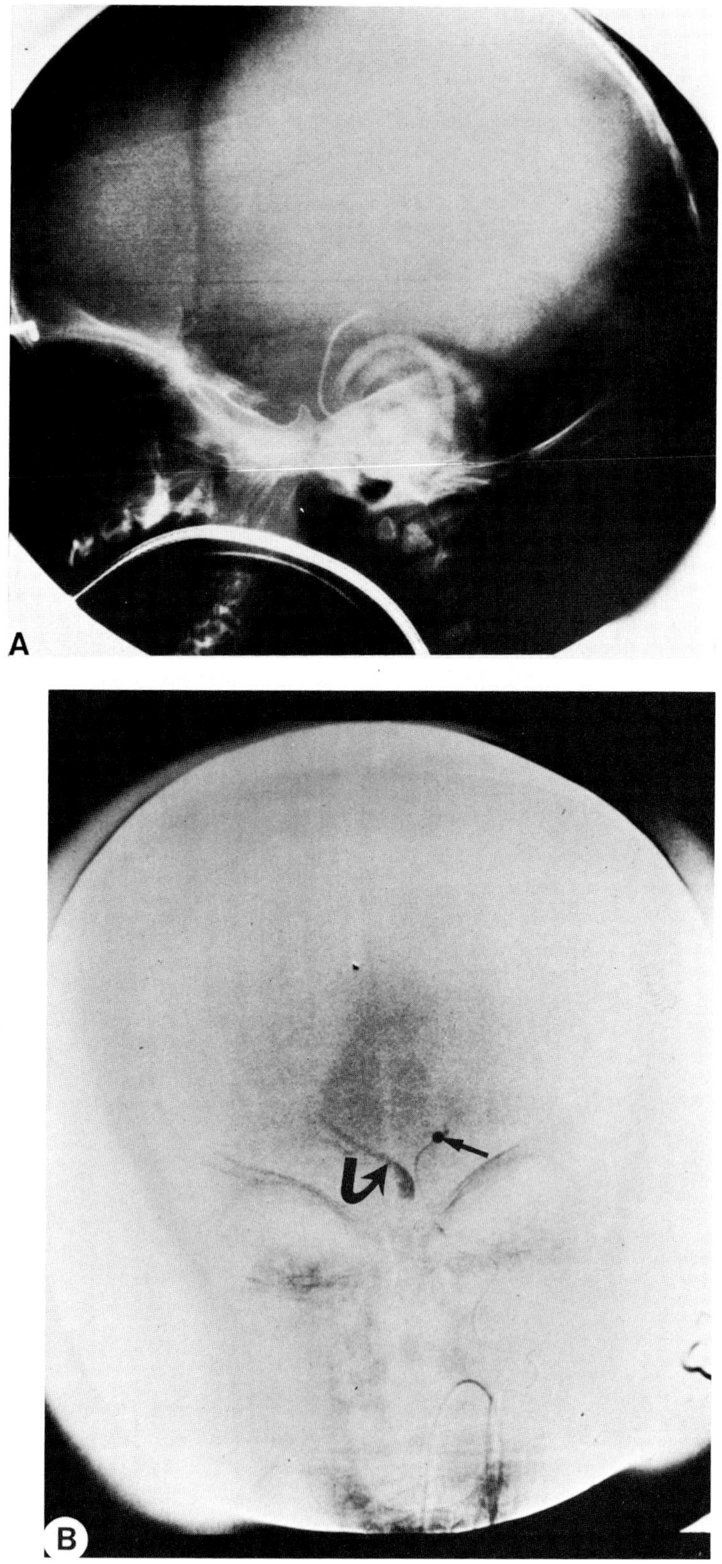

Figure 57-5. A. Lateral plain film shows the microcatheter position. The microcatheter was introduced following cutdown of the femoral artery via the vertebral basilar system. The balloon is not inflated. B. Frontal subtraction view during catheterization of the left feeding vessel via the left internal carotid artery. The arrow points to the balloon; the curved arrow points to the partially subtracted cast from the first embolization. C, D. Frontal and lateral plain film shows the IBCA cast following both embolizations. E. Lateral subtraction angiogram in midarterial phase of the vertebral injection immediately following the second embolization. Note the filling of the posterior fossa vessels via the "dominant" PICA that reconstitutes the AICA and superior cerebellar territories. F. Venous phase, lateral view. Note filling of the vein of Galen at the same time as the normal venous filling of the posterior fossa.

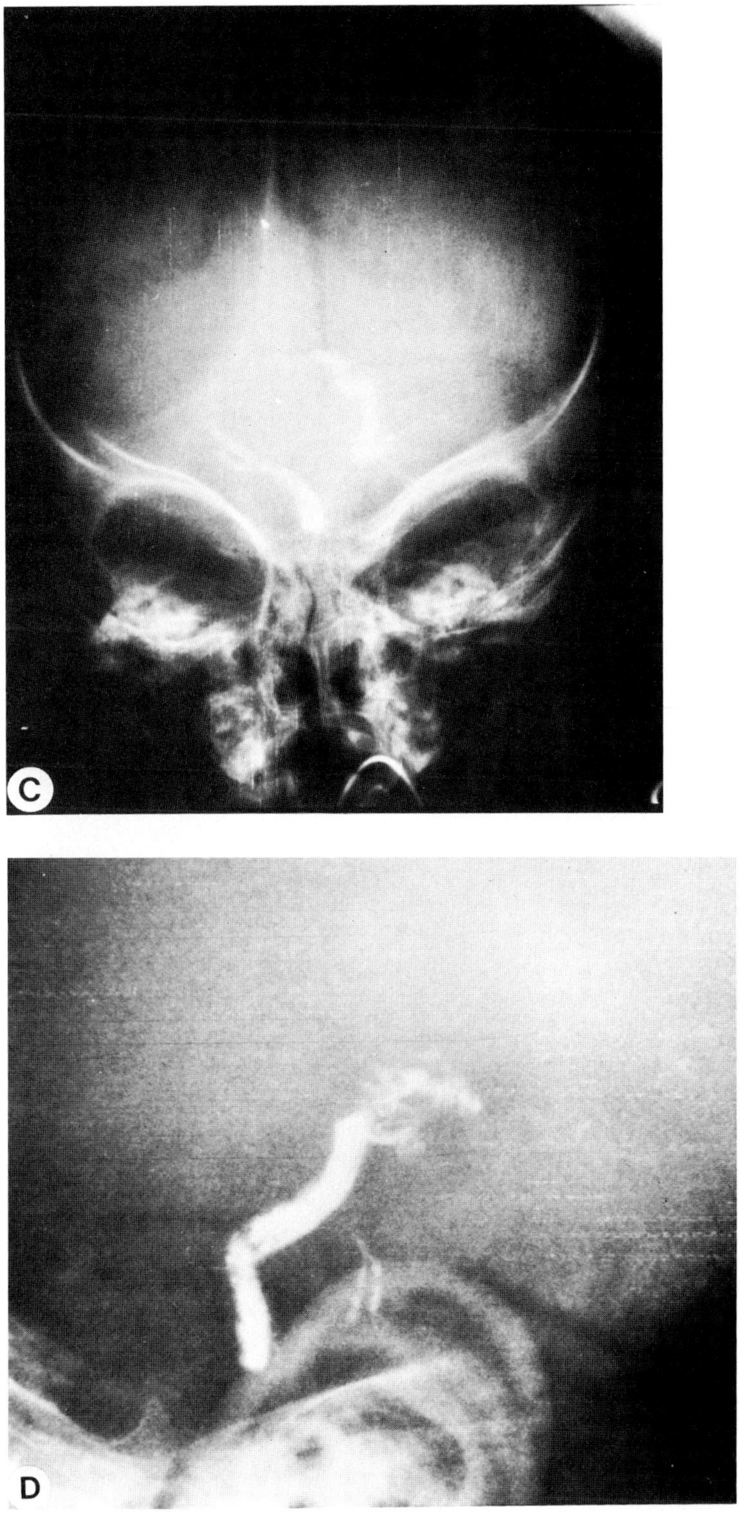
C
D

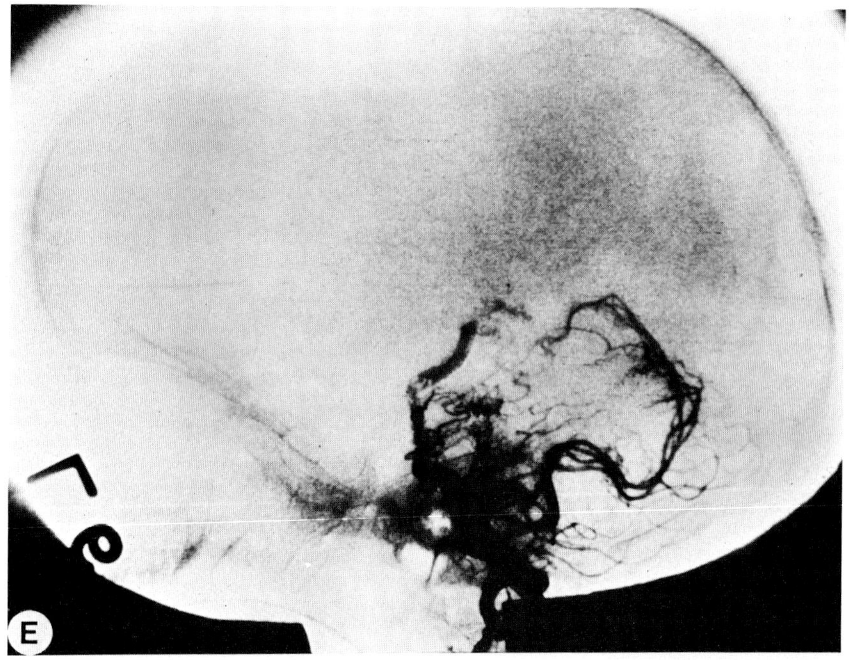

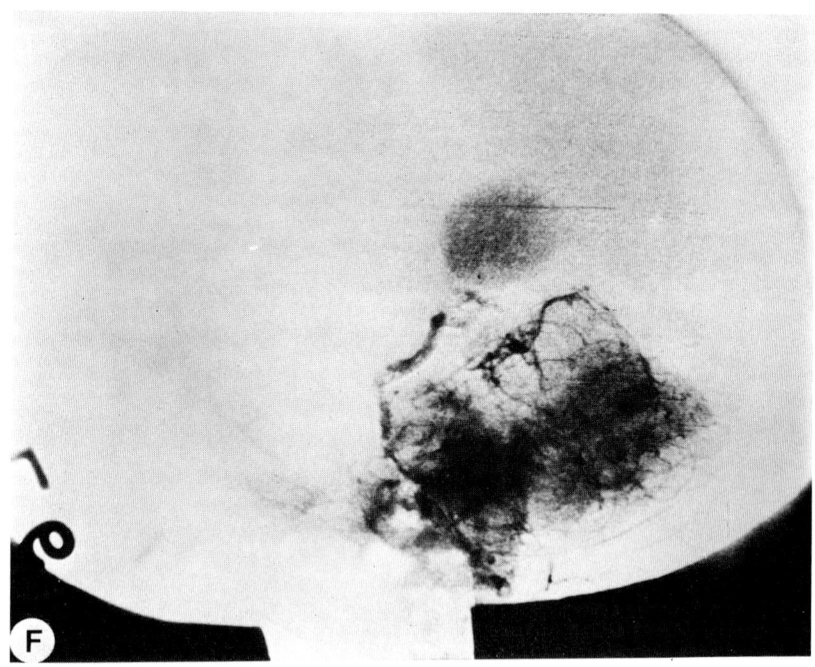

obvious that retraction and dissection of relatively ischemic brain contribute to the surgical hazard. Since many of these anomalies receive an arterial supply from the anterior cerebral arteries, it is technically simple to clip these vessels superficial to the corpus callosum, increasing the "sump" of the deeper posterior cerebral feeders, and thus making it possible for subsequent embolization to obliterate the remaining vascular supply.

On the basis of this very abbreviated experience, it would seem that embolization may be utilized in the neonate to permit surgery to be delayed, and in the infant, to make it less extensive. With improvement in catheter techniques, it is not beyond possibility that in the foreseeable future it may be feasible totally to obliterate the malformation and completely obviate surgery.

REFERENCES

1. Berenstein A, Kricheff II: Catheter and material selection for transarterial embolization. Technical considerations, I. Catheters. Radiology 132:619–631, 1979
2. Berenstein A, Kricheff II: Catheter and material selection for transarterial embolization: Technical considerations: II. Materials. Radiology 132:631–641, 1979
3. Kerber CW, Bank WO, Cronwell LD: Calibrated leak balloon microcatheter: A device for arterial exploration and occlusive therapy. AJR 132:207–212, 1979
4. Berenstein A: Technique for catheterization and embolization of the lenticulostriate arteries. J Neurosurg 54, 1981
5. Serbinenko FA: Balloon catheterization and occlusion of major cerebral arteries. J Neurosurg 41:125–145, 1974
6. Debrun G, Lacour P, Caron JP, et al: Inflatable and released balloon technique. Experimentation in dog—Application in men. Neuroradiology 9:267–271, 1975
7. Stein B, Wolpert S: Arteriovenous malformations of the brain. I: Current concepts and treatment. Arch Neurol 37:1–5, 1980
8. Stein B, Wolpert S: Arteriovenous malformations of the brain, II: Current concepts and treatment. Arch Neurol 37:69–75, 1980
9. Spitzler RF, Wilson CB, Weinstein P, et al: Normal perfusion pressure breakthrough therapy. Clin Neurosurg 25:651–672, 1978
10. Mullan S, Brown FD, Patronas NJ: Hyperemic and ischemic problems of surgical treatment of arteriovenous malformations. J Neurosurg 51:757–764, 1979

58. Hemophilia and Other Coagulopathies

Robin P. Humphreys

HEMOPHILIA

Hemophilia may have changed the course of Russian history, or as Kerensky once said, "If there had been no Rasputin, there would have been no Lenin."[15] Alexis, the son of Russian Czar Nicholas II and Alexandra, suffered from hemophilia. Alexandra sought the aid of a debauched "holy man" Rasputin, whom she regarded as a saint sent by God to save the throne and "holy Russia." Acting upon his advice, Alexandra altered the government administration, which became paralyzed. After the October Revolution, she, Nicholas, and their children were imprisoned by the Bolsheviks and later shot. Alexis therefore fell victim to political inopportunism and not his hemophilia.

As hemophilia may have influenced history, so the passage of time has witnessed considerable change in hemophilia diagnosis and treatment. The first report of intracranial hemorrhage in a probable hemophiliac was made in 1819 and it was not unusual through the first half of the 20th century to read of the numerous diagnostic and therapeutic frustrations with the neurologic consequences of hemophilia.[30] By the mid-1950s treatment programs improved when detailed knowledge of the particular deficiencies in the hemophiliac states became available. Subsequently replacement fractionated products were developed for quick and precise reestablishment of procoagulant activity.

Physiology

Factors VIII and IX are part of the intrinsic prothrombin activation system. Factor IX (having been activated by Factor XI), then reacts with Factor VIII, the resulting product bringing about activation of Factor X, which in a subsequent chain of activating events brings about the generation of thrombin.

Hemophilia (Factor VIII deficiency) and Christmas disease (Factor IX deficiency) are transmitted as sex-linked recessive characteristics. Hemophilia is found in its severe form in one per 25,000 population, but if the milder forms are

the treatment of intracranial hematoma in children and adults.[3,5–7,13,18–20,23,25,26–28] Our own experience reflects these advances (Table 58-1).

It is entirely feasible for a surgeon, therefore, to evacuate a life-threatening intracranial hematoma, or even operate electively on any other intracranial process in a hemophiliac, when this action is in concert with that of the hematologist.[17] Despite the advances of the past 20 years, however, many hemophiliacs who have suffered intracranial bleeding are left with severe neurologic residua—hemiparesis, visual and speech defects, epilepsy, retardation, and hydrocephalus.

Intraspinal Hemorrhage

As expected intraspinal hemorrhage is uncommon in hemophiliacs. Trauma precipitates bleeding in about one third of the cases and three quarters of patients have extramedullary bleeding. The treatment principles are those basic to the hematologic care of the hemophiliac and the neurosurgical care of the patient with an intraspinal mass.

Peripheral Nerve Lesions

Virtually all peripheral nerve lesions in hemophilia are due to external compression or traction on the nerve, particularly related to hemorrhage within closed tissue spaces such as the forearm or anterior compartment of the leg. Characteristically the femoral, ulnar, median, sciatic, or a cutaneous nerve of thigh is involved.[8] The syndrome is one of acute and often painful radiculopathy, perhaps associated with visible swelling and ecchymosis. The detection of the peripheral nerve lesion, however, may be masked by the muscle atrophy, areflexia, and contractures related to recurrent hemarthrosis and intramuscular bleeding. After appropriate replacement therapy has been given, the surgeon may consider evacuation of the hematoma or fasciotomy. Rehabilitation is difficult and prolonged.

DISSEMINATED INTRAVASCULAR COAGULATION

Disseminated intravascular coagulation (DIC) is a complication of a number of disease processes, of which head trauma may be one. The basic process is a stimulation of physiologic coagulation, which as it progresses brings about widespread intravascular blood coagulation. Eventually the coagulation factors are depleted, and with coincident activation of the fibrinolytic enzyme system that clears the fibrin and fibrinogen, a hypocoagulable state results.[14]

A variety of triggering mechanisms have been proposed, but it appears that a "thromboplastin-like" substance is released to initiate the coagulation. As brain has a high concentration of tissue thromboplastin, its release following cerebral trauma would not be unexpected. Disseminated intravascular coagulation has been documented after massive brain injury, but also in patients without significant damage of cerebral tissue.[12,29] Moreover patients with multisystem injuries may also suffer hypotension, anoxia, and acidosis, all of which are stimulants of DIC.[29] While the problem is not common in childhood brain injuries, it may occur more often than expected and escape detection unless coagulation studies have been performed.[12]

Finally, DIC with generalized bleeding is confirmed by laboratory findings of thrombocytopenia, low fibrinogen value and prolongation of the prothrombin time, and partial thromboplastin time. Treatment is directed against the triggering factor(s), with administration of heparin and replacement of the consumed blood clotting components.[29]

IDIOPATHIC THROMBOCYTOPENIC PURPURA

Idiopathic thrombocytopenic purpura (ITP) is a common disorder in children, frequently preceded by infection. The diagnosis is established by a platelet count of less than 100,000 per cubic millimeter, abundant megakaryocytes in the bone marrow, absence of associated hematologic changes other than those due to hemorrhage or infection, and absence of associated systemic illness except for infection. About 80 percent of patients with acute ITP of childhood recover spontaneously in the first few weeks of illness without any therapy. Aside from easy bruising and a petechial rash, most children are completely asymptomatic during that interval and restricted physical activity is the sole form of management.

Intracranial hemorrhage is the most serious complication of ITP, occurring in about 1 percent of children with the disorder. In 1976 the experience at the Hospital for Sick Children, Toronto, with spontaneous intracranial bleeding, which occurred in four children with this disorder, was reviewed.[10] As a result, a management program was developed. First the diagnosis of ITP, if not previously established, must be confirmed by bone marrow aspiration. Simultaneously, traditional methods to reduce cerebral edema using intravenous dexamethasone and mannitol (20 percent solution) should be started. In addition to its beneficial effect on cerebral edema (which in two of the children reported was severe), dexamethasone was administered during surgery and for a variable time thereafter to facilitate the platelet response. While steroids do not appear to shorten the course of ITP, their use may lessen bleeding by a direct vascular action or by improving platelet survival by blocking phagocytosis in the reticuloendothelial system. Lumbar puncture is contraindicated.

The subsequent surgical and investigative management, if necessary, can be conducted under a single anesthetic. Emergency splenectomy should be carried out and followed by infusion of platelet concentrates, which then seem to have more hemostatic effect. In our experience splenectomy for children with acute ITP is reserved for uncontrolled bleeding, since platelet transfusions alone seldom result in an increment in circulating platelet counts or ameliorate hemorrhage. Platelet survival generally increases following splenectomy, however, thereby permitting transfused platelets to effect hemostasis at that time.

In the original report,[10] it was proposed that cerebral arteriography be performed after splenectomy. With the availability of rapid scanning CT units, it is entirely feasible that such a scan can be obtained prior to splenectomy, and then, once the nature of the intracerebral clot is known, the patient's craniotomy can be performed under the same anesthetic in one operating room, after closure of the abdominal wound.

LEUKEMIC HEMORRHAGE

One of the penalties of successful chemotherapeutic treatment of acute childhood leukemia has been a marked rise in the neurologic manifestations of this disease. As the drug treatment of leukemia became more effective between 1948 and 1960, the incidence of central nervous system (CNS) manifestations increased from 4 to 40 percent, and it is now stated that over one half of children with acute leukemia can be expected to have neurologic involvement.[4,22] The type of CNS lesion may be quite variable, but the neurosurgeon's advice is most likely to be sought at the time of an acute and major neurologic event related to intracranial hemorrhage.

The latter has traditionally been the explanation for a leukemic patient's sudden demise. In 1960 intracranial hemorrhage was found to be responsible for 49 percent of deaths in an autopsy series of acute leukemia patients.[9] Hemorrhage may result from either the associated severe thrombocytopenia, or infiltration of white matter of the brain with leukemic cells. The latter plug small cerebral arteries and subsequently spread through the vessel walls, which become weakened and eventually rupture into cerebral parenchyma.

A leukemic patient who suddenly develops the clinical phenomena of a hemorrhagic stroke has usually suffered spontaneous intracranial bleeding. The CT examination will quickly certify the presence, site, and extent of the suspect intracranial bleeding in leukemic patients. The neurosurgeon can now accurately elucidate a prognosis for the disrupted cerebrum, and the hematologist can employ this information in an overview of the patient's primary illness and likely survival from it.

SUMMARY

The formulation of potent chemotherapeutic compounds and the purification of individual elements involved in the clotting process have presented fresh challenges to the surgeon handling the neurologic consequences of the primary hematologic upset. The hematologist must still act first, but by virtue of sophisticated diagnostic CT and pharmacotherapy, the surgeon will increasingly be expected to participate in a planned management program.

REFERENCES

1. Biggs R: Human Blood Coagulation, Haemostatis and Thrombosis (ed 2). Oxford Blackwell, 1976
2. Curless RG, Corrigan JJ Jr: Headache in classical hemophilia. The risk of diagnostic procedures. Child's Brain 2:187–194, 1976
3. Davies SH, Turner JW, Cumming RA, et al: Management of intracranial haemorrhage in haemophilia. Br Med J 2:1627–1630, 1966
4. Evans AE: Central nervous system involvement in children with acute leukemia. A study of 921 patients. Cancer 17:256–258, 1964
5. Ferguson GG, Barton WB, Drake CG: Subdural hematoma in hemophilia: Successful treatment with cryoprecipitate. J Neurosurg 29:524–528, 1968
6. Fessey BM, Meynell MJ: Haemorrhage involving the central nervous system in haemophilia: Account of the management of five cases. Br Med J 2:211–212, 1966
7. Guerth JH, Teng P, Goldenberg E: Surgery in a hemophiliac child with intracranial hemorrhage. Pediatrics 28:800–804, 1961
8. Gilchrist GS, Piepgras DG: Neurologic complications in hemophilia, in Hilgartner MW (ed): Progress in Pediatric Hematology/Oncology, Vol. I. Hemophilia in Children. Littleton, Mass., Publishing Sciences Group Inc., 1976
9. Groch SN, Sayre GP, Heck FJ: Cerebral hemorrhage in leukemia. Arch Neurol Psychiatr 2:439–451, 1960
10. Humphreys RP, Hockley AD, Freedman MH, et al: Management of intracerebral hemorrhage in idiopathic thrombocytopenic purpura. Report of four cases. J Neurosurg 45:700–704, 1976
11. Humphreys RP: Computed tomography and the early diagnostic lumbar puncture. Canad Med Assoc J 121:150–151, 1979
12. Jaap van der Sande J, Veltkamp JJ, Boekhout-Mussert RJ, Bouwhuis-Hoogerwerf ML: Head injury and coagulation disorders. J Neurosurg 49:357–365, 1978
13. Jones RK, Knighton RS: Surgery in hemophiliacs with special reference to the central nervous system. Ann Surg 144:1029–1034, 1956
14. Keith RG, Mahoney LJ, Garvey MB: Disseminated intravascular coagulation: An

important feature of the fat embolism syndrome. Canad Med Assoc J 105:74–76, 1971

15. Kerensky, Alexander: Russia and History's Turning Point. New York, Duell, Sloan & Pearce, 1965
16. Kerr CB: Intracranial haemorrhage in haemophilia. J Neurol Neurosurg Psychiatr 27:166–173, 1964
17. MacGee EE: Surgical treatment of arteriovenous anomaly in a hemophiliac patient. J Neurosurg 30:289–292, 1969
18. Moody RA, Mullen S: Factor VIII in hemophilia. Case report. J Neurosurg 29:520–523, 1968
19. Myles ST, Harris CEC, Hansebout RR: Epidural hematoma in hemophilia: Successful treatment. Canad Med Assoc J 104:51–52, 1971
20. Olsen ER: Intracranial surgery in hemophiliacs: Report of a case and review of the literature. Arch Neurol 21:401–412, 1969
21. Pailles JE, Boudouresques J, Tamalet J: Les hematomes intracraniens des hemophiles. Semaine Hop Paris 24:432, 1948
22. Pochedly C: Management of CNS leukemia in childhood: Outline of current concepts. Clin Pediatr 11:503–508, 1972
23. Potter JM: Head injury and haemophilia. Acta Neurochirurg 13:380–387, 1965
24. Raggio JR, Fleischer AS, Corley CC: Posterior fossa subdural hematoma in a hemophiliac. Neurosurgery 3:213–215, 1978
25. Seeler RA, Imana RB: Intracranial hemorrhage in patients with hemophilia. J Neurosurg 39:181–185, 1973
26. Silverstein A: Intracranial bleeding in hemophilia. Arch Neurol 3:141–157, 1960
27. Singer RP, Schneider RC: The successful management of intracerebral and subarachnoid hemorrhage in a hemophilic infant. A case report. Neurology 12:293–294, 1962
28. Travis RL, Mitchell OC, Youmans JR, et al: Intracranial surgery in hemophilia: Use of potent antihemophilic factor concentrate. Am Surg 34:602–604, 1968
29. Watts C: Disseminated intravascular coagulation. Surg Neurol 8:258–262, 1977
30. Wilson: Lectures to Royal College of Surgeons, 1819. Cited by Silverstein A

VII MISCELLANEOUS DISEASES

59. Epilepsy

Harold J. Hoffman

Epilepsy is a disorder consisting of episodic attacks, cerebral in origin and characterized by a disturbance in motor activity, sensation, emotion, or consciousness. Regarded in ancient times as a cursed affliction, epilepsy has resisted the sophistication of modern investigative tools and management techniques, and its basic physiologic mechanisms continue to remain a mystery.

ETIOLOGY OF CHILDHOOD EPILEPSY

Head Injury

Posttraumatic epilepsy is a common cause of seizures at all ages. Birth trauma accounts for some 25 percent of neonatal seizures.[1]

Beyond the neonatal period, seizures continue to be a common result of head injury. Seizures occurring within the first 24 hours after a closed head injury are usually related to the severity of the head injury and carry no prognostic significance in relation to development of posttraumatic epilepsy. In cases in which epilepsy occurs one day to one month after a head injury, however, there is a greater than 25 percent risk that posttraumatic epilepsy will develop. Late epilepsy can occur in as many as a third of all head injuries and is due to cicatrix formation in damaged brain. A family history of seizures and proximity of the damage to the Rolandic fissure will increase the likelihood of late epilepsy.

In cases of depressed skull fracture, if the dura is intact, the period of posttraumatic amnesia (PTA) is less than 24 hours, and there are no focal signs, the risk of epilepsy is less than 4 percent. By contrast if the dura and brain are torn, and there are focal signs and a prolonged PTA, the risk can be as high as 63 percent.[2]

Cerebral Neoplasm

Seizures resulting from a supratentorial brain tumor can be generalized, psychomotor, or focal motor and/or sensory in type. Seizures may be the initial symptom of a cerebral hemisphere neoplasm, sometimes persisting for years before development of any other signs. Computerized tomographic (CT) scan provides a benign method of investigating these "seizure" patients and finding those harboring intracranial tumors. In a series of supratentorial tumors at the Hospital for Sick Children, 63 out of 344 (18 percent) presented with seizures.[3]

Vascular Disease

With the advent of CT scanning, we are seeing small arteriovenous malformations (AVMs) which, through a small hemorrhage, have evoked a seizure disorder. Because of their small size and slow arterial flow, conventional cerebral angiography may fail to show evidence of a vascular malformation (Fig. 59-1).

Occlusive vessel disease of the moya-moya type can also present with a seizure-like disorder.

Febrile Seizures

Febrile seizures occur in 2 to 4 percent of children under 5 years of age. The recurrence rate of febrile seizures approaches an average of 33 percent. The child with febrile seizures has a sixfold increased risk of subsequently developing afebrile seizures as compared with the general population.[4]

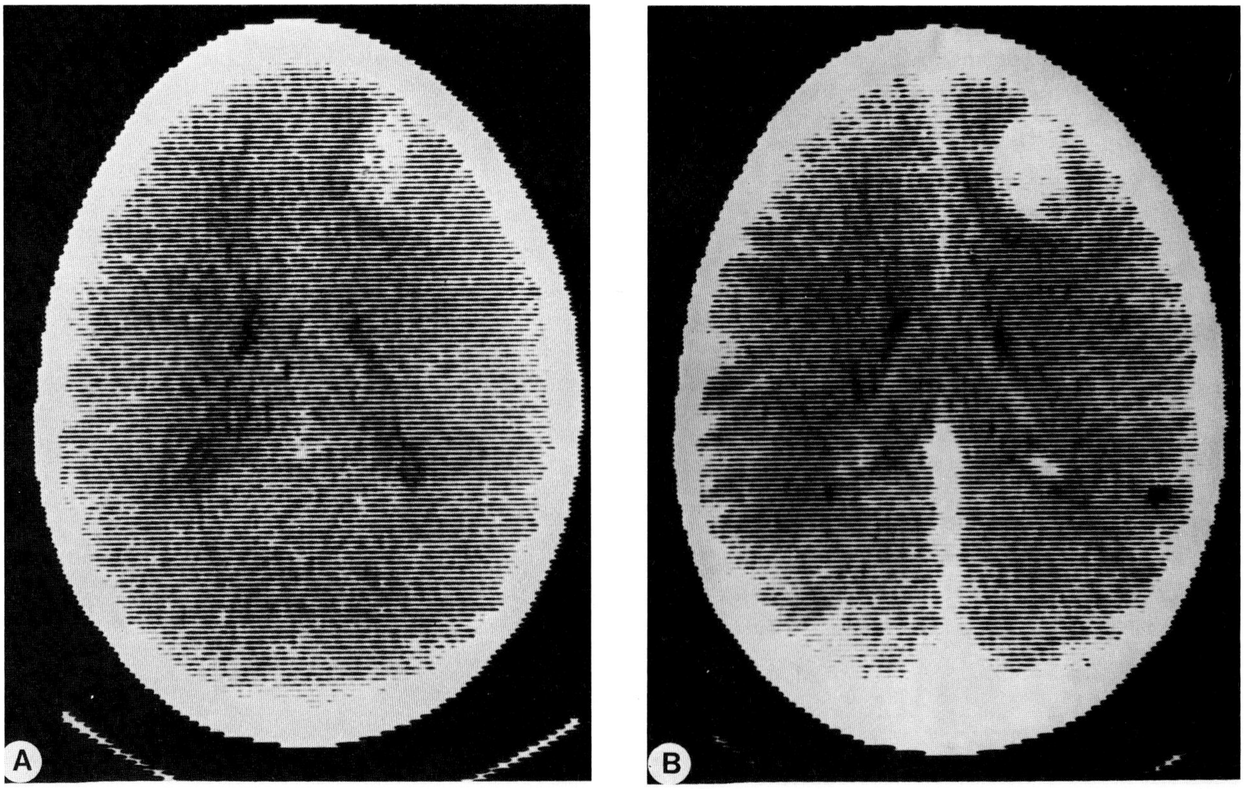

Figure 59-1. A. CT scan of 6-year-old with sudden onset of focal seizures showing hemorrhagic lesion in left frontal lobe. B. CT scan following contrast injection showing that lesion enhances. This child had normal angiogram. This lesion proved to be a cryptic arteriovenous malformation.

Falconer[5] found that some 20 percent of his patients with temporal lobe epilepsy had a history of prolonged febrile convulsions during the first four years of life. He hypothesized that the hypoxia generated by a prolonged febrile seizure induces mesial temporal sclerosis and thus establishes the pathologic substrate of temporal lobe epilepsy.

Other Causes

Seizures can also result from developmental disorders, infectious diseases, toxic metabolic states, and degenerative diseases.

CLINICAL SYMPTOMATOLOGY OF EPILEPSY

Grand Mal Epilepsy

A grand mal seizure may be preceded by prodromal symptomatology such as headache, irritability, mood changes, and unusual appetite. There may be an aura reflecting an abnormal focal electric discharge in the brain, which can consist of a focal motor seizure or focal sensory seizure.

The grand mal seizure usually begins with an epileptic cry. The patient becomes cyanotic, frequently froths at the mouth, and may empty the bladder. With loss of consciousness, the patient falls to the ground. Initially there is a phase of increased tone, which is then followed by a clonic phase lasting approximately two minutes. Following this there are a further five minutes of unarousable coma. Thereafter the patient can be wakened, but is confused and disorientated and usually prefers to sleep for a few hours.

Petit Mal Epilepsy

Petit mal epilepsy is a brief absence attack occurring almost always during childhood and associated with a classic electroencephalogram (EEG) abnormality of 3 Hz spike and wave activity. The child loses consciousness only for a matter of 5–10 seconds, during which time the eyes stir and there may be minor movements such as blinking or twitching of the face or arms. The child does not fall, and consciousness is regained in a matter of seconds, but there is total amnesia for the brief period of the attack.

Petit mal epilepsy starts before the age of 15 in nearly all cases and ceases at about the age of 20 in 80 percent or more cases. About 50 percent of those with petit mal seizures in childhood, however, will go on to develop grand mal attacks. Intelligence and development are typically normal in these children, but a small minority of those who develop severe grand mal epilepsy will have secondary intellectual deterioration.

Focal Motor Seizures

Initially described by Hughlings Jackson,[6] focal motor seizures are characterized by tonic spasm followed by repetitive twitching, which usually occurs in the area of the mouth, thumb, index finger, or great toe, and spreads in an orderly manner. The seizure is due to a discharge in the opposite motor cortex, and the spread reflects the topography of the body as represented in the motor strip. The convulsive movements may remain confined to the site of onset, may spread to involve one half of the body, or may terminate in a grand mal seizure with loss of consciousness. If the seizure arises in the dominant hemisphere, speech may be lost during the attack.

A prolonged period of paralysis of the affected limb can occur (Todd's paralysis). If the paralysis persists for more than 48 hours, some other etiology is usually implicated.

Focal Sensory Seizures

Somatosensory or visual seizures commence in the appropriate cerebral cortex and may manifest themselves as numbness, paresthesiae, or unformed visual phenomena. Visual disturbances in temporal lobe seizures may include various colors, scenes, or events.

Psychomotor Epilepsy (Temporal Lobe Epilepsy)

Hallucinations of olfaction or taste are frequent in temporal lobe epilepsy and may represent the aura of a generalized seizure. The odors and tastes are characteristically unpleasant.

Visceral sensations can also occur with a temporal lobe attack, often described as an epigastric constriction or discomfort that tends to rise to the throat and head, and may be accompanied by autonomic phenomena.

Auditory hallucinations such as buzzing, hissing, or whistling can occur, as can true epileptic vertigo. Involuntary micturition and, in rare instances, defecation can occur. Disorders of perception or motion are common, including déja vu. Jamais vu, less common, is characterized by a sense of familiar surroundings being unreal. Illusions of change in body size and distortion of time or sound can also occur. Emotional experiences, including fear, intense pleasure, depression, and rage, are also common.

Autonomic behavior may occur during a seizure, but usually takes place during the postictal phase and lasts less than five minutes. In these automatisms the individual retains control of posture or muscle tone and performs simple or complex movements and actions without being aware of what is happening. These include lip smacking, swallowing, or chewing, or more complex semipurposeful actions such as undressing, drinking, and running. Complex stereotype behavior can be well coordinated, but inappropriate. Aggression during automatism is rare, apart from the tendency to resist physical interference. Most automatisms are associated with epilepsy arising in the temporal lobe.

Many authors have found a high incidence of psychiatric illness in patients with temporal lobe epilepsy. Fifty percent of patients with anterior temporal EEG foci will display some type of personality disorder in contrast to the 10 percent of patients with foci elsewhere.[7] Interictal aggression is present in 36 percent of patients presenting for treatment of temporal lobe epilepsy.[8] Ervin, Epstein, and King[9] reported a diagnosis of schizophrenia in 81 percent of patients with temporal lobe epilepsy. In a series of 31 children treated at the Hospital for Sick Children by anterior temporal lobectomy for their seizures between 1966 and 1977, 25 (80.6 percent) had a behavioral problem frequently severe enough to secure expulsion from school and even imprisonment in reformatory.

INVESTIGATION

The initial step in the study of a child with a seizure disorder is documentation of the seizure. This may include the presence of an aura, focal motor activity, or automatisms. Relevant history, including febrile seizures in infancy, head injury, or birth trauma, must be sought and a proper physical examination carried out. Neurologic examination may reveal a deficit in keeping with a focal lesion. Integumentary review may show evidence of one of the phakomatoses, while an AVM's bruit may be auscultated or a skull defect palpated.

ELECTROENCEPHALOGRAM

The major use of the electroencephalogram today is in the diagnosis and follow-up of a seizure disorder. The EEG will differentiate diffuse encephalopathies from localized cerebral lesions in temporal lobe epilepsy. Routine electroencephalographic recording from the convexity of the head will sometimes miss seizure activity arising from the mesiobasal regions of the temporal lobe: the uncus, amygdala, and hippocampus. In order to detect these, pharyngeal and sphenoidal electrodes must be used.[10]

The interictal EEG is the most readily available electrographic evidence of a seizure focus in the epileptic patient. It is reasonable to assume that the interictal epileptiform abnormalities are closely related to the area giving rise to the patient's spontaneous attack; however, the interictal EEG may be misleading.

Ictal EEGs can be obtained by prolonged recording over many hours or by precipitating a seizure by intravenous injection of a convulsant drug such as pentylenetetrazol (Metrazol®—Knoll Pharmaceuticals, 30 North Jefferson Road, Whippany, New Jersey, 07981).[11] Sleep and hyperventilation are useful for activating interictal or ictal epileptiform abnormalities.

In 1963 Crandall, Walter, and Rand[12] pointed out that although conventional scalp and basal electroencephalograph recording showed bitemporal spiking, there could be a lateralized spike focus that was missed. They implanted depth electrodes in both temporal lobes and carried out prolonged recordings and stimulation in an effort to determine which patients were suitable candidates for temporal lobectomy.[12] Recently Delgado-Escueta, Nashold, Freedman, et al.[13] demonstrated the value of combining depth electrodes with videotaping of epileptic activity.

INTRACAROTID AMOBARBITAL TEST (WADA TEST)

The intracarotid amobarbital test, which was first introduced by Wada and Rasmussen[14] in 1960 to determine speech dominance, has become invaluable in the investigation of the patient with temporal lobe epilepsy. It can also be used to differentiate between primary and secondary bilaterally synchronous epileptiform abnormalities on the EEG by inhibiting each cerebral hemisphere independently.[15] Injection of the amobarbital into the internal carotid artery of the hemisphere with the primary focus not only abolishes the primary focus, but also the mirror focus in the contralateral hemisphere, whereas injection of amobarbital into the side of the mirror focus would have no effect on the primary focus. It has also been used to study memory function.[16] The usual examination of language function is performed, then a test of memory function is given as each hemisphere is anesthetized. In the face of unilateral hippocampal damage, the patient will exhibit memory loss with inhibition of the normal hippocampus. Such evidence of hippocampal disease on the side of the seizure disorder indicates mesial temporal sclerosis, and a good prognosis following temporal lobe resection.

NEUROPSYCHOLOGY

Neuropsychologic testing is invaluable in evaluating a patient with epilepsy for surgical consideration. In addition to providing a baseline of psychometric function prior to surgery, neuropsychologic testing can provide clues to lateralization. Verbal intelligence quotient is based on verbal and numerical tasks, whereas performance IQ is based on spatial and other perceptual tasks. When the performance IQ is seven or more points higher than the verbal IQ, a dominant hemisphere lesion should be suspected.[17] When the verbal IQ is higher than the performance IQ by a difference of more than 12 points, then a lesion in the nondominant hemisphere should be suspected.[18]

NEURORADIOLOGY

Neuroradiologic investigation is essential in the management of a patient with a seizure disorder. Plain x-rays can show evidence of raised intracranial pressure, pathologic calcification, or growing skull fractures. Signs of cerebral hemiatrophy such as asymmetry of the cranium, unilateral thickening of the vault, elevation of the sphenoid and petrous ridges, and enlarged nasal sinuses may be seen.

Computerized tomography will show evidence of atrophy, porencephaly, neoplasm, and pathologic vascularity. Recently Yang, Berger, Cohen, et al.[19] have shown that 52 percent of children with focal seizures will have an abnormal CT scan. Air encephalography is rarely used now in the investigation of epileptic surgical candidates and angiography is only considered if one wishes to study the vascularity of a pathologic area of brain as in AVMs.

MEDICAL TREATMENT

The aim of medical management of epilepsy is to achieve complete control of all seizures and allow the patient to live a normal life. More effective drugs are becoming available, and eventually the percentage of cases refractory to medical management will be very small.

Drug management in epilepsy is an empirical procedure (Table 59-1). The aim is to bring complete control of seizures with the minimum dosage and without side effects. On medical management relief can be provided in 60 percent of patients with generalized tonic-clonic seizures (grand mal), 50 percent of minor seizures (absences, atonic and akinetic seizures), and 30 percent of complex partial seizures (temporal lobe epilepsy).

Unfortunately uncontrolled seizures lead to deterioration in intellectual performance, perhaps because of subclinical seizure discharge or to anoxia. Seizures induced in neonatal rats have been shown to reduce the number of brain cells.[20]

PATHOLOGY OF EPILEPSY

Since the days of Hughlings Jackson,[6] it has been known that seizure activity arises in basically normal brain adjacent to a pathologic state such as tumor, infarct, or vascular lesion. The responsible lesion has no electrical properties, but only serves to kindle seizure activity in the adjacent tissue.

In a study of 506 surgical specimens removed at the Montreal Neurological

Table 59-1
Medical Treatment of Seizures

Seizure Disorder	Drug	Usual Daily Dose in Childhood	Rate	Doses/Day	Repeat Doses	Usual Therapeutic Serum Concentration
Major motor	Diphenylhydantoin (Dilantin®)*	4–8 mg/kg		1–3		10–20 mcg/ml
	Phenobarbital	3–6 mg/kg (8 mg/kg in infancy)		1–3		15–40 mcg/ml
	Primidone (Mysoline®)†	5–20 mg/kg		3–4		5–12 mcg/ml
Simple absences, myoclonic jerks	Valproic acid (Depakene®)‡	20–30 mg/kg		3–4		50–100 mcg/ml
	Ethosuximide (Zarontin®)§	20–40 mg/kg		1–3		40–100 mcg/ml
	Clonazepam (Rivotril®)‖	0.05–0.2 mg/kg		2–3		0.025–0.075 mcg/ml
	Nitrozepam (Mogedon®)#	0.6–1.2 mg/kg		2–3		
Psychomotor	Carbamazepine (Tegretol®)**	15–20 mg/kg		3–4		4–12 mcg/ml
	Primidone (Mysoline®)	5–20 mg/kg		3–4		5–12 mcg/ml
	Diphenylhydantoin (Dilantin®)	4–8 mg/kg		3–4		10–20 mcg/ml
			Rate		Repeat Doses	Max/24 Hrs.
Status epilepticus	Diazepam IV	0.5–15 mg/kg	1–5 mg/min		5–10 mg/q20–30 min	100 mg
	Diphenylhydantoin IV	10–15 mg/kg	30–50 mg/min		1.5 mg/kg/q30 min	20 mg/kg
	Phenobarbital IV	6 mg/kg	25–50 mg/min		3 mg/kg/q20 min	12 mg/kg

*Dilantin: Parke Davis, 2200 Eglinton Avenue East, P.O. Box 633, Station A, Scarborough, Ontario M1K 5C5
†Mysoline: Ayerst, 1026 Laurentian Boulevard, P.O. Box #6115, Montreal, P.Q. H4R 1J6
‡Depakene: Abbott, 5400 Cote De Liesse, P.O. Box 600, Station A, Montreal, P.Q. H3C 3K6
§Zarontin: Park Davis, 2200 Eglinton Avenue East, P.O. Box 633, Station A, Scarborough, Ontario M1K 5C5
‖Rivotril: Hoffmann La Roche Ltd., 1000 Boulevard Roche, Vandreuil, P.Q. J7V 6B3
#Mogedon: Hoffmann La Roche Ltd., 1000 Boulevard Roche, Vandreuil, P.Q. J7V 6B3
**Tegretol: Geigy Pharmaceuticals, 6860 Century Avenue, Mississauga, Ontario L5N 2W5

Institute in an effort to cure epilepsy, Matheson[21] found that 35.2 percent had no abnormality, 13.3 percent had hippocampal sclerosis, and 19.5 percent had gliomas, hamartomas, and vascular lesions. The remaining 32 percent of specimens demonstrated infarcts, tuberous sclerosis, Sturge–Weber malformation, and chronic encephalitis.

Destructive lesions occurring primarily within the territory of the middle cerebral artery are found in patients with infantile hemiplegia and intractable seizures. Five of our 9 patients with infantile hemiplegia who were treated by hemispherectomy had an atrophic lesion in the distribution of the middle cerebral artery.[22]

In 1953 Earle, Baldwin, and Penfield[23] studied the pathologic specimens of 157 cases of temporal lobe epilepsy and found that 63 showed changes in Ammon's horn, which they attributed to compression or anoxia at birth. They felt that with molding of the head, the hippocampal region herniated through the incisura and sustained vascular damage. They indicated that the uncus, the hippocampal gyrus, and the first temporal gyrus were the areas most frequently involved, and termed the entity "incisural sclerosis."

Falconer, Serafetinides, and Corsellis[24] preferred to call the pathologic lesion seen in temporal lobe epilepsy "mesial temporal sclerosis." They described the lesion as loss of nerve cells in the Sommer (H1) sector of the hippocampus together with gliosis of the amygdala (Fig. 59-2). The lesion was also associated with seizures dating from infancy or childhood, often with a history of a difficult birth or of febrile seizures. Twenty of our 31 children with temporal lobe epilepsy treated by anterior temporal lobectomy at the Hospital for Sick Children had mesial temporal sclerosis.

Neoplasms, usually of small size, in the temporal lobe can produce typical temporal lobe seizures.[25] This was true in 24 percent of Falconer et al.'s series of temporal lobe epileptics.[24]

The lesion in Sturge–Weber malformation[26] is a pial arteriovenous malformation. The involved vessels are capillaries and small veins that form tortuous folds, several layers deep, in the subarachnoid space, and thus give a purplish color to the leptomeninges (Fig. 59-3). Because of tremendous perfusion of blood through the angioma, there is little perfusion of adjacent brain. The resulting state of anoxia leads to early deposition of calcium, not only in the cortex, but in the white matter, progressively increasing in amount as the child grows older and

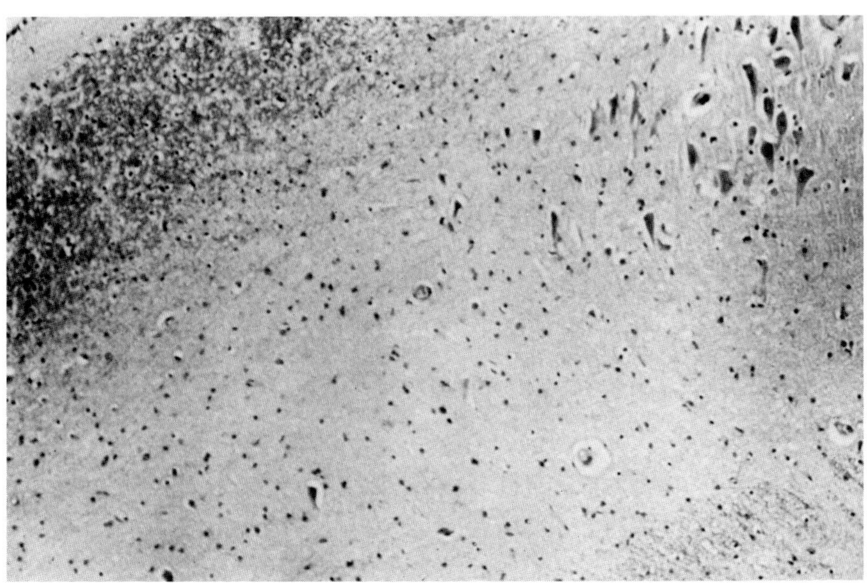

Figure 59-2. Hippocampus showing loss of neurons in Sommer (H1) sector removed from child. (H&E × 100)

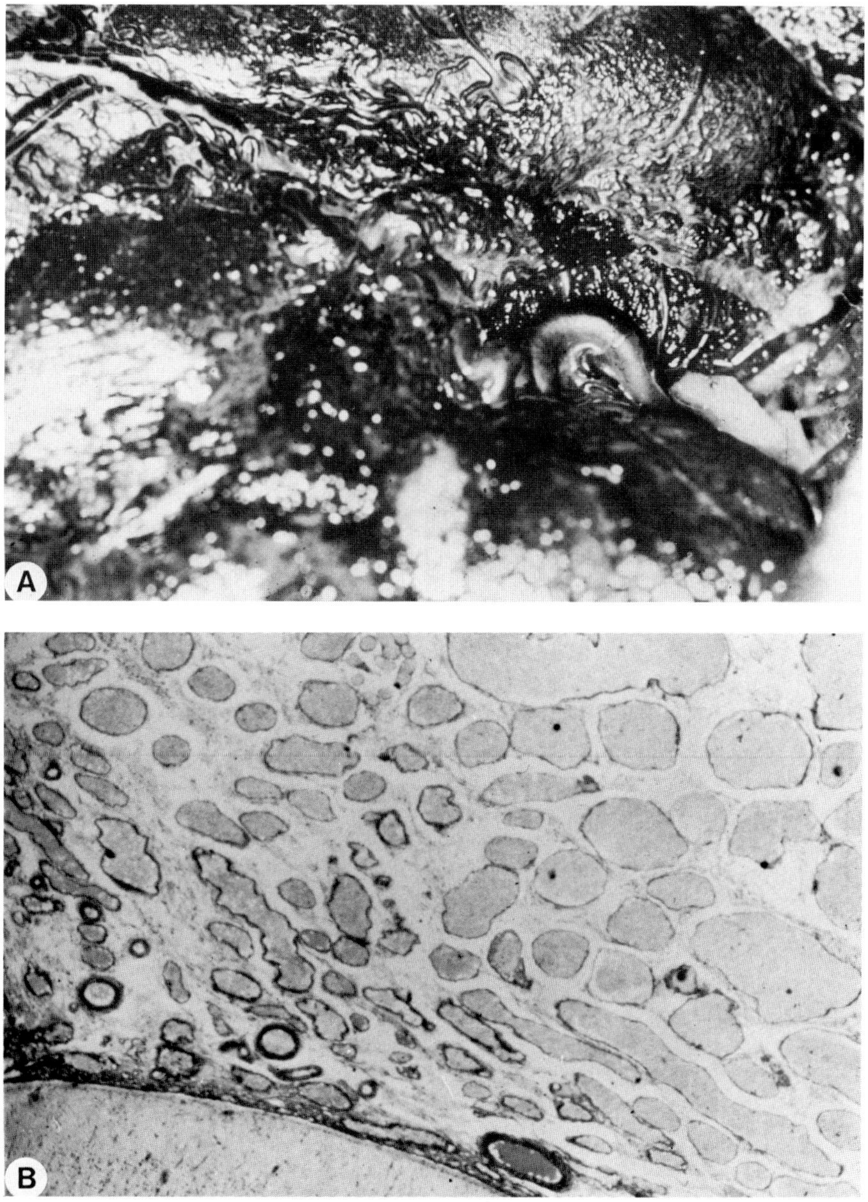

Figure 59-3. A. Cortical surface at sylvian fissure in child with Sturge–Weber syndrome showing tortuous pial vessels. (Reprinted with permission from Hoffman HJ: Hemispherectomy for Sturge–Weber syndrome. Child's Brain 5:233–248, 1979.) B. Histologic section through pia showing leptomeningeal AVM in hemisphere with Sturge–Weber involvement. (H&E × 100)

forming an epileptogenic focus. This calcification may be demonstrated by CT scanning, but conventional skull x-rays will fail to reveal calcification in a child younger than 2 years.

NEUROSURGICAL MANAGEMENT

Neurosurgical treatment should be considered whenever adequate medical treatment of the patient with focal epilepsy has failed to give satisfactory control and thus interferes significantly with the patient's ability to lead a normal or near-normal life. Although the aim of surgery is to cure the tendency for seizures, it may only be possible to decrease seizure frequency.

Goddard, McIntyre, and Leech[27] found that repeated electrical stimulation of the brain could lead to epileptiform discharging and eventually to spontaneous convulsive seizures. This sequence had actually been observed clinically after electroshock therapy.[28] They termed this phenomenon "kindling."

The possibility of kindling secondary and independent epileptic sites in normal brain suggests that any form of focal epilepsy should be aggressively treated early in childhood.

ELECTROCORTICOGRAPHY

Electrocorticography outlines the extent of the epileptogenic area during a neurosurgical operation. Large numbers of electrodes (at least 16) are required to cover the entire exposed cortical area. The electrodes must be movable so that they can be placed wherever necessary. The electrodes are silver wires with attached cotton wicks soaked in saline that are affixed to a horseshoe-shaped apparatus with ball joints that make each of the silver wires mobile (Fig. 59-4). The horseshoe can then be attached to the pin fixation head rest that keeps the patient's head in a fixed position during the procedure, a precaution that is particularly necessary because the operation is carried out under neuroleptic analgesia.

The patient is kept comfortable with the use of the neuroleptic agents Fentanyl® and Droperidol® (both manufactured by McNeil Laboratories, Stouffroille, Ontario, Canada), which exert no visible effect on the electrocorticogram. Abnormal activity in the electrocorticogram is essentially the same as in the scalp EEG, and frequently is seen much more clearly.

Electrical stimulation in the awake patient maps out areas concerned with motor or sensory functions as well as speech, and thus prevents inadvertent encroachment upon these areas by surgical excision.

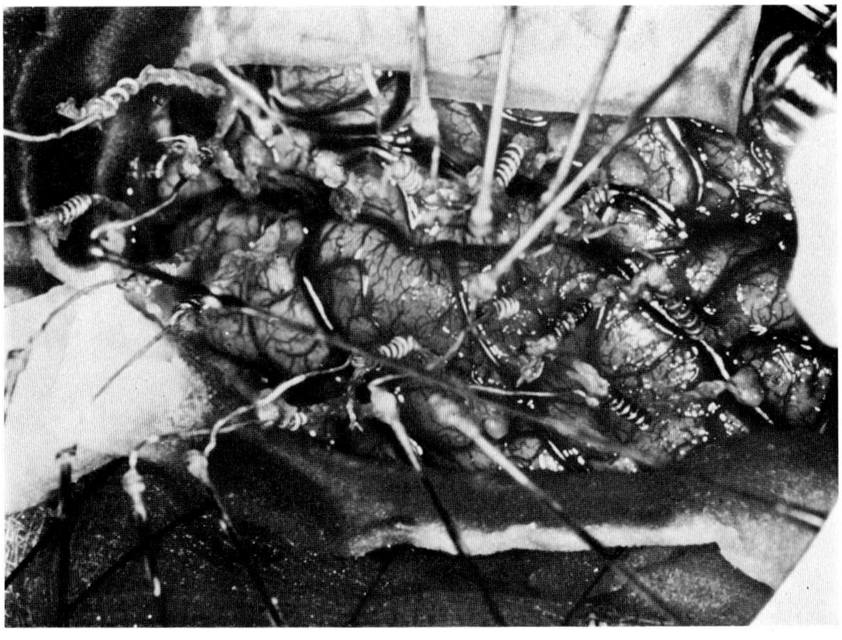

Figure 59-4. Electrocorticography, showing electrodes on cortical surface of brain.

Postexcision Electrocorticogram

The electrocorticogram should be repeated after excision of the epileptic area to determine whether all epileptiform abnormality has been eliminated. Recording of postexcision electrocorticograms is important because of the relatively unfavorable long-range prognostic significance of persistent epileptiform abnormality in the postexcision electrocorticogram. Further, it is possible to excise more cortex if an amenable resectable seizure focus is left in the remaining cortex.

SURGICAL TREATMENT OF TEMPORAL LOBE EPILEPSY

In 1950, Penfield and Flannigan[29] reported their initial findings on the beneficial effects of anterior temporal lobectomy for psychomotor epilepsy. Once regarded as a disease of adulthood, in recent years increasing evidence has come to the fore to show that temporal lobe epilepsy begins in childhood, and frequently during the first decade of childhood. In 1943 Gibbs, Gibbs, and Lennox[30] felt that temporal lobe epilepsy accounted for only 4 percent of the causes of seizures in children. More recent experience, however, suggests that some 10 percent of children with epilepsy have a temporal lobe origin for their seizures.[31]

In 1970 Falconer[32] commented on the need for earlier diagnosis in temporal lobe epilepsy: "From time to time, I have stressed the importance of earlier diagnosis, pointing out that had I been able to operate on these patients while they were still in their school years, and presuming that operation would achieve the same beneficial results in seizure release and social adaptation as it did in adult life, much physical and personal suffering would have been spared them and their families."*

Technique of Temporal Lobectomy

Temporal lobectomy is carried out as follows (Fig. 59-5). With the head positioned in a pin fixation head rest, an osteoplastic temporal flap is turned and the temporal lobe exposed 8 to 9 cm behind the temporal pole and slightly above the sylvian fissure. Once the dura is open, the electrodes are applied and electrocorticography carried out. The initial cortical incision is made parallel to the sylvian fissure along the convexity of the first temporal gyrus. At the desired distance posterior to the tip of the temporal lobe, the cortical incision is carried from the sylvian fissure downward to the floor of the middle fossa and continued across the inferior surface of the temporal lobe to the hippocampal gyrus. The incision in the cortex is deepened until the temporal horn is reached. It is at this point that Penfield, Lende, and Rasmussen[33] suggest removal of the lateral portion of temporal lobe. The remaining medial portion of the temporal lobe, including the amygdala and the hippocampus, are removed separately by suction and gross dissection. The hippocampal gyrus is sucked away from the underlying pia, which is left as a curtain to protect the structures in the basal cistern. Falconer et al.[24] emphasize that they remove the temporal lobe en bloc, which allows for more satisfactory pathologic examination of the specimen.

---

*Reprinted with permission from Falconer MA: Significance of Surgery for temporal lobe epilepsy in childhood and adolescence. J Neurosurg 33:233–252, 1970.

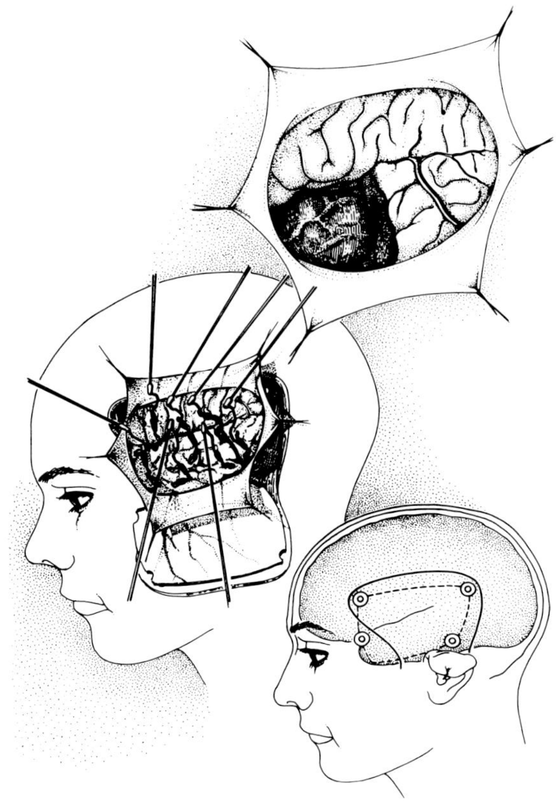

Figure 59-5. Operative steps in temporal lobectomy.

Results of Temporal Lobectomy

Davidson and Falconer[34] reported on 40 children treated by temporal lobectomy for temporal lobe epilepsy. They pointed out that the children differed from adults in that there were more children with mesial temporal sclerosis and there were no patients with scars or infarcts. Fourteen of the 24 children with mesial temporal sclerosis (58 percent) became seizure-free, usually without medication. The children in this group were operated upon primarily for epilepsy, but improvement in behavior occurred as a bonus. All but one of the children were aggressive to some extent, and many exhibited bizarre behavior.

Green[35] treated 28 children by temporal lobectomy for temporal lobe epilepsy between 1949 and 1973. Twenty-six of these procedures had a satisfactory result; 5 patients were seizure-free without medication and 12 had no seizures but were still maintained on medication. He also demonstrated an improvement in behavior. Seven of 11 aggressive and destructive children in this group became normal.

Rasmussen[36] found that 10 percent of 760 patients with temporal lobe epilepsy treated up to 1973 at the Montreal Neurological Institute were children. Of these 77 patients, 31 (43 percent) became seizure-free and 22 (30 percent) had a significant reduction in seizure tendency.

In our own series of 31 children with temporal lobe epilepsy treated by temporal lobectomy, 12 are seizure-free and off medication and four are seizure-free but still on medication. Preoperative scalp EEG studies showed a clearcut spike focus in one temporal lobe in all the patients who were seizure-free. A homonymous superior quadrantic visual field defect, usually incongruous in nature, was found in all patients postoperatively. Rarely was it complete and usually it was minimal. Of the 25 patients who displayed behavioral abnormalities preoperatively, 23 have improved. In many of these, the improvement was so dramatic that they could be rehabilitated to the point of resuming school or eventually obtaining a job.

HEMISPHERECTOMY

Dandy reported the first hemispherectomy[37] in a patient with a glioma. Ten years later McKenzie[38] carried out the first hemispherectomy for control of seizures. In 1950 Krynau[39] reported encouraging results in 12 patients in whom he had carried out a hemispherectomy for epilepsy. He clearly demonstrated the benefits resulting from excision of the atrophic hemisphere in children with infantile hemiplegia associated with uncontrolled seizures and personality problems. In 1969[22] we reported our results of 17 children treated by hemispherectomy; in three of these the pathology was Sturge–Weber syndrome and in 14 there were gross destructive lesions in the hemisphere.

Operative Procedure for Hemispherectomy

A large frontoparietal bone flap is turned, approaching the midline over the convexity and posteriorly and extending low enough posteriorly almost to reach the tentorium and the floor of the middle fossa.

In patients with infantile hemiplegia, there is usually a large atrophic lesion in the central portion of the hemisphere in the area perfused by the middle cerebral artery (Fig. 59-6). The ventricle is typically dilated so that with withdrawal of cerebrospinal fluid (CSF) a small shrunken hemisphere is visualized. On the other hand, in infants with the Sturge–Weber syndrome, the hemisphere early in infancy is not atrophic but of normal size and typically engorged with blood. In either case, it is important to deal with the arterial supply to the hemisphere as the initial step prior to obliterating the venous drainage. The sylvian fissure is then exposed and the bifurcation of the internal carotid artery is dissected free. The anterior and middle cerebral arteries are clipped and divided. This allows for reduction of blood supply to the affected hemisphere and one can thus quite safely approach the parasagittal draining veins and, after bipolar coagulation, divide them. The hemisphere is then retracted away from the falx, the corpus callosum is exposed and transected, and the lateral ventricle is entered. The incision is then carried from just above the caudate nucleus through the central white matter and the putamen down to the temporal horn. The incision in the corpus callosum is extended anteriorly to the genu and carried through the frontal lobe cortex immediately anterior to the optic chiasm and the optic nerve. The draining veins under the temporal lobe and over the medial side of the occipital lobe are divided. The incision is then carried down through the medial portion of the temporal lobe, taking the hippocampus and uncus. The posterior cerebral artery is clipped and divided as it enters the calcarine sulcus just beyond its origin. The splenium of the corpus callosum is divided and the entire cerebral cortex is removed en bloc, leaving the basal ganglia and thalamus intact. The choroid plexus is removed, particularly in cases of Sturge–Weber syndrome where the choroid plexus is hypertrophied. Care is taken to leave the foramen of Monro open to allow for irrigation of the hemicranium by CSF (Fig. 59-7).

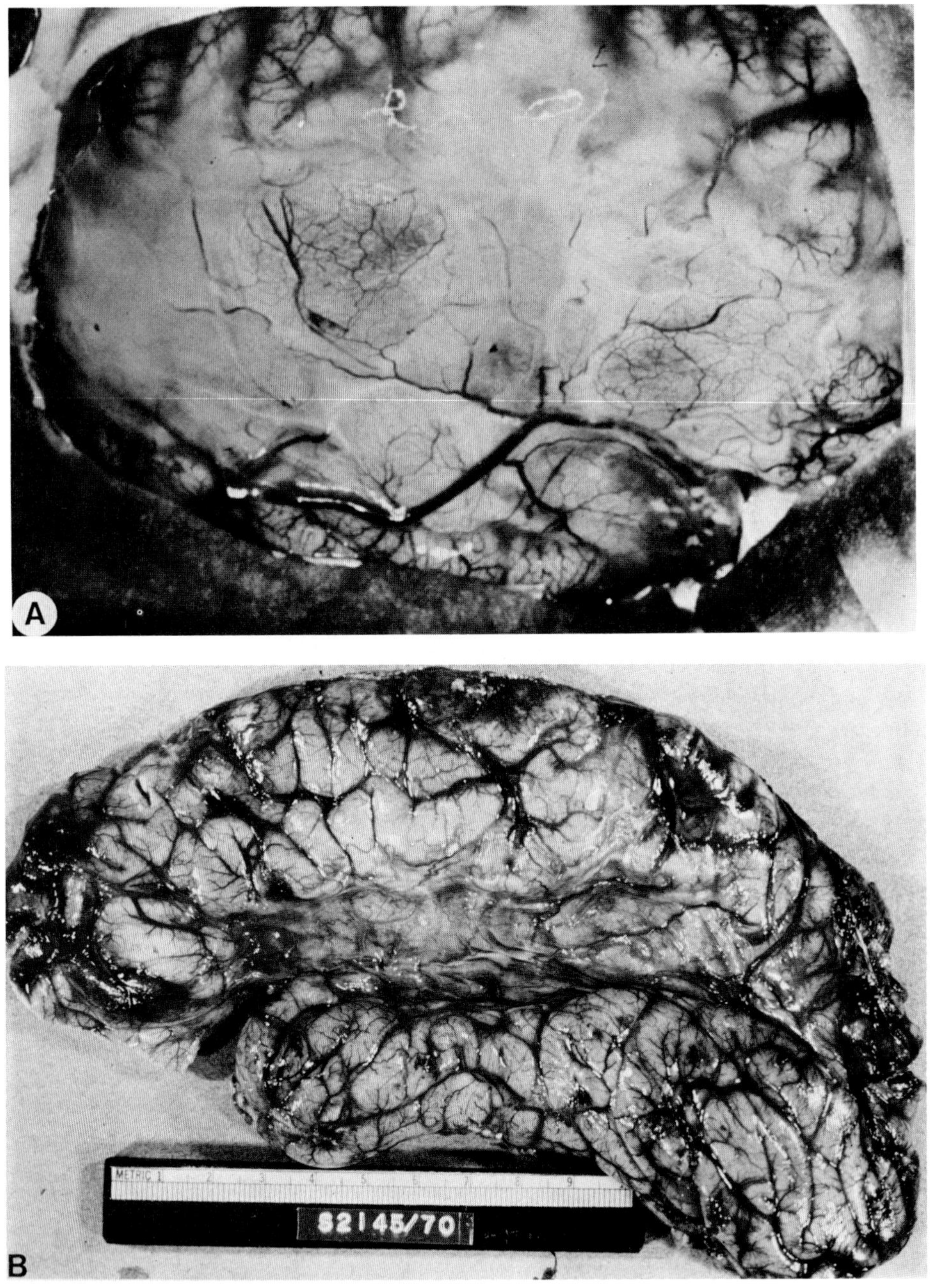

Figure 59-6. A. Hemisphere in child with infantile hemiplegia showing gliosis in distribution of middle cerebral artery. B. Removed hemisphere showing shrunken gliotic area in distribution of middle cerebral artery.

Results of Hemispherectomy

The results of hemispherectomy in properly selected cases of the Sturge–Weber syndrome have been gratifying. Five of the 7 patients treated at our insitution by hemispherectomy are seizure-free and taking no anticonvulsants.[26] All of our patients who underwent hemispherectomy in infancy have a normal IQ, and the IQ seems directly to be related to the time of hemispherectomy after the onset of seizures.

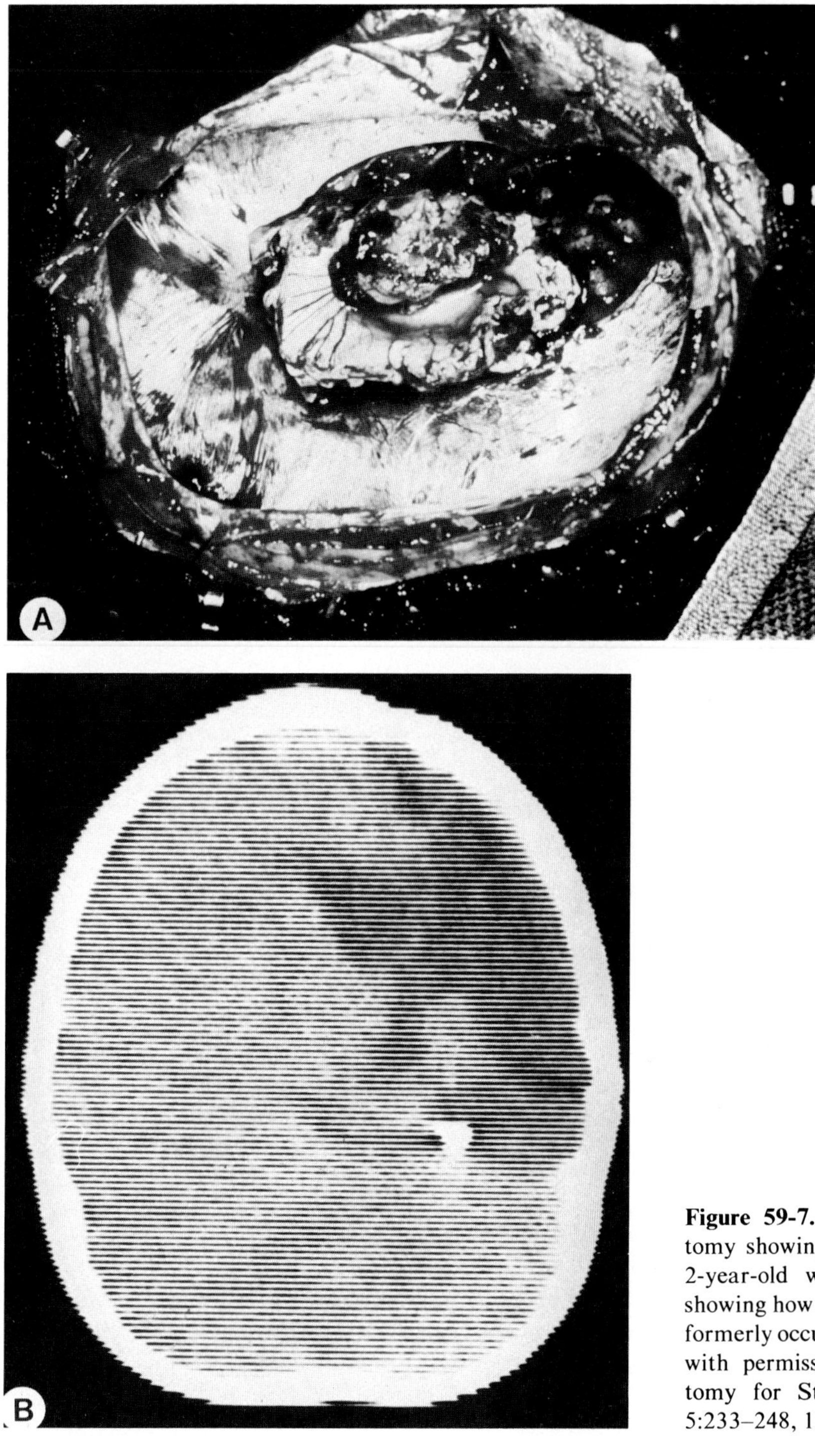

Figure 59-7. A. Surgical field after hemispherectomy showing empty hemicalvarium. B. CT scan in 2-year-old who had hemispherectomy as neonate showing how normal hemisphere has moved into space formerly occupied by diseased hemisphere. (Reprinted with permission from Hoffman, HJ: Hemispherectomy for Sturge–Weber syndrome. Child's Brain 5:233–248, 1979.)

Rasmussen and Gossman[40] carried out hemispherectomy for gross destructive brain lesions in a group of 17 patients and were able to abolish seizures in 10 patients (59 percent) and to achieve a marked reduction in seizure tendency in 5 patients (29 percent).

CORTICAL RESECTION FOR EPILEPSY

Cortical resection for epilepsy was done as long ago as 1886 by Horsley.[41] Modern use of cortical resection for epilepsy began with the work of Foerster,[42] and finally culminated in the modern application of surgery for epilepsy in the work of Penfield and Jasper in 1954.[43] The surgery is carried out under local anesthesia supplemented by neuroleptic analgesia. We have done this in children as young as 7 years. Electrocorticography is essential in mapping the area to be resected.

Technique of Cortical Excision

The pia-arachnoid over the convolutions of brain in the area to be excised is coagulated by bipolar cautery and then sharply incised with fine scissors. The incision is carried down into white matter using a blunt dissector. Larger arteries are clipped as well as coagulated, and the block of cortex and subcortical white matter is removed.

Results of Cortical Excision

Rasmussen reported on 1267 patients who had undergone cortical excision for nontumoral epileptogenic lesions up to 1971 at the Montreal Neurological Institute. He found that 416 (36 percent) were seizure-free and 320 (28 percent) were improved.[44]

SURGERY OF EPILEPSY ASSOCIATED WITH BRAIN TUMORS

The incidence of epilepsy as a symptom in patients with brain tumors has been documented at 35 percent in a number of studies. Of 1702 patients treated surgically for epilepsy at the Montreal Neurological Institute between 1928 and 1973, 19.2 percent had tumors and 1 percent had vascular malformations.[45] In such patients the use of electrocorticography and excision of the seizure focus as well as of the neoplasm has been the practice in our institution as suggested by Gonzales and Elvidge.[46]

CENTRAL LESIONS IN THE BRAIN FOR CONTROL OF EPILEPSY

Stereotactic surgery for epilepsy remains largely an experimental effort in the management of patients who cannot be managed medically and who do not meet the indications for the usual cortical resection. The thalamic nuclei have been favored targets for stereotactic intervention in seizure disorders, particularly because of the suspected relationship between the thalamic nuclei and the bilateral synchronous 3 cycles per second spike and wave discharge. Lesions have been made in the ventroanterior[47] and the centromedian nuclei[48] of thalamus, in Forel's fields,[49] in the posterior medial area of the hypothalamus,[50] in the cingulate gyrus,[51] in the amygdala,[52] and in the midbrain.[53]

CEREBRAL COMMISSUROTOMY

Cerebral commissurotomy, a procedure in which the major commissural pathways between the hemispheres are divided, is carried out to diminish the spread of seizure discharge between the hemispheres. In 1940 Van Wagenen and Herren[54] sectioned portions of the corpus callosum by open craniotomy in 27 patients. Postoperatively 12 patients had seizures restricted to only one side and did not lose consciousness, in contrast to their preoperative seizures. More recently Bogen, Sperry, and Vogel[55] reported a series of 10 patients in whom the corpus callosum, anterior commissure, and hippocampal commissure were divded; 9 of these patients stopped having grand mal seizures.

CEREBELLAR STIMULATION

Cooper, Crighel, and Amin[56] in 1973 reported on 32 patients with intractable epilepsy treated by chronic cerebellar stimulation and found significant suppression of seizures in 18 of 27 surviving patients. The stimulating electrodes were placed over the superior and posterior surfaces of cerebellum on either side of midline.

Van Buren, Wood, Oakley, et al.[57] used a double blind technique to study the effectiveness of chronic cerebellar stimulation in the treatment of epilepsy. Objective testing showed that cerebellar stimulation made no difference in seizure frequency whether the machine was on or off. None of the patients were rendered free of seizures, but despite the lack of objective evidence on clinical testing, the families insisted that the patients functioned better and had increased alertness and interest in their surroundings. They felt that the seizures seemed less severe, of shorter duration, and less debilitating, and they cited a reduction in frequency.

CONCLUSIONS

Prior to the discovery of the present armamentarium of anticonvulsant drugs, neurosurgical management was effectively the only means of controlling many of the epileptic disorders of childhood. With the increased availability and effectiveness of anticonvulsant drugs, however, some authorities have stated that the surgical treatment of epilepsy in childhood should be undertaken reluctantly and only after all reasonable attempts at medical management have failed. There is a group of epileptic disorders, however, that do not respond to medical management and are remarkably amenable to surgical therapy. Further, ablative surgery carried out early in childhood allows for excellent adaptation of the remaining brain. There is no doubt that improved medical and surgical management of epilepsy will control this disorder in childhood and spare these children the ill effects of a seizure diathesis during their growing and formative years.

REFERENCES

1. Rose AL: Neonatal Seizures, in Blow ME, Rapin I, Kinsbourne, M (eds): Topics in Child Neurology. New York, Spectrum, 1977, p 72
2. Jennett B: Epilepsy After Non-Missile Head Injuries. Chicago, Year Book Medical Publishers, 1975, p 170

3. Hoffman HJ: Supratentorial tumors in childhood, in Youmans J (ed): Neurological Surgery. Philadelphia, W.B. Saunders (in press)
4. Fishman MA: Febrile seizures: The treatment controversy. J Pediatr 94:177–184, 1979
5. Falconer MA: Genetic and related aetiological factors in temporal lobe epilepsy. Epilepsia 12:13–31, 1971
6. Jackson JH: On the scientific and empirical investigation of epilepsies. Med Press Circular 18:475, 1874
7. Gibbs FA: Ictal and non-ictal psychiatric disorders in temporal lobe epilepsy. J Nerv Ment Dis 113:522–528, 1951
8. Falconer MA: Reversibility by temporal lobe resection of the behavioral abnormalities of temporal-lobe epilepsy. N Engl J Med 289:451–455, 1973
9. Ervin F, Epstein AW, King HE: Behavior of epileptic and nonepileptic patients with "temporal spikes." AMA Arch Neurol Psychiatr 74:488–497, 1955
10. Rovit RL, Goor P, Rasmussen T: Sphenoidal electrodes in the electrographic study of patients with temporal lobe epilepsy. J Neurosurg 18:151–158, 1961
11. Cure C, Rasmussen T, Jasper H: Activation of seizures and electroencephalographic disturbances in epileptic and in control subjects with "Metrazol." Arch Neurol Psychiatr 59:691–717, 1948
12. Crandall PH, Walter RD, Rand RW: Clinical applications of studies on stereotactically implanted electrodes in temporal-lobe epilepsy. J Neurosurg 20:827–840, 1963
13. Delgado-Escueta AV, Nashold B, Freedman M, et al: Videotaping epileptic attacks during stereoelectroencephalography. Neurology 29:473–489, 1979
14. Wada J, Rasmussen T: Intracarotid injection of sodium amytal for the lateralization of cerebral speech dominance: Experimental and clinical observations. J Neurosurg 17:266–282, 1960
15. Rovit R, Gloor P, Rasmussen T: Intracarotid amobarbital in epileptic patients. Arch Neurol 5:606–626, 1961
16. Blume WT, Grabow JD, Darley FL, et al: Intracarotid amobarbital test of language and memory before temporal lobectomy for seizure control. Neurology 23:812–819, 1973
17. Meyer V, Jones HG: Patterns of cognitive test performance as functions of the lateral localization of cerebral abnormalities in the temporal lobe. J Ment Sci 103:758–772, 1957
18. Milner B: Psychological defects produced by temporal lobe excision. Res Publ Assoc Neur Ment Dis 36:244–257, 1958
19. Yang PJ, Berger PE, Cohen ME, et al: Computed tomography and childhood seizure disorders. Neurology 29:1084–1088, 1979
20. Wasterlain C: Developmental effects of seizures: Role of malnutrition. Pediatrics 57:197–200, 1976
21. Matheson G: Pathologic aspects of epilepsy with special reference to the surgical pathology of focal cerebral seizures, in Purpura DP, Penry JK, Walter RD (eds): Neurosurgical Management of the Epilepsies. New York, Raven Press, 1975, p 114
22. Hendrick EB, Hoffman JH, Hudson AR: Hemispherectomy in children. Clin Neurosurg 16:315–327, 1969
23. Earle KM, Baldwin M, Penfield W: Incisural sclerosis and temporal lobe seizures produced by hippocampal herniation at birth. Arch Neurol Psychiatr (Chicago) 69:27–42, 1953
24. Falconer MA, Serafetinides EA, Corsellis JAN: Etiology and pathogenesis of temporal lobe epilepsy. Arch Neurol 10:233–248, 1964
25. Steegman AT, Winer B: Temporal lobe epilepsy resulting from ganglioglioma. J Neurosurg 18:406–412, 1961
26. Hoffman HJ, Hendrick EB, Dennis M, et al: Hemispherectomy for Sturge–Weber syndrome. Child's Brain 5:233–248, 1979
27. Goddard GV, McIntyre DC, Leech CK: A permanent change in brain function resulting from daily electrical stimulation. Exp Neurol 25:295–330, 1969
28. Assael MI, Halperin B, Alpern S: Centrencephalic epilepsy induced by electrical convulsive treatment. Electroenceph Clin Neurophysiol 23:193–196, 1967

29. Penfield W, Flannigan H: Surgical therapy of temporal lobe seizures. Arch Neurol Psychiatr 64:491–500, 1950
30. Gibbs FA, Gibbs EL, Lennox WG: Electroencephalographic classification of epileptic patients and control subjects. Arch Neurol Psychiatr 5:111–128, 1943
31. Falconer MA, Davidson S: The rationale of surgical treatment of temporal lobe epilepsy with particular reference to childhood and adolescence, in Harris P, Maudsley C (eds): Epilepsy. Edinburgh, Churchill Livingstone, 1974, p 209
32. Falconer MA: Significance of surgery for temporal lobe epilepsy in childhood and adolescence. J Neurosurg 33:233–252, 1970
33. Penfield W, Lende RA, Rasmussen T: Manipulation hemiplegia: An untoward complication in the surgery of focal epilepsy. J Neurosurg 18:760–776, 1961
34. Davidson S, Falconer MA: Outcome of surgery in 40 children with temporal lobe epilepsy. Lancet 1:1260–1263, 1975
35. Green JR: Surgical treatment of epilepsy during childhood and adolescence. Surg Neurol 8:71–80, 1977
36. Rasmussen TB: Surgical aspects: Temporal lobe seizures in childhood, in Blow ME, Rakin I, Kinsbourne M (eds): Topics in Child Neurology. New York, Spectrum, 1977, pp 143–157
37. Dandy WE: Removal of right cerebral hemisphere for certain tumors with hemiplegia. JAMA 90:823–825, 1928
38. McKenzie KG: The present status of a patient who had the right cerebral hemisphere removed. JAMA 3:168–183, 1938
39. Krynau RA: Infantile hemiplegia treated by removal of one cerebral hemisphere. J Neurol Neurosurg Psychiat 13:243–267, 1950
40. Rasmussen T, Gossman H: Epilepsy due to gross destructive brain lesions: Results of surgical therapy. Neurology 7:659–669, 1963
41. Horsley V: Brain surgery. Br Med J 2:670–675, 1886
42. Foerster O: Zur Pathogenese und chirurgeschen behandlung der epilepsie. Zentralbl Chir 52:531–549, 1925
43. Penfield W, Jasper HH: Epilepsy and the Functional Anatomy of the Human Brain. Boston, Little, Brown, 1954
44. Rasmussen T: Cortical resection in the treatment of focal epilepsy. Advances in neurology, in Purpura DP, Penry JK, Walter RD (eds): Neurosurgical Management of the Epilepsies, vol 8. New York, Raven Press, pp 139–154
45. Rasmussen T: Surgery of epilepsy associated with brain tumours. Advances in neurology, in Purpura DP, Penry JK, Walter RD (eds): Neurosurgical Management of the Epilepsies, vol 8. New York, Raven Press, 1975, pp 227–239
46. Gonzalez D, Elvidge AR: On the occurrence of epilepsy caused by astrocytomas of the cerebral hemispheres. J Neurosurg 19:470–482, 1962
47. Mullan S, Vailati G, Karasick J, et al: Thalamic lesions for the control of epilepsy. Arch Neurol 16:277–285, 1967
48. Kalyanaraman S, Ramamurthi B: Stereotaxic surgery for generalized epilepsy. Neurol India 18 (suppl 1):34–41, 1970
49. Jinnai D: Clinical results and significance of Forel-H-Tomy in the treatment of epilepsy. Confin Neurol 27:129–136, 1966
50. Sano K, Maganaji Y, Sekino H, et al: Results of stimulation and destruction of the posterior hypothalamus in man. J Neurosurg 33:689–707, 1970
51. Diemath H, Heppner F, Engl S, et al: Die stereotakische vordere cingulotomie dei therapieresistenter generalisierter Epilepsie. Confin Neurol 27:44, 1966
52. Naraboyashi H, Mizutani T: Epileptic seizures and the stereotaxic amygdalotomy. Confin Neurol 32:289–297, 1970
53. Sano K: Upper mesencephalic reticulotomy in epilepsy and behaviour disorders. Neurol Med Chir 2:138–146, 1960
54. Van Waganen W, Herren R: Surgical division of commissural pathways in the corpus callosum. Arch Neurol Psychiatr 44:750–759, 1940
55. Bogen J, Sperry R, Vogel P: Addendum: Commissural section and propagation of seizures, in Jasper H, Ward A, Pope A (eds): Basic Mechanism of the Epilepsies. Boston, Little, Brown, 1969

56. Cooper IS, Crighel E, Amin I: Clinical and physiological effects of stimulation of the paleocerebellum in humans. J Am Geriat Soc 21:40–43, 1973

57. Van Buren JM, Wood JH, Oakley J, et al: Preliminary evaluation of cerebellar stimulation by double-blind stimulation and biological criteria in the treatment of epilepsy. J Neurosurg 48:407–416, 1978

60. Spasticity and Involuntary Movements in Children

Sanford J. Larson

Spinal cord injury is uncommon in children, and with the exception of dystonia musculorum deformans, the treatable progressive disorders of involuntary movement are restricted to adults. The treatment of spasticity and involuntary movements in children, therefore, is almost exclusively the treatment of cerebral palsy. The term "cerebral palsy" encompasses a group of disorders characterized by abnormalities of posture and movement, present from birth, and persistent throughout life. Although the abnormal postures and movements may be modified to some extent by maturation and training, the basic physiologic and anatomic deficits persist without change. The physiologic abnormalities, however, have not been quantitatively defined, and the anatomic spectrum extends from brains that appear normal to those that are severely malformed. The etiologic factors are similarly variable. Although antenatal or perinatal events such as anoxia, physical injury, and kernicterus have been considered to be the major causes of cerebral palsy, there is evidence that many cases are a result of genetically determined maldevelopment or arrested development.[1,20,33] As in other disorders of involuntary movement, clinical findings often cannot be correlated with an anatomic substrate.

Since it has not been possible to describe patients with cerebral palsy on anatomic or quantitative physiologic grounds, the dominant clinical manifestation has been used as a basis for classification. The most commonly used terms include spastic quadriplegia (double hemiplegia), spastic diplegia (lower limbs more severely affected than the upper limbs), spastic paraplegia, and athetosis (double athetosis). Although some patients are almost exclusively spastic and others are athetoid, most display a mixture with one functional abnormality being dominant.

Because classification and definition of physiologic abnormalities have been qualitative, because severity of disability fluctuates and is significantly influenced by emotional factors, and because overall performance usually improves with increasing age, the evaluation of treatment has been difficult. It is safe to say, however, that pharmacologic treatment has been ineffective. Physical therapy has been useful in limiting contractures and improving gait in patients with spasticity, but has had little effect on ultimate function in patients with athetosis.[36] Surgical treatment has largely been equated with orthopedic operations such as arthrodesis, osteotomy, and tenotomy.

Both physical therapy and orthopedic surgery are attempts at adaptation to a fixed physiologic abnormality. Neurosurgical treatment, although not widely applied, represents an effort toward modification of this abnormality with a view of releasing function obscured by the spasticity or athetosis. Neurosurgical treatment has had three major directions: interruption of motor pathways, interruption of sensory pathways, and interruption of cerebello-thalamo-cortical pathways.

INTERRUPTION OF MOTOR PATHWAYS

Horsley[28] was perhaps the first to treat athetosis by resection of motor cortex that had been identified by electrical stimulation. Following surgery the patient not only had paralysis of the contralateral upper limb, but also a profound reduction in sensory perception. From this Horsley concluded that the precentral gyrus was essential for perception of sensation, although it is likely that the resection was more extensive than anticipated. In any event the patient recovered some sensory perception and motor function, but the involuntary movements were almost completely obliterated. A number of years later, this procedure was revived.[8,9]

Based on the hypothesis that involuntary movements were generated in premotor cortex and transmitted over extrapyramidal corticifugal pathways, attempts were made to spare area 4. In these operations, however, the resection had been carried down to the lateral ventricle and the patient had severe postoperative weakness, suggesting that motor as well as premotor fibers were involved. Nevertheless involuntary movements were satisfactorily relieved, and the motor function that reappeared after several weeks was unimpeded by involuntary movements, and thus significantly more useful than prior to operation. These operations, however, could only be applied unilaterally and for involuntary movements of the upper limb. To improve function in those patients with bilateral involvement of upper and lower limbs, Putnam[38,39] advocated anterior cordotomy to interrupt tracts considered extrapyramidal, such as the reticulospinal, tectospinal, and vestibulospinal. This procedure was performed at a single stage bilaterally at the C2 and C3 level. Following surgery most had a profound quadriparesis, indicating corticospinal tract involvement, with loss of sphincter control and difficulty with ventilation. After several weeks motor function recovered substantially, and involuntarily movements returned but not with the preoperative intensity.

Although the net effect of these operations on motor pathways was positive, they were not widely applied and eventually were abandoned.

INTERRUPTION OF AFFERENT PATHWAYS

The treatment of spasticity by dorsal rhizotomy is effective, but in patients with cerebral palsy total deafferentiation of a limb is unacceptable. Consequently subtotal rhizotomy has been applied, particularly for spastic diplegia. In these procedures either two thirds of three fourths of each root is divided or the afferent fibers involved in the stretch reflex are identified electrophysiologically and cut.[18,19] After lumbar rhizotomy spasticity has been reported to be substantially decreased in the lower limbs and to a lesser extent in the upper limbs. Although communication with many of these patients was difficult, sensory perception was apparently not significantly affected. Subtotal rhizotomy has also been done to relieve spasticity in the upper limbs and has been effective without producing a significant sensory deficit.[2,22] Bilateral dorsal rhizotomy of C1 through C3 has been performed in an effort to abolish tonic neck reflexes and the severity of spasticity and involuntary movements have been reduced in the upper and lower limbs.[26] The improvement, although significant, was not dramatic. Complications were minimal. When the procedure was extended to include C4, C5, and C6, however, more than 50 percent of patients had respiratory problems.[22] Other operations designed to interrupt afferent pathways have included the creation of stereotactic lesions in the thalamocortical radiation.[16] Although involuntary movements were reduced and permanent significant loss of sensory perception was not observed, the improvement appeared related to the degree of sensory deficit seen immediately following surgery.

The reduction of spasticity and of involuntary movements without disabling sensory loss after a considerable interruption of afferent pathways reflects the redundancy of the nervous system and the relative crudeness of the clinical evaluation, and suggests that involuntary movements depend upon intact afferent pathways.[3,15,29]

INTERRUPTION OF CEREBELLO-THALAMO-CORTICAL CIRCUITS

The gratifying results of stereotactic procedures directed at the globus pallidus and the ventrolateral nucleus of the thalamus in patients with Parkinson's disease and other dyskinesias led to the application of these operations to patients with cerebral palsy.[11,34] Except for the relatively few almost purely athetoid patients with cerebral palsy, however, the relief from involuntary movements and posture was not nearly as striking as in dystonia musculorum deformans, and the effect upon spasticity and was not significant.[11,24] Because of the known hypotonia associated with large cerebellar lesions or with lesions of the dentate nucleus or superior cerebellar peduncle, attention was directed to the cerebellum. Schneider and Crosby[41] reported delayed but substantial bilateral reduction in spasticity following extensive unilateral cerebellar resection in a patient with cerebral palsy. They indicated, however, that this procedure probably could not be widely applied because of the difficulty in determining precisely how much cerebellum should be resected to achieve a satisfactory reduction of spasticity without an undesirable degree of hypotonia. Subsequently stereotactic dentatotomy was introduced, and although considered relatively effective, the postoperative improvement was significant but not striking.[21,24,25,42]

The application of electric current to the cerebellum for relief of involuntary movements and spasticity was proposed by Cooper and Riklan with Amin et al.[12] and with Tabaddor et al.[13] Others have also observed a reduction in spasticity and in severity of involuntary movements associated with cerebellar stimulation.[31,38,43,44] The major problem associated with evaluation of the effects of cerebellar stimulation in cerebral palsy (and this is true of all types of treatment of this disorder) is that the observed changes are difficult to express quantitatively. The temporal variation in severity and the significant influence of emotional stress upon spasticity and involuntary movements compound the problem. Recording of somatosensory evoked potentials, however, while not necessarily related to changes in spasticity or involuntary movements, nevertheless represents an objective and quantitative means of assessing the effects of application of current to the cerebellum. In both humans and monkeys, the amount of current required to produce a functional change is approximately the same as that required to produce a significant reduction in amplitude of the somatosensory evoked potential.[27,30,31,40,43,44] Application of current to the animal cerebellum at intensities similar to that used clinically is associated with the firing of Purkinje cells at a rate synchronous with the applied current.[4-6] Furthermore Purkinje cells remote from the locus of applied current are driven at latencies suggestive of activation by axon collaterals of inferior olivary neurons. This factor may account for the changes observed in both involuntary movements and evoked potentials with directly effective application of current to only a relatively small portion of the cerebellar neuronal population.[30] Since the dentate and other cerebellar subcortical neurons have a tonic facilitatory effect on those neurons with which they synapse,[17] an increase in Purkinje cell activity would have a dysfacilitatory effect. Consequently the improvement in spasticity and involuntary movements and the reduction in somatosensory evoked potential amplitude could well be causally related.

Questions have been raised regarding the safety of cerebellar stimulation and damage to the cerebellar cortex associated with application of current has been reported.[7,14] Evidence, however, is available to the effect that currents applied at levels sufficient to reduce spasticity, involuntary movements, and the amplitude of evoked potentials do not produce significant injury.[27,30,31] Neuronal loss observed has been superficial and related to mechanical injury. When currents were applied through the cerebellum from negative electrodes on one surface to positive electrodes on another, substantially greater effects were observed as compared with application through electrodes of alternate polarity, and the levels of current were well below those found to cause neuronal damage.[31,40] Furthermore, in those patients who have shown significant clinical changes and significant reduction in evoked potential associated with currents, the amount of current required to produce these changes has not increased with the passage of time as would be expected with progressive injury to the cerebellum.[31]

As indicated previously the major problem associated with evaluation of the treatment given patients with cerebral palsy is the lack of objective, quantitative means of assessment of physiologic function. The systems that have been employed for this purpose evaluate functional improvement related to education, both physical and intellectual. In many patients with cerebral palsy, useful function may be present but masked by spasticity and involuntary movements. If these impediments can be relieved, then education should be more effective. In children who already have neuromuscular disability, the imposition of an additional deficit associated with an anatomic lesion is undesirable. There is evidence that the effects of thalamotomy and dentatotomy can be reversibly reproduced by cerebellar stimulation and without significant anatomic damage. Despite the encouraging results that have been reported, quantitative, objective means of assessing neurologic disability must be developed to determine the usefulness of cerebellar stimulation. Preliminary observations suggest that such methods are feasible.[23,32,37,44]

The association of prematurity and cerebral palsy is well known. With the development of neonatal intensive care units, increasing numbers of prematurely born children survive and, therefore, an increasing number of patients with cerebral palsy can be anticipated. Although the various surgical procedures employed have been shown to have some beneficial effect, all those that involve tissue destruction share this as a common defect. Therapeutic application of current to various portions of the nervous system is in its infancy; however, this technique, whether applied to the cerebellum or other portions of the nervous system, has the advantage of reversibility and minimal anatomic disruption. Consequently continued efforts in this direction appear justified.

REFERENCES

1. Alexander L: The fundamental types of histopathologic changes encountered in cases of athetosis and paralysis agitans. Res Publ Assoc Res Nerv Ment Dis 21:334–493, 1942
2. Benedetti A, Carbonin C, Columbo F: Extended posterior cervical rhizotomy for severe spastic syndromes with dyskinesias. Appl Neurophysiol 40:41–47, 1978
3. Bertrand C: Anatomy and physiology of extrapyramidal diseases. J Neurosurg 24:233, 1966
4. Bilof R, Boehmer R, Sances A Jr, et al: On the relationship between cerebellar cortical current application and the underlying cellular activity, in Proceedings of the 29th Annual Conference on Engineering in Medicine and Biology, 1976, p 450
5. Boehmer RD: Distribution of applied electrical current in the cerebellum and its effect on Purkinje cell activity. Ph.D. dissertation, Marquette University, Milwaukee, April 1979
6. Boehmer RD, Bilof RM, Sances A Jr, et al: Recording from Purkinje cells during cerebellar stimulation in Proceedings, 14th Annual AAMI Meeting, Las Vegas, May 20–24, 1979, p 30
7. Brown WJ, Babb TL, Soper HV, et al: Tissue reaction to long-term electrical stimulation of the cerebellum in monkeys. J Neurosurg 47:366–379, 1977
8. Bucy PC, Buchanan DN: Athetosis. Brain 55:479–492, 1932
9. Bucy PC, Case TJ: Athetosis—II. Surgical treatment of unilateral athetosis. Arch Neurol Psychiatr 37:983–1020, 1937
10. Carpenter MB: Athetosis and the basal ganglia. Arch Neurol Psychiatr 63:875–901, 1950
11. Cooper IS: Involuntary Movement Disorders. New York, Harper & Row, 1969, p 410
12. Cooper IS, Riklan M, Amin I, et al: Chronic cerebellar stimulation in cerebral palsy. Arch Neurol 26:744–753, 1976
13. Cooper IS, Riklan M, Tabaddor K, et al: A long term follow up study of chronic cerebellar stimulation for cerebral palsy, in Cooper IS (ed): Cerebellar Stimulation in Man. New York, Raven Press, 1978, pp 59–99
14. Dauth GW, Defendin R, Gilman S, et al: Long-term surface stimulation of the cerebellum in the monkey—I. Light microscopic, electrophysiologic and clinical observations. Surg Neurol 7:377–384, 1977
15. Denny-Brown D: The Basal Ganglia. London, Oxford University Press, 1962, 144 pp
16. Dierssen G: Treatment of dystonic and athetoid symptoms by lesions in the sensory portion of the internal capsule. Confin Neurol 26:404–406, 1966
17. Eccles JF, Ito M, Szentagothai J: The Cerebellum as a Neuronal Machine. New York, Springer-Verlag, 1967, p 335
18. Fasano VA, Broggi G, Barolat-Romana G, et al: Surgical treatment of spasticity in cerebral palsy. Child's Brain 4:289–305, 1978
19. Fasano VA, Barolat-Romana G, Zeme S, et al: Electrophysiological assessment of spinal circuits in spasticity by dorsal root stimulation. Neurosurgery 4:146–151, 1979
20. Ford FR: Diseases of the Nervous System in Infancy, Childhood, and Adolescence (ed 6). Springfield, Charles C Thomas, 1973
21. Fraioli B, Guidetti B: Effects of stereotactic lesions of the dentate nucleus of the cerebellum in man. Appl Neurophysiol 38:81–90, 1975
22. Fraioli B, Nucci F, Baldassarre L: Bilateral cervical posterior rhizotomy: Effects on dystonia and athetosis on respiration and other autonomic functions. Appl Neurophysiol 40:26–40, 1978

23. Harris GF, Sances A Jr, Ackmann JJ, et al: Biomechanical quantification of passive resistance to motion in patients with cerebral palsy: Before and after cerebellar implant, in Proceedings of the Second Annual Meeting, American Society of Biomechanics, Ann Arbor, Mich., October 25–27, 1978
24. Heimburger RF, Whitlock CC: Stereotaxic destruction of the human dentate nucleus. Confin Neurol 26:346–358, 1965
25. Heimburger RF: The role of the cerebellar nuclei in spasticity. Confin Neurol 32:105–113, 1970
26. Heimburger RF, Slominski A, Griswold P: Cervical posterior rhizotomy for reducing spasticity in cerebral palsy. J Neurosurg 39:30–34, 1973
27. Hemmy DC, Larson SJ, Sances A Jr, et al: The effect of cerebellar stimulation on focal seizure activity and spasticity in monkeys. J Neurosurg 46:648–653, 1977
28. Horsley V: The function of the so-called motor area of the brain. Br Med J 2:121–132, 1909
29. Larson SJ, Sances A Jr: The specific somatosensory system and dyskinesia. Arch Neurol 18:543–548, 1968
30. Larson SJ, Sances A Jr, Cusick JF, et al: Cerebellar implant studies. IEEE Trans Biomed Eng 23(4):319–328, 1976
31. Larson SJ, Sances A Jr, Hemmy DC, et al: Physiological and histological effects of cerebellar stimulation. Appl Neurophysiol 40:160–174, 1978
32. Larson SJ, Harris GF, Millar EA, et al: Quantitative evaluation of cerebellar stimulation, in Proceedings of the 14th Annual AAMI Meeting, Las Vegas, May 20–24, 1979, p 158
33. Miller JQ: Lissencephaly in two siblings. Neurology 13:841–850, 1963
34. Mundinger F, Riechert T, Disselhoff J: Long-term results of stereotaxic operations on extrapyramidal hyperkinesia (excluding Parkinsonism). Confin Neurol 32:71–78, 1970
35. Narabayashi H: Stereotaxic surgery for athetosis or the spastic state of cerebral palsy. Confin Neurol 22:364–367, 1962
36. Paine R: On the treatment of cerebral palsy: The outcome of 177 patients, 74 totally untreated. Pediatrics 29:605–616, 1962
37. Penn RD, Gottlieb GL, Agarwal GC: Cerebellar stimulation in man: Quantitative changes in spasticity. J Neurosurg 48:779–786, 1978
38. Putnam TJ: Treatment of athetosis and dystonia by section of extrapyramidal motor tracts. Arch Neurol Psychiatr 29:504–521, 1933
39. Putnam TJ: Results of treatment of athetosis by section of extrapyramidal tracts in the spinal cord. Arch Neurol Psychiatr 39:258–275, 1938
40. Sances A Jr, Larson SJ, Myklebust J, et al: Evaluation of electrode configurations in cerebellar implants. Appl Neurophysiol 40:141–159, 1978
41. Schneider RC, Crosby EC: The interplay between cerebral hemispheres and cerebellum in relation to tonus and movements. J Neurosurg 20:188–198, 1963
42. Siegfried J, Esslen E, Gretener U, et al: Functional anatomy of the dentate nucleus in the light of stereotaxic operations. Confin Neurol 32:1–10, 1970
43. Upton AR, Cooper IS: Some neurophysiological effects of cerebellar stimulation in man. Canad J Neurol Sci 3:237–253, 1976
44. Wong PKH, Hoffman HJ, Froese AB, et al: Cerebellar stimulation in the management of cerebral palsy: Clinical and physiological studies. Neurosurgery 5:217–224, 1979

VIII DIAGNOSTIC IMAGING

61. Pediatric Neuroradiology: Techniques and Complications

Roy D. Strand

This chapter may be faulted by having the practices of one hospital as its basis. An effort has been made to indicate alternative methods in a few areas in which controversy might arise.

Cranial computed tomography (CCT) has had a huge effect in reducing pneumoencephalography, angiography, and ventriculography (Table 61-1). The Hospital for Sick Children, Toronto, has had much less reduction in angiography than is our experience in Boston. Children's hospitals vary somewhat in their typical practices with respect to special procedures and readers are encouraged to use the definitive book in pediatric neuroradiology by Harwood-Nash and Fitz.[1] Winston[2] has studied the changing patterns in neurodiagnostic tests in children with brain tumors and associated costs.

Table 61-2 is an attempt to stereotype further radiologic procedural requirements, given certain CCT findings. Reasonable thought requires the addition of clinical information as part of the assessment in determining whether to do angiography or other radiologic special procedures in addition to CCT. The presentation determines the urgency of preoperative workup, such as failing vision in the setting of hydrocephalus, or craniopharyngioma. Other tactical factors will be discussed in the sections devoted to the specific examinations.

Complications for neuroradiologic procedures should be very few. If conservative practices are followed, nonsuccess of the procedure is an acceptable complication, certainly preferred to something more serious as a result of overzealous pursuit, when things are going poorly.

The author wishes to acknowledge the doctors who encouraged his entering neuroradiology and who were important influences on his training and development. These include Donald D. Matson, Edward B. D. Neuhauser, Richard Hoare, Kenneth Till, Per Amundsen, John Shillito, Jr., and Keasley Welch.

tive of malignancy, may be identified more convincingly with stereo filming.[3] Stereo filming is useful in the study of aneurysms and arteriovenous malformations as well.

Indications

Prior to the availability of CCT, the indications were those of suspected tumor, arteriovenous malformation, or aneurysm, and suspected hydrocephalus or subdural effusions. Now, in the minds of many, the indications are in those patients in whom a vascular lesion or a highly vascular tumor is suspected. Occasionally angiography is still indicated when a subdural effusion is suspected but cannot be confirmed by CCT. An unfortunate fact is that a long, thin subdural effusion may be undetectable by CCT, particularly in early infancy. Angiography may be avoided with the prudent use of subdural taps in some such situations.

Technique

The general considerations with regard to technique are the route of the delivery of the contrast material and the form of sedation or anesthesia. It is hardly a point of discussion now as to the route, with percutaneous femoral catheterization the method of choice. The transfemoral approach allows multiple vessel injections, which is a common requirement in infants and children, and also permits relatively uncontrolled head motion in a sedated child when filming is not being carried out. Anesthesia has been advocated by others as necessary in most young children, but it is generally not necessary. A local or departmental pattern that includes anesthesia being readily available may continue to make that option tempting; see the appendix on premedication, sedation, and anesthesia.

Once the procedure is underway, positioning of the patient becomes critical to the success of the study. The groin must be elevated to the production of an arch that tends to present the femoral artery for palpation and puncture (Fig. 61-2). It is recommended that local anesthetic used prior to puncture be small in amount and be injected immediately adjacent to both sides and over the femoral artery that is being palpated during the infiltration. Then a very small skin incision is made directly over the femoral artery 1 to 2 cm below the inguinal crease. The puncture itself should be done at approximately 45 degrees to the skin. It is useful in children to have the first two fingers of the left hand in a vertical position directly over the vessel at the inguinal crease. The femoral artery should be entered just below the inguinal ligament. The 45-degree angle approach provides a larger luminal target and the oblique path through the vessels closes off once the needle and catheter have been removed (Fig. 61-3).

The puncture generally has to go through both walls of the vessel and then be withdrawn into the lumen with the stilette removed. When freely pulsating blood flows through the needle, a flippy tipped guide wire is inserted to a level between the aortic bifurcation and the diaphragm. There should be negligible resistance to the insertion of the guide wire if subintimal dissection is possible. The leading end of the guide wire or catheter should be viewed by fluoroscopy whenever it is advanced. This assures that the operator knows exactly where the leading tip is and that it is free within the lumen.

All doubt should be eliminated as to the identity of the vessel injected and to the adequacy of flow or runoff. The estimate of the flow during the test injection is a determining factor in the injection delivery rate and final volume. The injection volumes for the vertebral studies range from 1.5 cc in early infancy to

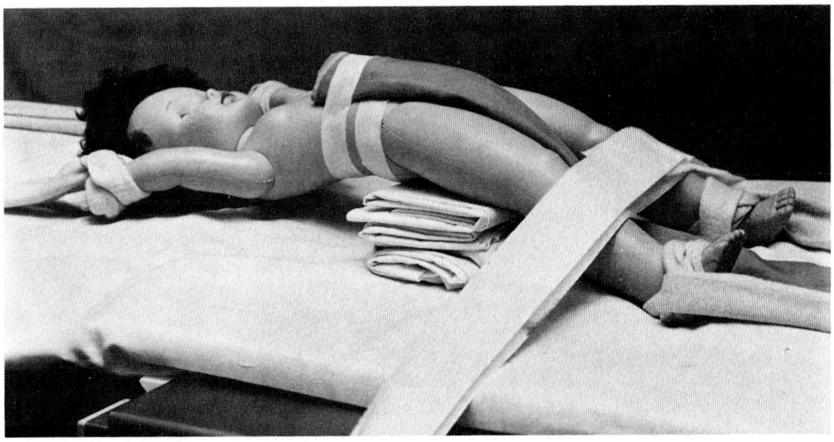

Figure 61-2. Positioning of the patient for puncture. This photograph of a doll is to dramatize, by slight exaggeration, the importance of arching the pelvis over supporting towels. This positioning presents the femoral artery for easier punctures than when pelvic arching is not employed. The hand restraints are only tight enough to keep the hands from reaching down to the groin. The ankle restraints are firm, not tight. The important straps over the legs, extending from the side of the angiographic table, usually include those seen here plus another, similar combination of Velcro® extended over the thighs, just above the knees.

4–5 cc in late childhood. Carotid injection volumes range, conservatively, from 4 to 8 cc, depending on age. The injections should be delivered in approximately one second.

The left carotid is catheterized by one of the three methods: (1) with the guide wire ahead of the catheter, the two being withdrawn together, from the innominate into the left carotid; (2) with the combination of catheter and guide wire at the same level being drawn into the left carotid from the innominate; (3) with the vessel being catheterized directly from the aortic arch with some combination of the catheter and guide wire.

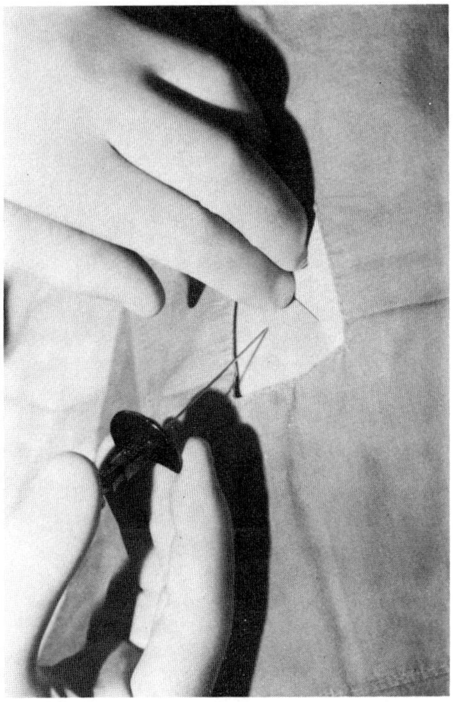

Figure 61–3. Femoral puncture. The important features here are the relatively low angle of approach of the puncture needle, its point of entry approximately a finger's width below the inguinal crease, and an effort to have two fingers of the nonpuncturing hand lined up over the femoral artery at the inguinal crease.

Approximately 15 percent of the time there is some delay in catheterizing the left common carotid artery and patience is required in those instances. The use of a catheter tip of a reduced degree of curve to approximate the curve of a hockey stick, or a tip even slightly less acutely angled, is one of the more helpful suggestions (Fig. 61-4). A variable-stiffness guide wire[5] adjusted toward "stiff" is an aid in going from the innominant artery into the origin of the left common carotid.

Various x-ray tube and film changer combinations are available. One with parallel linkage between the two is suggested[6] as desirable.

The catheterization of the left vertebral artery is the most straightforward method of all, as a straight catheter or guide wire, when it is advanced up the descending aorta, will tend to course naturally into the left vertebral artery. When a slightly curved catheter is used, it is pointed toward the left shoulder into the left subclavian, and then the curve is reversed to a medial orientation and the catheter advanced into the proximal left vertebral. C6 or C5 at the highest is the recommended injection level. Higher catheter placements tend to cut down the flow in the vertebral artery and consequently are dangerous. If the catheter/guide wire combination tends to course repeatedly into the thyrocervical trunk, a small curved guide wire directed medially as soon as one is in the subclavian usually gets around this problem. Less than 1 percent of the time, the left vertebral will be a separate branch from the aorta just distal to the origin of the left common carotid.

Complications in cerebral angiography involving the brain are, and should be, rarer than in adults. Spasm is less likely in childhood, but it may occur transiently at the catheter tip. Loss of the femoral pulse due to thrombosis or spasm is the source of primary alert. This complication should be very rare and is

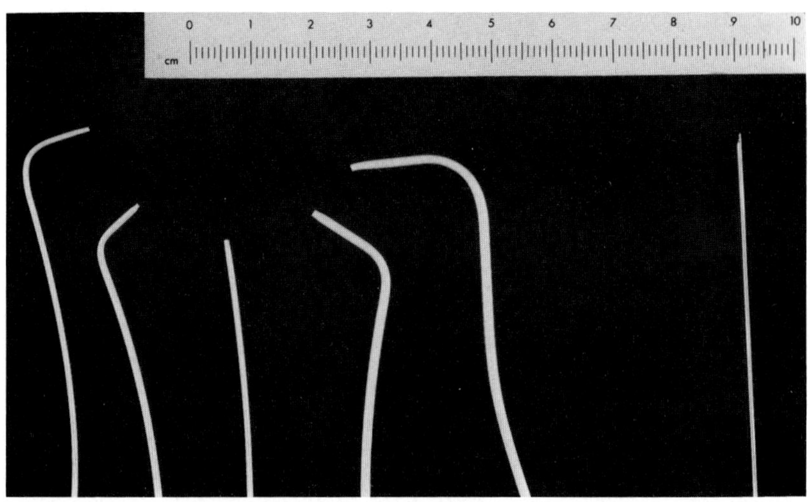

Figure 61-4. Catheter shapings for angiography. Essentially only two shapes are required for all pediatric ages. The two catheters pointed toward each other on the outside of the cluster of five catheters are shaped into a near right angle. These are called "right" catheters and are suitable for easily going around the aortic arch and into the right carotid system. The inner facing pair are shaped into a lesser curve similar to that of a hockey stick and are called "left" catheters. These are more suitable for catheterizing the left carotid system. The central single catheter is straight and is used as an introducer to dilate the vessel to size. The smallest catheter on the far left has an inner diameter of 0.025 inch. The next "left" catheter has an inner diameter of 0.037 inch and the two catheters to the right of the straight one have inner diameters of 0.045 inch. The "spear"-type puncture needle shaft and tip are seen far to the right.

minimized by the use of spear-type needles, rather than beveled ones. Other considerations in complications during or subsequent to angiography have been listed elsewhere.[7–14]

VENTRICULOGRAPHY

Indications

The usual indication is in obstructive hydrocephalus when the cause of the obstruction is poorly understood. This is much more commonly due to lesions in relationship to the third ventricle, notably at the foramina of Monro or along the aqueduct. In hydrocephalus without suspected solid tumor, ventriculography may be useful in proving that certain communications exist that may be ambiguous by CCT. This would include congenital malformations such as aqueduct stenosis, Dandy–Walker malformation, or retrocerebellar cysts. Ordinarily hydrocephalus that presumably has free communication through the entirety of the ventricular system to the cisterna magna, or "communicating hydrocephalus," does not require ventriculography. If tumor is not regarded as likely and a ventricular shunt is planned, the question of patency of the aqueduct may go unanswered.

The use of water-soluble contrast material in ventriculography is going into its second decade.[15] The past 10 years have seen progress in the tri-iodinated nonionic contrast material to provide increasingly safe positive contrast ventriculography.[16,17] In the circumstances of ventricular obstruction, any of the historic preparations appear to be safe as complications tend to arise when the material reaches the subarachnoid space. Separate from the selection of the contrast material is the fact that passing a ventricular needle through the brain is not an entirely benign manipulation.[18]

Cerebellopontine angle tumors rarely obstruct the ventricular system and hence are more likely to be studied by CCT, with or without angiography or pneumoencephalography (now both rare) or metrizamide cisternography. The usefulness and application of metrizamide cisternography are expected to grow.[19] A small lumbar dose of 2–3 cc of the isomolar solution of metrizamide is adequate (Fig. 61-5).

Tumors that protrude into the lateral ventricles, such as choroid plexus tumors, ependymomas, or meningiomas (rare), may be better delineated by ventriculography than by CCT alone.

Computed cranial tomography has been sufficiently revealing of the gross

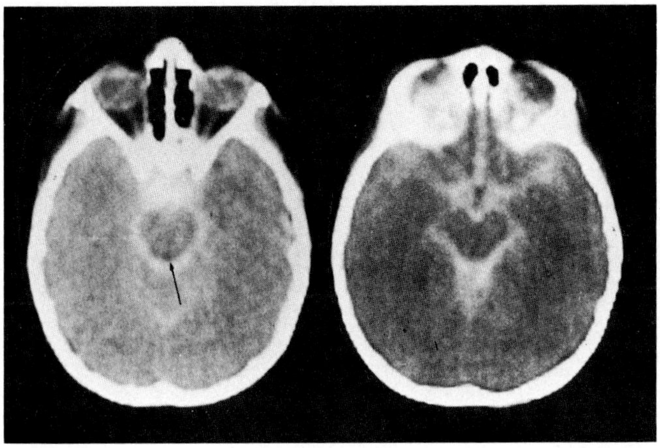

Figure 61-5. Metrizamide cisternography using CCT. Two cubic centimeters of an isoosmolar solution of the water-soluble contrast material were placed by the lumbar route and tilted into the head in the prone position. The patient had then been turned into the supine position for approximately half an hour before the CT. The image on the left is through the level of the upper pons and most rostral fourth ventricle (arrow). The pons is slightly expanded. The image on the right is through the level of the midbrain, which is not detectably expanded. The Amipaque can be seen anteriorly in the prepontine and interpeduncular cisterns, through the ambient cisterns to the quadrigeminal plate cistern posteriorly.

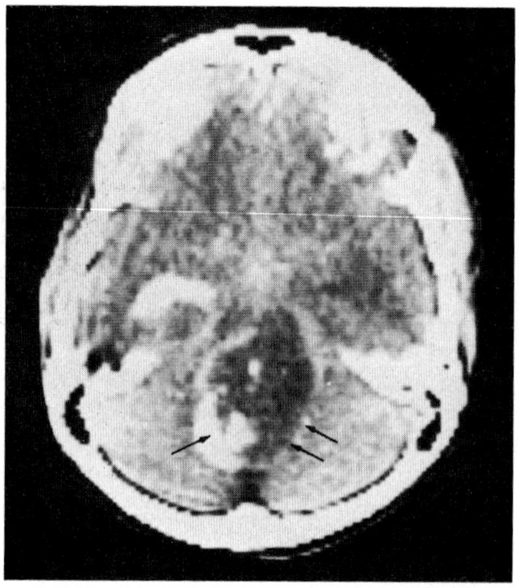

Figure 61-6. Posterior fossa tumor by ventriculography in combination with CCT. The patient had had one partial removal of a benign cerebellar tumor and the question was whether or not the residual mass was attached to the floor of the fourth ventricle. This image shows free flow of contrast material around one side of the dilated fourth ventricle (single arrow) and the lack of such precommunication and likely deep attachment of the tumor on the opposite side (double arrows). At surgery the mass was seen to be firmly attached to the floor of the fourth ventricle.

anatomy of posterior fossa masses and so ventriculography is used less often in this instance than it was in the past. When an obstruction in the posterior fossa, as observed by CCT, cannot be determined to be free from the brain stem, ventriculography may be useful. Ventriculography in conjunction with CCT can be an aid in assessing lateral ventricular tumors or posterior fossa tumors that may be attached to the brain stem (Fig. 61-6).

Technique

The use of water-soluble positive contrast material is popular at this time. Gas, either air or oxygen, should be remembered as a very useful and inexpensive agent. With CCT usually preceding ventriculography, the examination often has a target that is likely to be more sharply delineated by water-soluble contrast material than by gas.

Oily positive contrast material largely has fallen into disuse because of its slow resorption and the possibility that it will set up an obstructive reaction of its own. The key to ventriculography, as in most procedures, is to have specific objectives.

The usual routine is an approach in early infancy, to go through the anterior fontanel laterally when the coronal sutures are separated. The smallest bore needle that can readily be manipulated (no. 20 or no. 22 gage) is recommended. When the fontanel and suture are not available, from later infancy on, a small burr hole is made in close relationship to the coronal suture at the midpupillary line.

In the ventricular puncture, a CCT of the subject is used as a guide in determining the preferred angle, which may vary from an approach directed toward the ipsilateral inner canthus to the contralateral inner canthus (Fig. 61-7). Following the exchange into the anterior horn with gas, the next maneuver is usually the hanging head lateral to clarify the anatomy of the anterior third ventricle, filmed only in lateral, which is immediately followed by the completion of the backward somersault to the brow-down position for the filling of the back end of the third ventricle, aqueduct, and fourth ventricle. For the brow-down projections, there needs to be either manual support of the shoulders or shoulder pads placed anteriorly to free the face from the filming surface, and the head rests on a pad at the forehead.

Gas ventriculography, as described, is probably most useful in early infancy, delineating or excluding an intraventricular obstruction.

Neurosurgical practice is such now that a ventricular catheter commonly is

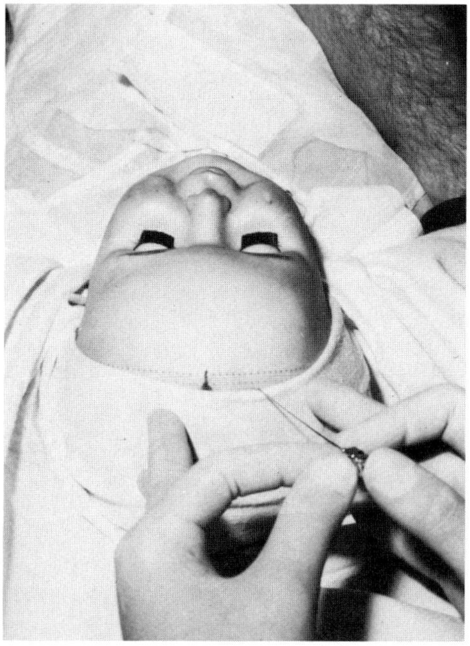

Figure 61-7. Ventricular puncture for ventriculography in an infant. The puncture is carried out through the coronal suture just lateral to the anterior fontanel (depicted here along a line of incidental stitch marks on the doll's head). The precise degree of medial angulation, with the needle in this instance directed at the opposite inner canthus, is determined from study of the ventricular position by CCT.

placed in the anterior horn, as part of the completed shunting procedure, or as a safeguard in a patient at high risk of ventricular obstruction. The shunt or catheter reservoir is then the route of administration of a water soluble contrast material.*

For the usual third-to-fourth ventricular study, the patient is supported in an exaggerated prayer position prior to the placement of contrast material. Once flow from the ventricle is established, 2–3 cc of a slightly hyperosmolar solution of contrast material is injected slowly in exchange for the same amount withdrawn, if the patient does not have a functioning shunt. Then a lateral film is exposed and the proper placement of the contrast material in the anterior horn and the third ventricle is confirmed (Fig. 61-8) and the final volume of contrast material to be used is determined. The usual final dose ranges from 4 to 6 cc of a 170–200 mg iodine/cc solution.

From the filling position, the patient is moved to a more directly upright position for the lateral and, if necessary, frontal filming. This position is maintained only briefly and then the patient is further rotated toward the supine position for final filming. The lateral projection is, by far, the most useful and anteroposterior or Townes' projections are usually done only once, to show any lateral shift or deformity to the ventricles.

PNEUMOENCEPHALOGRAPHY

Indications

The indications have been reduced considerably. The question of atrophy and porencephaly have largely been relegated to CCT. Some patients with hemispheric tumors, particularly those in the temporal lobe (Fig. 61-9), are studied by pneumoencephalography (PEG) to determine in detail, the extent of tumor and its relationship with the adjacent ventricle. Small or even suspected

*Metrizamide (Amipaque®), Sterling-Winthrop Research Institute, A Division of Sterling Winthrop Drug Inc., Rensselaer, N.Y. 12144.

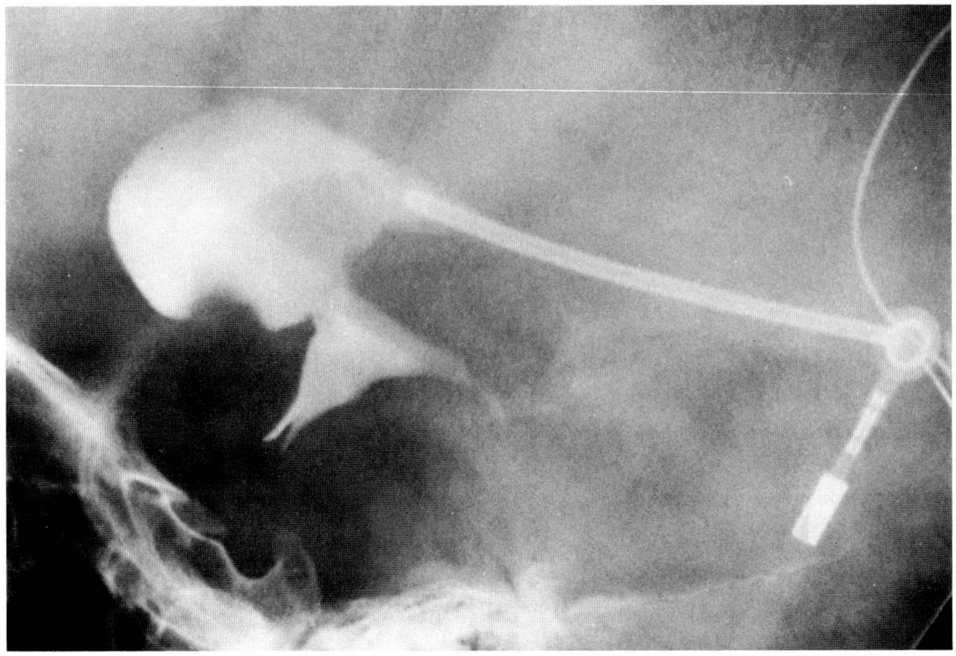

Figure 61-8. Ventriculography by way of a ventricular catheter with reservoir. The patient had been placed in a forward leaning position so that the contrast material fell into the anterior horn and anterior third ventricle. This film was made after the injection of 3 cc of material and would be adequate for any study of the third or fourth ventricle. The injecting needle and small connecting tubing can be seen overlying the reservoir. When the ventricular pressure is low, the patient should not be in the erect position or air may be introduced into the ventricular system.

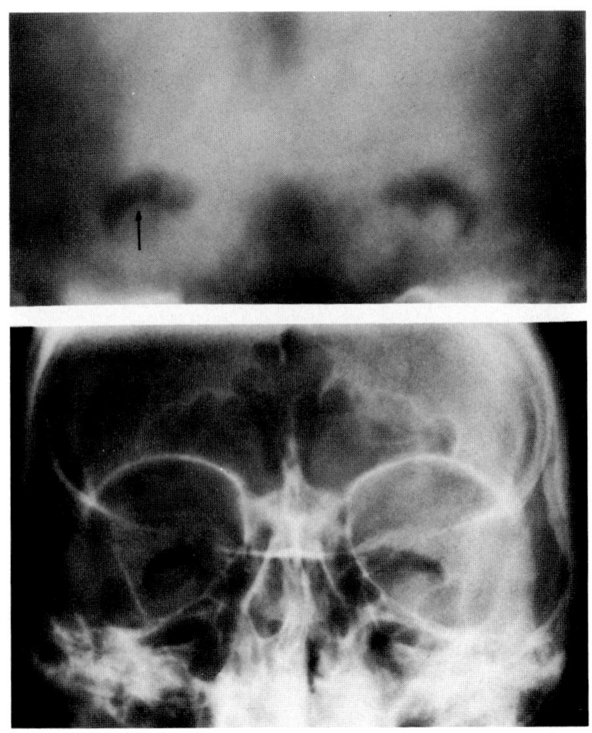

Figure 61-9. PEG for temporal horn visualization. The lower projection is the plain film transorbital brow-up projection, following full forward somersault. Filling the two temporal horns simultaneously allows direct comparison. The upper frame with polytomography, with the patient in the same position, reveals a subtle elevation of the right temporal horn (arrow) associated with minor temporal horn deformity, caused by a medial, anterior temporal lobe mass.

masses in relationship to the third ventricle, such as craniopharyngioma, germinoma, pinealoma, colloid cyst, or glioma, are still sometimes studied for the purposes of surgical or other therapeutic planning. When a mass is seen on CCT but the question of whether or not it is intrinsic to brain cannot be settled, PEG may be necessary. It is relatively contraindicated in the setting of increased intracranial pressure. The technique may be delayed until after shunting in certain cases of obstruction, most notably in relationship to the pineal region and aqueduct of Sylvius. It is contraindicated in patients suspected of having a posterior fossa tumor.

Technique

Initial positioning is the most crucial single factor in obtaining a diagnostic pneumoencephalogram. The posture of the patient is that of sitting, with the back leaning forward and the head flexed so that the mentum of the chin and the vertex of the skull are vertical. This produces a smooth curve to the course of the spinal axis and promotes gas filling of the cisterna magna first, rather than the anterior basal cisterns.

The ventricular system begins to fill when the cisterna magna has been completely filled down to the foramen of Magendi. The lumbar puncture is done through the most palpable interspace above the level of the iliac crests. This is usually L2–3 or L3–4. Below this level the subarachnoid space narrows and above L2 there is the risk of interfering with the conus medullaris. A no. 22 spinal needle is a reasonable compromise of small bore size and shaft stiffness to facilitate a successful puncture.

Good needle puncture technique requires the thumb and forefinger of each hand to be the needle hub, with both little fingers resting against the skin of the patient's back. This combination starts the needle straight and keeps it straight through the completion of the puncture. The fingers do not touch the shaft of the needle. Small adjustments to the course that the needle is taking during its advance are made by changing the direction of the needle bevel.

When the needle tip is in place in the estimated center of the arachnoid space, sufficient fluid is collected for the usual tests of protein, sugar, and cells, and it is recommended that an additional 2 cc be collected and refrigerated for tests that are suggested later in the day. For proper PEG no fluid need be removed, generally speaking. Certainly nothing like an exact exchange of gas for cerebrospinal fluid is ever indicated. If the cervical–medullary junction is part of the target to be filmed, a combination of exaggeration of the forward leaning of the patient and further flexion at the neck to just above the horizontal plane, plus the removal of 10–12 cc of fluid, may be helpful. Filling is generally done with oxygen in 7 cc amounts of either film of fluoroscopic control to a volume of 28–35 cc.

The problem orientation of the examination determines the remainder of the procedure in technique and duration. The examination is over when the clinical queries have been satisfied, even if all of the ventricular system has not been demonstrated.

If the question is about brain-stem dimension and detail about patency or deformity around the aqueduct, lateral tomography in the upright filling postion is required. The films should include exposure from C1 to the third ventricular level. If the lateral tomography is normal, frontal tomography is usually not required. Frontal tomography is done to confirm any asymmetry and to assist in determining whether an identifiable expansion from the lateral is intrinsic or extrinsic to brain.

When subarachnoid filling is required along the anterior brain stem, the

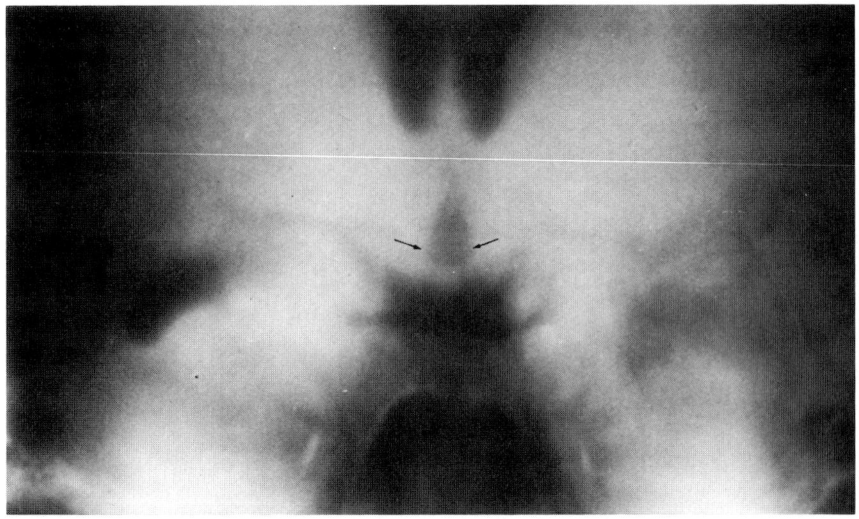

Figure 61-10. PEG for anterior third ventricle and chiasmatic cistern. Brow-up projection with polytomography following enough momentary backward tilting of the head so that the third ventricle is filled from the lateral ventricles. The tear-shaped anterior-most third ventricle at the optic recess is seen between the arrows. The optic chiasm and chiasmatic cistern are directly beneath the optic recess. Also seen are the two anterior horns and right temporal horn of the lateral ventricles. The ventricular system is slightly dilated.

cistern of the quadrigeminal plane, or chiasmatic cisterns, approximately 6 cc of room air is injected after the ventricular filling has been completed and the patient has been rotated backward so the gas will flow up along the clivis. The needle is removed and the rotation to the brow-up position is then completed.

If the suprasellar cisterns and anterior recesses of the third ventricle are to be studied, the patient is rotated briefly 20 degrees beyond the horizontal or the head is tilted back briefly to ensure third ventricular filling. Lateral, brow-up tomography then ensues with the head in a horizontal plane (Reid's baseline vertical). A general rule is to have a good-quality plain film at any position in which one is doing tomography. If the target is the pituitary fossa or chiasm, lateral tomography is followed by frontal tomography—the latter after the patient has been moved from the PEG chair to the tomographic table in most instances. The chiasm and anterior third ventricle are usually well seen on cuts that are on a plane 7.5 to 8.5 cm posterior to the nasion (Fig. 61-10).

Three classic articles delineate the normal third ventricular appearance, the subarachnoid cisterns, and ventricular anatomy.[20–22] The patterns of alteration in the appearance of the third ventricle in communicating hydrocephalus have been described by Hoare and Strand.[23]

MYELOGRAPHY

General Considerations in Choice of Agent

As CCT has changed the scene in cranial and spinal neuroradiology in general, the demonstrated safety of water-soluble positive contrast material has significantly altered and improved the established practices in myelography. Water-soluble positive contrast myelography has improved the accuracy and ease of diagnosis in disk disease, and the identification of other extradural expansions, and of most intradural lesions, including those of occult spinal dysraphism (Fig. 61-11).

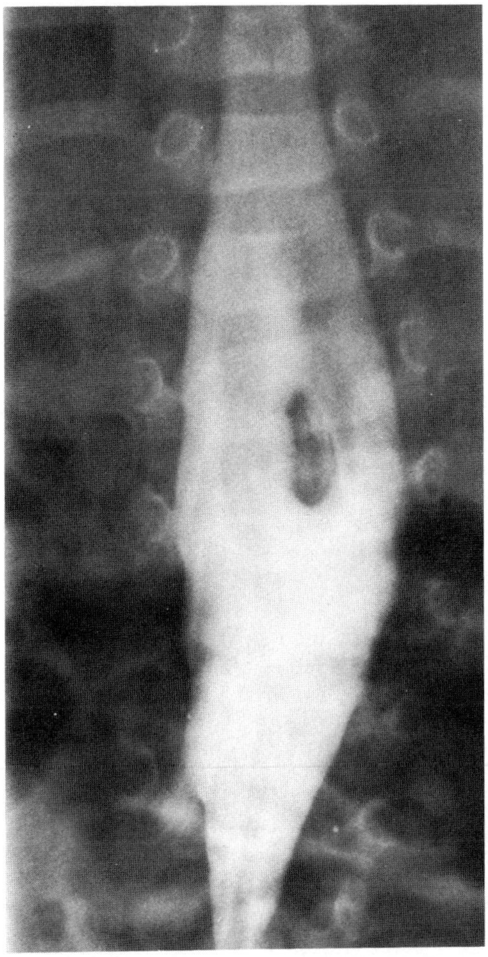

Figure 61-11. Occult spinal dysraphism—diastematomyelia. Metrizamide myelography with the material introduced through the cisterna magna in a 6-month-old. The central dural defect and bony spur are seen at the L1–2 level. The cord is seen to extend to just below the level of the diastematomyelia terminating in a fat filum terminale.

There are disadvantages and hazards to positive contrast myelography. One disadvantage is that complete myelography in an adult-sized patient is likely not to be optimal at all levels as a result of dilution. Lumbar-thoracic or cervical-thoracic studies are usually satisfactory, but the third spinal level may be lacking in fine detail. The dilution problem can be largely reduced to not being a clinical problem if certain techniques are followed. The risk of seizure production and other transient central nervous side effects is small, but is nonetheless a disadvantage to be dealt with. Drugs that are known to lower the threshold to seizure (phenothiazine derivatives) or those drugs occasionally thought to be epileptogenic are not recommended for use two days before or the day after the myelography. The contraindication for phenothiazine use is largely based on one case[24] in which the drug had been used long-term in a patient.

A number of articles discuss the use of water-soluble agents in myelography.[25–34]

There is considerable experience that the single-dose use of promethazine in combination with meperidine may be used for purposes of sedation without the production of seizures. Other disadvantages of the use of water-soluble contrast material, as it is available today, is that it is in a powder form that must be mixed with a diluent immediately before use, and that it is expensive.

Some of the advantages of the use of water-soluble contrast material include its ease of administration, once it has been mixed, the small needle bore through which it can be delivered, and the fact that the material need not be removed by aspiration. Its intermediate density allows one to see through material, so to speak, as well as to appreciate the clearcut delineation of normal and pathologic structures. Its lesser surface tension allows it to penetrate the subarachnoid space more completely than did the oily contrast agents, particularly with respect to the root pouches.

Gas myelography is still a useful technique to have at one's disposal. It is an excellent way to delineate the spinal canal and cord injury secondary to trauma, either by itself or in combination with positive contrast material. Gas is the only agent to consider in myelography with patients known to be allergic to iodine. The technique of gas myelography is discussed briefly below, and more extensively elsewhere.[35]

Oily positive contrast material is still an occasional consideration and its use is expected to continue, although markedly less than in the past. In patients with malignancy, in whom an extradural compression is suspected, the use of oily material is reasonable and its failure to absorb readily becomes an advantage in follow-up. Arachnoiditis has been an occasional complication from oily water-soluble contrast material, even in the absence of blood in the subarachnoid space, and this complication has not yet been reported with the clinically recommended doses for myelography with the water-soluble positive contrast material.

The use of CCT is being actively assessed and eagerly pursued by a number of medical centers. Determination of the presence of spinal fracture is an obvious superb use of CCT. Unfortunately the visualization of the spinal cord, without the addition of contrast material in the subarachnoid space, is at the threshold of what can be visualized by even the most advanced present-day CT scanner.

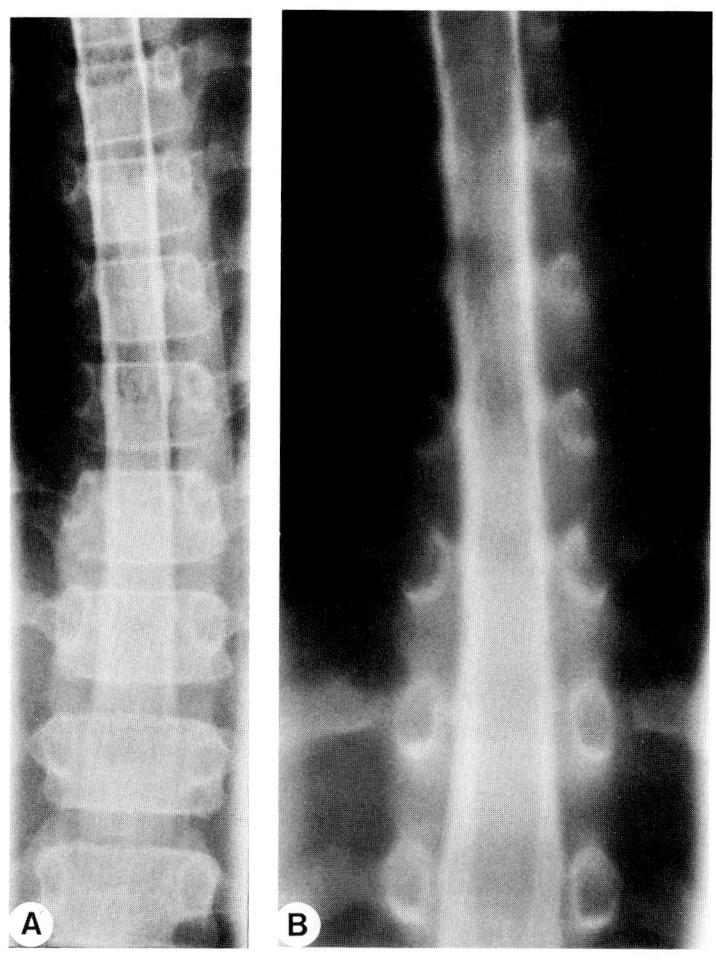

Figure 61-12. Positive contrast myelography. A. Without tomography. B. With polytomography. For many purposes the nontomographic presentation is adequate. When more details about a cord dimension and the placement of the conus medullaris are needed, multidirectional tomography is useful. The upper one quarter of the thoracic cord, seen here, is expanded by an intermedullary tumor, difficult to appreciate without polytomography.

Dysraphic states are also an obviously worthwhile area for the use of CCT. The delineation of the extent of a subcutaneous lipoma that extends intradurally and the demonstration of a diastematomyelia bony spur are suitable for CCT. Chiari malformation Type I, or the occasional acquired form, is also an intriguing possibility for this still relatively new technique. The combination of water-soluble contrast material, conventional myelographic filming, and CCT no doubt will be employed in certain circumstances.

It should be kept in mind that sometimes a simple combination of plain film and traditional myelography will handle straightforward problems, and so the overuse of certain appealing new technical advances should be avoided. Complex motion tomography (polytomography), as an addition to plain film study, has been a very useful means of clarifying the anatomy, particularly in gas myelography, but now with water-soluble myelography as well (Fig. 61-12).

Indications

Applications of myelography in patients suspected of having herniated disk disease, extradural pathology adjacent to spinal fracture, or other bony abnormality, or in those suspected of having a cord tumor, are all quite straightforward. Suspected transverse myelitis requires myelography, in most instances, for the confirmation of the diagnosis. The use of myelography in scoliosis is a little difficult to typify, except in those who, based on the character of the plain film abnormalities, particularly any spinal canal widening, are suspected of having an underlying intrathecal mass. Scoliosis of a degree that requires instrumentation also requires preoperative myelography in the view of many orthopedic surgeons. Complicated combinations of scoliosis and kyphosis are now subject to exceedingly complex orthopedic surgery to achieve normality, including anterior and posterior release of bony and soft tissue elements prior to fusion. These cases, when they contain plain film elements that are poorly understood, are reasonable subjects for myelography.

Complex kyphoscoliosis was never suitable for gas myelography and Pantopaque myelography has been very difficult to carry out in this case because of the acute bends. This is an instance in which water-soluble material with its greater penetration of the subarachnoid space has shown real value. When intradural tumor is suspected, the localization is good enough that water-soluble contrast can be directed to the proper level with safety and without dilutional problems. Tomography, preferably multidirectional or complex motion tomography, is a useful supplementary technique in further delineating the pathology in abnormal cases.

Techniques

Lumbar

The traditional technique of lumbar myelography with oily positive contrast material largely applies with a few additional notes. L3–4 is the most reliable level for the puncture, unless the pathology is suspected at that site. We prefer having the patient prone for the puncture with padding under the pelvis and abdomen to reduce the lumbar lordosis. A spinal needle of no. 22 gage or smaller should be used, with particular care directed at maintaining the midline position for the puncture, and an attempt should be made to direct the needle tip toward the midbody of the segment above the puncture site, after just having slipped under the lamina of the segment above the puncture site.

It is generally advisable to have a single coned-down lateral horizontal beam exposure when the needle is thought to be at the proper level, if there is any doubt as to its positioning. This ensures the success of the procedure and also serves as a preliminary film for both exposure factors and anatomic abnormalities. A table tilt of approximately 15 degrees with the head up is desirable both for the puncture and the initial placement of the positive contrast material. Once sufficient fluid has been removed for the requirements of laboratory study, a freshly mixed solution of water-soluble contrast material that is approximately 190 mg iodine/ml in the larger children, and down to the isosmolar solution of 170 mg iodine/ml in patients 4–5 years of age and younger, is used. When filling is seen by fluoroscopy to be progressing satisfactorily, the volume of the contrast material in the subarachnoid space is brought up to 8 cc and then an estimate is made as to how much additional volume is necessary. An application of 10 to 12 cc is typical for a mid-teenager, and complete lumbar myelography has been done in 8–10-year-olds with just 8 cc; 4 to 6 cc are used in infants over, and even less under, 6 months of age (Fig. 61-13).

Routine filming is that of a straight PA after the patient has been tilted into a more erect position for better filling of the root sleeves, and then both oblique projections and a horizontal beam lateral are used.

If there is some question about the root sleeves on a particular side, that-side-down lateral decubitus is done, sometimes followed by a delayed PA straight view, which again may have more detail because the material has had more time to invest the roots. The needle is left in place until the patient is about to be turned supine, as leak will ensue. Unless it is clearly not necessary, we

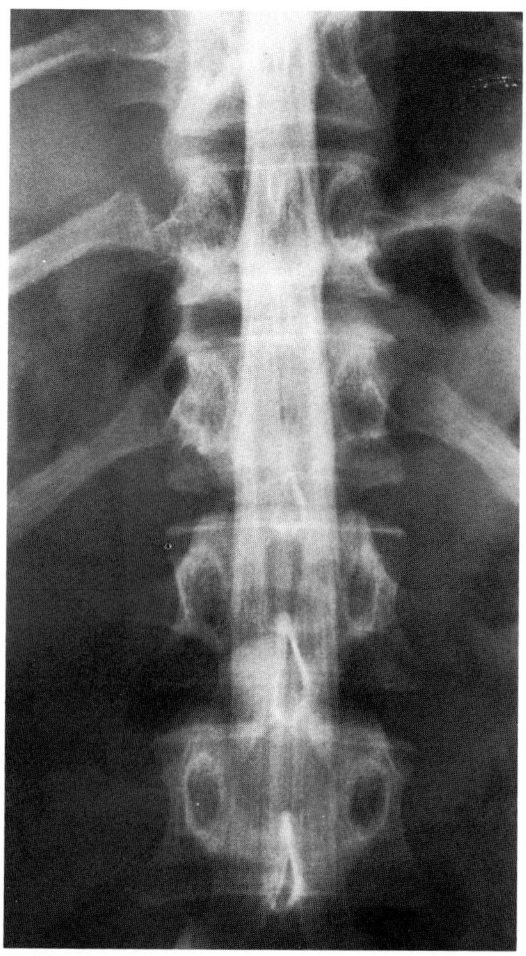

Figure 61-13. Metrizamide myelography for the lower cord and conus without tomography. This examination was done by lumbar puncture in an 18-year-old with 190 mg iodine per cubic centimeter of material. This normal conus is seen to terminate near the midportion of L1 and the lower thoracic cord is normal.

commonly take a single supine film of the lower half of the thorax and lumbar levels with the knees flexed. This gives a very good incidental low cut in the lower half of the cord, and the conus, and a final view at the lumbar root sleeves. Having the knees and hips flexed in the supine position is an important feature of successful lumbar myelography.

THORACIC MYELOGRAPHY

The thorax has been difficult to study at times with either gas or oily positive contrast material. It is generally very straightforward with water-soluble contrast material, when one uses the usual thoracic kyphosis to advantage. The material is placed in the midlumbar space as described above, with the exception of the table tilting. The table should be nearly flat and only the upper lumbar segments are opacified. Again, approximately 8 cc of material of from 170 to 190 mg iodine/ml is placed, with intermittent fluoroscopic control. With the final volume in place, the patient is tilted toward the head-down position, prone as long as a good column can be seen. PA filming must be done quickly in this situation (Fig. 61-14).

When the material is approximately halfway through the thoracic levels, the patient is placed in the lateral decubitus position, with the head and neck supported so that the upper cervical levels are higher than the upper thoracic levels to prevent significant spill of contrast material into the head.

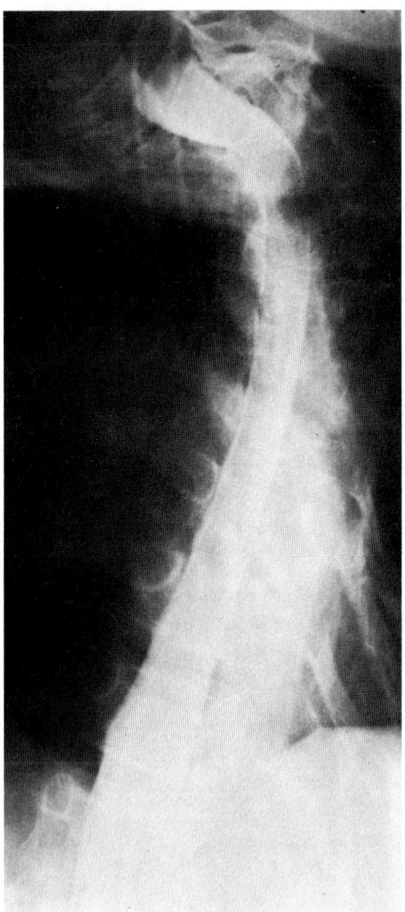

Figure 61-14. Thoracic myelography with kyphoscoliosis. This 12-year-old had myelography prior to instrumentation. The water-soluble contrast material readily demonstrates the configuration of the cord through the upper thoracic kyphoscoliosis in a much easier manner than would have been achieved with oily contrast material. Gas myelography would also not have been suitable, as the gas would have been too difficult to identify in plain film and tomography would not have been satisfactory because of the spinal canal curving in and out of the tomographic planes.

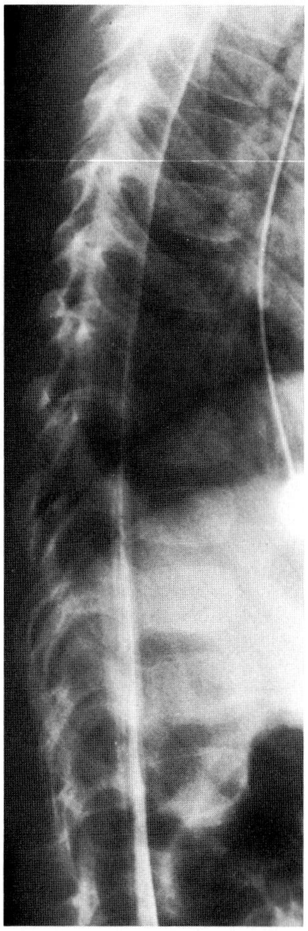

Figure 61-15. Lateral thoracic myelography with metrizamide. For general screening of the location of the anterior dural surface, the projection without tomography is quite satisfactory. Only if fine details about the dimensions of the thoracic cord were required, would polytomography need to be used. This study was done with 9 cc of the isoosmolar, 170 mg iodine/cc material by lumbar injection. The patient was 2 years and 3 months old. There was no abnormality.

With the material extending over the thoracic levels, plain lateral filming is done (Fig. 61-15). Tomography is generally not carried out in this position if the plain film examination is normal. The supine position affords trapping of the contrast material and excellent examination of thoracic subarachnoid space up to T3–4. When the upper several thoracic segments or the cervical thoracic junction are desired, this is best done, as with oily positive contrast material, by bringing the material down from the cervical region into upper thoracic levels in the prone position.

CERVICAL MYELOGRAPHY

Age is a big factor here. Up to the age of 10–12 years, the shorter vertical dimension of the spinal canal and the usually mild upper thoracic kyphosis will allow lumbar puncture for cervical studies. The material should be brought up from the lumbar needle puncture site directly to the cervical canal in the prone position. Teenagers and older patients may be best examined by C1–2 puncture with the guide of lateral horizontal beam fluoroscopy. In most departments there will be a C-arm portable unit that can be placed at the end of the myelographic table (Fig. 61-16).

The puncture is done with a no. 22 gage spinal needle. The needle is not angled but placed straight into the posterior subarachnoid space (Fig. 61-17). Careful review of the direct lateral plain film is the best guide. When the estimated sagittal C1–2 spinal canal is divided into thirds, the proper target is the middle of the posterior third.

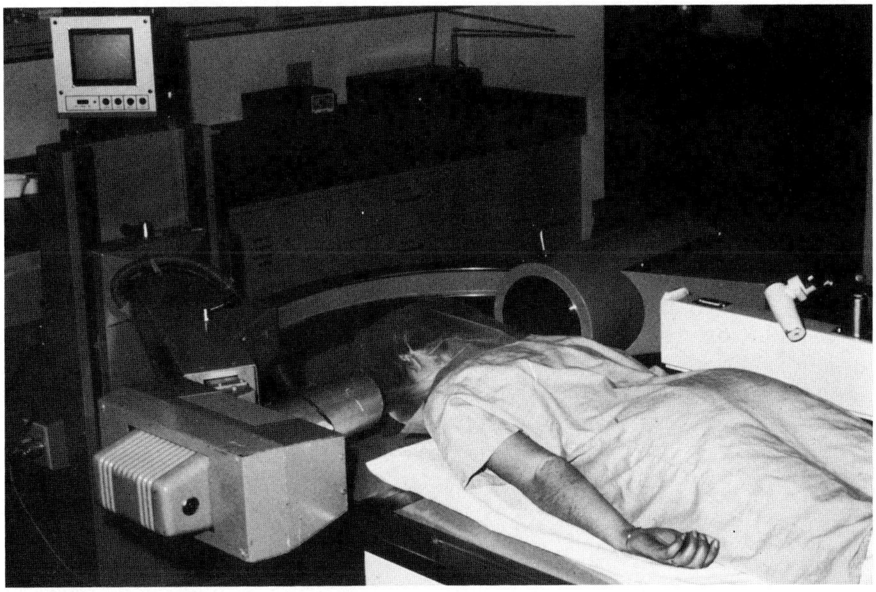

Figure 61-16. Cervical myelography: positioning for lateral C1–C2 puncture. So that the injected material will drop down into the cervical lordosis and thus be easily controlled, the patient needs to be in the prone position. Few departments have horizontal-beam lateral fluoroscopy as part of the table arrangement, so a portable "C arm" is the usual solution. In this example the portable device is placed at the end of the polytomography table. Following the completion of successful puncture, injection, and removal of the needle, the patient is pulled down into the center of the x-ray table for the regular and tomographic filming.

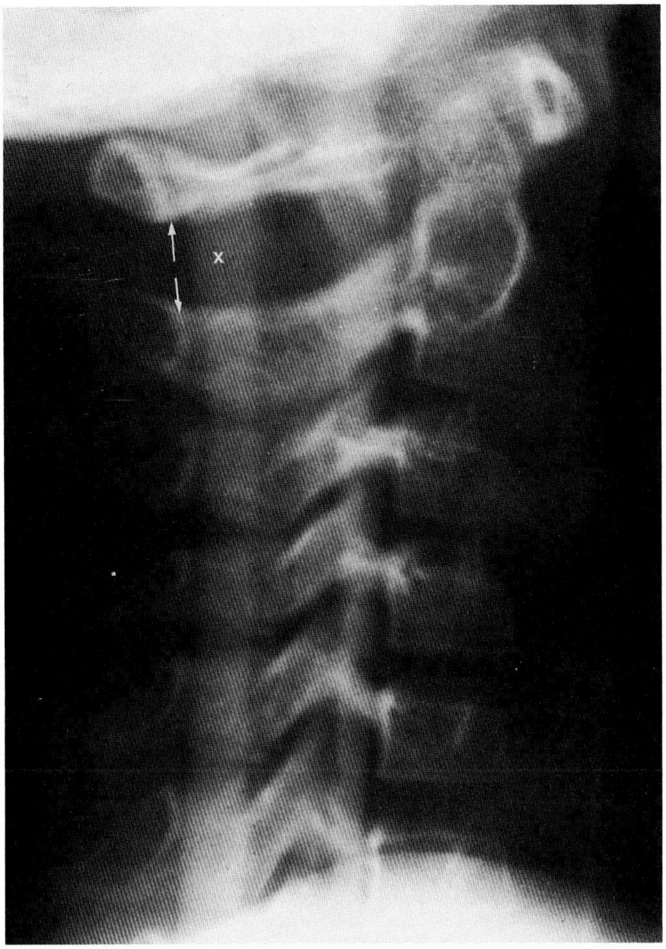

Figure 61-17. Cervical myelography with metrizamide. This material was placed by the lumbar route and tilted into the cervical level. There is very little lordotic curve in the 6-year-old and more material than is desirable drifted intracranially during the tilt. The visualization of the cervical cord, as seen, was quite satisfactory. The site for lateral C1–C2 puncture, the alternative route, is marked by the X. This site is estimated by dividing the spinal canal into thirds and puncturing near the middle of the posterior third, or alternatively 2–3 mm anterior to the posterior margin of the bony spinal canal (divergent arrows).

Alternatively the level of the dura can be predicted from viewing the posterior lamina and merely directing the needle just inside the estimated posterior dural surface. Minor changes in needle direction should be made by turning the bevel of the needle. For major alterations the needle should be withdrawn to just under the skin and a straight approach redone.

Complications from myelography by any means, but particularly by water-soluble agents, should be few, but a number of reports have appeared in the literature.[36–46] The obvious conclusion is that no agent is 100 percent safe at all dilutions, and that the prudent use of reasonably dilute solution under control conditions will result in satisfactory examinations with a very low complication rate. Though there is such a thing as legitimate complication, a significant number of complications can be traced to a breakdown in technique that includes an unnecessarily high concentration or volume of contrast material. With regard to other considerations, although most of the material already presented in this chapter is devoted to the older and more traditional procedures, the overwhelming activity at present is in the area of computed tomography. Little space is required in the consideration of techniques and complications. Anesthesia is probably not a requirement in 90 percent of the cases through infancy and childhood. Sedation in the same manner or formula as dictated by angiography should suffice (see the appendix). Although it is an exceedingly sensitive diagnostic modality CCT has varying degrees of specificity in the categories of brain tumors, enhancing lesions, and hydrocephalus.[47–49]

A prominent area of recent interest is the evaluation of neonatal intracranial hemorrhage in the mature and the premature.[50–54] This is a setting in which the evaluation of intracranial structures by ultrasound has its most obvious application.[55–56] As ultrasound has clearly improved in recent years, it would appear to be a very reasonable method for the early nursery evaluation of questions in neonatal hydrocephalus and hemorrhage. Usually more definition can then be obtained by CCT and follow-up done as a combination of ultrasound and CCT as the process is studied in resolution or progression. The advantages of the mobility of the ultrasound unit and its improving resolution will no doubt increase.

Not covered except by reference is the consideration of petrous bone tomography, particularly in the setting of trauma. The consideration of sedation in infancy and childhood is the same as that for angiography, and the filming

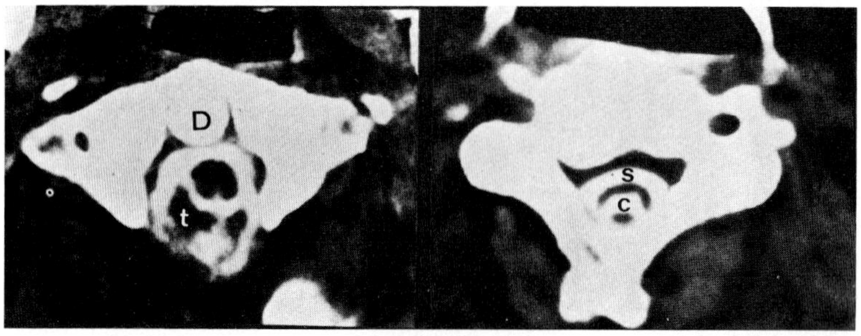

Figure 61-18. Hydromyelia by CT following ventriculography. Caudal migration of the hindbrain had been diagnosed in this 20-year-old a year earlier and decompression at the foramen magnum and posterior arch of C1 was done. Symptoms of syringomyelia ensued. The study is CT of the upper cervical spine following injection of the contrast material into a lateral ventricle. The frame on the left through the laminectomized C1 level demonstrates the low-placed tonsils (t) posterior to the upper cervical cord. The dens identifies the level (D). The frame at the right is at the C3 level demonstrating contrast material in the dilated central canal (c), the very thin spinal cord, and the subarachnoid space (s).

considerations are the same as those for adults. One change that is taking place is that a CCT probably will deplant much of the traditional use of film tomography, including multidirectional or polytomography, as the patient is evaluated for both intracranial abnormality and the possibility of petrous bone fracture.

Because of its rarity of application and because of the author's inexperience and reluctance in engaging in the activity, spinal cord angiography has not been considered in this chapter. Arteriovenous malformation is a rare condition in childhood, and when encountered the diagnostic investigation should be carried out as in adult procedures but with extreme caution. The selection for such cases prior to angiography may be screened by radionuclide studies.[62]

Computerized tomography of the spine, with and without water-soluble contrast material in the subarachnoid space, is an activity of current growth and interest. The technique is useful from the level of the foramen magnum and C1 (Fig. 61-18) to the cauda equina. Fracture of the spine that may include encroachment on the spinal canal is another example of proper utilization of CT.

REFERENCES

1. Harwood-Nash DC, Fitz CR: Neuroradiology in Infants and Childhood, vol 1. St. Louis, CV Mosby, 1976, p 1
2. Winston KR: Neurodiagnostic tests in children with brain tumors: Changing patterns of use and impact on cost. Pediatrics 61:847–852, 1978
3. Stein RL, Rosenbaum AE: Deep supratentorial veins. I. Normal deep cerebral venous system, in Newton TH, Potts DG (eds): Radiology of the Skull and Brain, vol 2, book 3. St. Louis, CV Mosby, 1974, p 1999
4. Haughton VM, Rosenbaum AE: The normal and anomalous aortic arch and brachiocephalic arteries, in Newton TH, Potts DG (eds): Radiology of the Skull and Brain, St. Louis, CV Mosby, 1974
5. Willson JKV: A new technique for cerebral angiography: The variable stiffness guidewire. Radiology 134:427–430, 1980
6. Fellows KE, Strand RD: Arteriography in children using an isocentric parallelogram. Tech Notes 128:824, 1978
7. Mishkin MM: Petechial reactions in angiography. Acta Radiol Diag 5:413–423, 1966
8. Howieson J, Megison LC Jr: Complications of vertebral artery catheterization. Radiology 91:1109-1111, 1968
9. Rosenthal A, Anderson M, Thomson SJ, et al: Superficial femoral artery catheterization: Effect on extremity length. Am J Dis Child 124:240–242, 1972
10. Mani RL, Eisenberg RL, McDonald EJ, et al: Complications of catheter cerebral arteriography: Analysis of 5,000 procedures. I. Criteria and incidence. Am J Roentgenol 131:861–865, 1978
11. Mani RL, Eisenberg RL: Complications of catheter cerebral arteriography: Analysis of 5,000 procedures. II. Relation of complication rates to clinical and arteriographic diagnoses. Am J Roentgenol 131:867–869, 1978
12. Hansen PE, Stenbjerg S: Possible increased tendency to thrombosis after cerebral angiography. Acta Neurol Scand 59:148–153, 1979
13. Huckman MS, Shenk GI, Neems RL, et al: Transfemoral cerebral arteriography versus direct percutaneous carotid and brachial arteriography: A comparison of complication rates. Radiology 132:93–97, 1979
14. Enzmann DR, Miller DC, Olcott C, et al: Carotid back pressures in conjunction with cerebral angiography. Radiology 134:415–419, 1980
15. Raimondi AJ, Samuelson GH, Yarzagaray L: Positive contrast serial ventriculography in the normal and hydrocephalic infant. Radiology 94:714, 1970
16. Strand RD, Baker RA, Ordia IJ, et al: Metrizamide ventriculography and computed tomography in lesions about the third ventricle. Radiology 128:405–410, 1978

17. Swick HM, Sty JR: Pediatric metrizamide ventriculography. Arch Neurol 37:582–584, 1980
18. Lorber J, Grainger RG: Cerebral cavities following ventricular punctures in infants. Clin Radiol 14:98–109, 1963
19. Drayer BP, Rosenbaum AE, Higman HB: Cerebrospinal fluid imaging using serial metrizamide CT cisternography. Neuroradiology 13:7–17, 1977
20. Bull J: The normal variations in the position of the optic recess of the third ventricle. Acta Radiol 46:72–80, 1956
21. Liliequist B: The subarachnoid cisterns; An anatomic and roentgenologic study. Acta Radiol Supp 185:5–108, 1959
22. DiChiro G: An Atlas of Detailed Normal Pneumoencephalographic Anatomy (ed 2). Springfield, Charles C Thomas, 1971
23. Hoare RD, Strand RD: The third ventricle in hydrocephalus due to basal cistern block. Pediatri Radiol 2:15–22, 1974
24. Hindmarsh T, Grepe A, Widen L: Metrizamide–phenothiazine interaction. Report of a case with seizures following myelography. Acta Radiol Diag 16:129–132, 1975
25. Skalpe I, Amundsen P: Thoracic and cervical myelography with metrizamide. Radiology 116:101–106, 1975
26. Grainger RG, Kendal BE, Wylie IG: Lumbar myelography with metrizamide—A new non ionic contrast medium. Br J Radiol 49:996–1003, 1976
27. Fitz CR, Harwood-Nash DC, Barry JF, et al: Pediatric myelography with metrizamide. Acta Radiol Supp 355:182–192, 1977
28. Irstam L: Lumbar myelography with Amipaque. Spine 3:70–82, 1978
29. Leo JS, Bergeron RT, Kricheff II, et al: Metrizamide myelography for cervical spinal cord injuries. Radiology 129:707–711, 1978
30. Sackett JR: Cervical and lumbar routes for metrizamide cervical examination. Neuroradiology 16:273–274, 1978
31. Kieffer SA, Binet EF, Esquerra JV, et al: Contrast agents for myelography: Clinical and radiological evaluation of amipaque and pantopaque. Radiology 129:695–705, 1978
32. Sty JR, Babbitt DP: Cervical metrizamide by lumbar puncture. Pediatr Radiol 7:133–135, 1978
33. Amundsen P, Weber H, Hoel L, et al: Excretion of metrizamide (amipaque) in humans following lumbar subarachnoid injection. Acta Radiol Diag 20:401–409, 1979
34. Scotti G, Musgrave MA, Harwood-Nash DC, et al: Diastematomyelia in children; Metrizamide and CT metrizamide myelography. Am J Neurol Radiol 1:403–410, 1980
35. Baker RA, Rosenbaum AE, Strand R: Gas myelography. Med Radiogr Photogr 53:42–60, 1977
36. Eldevik OP, Haughton VM: Risk factors in complications of aqueous myelography. Radiology 128:415–416, 1978
37. Eldevik OP, Haughton VM: The effect of hydration on the acute and chronic complications of aqueous myelography. Radiology 129:713–714, 1978
38. Bastow M, Godwin-Austen RB: Cervical myelopathy after metrizamide myelography. Br Med J 17:1262–1263, 1979
39. Hansen EB, Fahrenkrug A, Praestholm J: Late meningeal effects of myelographic contrast media with special reference to metrizamide. Br J Radiol 51:321–327, 1978
40. Laasonen EM, Servo A, Soini J, et al: A new relative contraindication for lumbar myelography. Neuroradiology 16:367–368, 1978
41. Seyfert S, Mager J: Abducens palsy after lumbar myelography with water soluble contrast media. J Neurol 219:213–220, 1978
42. King AY, Khodadad G: Intravasation of Pantopaque during myelography. Surg Neurol 11:3–4, 1979
43. Zito JL, Schellinger D: Nontraumatic intravasation of myelographic contrast medium. Am J Roentgenol 132:795–797, 1979
44. Kelley RE, Daroff RB, Sheremata WA, et al: Unusual effects of metrizamide lumbar myelography. Arch Neurol 37:588–589, 1980

45. Rolfe EB, Maguire PD: The incidence of headache following various techniques of metrizamide myelography. Br J Radiol 53:840–844, 1980
46. Paling MR, Quindlen EA, DiChiro G: Spinal seizures after metrizamide myelography in a patient with a spinal block. Am J Neurol Radiol 1:473–474, 1980
47. Butler AR, Horii SC, Kricheff II, Shannon MB, et al: Computed tomography in astrocytomas. Radiology 129:433–439, 1978
48. Norman D, Stevens EA, Wing SD, et al: Quantitative aspects of contrast enhancement in cranial computed tomography. Radiology 129:683–688, 1978
49. Robertson WC Jr, Gomez MR: External hydrocephalus. Early finding in congenital communicating hydrocephalus. Arch Neurol 35:541–544, 1978
50. Krishnamoorthy KS, Fernandez RA, Momose KJ: Evaluation of neonatal intracranial hemorrhage by computerized tomography. Pediatrics 59:165–172, 1977
51. Donat JF: Intraventricular hemorrhage in full-term and premature infants. Mayo Clinic Proc 7:437–441, 1978
52. Volpe JJ: Neonatal intracranial hemorrhage; Pathophysiology, neuropathology, and clinical features. Clin Perinatol 4:77–102, 1977
53. Volpe JJ: Neonatal periventricular hemorrhage: Past, present, and future. J Pediatr 92:693–696, 1978
54. Pape K, Wigglesworth JS: Clinical aspects of intraventricular hemorrhage, in Clinics in Developmental Medicine no 69/70, 1979, p 149
55. Lees RF, Harrison RB, Sims TL: Gray scale ultrasonography in the evaluation of hydrocephalus and associated abnormalities in infants. Am J Dis Child 132:376–378, 1978
56. Johnson ML, Rumack CM: Ultrasonic evaluation of the neonatal brain. Radiol Clin N Am 18:117–131, 1980
57. Kaseff LG: Tomographic evaluation of trauma to the temporal bone. Radiology 93:321–327, 1969
58. Harwood-Nash DC: Fractures of the petrous bone in children; A tomographic study of 35 cases. Am J Roentgenol Radium Ther Nucl Med 110:598–607, 1970
59. Tos M: Course of the sequelae to 248 petrosal fractures. Acta Otolaryngol 75:353–354, 1973
60. Fitz CR, Harwood-Nash DC: Radiology of the ear in children. Radiol Clin N Am 12:553–570, 1974
61. Wright JW Jr: Trauma of the ear. Radiol Clin N Am 12:527–532, 1974
62. Obayashi T, Furuse M, Nakama M: Radionuclide angiography of vascular lesions of the spinal cord. Arch Neurol 37:572–574, 1980

APPENDIX: PREMEDICATION, SEDATION, AND ANESTHESIA

For CCT, spinal CT, angiography, ventriculography, and polytomography, general anesthesia, in our opinion, is rarely required. The exceptions are in the profoundly retarded, and in patients with severe behavior disorders and special requests. When anesthesia is not being employed, the guidelines cited below are followed.

Preparation

Hydration is promoted, particularly during infancy. Infants are held NPO for two hours prior to any study that may include contrast material injections. Older children are held NPO for four to six hours, depending on age.

Sedation

For infants under 1 year of age, morphine sulfate, IM, at the rate of *0.1*–0.2 mg/kg is used.

For all children over 1 year of age, a Demerol Compound is used at a rate of 1 cc/15 kg, and fractions thereof, with a maximum of 2 cc. Demerol Compound is prepared beforehand in the hospital pharmacy by the following formula. Each cubic centimeter contains 25 mg meperidine (Demerol), 6.25 mg chlorpromazine (Thorazine), and 6.25 mg promethazine (Phenergan).

When the foregoing fails to sedate the patient in 45–60 minutes, chloral hydrate, by mouth, is added, at a rate of 30 mg/kg. When chloral hydrate is considered as the only form of sedation, the dose is 40 to 50 mg/kg. Chloral hydrate is very useful as a supplement or as the primary agent when injection is refused or regarded as probably unnecessary.

Plain morphine is proposed in the first year of life because it is reversible with naloxone (Narcan®—1000 Stewart Avenue, Garden City, New York, 11530). Narcan® is effective in reversing Demerol Compound as well.

When an anesthetist or anesthesiologist is available, a mixture of low-dose combination morphine and Valium intravenously can be useful in patients who have a history of being refractory to prior attempts at sedation.

The use, dosage, and control of ketamine (Ketalar®—Parke-Davis, 201 Tabor Road, Morris Plains, New Jersey, 07950), methohexital (Breuital®—Eli Lilly and Company, 307 East McCarty, P.O. Box 618, 46206, Indianapolis, Indiana, 46225), and other fast-acting agents should be in the hands of an anesthesiologist. The determination of the details of intubation anesthesia is also clearly up to the habits, bias, and policy of each anesthesia department.

General anesthesia is advocated for pneumoencephalography through all pediatric ages. Myelography is better done with anesthesia up to the age of 8 to 11 years, depending on the patient and the anticipated morbidity of the myelography planned.

62. Ultrasonography of the Head

Diane S. Babcock
Bokyung K. Han

The history of sonography in neuroradiology goes back to 1956 when Leksell[1] described the use of A-mode or one-dimensional ultrasonography for cranial imaging and recommended its use to determine the position of the midline of the brain. B-mode or two-dimensional ultrasonography was developed in the middle 1950s, but while the potential usefulness of B-mode ultrasonography for examining the infant's head was demonstrated in images published as early as 1973, it was not until the late 1970s, when technical advances in ultrasound equipment resulted in high-quality gray scale images, that enthusiasm for the technique developed.

Diagnostic ultrasonography is an imaging modality that uses high-frequency sound waves beyond the audible range of the human ear to visualize structures within the body. The sound waves are produced in the transducer by the piezoelectric effect, and are projected into the patient's body and the returning sound waves or echoes are picked up by the transducer and then converted into an image on an oscilloscope screen.[2] The intensity of the returning echo is determined by the type of tissue being scanned. The ultrasound beam is partially attenuated by bone because of the strong interface between the soft tissue and the bone, but the infant skull is thinner and contains less organic material, and the infant has openings in the calvarium (sutures and fontanels) allowing access to the brain.

The indications for head ultrasonography in infants include increased head size, seizures, abnormal neurologic examination, apnea, screening of premature infants at risk for intracranial hemorrhage, meningitis not responding to therapy, congenital anomalies associated with known brain anomalies such as patients with meningomyelocele or facial cleft defects, and trauma.

INSTRUMENTATION AND SEDATION

Three basic types of ultrasound equipment are currently used for head scanning: contact scanners, real-time scanners, and automated water-delay scanners. With contact scanning the transducer is manually moved over the baby's head, producing the image (Fig. 62-1). Optimal resolution and panoramic images of the entire head can be obtained with this type of scanner. Disadvantages include nonportability, the longer time necessary for performing an examination, and, the fact that more technical expertise and experience are required. Real-time scanners allow dynamic presentation of sequential images, at frame rates of up to 60 per second, which results in a movie of structures as they change position with time. In real time the ultrasound beam is moved in space, either mechanically or electronically, producing automated imaging that is largely independent of the manual skill of the sonographer. The resolution, though adequate, is not as good as can be seen with current contact scanners. In addition the image produces an incomplete sector of a portion of the head and those observers not familiar with the anatomy find the images more difficult to understand. The advantage of real time is that most machines are portable and can be taken to the intensive care unit and the baby scanned in the incubator. This is particularly important with unstable premature infants. The automated water-delay scanners have an array of transducers in a water bath. The patient lies on a plastic membrane covering a water tank. This technique has advantages in that generally infants or small children are lulled to sleep on the warm water bed and require no sedation. Panoramic images of the entire head comparable to those obtained with computerized tomography (CT) are obtained. The resolution with the current equipment, however, is somewhat less than that possible with contact scanners using higher frequency transducers. Also, this equipment is significantly more expensive than other types of ultrasound equipment.

Sedation is not usually necessary with real-time scanning or water-delay scanning. With contact scanning infants between 3 months and 3 years of age

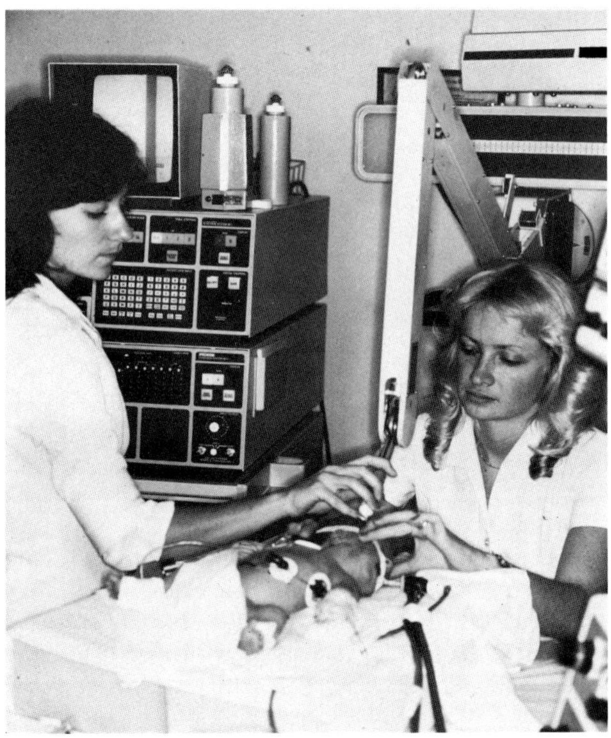

Figure 62-1. Sonographer scanning baby's head with contact scanner. Transducer manually moved over baby's head, producing image. Sector scans performed through open sutures and fontanel. (Reproduced with permission from Babcock DS, Han BK: Cranial Ultrasonography of Infants (ed 1). Baltimore, Williams & Wilkins, 1981.)

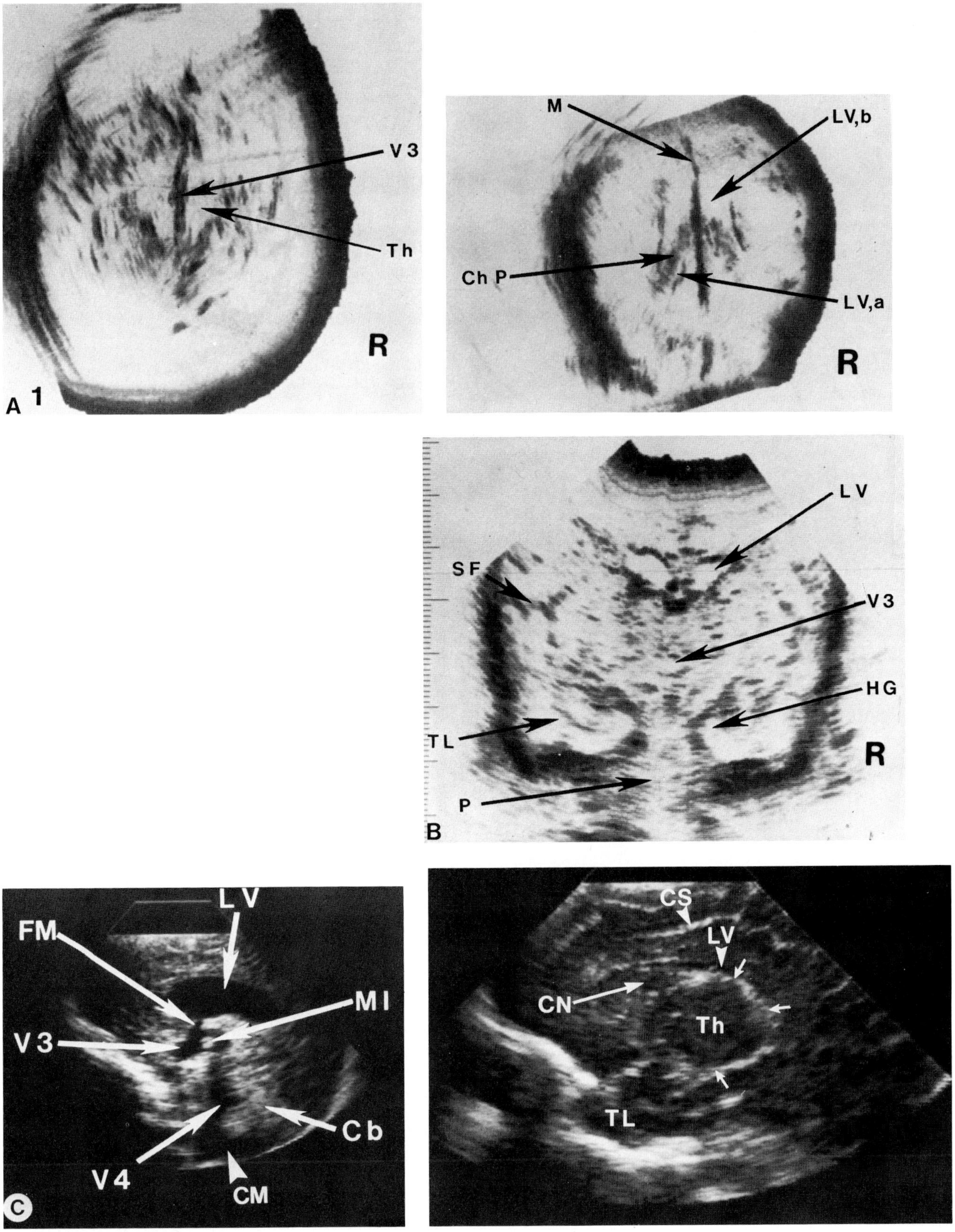

Figure 62-2. See legend on page 710.

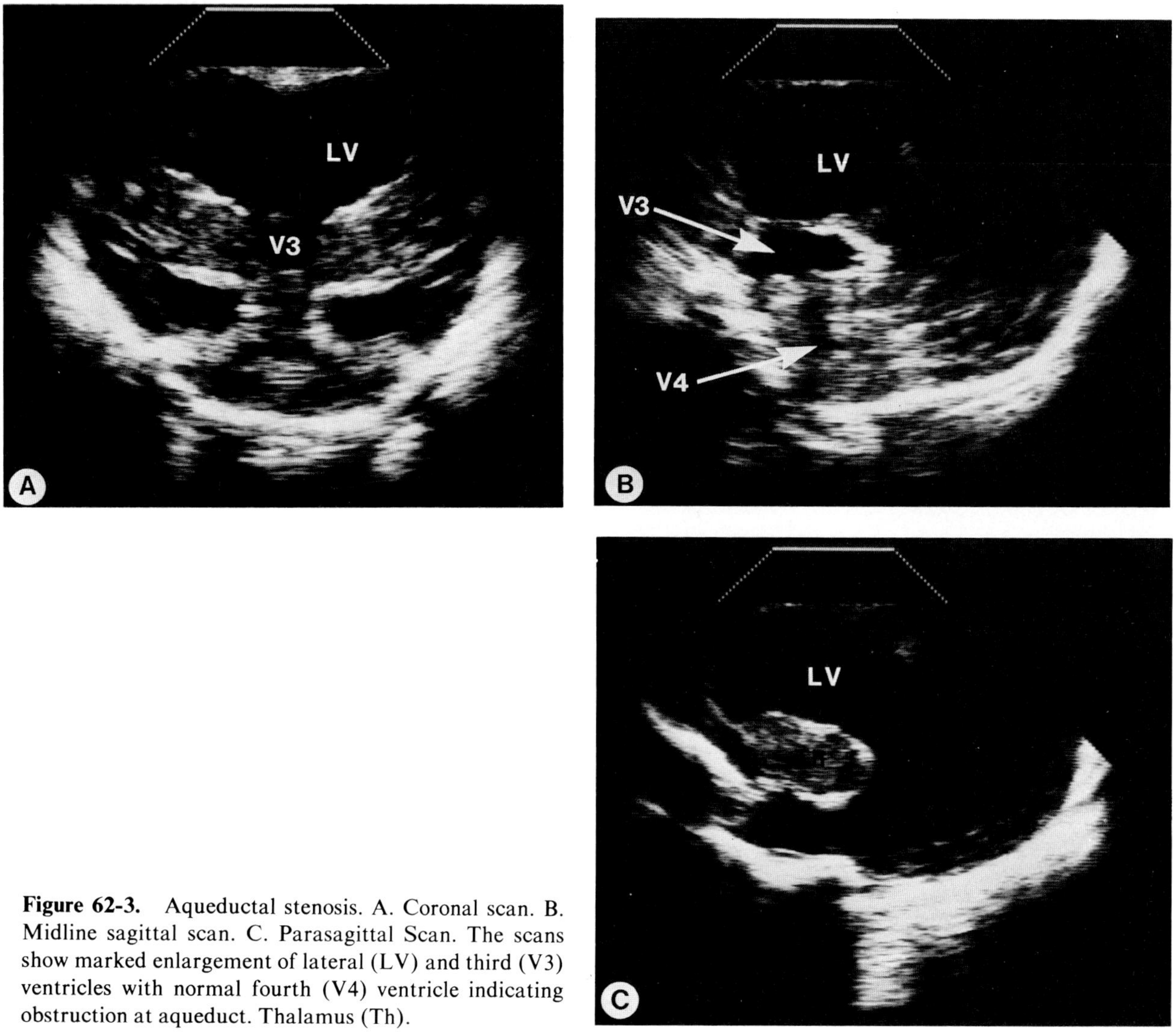

Figure 62-3. Aqueductal stenosis. A. Coronal scan. B. Midline sagittal scan. C. Parasagittal Scan. The scans show marked enlargement of lateral (LV) and third (V3) ventricles with normal fourth (V4) ventricle indicating obstruction at aqueduct. Thalamus (Th).

Figure 62-2. Normal head scan. A. Axial scan: left shows through level of third ventricle (V3) and thalamus (Th), and right shows at level of bodies (LV,b) and atria (LV,a) of lateral ventricles. Midline strong linear echoes represent falx cerebri and septum pellucidum (M). Choroid plexuses (ChP) seen as echogenic structures in floor of lateral ventricles. B. Coronal scan through lateral (LV) and third (V3) ventricles. Temporal lobes (TL) with most medial gyrus, hippocampal gyrus (HG), pons and midbrain (P) inferior. Sylvian fissure (SF). (Case with mild hydrocephalus). C. Sagittal scan: left shows sector real-time midline sagittal scan. Third ventricle (V3). Portion of slightly dilated lateral ventricle (LV). Massa intermedia (MI) seen as dot in third ventricle. Foramen of Monro (FM) connects third ventricle to lateral ventricle. Fourth ventricle (V4) demonstrated inferiorly with echogenic cerebellum (Cb) forming roof. Cisterna magna (CM) seen as sonolucent space inferior to cerebellum. Right shows sector real-time parasagittal scan through lateral ventricle with choroid plexus (arrows) beginning at foramen of Monro and coursing along floor of lateral ventricle into atrium and temporal horn. Moderately echogenic head of caudate nucleus (CN) lies inferior to frontal horn of lateral ventricle and anterosuperior to thalamus (Th). Thalamus (Th) lies inferior to body of lateral ventricle (LV). Temporal lobe (TL). Cingulate sulci (CS). A and B are reproduced with permission from Babcock DS, Han BK, LeQuesne GW: B-mode gray scale ultrasound of the head in the newborn and young infant. Am J Roentgenol 134:457–468, 1980. C is reproduced with permission from Babcock DS, Han BK: The accuracy of high resolution, real-time ultrasonography of the head in infancy. Radiology 139:665–676, 1981.)

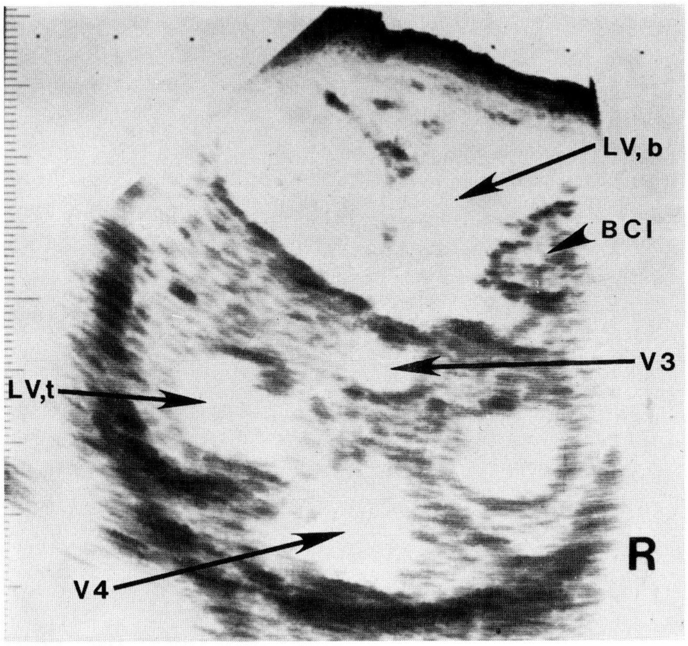

Figure 62-4. Communicating hydrocephalus secondary to intraventricular hemorrhage. The 60-degree coronal scan shows moderate enlargement of all ventricles. Body (LV,b), and temporal horn (LV,t) of lateral ventricle. Third ventricle (V3). Fourth ventricle (V4). Blood clot from previous intraventricular hemorrhage (BC1) seen within right lateral ventricle. (Reproduced with permission from Babcock DS, Han BK, LeQuesne GW: B-mode gray scale ultrasound of the head in the newborn and young infant. Am J Roentgenol 134:457–468, 1980.)

frequently require sedation and we routinely use chloral hydrate in an oral dose of 50 mg/kg. Other patients can be examined using immobilization, such as wrapping the infant in a sheet, placing sandbags on the legs, and having a helper hold the infant's head in place.

NORMAL ANATOMY

The patients are routinely scanned in several projections including axial, coronal, and sagittal views. Representative scans showing normal anatomy in these planes are seen in Figure 62-2. The walls of the ventricles are easily seen because of their strong reflective surfaces. More subtle differences in the echogenicity of various anatomic structures within the brain parenchyma allow identification of these structures.

HYDROCEPHALUS

Ultrasonography is highly sensitive for detection of even mild degrees of hydrocephalus[3] and is the procedure of choice to determine the presence or absence of a dilated ventricular system in an infant. The type of hydrocephalus (communicating or noncommunicating), as well as the etiology, often can be determined by sonography. With hydrocephalus secondary to aqueductal stenosis, the lateral and third ventricles are dilated, whereas the fourth ventricle is normal in size (Fig. 62-3). With communicating hydrocephalus such as occurs in premature infants as a sequelae of intraventricular hemorrhage, there is enlargement of all the ventricles (Fig. 62-4). Clotted blood frequently can be demonstrated in the ventricles as well.

Ultrasonography has proved useful in evaluating for possible shunt malfunction, particularly when shunted infants present with nonspecific symptoms,

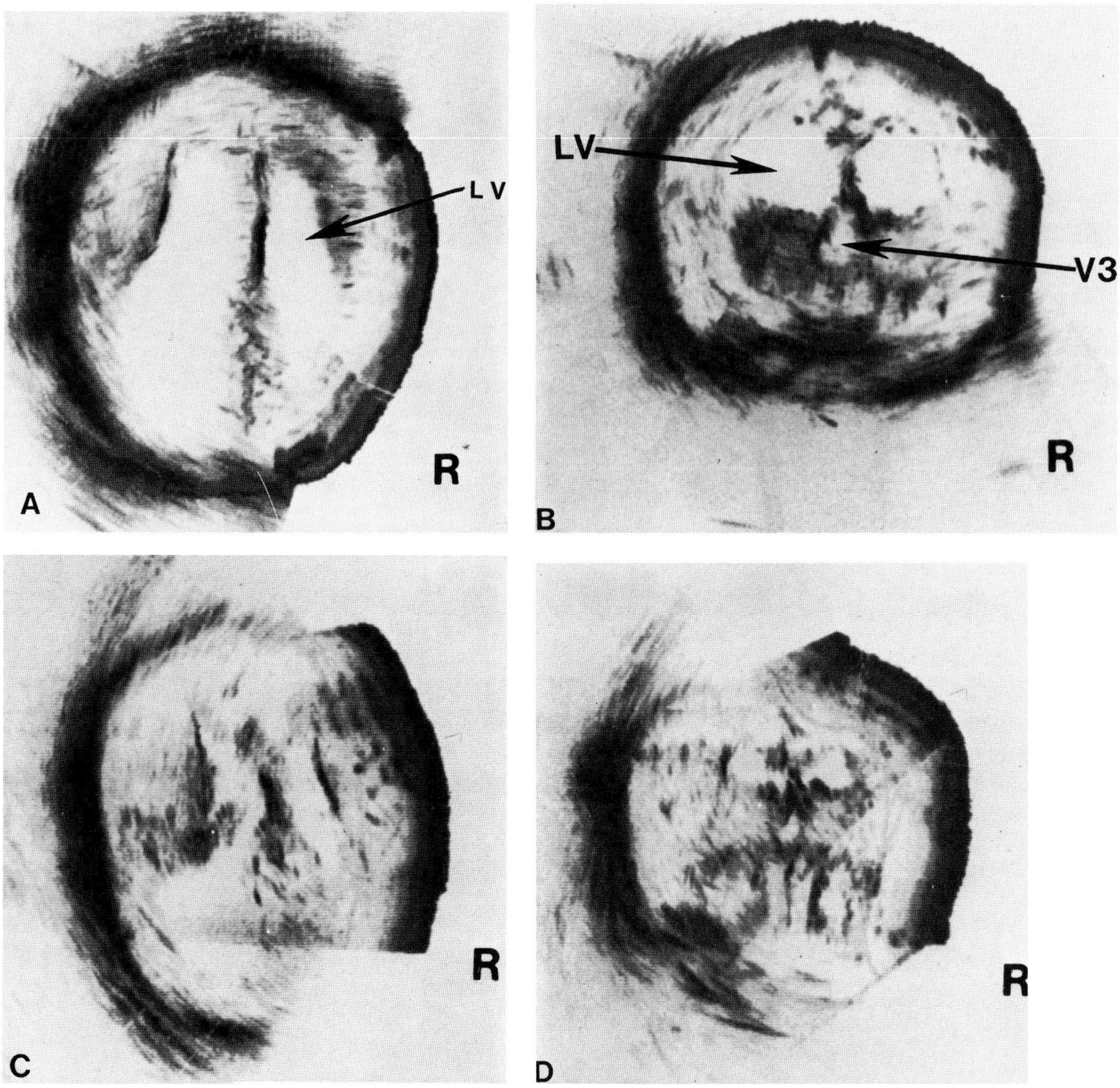

Figure 62-5. Ventricular shunt function. A 37-week-old gestation newborn with meningomyelocele and mild head enlargement. A. Axial scan at age 2 days. B. Coronal scan at age 2 days. These scans show moderate-to-severe dilatation of lateral (LV) and third (V3) ventricles with rounding of ventricular angles. Atria and occipital horns dilated more than frontal horns. C, D. Follow-up examination nine days later after temporary ventricular shunt. Lateral and third ventricles diminished, although still mildly enlarged. Ventricular angles less rounded. E, F. Two-week follow-up for increasing head size. Increased ventricular size and rounded ventricular angles shown indicating shunt (S) malfunction. Malfunctioning shunt was replaced. G, H. Postoperative examination one month later. Ventricles collapsed and slit-like. (Reproduced with permission from Babcock, DS, Han BK, LeQuesne GW: B-mode gray scale ultrasound of the head in the newborn and young infant. Am J Roentgenol 134:457–468, 1980.)

such as irritability, and the clinician cannot readily differentiate between shunt malfunction and other diseases of childhood. After ventricular shunting the ventricles decrease in size and the angles become less rounded, although they may not return to normal size. The ultrasound examination in the case of shunt malfunction will demonstrate increasing ventricular size and aid in making a proper diagnosis (Fig. 62-5).

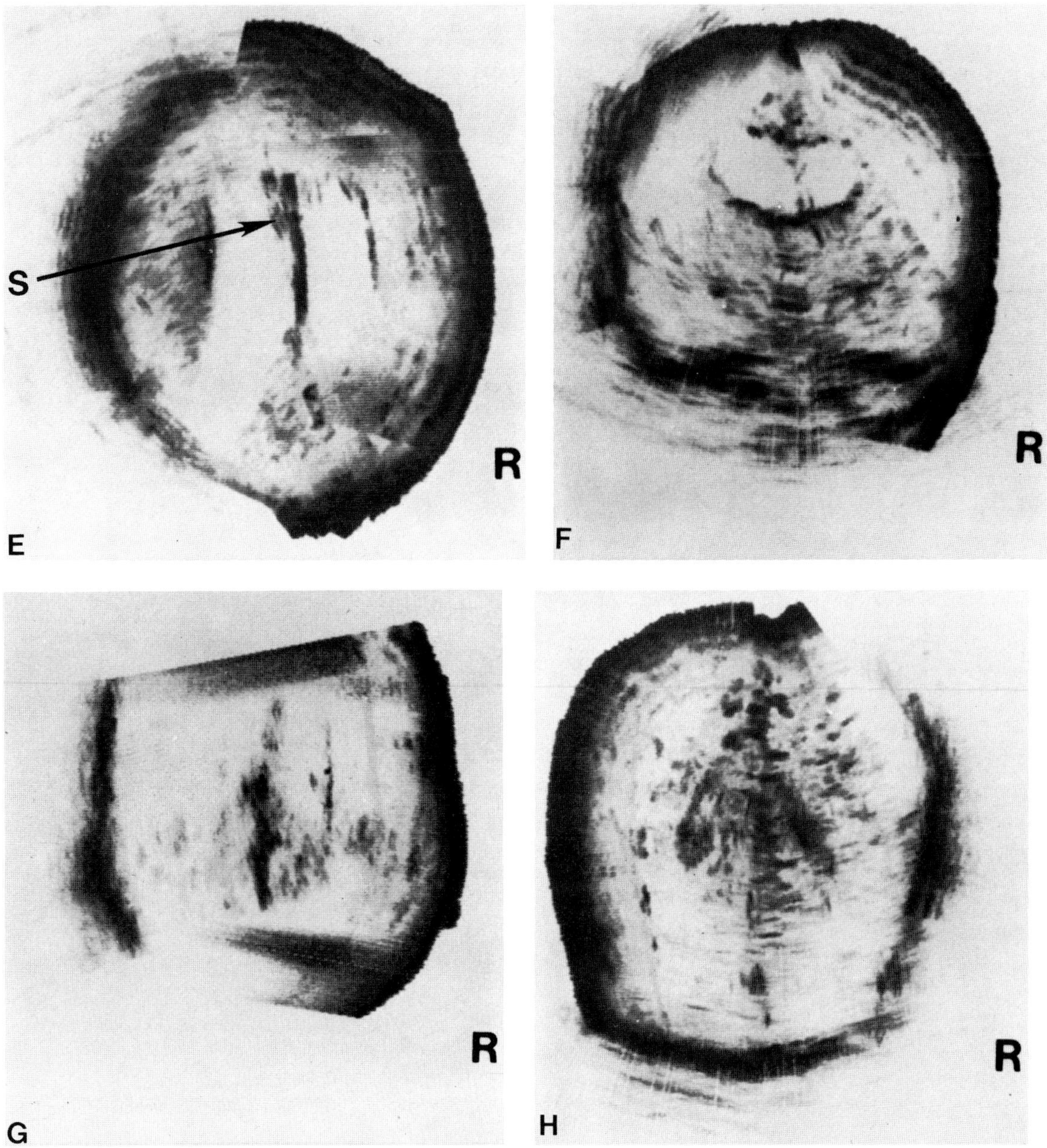

CONGENITAL ANOMALIES

Ultrasonography has proved useful in evaluating congenital malformations of the brain that have altered macroscopic morphology. Cystic malformations are particularly well demonstrated by ultrasonography because of the impedance mismatch between the brain and fluid.

Ultrasonography of a Dandy–Walker cyst demonstrates (Fig. 62-6) a large posterior fossa cyst continuous with a dilated fourth ventricle. The cerebellum is small and displaced anterolaterally. The lateral and third ventricles may be dilated to varying degrees and the occipital horns of the lateral ventricle show a typical divergence due to displacement by the posterior fossa cyst and elevated tentorium. The differential diagnosis would include a posterior fossa arachnoid cyst that could look very similar but does not communicate with the fourth ventricle. Cranial computed tomography, (CCT) or contrast material injection is sometimes necessary to differentiate between these two.

Meningomyelocele patients with the Chiari II malformation show a variety of findings that can be demonstrated on cranial ultrasonography.[4] Ventricular enlargement of varying degrees occurs in these infants. There is a characteristic anterior pointing and medial convexity of the frontal horns of the lateral ventricle on axial view and inferior pointing on the coronal view resulting from prominence of the caudate nuclei that bulge medially into the lateral walls of the lateral ventricles. The septum pellucidum is frequently absent. The massa intermedia is often prominent. The posterior fossa is relatively small and the tentorium cerebelli appears relatively low in position.

Other anomalies such as hydrancephaly, porencephalic cyst, encysted ventricles, agenesis of the corpus callosum, holoprosencephaly, and arteriovenous malformations have been demonstrated by ultrasound.[5]

CRANIAL HEMORRHAGE

Craniocerebral hemorrhage is a relatively common problem in infancy and accounts for a large percentage of cranial sonograms at our institution. It may occur as a result of trauma, spontaneously in normal infants or infants with bleeding diathesis, or in premature infants for as yet incompletely understood reasons.

Hemorrhage into the brain parenchyma and into the ventricles occurs particularly in premature infants of less than 32 weeks' gestation and is a common central nervous system abnormality in neonatal autopsies. Recent

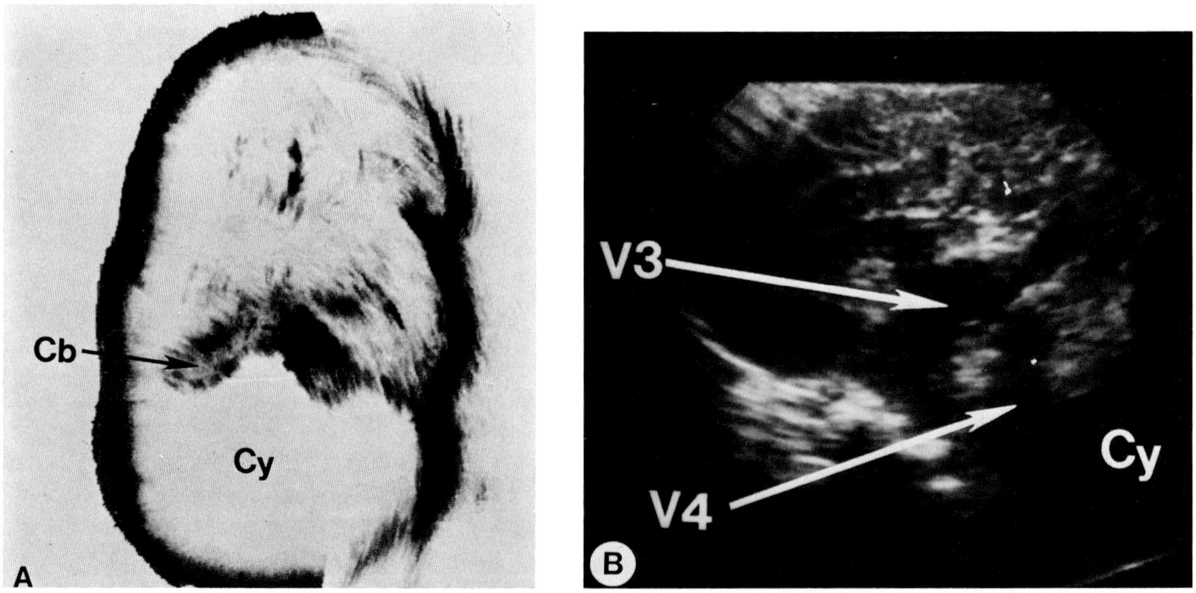

Figure 62-6. Dandy–Walker cyst (unproven). Two-day-old infant with dysmorphic features and increasing head size with prominent fontanels. A. Axial scan. B. Sagittal scan. These scans show large cyst (Cy) in posterior fossa tapering anteriorly into fourth ventricle (V4). Hypoplastic cerebellum (Cb) seen laterally and anteriorly. Slight dilatation of lateral (not shown) and third ventricles (V3) present. (A is reproduced with permission from Swischuk LE: Radiology of the Newborn and Young Infant (ed 2). Baltimore, Williams and Wilkins, 1980, p 771. B is reproduced with permission from Babcock DS, Han BK: The accuracy of high resolution, real-time ultrasonography of the head in infancy. Radiology 139:665–676, 1981.)

studies using CT and ultrasonography prospectively to evaluate this problem have shown an incidence of 40 to 60 percent in this group.[6] The hemorrhage usually originates in the subependymal germinal matrix in the caudathalamic groove. The germinal matrix is largest at 24 to 32 weeks' gestation and then involutes so that it is virtually absent in the full-term infant.[7] Currently there are much interest and research on the pathogenesis, etiologic factors, and treatment of this problem. The prospective studies have shown that clinical methods are inaccurate and underestimate the incidence. Cranial CT and ultrasonography

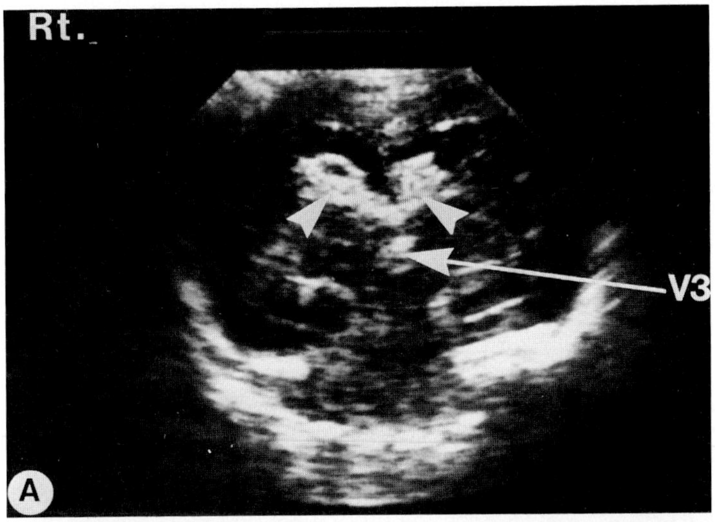

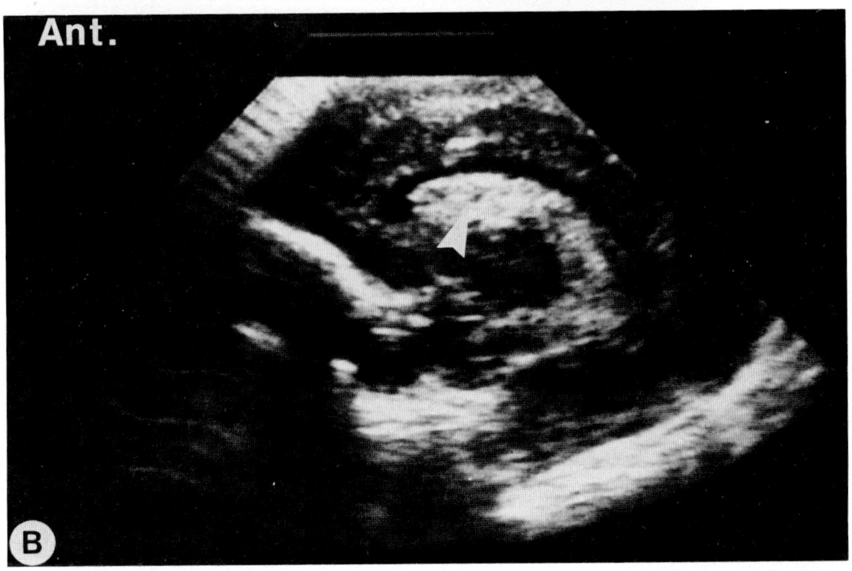

Figure 62-7 *(continued on page 716).* Subependymal hemorrhage with slight intraventricular extension. Infant weighing 1500 grams, 30 weeks' gestation, with respiratory distress syndrome and seizures. A. Coronal scan. B. Sagittal scan. These scans show bilateral small subependymal hemorrhages (arrowheads) in the region of heads of caudate nuclei. Mild ventricular dilatation and echogenic cast clots within lateral and third ventricles (V3) represent intraventricular extension. C. Brain section shows intraventricular hemorrhage with bilateral asymmetric subependymal hemorrhage (arrowheads) and subarachnoid hemorrhage (open arrows.) (Reproduced with permission from Babcock DS, Han BK: Cranial Ultrasonography of Infants (ed 1). Baltimore, Williams & Wilkins, 1981, 210–211.)

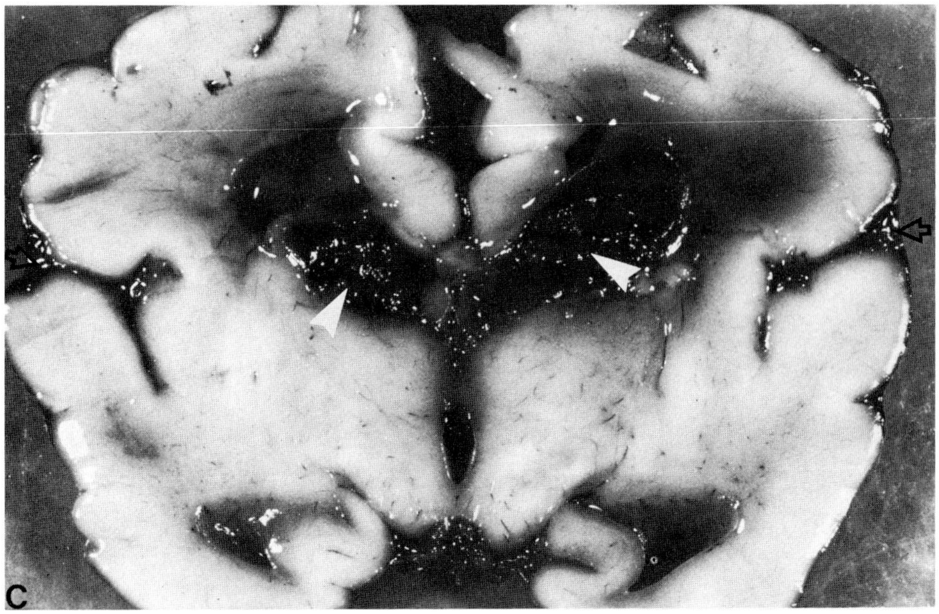

have proved accurate for diagnosing intracranial hemorrhage. Ultrasound has advantages over CT in that it uses nonionizing radiation, it can be performed portably in the incubator in the intensive care unit with the newer real-time equipment, and the examination is less expensive.

Subependymal hemorrhage is seen on ultrasonography as an area of increased echogenicity in the wall of the lateral ventricle, most frequently in the region of the head of the caudate nucleus (Fig. 62-7). The diagnosis of intraventricular extension of the hemorrhage through the ependymal lining can be made when echogenic clot is seen within the ventricles. The ventricles frequently enlarge and are seen as fluid-filled or echogenic clot-filled, rounded structures. The ventricular dilatation may be mild, moderate, or marked, and remain stable, regress, or progress with time and require permanent ventricular shunting. With intraparenchymal extension of the hemorrhage, an area of increased echoes is seen not only in the immediate periventricular germinal matrix region, but extending diffusely into the brain parenchyma—the cerebral hemispheres or basal ganglia (Fig. 62-8). Over a several-week period, the echogenic intraparenchymal hemorrhage becomes partially anechoic with liquification and retraction of the clot and eventual cavitation of that portion of the brain resulting in porencephaly.

Ultrasonography has proved useful for the diagnosis and follow-up of intracranial hemorrhage and its sequelae, particularly in premature infants. It has become a routine part of patient care in these infants.

INTRACRANIAL TUMORS

Ultrasonography can be used as a screening procedure in infants with neurologic abnormalities, including suspected tumors. The echogenicity of the tumor is frequently different than that of the normal brain tissue and its mass effect on normal structures, with resulting hydrocephalus, can be demonstrated (Fig. 62-9). Further investigation with CT and angiography is usually necessary for a more specific diagnosis.

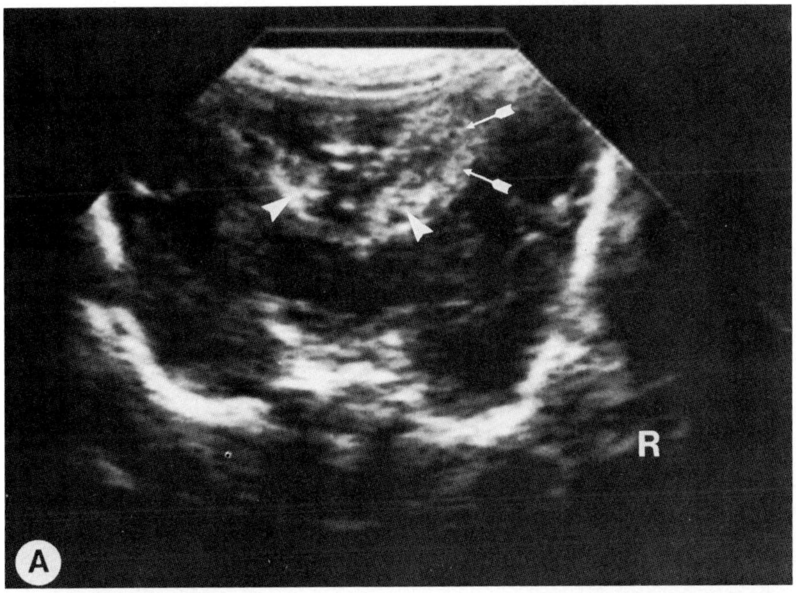

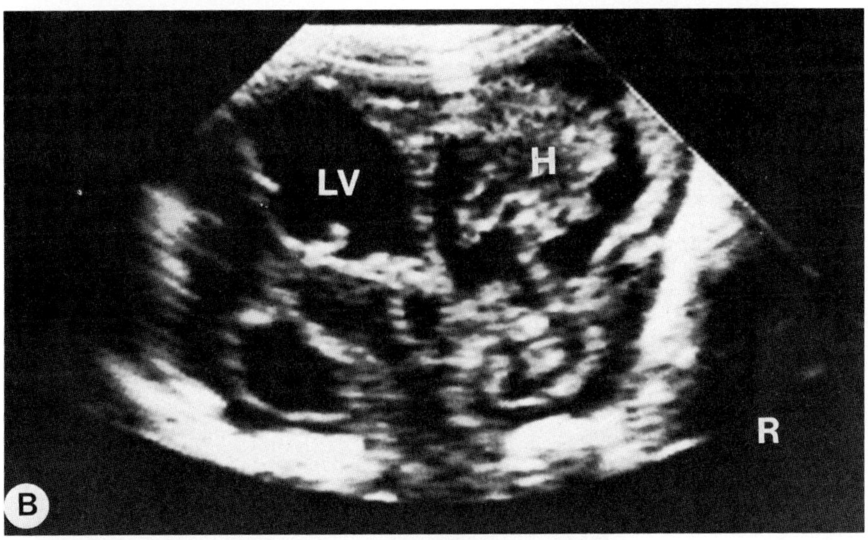

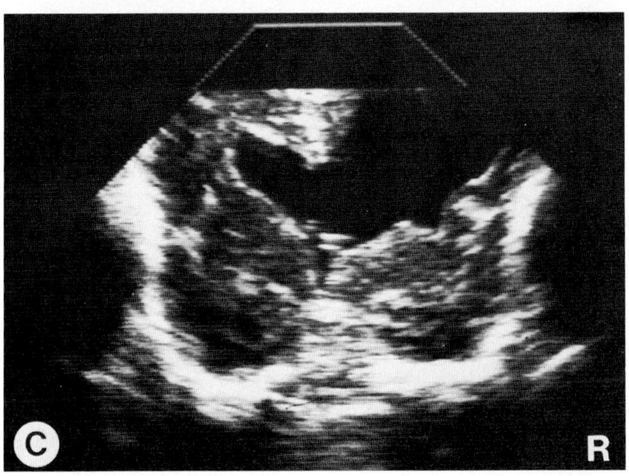

Figure 62-8. Subependymal, intraventricular, and intraparenchymal hemorrhage with secondary porencephaly. A 1020-gram 27-week-gestation infant with full fontanel and metabolic acidosis. A. Coronal scan on first day of life shows bilateral small subependymal hemorrhages (arrowheads) with slight parenchymal extension (arrows) on right. B. Three weeks later, coronal scan. Periventricular parenchymal hematoma (H) sloughed off into ventricle, which results in porencephalic dilatation of right lateral ventricle (LV). Ventricles moderately enlarged. C. Coronal scan, four months later. Hematoma liquified and absorbed resulting in porencephaly. (Reproduced with permission from Babcock DS, Han BK: Cranial Ultrasonography of Infants (ed 1). Baltimore, Williams & Wilkins, 1981, pp 220–221.)

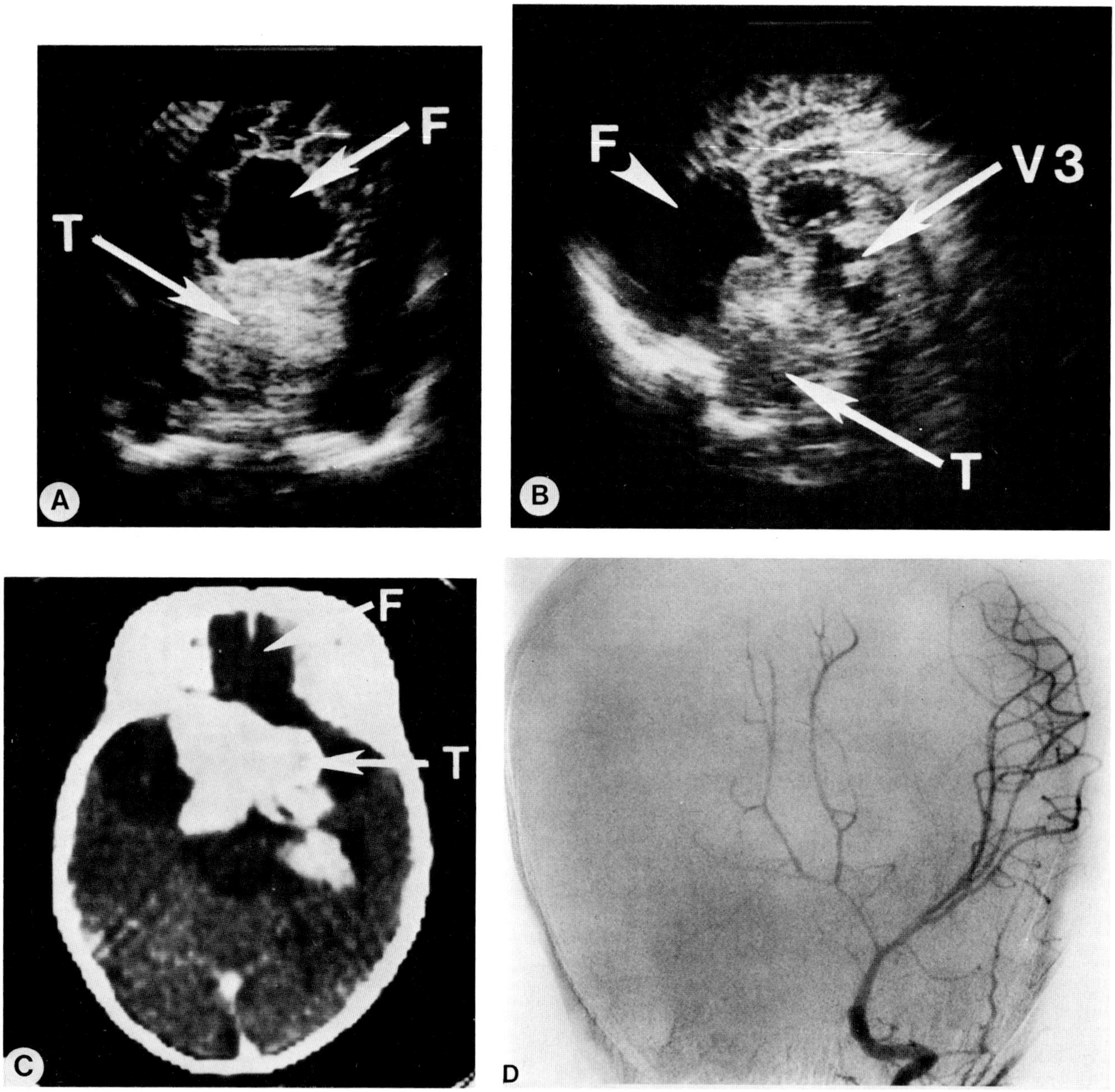

Figure 62-9. Chiasmatic astrocytoma. Six-month-old infant with macrocrania and searching nystagmus. A. Coronal scan. B. Sagittal scan. Third ventricle (V3) is displaced superiorly and posteriorly by suprasellar tumor (T) and loculated fluid collection (F) between frontal lobes. C. CT scan shows enhancing tumor in chiasmatic hypothalamic/thalamic region with fluid (F) in interhemispheric fissure between frontal lobes and under tip of both temporal lobes. D. Brain angiography shows slightly vascular mass with vessel displacement. Biopsy proved pilocytic astrocytoma with secondary pseudocyst. (Reproduced with permission from Babcock DS, Han BK: The accuracy of high resolution, real-time ultrasonography of the head in infancy. Radiology 139:665–676, 1981.)

INTRAOPERATIVE USES OF ULTRASOUND

With the development of high-resolution real-time scanners, ultrasonography can now be used portably in the operating room to aid in neurosurgical procedures. Sterile coverings are available for the transducers allowing direct scanning of the brain or the anterior fontanel can be used as a window to observe the intracranial contents as a shunt catheter or needle is inserted through a burr

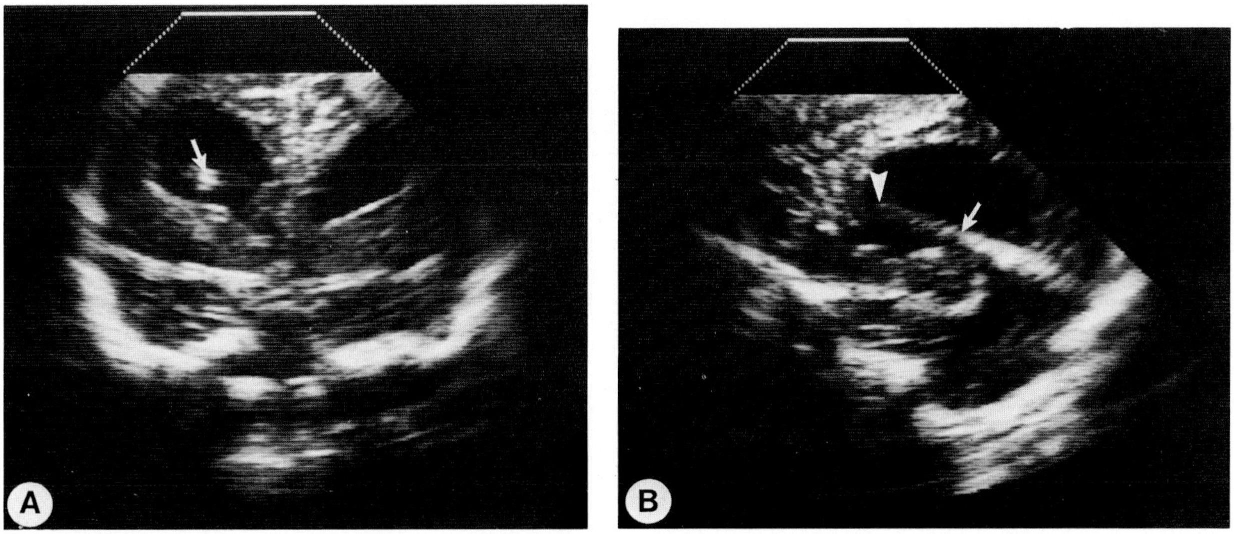

Figure 62-10. Intraoperative real-time ultrasound for shunt placement. A. Coronal scan. B. Sagittal scan. Scans show moderately dilated lateral ventricles. Shunt tube (arrows) seen in right lateral ventricle. Shunt tip indicated (arrowhead).

hole in a remote site. Ultrasonography has been used to monitor the placement of ventricular shunt catheters (Fig. 62-10). It has also been used for the localization of tumors for needle biopsy and as an aid in the aspiration of intracranial cysts and abscesses.

CONCLUSIONS

Ultrasonography has proved useful for diagnosing and following a variety of abnormalities of the brain of infants. It has advantages over other modalities such as angiography, CCT, and pneumoencephalography in that it is noninvasive, frequently requires no sedation, can be performed portably, and is less expensive than other techniques.

REFERENCES

1. Leksell L: Echoencephalography: Detection of the intracranial complications following head injury. Acta Chir Scand 110:301–315, 1956
2. Ziskin MC: Basic principles: Instrumentation, in Goldberg DB, Cotler MN, Ziskin MC, Waxham RD (eds): Diagnostic Uses of Ultrasound. New York, Grune & Stratton, 1975, pp 1–69
3. Garrett WI, Kossoff G, Warren PS: Cerebral ventricular size in children: A two-dimensional ultrasonic study. Radiology 136:711–715, 1980
4. Babcock DS, Han, BK: Cranial ultrasound findings in patients with meningomyelocele. Am J Roentgenol 136:563–569, 1981
5. Babcock DS, Han BK: Cranial Ultrasonography of Infants. Baltimore, Williams & Wilkins, 1981
6. Fleischer AC, Hutchison AA, Kirchner SG, et al: Cranial sonography of the preterm neonate. Diag Imag 3:20–28, 1981
7. Friede RL: Developmental Neuropathology. New York, Springer, 1976, pp 1–37
8. Babcock DS, Han BK: The accuracy of high resolution, real-time ultrasonography of the head in infancy. Radiology 139:665–676, 1981

IX METABOLISM, ANESTHESIA, AND INTENSIVE CARE

63. Neuroendocrinology

Jack Holland
Robert M. Ehrlich

STRUCTURE AND FUNCTION OF THE HYPOTHALAMIC–PITUITARY AXIS

During the past 40 years, the innovative techniques focused on the hypothalamus by anatomist and physiologist, endocrinologist, and biochemist have yielded enormous details on the mechanism of neuroendocrine regulation, culminating in the isolation and characterization of the hypothalamic hypophysiotropic factors. It is now known that the hypothalamus is the final common pathway subserving neuroendocrine, autonomic, behavioral, and emotional function in man and the lower animals.[1]

This chapter reviews current knowledge regarding hypothalamic structure and function, with particular reference to neurologic and endocrinologic problems arising from abnormalities in this area.

The Hypothalamic–Anterior Pituitary Axis

Anatomy

In early embryologic development, the structures destined to become the hypothalamus are an integral part of the neuroectoderm of the prosencephalon or forebrain, which gives origin to all the central nervous system cranial to the midbrain. During the seventh week of development, the anterior forebrain enlarges to form the cerebral hemispheres, which extend outward and downward to envelop the remaining portion, now termed the diencephalon. From its walls are derived the thalamus and its associated nuclei. Its floor gives rise to the hypothalamus and pars nervosa of the pituitary gland, and its roof gives origin to the choroid plexus of the third ventricle and the pineal gland. Simultaneous with early cerebral hemispheric development is the external appearance of the primitive mouth, together with the maxillary and mandibular processes and the olefactory pits. The anterior pituitary gland is formed from an outpouching of ectoderm from the roof of the mouth, Rathke's pouch. The pouch makes contact with the infundibulum from the floor of the hypothalamus, while constricting its

Table 63-1
The Principal Nuclei of the Hypothalamus,
Grouped According to Their Anatomic Location

Anterior–Hypothalamic	Tuberoinfundib	Posterior–Hypothalamic
Supraoptic	Dorsomedial	Mammillary
Paraventricular	Ventromedial	Posterior hypothalamic
Preoptic	Ventrolateral	
Suprachiasmatic*	Arcuate	

*The suprachiasmatic nucleus has been identified only in the rat brain. Its existence in the human brain is uncertain.

attachment to the pharyngeal roof. Proliferation of the cells in the anterior wall establishes the pars anterior, its upper extension eventually enveloping the pituitary stalk as the pars tuberalis. The pouch lumen becomes almost obliterated, leaving a narrow pars intermedia in contact with the posterior pituitary. The cells of the anterior hypophysis later assume specific morphologic and staining characteristics as their endocrine function become established. The close anatomic and developmental relationship between the hypothalamic–pituitary axis and the forebrain is of major clinical importance (see below).

Within the hypothalamus cell clusters become aggregated and can be identified as discrete nuclei. From a functional and anatomic point of view they can be described according to their position within the hypothalamic boundaries (Table 63-1).

Multiple neural pathways have been identified within the hypothalamus. Major efferent tracts include the fornix, or corticomammilary tract, which contains fibers originating in the hippocampus and terminating in the ventromedial and arcuate regions; the stria terminalis, which transmits fibers from the amygdaloid nucleus to the anterior hypothalamus and the nuclei of the medial basal hypothalamus; and the medial forebrain bundle, which mediates olfactory information to the preoptic and lateral hypothalamic areas. Among the principal efferent tracts are the hypothalamo–hypophysial tracts, carrying the neurosecretory fibers from the supraoptic and paraventricular nuclei to the pars nervosa of the pituitary; the medial forebrain bundle, with efferents to the midbrain nuclei and reticular formation; and the dorsal longitudinal fasciculus, carrying further fibers from the hypothalamus and the reticular formation of the midbrain. The functional aspects of these pathways, and of aminergic and peptidergic neurons, are discussed in some detail later in this chapter.

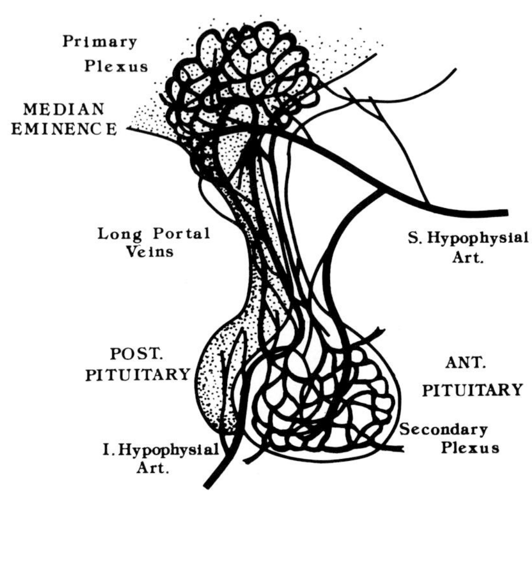

Figure 63-1. Blood supply of the hypothalamic–pituitary axis. Blood from the primary venous plexus drains the median eminence, and reaches the distal anterior pituitary gland via the long portal veins.

Blood Supply to the Hypothalamus and Hypophysis

During its development the pars anterior of the pituitary gland becomes richly vascularized and its cells become arranged in columns surrounding the blood vessels. A primary and a secondary complex of veins occupying the superior and inferior portions of the gland unite by midgestation to form a system of portal vessels, permitting rapid transport of blood throughout the entire gland (Fig. 63-1). The vessels of the primary complex are intimately connected with nerve terminals of the tuberoinfundibular neurons in the median eminence, whose secretions, directly into the portal venous system of the pars anterior, profoundly affect anterior pituitary activity. The arterial blood supply is derived from the superior hypophysial artery, which branches from the internal carotid artery. The posterior pituitary gland is supplied largely from the inferior hypophysial artery, and until recently it was felt that there was little intermixing of these two circulations. The possibility of retrograde flow from pituitary to median eminence has been renewed, however, with the demonstration of high concentrates of pituitary hormones in portal blood, and vascular connections between the posterior pituitary and the median eminence.[2]

The Median Eminence and the Circumventricular Organs

Several ependymal sites have been identified in animal models as having a morphology suggestive of possible endocrine function.[3] These areas include the median eminence, the subfornical organ, the organum vasculosum of the lamina terminalis (OVLT), the subcommissural organ, the area postrema, and the pineal gland (Fig. 63-2). Histologically the characteristic finding consists of synaptic nerve endings abutting onto specialized ependymal cells, or tanycytes. These cells may permit direct transfer of peptides to or from the cerebrospinal fluid (CSF), and are relatively permeable to passage of large-molecular-weight materials otherwise denied access by the blood–brain barrier.

The median eminence extends from the optic chiasma to the infundibulum beneath the floor of the third ventricle. It is the site of contact between the capillaries of the primary complex of the hypophysial system, the terminal fibers of the tuberoinfundibular neurons, and the tanycytes. It therefore represents the final common pathway by which neural, limbic, and extrahypothalamic influences regulate anterior pituitary function, and contains neurotransmitters, catecholamines, enzymes, hormones, and other substances of uncertain function, in higher concentrations than in any part of the nervous system. It can be divided

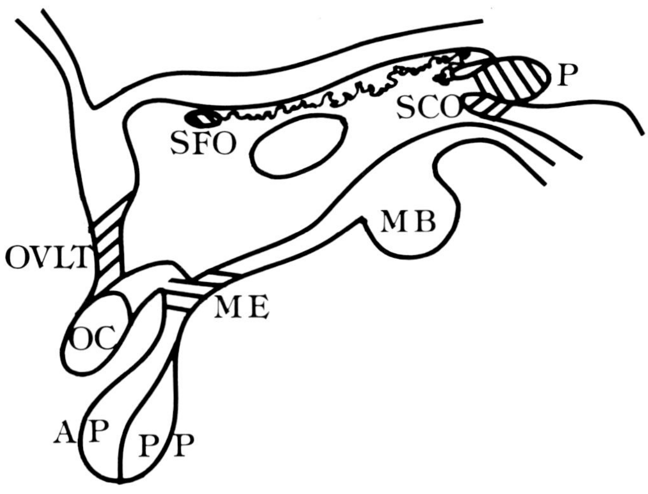

Figure 63-2. The circumventricular organs of the human brain. Abbreviations: PP, posterior pituitary; AP, anterior pituitary; OC, optic chiasm; OVLT, organum vasculosum of the lamina terminalis; SFO, subfornical organ; P, pineal; SCO, subcommissural organ; MB, mammillary body. Not shown is the area postrema, situated near the inferior aspect of the fourth ventricle.

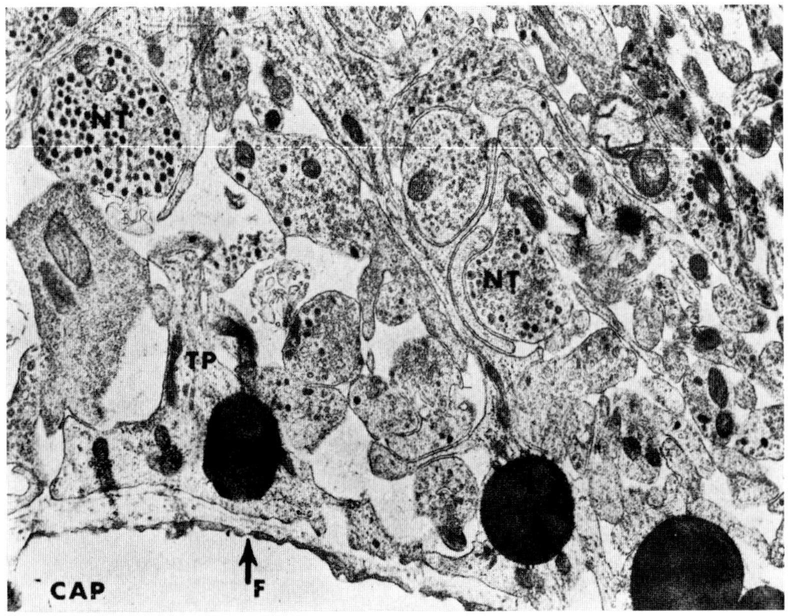

Figure 63-3. Electron microscopy of the rat median eminence. A capillary lumen (CAP) is present in the lower part of the figure. Fenestrations (F, arrow) can be identified. Tanycyte processes (TP) and nerve terminals (NT) abut on the capillary. Neurosecretory neurons (NT) contain dense core and synaptic vesicles, containing peptidergic hormones and neurotransmitters. (Reprinted with permission from Reichlin S, Martin J, Brown G: Contemporary Neurology Series: Clinical Neuroendocrinology. Philadelphia, FA Davis Co, 1977.)

anatomically into an outer zone strongly positive for dopamine[4] and an inner zone, lining the third ventricle which by contrast contains high concentrations of norepinephrine.[5] Running between these layers are the fibers of the neurohypophysial tracts.

The outer zone of the median eminence contains terminal fibers of nerves whose cell bodies appear to be largely situated in the periventricular and arcuate nuclei.[6] On electron microscopy neurosecretory granules can be demonstrated adjacent to the basement membrane that separates synapse and capillary endothelium (Fig. 63-3). Some of these granules have been shown to contain monoamines, and thus resemble those previously identified in the autonomic nervous system. Others contain the hypothalamic-releasing hormones, of which three have been isolated and characterized, and made available for clinical studies (Fig. 63-4).

pyro — GLu — His — Pro — NH_2

THYROTROPIN RELEASING HORMONE (TRH)

pyro—Glu —HIS—TRP—SER—TYR—GLY—LEU—ARG—PRO—GLY—NH_2

GONADOTROPIN RELEASING HORMONE (LH—RH)

H—ALA—GLY—CYS—LYS—ASN—PHE—PHE—TRP—LYS—THR—PHE—THR—SER—CYS—OH

GROWTH HORMONE RELEASE—INHIBITING HORMONE (GIF, SOMATOSTATIN)

Figure 63-4. The hormones of the hypothalamic-hypophysial peptidergic system, so far identified.

Thyrotropin-releasing hormone (TRH) is a tripeptide, first identified by Schally and Guillemin and their respective co-workers.[7,8] It causes release and synthesis of thyroid-stimulating hormone[9] from the thyrotropes of the anterior pituitary. It also causes brisk release of prolactin,[10] although it is uncertain whether this effect is a truly physiologic one. The second peptidergic hormone to be isolated was luteinizing hormone-releasing hormone (LH-RH), identified by Schally in 1971.[11] Intravenous injection of LH-RH causes release of both luteinizing hormone (LH) and follicle-stimulating hormone (FSH), although there may be an additional releasing hormone for FSH.[12,13] Somatostatin, or growth hormone release-inhibiting hormone (GIF), is a linear peptide of 14 amino acids isolated and characterized by Brazeau and Guillemin,[14] which inhibits not only growth hormone release from the pituitary, but also the TSH response to TRH in vivo and in vitro.[15] In addition to these three neurohormones, there are several others that await isolation and characterization from biologically active fragments of hypothalamic tissue. These include corticotropin-releasing factor (CRF), growth-hormone-releasing factor (GRF), prolactin-releasing hormone (PRF), and regulating hormones for control of melanocyte-stimulating hormone. All are thought to be low MW peptides, and like TRH and LH-RH, to react with respective receptors in the anterior pituitary by an adenyl cyclase dependent mechanism.

The Organum Vasculosum of the Lamina Terminalis

In the rat the structure of the OVLT bears a startling resemblance to that of the median eminence. Situated in the midline of the lamina terminalis with its internal surface in contact with the CSF of the third ventricle, its histologic appearance consists of neurosecretory nerve endings terminating on the basement membranes surrounding fenestrated capillary loops.[16,17] Immunohistologic techniques and radioimmunoassay of OVLT extracts have revealed the presence of high concentrations of LH-RH.[18,19] Since there appear to be no vascular connections between the OVLT and the pituitary capillaries, any functional activity of LH-RH peptidergic neurons must therefore depend on secretion directly into the capillaries surrounding the OVLT or on direct transport to the CSF via tanycytes.[20]

The Subfornical Organ

The subfornical organ, situated at the junction of the lamina terminalis and the choroid plexus of the third ventricle beneath the fornices of the hippocampus (Fig. 63-2), shares the general histologic structure common to the circumventricular organs. This area is of interest because of the observation that stimulation of drinking behavior and release of antidiuretic hormone (ADH) follows injection of angiotensin II into this region.[21]

The Subcommissural Organ and the Area Postrema

Little is known about the functional significances of these two structures (Fig. 63-2). Vomiting reflexes may be induced by certain drugs or by structural changes at the level of area postrema, or by pressure changes in the fourth ventricle or adjacent brain stem.

The Pineal Gland

Although apparently remote from the median eminence and hypophysis, the pineal gland exerts a unique influence on neuroendocrine function because of its intimate involvement with light–dark cycles and its production of melatonin, which may be an important modulator of reproductive behavior. Reference has been made previously to the conceptualization of pineal regulation as a model of hypothalamic activity.[1]

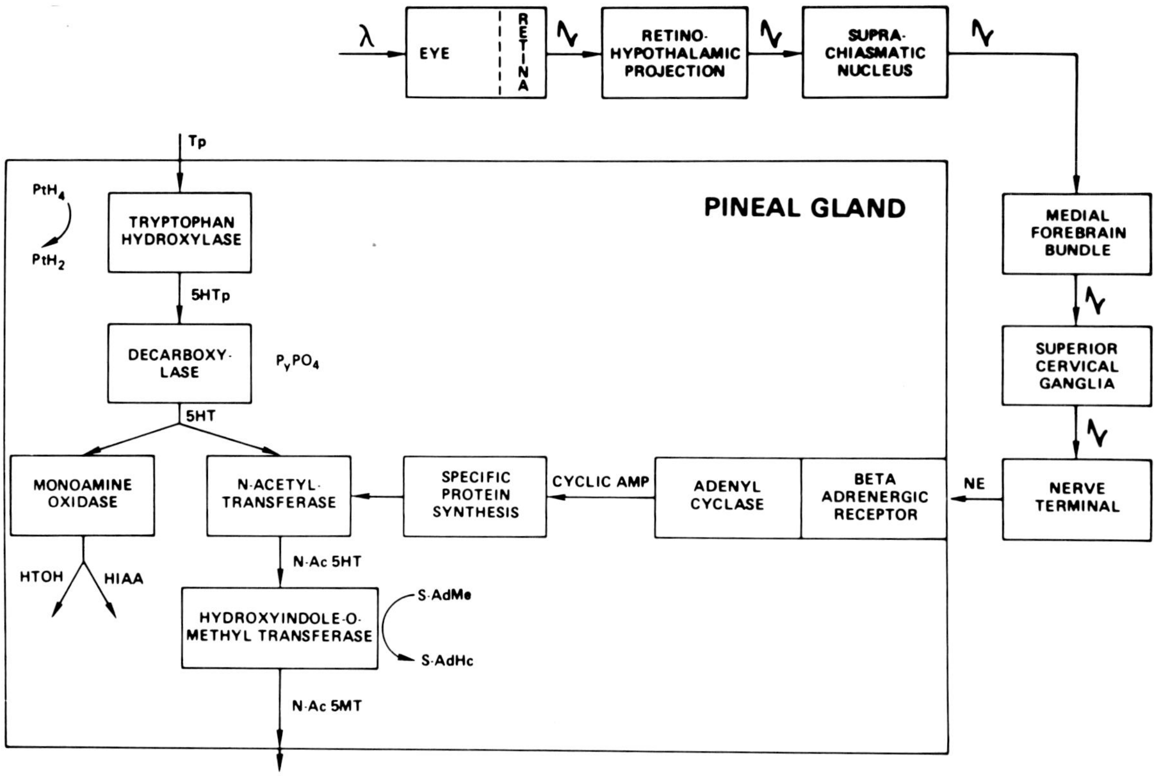

Figure 63-5. Diagram of pineal innervation. Norepinephrine (NE) released from nerve terminal combines with β-adrenergic receptor to activate adenyl cyclase. Increased cyclic AMP stimulates specific protein synthesis which leads to increase in N-acetyltransferase activity and formation of melatonin (Reprinted with permission from Klein DC, Parfitt A. in Weiss B (ed): Cyclic AMP in Disease. Baltimore, University Park Press, 1976.)

Studies, chiefly in rats, have shown that in response to dark exposure, impulses are transmitted from the retina to the contralateral suprachiasmatic nucleus and conveyed to the inferior accessory tract in the midbrain via the median forebrain bundle. Secondary fibers travel to the superior cervical ganglion, from which sympathetic fibers pass to the pineal gland. Through production of cyclic AMP and induction of protein synthetic enzymes, melatonin is formed from its serotonin (5-HT) precursor (Fig. 63-5). There is thus a reciprocal relationship between 5-HT and melatonin, during exposure to both light and darkness. For further information the reader is referred to the excellent review by Klein.[22] Apart from melatonin indoleamines and their precursors, and enzymatic markers, other substances have also been found in the pineal gland. These include TRH, LH-RH, and GIF and arginine vasotocin, a substance with antigonadal and antiadrenal properties. Pinealectomy has been reported to cause adrenal hypertrophy and elevation of plasma corticosteroids, while blindness may produce the opposite effect.[23]

The regulation of pineal function, although apparently complex, can be viewed in fairly simple, fundamental terms. Afferent information (light–dark) is transported by specific neural pathways (retinohypothalamic projection/median forebrain bundle) to the pineal gland via monoaminergic intermediate neurons (postganglionic sympathetic), where melatonin is formed by interaction with specific cell membrane receptors. Modulating the neuronal–receptor interaction is the overriding influence of inherent biologic rhythms generated by the suprachiasmatic nucleus. If these mechanistic principles are to be applied to

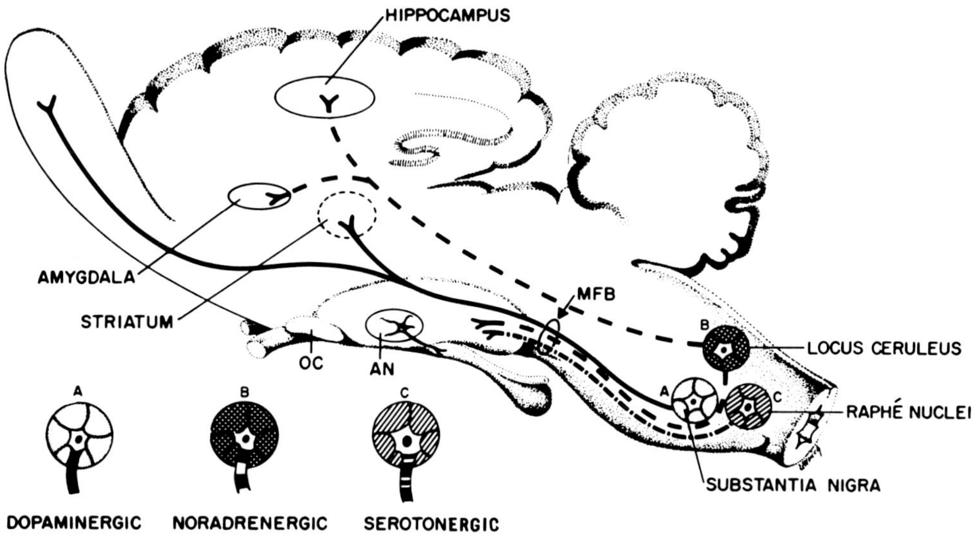

Figure 63-6. Monoaminergic pathways in mammalian brain. The principal localization of the neurons containing norepinephrine, dopamine, and serotonin. Axons of these cells are distributed to widespread areas of cortex, limbic system, and striatum, with the exception of the dopaminergic system localized to the arcuate. Abbreviations: MFB, medial forebrain bundle; AN, arcuate nucleus; OC, optic chiasm. (Reprinted with permission from Reichlin S, Martin J, Brown G: Contemporary Neurology Series: Clinical Neuroendocrinology. Philadelphia, FA Davis Co, 1977.)

hypothalamic–anterior pituitary regulation, as implied by Reichlin,[1] then it would be expected that there would be precise anatomic relationships between the aminergic neural pathways and the neurosecretory (peptidergic) neurons in their distribution within the hypothalamus, and that functionally they too may be influenced by the endogenous body rhythms.

Distribution of Hypothalamic Biogenic Amines

With the technological advances in identifying tissue monoamines and indoleamines, together with the use of specific pharmacologic receptor agonists and antagonists, the distribution of monoaminergic pathways has been fairly well-defined (Fig. 63-6), at least in the rat brain. As discussed previously, the external layer of the median eminence has a high concentration of dopamine, and almost all of it is contained in neurons originating in the arcuate-periventricular areas. These constitute the tuberoinfundibular dopaminergic system.[24] The major site of origin of the dopaminergic tracts, however, is the substantia nigra of the brain stem. Fibers are distributed to the corpus stratum and forebrain via the median forebrain bundle.[25]

Noradrenergic neurons sweep anteriorly from their origin in the locus ceruleus to terminate in the inner zone of the median eminence and in the parachiasmatic areas of the anterior hypothalamus, as well as parts of the basal hypothalamus, including the ventromedial nucleus.[26]

The distribution of serotonergic pathways is less well-defined. Cell bodies can be identified in the pontine raphe nuclei and in the ventromedial reticular formation. Neurons terminate in the cortex and hippocampal areas of the limbic system, but a major site of 5-HT fluorescence is found in the suprachiasmatic nucleus and, to a lesser extent, in the septal and preoptic areas of the hypothalamus.[27] Nerve terminals have also been demonstrated between ependymal cells, presumably discharging 5 HT into the CSF of the third ventricle.[28,29]

Distribution of Peptidergic Neurons

TRH has been shown to be widely distributed throughout the nervous system, including the cerebral cortex and spinal cord, suggesting that it has functions other than that of TSH and prolactic regulation.[30,31] TRH possibly may act as a modulator of synaptic activity in a number of different neural systems. In the hypothalamus TRH-containing neurons are found in highest concentration in the external layer of the median eminence with cell bodies situated in the dorsomedial nucleus. A significant TRH-positive zone lies in the anterior hypothalamus in an area close to the wall of the third ventricle. Fibers are also seen in the median forebrain bundle and in the upper brain stem.[32-34]

LH-RH, identified by immunohistochemical methods and by radioimmunoassay, has been found in cell bodies in the suprachiasmatic area and in fibers extending from the prechiasmatic area to the median eminence. Nerve terminals in the external layer of the median eminence, in the inferior floor of the third ventricle, and in the OVLT have numerous LH-RH positive granules.[35,36] In the median eminence these are in close association with dopamine at storage sites.

GIF, initially isolated in the hypothalamus, has now been demonstrated in the D-cells of the pancreas, in the gastrointestinal tract, and in the thyroid gland.[37,38] Within the CNS its main distribution is similar to that of LH-RH, with GIF-containing cell bodies in the anterior periventricular area, and nerve tracts leading to the median eminence, which stains strongly for GIF. GIF-positive nerve terminals are also present in the arcuate-ventromedial nuclei, the suprachiasmatic nucleus, and in the OVLT. GIF has also been found in the pineal gland, hippocampus, and corticomedial amygdala.

Other brain peptides of uncertain function have been identified, including enkephalin,[39] endorphin,[40] substance-P,[41] and neurotensin.[42] It is quite certain that further details regarding their role in cerebral function or hypothalamic–pituitary regulation will soon emerge.

Endocrine Function

Coupled with the advances leading to the present state of knowledge in the chemistry and microanatomy of the hypothalamus and the adenohypophysis, there has been a parallel surge in the understanding of the functional relationships of the hypothalamic–pituitary axis.

The Hormones of the Anterior Pituitary Gland

Electron microscopy, histologic staining techniques, and use of peroxidase-labeled antibodies have shown that the hormones of the adenohypophysis are secreted by specific cell types, each from broadly regionalized anatomic areas within the pars distalis. All are composed of peptide chains, with LH, FSH and TSH, the glycoprotein hormones, secreted in linked subunits. The alpha subunit is immunologically common to all three hormones (and, for that matter, to the placental hormone chorionic gonadotropin), although it is biologically inactive. Biologic activity and immunologic specificity are dependent on the beta subunit of each of these hormones.[43,44]

Hormone secretion or inhibition of secretion is effected through the influence of the hypophysiotropic or peptidergic hormones, previously described, transmitted directly by the capillaries of the portal system to their target cells in the pituitary gland. The hormones of the anterior pituitary and their regulatory hormones are shown in Table 63-2.

β-Lipotropin (LPH) was identified as a pituitary hormone several years ago by C. H. Li and his coworkers,[45] but interest in this 91-amino-acid molecule has been recently renewed with the discovery of enkephalin[46] and β-endorphin,[47]

Table 63-2
Functional Relationship of the Hormones of the Hypothalamic–Pituitary Axis

Hypophysiotropic Hormone	Pituitary Tropic Hormone	Pituitary Target Organ	Target Organ Response
Growth hormone-releasing-factor/somatostatin	Growth hormone	Liver, kidney ? Other tissues	Somatomedin ± Other growth factors
Prolactin-releasing hormone/ inhibiting hormone	Prolactin	Breast, gonad ? Other tissues	Lactation
Gonadotropin-releasing hormone	Luteinizing hormone, follicle-stimulating hormone	Leydig/thecal cells Gonadal germ cells	Sex steroids Inhibin, sperm
Thyrotropin-releasing hormone/somatostatin	Thyroid-stimulating hormone (prolactin)	Thyroid gland	Thyroid hormone
Corticotropin-releasing hormone	Lipotropic hormone (LPH) endorphin/enkephalin	CNS, pituitary	Analgesia ? Prolactin ? growth hormone
	Adrenocorticotropic hormone	Adrenal	Adrenal steroids
	Melanocyte-stimulating hormone	Skin	Melanin

endogenous morphinelike peptides, whose amino-acid sequences are incorporated within the LPH molecule, as characterized by Li. This has led to the speculation that LPH may serve as a prohormone for these and other related peptides.[48]

Rhythmic Secretion of Anterior Pituitary Hormones

Many of the anterior pituitary hormones have specific patterns of secretion that are linked to the various phases of sleep. In addition there are endogenous biologic rhythmic patterns that are influenced by light–dark cycles. From work in experimental animals, the site of this endogenous "biologic clock" is felt to be the suprachiasmatic nucleus (SCN.) The importance of the SCN has been discussed previously in connection with the regulation of pineal function. In rats exposure to light increases the electrophysiologic firing rate of the SCN, increasing neuronal activity of its afferent connections and decreasing melatonin production.[49,50] Lesions in the SCN by contrast lead to loss of rhythmic secretion by melatonin, adrenocortical steroids, and gonadotropins.[51,52] The ACTH levels in the peripheral circulation reach their maximum at about 0400–0500 hours in normal individuals with well-established sleep patterns. Such episodic, minute-to-minute secretion is of neural origin and is not inhibited by the usual feedback regulation. Episodic secretion, is seen with ACTH, GH, prolactin, and the gonadotropins, and is responsible for variations noted in random meausrements of these hormones.

In contrast to the diurnal rhythm exhibited by ACTH and related peptides (LPH, MSH, and endorphin), the remaining anterior pituitary hormones show patterns of secretion that bear a direct relationship to sleep itself. The large episodic bursts of activity noted within the first two hours of sleep with GH[53] and prolactin[54] can be aborted by interruption of sleep, and can be reproduced by daytime naps. The magnitude of these sleep-related secretory discharges increases with advancing maturity from childhood to early adult life. Of interest in this regard is the appearance of nocturnal surges of gonadotropins immediately prior to the clinical onset of puberty and their disappearance after the attainment of full puberty development.[55] The mechanisms of sleep-induced modulation of hormonal secretion are not clearly understood, but serotonergic input may be important, since 5-HT neurons from the raphe nuclei play a prominent role in the activity of the SCN, the "biologic clock," and since 5-HT receptors have been implicated in the regulation of GH[56] and prolactin,[57] and in slow-wave sleep itself.[58]

Regulation of Anterior Pituitary Hormone Secretion

The basic mechanism of regulation, common to all the anterior pituitary hormones, involves the interaction of an appropriate stimulus and specific neuronal cell bodies in hypothalamic or extrahypothalamic sites. The initiating stimulus can be significantly modulated by a great variety of hypothalamic and extrahypothalamic influences—exercise, stress, sleep, feeding patterns, temperature, pharmacologic agents—but the most prominent component in the regulation of hormone secretion is feedback control. Feedback control is effected through the inhibition of the hypothalamus or pituitary, by the products of end-organ stimulation (Table 63-2)—"long-loop" feedback, and by direct actions of the pituitary trophic hormones themselves on the hypothalamus—"short-loop" feedback control.

Growth Hormone

Peptidergic neurons for GH are both stimulatory and inhibitory. Only the inhibitory neurohormone, GIF, has been isolated so far.[14] In humans, GH release—by exercise, hypoglycemia, and glucagon—is mediated through a noradrenergic receptor, whereas stimulation of β-sympathetic receptors causes inhibition of GH secretion. Dopaminergic and serotonergic receptors have also been implicated in GH release, and recent investigations in rats indicate that the opiate receptor may also play a facilitatory role.[59,60,61] Short-loop and long-loop feedback regulation are mediated through GH, and possibly somatomedin,[62] acting on either GIF or GRF neurons in the hypothalamus.

Prolactin

The control of prolactin (PRL) differs from that of the other pituitary hormones in that it is predominantly inhibitory. Prolactin inhibitory factor (PIF) has not been characterized, but is thought by many researchers to be dopamine, secreted by tuberoinfundibular neurons. Stress, sleep, and, most important, stimulation of the breast are strong positive factors leading to PRL secretion, presumably via prolactin-releasing factor (PRF).

Estrogen sensitizes pituitary lactotropes, and therefore is the cause of hyperprolactinemia in pregnancy and in the newborn infant and in subjects taking exogenous estrogens. Paradoxically, estrogen inhibits the PRL effect on the breast, and galactorrhea therefore is usually found in states characterized by high PRL levels and falling estrogen levels (for example, postpartum).

Prolactin exerts a short-loop feedback control on its secretion. Although prolactin receptors are found in the corpus luteum and the lung, the functional role of PRL in the sites and of their involvement in possible long-loop feedback is unknown.

Corticotropin, LPH, MSH, and Endorphins

Corticotropin-releasing factor mediates the diurnal rhythm of ACTH and also the ACTH output in response to stress. Aminergic mechanisms involved include an inhibitory noradrenergic pathway, and cholinergic and serotonergic pathways that serve diurnal and stress-induced ACTH release respectively.

Gonadotropins

The episodic discharge of LH and FSH from pituitary gonadotropes is thought to result from the activity of LH-RH secretory neurons arising in the anterior hypothalamus, although a separate system for FSH secretion may also exist.[12] In birds and lower animals, olfactory sensations and changing light exposure may promote sexual activity or breeding behavior, possibly through alteration in melatonin production.

The OVLT, rich in LH-RH neurosecretory granules, is thought to be the site of cyclic gonadotropin production in rodents, but this has not been demonstrated in higher animals. Both tonic and cyclic secretion appear to be controlled at the level of the medial basal hypothalamus in the primate.

Thyrotropin

Release of TSH is produced by stimulation of TRH-containing neurons in the anterior paraventricular area of the hypothalamus.[7] Inhibitory control is mediated through GIF, and perhaps a specific thyrotropin inhibitory hormone. Stress and exposure to cold are important stimuli for TSH release.[63,64]

Glucocorticoids in high dosage inhibit TSH production at the level of the pituitary,[65] and GH also acts as an inhibitor, probably through secondary increase in GIF activity. Estrogens, on the other hand, sensitize thyrotropes to stimulation by TRH. Clinically this leads to increased TSH responses to exogenous TRH in the late follicular phase of the menstrual cycle.[66] Long-loop feedback regulation is maintained by thyroxine and its metabolically active metabolite, triidothyronine (T_3). The relationship between the hormones of the hypothalamic–pituitary–thyroid axis is an extremely sensitive one, such that small increases in circulating thyroid hormones outside the normal physiologic range will produce marked inhibition of basal TSH and of TRH-induced TSH release.

The Hypothalamic–Posterior Pituitary Axis

Anatomy

The embryologic development of the neurohypophysis was described earlier. The components of the hypothalamic–neurohypophysial system consist of two anteriorly placed nuclei, the supraoptic nucleus (SON) and the paraventricular nucleus (PVN), the neurohypophysial tract, and the posterior pituitary gland.

The SON in the human is situated over the optic tract, which forms an almost complete division between its anterior and posterior parts.[67] The PVN is a long vertical structure in the anterolateral wall of the third ventricle. Application of immunohistochemical techniques has demonstrated the presence of the two hormones, antidiuretic hormone (ADH) and oxytocin (OT), each composed of nine amino acids. Each hormone is bound to a specific carrier protein of MW$\sim$10,000 daltons, termed neurophysin, the complex contained within secretory granules that are ultimately transported from the perikarya to nerve terminals where their contents are discharged by a process of exocytosis into perivascular spaces.[68,69] Both ADH and OT are found in both nuclei, although each has separate regulatory mechanism. In humans the ratio of ADH:OT containing neurons is $\sim$2.5:1, with the greater concentration of ADH (and its neurophysin) found in cells originating in the SON.[67] Nerve fibers from the PVN merge with those from the SON and together pass between the inner and outer layers of the median eminence to terminate on capillaries of the systemic circulation situated along the posterior pituitary. Granules of ADH, however, have been identified in the zona externa of the median eminence itself, and ADH and its neurophysin have been found in high concentration on the portal vessels of the anterior pituitary.[70] This finding has supported the belief that ADH may function as a corticotropin-releasing factor, a belief further strengthened by the observation that serum ADH is increased after adrenalectomy.[71] It also helps to explain why simple stalk section of the pituitary fails to produce permanent diabetes insipidus.

Endocrine Function

Regulation of Salt and Water Metabolism

The maintenance of plasma osmolality within normal limits is dependent on the delicate relationship between water intake, induced by thirst, and water excretion through the renal tubules. Receptors in the supraoptic region respond to changes in extracellular osmolality by altering the firing rate of the SON and PVN, and thus the secretion of antidiuretic hormone. A 3 percent change in plasma osmolality will result in inhibition of full diuresis and initiation of antidiuresis.[72] Changes in blood volume are detected by stretch receptors in the left atrium and the wall of the vena cava, and by aortic baroreceptors, and this information is conveyed to central pathways via the vagus nerve and nerves from the carotid sinus. A third mechanism by which ADH secretion is influenced is through the direct stimulating effects of angiotensin II. Renin, secreted from afferent renal arterioles in response to reduced renal blood flow or hyponatremia, catalyzes the initial step in the formation of angiotensin II from an α_2-globulin, angiotensinogen. Apart from stimulating ADH output, angiotensin II increases aldosterone production from the adrenal, contracts peripheral arterioles, and also stimulates thirst, possibly via the subfornical organ.[73,75] Maintenance of normal circulation following dehydration or blood loss thus is the end result of water conservation mediated by ADH release, sodium retention, and stimulation of the thirst center. Under normal conditions, ADH is regulated by osmoreceptors, but with significant hypovolemia, osmotic changes play a minor role as compared with the potent effects induced through stretch receptors and the renin–angiotensin mechanism.[72]

Central Regulating Mechanisms

In addition to mechanisms arising from changes in the systemic circulation, ADH is also influenced by suprahypothalamic factors and by biogenic amines. Emotional stress, pain, and anxiety cause ADH release,[76] and, as with hormones of the anterior pituitary, a diurnal rhythm of ADH secretion has been described, with antidiuresis during the hours of sleep.[77] Cholinergic activation via a nicotinic receptor stimulates ADH secretion, and alpha-adrenergic agonists and a number of drugs, including morphine, barbiturates, chlopropamide, and clofibrate, also promote ADH release. By contrast alcohol, beta-adrenergic agonists, and diphenylhydantoin inhibit secretion.[77] Furthermore, studies indicate that ADH may inhibit its own secretion by a short-loop feedback system effected by recurrent collateral inhibition, analogous to the action of the Renshaw cell in the spinal cord.[78] This observation might explain the occurrence of sustained ADH release following lesions close to but sparing the SON and PVH.

Regulation of Oxytocin Secretion

Oxytocin is structurally similar to antidiuretic hormone, but control mechanisms for these two hormones and their neurophysins are separate. Oxytocin secretion is not significantly affected by changes in hypothalamic osmoreceptors or by nicotinic stimulation, although both oxytocin and ADH are inhibited by alcohol and beta-adrenergic agonists.

The major stimulus for oxytocin release is suckling of the breast, particu-

Table 63-3
Anatomic Distribution within the Hypothalamus and Brain Stem of the Putative Major Sites Involved in Nonendocrine Hypothalamic Function: Bilateral Destruction of Such Sites Results in Loss of Corresponding Function

	Hypothalamic Regionalization			
Function	Anterior	Medial-Basal	Posterior	Mid-Brain
Temperature	Receptors for hot–cold recognition	Efferents via median forebrain bundle to posthypothal	Effector for temperature regulation	
Consciousness	"Sleep" center		"Wake" center	Ascending reticular activity
Appetite		Ventrolateral "hunger center" Ventromedial "satiety" center		Substantia nigra "Satiety center"
Memory		Ventromedial area	Premammillary area	

larly when estrogen levels are elevated. Estrogen stimulates oxytocin-associated neurophysin release[79] and also sensitizes the myoepithelial cells of the breast, and the smooth muscle of the uterus, to the effects of oxytocin. It is uncertain whether oxytocin deficiency, either isolated or in association with diabetes insipidus, causes significant physiologic dysfunction. The role of oxytocin in sperm mobility and orgasm in women is not clear.

The Hypothalamic–Pituitary Axis

Nonendocrine Function

Previous discussion has centered on the hypothalamus as a neuroendocrine unit, but in addition, through its interaction with brain stem and limbic system, the hypothalamus acts as the final integrator of several specific aspects of behavior. Important functions include the regulation of (1) temperature, (2) sleep and level of consciousness, (3) appetite for food and water, (4) memory and other cognitive functions, and (5) emotional behavior (Table 63-3).

Studies in animals would suggest that the major locus for temperature recognition lies in the anterior hypothalamus in the preoptic area that contains receptors responsive to either heat or cold. The posterior hypothalamus receives this information via the medial forebrain bundle and coordinates this with thermal signals from other sites, to activate appropriate physiologic mechanisms to either conserve or dissipate heat. The posterior hypothalamus therefore acts as the integrator and effector in temperature regulation and significant lesions in this area thus result in large fluctuations in body temperature.[80]

Similar experimental approaches in laboratory animals, and clinicopathologic observations in humans with discrete hypothalamic lesions, have identified the anterior hypothalamus as the "sleep center." It appears to function primarily through cyclic inhibition of ascending reticular activity from the brain stem (RAS). Conversely a "wake center" is situated in the posterior hypothalamus, and normal sleep wake cycles are dependent on the coordination of anterior and posterior activity and net influence on the RAS.[81]

The concept of a ventromedial (VM) "satiety center" and a ventrolateral (VL) "hunger center" has been established for many years.[82] Extensive studies, however, have indicated the existence of more complex and less anatomic discrete mechanisms for regulation of food intake. The classic hunger center may represent only part of a neural pathway, connecting the substantia nigra with the globus pallidus. Many of its fibers may be dopaminergic, since dopamine depletion or interference with striatal function may significantly depress food intake.[83]

Loss of short-term memory with retention of memory for distant events are the typical defects associated with hypothalamic disease. Identical patterns of memory loss are found in the mammillary and premammillary lesions of the Wernicke–Korsakoff syndrome,[84] and, indeed, observations in patients with discretely distributed hypothalamic tumors, and in laboratory animals, would suggest that the ventromedial and premammillary areas are essential in memory function.[85,86] The hippocampus, and its projections to the ventromedial hypothalamus, are also important.[87] Hypophysectomy may result in problems with memory retention, which can be corrected by administration of ADH or ACTH[88] or by fragments of ACTH which have no tropic effect on the adrenal glands.[89] Furthermore, subsequent studies have shown similar properties for endorphin and other fragments of lipotropic hormone. With the realization that retrograde portal blood flow may occur, it is therefore possible that hormones, secreted by pituitary cells, or from peptidergic neurons within the brain, may play a significant role in the process of learning and memory.

Emotions are the subjective feelings resulting from neurochemical activity within the limbic system and its connections. Emotional behavior is expressed through outbursts of autonomic, motor, and endocrine activity that are appropriate for the emotion aroused. The hypothalamus acts to coordinate this activity, and anatomic or surgical lesions may therefore result in behavior that is inappropriate in its type and intensity. Euphoria is usually seen in young subjects with destruction of the anterior hypothalamic region of interference with pathways arising from the frontal cortex. Conversely posterolateral hypothalamic damage may result in a state of apathy.[90,91] Rage reactions, again inappropriate for the given stimulus, are most often seen following lesions to the VM hypothalamus, and often accompany the disorders in food intake seen in such patients.[92]

Clinical Implications

The complexity of the neurovascular connections of the hypothalamic–pituitary axis is such that a relatively small lesion may result in devastating abnormalities in function. Several principles emerge, however, which may facilitate clinical evaluation of neuroendocrine disorders.

Congenital Versus Acquired Disease

Reference was made previously to the close relationship between the embryologic development of the forebrain, facial and olefactory structures, and the hypothalamus. It is not surprising, therefore, that neuroendocrine disturbances have been described with high frequency in association with (1) abnormalities of the forebrain: holoprosencephaly, absent corpus callosum and septum pellucidum, and distortion of the third ventricle: (2) abnormalities of the eyes and/or optic nerves: septo-optic dysplasia, hypertelorism, congenital absence of the eye;[93] (3) maxillary abnormalities: cleft lip and palate, single central incisor;[94] and (4) nasal and olefactory abnormalities: choanal atresia and impaired sense of smell.[95] Additional findings of micropenis and undescended testes, or persistent neonatal hypoglycemia, might also suggest congenital deficiency or LH-RH, and of GH and/or ACTH respectively. Apart from diabetes insipidus, or acute symptoms of hypoglycemia, congenital hypothalamic–pituitary disorders tend to give rise to chronic dysfunctional problems and therefore tend to present clinically relatively late. By contrast acquired disorders, whether inflammatory, neoplastic, or vascular, usually announce themselves relatively acutely, with symptoms stemming directly from the close anatomic relationship of hypothalamus, third ventricle, and optic nerves—that is, raised intracranial pressure and/or visual field abnormalities.

Clinicopathologic Correlation

The hypothalamus differs functionally from the remainder of the nervous system in that both right and left halves appear to be of equivalent functional importance, such that bilateral (but not necessarily symmetric) lesions are required to produce clinical deficits. Consequently areas most commonly involved are the paired structures of the medial basal hypothalamus—the VM nucleus, arcuate nucleus, and median eminence, which are closely opposed to the inferolateral walls of the third ventricle. Specific clinical syndromes may correlate well with lesions in the principal sites in which peptidergic or aminergic neurons are known to be distributed (Table 63-1). In general terms acute or rapidly enlarging lesions tend to produce the most profound changes, particularly in levels of consciousness, temperature regulation, and autonomic function. Smaller, more chronic destruction, by contrast, may result in endocrine, memory, and cognitive dysfunction.

Laboratory Evaluation of Hypothalamic-Pituitary Disease

The spectrum of neurosurgical problems of childhood and adolescence, and their clinical presentation, have been discussed in detail elsewhere. Diagnosis and optimal perioperative and postoperative management results from (1) accurate and pertinent history-taking; (2) physical examination, with particular attention to potential neurologic deficits and evidence of visual and endocrine dysfunction; (3) appropriate radiological assessment; and (4) specific neuroendocrine evaluation. A reasonable approach to assessment of the hypothalamic-pituitary axis follows.

Anterior Pituitary Function

ACTH: Hyperfunction. Autonomous overproduction of ACTH by a pituitary adenoma (Cushing's disease) is reflected by continuous excessive secretion of cortisol. This may be assessed by demonstration of increased plasma cortisol and its urinary metabolite, 17-hydroxysteroid, and by increased excretion of urinary free-cortisol. An early biochemical sign is loss of diurnal variation in plasma cortisol. Plasma levels of ACTH may be significantly elevated, although laboratory measurement is technically difficult and results may not be diagnostic.

Differentiation of Cushing's disease from adrenal tumors (or rarely ovarian tumors) can be made by demonstrating lack of ACTH dependence using the dexamethasone suppression test. This potent glucocorticoid inhibits pituitary ACTH secretion yet does not contribute significantly to measurements of either plasma cortisol or urinary excretion products. Persistence of high secretion rates in the face of dexamethasone therapy therefore indicates that production of cortisol (or of other adrenal steroids) is independent of ACTH stimulation. The test may be performed by giving (1) dexamethasone 1 mg at midnight and measuring plasma cortisol at 08.00 hours, or (2) dexamethasone 20 $\mu g/kg$ (or 1.25 mg/m^2 surface area) per day, divided into six-hourly doses for two to three days, with measurement of urinary 17-hydroxysteroids and 17-ketosteroids and urinary free-cortisol prior to and on each day of the test—a regime that will produce suppression of adrenal steroid output in obese individuals or in stressed patients or in patients with congenital adrenal hyperplasia but not in Cushing's disease or adrenal carcinomas; (3) dexamethasone 80 $\mu g/kg$ (or 3.75 mg/m^2) per day (high-dose test), which will suppress adrenal output in ACTH-producing pituitary adenoma, but not in adrenal carcinoma.

ACTH: Hypofunction. Hypothalamic–pituitary insufficiency may be a frequent preoperative finding and this clearly should be borne in mind if major diagnostic procedures such as carotid angiograms or pneumoencephalograms are to be undertaken. A deficiency in ACTH is almost invariable following total removal of a craniopharyngioma, and perioperative management should be planned accordingly. Low cortisol levels, with lack of diurnal variation, is suggestive of ACTH deficiency, but to establish definitively this diagnosis it is necessary to carry out one or more stimulation tests.

1. ACTH stimulation. In this test 250 $\mu g/m^2$ of synthetic β^{1-24}-corticotrophin (Synacthen or Cortrosyn) is given by intravenous injection, and blood is taken at time 0, +30, and +60 minutes after injection for cortisol determination. With normal adrenal function, cortisol usually increases by > 7 $\mu g/100$ ml over baseline values. Absent or blunted responses indicate either primary adrenal failure, or long-standing hypothalamic–pituitary disease.[96]
2. Insulin hypoglycemia. Cortisol may be measured 30 minutes after obtaining hypoglycemia in the insulin tolerance test. Insulin, 0.05 U/kg, or 0.025 U/kg in individuals with a documented history of hypoglycemia, is given intravenously, and blood taken at time 0, +30, +45, +60, and +90 minutes after injection. Significant hypoglycemia is defined as a 50 percent decline of blood glucose from baseline values, and occurs usually at +30 minutes after insulin treatment. Because of its potential dangers, this test should be performed only under direct medical supervision, and with 50 percent glucose available for correction of symptomatic hypoglycemia.

Growth hormone: Hyperfunction. Growth-hormone-secreting tumors are extremely rare in the pediatric age group. Diagnosis can be made on clinical grounds, in combination with elevation of basal concentrations of plasma growth hormone and somatomedin. Somatomedins are small MW peptides, which are thought to be the mediators of the biologic actions ascribed to growth hormone. Autonomous production of growth hormone is demonstrated by failure of suppression by glucose infusion during the glucose tolerance test, using 1.75 g glucose/kg body weight as an oral dose. Normally growth hormone is suppressed to <2 ng/ml by 30 minutes to 60 minutes after glucose ingestion.

Growth hormone: Hypofunction. Standard tests of growth hormone reserve are performed in the fasting state and include the following.

1. Insulin hypoglycemia. This is performed as described earlier. With significant hypoglycemia, growth hormone levels should increase by 5 ng/ml, or to an absolute level of >7 ng/ml.
2. Arginine stimulation. Arginine hydrochloride 0.5 g/kg, up to a maximum of 30 grams, is given in saline by a 30-minute intravenous infusion. Because it is acidic, the solution should be neutralized by sodium bicarbonate prior to infusion. Maximum growth hormone responses usually occur at 30–60 minutes of the test.
3. Exercise. After 15 minutes of strenous exercise in compliant cases,

> sufficient to produce tachycardia, increased respiratory rate, and sweating, large incremental changes in growth hormone can be measured in samples taken at 30 or 45 minutes from the onset of exercise. This can be a useful outpatient testing procedure.

In each of these tests, there can be false negative results in approximately 12 percent, and for that reason, two independent tests are required before the diagnosis of growth hormone deficiency can be accepted. This rate of false negatives can be lowered with the use of either propranolol (which blocks the inhibitory tone on growth hormone release) or estrogens (which increase hypothalamic–pituitary sensitivity to provocative stimuli) prior to the testing procedure.

Prolactin: Hyperfunction. Because of the inhibitory regulatory mechanisms in the control of prolactin secretion, significant hypothalamic lesions and stalk section will cause hyperprolactinemia. In addition estrogens and dopaminergic antagonists and prolactin-secreting adenomas of the pituitary gland will cause elevation in prolactin levels. In all cases basal concentrations of plasma prolactin are above normal, with highest levels seen in pituitary macroadenomas. In almost all cases, irrespective of cause, prolactin secretion can be inhibited by dopamine agonist treatment (L-dopa, bromocryptine, pimozide) but as diagnostic procedures, they are not helpful in differentiating tumor from other causes. Similarly with stimulation by TRH, or with a dopamine antagonist (chlorpromazine), results do not provide definitive data to identify prolactin-secreting tumors.

Prolactin: Hypofunction. Prolactin levels can be at the lower limit of detection (>1 ng/ml) in healthy normal individuals, but failure of response to thyrotropin-releasing hormone is indicative of pituitary disease.

Intravenous TRH (7 μg/kg) will produce peak increases in prolactin of twofold to 10-fold at 30 minutes after injection in normal children.

Thyroid-stimulating hormone (TSH): Hyperfunction. Elevation of serum TSH in childhood is invariably due to primary hypothyroidism: TSH-secreting tumors are extremely rare.

Thyroid-stimulating hormone: Hypofunction. Hypothalamic–pituitary disease will produce the symptoms and signs of hypothyroidism. The TRH stimulation test will separate primary pituitary insufficiency from hypothalamic dysfunction, by showing absence of TSH response to TRH in pituitary disease. The test is performed as described previously. Absence of TSH response also occurs in active hyperthyroidism, in thyroxine ingestion, and if thyroid-stimulating immunoglobulins are present in the circulation.

Gonadotropins (LH and FSH): Hyperfunction. In childhood excessive production of gonadotropins produces precocious sexual development, and in the majority of cases is secondary to hypothalamic dysfunction. In girls the cause is most often "idiopathic," in which there is premature maturation of normal pubertal control mechanisms. In a high proportion of males, however, a specific hypothalamic lesion will be found. In either case intravenous injection of 100 μg synthetic gonadotropic–releasing hormone (LH-RH) will produce a "pubertal" type of response, with a fourfold increase in plasma LH by 30–45 minutes,[97] in contrast to the usual modest rise seen in the normal prepubertal child. Exceptions to this are found in situations in which the causative lesion is an actively functioning endocrine unit. Typical examples are the hCG-secreting dysgerminoma and the LH-RH-secreting hamartoma. Here "LH-like" activity is high, and there will be suppression of the normal response to exogenous LH-RH.

Elevated LH and FSH also are seen, of course, in primary hypogonadism.

Gonadotropins: Hypofunction. The LH-RH stimulation test will produce a "flat" LH response in significant pituitary disease, and in long-standing hypothalamic insufficiency. In the latter situation, continuous four-hour LH-RH infusion, or repeated LH-RH injections given over a four-day period, will produce increasing increments in LH response.

Posterior Pituitary Function

The diagnosis of diabetes insipidus is usually straightforward, and based on clinical history, and the finding of low urine specific gravity (usually <1.005) in an early morning sample. Occasionally a formal water-deprivation test is required.

Water-deprivation test. After a light fluid-free breakfast at 08.00 hours, the patient is asked to void, is weighed, and has blood taken for measurement of electrolytes, osmolality, BUN, and hematocrit.

Administered under strict supervision, no further water is permitted by mouth for the duration of the test, and urine volume, osmolality, and body weight are measured at hourly intervals.

After seven hours, or if 3 percent weight loss has occurred, blood measurements are repeated, and if two consecutive urine samples indicate a change in osmolality of <30 mOsm, pitressin is given and measurements repeated on urine and blood one hour later. Pitressin is usually given as aqueous vasopressin, 5 units by subcutaneous injection, but we have also used nasal DDAVP (D-desaminoarginine vasopressin) and found it very satisfactory.

In the normal individual, blood osmolality, electrolytes, and hematocrit should remain unchanged, and the urine osmolality should be at least twice that of the blood. With diabetes insipidus of central nervous system origin, urine osmolality fails to rise significantly, and there are inappropriate continued diuresis and serum osmolality, sodium, BUN, and hematocrit increases. With ADH treatment, there is an immediate reduction in urine output, and urine osmolality increases by more than 9 percent.

CLINICAL MANAGEMENT OF NEUROSURGICAL LESION OF THE HYPOTHALAMUS AND PITUITARY IN CHILDREN

Recent advances in neurosurgery have improved the prognosis and outlook for patients with disease in the hypothalamic–pituitary region. New knowledge of neuroendocrinology and improved hormonal therapy have decreased morbidity and altered the postoperative outlook of these surviving patients. Modern management requires cooperation between the neurosurgeon and the endocrinologist. This team approach to the patients with neuroendocrine disorders has improved the preoperative and postoperative care and improved the long-term outlook of patients.

Neurosurgical lesions of the hypothalamic and pituitary region are primarily tumors. Occasionally granulomas due to histiocytosis X, arterial aneurysms, pyogenic abscesses, and primary and secondary malignancies occur. Severe head injuries can also damage the hypothalamus and/or the pituitary gland. Lesions in this area may interfere with the normal functioning of the hypothalamic–pituitary–target organ axis by direct interference with the secretion of releasing hormone from the hypothalamus or the trophic hormone from the pituitary. In addition most tumors produce symptoms of increased intracranial pressure (headache and vomiting), visual disturbance (decreased acuity, field defects), or endocrine disturbances. The endocrine disturbances are mainly those of hormonal deficiency; however, some tumors, notably hamartomas of the tubercinereum, may secrete releasing hormones, resulting in hyperpituitarism.

Endocrine symptoms include short stature or slow growth, polyuria, polydipsia, delayed sexual maturation, sexual precocity, and, very rarely, acromegagly. Some children have no endocrine symptoms or signs preoperatively, the tumor presenting only with visual symptoms or increased intracranial pressure. Galactorrhea and amenorrhea may also occur.

The most common tumor in the region is a craniopharyngioma.[98] Others include optic gliomas, hypothalamic gliomas, hamartomas, and pineal tumors. Pituitary adenomas are rare in childhood, as are pituitary abscesses.

The *diagnosis* of hypothalamic and pituitary tumors is usually made on the basis of a history, physical examination with particular emphasis on the eyes, visual fields, and appropriate radiographic studies.

The *endocrine assessment* should include an accurate height and weight, and the assessment of sexual development scored according to the method of Tanner.[99] Since operative intervention may be of some urgency, only simple preoperative laboratory investigations are usually indicated. Most, if not all, tests will have to be repeated postoperatively. The 24-hour urine volume, specific gravity or osmolality (random or first morning sample), serum electrolytes, thyroxine, thyrotropic hormone, and diurnal cortisol levels can usually be obtained within 24 hours. If children are in the pubertal age range or show evidence of early sexual development, gonadotropic hormone, estradiol, and testosterone levels should also be obtained. Pituitary stimulation tests are usually not indicated preoperatively unless acromegaly is suspected. If acromegaly is present, the child usually demonstrates excessive growth in height as well as acromegalic features, such as thickening of the hands and coarsening of the facial features. If a pituitary adenoma is suspected, prolactin levels should also be obtained.

Children with lesions in the hypothalamic pituitary area may have no symptoms or signs of adrenal insufficiency, but with stress (e.g., induction of anaesthesia) may become hypotensive and go into shock. It is mandatory that glucocorticoids be given during such investigative procedures. Soluble hydrocortisone 100 mg IV during induction and 100 mg in divided doses over the next 24 hours is usually satisfactory. Depending on subsequent plans, the hydrocortisone can be safely discontinued after 24 hours without tapering the dose as long as the child remains well. Many patients are on dexamethasone to control cerebral edema. In our experience this drug seems satisfactory to cover any stress on the hypothalamic–pituitary–adrenocortical axis.

Preoperative Management

Most children require little preoperative therapy if they are asymptomatic. If hypothyroidism is diagnosed, L-thyroxine, 0.1 to 0.2 mg/day, is given orally as replacement. If diabetes insipidus is diagnosed, (low specific gravity, high-volume urine), DDAVP (1-desamino-8-D-arginine vasopressin, a synthetic analog of vasopressin) 0.05 to 0.1 ml, can be given intranasally over 12 to 24 hours. Any ACTH deficiency is adequately managed by dexamethasone. The replacement of growth hormone and sex steroids should await complete postoperative recovery.

require DDAVP three times a day and in larger doses. Seasonal nasal allergies and upper respiratory tract infections may interfere with the absorption of DDAVP for short periods of time.

The assessment of anterior pituitary function should be delayed at least six months. This allows the child to recover from the surgery and any subsequent radiation. It is the minimum time in which growth velocity can be measured accurately. By this time it will be obvious whether cortisone is necessary. The assessment thus is mainly for growth hormone and the gonadotropins.

Endocrine Deficit

Most children, except those with very small tumors that are totally removed, have some evidence of endocrine deficit. Hypothyroidism (serum thyroxine less than the normal range) can be treated easily with L-thyroxine, 0.1 to 0.2 mg/day by mouth. Cortisol lack secondary to ACTH deficiency can be replaced using cortisone acetate, 20–25 $mg/m^2/day$ or less. As discussed above many children can get by with lower doses except at times of stress when the maintenance dose should be tripled. Gonadotropic hormone deficiency can be treated with oral testosterone or estrogens. If growth hormone deficiency is present and the child is significantly short, then administration of the sex hormone should be delayed until the full growth potential using therapeutic growth hormone has been achieved.

If growth hormone deficiency is diagnosed (growth velocity less than 4 cm per year with low or undetectable levels of growth hormone in the plasma following stimulation tests), growth hormone extracted from human pituitary glands is available for therapy. Normal growth and the attainment of a respectable adult height are now achievable.[103] Growth hormone soon may be available in larger quantities due to advances in recombinant DNA research. Every child with growth hormone deficiency thus should now be able to receive adequate treatment.

The management of children with multiple pituitary hormone deficiencies usually requires the expertise of an endocrinologist in order to use optimally the hormone preparations available.

Radiation and Intracranial Tumors

It has recently been reported that isolated growth hormone deficiency has developed in children with intracranial lesions following external radiation.[67] These tumors need not be in the pineal, hypothalamic, or pituitary region. Isolated growth hormone deficiency has developed even when the pituitary gland has been shielded from the radiation. The mechanism of this isolated growth hormone deficiency is not clear. The growth of all children who have had radiation to lesions in the cranium thus should be carefully followed.

INAPPROPRIATE ANTIDIURETIC HORMONE SECRETION

The physiologic regulation of antidiuretic hormone secretion (ADH) was discussed earlier in this chapter. There are a number of pediatric conditions associated with inappropriate or nonphysiologic secretion of ADH.[104] Infections of the central nervous system, notably bacterial meningitis, encephalitis, or trauma, are the conditions usually associated with excess ADH.[105] Malignant neoplasms that produce ADH-like peptides are very rare in children. Head injuries with or without skull fractures may be associated with both ADH deficiency or inappropriate secretion,[106] and subdural hematomas and diffuse cerebrovascular disease can also be associated with inappropriate ADH secretion.[107,108]

Normally ADH is secreted during surgery as a result of a number of factors, including the stress of surgery, preoperative medications, relative fluid restriction, and the anesthesia.[109] This antidiuresis is usually short lived, and with judicious fluid administration, careful monitoring of urine flow, and serum electrolytes, rarely causes difficulty.

Inappropriate ADH secretion is diagnosed when the following criteria are present: (1) hyponatremia and plasma hypo-osmolality, (2) inappropriate high urine osmolality, (3) continuing sodium loss in the urine, (4) a normal or expanded blood volume, and (5) normal renal and adrenal function.[110]

The excess ADH, together with continued normal water intake, causes renal retention of water and expansion of the extracellular fluid, with resultant hyponatremia. The ADH effect on the kidney causes a fall in urine volume and a rise in urine osmolality. The extracellular fluid expansion results in continued urinary sodium excretion.

In mild cases (serum sodium between 120 and 130 mEq/l) and plasma osmolality above 240 mOsm/kg of water) no symptoms may occur. When the serum sodium level falls below 120 mEq/l, nausea, anorexia, and vomiting may occur. Below 110 mEq/l neurologic symptoms, notably lethargy, sleepiness, and seizures develop. Neurologic symptoms can occur at any level of serum sodium. The more rapid the fall in serum sodium, the more likely symptoms are to occur.

Management of Inappropriate ADH Secretion

Postoperative hyponatremia of a mild degree is usually due to the inadvertent administration of excess hypotonic fluid and the normal secretion of ADH that occurs with surgery. Careful attention to fluid administration following surgery will prevent hyponatremia. If hyponatremia does occur, restricting fluids to a volume equal to the calculated insensible losses until the excess water is excreted and the serum sodium returns to normal is usually sufficient to correct the problem.

Acute or chronic inappropriate ADH secretion occurring during intracranial disease is best handled by treating the underlying condition (e.g., meningitis) and by restricting fluids to two thirds or three quarters of maintenance values. Saline infusions are not beneficial in these cases. The sodium load is rapidly excreted because of the extracellular volume expansion present.

If acute hyponatremia develops or neurologic symptoms occur, fluid restriction alone may be too slow to raise the plasma sodium. Hypertonic saline infusions calculated to raise the serum sodium approximately 10 mEq may help. If used in conjunction with furosamide, a loop diuretic, the serum sodium level can usually be raised. Lithium chloride and demeclocycline, renal antagonists of ADH, have also been used.[111]

Serious hyponatremia can be prevented by fluid restriction in the clinical settings likely to be associated with ADH secretion. Severe hyponatremia with neurologic symptoms may be helped by hypertonic saline, diuretics, or ADH antagonists.

REFERENCES

1. Reichlin S, in Reichlin S, Baldessarini RJ, Martin JB (eds): The Hypothalamus. New York, Raven Press, 1978, p 1
2. Daughaday WH: The adenohypophysis, in Williams RH (ed): Textbook of Endocrinology. Philadelphia, WB Saunders Co., 1982
3. Knowles F: Ependymal secretion, especially in the hypothalamic region. J Neurovisc Relations 14(suppl):97–101, 1969
4. Lichensteizer W, Langemann H: Uptake of exogenous catecholamines by monoamine-containing neurons of the CNS. J Pharmacol Exp Ther 151:400–402, 1966
5. Jonsson G, Fuxe K, Hokfelt T: On the catecholamine innervation of the hypothalamus with special reference to the median eminence. Brain Res 40:271–274, 1972
6. Bjorklund A: Identification and terminal distribution of the tuberohypophysial monoamine fiber systems in the rat. Brain Res 17:1–23, 1970
7. Nair RMG, Barrett JF, Bowers CY, et al: Structure of porcine TRH. Biochemistry 9:1103–1106, 1970
8. Burgus R, Dunn TF, Desiderio D, et al: Characterization of ovine hypothalamic hypophysiotropic TSH-releasing factor. Nature 226:321–325, 1970
9. Fleisher N: Synthetic TRH as a test of pituitary thyrotropin reserve. J Clin Endocrinol 34:617–619, 1972
10. Gautvik KM: Serum prolactin and TSH: Effects of nursing and pyro. Glu-His-Pro-NH to postpartum women. J Clin Endocrinol 37:135–138, 1973
11. Schally, AV, Arimura A, Kastin AJ, et al: Hypothalamic regulatory hormones. Science 179:341–343, 1973
12. Franchimont P: Effects of LH-RH on plasma gonadotropin levels in normal subjects. Clin Endocrinol 3:27–30, 1974
13. Schally AV, Kastin AJ, Arimura A: FSH regulatory hormones. Science 179:341–344, 1973
14. Brazeau P, Vale W, Burgus R, et al: Hypothalamic polypeptide that inhibits the secretion of immunoreactive pituitary growth hormone. Science 179:77–79, 1973
15. Martin JB: Brain regulation of GH secretion, in Martini L, Ganong WF (eds): Frontiers of Neuroendocrinology, vol. 4. New York, Raven Press, 1976, p 129
16. Leveque TF, Slutinsky F, Porte A, et al: Ultrastructure of the medial prechiasmatic gland in the rat and mouse. Neuroendocrinology 2:56–59, 1967
17. Weindl A: Neuroendocrine aspects of the circumventricular organs, in Ganong WF, Martini L (eds): Frontiers in Neuroendocrinology. Oxford, Oxford University Press, 1973, p 3
18. Barry J, Dubois MP: Etude en immunofluorescence des structures hypothalamiques a competence gonadotrope. Ann Endocrinol 34:735–742, 1973
19. Kizer JS, Palkovits M, Brownstein M: Releasing factors in the circumventricular organs of the rat brain. Endocrinology 98:311–321, 1976
20. Joseph SA, Sorrentino S, Sundberg DA: Releasing hormones LRF and TRF in the CSF of the third ventricle, in Knigge KM, Scott DE, (eds): Brain Endocrine Interactions II. Basel, Karger, 1975, p 306
21. Simpson JB, Routtenberg A: Subfrontal organ site of drinking elicitation of angiotensin II. Science 173:1172–1174, 1970
22. Klein DC: The pineal gland: A model of neuroendocrine regulation, in Reichlin S, Baldessarini RJ, Martin JB (eds): The Hypothalamus. New York, Raven Press, 1978, p 303
23. Vaughan MK: Arginine vasotocin: Structure activity relationships and influence on gonadal growth and function. Am Zool 16:25–29, 1976
24. Fuxe K: Cellular localization of monoamines in the median eminence and in the infundibular stem. Acta Phys Scand 58:383–388, 1963
25. Fuxe K, Hökfelt T: Catecholamines in the hypothalamic and the pituitary gland, in Ganong WF, Martin L (eds): Frontiers in Neuroendocrinology. New York, Oxford Univ Press, 1969
26. Anden NE, Dahlstron A, Fuxe K, et al: Ascending monoamine neurons in the telencephalon and diencephalon. Acta Physiol Scand 67:313–326, 1966

27. Fuxe K, Jonsson G: Further mapping of central 5 HT neurons. Adv Biochem Psychopharm 10:1–9, 1974
28. Richards JG, Lorex HP, Tranzer JP: Indealkyleamine nerve terminals in cerebral ventricles. Brain Res 57:277–281, 1973
29. Richard JG, Tranzer JP: The characterization of nonaminergic nerve terminals in the brain by few structural chemistry, in Knowles F, Volbrath L (eds): Neurosecretion: The Final Neuronendocrine Pathway. Berlin, Springer-Verlag, 1974
30. Hökfelt T, Fuxe K, Johansson O, et al: Distribution of TRH in the CNS as revealed by immunohistochemistry. Eur J Phar 34:389–392, 1975
31. Hökfelt T, Fuxe K, Johansson O, et al: TRH containing nerve terminals in certain brain stem nuclei and in the spinal cord. Neuroscience Lett 1:133–139, 1975
32. Köves K, Magyar A: On the location of TRH producing neurons. Thyroid response to PTU treatment after stereotoxic interventions in hypothalamus. Endocrine Exp 9:247–257, 1975
33. Palkovits M, Brownstein M, Kizer SJ: Effect of total hypothalamic differentiation on releasing hormones and neurotransmitter concentration in the medial basal hypothalamus in the rat, in Endroczy E (ed): International Symposium of Neuroendocrinology Processes, Budapest, Akodemiai Kiado, 1975, p 575
34. Reichlin S: Thyroid function, body temperature regulation and growth in rats with hypothalamic lesions. Endocrinology 66: 340–354, 1960
35. Setalo G, Vigh S, Schally AV, et al: Immunohistochemical study of the origin of LH-RH containing nerve fibers of the rat hypothalamus. Brain Res 103:597–602, 1976
36. Zimmerman EA, Hsu KG, Ferin M, et al: Localization of LH-RH in the hypothalamus of mouse by immunoperoxidase technique. Endocrionology 95:1–8, 1974
37. Erlandsen SL, Hegre OD, Parsons JA, et al: Pancreatic islet cell hormones. Evidence for the presence of SRIF and gastrin within the D-cell. J Histochem Cytochem 24:883–897, 1976
38. Orci L, Baetens D, Dubois MP, et al: Evidence for the D-cell of the pancreas secreting somatostatin. Hormon Metab Res 7:400–402, 1975
39. Hughes I, Smith TW, Kosterlitz HW, et al: Identification of two related pentapeptides from the brain with potent opiate agonist activity. Nature 258:577–579, 1975
40. Guillemin R, Ling N, Burgus R: Endorphins, peptides, d'origini hypothalamique et neurohypophysaire a activite morphinomimetique. Isolement et structure moleculaire de l'u-endorphine. CR Acad Sci, Paris 282:783–785, 1976
41. Powell D, Leeman SE, Tregear GW, et al: RIA for substance P. Nature 241:252–254, 1973
42. Carraway R, Leeman S: Radioimmunoassay for neurotensin, a hypothalamic peptide. J Biol Chem 251:7035–7044, 1976
43. Baker BL: In Greep RO, Asywood EB (eds): Handbook of Physiology. Section 7: Endocrinology, Vol. 4, Part I, American Physiology Society. Baltimore, Williams & Wilkins, 1974, p 45
44. Martin JB, Reichlin S, Brown GM (eds): Clinical Neuroendocrinology. Philadelphia, FA Davis, 1974, p 13
45. Li CH, Barnafi L, Chretien M, et al: Isolation and amino acid sequence of n-LPH from sheep pituitary glands. Nature 208:1093–1094, 1965
46. Hughes J, Smith TW, Kosterlitz HW, et al: HR with potent opiate agonist activity. Nature 258:577–579, 1975
47. Cox BW, Goldstein A, Li CH: Opioid activity of a peptide, n-LPH (61–91) derived from n-LPH. Proc Natl Acad Sci USA 73:1821–1823, 1976
48. Lazarus LH, Ling N, Giullemin R: n-LPH as a prohormone for the morphinomimetic peptides, endorphins and encephalins. Proc Natl Acad Sci USA 73:2156–2159, 1976
49. Klein DC, Weller JL: Indole metabolism in the pineal gland. A circadian rhythm in N-acetyl transferase. Science 169:1093, 1970
50. Klein DC, Weller JL: A rapid light-induced decrease in pineal serotonin N-acetyltransferase activity. Science 177:532–533, 1972

51. Koizumi K, Hishina H, Colman D: The suprachiasmatic nuclei and circadian rhythms, in Neuroscience Abstracts, fifth Annual Meeting, Society for Neuroscience, 1975, p 446
52. Smalstig EB, Clemens JA: The role of the suprachiasmatic nuclei in reproductive cyclicity, in Neuroscience Abstracts, Fifth Annual Meeting, Society for Neurosciences, 1975, p 434
53. Sassin JF, Parker DC, Mace JW, et al: Human growh hormone secretion release: Relation to slow-wave sleep and sleep-walking cycles. Science 165:513–516, 1969
54. Parker DC, Rossman LG, Vander Loon EI: Sleep related nucleothermeral and briefly episodic variation in human plasma prolactin concentrations. J Clin Endocrinol 36:1119–1124, 1973
55. Boyar R: Synchronization of augmented LH secretion with sleep during puberty. N Eng J Med 287:582–585, 1972
56. Imura, H., Nakai Y, Yoshima T: Effects of 5HTP on growth hormone and ACTH release in man. J Clin Endocrinol 36:204–206, 1973
57. MacLeod, RM: Regulation of prolactin secretion, in Martini L, Ganong WF (eds): Frontiers in Neuroendocrinology, vol 4. New York, Raven Press, 1975, p 168
58. Martin JB: Regulation in GH secretion, in Martini L, Ganong WF (eds): Frontiers in Neuroendocrinology, vol. 4. New York, Raven Press, 1975
59. Martin JB: Regulation in GH secretion, in Martini L, Ganong WF (eds): Frontiers in Neuroendocrinology vol 4. New York, Raven Press, 1975
60. Chambers JW, Brown GM: Neurotransmitter regulation of growth hormone and ACTH in the rhesus monkey: Effects of biogenic amines. Endocrinology 98:420–428, 1976
61. Rivier C, Brown M, Vale W: Effect of neurotensin substance P and morphine sulfate on the secretion of prolactin and growth hormone in the rat. Endocrinology 100:529–533, 1977
62. Van Wyk JJ, Underwood LE: Relation between GH and somatomedin. Ann Rev Med 26:427–438, 1975
63. Martin JB, Reichlin S: Neural regulation of the pituitary thyroid axis, in Kenny AD, Anderson RR (eds): Proceedings, Sixth Midwest Conference on the Thyroid. New York, Columbia University Press, 1970, p 1
64. Mason JW: A review of psychoendocrine research on the pituitary-thyroid system. Psychosom Med 30:666–669, 1968
65. Hershman JM, Pittman JA Jr: Control of TSH in man. N Engl J Med 285:997–999, 1971
66. Hall R: The TRH test in diseases of the pituitary and hypothalamus. Lancet 1:759–861, 1972
67. Defendini R, Zimmerman E: The magnocellular neurosecretory system of the mammalian hypothalamus, in Reichlin S, Baldessarini R, Martin JB (eds): The Hypothalamus. New York, Raven Press, 1978, p 137
68. Van Dyke HB, Chow BF, Greep RO et al: The isolation of a protein from pars neuralis of the ox pituitary with constant oxytocic, pressor and diuresis-inhibiting effects. J Pharmacol (Kyoto) 74:19–209, 1941
69. Douglas WW: Mechanism of release of neurohypophysial hormones, in Knobil E, Sawyer WH (eds): Handbook of Physiology, sect. 7, Washington, DC, American Physiological Society, 1974
70. Zimmerman EA, Carmel PW, Hussain MK, et al: Vasopressin and neurophysin. Science 182:925–927, 1973
71. Zimmerman EA, Stillman MA, Recht LA, et al: Vasopressin and CRF. Ann NY Acad Sci 297:405–419, 1977
72. Moses AM: Diabetes insipidus and ADH regulation, in Kreiger DT, Hughes JC (eds): Neuroendocrinology. Sunderland, Massachusetts, Sinauer Associates, 1980, p 141
73. Reid IA, Morris BJ, Ganong WF: The renin–angiotensin system. Ann Rev Physiol 40:377–380, 1978
74. Reid IA, Ramsay DJ: The effects of intracerebroventricular administration of renin on drinking and blood pressure. Endocrinology 97(3):536–538, 1975

75. Simpson JB, Epstein AN, Camardo JS Jr: Localization of receptors for the dipsogenic action of angiotensin II in the subfornical organ of the rat. J Comp Physiol Psychol 92(4):581–584, 1978
76. Hayward JN: The amygdaloid nuclear complex and mechanisms of release of vasopressin from the neurohypophysis, in Eleftherion BE (ed): Neurobiology of the Amydala. New York, Plenum Press,1972, p 685
77. Martin JB, Reichlin S, Brown GH: Clinical neuroendocrinology, in Contemporary Neurology Series. Philadelphia, FA Davies, 1977, chap 4
78. Nicoll RA, Barker JL: The pharmacology of recurrent inhibition in the supraoptic neurosecretory system. Brain Res 35:501–504, 1971
79. Robinson AG: Isolation and secretion of individual human neurophysin. J Clin Invest 55:360–367, 1975
80. Hensel H: Neural processes in thermoregulation. Physiol Rev 53:948–1017, 1973
81. Plum F, Posner J: The Diagnosis of Stupor and Coma (ed 2). Philadelphia, FA Davis, 1972
82. Hetherington AW, Ranson SW: Experimental hypothalamico–hypophyseal obesity in the rat. Proc Soc Exp Biol Med 41:465–466, 1939
83. Grossman SP: The neuroanatomy of eating and drinking behavior, in Kreiger DT, Hughes JC (eds): Neuroendocrinology. Massachusetts, Sinauer Associates, 1980, p 141
84. Brierley JB: The neuropathology of amnesic states, in Whitty CWM, Zangwill OL (eds): Amnesia. London, Butterworths, 1966, pp 150–180
85. Kahn E, Crosby EC: Korsakoff's syndrome associated with surgical lesions involving the mammillary bodies. Neurology (Minneapolis) 22:117–125, 1972
86. Reeves AG, Plum F: Hyperphagia, rage and dementia accompanying a ventromedial hypothalamic neoplasm. Arch Neurol 20:616–624, 1969
87. Penfield W, Milner B: Memory deficit produced by bilateral lesions in the hippocampal zone. Arch Neurol Psychiatr 79:475–497, 1958
88. van Ree JM, Bohus B, Versteeg DHG, et al: Neurohypophyseal principles and memory processes. Biochem Pharmacol 27:1793–1800, 1975
89. de Wied D: Effects of peptide hormones on behavior, in Ganong WF, Martinin L (eds): Frontiers in Neuroendocrinology, New York, Oxford Press, 1969
90. Brown FC Jr, Forney WR: Diencephalic syndrome of early infancy associated with brain tumor. Pediatrics 24:609–615, 1959
91. Bernard JD, Aguilard MJ: Localized hypothalamic histiocytosis X. Arch Neurol 20:368–372, 1969
92. Wortis H, Maurer WS: "Sham rage." Man Am J Psychol 98:638–644, 1942
93. Kaplan S, Grumbach M: A syndrome of hypopituitary dwarfism, hypoplasia of optic nerve and malformation of the prosencepholan. Pediat Res 4:480, 1970 (Abst)
94. Rudman D: Growth hormone deficiency with cleft lip or palate. J Pediat 93:3, 378–379, 1978
95. Rimoin DL, Schimke RN: Anterior pituitary in genetic disorders of endocrine glands. St. Louis, CV Mosby, 1971, pp 11–65
96. Crieg WR, Boyle JA, Maxwell JD, et al: Criteria for distinguishing normal from subnormal adrenocortical function using ACTH. Postgrad Med J 44:307, 1969
97. Grumbach MM, Roth JC, Kaplan SC, et al: Hypothalamic-pituitary regulation of puberty in man, in Grumbach MM, Grave GD, Mayer FE (eds): The Control of the Onset of Puberty. New York, Wiley, 1974
98. Banna M, Hood RD, Stanley P, et al: Craniopharyngioma in children. J Pediatr, 83:781–785, 1973
99. Tanner JM: Growth at Adolescence (ed 2). Oxford, Blackwell, 1962
100. Hoffman HJ, Hendrick EB, Hymphreys RP, et al: Management of craniopharyngioma in children. J Neurosurg 47:218–227, 1977
101. Daneman D, Ehrlich RM, Bailey JD: Postcraniotomy diabetes mellitus. Treatment with DDAVP a synthetic analog of vasopressin. J Pediatr 93:879–880, 1980
102. Bode BH, Harley BM, Crawford JD: Restoration of normal drinking behavior by chlorpropamide in patients with hypodipsia and diabetes insipidus. Am J Med 51:304–313, 1971

103. Guyda H, Fraser H, Bailey JD, et al: Medical Research Council of Canada therapeutic trial of human growth hormone: First five years of therapy. Can Med Assoc J 112:1301–1306, 1975
104. Mendoza S: Syndrome of inappropriate antidiuretic hormone secretion. Paed Clin NA, 23:681–690, 1976
105. Mangos JA, Lobeck CC: Studies of sustained hyponatremia due to central nervous system infection. Pediatrics 34:503–510, 1964
106. Haden HT, Knox GW: Cerebral hyponatremia with inappropriate antidiuretic syndrome. Am J Med Sci 249:381–390, 1965
107. Goldberg M: Hyponatremia and inappropriate secretion of antidiuretic hormone. Am J Med 35:293–298, 1963
108. Maroon JC, Campbell RL: Subdural hematoma. AMA Arch Neurol 22:234–239, 1970.
109. Klenk EL, Winters RW: Inappropriate secretion of antidiuretic hormone, in Winters RW (ed): The Body Fluids in Pediatrics. Boston, Little, Brown, 1973, p 429–436
110. Bartter FC, Schwartz WB: The syndrome of inappropriate secretion of antidiuretic hormone. Am J Med 42:790–801, 1967
111. Friedman AL, Segar WE; Antidiuretic hormone excess. J Pediatr 94:521–526, 1979

64. Nutrition, Volumes, Ions, and Radicals

A. Loren Amacher
Rolando F. Del Maestro

Among the pitfalls confronting the clinician charged with the care of a sick child, preoperatively or postoperatively, neurosurgically or otherwise, the deepest and most difficult from which to extract oneself involves the commonly interlaced abnormalities of nutritional status, body volumes, electrolyte balance, and free radical generation. In general the older the child, the less difficult it is to anticipate and treat such abnormal states. In the case of oxygen-derived free radical generation, we are just beginning to comprehend the pathophysiology involved, particularly as it relates to the sick central nervous system.

In this chapter we outline normal requirements and values in the well child, the changes that may occur in selected pathologic states, current concepts of management, and common pitfalls.

NUTRITION

The growing child has extraordinary requirements, compared with the mature adult, for all nutritional materials. Table 64-1 is an outline of the necessities for maintenance of an anabolic state in children, for calories, protein, fats, and carbohydrates. Vitamin and mineral requirements vary with age, and the reader is referred to any current textbook on pediatrics or nutrition. Demands change with age, and increase—often vastly—in times of stress such as trauma, postoperatively, with sepsis, or tissue loss, especially burns. While the normal child can tolerate short periods of starvation without ill effect, the child in a catabolic state is doubly at risk if caloric and protein requirements are withheld for even a few days. The protein-sparing effect of adequate caloric intake is recognized, but loss of more than 30 percent of lean body mass (principally muscle) is irreplaceable by oral intake, and carries a very poor prognosis concerning adequate recovery, even survival. While infusions of lipid and carbohydrate can provide caloric requirements, they will not protect protein synthesis during catabolic states. Most seriously the maturing nervous system requires a constant supply of energy substrate (glucose), amino acids, and oxygen if it is to reach its functional potential.

Table 64-1
Daily Requirements in Children

	Newborn	Infant	Child	Adolescent
Calories	120 kcal/kg	110 kcal/kg ⟶		50 kcal/kg
Protein	2.5–3.5 g/kg	2.0–3.0 g/kg	2.0 g/kg	1.5 g/kg
Fat	⟵ Must contain linoleic and arachidonic acid ⟶			
Carbohydrate	⟵ To make up caloric value. Protein-sparing effect ⟶			
Water	100 ml/kg	100 ml/kg	75 ml/kg	50 ml/kg

As soon as possible following any major stress to the child, nutritional requirements should be restored. The gastrointestinal (GI) tract is the best alimentary mechanism known, and in the absence of major abdominal trauma, abdominal sepsis, or ileus, should be used for oral, tube, gastrostomal, or jejunostomal feedings. To counteract poststress catabolism, daily requirements of calories and protein should be oversupplied by at least 50 percent. When feedings are provided by any of the tube methods, continuous infusion may help prevent stress ulcers of the GI tract. Protein losses may be excessive in some renal, hepatic, and GI conditions such as nephrosis, cirrhosis-ascites, and protein-losing enteropathies—all of which, incidentally, may occur iatrogenically—and should be replaced.

When the GI tract cannot be used for alimentation, as may be the case in association with abdominal trauma, sepsis, postshock states, or the ileus that may accompany any major stress, an intravenous method is next best. Hyperalimentation solutions are readily available commercially, and will supply adequate nutrition. Intravenous vitamins should be given liberally, especially vitamin C and the fat-soluble members of the B complex. Peripheral venous hyperalimentation may suffice for short periods such as several days, but for prolonged therapy, delivery of the solution by central lines is mandatory.

Nor is such therapy without risk. Sepsis is the most serious danger, but fatty degeneration of the liver, cholestasis (even with empyema), and nephropathy are encountered with disturbing frequency. Hyperalimentation may make the control of inappropriate secretion of antidiuretic hormone (ADH) (ISADH) very difficult.

It is well to remember that prolonged antibiotic therapy, by any route, may lead to serious dysfunction of the GI and renal systems. There are few more difficult management problems in all of surgery than the child with multiple organ injury, with recurrent bouts of sepsis requiring intravenous antibiotics, needing central hyperalimenatation for protection against a rampant catabolic state, and most particularly if the child is unconscious.

VOLUMES

It is very easy and extremely dangerous to miscalculate or misappreciate the delicate balance between and small quantities involved in intravascular, extracellular, and intracellular volumes, especially in the infant. Further, the younger the child, the less mature is the autonomic nervous system and the more likely are sudden stresses to induce abnormalities in temperature control and in water and ionic balances. Loss of temperature control and dehydration are often lethal in infants.

BLOOD VOLUME

The premature neonate is at greatest risk. For example, a 2500-gram infant has 200 ml of *total* blood volume (80 ml/kg). In such a patient, 50 ml of blood loss is very likely to induce sudden hemodynamic collapse. Major blood loss in children tends to creep up on the unwary surgeon, especially the slow low-pressure ooze from open bone channels or extensive subcutaneous exposures. The insidious leakage of blood from incisional vessels, if uncontrolled easily can result in a vascular volume loss of 10 percent over the course of a one-hour procedure. For this reason, many pediatric surgeons infiltrate all incisional lines with a weak epinephrine solution (1:200,000 solution is effective) a few minutes prior to opening the incisions. The epinephrine assists in closing down the small subcutaneous vessels.

In addition to the agonal state, there are certain posthead injury situations in young children that may be associated with hemodynamic shock.

1. Scalp artery laceration, especially the superficial temporal, occipital, supratrochlear, and supraorbital arteries.
2. Intracranial bleeding, especially in infants. We have seen a 400-ml epidural hematoma in a 10-kg infant—50 percent of blood volume. Such risk is increased in a hydrocephalic child with a functioning shunt, because all intracranial tamponade effects are negated when cerebrospinal fluid (CSF) can simply run through a pressure-dependent valve more quickly. As an addendum the premature neonate with ventricular haemorrhage quite regularly experiences a sudden drop in hematocrit of 50 percent.
3. Sudden release of intracranial pressure. Occasionally this will induce a shock-like state, with peripheral vasoconstriction, sweating, tachypnoea, and tachycardia. This response may be profound in the infant and probably is related to immaturity of the autonomic nervous system. Further, we have seen sudden release of ICP cause multiple subcortical and deep nuclear hemorrhages, associated with hemodynamic collapse.

EXTRAVASCULAR AND INTRACELLULAR VOLUMES

The interchange of water, electrolytes, and nutritional or waste product molecules between vascular, extracellular, and intracellular spaces is controlled by several factors. These include:

1. The integrity of the capillary endothelium and, in the case of the central nervous system (CNS), the blood–brain barrier (endothelial tight junctions and the basement membrane–astrocytic footplate complex).
2. The hydrostatic and osmotic pressure gradients along the capillary–extravascular interface, gradients that follow Starling's principles.
3. The integrity of cellular membrane pumping mechanisms that maintain ionic concentrations essential for the function of both the cell and its membrane. Using the neurone as an example, the membrane pump must maintain intracellular ion concentrations in the face of adverse transmembrane gradients, must maintain intracellular hydrogen ion (proton) concentration within very narrow limits, and must eliminate a wide range of toxic end products of metabolism and enzymatic action. One of the principal effects of anaerobic metabolism (glycolysis) in

neurones is the failure of glycolytic processes to provide sufficient energy in the form of adenosine triphosphate (ATP) to keep the membrane pumps running at full efficiency. Failure to maintain intraextracellular ionic gradients soon leads to neuronal swelling and membrane depolarization.

4. The specific activity of certain hormones upon renal membranes, especially the effect of antidiuretic hormone (ADH) upon the renal collecting tubules.

ISADH

The output of ADH increases in any stressful condition, and water is retained as an automatic mechanism to increase intravascular volume. Occasionally, and particularly in association with a host of acute CNS abnormal states ranging from uncomplicated surgical procedures to intracranial sepsis and intracranial pressure (ICP) decompensation, ADH secretion is inappropriately vigorous. The resulting excessive retention of water overwhelms the ability of normal membranes and membrane pumps to maintain water balance within and without cells. This syndrome, inappropriate secretion of ADH (ISADH), is very common and frequently missed. It may be accompanied by deterioration in the level of consciousness, seizures where serum sodium falls precipitously or to levels less than 120 mEq/1, or death when serum sodium is less than 110 mEq/1. The diagnosis is suggested whenever the serum sodium concentration falls below 130 mEq/1 while urine volume remains reasonably normal. The diagnosis is confirmed by finding a serum osmolarity of less than 275 mOsm, a urine osmolarity in excess of 300, a spot urine sodium in excess of 40 mEQ/1, and normal urine volume. There are two methods of treatment:

1. Simple water restriction, 100–600 ml/24 hr depending upon the size and age of the child. This method usually takes several days to restore proper water balance.
2. Normal saline infusion at daily minimum requirement levels, combined with furosemide therapy at 5 to 40 mg three or four times daily. Whereas furosemide induces a sodium diuresis that carries along an obligatory and passive water load, the sodium infusion is more than sufficient to maintain and restore normal total body sodium. Twice-daily serum electrolytes and daily serum and urine osmolarities are necessary for proper monitoring of treatment. This regime usually provides correction of the electrolyte concentrations within 24 to 36 hours, though the resolution of the ISADH may require the passage of several days. In general this treatment method should be reserved for severe cases of ISADH.

DIABETES INSIPIDUS

When ADH secretion is prevented by such diverse mechanisms as pituitary infarction with meningitis or severely increased ICP, section of the pituitary stalk with trauma or intentionally at operation, or stalk section by a tumor such as craniopharyngioma, water diuresis may reach tremendous volumes of 1 to 10 liters per day, depending upon the size of the patient. Frequently the condition is transient, but such water losses must be replaced. Replacement of ADH makes management in such situations easier, but there are risks. Early on, and especially in small patients, aqueous pitressin 0.5 to 1 unit as necessary is the safest agent, because the drug is well mixed and there is much less danger of having unused depot drug in the patient if the pituitary suddenly begins secretion of endogenous ADH. In the latter situation, water intoxication may supervene very quickly.

WATER INTOXICATION

While the effects of water intoxication mimic those of ISADH, it usually arises because of excessive infusion of hypo-osmolar solutions. Compartmental distribution of the water load produces a functional reduction in intracellular osmotic concentrations compared with the extracellular space, simply because of the much greater volume involved. Eighty percent of total body volume is intracellular, 15 percent is extracellular, and 5 percent is intravascular. The treatment, quite simply, is vigorous fluid restriction.

STRESS DIURESIS

Children may develop an inordinate water diruesis in association with severe general body stress such as occurs with multiple organ trauma. It seems that, regardless of the amount of ADH secreted, the collecting tubules fail to respond to the ADH stimulus properly, for reasons that are not well understood.

DEHYDRATION HYPOXEMIA

An unusual response, seen principally in patients with pulmonary injury or neurogenic pulmonary edema in whom dehydration therapy has been vigorous, is that of hypoxemia while total body volume is substantially reduced as with treatment of cerebral swelling. It seems that one response of the pulmonary vasculature to certain critical reductions in vascular volume is to open arteriovenous shunts within the pulmonary bed. Restoration of vascular volume corrects the hypoxemia and, interestingly, does not induce a rise in intracranial pressure. This phenomenon constitutes a little-recognized hazard of dehydration therapy.

IONS AND RADICALS

An *ion* is an atom with an excess or deficiency of electrons as compared with the number of protons, so that the atom carries a net electric charge. A *radical* is an atom or molecule with a single electron in its outer orbital. An *isotope* is a particular nuclear configuration of any atom. Which element an atom represents depends upon the number of protons the nucleus contains. Which isotope of the given element is present depends upon the total number of nuclear particles (protons plus neutrons). Carbon 13 contains six protons and seven neutrons; nitrogen 13 contains seven protons and six neutrons.

An ion is reactive because of its charge, a radical because of its solitary outer electron, and an isotope because of its unstable nuclear configuration. Radicals may or may not be ions, and not all ions are radicals. In human biology isotopes are important principally in diagnosis and treatment. Ions and radicals, however, are of constant interest to the cell.

In solution all molecules ionize to some extent, depending upon other elements in the vicinity, the degree of solubility, and the type of atomic bonding employed by the molecule. Membranes pass or exclude molecules principally on the basis of the size of the hydrated molecule. With ions, however, the additional factors of electric charge and specific pump mechanisms are operational. Ionic transfer across membranes frequently requires energy input and intact membrane anatomy. Abnormal concentrations of ions may be "toxic" because they carry excess water into or out of the cell, they change the pH, they change membrane polarization, or because they are radicals. Usually such toxicity is a concentration phenomenon. Many enzyme systems depend upon ionic catalysts, principally calcium, and certain trace elements such as cobalt, copper, magnesium, manganese, and zinc.

Radicals, on the other hand, may be toxic simply because they are present. Most current interest is centered upon the oxygen-derived activated species, hydrogen peroxide (H_2O_2), superoxide anion radical (O_2-), and hydroxyl radical ($OH\cdot$). The $OH\cdot$ radical may be the most toxic substance in all of biology. Much of cellular evolution has had to do with the ability to deal with oxygen and its derived radicals. Within the CNS, oxygen-derived free radicals are felt to be of enormous importance in mechanisms of vascular permeability, cell ischemia, and cellular response to radiotherapy. A group of enzymes called superoxide dismutases, along with peroxidases and catalases, are recognized increasingly as one of the body's principal detoxifying chemicals.[1]

Within the cell the mitochondrion is equipped to deal with oxygen quickly enough to prevent oxygen toxicity and cell death. The cytochrome oxidase system, rapidly detoxifying oxygen and extracting energy in the process, resides exclusively within the mitochondrion. Aerophobic bacteria, lacking a cytochrome oxidase chain, cannot survive in an oxygen-rich environment. Under anaerobic conditions lasting more than a few minutes, the mitochondrion stops functioning and begins to swell because its membrane pumps shut down. Without the energy production from the citric acid cycle mechanism, which is also confined to the mitochondrion, the rest of the cell must rely upon glycolysis for its energy requirements. For the neurone this process is insufficient to maintain function. Within the cytoplasm oxygen is reduced by adding one electron at a time (the univalent pathway) compared with four-electron increments provided by the cytochrome oxidase system (Figure 64-1). When normal oxygen flow is restored, the mitochondrion may take some time to get back into action. During this interval the cell may be unable to deal with the oxygen it receives and cell damage may occur, paradoxically, because of too much oxygen. Such considerations may be of paramount importance during postischemia resuscitation.

Similarly, radiation damages a cell by inducing formation of oxygen-derived free radicals, especially the $OH\cdot$ radical.[2] Of course normal cells may be destroyed as well, both by intracellular and extracellular appearance and persistence of free radicals. The hope is that tissue surrounding a focus to be destroyed may be protected by introduction of chemicals capable of soaking up,

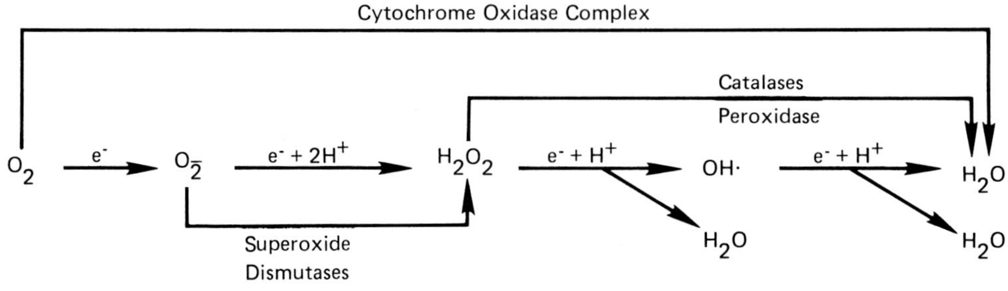

Figure 64-1. The univalent and quadrivalent electron pathways for the reduction of molecular oxygen.

or "scavenging," free radicals, permitting the delivery of much higher doses to the malignant focus.

Perhaps the most exciting aspect of free radical chemistry for the neurosurgeon is in the area of microvascular permeability and cerebral swelling. It appears that the hydroxyl radical (OH·) has a profound effect upon the integrity of the postcapillary venule endothelium, inducing a severe and persistent fluid leak into the surroundings.[3] Hydroxyl radical concentration increases in the extracellular fluid under conditions of hypoxia, ischemia, and superoxide dismutase (SOD) depletion. Suspicion is growing that some of the beneficial effects that may occur with the use of high-dose steroids, or barbiturates, may accrue from their ability to neutralize free radicals. The search for free radical scavengers may become the most important part of neurologic pharmacology in the future.

REFERENCES

1. Fridovich I. The biology of oxygen radicals. Science 201:875–880, 1978
2. Benon H, Bielski J, Gebicki JM. Application of Radiation Chemistry to Biology, in Pryor W (ed): Free Radicals in Biology, vol 3. New York, Academic Press, 1977, pp 1–51
3. Del Maestro RE: The influence of oxygen derived free radicals on in vitro and in vivo model systems. Interactions of superoxide anion radical, hydrogen peroxide and hydroxyl radical. Diss. Acta, Universitatis Upsaliensis, Uppsala, 1979, Abstract 340

Table 65-1
Neurosurgical and Neuroradiology Procedures: Performed under General Anesthesia (Children's Hospital of Pittsburgh 1978–1979)

Operative Procedures	
• Insertion intracranial monitor (isolated procedure)	33
• Craniotomy for subdural or epidural bleeding	15
• Craniotomy for tumor/vascular	45
• Elevation depressed skull fracture	18
• Repair encephalocele	3
• Repair meningomyelocele	13
• Craniectomy (synostosis)	14
• Shunt/shunt revision	230
• Lumbar/cervical laminectomy	18
• Neuroradiology procedures	
Myelography	35
Cerebral angiography	41
CT scan	30
Pneumoencephalography	5

PHYSIOLOGIC AND PHARMACOLOGIC FACTORS THAT INFLUENCE ANESTHESIA IN THE INFANT

Physiologic Factors

The head of the young infant is large and poorly supported on the trunk by a short, weak neck. The tongue is large and the teeth, of course, have not developed. To maintain a patent airway in the unconscious infant, the head is extended largely by arching the back. The head, particularly in the child with hydrocephalus, should be stabilized during anesthesia by placing the crown of the head in a head ring. The body of the child with severe hydrocephalus can be supported on several blankets in order to maintain the airway and to facilitate endotracheal intubation. Heat loss from the large head can be minimized prior to surgery by the use of a stocking cap or a plastic bag.

The infant larynx is funnel-shaped, the narrowest portion being not at the glottis but at the cricoid ring below the glottis. In the infant the diameter of the airway at the cricoid ring thus determines the size of endotracheal tube that may be passed. The larnyx, which is small in the absolute sense, is easily obstructed by edema. For this reason we are reluctant to perform endotracheal anesthesia on consecutive days.

The various lung volumes and capacities are generally comparable to those of an adult on a percentage basis (Table 65-2). Lung compliance is low in the newborn since it is a function of the size of the patient, but distensibility of the infant's lung is comparable to that of the adult on a unit per body weight basis. The same pressures are required to inflate the lungs of the infant and the adult to achieve a tidal volume. The functional respiratory surface area of the infant's lung is small per unit of lung volume or body weight.

The breathing of the newborn is largely diaphragmatic, the intercostal muscles being relatively ineffective. The ribs lie in an almost horizontal position, and the sternum offers little fixation against diaphragmatic contraction. Sternal and suprasternal retraction therefore is common in exaggerated breathing. The pattern of normal respiration is shallow and frequently irregular. Oxygen consumption per kilogram in the infant is nearly twice that of the adult (6.2

Table 65-2
Normal Values for Lung Functions

	Newborn	Adult
FRC (ml)	75	3030
VC (ml)	100	4620
V_E (ml/min)	550	6000
V_T (ml)	17	500
f (frequency)	34	12
V_A (ml/min)	385	4140
V_D (ml)	7.5	150
C_l (ml/cm H_2O)	5	163
Peak flow rates (l/min)	10	457
R (cm H_2O/l/sec)	29	2

mg/kg/min); therefore, the infant must move twice the amount of air per kilogram. This increased work is accomplished mainly through an increased respiratory rate that is nearly double that of the adult. Because of the relatively greater effort required to achieve normal respiration, the infant's ventilation is easily compromised by drugs, hypothermia, or hypoxia.

The cardiovascular system of the infant functions at lower pressures and at higher pulse rates than those of the adult. Both pulse and blood pressure are quite labile and may increase markedly with crying, straining, or even minor stimuli. On the other hand, the heart is particularly sensitive to vagal stimulus, and the rate may slow alarmingly with hypoxia or certain parasympathomimetic drugs. Normal cardiovascular values are given in Table 65-3. Cardiovascular compensation in response to blood loss or hypovolemia is accomplished mainly through intense vasoconstriction. Circulatory collapse, when it occurs, develops suddenly and without the premonitory signs usually seen in the adult.

Homeostatis of Body Heat

The infant, who has a relatively large surface area per unit of weight, is unable to maintain normal body temperature in a cool environment. Diminished muscle tone and peripheral vasodilatation caused by general anesthetics and muscle relaxants further contribute to the risk of hypothermia. Ideally, therefore, the temperature of the operating room itself should be increased to 25–27°C. During preparation for surgery, the infant should be kept as closely covered as possible with blankets. A transparent plastic bag that encloses the body except for the head and neck makes an effective device to prevent heat loss. A circulating warm water mattress covered with a single layer of drapes should be used. The mattress temperature should be carefully monitored and maintained at

Table 65-3
Normal Cardiovascular Values for Infants and Adults

Comparison	Newborn	Adult
SA (m^2)	0.25	1.75
Weight (kg)	3.2	70
Arterial BP (mm Hg)	70/40	120/80
Rate (/min)	120/140	70
Cardiac output (l/min)	0.5/0.6	5–6.0
Stroke vol (cc/beat)	4–6	60–80
Total peripheral resistance	+ + +	+
Circulation time arm to eye (sec)	10.2 (5–14)	10 (70–15.6)

no more than 37°C to prevent burns. Radiant heat lamps are also very effective in reducing heat loss. Anesthetic gases should be heated and humidified if non-rebreathing techniques are used. Antiseptic solutions used for surgical preparation should be warmed.

The danger of hypothermia is best seen at the conclusion of anesthesia and surgery when such patients normally can be expected once again to maintain their own airways and sustain normal spontaneous ventilation. Hypothermic infants, however, remain lethargic and have poor muscle tone, and thus are less able to rewarm themselves. Spontaneous ventilation is depressed or nonexistent. The additive effects of hypoventilation, hypoxia, and the hypothermia itself engender both metabolic and respiratory acidosis. The acidosis, in turn, leads to less forceful myocardial contraction and, if not treated, to circulatory collapse. These hazards of cold stress underline the importance of careful temperature monitoring and efforts to prevent heat loss during anesthesia. In the event body temperature does fall more than a degree, active measures for rewarming and respiratory support must be instituted in the operating room until temperature returns to normal.

Pharmacologic Differences

The young infant, especially during the neonatal period, differs from the adult in the quantitative responses to many anesthetic drugs and adjuncts.[5] During the first several months of life, there are rapid physical growth and rapid maturation and change in the factors involved in the uptake, distribution, redistribution, metabolism, and excretion of drugs. Important differences in these processes between the infant and adult have been identified to explain the young infant's altered response to many drugs. In addition variations in penetration of the blood–brain barrier and in receptor sensitivity have been observed in infants for some anesthetics.

Several factors make the use of potent inhalation anesthetics less suitable for neonates and young infants than for older children and adults:

1. The neonate requires higher alveolar anesthetic concentrations than the adult for a given surgical stimulus. For example in neonates the minimum alveolar concentration (MAC) of halothane is 30–50 percent higher than that of a young adult.

Table 65-4
Pharmacologic Differences: Differences in Body Composition

Body Compartment	Premature (1.5 kg)	Full Term (3.5 kg)	Adult (70 kg)
Total body water (% body weight)	83	73.0	60.0
ECF (% body weight)	62	44	20.0
Blood volume (ml/kg)	60	85–105	70
ICW (% body weight)	25	33	40
Muscle mass (% body weight)	15	20	50
Fat (% body weight)	3	12	18

Adapted from Friss-Hansen, B: Body composition during growth. Pediatrics 47:264–274, 1971.

2. The rate of rise of alveolar levels of inhalation anesthetic agents toward equilibrium, at constant inspired concentrations, is more rapid in infants and children than in adults. Markedly larger alveolar ventilation relative to the functional residual capacity in the neonate as compared with the adult allows more rapid equilibration of alveolar tension in the neonate than in the adult. In addition greater perfusion and ventilation on a weight basis, the low fat and muscle content, and diversion of a greater fraction of the cardiac output to highly perfused tissues in the neonate also explain these differences in uptake.
3. Unfortunately, at equal MAC levels of halothane, myocardial contractility seems more easily depressed in the neonate than in the adult. The therapeutic ratio thus is less in the neonate. Significant hypotension and cardiac arrest are more common in neonates than adults when potent anesthetics are used. The pediatric anesthetist therefore depends heavily upon the use of muscle relaxants and narcotics as adjuncts to nitrous oxide/oxygen anesthesia in order to eliminate or reduce the need for high concentrations of potent inhalation anesthetics.

In the neonate, differences in the size of the body fluid compartments, relatively smaller muscle mass and fat stores, and presumably greater blood flow per unit of organ weight influence the distribution of drugs to their active sites and secondary redistribution. Total body water, extracellular fluid, and body volume of the neonate are larger on a weight basis than those of an adult (Table 65-4). The initial larger volume for distribution of a parenterally administered drug may explain, in part, why neonates appear to require larger amounts of some drugs on a milligram-per-kilogram basis to produce a given effect. Differences in fat stores and muscle mass at different ages are shown in Table 65-4. Smaller muscle and fat stores provide less uptake to inactive sites and tend to keep plasma concentration higher. The smaller amount of fat tissue in neonates provides a relatively small reservoir for fat-soluble drugs. Little is known about the blood flow per unit mass of various organs in neonates.

Neonatal hepatic enzyme systems responsible for the metabolism of drugs are incompletely developed or absent. The activity of oxidative and reductive enzymes, however, increases to adult levels within a few days of life. The ability to conjugate with acetate develops by 1 month of age, with glucuronide by 2 months, and with amino acids by 3 months. The activity of all these enzyme systems can be increased by known enzyme inductors such as benzpyrene or phenobarbital. The low enzyme activity for various substrates thus reflects lack of stimulation rather than inability of the enzyme system to be stimulated. The age from birth is important for maturation of these enzyme systems, not the duration of gestation. Premature infants and mature-born infants develop the ability to metabolize drugs to the same degree at the same time period after birth.

Since many drugs or foreign substances are simply filtered by the kidney, glomerular filtration rate (GFR) influences drug excretion and action. Inulin and thiosulfate clearances that reflect GFR are lower in newborns and young children than in adults. Volume clearance, when related to surface area, approaches adult values at about 3 months of age. If, on the other hand, clearance is related to weight, adult values are reached in about 10 days to two weeks. The time-clearance method eliminates this choice of what basis to select. The elimination half-life for thiosulfate is about three times slower in newborns than in older children or adults; by 3 weeks of age these differences disappear. The maturation of glomerular function may be related to changes in the permeability of the glomerular membrane of conversion of nonfunctional glomeruli to functional participants in the process of filtration. Proximal tubular secretion assumes adult values in the first 4 to 5 months of age.

There thus is rapid maturation in the infant's ability to metabolize and excrete drugs. This pharmacologic maturation combined with gradual physiologic maturation lessens the anesthetist's concerns about immaturity.

EVALUATION OF THE NEUROSURGICAL PATIENT

Assessment of the Patient

The neurosurgical patient should be evaluated in a three-step approach:

1. The neurosurgical problem itself, its nature, severity, and duration.
2. The general medical condition, especially those organ systems of particular concern to the anesthetist, for example, the state of consciousness, the airway, the cardiovascular status, ventilation, medications, and laboratory findings.
3. The patient as a candidate for anesthesia—reaction to the illness and to hospitalization, anxiety, and degree of comprehension.

Much of this information can be gleaned from the patient's record and from the surgeon, but is incomplete without direct contact with the patient and, when possible, with the parents. Baseline values of blood pressure, pulse, temperature, respiration, level of consciousness, and focal neurologic signs, if any, should be ascertained and recorded. The level of consciousness or the response of the patient to commands, painful stimuli, and the like should be recorded.

PREOPERATIVE PREPARATION AND PREMEDICATION

Preoperative Preparation

Pediatric patients, because of their age, background, awareness, or previous hospitalization, differ widely in their reactions to a discussion of anesthesia. Parents, too, depending on their education and experience, present a wide range of response. The child or parent who expresses more than minimal interest in or anxiety about the anesthetic deserves honest and straightforward, if not too detailed, answers to any questions. Where no such interest is evident, detailed explanations may create anxiety where none previously existed. Ordinarily the best policy is a simple explanation of what may be expected before induction; this reduces the element of surprise. In the case of the alert, older child, this preanesthetic discussion establishes a degree of rapport between patient and anesthetist and permits the child to identify a familiar face in the strange atmosphere of the operating room. The anesthetist may choose to show a mask and "balloon" to the child and have the child practice breathing.

In recent years increasing emphasis has been placed on better emotional preparation of the child for anesthesia and surgery through teaching. This teaching can best be done by the anesthetist, or even more efficaciously by parents, if they are able. This is not always possible, however. Many hospitals have instituted preanesthetic group teaching sessions where films are shown and the equipment handled and "tried out" by the patient. The effects of this preanesthetic teaching have yet to be critically evaluated.

Preanesthetic Medication

Traditionally sedative-hypnotic, narcotic, or ataractic drugs together with a belladonna preparation are administered before anesthesia, primarily to allay anxiety, but also to facilitate induction, to control secretions, and to obtund vagal reflexes evoked by anesthetic drugs and surgical stimuli. Nowhere has this been considered more important than in the pediatric age group because of the child's relative inability to cope with fear, but also because the child, and particuarly the infant, is most vulnerable to vagal stimulus.

The ideal drug or combination of drugs for this purpose has not been found; preferences vary widely. Many of the most commonly used drugs have disadvantages in that they are long acting both in onset and duration, and may cause respiratory depression or undesired dizziness or restlessness. Recently, partly for these reasons and because greater emphasis has been placed on psychologic rather than pharmacologic preparation of the pediatric patient, many anesthesiologists have abandoned or greatly reduced the use of preanesthetic medication for children. Definitive studies, as mentioned above, have yet to be devised accurately to evaluate the effectiveness of either approach.

Even without the availability of such data, however, one cannot but be impressed with the quiescence or drowsiness of the properly sedated child at the time of induction of anesthesia. The fully alert, unsedated child, or course, may not manifest anxiety by crying or other untoward behavior, but may nonetheless be unduly frightened. The use of preoperative medication in those patients who are not at risk because of cortical depression, or central or peripheral respiratory impairment, therefore seems justified and desirable.

Atropine and Scopolamine

Atropine or scopolamine is virtually always a part of preanesthetic medication in pediatrics. Of the two drugs, atropine is the superior vagolytic agent and scopolamine is more effective in controlling airway secretions. The choice between the two drugs depends on the principal effect desired and, to some extent, on personal preference. Atropine is administered preoperatively to prevent the bradycardia that may be caused by certain anesthetic agents or surgical stimuli; however, it has a relatively short duration of action, and is ineffective 30 minutes after intramuscular or subcutaneous injection. It is, therefore, often given intravenously at the time of the induction of anesthesia.

At the age when sedative drugs are indicated, we prefer scopolamine to atropine because of its contribution of additional sedation, amnesia, and effective suppression of secretions in the airway. The usual dose is approximately half that of atropine.

Sedative and Narcotics

Sleep (or quiescence) and freedom from apprehension are desirable for the child who is to undergo anesthesia and surgery; however, such a state is achieved at the price of some degree of respiratory depression. The anesthetist must decide not only the degree of sedation desired for the patient, but also how much sedation the patient can "afford." The child with increased intracranial pressure, obtunded consciousness, respiratory depression from any cause, or any impairment of the airway or airway reflexes should receive no preanesthetic sedation whatsoever.

The ideal choice of sedative drugs for children remains a matter of controversy. The barbiturates are by far the most commonly used and for the most part are the safest. The child given barbiturates alone, however, often

Table 65-5
Preoperative Medication Table

Age	Weight (kg)	Morphine-Im-Atropine or Scopolamine (mg)	Scopolamine (mg)	Seconal (Intramuscular) [mg(cc)]	
Premature	Under 2.5		Atr. 0.075		
0–1 month	2.6–3.5		Atr. 0.1		
2–3 months	3.6–5.5		Atr. 0.15		
4–5 months	5.6–7.0		Atr. 0.2		
6–7 months	7.1–8.5	0.5	Scop. 0.1	15	(0.3)
8–11 months	8.6–10.0	0.6	Scop. 0.1	20	(0.4)
12–18 months	10.1–11.5	0.8	Scop. 0.15	25	(0.5)
19–24 months	11.6–13.0	1.0	Scop. 0.15	30	(0.6)
2–3 years	13.1–15.0	1.5	Scop. 0.15	40	(0.8)
4–5 years	15.1–20.0	2.0	Scop. 0.15	50	(1.0)
6–8 years	20.1–30.0	3.0	Scop. 0.2	75	(1.5)
9–10 years	30.1–40.0	4.0	Scop. 0.2	75	(1.5)
11–12 years	40.1–50.0	5.0	Scop. 0.3	100	(2.0)
13–14 years	50.1–60.0	8.0	Scop. 0.3	100	(2.0)
Over 14 years	Over 60.0	10.0	Scop. 0.3	100	(2.0)

complains of dizziness. With larger doses the sleep induced is frequently fitful. A sleeping child thus may suddenly become resistive and uncooperative when aroused by being picked up, by the prick of a needle, or by the application of a mask. For this reason narcotics (preferably morphine) are often given with the barbiturate. Diazepam in *oral* doses of 0.1–0.15 mg/kg is an excellent substitute for the barbiturate.

Many drugs and combinations of drugs have been tried, but in our experience they are little better than the combination of narcotic, sedative, and scopolamine. Table 65-5 shows a dosage schedule that may be used as a guide.[6] The doses of sedative and narcotic in this table are quite conservative. With scopolamine, however, they provide adequate sedation in most situations. Either the narcotic or the barbiturate, however, may be safely increased several degrees, or even doubled for the particularly apprehensive child, if heavier sedation is desired.

Route of Administration

Preanesthetic medication may be given orally or by rectum as well as by intramuscular injection. A number of commonly used barbiturates and sedatives are available as suppositories or flavored syrups. In general, however, the results are less satisfactory, except in the hands of those accustomed to this practice. Absorption from the rectum is uneven and unpredictable, and oral preparations may be refused or vomited. Unless the child has an intense fear of needles or requires frequent injections, the intramuscular route does not appear to be unduly traumatic and is by far the most reliable.

Time of Injection

Sedative drugs can be effective only if sufficient time is allowed for them to achieve their full effect. The various drugs used reach their maximum effect at different times and, therefore, theoretically should be given separately. In most cases, however, this is impractical, and usually all drugs are administered at the same time. They should be given at least 45 minutes to one hour before anesthesia. It is our practice that each patient is called twice: one hour before operation for medication, and a second time just before anesthesia is to be begun. This requires planning and cooperation of the surgical, nursing, and anesthesia staffs. It is well worth the effort, however, since the sedation is more effective and anesthetic inductions are made easier for patient and anesthetist alike.

ANESTHETIC DRUGS AND TECHNIQUES

For most pediatric neurosurgical procedures, general endotracheal anesthesia is required. The choice of anesthetic agents and adjuncts will be dictated by the nature of the neurosurgical problem and the age and associated problems of the patient. Likewise, for most procedures controlled ventilation is mandatory, either to facilitate control of intracranial pressure or to reduce the work of breathing in infants or those in the prone position. Appropriate, intensive monitoring of the pediatric neurosurgical patient is now feasible because of satisfactory miniaturization of adult equipment.

Endotracheal Intubation

Because most neurosurgical procedures involve unusual positions, distortion of the airway, or conditions in which the anesthetist does not command access to the airway, endotracheal intubation is an indispensable part of all neurosurgical procedures. For procedures involving extreme flexion of the head and neck or other situations in which the endotracheal tube might be kinked, we prefer wire-reinforced endotracheal tubes. Routine intubation of infants and children can be achieved with an exceedingly low incidence of laryngeal edema or other sequelae.

Movement of the head and use of wire-reinforced tubes, however, does increase the incidence of postintubation croup in neurosurgic patients. Trauma in intubation can be minimized by gentleness and by assuring adequate relaxation, either with a sufficiently deep plane of anesthesia or with muscle relaxants. The choice of the proper size of endotracheal tube is of utmost importance; it should be as large as possible but should pass the glottis and cricoid without resistance. At most there should be only a slight air leak. Table 65-6 provides a guide to proper selection. In general the use of cuffed endotracheal tubes in children under 10 years of age is neither necessary nor good practice.

Table 65-6
Approximate Size of Endotracheal Tubes

Age	Weight (kg)	French No.	ID (estimated) (mm)
Premature	1.0–2.3	12	3
Newborn–3 months	2.3–5.0	14	3.5
6 months	6	16	4
9 months	9	18	4.5
9 months–18 months	9–11	20	5
2 years	11–15	22	5.5
4 years	16	24	6
6 years	20	26	6.5
8 years	26	28	7
10 years	30	30	7.5

Effects of Anesthetics on Intracranial Pressure

Most anesthetic agents can effect direct or indirect changes in cerebral blood flow either by influencing $PaCO_2$ and PaO_2, and blood pressure, or by direct vasodilation effects of the anesthetics themselves, independent of changes in $PaCO_2$.[7–11] Anesthetic techniques can also influence cerebral venous flow (e.g., cerebral venous flow can be affected by posture or surgical positioning, by positive pressure ventilation, especially CPPV, and by changes in blood volume). In the patient with reduced brain compliance, such increases in cerebral blood flow or retardation of cerebral venous flow can dramatically raise intracranial pressure.

In a normal awake person, there is an inverse linear relationship between cerebral blood flow and $PaCO_2$ over the range of 20 to 60 torr; below 20 torr little reduction in cerebral blood flow occurs; and above 60 torr cerebral blood flow tends to be fixed at a high level. Since $PaCO_2$ has such a profound affect on cerebral blood flow, the specific drug effects of anesthetics on cerebral blood flow can only be determined if $PaCO_2$ is controlled. Table 65-7 notes the percent change in cerebral blood flow and cerebral oxygen consumption at normocapnia produced by various intravenous induction agents, narcotics, and inhalation anesthetics.[12–20] High doses of sedative-hypnotics, narcotics, or general anesthesia with spontaneous respiration can all raise $PaCO_2$ and thus indirectly increase cerebral blood flow. When arterial oxygen tension is decreased below 40 to 50 torr, cerebral vascular dilatation begins to occur; little or no change in cerebral blood flow occurs with hyperoxia at one atmosphere.

Intravenous induction agents such as thiopental or diazepam can be safely used in all age groups. In patients with suspected increased intracranial pressure, an intravenous induction with thiopental is preferable to an inhalation induction. When starting an infusion provokes crying and struggling, however, an inhalation induction appears to be a lesser evil than to persist with attempts at venipuncture. Unfortunately no data exist to clarify this issue.

The use of halothane for intracranial surgery is somewhat controversial because it increases cerebral blood flow at normocapnia. But when preceded by intravenous thiopental and hyperventilation, halothane seldom raises cerebral

Table 65-7
Effect of Sedative-Hypnotics, Narcotics, Neuroleptanalgesics, and Volatile Anesthetics on Cerebral Blood Flow (CBF), and Oxygen Consumption ($CMRO_2$)

Anesthetic (Dose)	Species	CBF (% Change)	$CMRO_2$ (% Change)
Thiopental (35 mg/kg)	Human	−35	−35
Diazepam (0.25 mg/kg)	Dog	−17	−17
Althesin (0.1 mg/kg + 0.3 ml/kg/hr)	Human	−40	−50
Ketamine (2 mg/kg)	Human	+80	+16
Droperidol (0.3 mg/kg)	Dog	−40	0
Fentanyl (0.006 mg/kg)	Dog	−47	−18
Morphine (2 mg/kg)	Human	0	0
Nitrous oxide (70%)	Human	+2	−23
Halothane (1.2%)	Human	+23	−7 to −26
Halothane (1.0%)	Human	+27	−26
Ether (2.4%)	Human	−6	−34 to −40
Ether (4.5%)	Human	+35	−12
Enflurane (0.85%)	Human	−5	−25
Enflurane (2.0%)	Human	+2	−33
Enflurane (3.0%)	Human	−3	−50
Enflurane (3.2%)	Human	+2	−40

blood flow or intracranial pressure. The use of halothane in low concentration during intracranial procedures allows easier control of blood pressure without resorting to nitroglycerin, nitroprusside, or trimethaphan. Similarly, enflurane may be used in low concentration to reinforce anesthesia since there is little or no change in cerebral blood flow or cerebral oxygen consumption; however, high-dose enflurane in association with hyperoxia has been associated with electroencephalogram (EEG) seizure activity.

The non-neuromuscular blocking side effects of the muscle relaxants must be considered in the neurosurgical patient. Succinylcholine can produce significant hyperkalemia in the patient with peripheral neuropathy. Its effects on cerebral blood flow and intracranial pressure appear to be minimal. Pancuronium, particularly in high doses, often produces tachycardia and hypertension. In our view this feature often complicates rather than facilitates nitrous oxide/narcotic anesthesia. Although D-tubocurarine (dtc) occasionally liberates histamine that can produce cerebral vasodilation, in most situations minimal falls in blood pressure and no changes in heart rate are observed following dtc. Metocurine has few non-neuromuscular blocking effects; it is perhaps the ideal muscle relaxant for neuroanesthesia.

MONITORING

Although most pediatric surgical patients can be adequately monitored by the intelligent use of a few simple devices, the advent of more sophisticated equipment allows moment-to-moment monitoring of blood pressure, electrocardiogram (ECG), central venous pressure (CVP), intracranial pressure (ICP), and end-tidal gases in the neurosurgical patient.

The infant or child should be monitored continuously with a precordial or esophageal stethoscope. The anesthetist can thus detect changes in the rate, quality, and intensity of the heart sounds that may be helpful in evaluating blood loss, depth of anesthesia, or failing circulation, or in diagnosing air emboli. Plethysmographic monitors attached to the finger or toe are helpful but are subject to artefacts and are frequently unreliable in the very young. Doppler monitors (discussed in the section on blood pressure) are most reliable as audible pulse indicators.

Electrocardiographic monitoring is useful in determining pulse rate and the presence of cardiac arrhythmias. The value of the ECG tracing in evaluating cardiac function is limited, however, since it indicates only electrical activity and gives no indication of cardiac output.

Blood Pressure

Systolic blood pressure may be determined in virtually all patients by the oscillometric method with use of a suitable cuff and an aneroid manometer. Several relatively simple electronic devices, however, have greatly facilitated the indirect determination of blood pressure in small patients. A radio-frequency signal is transmitted through a transducer into a peripheral artery. The reflected signal (by the Doppler principle) is returned at a lower frequency. The differential frequency is integrated and amplified to an audible signal of the peripheral pulse. This is the basis of the Parks Transcutaneous Doppler (Parks Electronics Laboratoy, Beaverton, Oregon, 97005) and the Arteriosonde (Hoffman-La Roche, Inc. Medical Electronics Division, Cranbury, New Jersey 08512). With the Parks Doppler the transducer must be placed separately over an artery; it may thus serve as a pulse monitor, if desired. The transducer of the Arteriosonde is incorporated into a specially provided blood pressure cuff.

Cannulation of the radial artery or dorsalis pedis artery allows continuous measurement of blood pressure and permits frequent serial determinations of blood gases and pH, hematocrit, serum solids, electrolytes, and osmolality determinations. With a translumination technique, either 22 or 24 gage plastic cannulae can be placed percutaneously in infants; rarely, a cutdown may be necessary. The transducer should be "zeroed" at the level of the head rather than at the heart in order to estimate cerebral perfusion pressure.

Central Venous Pressure Monitoring

Central venous pressure catheters can be used to estimate mean intrathoracic pressure during mechanical ventilation, to estimate adequacy of blood replacement or venous return, and to extract air embolism from the right heart.

Catheters can be inserted from the antecubital fossa, external jugular, or internal jugular vein. Since the position of the catheter is critical if the catheter is to be used to extract air, a chest x-ray must be taken to confirm its position. Monitoring changes in the P-waves of the electrocardiograph can assist in correct placement of a right arterial catheter.

Respiration

The anesthetist has few direct aids to measure tidal volume in infants and must depend to a large extent on clinical observation. Standard ventilation meters such as the Wright Respirometer are useful for older children, but they either do not respond or are grossly inaccurate in the ranges required for infants. When available arterial pH, PCO_2, and PO_2 determinations are the most reliable indexes of adequate ventilation.

Temperature

The thermistor thermometer has greatly facilitated continuous temperature determination during anesthesia. The hazards of elevated temperature as well as hypothermia in the infant have already been mentioned. We feel that temperature monitoring should be routine in virtually all surgical patients. Its importance is unquestioned in the management of all infants, and in major cases at any age.

Doppler Ultrasonic Bubble Detector

Continous-wave Doppler ultrasound produces a characteristic signal when reflected from moving red cells. Since ultrasound is much better reflected from an air–blood interface, a higher pitched, easily recognized, and distinctly diagnostic audible signal is produced during air embolism. To monitor right heart flow, such detectors should be placed in the right third to fifth intercostal space along the sternum. The lower limit of response of such detectors is 0.25 to 0.5 ml.

End-Tidal CO_2 Detectors

Monitoring of end-tidal CO_2 will reflect alveolar carbon dioxide and serve as a secondary detector for air embolism. Unfortunately, most detectors are too heavy and the high vacuum flow precludes their routine use in small infants and children.

Estimation of Blood Loss

Accurate estimation of blood loss during surgery is the most difficult and least satisfactory aspect of patient monitoring. The smaller the patient, the less accurate are the usual methods of weighing sponges or determining the hemoglobin content of the sponges and drapes. The use of small graduated bottles in the suction system, however, greatly improves the accuracy of measuring this aspect of the blood loss. One can only make the estimates by whatever methods are available as accurately as possible and then recognize their limitations. The final estimation of loss and requirements for replacement must rest on careful evaluation of the clinical signs together with whatever information can be gleaned from the measured loss.

ANESTHESIA FOR NEURORADIOLOGY

Children and infants, unlike their adult counterparts, frequently require general anesthesia or heavy sedation for neuroradiologic diagnostic and therapeutic procedures. Although some of these procedures are painful, at least during part of the procedure, the principal indication for anesthesia is the inability of the young patient or combative patient to cooperate and to maintain the necessary immobility for extended periods; rigid restraints are strong stimuli for struggling and movement in infants, the semiconscious, and otherwise uncooperative patients.

A major problem common to all these procedures is that they must be performed in a location not usually designed for the administration of anesthesia and which is remote from the operating rooms and recovery facilities. All or most of the equipment must be transported to the radiology department. The situation is often further complicated by the fact that in many institutions these facilities are shared by both adult and pediatric patients, and generally it is the pediatric patient who is the exception; thus the radiology staff is less likely to be able to deal with the special needs of infants and children. Finally, at the conclusion of the procedure, the anesthetized infant or child must be transported over long distances to the recovery area. Portable oxygen equipment, including a bag/mask/valve unit and a portable ECG monitor, must be available during transportation to the recovery area.

Anesthesia or Sedation

Since the anesthetic requirement for most of these procedures is minimal, the question frequently arises as to whether sedation may be substituted for formally administered general anesthesia. In our experience sedation has been effective in only a small percentage of these patients—generally the older, cooperative children undergoing angiography or those undergoing studies that require immobility only for short periods of time. Difficulties encountered with sedation as a substitute for general anesthesia have been numerous. Even moderately heavy sedation with a combination of narcotics and sedatives has not provided adequate quiescence and immobility when the child was firmly restrained or placed in an unnatural position. There has been a wide and unpredictable variation in the effectiveness of the drugs even at comparable ages and dosages. The large doses of these drugs by either the intramuscular or intravenous route (or a combination of both) required to achieve quiescence have led to respiratory depression and increased arterial carbon dioxide tension and cerebrovascular dilatation. The dilatation in turn increased ICP and interfered with successful angiography. Sedation, effective or not, which was heavy enough to induce unconsciousness and respiratory depression, in fact became a form of general anesthesia in which the anesthetist had no direct control of airway or ventilation. The effects of the sedative drugs, not all of which could be satisfactorily reversed, far outlasted the duration of the procedure. For all of these reasons, endotracheal inhalation anesthesia in our experience has proved to be far safer, more flexible, and more predictable. The rare exception is the older, already cooperative child for whom "conscious sedation" may be all that is required.

Technique of Anesthesia

The type of anesthesia used for these procedures differs little in principle from that for neurosurgical patients of comparable age. The choice of anesthetic agents and relaxants is usually of secondary importance. Endotracheal intubation is mandatory since the anesthetist may not have access to the head and because the patient may be turned into one (or more) difficult positions.

Routine monitoring of pulse, respiration, blood pressure, ECG, and temperature is essential. Special efforts to maintain normal body temperature, particularly in the very young, are essential but may prove difficult since it is frequently impossible to regulate the temperature of the room, and because the use of the circulating warm water mattress may interfere with radiography. Radiant heat lamps, wrapping of the extremities, a plastic bag about the head (when possible), and of heated, humidified anesthetic gases are effective means that are available to combat heat loss.

Cerebral Angiography

The anesthetist must be aware of the volume and type of fluids used in conjunction with angiography and adjust the administration of fluids accordingly. In general the total volume of Hypaque® Sodium (Wintrop Laboratories, New York, New York) should be limited to 4–6 ml/kg.

Following hyperosmolar contrast materials, there is an initial increase in blood viscosity and a decrease in hematocrit followed by a translocation of fluid that increases circulating blood pressure, cardiac output, and usually urine flow. Occasionally anaphylactoid reactions with angioneurotic edema, hypotension, and bronchospasm may occur. In addition severe dehydration has occurred in some patients receiving contrast material. Mass lesions of the brain associated with loss of autoregulation may be enhanced by hyperventilation, which decreases cerebral blood flow to normal brain tissue; in general, however, hyperventilation results in enhanced angiograms.

Air Studies

The introduction of gas into the ventricles or subarachnoid space for air myelography, pneumoencephalography, and ventriculography complicates the use of general anesthesia. Nitrous oxide, which is often used for this type of procedure, is contraindicated since, because of its relatively greater solubility than nitrogen in blood, it will accumulate in the closed gas-filled compartments and raise their pressure.[21] The exception is, of course, when nitrous oxide itself is used by the radiologist as the contrast gas instead of air or oxygen.

The anesthetist must be aware and informed of the volumes of cerebrospinal fluid removed and the volumes of gas injected. Changes in pulse and blood pressure as fluid and gas are exchanged must be watched for, recorded, and communicated immediately to the radiologist. In all of these procedures, but particularly during pneumoencephalography, the patient may have to be moved into a variety of unnatural positions that may affect the circulation and present technical problems with anesthetic and monitoring equipment attached to the patient.

Radiation Therapy

The greatest number of technical problems for the anesthetist present with the infant or child who is to undergo radiation therapy. These include those common to the infant and the neurologic disease, the need for absolute immobility, lack of access to the patient, and, in addition, the need for daily serial anesthetics, frequently on an outpatient basis. Sedation, regardless of the combinations and doses of drugs or their route of administration, has proved unsatisfactory for radiation therapy because it does not assure the absolute immobility required and because of the long duration of action of the drugs used. Inhalation anesthetics are unsatisfactory because of the hazards either of airway obstruction without intubation, or of multiple intubations. The technical difficulties inherent in securing an intravenous infusion in a small infant on so many successive occasions virtually precludes the use of intravenously administered drugs.

The following technique, which admittedly involves a degree of compromise, has proved successful.[22] On each treatment day, the fasting infant, preferably accompanied by a parent, is brought to a quiet room adjacent to the radiation laboratory a few minutes before the scheduled treatment. When the radiation team is completely ready, the infant is given a single intramuscular injection containing atropine 0.02 mg/kg and ketamine 5 mg/kg. Upon becoming quiescent, the infant is quickly taken to the laboratory and positioned by the radiation therapist and anesthetist. Monitoring equipment is attached, supplemental oxygen begun, and the patient carefully observed for adequate airway and respiration. Radiation treatment is then begun without delay. Following treatment the infant is taken to the recovery room by the anesthetist.

Careful prior planning and communication are absolutely essential for the success of this deceptively simple technique. All necessary equipment must be available. Since the anesthetist must leave the patient during the therapy, special arrangements for remote monitoring and unobstructed viewing of the patient must be available. The radiation and anesthesia teams must thoroughly understand each other's problems. The short duration of effective anesthesia necessitates the avoidance of any delay once the injection is made. A plan for abortion of therapy in the event of complications must be agreed upon.

Usually slight increases in ketamine dosage will be required with successive treatments. In a few cases, however, the infant seems to adapt to the daily routine and will remain quiescent on progressively smaller dosage. In addition to the usual anesthetic record, a simple tabular log showing date, dosage, effect, and complications should be kept to indicate these trends.

SUPPORTIVE CARE OF HEAD-INJURED PATIENTS OR POSTCRANIOTOMY PATIENTS

Many neurosurgical patients, particularly those with head injuries or following major craniotomies, may require short- or long-term respiratory care, nutrition, and long-term control of intracranial pressure. In many instances attention to these aspects of care will decide the degree of morbidity and eventual outcome.

Table 65-8
Indications for Intubation and Ventilation

Clinical signs of elevated ICP
Pulmonary insufficiency
$PaCO_2 > 45$ torr with elevated ICP
$PaO_2 < 60$ torr, by face mask, $F_IO_2 > 0.60$
Absent cough or gag reflexes
Anatomical airway obstruction
Spontaneous hyperventilation
$PaCO_2 < 20$ mg Hg
Progressive deterioration of neurologic status

Respiratory Support

Intubation and ventilatory support are often required in neurosurgical patients to relieve upper airway obstruction, to maintain adequate oxygenation by protecting the lung from aspiration of secretions, to provide means for tracheobronchial toilet and artificial sighing or coughing, and to provide an adjunct to ICP control by manipulation of $PaCO_2$.

Table 65-8 lists major indications for intubation and ventilatory support. Sedation with intravenous thiopental, lidocaine, or small doses of narcotics can be used to diminish ICP, and muscle relaxants used to prevent coughing during endotracheal intubation and during suctioning. In the absence of a basal skull fracture or rhinorrhea, nasal intubation is preferable since it facilitates oral hygiene and nasal tubes are easier to secure. Uncuffed endotracheal tubes are adequate for ventilating children under 9 or 10 years of age.

Airway Care

Heated humidification of inspired gases through an artificial airway is indispensable to maintain ciliary function and mucus flow, to prevent thickening of secretions, and to minimize heat loss. Inspired gases saturated with water vapor at 32°C provide about 70 percent relative humidity when they reach body temperature in the lung; this is sufficient humidity to prevent cellular damage of the upper airways without causing unwanted heat gain or causing damage to the respiratory mucosae.[23]

Sterile endotracheal suctioning combined with reexpansion of alveoli and reoxygenation is routinely required at least every two hours. Small amounts (0.2–2 ml, depending on the size of the patient) of sterile saline solution are instilled through the endotracheal tube to facilitate the removal of secretions.

Arterial PO_2 should be kept at 100–150 torr to guarantee complete hemoglobin saturation and to provide some leeway in oxygenation if a pulmonary setback should occur; ideally, inspired oxygen should be no more than 50 percent. All intubated patients should have a small amount of positive end tidal pressure (PEEP) (2–4 cm H_2O) to facilitate gas exchange and to maintain an adequate functional residual capacity. In high levels (greater than 8–10 cm H_2O), PEEP can occasionally raise ICP by impeding cerebral venous return.[24] This modality therefore, should be used cautiously. Elevation of the head of the bed 30 degrees both facilitates gas exchange and helps to counteract the effects of PEEP.

Mechanical Ventilation

The difference in tidal volume and respiratory rate between infants and older children makes it difficult to use the same ventilator for all age groups. In some instances one may modify an adult ventilator for infants. On the other hand, a ventilator used exclusively for infants may be unsatisfactory for older children. An ideal pediatric ventilator should allow accurate control of a wide range of tidal volumes with small internal compliance, inspiratory and expiratory times, inspiratory flow rates, and inspired oxygen concentrations. An adjustable high-pressure relief valve should be included. There should be access to the exhalation valve to provide PEEP. In addition there should be a mechanism to allow the patient to inspire out of phase with the mechanical ventilator (IMV). The choice of ventilators in any intensive care unit probably should not exceed two or three types. This limitation permits technicians, nurses, and physicians to become thoroughly familiar with their use and idiosyncrasies. The inflation pressure generated by the ventilator should be monitored. Changes in the patient's lung compliance will be reflected by this pressure. Pressure alarms must be added to all ventilators to warn if pressure limits are exceeded or if minimal pressure is not reached in a definite time. The latter then serves as a disconnect alarm. This is imperative since many patients are paralyzed to facilitate ventilator care.

Extubation requires the fulfillment of specific criteria. Table 65-9 lists the criteria using the mnemonic SOAP. Secretions should be minimal, oxgenation should be adequate ($PO_2 > 65$ torr with F_IO_2 0.45, PEEP 2–4 cm H_2O), the airway must be protected with presence of cough and gag reflexes, and parameters must be met. The parameters should include a resolving or stable neurologic status and an inspiratory force of more than -25 cm H_2O.

Prolonged intubation, especially with the use of a ventilator, has been associated with laryngeal edema, ulceration, glottic granulomas, and subglottic stenosis. Subglottic stenosis is seen in 2 to 8 percent of patients surviving long-term endotracheal intubation.[25,26] It is difficult to predict how long an endotracheal tube may be kept safely in place. The patient's age, duration of intubation, number of tube changes, relative tube size, use of mechanical ventilation, effective fixation of the tube, nasal or oral intubation, type and material of the tube, and presence and type of cuff are all contributing factors to glottic and subglottic injury.

Tracheostomy should be considered in infants and children when the need for intubation exceeds one week. Ideally all tracheostomies should be performed in the operating room under controlled sterile conditions. We prefer tracheostomies to be done between the second and third tracheal rings when possible. Low tracheostomies, particularly in the infant, increase the incidence of pneumothorax and endobronchial cannulation. A longitudinal tracheal incision without a wedge-shaped flag is used.[27] Stay sutures are placed in both sides of the tracheostomy site. Tracheostomy tubes that have universal male connectors for attachment onto ventilator tubing are now available in all sizes. In children under 10 years of age, uncuffed tracheostomy tubes are preferable.

Table 65-9
Criteria for Extubation

S—Minimal Secretions
O—Adequate Oxygenation
A—Protected Airway
P—Other Parameters

Fluids and Nutrition

Neurosurgical patients require frequent adjustments in fluid management to maintain a mean arterial pressure of at least 60 torr and venous pressures in the low to mid-normal range (4–8 torr). Initial fluid rates should provide one half to two thirds of the normal calculated maintenance requirements. If the perfusion pressure cannot be maintained despite adequate volume therapy, the use of vasoactive agents such as dopamine or dobutamine is indicated. In the choice and amount of fluids, neurologic function takes precedence over renal function. Central venous or pulmonary artery catheters provide important information that can be used in managing fluid therapy.

The syndrome of inappropriate antidiuretic hormone secretion (SIADH) is a clinical complex consisting of serum hyponatremia and hypo-osmolality in conjunction with a high urine sodium and osmolality. This problem frequently follows head injury and should be carefully looked for. It is normally a transient phenomenon lasting 24 to 48 hours and is, in the vast majority of cases, successfully treated by fluid restriction. In cases of severe hyponatremia (<125 mEq/l), the use of a potent loop diuretic and hypertonic NaCl (3N) will facilitate a more rapid correction of the hyponatremic state.

Diabetes insipidus often follows operations or injury involving the pituitary and hypothalamus. The diagnosis is based on the presence of a rising serum sodium and osmolality in association with the excretion of large volumes of dilute urine. Early after fluid resuscitation or operation, the diagnosis may be in doubt since the large volumes of urine may represent excretion of excess water given during the operative procedure; however, in this case the serum $Na+$ and osmolality are generally within the normal ranges. Treatment consists of hourly replacement of urine output using 0.2 to 0.3 NaCl solutions. If the urine output is greater than 1 percent of body weight per hour, subcutaneous aqueous pitressin is recommended. The beginning dose is one unit. Incremental doses of one unit are then added until the desired effect is seen.

Fluid losses from nasogastric drainage can be significant, and if untreated, can lead to hyponatremia and metabolic alkalosis. Such losses should be replaced with equal volumes of 0.45 N or 0.9 N saline solutions.

In the neurosurgical patient, as with any other critically ill child who is in a catabolic state, weight loss is progressive and significant. Caloric intake should be no less than 100 cal/kg of body weight for the first 10 kg, and 25–50 cal/kg for each subsequent kilogram of body weight. Peripheral alimentation with 10 percent dextrose and a 2.5 percent amino acid solution with vitamins should be started within 24 to 48 hours after admission to the intensive care unit. Enteral feedings of an elemental high-caloric, iso-osmolar formula can be given if the gastrointestinal system will tolerate them. If it will not, central hyperalimentation should be instituted within five to seven days after injury. Lipid-containing solutions can be easily given peripherally, both to supplement caloric intake and to provide essential fatty acids. Liver and renal function, mineral levels, and serum triglyceride levels should be regularly checked when central hyperalimentation and lipid solutions are used. Adequate nutrition can frequently decrease morbidity associated with neurosurgical injuries, and should be viewed as an integral part of the management in these patients.

SPECIFIC NEUROLOGIC THERAPY AND ICP CONTROL

The desired result of all therapy is the preservation of normal cerebral function. The ultimate success of therapy during the acute stages of neurologic injury may lie in the control of intracranial pressure. The unique volume compliance relationship of the brain indicates that very small changes in volume can lead to very rapid and significant changes in intracranial pressure. Changes in neurologic status as determined by clinical examination can lag behind these changes in ICP by hours. For this reason direct measurement of ICP is an essential part of therapy in severely brain-injured patients. The two most commonly used techniques are the Richmond subarachnoid screw, and the intraventricular catheter. Both techniques accurately reflect intracranial pressure. The subarachnoid screw may be inserted while the child is in the intensive care unit. Its stability, however, requires a cranial bone that is thick enough to support the apparatus, and is therefore generally used only for children older than 2 years of age. Catheters have the added advantage of offering CSF drainage capabilities, but are more invasive and therefore not favored in some centers.

Techniques for measuring cerebral function such as evoked potentials and bedside measurement of regional blood flow are promising adjuncts for following the course of therapy, but are at present in the developmental stages and are not readily available.

Blood pressure as well as ICP must be considered. The cerebral perfusion pressure is determined by the difference between the mean arterial pressure and the ICP. Perfusion to the brain thus is diminished by either arterial hypotension or intracranial hypertension. In normal brain cerebral blood flow remains normal until the perfusion pressure falls below 40–45 mm Hg. In damaged brain, however, cerebral blood flow is more pressure sensitive and the minimal perfusion pressure may need to be higher.[28,29] Data are not readily available concerning cerebral perfusion pressure in children. Nevertheless, it is important to maintain an adequate blood pressure (mean arterial pressure between 55 mm Hg and 110 mm Hg), especially in the presence of increased ICP.

Specific treatment modalities for increased ICP include hyperventilation, corticosteroid use, osmotherapy, hypothermia, barbiturate therapy, and craniectomy. Use of each is intended to affect ICP by decreasing the volume of one or more of the three types of tissue contained in the cranium. Table 65-10 summarizes these modalities and the tissue matter each is designed to affect.

Hyperventilation

Hypocapnia of $PaCO_2$ levels of 25–30 torr decreases cerebral blood volume by causing constriction of cerebral vasculature.[30,31] How long cerebral vessels continue to constrict in the presence of hypocarbia of more than a few hours duration is unclear. It is also unclear what the effect of hypocarbia is upon regional blood flow in areas of the brain with altered or lost autoregulation.

Corticosteroids

Despite the absence of any accepted explanation of how they work, corticosteroids have enjoyed a tremendous popularity as therapeutic agents for brain injury. The indications for their use are controversial. High-dose dexa-

Table 65-10
Treatment Modality and Altered Tissue Volume

Blood	CSF	Brain Tissue	Cranium
Hyperventilation	Steroids	Steroids	Frontal craniectomy
Osmotherapy	Furosemide	Osmotherapy	
Barbiturates	Diamox	Hypothermia	
	Catheter Drainage	Barbiturates	

methasone 1–1.5 mg/kg/day) therapy has become popular. Initial results indicated potential advantages over conventional low-dose therapy (0.25–0.5 mg/kg/day).[32,33] Recent studies, however, also question the efficacy of high-dose steroid therapy.[34,35] Despite questions regarding their usefulness, steroids are often used for five to seven days following the injury and are then tapered over a similar period of time.

Osmotherapy

Treatment of cerebral edema with osmotic agents has remained an important mode of therapy. Mannitol, presently the most popular agent, is presumed to work by causing extravascular dehydration by establishing an osmotic gradient across the blood–brain barrier. A desired serum osmolality is approximately 320 mOsm/l. Small doses (0.25 g/kg) appear to have the same desired effect as higher doses of 1 g/kg.[36] Continuous versus bolus therapy is controversial.

Osmotherapy has been challenged on several grounds. Brain injury in the pediatric patient appears to involve an early hyperemic phase.[37,38] The transient hypervolemia that may occur following osmotherapy could aggravate this phase. The effectiveness of mannitol requires an intact blood–brain barrier. Disruption of this partition for whatever reason would allow the osmotic agent to escape into extravascular spaces and possibly establish a reverse osmotic gradient. This would result in a worsening of cerebral edema. For these two reasons some people now recommend osmotherapy only as a temporizing measure, using other modes of therapy as definitive treatment.

Furosemide, a loop diuretic, may be useful in the treatment of cerebral edema.[39] It is believed to work by altering cellular ion exchange pumps with a resulting decrease in CSF production.[40] It does not work by creating a diuresis, although this may be a side effect. This diuresis should be replaced if massive.

Hypothermia

Hypothermia lowers cerebral oxygen consumption approximately 4 to 5 percent per degree Celsius. Rapid cooling can be established with judicious use of chlorpromazine in conjunction with a cooling blanket. Shivering should be avoided by using muscle relaxants. Mild levels of hypothermia, 31–32°C, can be a useful adjunct in the treatment of increased ICP. Levels lower than this, near 28°C, increase the risk of spontaneous ventricular arrhythmias, including ventricular fibrillation. It is debatable whether hypothermia alters the course of the treated disease and it is not used consistently for this reason.

Barbiturate

Barbiturates, both short acting and moderately long acting, may be useful agents in the treatment of increased intracranial pressure. Barbiturates appear to decrease both cerebral metabolism and cerebral blood flow.[41,42] In many centers pentobarbital currently is being given to reach blood levels of 2.5–3.5 mg/dl in an attempt to control ICP if hyperventilation and osmotherapy have failed to do so.[43] A more controversial issue has been the proposed use of barbiturates to preserve ischemic or hypoxic brain tissue. At the present time, more information has to be obtained before any conclusion can be drawn. Whenever barbiturates are used, the cardiovascular system must be closely monitored.

Bifrontal Craniectomy

Bifrontal craniectomy has generally been reserved for cases refractory to all other therapy. In most centers results with this technique have been disappointing. It may be that more success could be obtained by performing this procedure at an earlier point in the course of the disease.

REFERENCES

1. Michenfelder JD, Gronert GA, Rehder K: Neuroanesthesia. Anesthesiology 30:65–100, 1969
2. Geevarghese KP (ed): Anesthesia for Neurological Surgery. International Anesthesiology Clinics, vol 15, no 3. Boston, Little Brown, 1977
3. Gordon E (ed): A Basis and Practice of Neuroanesthesia. New York, Excerpta Medica, 1975
4. McComish PB, Bodley PO: Anaesthesia for Neurological Surgery. Chicago, Year Book, 1971
5. Cook DR: Pediatric pharmacology: A Review. Drugs 12:212, 1976
6. Marcy JH, Cook DR: Pediatric anesthesiology, in Practice of Surgery, General Surgery Introduction. Hagerstown, Harper & Row, 1974
7. Smith AL, Wollman H: Cerebral blood flow and metabolism: Effect of anaesthetic drugs and techniques.Anesthesiology 36:378–400, 1972
8. McDowall DG (ed): Cerebral Circulation. International Anesthesiology Clinics, vol 7, no 3. Boston, Little Brown, 1969
9. McDowall DG: Pharmacology of the cerebral circulation. Int Anesthesiol Clin 7:557–578, 1969
10. McDowall DG: Fluid dynamics of the cerebral circulation, in Scurr C, Teldman S (eds). Scientific Foundation of Anaesthesia. Chicago, Year Book, 1974
11. Smith AL, Neigh JL, Hoffman JC, et al: Effects of general anesthesia on autoregulation of cerebral blood flow in man. J Appl Physiol 29:665–669, 1970
12. McDowall DG, Harper AM, Joacobson I: Cerebral blood flow during halothane anesthesia. Br J Anaesth 35:394–401, 1963
13. McDowall DG: The effects of general anesthetics on cerebral blood flow and cerebral metabolism. Br J Anaesth 37:236–245, 1965
14. McDowall DG, Harper AM: Blood flow and oxygen uptake of the cerebral cortex of the dog during anaesthesia with different volatile agents. Acta Neurol Scand 41 (suppl 14): 146–151, 1965
15. Michenfelder JD, Theye RA: Effects of fentanyl, droperidol, and innovar on canine cerebral metabolism and blood flow. Br J Anaesth 43:630–635, 1971
16. Michenfelder JD, Cucchiara RF: Canine cerebral oxygen consumption during enflurane anesthesia and its modification during induced seizures. Anesthesiology 40:575–580, 1974
17. Takeshita H, Okuda Y, Sari A: The effects of ketamine on cerebral circulation and metabolism in man. Anesthesiology 36:69–75, 1972
18. Theye RA, Michenfelder JD: The effect of nitrous oxide on canine cerebral metabolism. Anesthesiology 29:1119–1124, 1968
19. Theye RA, Michenfelder JD: The effect of halothane on canine cerebral metabolism. Anesthesiology 29:1113–1118, 1968
20. Jobes DR, Kennell E, Bitner R, et al: Effects of morphine-nitrous oxide anesthesia on cerebral autoregulation. Anesthesiology 42:30–34, 1975
21. Saidman LJ, Eger EL: Change in cerebrospinal fluid pressure during pneumoencephalography under nitrous oxide anesthesia. Anesthesiology 26:67–72, 1965
22. Marcy JH: Commentary in "The Experts Opine," Surv Anesthesiol. 24:2:124–125, 1980
23. Forbes A: Temperature, humidity and mucus flow in the intubated trachea. Br J Anaesth 46:29–34, 1974
24. Aidinis S, Lafferty J, Shapiro H: Intracranial responses to PEEP. Anesthesiology 45:275–286, 1976

25. Abbott T: Complications of prolonged nasotracheal intubation in children. Br J Anaesth 40:347, 1968
26. Allen T, Stevens I: Prolonged endotracheal intubation in infants and children. Br J Anaesth 37:566, 1965
27. Stool S, Campbell J, Johnson D: Tracheostomy in children: The use of plastic tubes. J Pediatr Surg 3:402, 1968
28. Fitch W, Mackenzie ET, Harper AM: Effects of decreasing arterial blood pressure on cerebral blood flow in the baboon. Circ Res 37:550, 1975
29. Purves MJ: Control of cerebral blood vessels: Present state of the art. Ann Neurol 3:377, 1978
30. Phelps ME, Grubb RL, Ter-Pogossian MM: Correlation between $PaCO_2$ and regional blood volume by x-ray fluorescence. J Appl Physiol 35:741, 1973
31. Reivich M: Arterial PCO_2 and cerebral hemodynamics. Am J Physiol 206:25, 1964
32. Faupel G, Reulen HJ, Muller D, et al: Double-blood study on the effects of steroids on severe closed head injury, in Pappius HM, Feindel W (eds): Dynamics of Brain Edema. Berlin/Heidelberg/New York, Springer Verlag, 1976, pp 337–343
33. Gobiet W, Bock WJ, Liesegang J, et al: Treatment of acute cerebral edema with high dose of dexamethasone, in Becks JWF, Bosch DA, Brock M (eds): Intracranial Pressure III. Berlin/Heidelberg/New York, Springer Verlag, 1976, pp 231–235
34. Gudeman S, Miller J, Becker D: Failure of high-dose steroid therapy to influence intracranial pressure in patients with severe head injury. J Neurosurg 51:301–306, 1979
35. Cooper P, Moody S, Drone W, et al: Dexamethasone and severe head injury; a prospective double-blind study. J Neurosurg 51:307–316, 1979
36. Marshall L, Smith R, Rauscher L, et al: Mannitol dose requirements in brain-injured patients. J Neurosurg 48:169, 1978
37. Bruce D, Gennarelli T, Langfitt T: Resuscitation from coma due to head injury. Crit Care Med 6:254–269, 1978
38. Obrist W, Gennarelli T, Langfitt T, et al: Relation of cerebral blood flow to neurological status and outcome in head-injured patients. J Neurosurg 51:292–300, 1979
39. Cottrell J, Robustelli A, Post K, et al: Furosemide and mannitol—Induced changes in intracranial pressure and serum osmolality and electrolyte. Anesthesiology 47:28–30, 1977
40. Kimelberg H: Glial enzymes and ion transport in brain swelling, in Popp AJ (ed): Neural Trauma. New York, Raven Press, 1979, p 137
41. Pierce EC Jr, Lambertson C, Datsch S, et al: Cerebral circulation and metabolism during thiopental anesthesia and hyperventilation in man. J Clin Invest 41:1164–1671, 1962
42. Price M, Price H: Effects of general anesthetics on contractile responses of rabbit aortic strips. Anesthesiology 23:16, 1962
43. Rockoff M, Marshall L, Shapiro H: High-dose barbiturate therapy in humans: A clinical review of 60 patients. Ann Neurol 6:194, 1979

Index

Page numbers in *italics* indicate illustrations. Page numbers followed by *t* indicate tables.

a
2 b
3 c
4 d
5 e
6 f
7 g
8 h
9 i
8 0 j